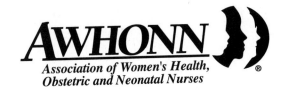

AWHONN
Association of Women's Health,
Obstetric and Neonatal Nurses

Perinatal Nursing

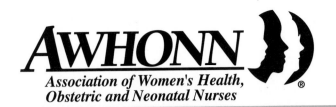

AWHONN
Association of Women's Health,
Obstetric and Neonatal Nurses

Perinatal Nursing

THIRD EDITION

Kathleen Rice Simpson, PhD, RNC, FAAN
Perinatal Clinical Nurse Specialist
St. John's Mercy Medical Center
St. Louis, Missouri

Patricia A. Creehan, MSN, RNC
Manager of Clinical Operations, Labor and Delivery
Advocate Christ Medical Center
Oak Lawn, Illinois

Wolters Kluwer | Lippincott Williams & Wilkins
Health
Philadelphia • Baltimore • New York • London
Buenos Aires • Hong Kong • Sydney • Tokyo

Senior Acquisitions Editor: Margaret Zuccarini
Managing Editor: Susan Rainey
Editorial Assistant: Kenya Flash
Production Project Manager: Cynthia Rudy
Director of Nursing Production: Helen Ewan
Senior Managing Editor / Production: Erika Kors
Design Coordinator: Holly Reid McLaughlin
Cover Design: Melissa Walter
Manufacturing Coordinator: Karin Duffield
Production Services / Compositor: Aptara, Inc.

3rd edition

9 8 7 6 5 4 3 2 1

Library of Congress Cataloging-in-Publication Data
Perinatal nursing / [edited by] Kathleen Rice Simpson, Patricia A. Creehan.
– 3rd ed.
    p. ; cm.
Includes bibliographical references and index.
ISBN-13: 978-0-7817-6759-0 (alk. paper)
ISBN-10: 0-7817-6759-8 (alk. paper)
1. Maternity nursing. I. Simpson, Kathleen Rice. II. Creehan, Patricia A.

[DNLM: 1. Maternal-Child Nursing. 2. Neonatal Nursing. 3. Perinatal Care.   WY 157.3 P4457 2008]
RG951.A985 2008
618.2'0231–dc22

2007017165

Care has been taken to confirm the accuracy of the information presented and to describe generally accepted practices. However, the authors, editors, and publisher are not responsible for errors or omissions or for any consequences from application of the information in this book and make no warranty, expressed or implied, with respect to the currency, completeness, or accuracy of the contents of the publication. Application of this information in a particular situation remains the professional responsibility of the practitioner; the clinical treatments described and recommended may not be considered absolute and universal recommendations.

The authors, editors, and publisher have exerted every effort to ensure that drug selection and dosage set forth in this text are in accordance with the current recommendations and practice at the time of publication. However, in view of ongoing research, changes in government regulations, and the constant flow of information relating to drug therapy and drug reactions, the reader is urged to check the package insert for each drug for any change in indications and dosage and for added warnings and precautions. This is particularly important when the recommended agent is a new or infrequently employed drug.

Some drugs and medical devices presented in this publication have Food and Drug Administration (FDA) clearance for limited use in restricted research settings. It is the responsibility of the health care provider to ascertain the FDA status of each drug or device planned for use in his or her clinical practice.

CONTRIBUTORS

Debbie Fraser Askin, MN, RNC
Associate Professor, Faculty of Nursing
Neonatal Nurse Practitioner
University of Manitoba
Winnipeg, Manitoba
*Chapter 11: Newborn Adaptation to
Extrauterine Life*

Mary Lee Barron, PhD(c), APRN, BC, FNP
Associate Professor
Saint Louis University School of Nursing
St. Louis, Missouri
Chapter 5: Antenatal Care

Susan Tucker Blackburn, RN, PhD, FAAN
Professor, Family and Child Nursing
University of Washington
Seattle, Washington
Chapter 3: Physiologic Changes of Pregnancy

Nancy A. Bowers, RN, BSN, MPH
President
Marvelous Multiples, Inc.
Birmingham, Alabama
*Chapter 6: High-Risk Pregnancy—Multiple
Gestation*

Lynn Clark Callister, RN, PhD, FAAN
Professor
Brigham Young University College of Nursing
Provo, Utah
*Chapter 2: Integrating Cultural Beliefs and Practices
When Caring for Childbearing Women and
Families*

Patricia A. Creehan, MSN, RNC
Manager of Clinical Operations, Labor and Delivery
Advocate Christ Medical Center
Oak Lawn, Illinois
*Chapter 9: Pain Relief and Comfort Measures
in Labor*
Chapter 12: Newborn Physical Assessment

Carol A. Curran, RNC, MS, OGNP
Perinatal Clinical Nurse Specialist
Clinical Specialist Consulting, Inc.
Virginia Beach, Virginia
Chapter 6: High-Risk Pregnancy—Cardiac Disease

Jeanne Watson Driscoll, PhD, APRN, BC
Private Practice, and Member of Mica Collaborative
Psychotherapy/Consultation/Education
JWD Associates, Inc.
Boston, Massachusetts / Wellesley, Massachusetts
*Chapter 4: Psychosocial Adaptation to Pregnancy
and Postpartum*

Margaret Comerford Freda, EdD, RN, CHES, FAAN
Professor of Clinical Obstetrics & Gynecology and
Women's Health
Albert Einstein College of Medicine, Montefiore
Medical Center
Bronx, New York
Chapter 6: High-Risk Pregnancy—Preterm Labor

Dotti C. James, PhD, RNC
Associate Professor and Coordinator of Perinatal
Graduate Specialty
Doisy College of Health Sciences School of Nursing,
Saint Louis University
St. Louis, Missouri
Chapter 10: Postpartum Care

Jill Janke, RNC, DNSc
Professor
University of Alaska, Anchorage
Anchorage, Alaska
Chapter 13: Newborn Nutrition

Cynthia F. Krening, RNC, MS
Perinatal Clinical Nurse Specialist
Littleton Adventist Hospital
Littleton, Colorado
*Chapter 6: High-Risk Pregnancy—Pulmonary
Complications*

Patricia L. Nash, MSN, RNC, NNP
Neonatal Nurse Practitioner
Cardinal Glennon Children's Medical Center
St. Louis, Missouri
Chapter 14: Common Neonatal Complications

Judith H. Poole, PhD, RNC
2007 AWHONN President
Nurse Manager, Birthing Care & Special
    Maternity Care
Presbyterian Hospital
Charlotte, North Carolina
Chapter 6: High-Risk Pregnancy—Hypertension

Kathleen Rice Simpson, PhD, RNC, FAAN
Perinatal Clinical Nurse Specialist
St. John's Mercy Medical Center
St. Louis, Missouri
*Chapter 1: Perinatal Patient Safety and Professional
    Liability Issues*
Chapter 7: Labor and Birth
Chapter 8: Fetal Assessment During Labor

Julie Slocum, RN, MS, CDE
Diabetes Nurse Clinician
Department of Maternal–Fetal Medicine, Women &
    Infants' Hospital
Providence, Rhode Island
Chapter 6: High-Risk Pregnancy—Diabetes

Joan Renaud Smith, RNC, MSN, NNP
Neonatal Nurse Practitioner
St. Louis Children's Hospital
St. Louis, Missouri
Chapter 14: Common Neonatal Complications

Mary Ellen Burke Sosa, RNC, MS
President, Perinatal Resources
Per Diem Staff Nurse, Labor/Delivery/Recovery
Women & Infants' Hospital
Providence, Rhode Island
*Chapter 6: High-Risk Pregnancy—Bleeding,
    Maternal Transfer*

REVIEWERS

Nancy O'Brien Abel, MN, RNC
Perinatal Nurse Specialist
Center for Perinatal and Pediatric Excellence
Swedish Medical Center
Seattle, Washington

Julie M. R. Arafeh, RN, MSN
Perinatal Outreach Coordinator
Assistant Director of Center for Advanced Pediatric
    Education
Division of Neonatal and Developmental Medicine,
    Department of Pediatrics
Stanford University
Palo Alto, California

Kathleen R. Beebe, RNC, PhD
Assistant Professor of Nursing
Dominican University of California
San Rafael, California

Cheryl Beck, DNSC, CNM, FAAN
Professor
University of Connecticut
Storrs, Connecticut

Laurie Caton-Lemos, RN, MS
Instructor
University of Southern Maine College of Nursing
    and Health Professions
Portland, Maine

Joanne E. Foresman, RNC, MSN
Nurse Clinician, Family Focused Care
St. John's Mercy Medical Center
St. Louis, Missouri

Ann C. Holden, RN, BScN, MSc(T), PNC
Perinatal Consultant, Manager, Clinical Lecturer
Family Birthing Centre at St. Joseph's Health Centre
McMaster University, School of Nursing
Toronto, Canada

Tara Hulsey, RN, BSN, MSN, PhD
Associate Dean for Faculty and Associate Professor
Medical University of South Carolina, College of
    Charleston
Charleston, South Carolina

Maribeth Inturrisi, RN, MS, CNS, CDE
Coordinator and RN Educator Consultant
California Diabetes and Pregnancy Program
Family Health Care Nursing
Associate Professor
University of California, San Francisco
San Francisco, California

Teresa Johnson, PhD, RN
Professor
College of Nursing at the University of Milwaukee
Milwaukee, Wisconsin

Dawn Kuerschner, MS, NNP, RNC
Associate Professor of Nursing
Oakton Community Colleges
Des Plaines, Illinois

Audrey Lyndon, RN, PhD, CNS
Betty Irene Moore Fellow, Department of Family
    Health Care Nursing
University of California San Francisco School of
    Nursing
San Francisco, California

Mary Ann Maher, RNC, BSN
Nurse Clinician Labor & Delivery/Women's
    Evaluation Unit
St. John's Mercy Medical Center
St. Louis, Missouri

Linda J. Mayberry, RN, PhD, FAAN
Associate Professor and Director of Research
New York University
New York, New York

Mary Lou Moore, PhD, RN, FACCE, FAAN
Associate Professor
Wake Forest University School of Medicine
Winston-Salem, North Carolina

Merry-K. Moos, RN, FNP, MPH, FAAN
Professor
Maternal Fetal Medicine Division
Department of Obstetrics and Gynecology
University of North Carolina
Chapel Hill, North Carolina

Barbara O'Brien, RN, BSN
Coordinator, Office of Perinatal Continuing
    Education
The University of Oklahoma Health Sciences Center,
    Department of OB/GYN
Oklahoma City, Oklahoma

Virginia B. Pearson, BSN, MSN, RN
Maternal–Child Nursing Instructor
The University of Southern Mississippi
    School of Nursing
Ellisville, Mississippi

Judith H. Poole, PhD, RNC
2007 AWHONN President
Nurse Manager, Birthing Care and Special
    Maternity Care
Presbyterian Hospital
Charlotte, North Carolina

R. Jeanne Ruiz, PhD, RNC, WHCNP
Associate Professor
University of Texas Medical Branch
Galveston, Texas

Teresa J. Martin Stanfill, RNC, MSN
Clinical Instructor, Maternity Services
St. Luke's Regional Medical Center
Boise, Idaho

Terry Tobin, RN, MSN, MPH
Associate Professor
Marquette University
Milwaukee, Wisconsin

Carol W. Trotter, PhD, NNP, RNC
Research Nurse/Neonatal Nurse Practitioner;
    Clinical Assistant Professor
St. John's Mercy Medical Center;
    University of Missouri
St. Louis, Missouri/Kansas City, Missouri

Lyn Vargo, PhD, RNC, NNP
Clinical Assistant Professor
University of Missouri
State University of New York–Stony Brook
Kansas City, Missouri/Stony Brook, New York

Sheila M. Weibert, RNC, WHNP, MSN
Women's Health Nurse Practitioner
Naval Medical Center, San Diego
San Diego, California

Patricia M. Witcher, RNC, MSN
Operations Manager, Labor and Delivery
Northside Hospital
Atlanta, Georgia

FOREWORD

THE specialty of perinatal nursing is dynamic in nature. Research, practice, and education are integrated to define and refine healthcare provided to women and newborns. As a result of technology, science, and changes in the healthcare environment, nurses today are being challenged to meet many demands within the healthcare delivery system, yet provide excellent care.

To achieve excellence in care, perinatal nurses are expected to be highly skilled, well-prepared, and competent. The knowledge base from which nurses function is multidimensional, incorporating the basic sciences and the art of caring. Perinatal nurses have the unique opportunity to make an impact on the lives of their patients, and their patients' families, in ways other specialties cannot. Attending the birth of a baby is a privilege that is shared within the profession.

In response to the needs of the perinatal nursing population, AWHONN is pleased to present the third edition of *Perinatal Nursing,* an important resource for the continued intellectual and professional growth of the specialty. Through the promotion of excellence in nursing practice, the association's mission of promoting and improving the health of women and newborns is realized. It is my hope that you will find this book an invaluable source of information as you aspire to excellence in providing their care.

Judith H. Poole, PhD, RNC
2007 AWHONN President

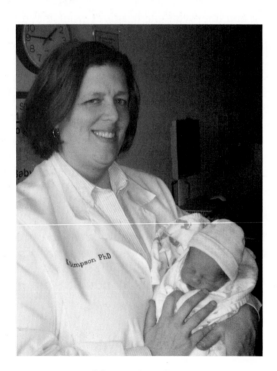

Kathleen Rice Simpson

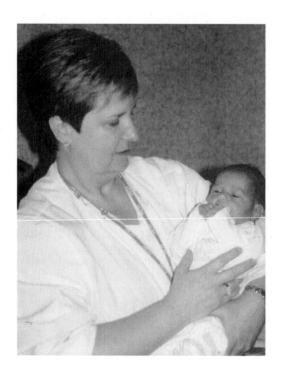

Patricia A. Creehan

PREFACE

OUR goal for *AWHONN's Perinatal Nursing* is to provide perinatal nurses with the latest evidence to promote the best possible outcomes for mothers and babies. The content reflects the philosophy that pregnancy, labor, and birth are natural processes for most women. Healthy women do well with minimal selected interventions within the context of a well-designed safety net (ie, the ability to intervene when necessary in a clinically timely manner). It is important to remember that unnecessary interventions increase the risk of iatrogenic patient harm. We have attempted to present pregnancy, labor, and birth as healthy life events rather than medical interventions. However, effective strategies for providing comprehensive nursing care to mothers and babies when complications arise also are covered. As perinatal nurses, we must critically examine the continued medicalization of the childbirth process. The benefits of supportive care and "being there for the woman" must not be overlooked when using the latest technology.

The best hope for advocating for safe and effective perinatal nursing care is a firm commitment to providing care based on the cumulative body of available evidence. This commitment involves making an effort to become educated about how to critique research and apply the evidence to everyday clinical practice. Perhaps some nurses will be inspired to conduct original research to answer some of the many unanswered questions about routine perinatal practices. Knowledge is power. This power is within all perinatal nurses who arm themselves with the skills required to have clinical discussions with physician colleagues and hospital administrators based on rigorous evidence and to become true partners in determining the best practices for caring for mothers and babies. When practices are identified that are not consistent with current evidence, standards, or guidelines, knowledge of the latest data provides the foundation to suggest changes. Instead of "going along to get along," we can use our current knowledge as the catalyst to develop effective strategies to move forward with necessary practice modifications.

We were fortunate to have many expert nurses collaborate with us as contributors and reviewers. This edition reflects the collective work of all of these professionals and we are truly grateful for their participation. We are often told that this book is used as a reference to guide perinatal unit policy, protocols, and practices. With this knowledge we are aware of the substantial responsibility to make sure that the content is accurate, practical, and supported by the best science available. We did our best to live up to the high expectations of those who use this book as a resource to care for mothers and babies. We sincerely hope our fellow AWHONN members and all perinatal nurses will continue to find this text practical and useful in the clinical setting.

Kathleen Rice Simpson, PhD, RNC, FAAN
Patricia A. Creehan, MSN, RNC

ACKNOWLEDGMENTS

The authors gratefully acknowledge Jennifer Plaat, Mayris Woods, Kathy Alsup, and Judy Duffy, medical librarians at St. John's Mercy Medical Center in St. Louis, Missouri, who spent many hours locating resources and checking references. They are amazing professionals who were invaluable to the process.

CONTENTS

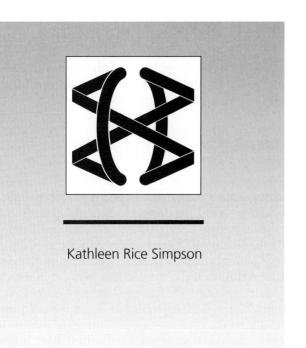

Kathleen Rice Simpson

CHAPTER **1**

Perinatal Patient Safety and Professional Liability Issues

CREATING a safe clinical environment during labor and birth requires effective leadership, a shared philosophy, professional behavior, and excellence in key clinical practices (Simpson & Knox, 2006). Ideally, there are established processes for ongoing monitoring of quality of care that include structure, process, and outcome measures (Simpson, 2006). This chapter provides recommendations for creating conditions that provide the safest care possible for mothers and babies using a framework that includes each of these essential criteria. Suggestions to minimize risk of professional liability are also provided. The recommendations are based on data concerning the most common causes of preventable injuries to mothers and babies during labor and birth. Data include the Joint Commission on Accreditation of Healthcare Organizations (JCAHO, 2004) sentinel event alert *Preventing Infant Death and Injury During Delivery*, the American College of Obstetricians and Gynecologists' (ACOG, 2004a) *2003 ACOG Survey of Professional Liability*, the Jury Verdict Research (2004) report *Current Award Trends in Personal Injury*, reports from professional liability insurance company claims (Greenwald & Mondor, 2003), and experience working with hospitals and healthcare systems to reduce risk of perinatal patient harm and to promote patient safety.

Inpatient obstetric care results in more than 50% of obstetrics and gynecology claims (White, Pichert, Bledsoe, Irwin, & Entman, 2005). The number and severity of successful obstetric liability claims and jury awards have steadily increased over the years (Jury Verdict Research, 2004). And although the number of obstetric claims typically represents only about 5% of

all malpractice claims, the dollar amount reserved for current and future payment is usually 25% to 35% of the total financial liability cost to hospitals and healthcare systems. Increasing patient safety decreases institutional and professional liability risk. Although all adverse outcomes cannot be prevented, defensibility is enhanced when care is consistent with current evidence and national standards and guidelines.

LEADERSHIP

Without effective leaders, staff members are challenged to implement essential criteria for safe care. The leadership team, composed of top hospital administrators, physician department chairs, unit nurse managers, clinical nurse specialists, and charge nurses, must be enthusiastic participants actively engaged in promoting safe care as the number-one priority (Partnership for Patient Safety, 2002). The fundamental goal of keeping patients safe from harm is worthy of sustained leadership attention and focus. Patient safety is a matter of integrity (Ryan, 2004). Leaders must be fully committed and have the will to do the right thing for mothers and babies, their families, their caregivers, and the institution, even when faced with the pressures of economics, productivity, and perceived provider convenience. This includes insisting on research-based, safe clinical practices and a professional environment where physicians and nurses are encouraged to work as a team, interact as colleagues, and collaborate on clinical solutions in a respectful manner. Our moral and ethical responsibility to do the right thing is discussed in detail in the *Code of Ethics for Nurses*

(American Nurses Association [ANA], 2001). Adequate financial and personnel resource allocation and support for practices based on research findings that demonstrate safe and effective care are critical foundations of our moral and ethical responsibility to patients (ANA, 2001; Ryan, 2004).

SHARED PHILOSOPHY OF CARE

In a high-reliability unit, there is an agreement that clinical practice will be based on the cumulative body of evidence and national standards and guidelines (Knox, Simpson, & Townsend, 2003). This shared philosophy should serve as a guide to develop unit policies and protocols and, ultimately, for how perinatal care is provided daily. An interdisciplinary practice committee should have a standing agenda item each month to review the most recently published science and standards and guidelines from professional organizations and regulatory agencies such as the Association of Women's Health, Obstetric and Neonatal Nurses (AWHONN); the American College of Nurse Midwives (ACNM); ACOG; the American Academy of Pediatrics (AAP); the American Society of Anesthesiologists (ASA); JCAHO; the Centers for Disease Control and Prevention (CDC); and the Food and Drug Administration (FDA). Discussion during these committee meetings should focus on how and when new standards and guidelines will be incorporated into unit operations and daily practice.

Patient safety must take priority over convenience, productivity, and costs. Standard unit polices and protocols should be in place for key clinical practices that are known to be associated with risk of adverse outcomes (Knox et al., 2003). These include cervical ripening, labor induction, fetal monitoring, perinatal group B streptococcus (GBS) prophylaxis, second-stage labor care, vaginal birth after cesarean birth (VBAC), operative vaginal birth, emergent cesarean birth, neonatal resuscitation, etc. All members of the interdisciplinary team must adhere to the unit policies. In rare cases where there may be a need to practice outside of unit policy, interdisciplinary discussion should occur, medical record documentation should be appropriately descriptive, and the case should be evaluated through the quality review process. Patient safety is created through accountability based on standardization, simplification, and clarity, as supported by the principles of safety science (Kohn, Corrigan, & Donaldson, 1999). While standardization of unit practices and policies may be perceived as an inconvenience to some team members, it should be acknowledged that the collective good of mothers and babies is the primary concern. A conservative approach to perinatal practice based on cumulative evidence and published professional standards creates conditions that promote safer care and decrease the probability of preventable adverse outcomes.

PROFESSIONAL BEHAVIOR

Professionals should conduct themselves in a professional manner at all times. Expectations for professional behavior should be outlined explicitly in institutional policies for good citizenship and reaffirmed both by the leaders as well as each team member annually during contract renewal and performance reviews. Respectful, collegial interactions between nurses and physicians and with patients are the bedrock of the unit culture. The *different but equal* contribution of nurses to the care process and ultimate clinical outcomes should be recognized and valued. Poor behavior (eg, throwing instruments, having temper tantrums, or making demeaning comments) should not be defined or qualified by discipline. Exceptions should not be made because "the individual is a good colleague otherwise," "we need his patient volume," or "she's one of the few who is always willing to work overtime."

Disruptive behavior can be overt, such as yelling, using profanity, throwing instruments, slamming charts, physically threatening or abusing others, berating someone, or displaying a rude, demeaning attitude (Porto & Lauve, 2006). More subtle examples are disrespect, nonverbal devaluation, eye rolling when a colleague makes a suggestion, gender discrimination, or sexual innuendo (Weber, 2004). Disruptive behavior is a significant threat to patient safety. After an experience with a disruptive clinician, many victims intentionally avoid additional interactions to minimize further opportunities for abuse (Rosenstein & O'Daniel, 2005). During labor, this can involve the nurse not calling the physician about a nonreassuring fetal heart rate (FHR) pattern because the last time they interacted, the nurse felt berated and demeaned (Simpson, James, & Knox, 2006). Nurses may feel pressured to increase oxytocin rates during hyperstimulation and avoid speaking up to prevent another unpleasant encounter with the physician who believes more oxytocin will speed labor. A nurse may be reluctant to seek advice from a nurse colleague concerning FHR interpretation because of past inferences of inadequacy during similar consultation. Because most (but not all) nonreassuring FHR patterns are not the result of fetal acidemia and most (but not all) hyperstimulation will not cause maternal or fetal harm, these avoidance strategies will work for some time, until the inevitable adverse outcome occurs.

Respectful, collegial, professional behavior should be valued equally to competent clinical practice and patient volume. Processes for reporting disruptive behavior should be widely disseminated and their use actively encouraged and supported by the leadership team. There should be accountability for individual actions and meaningful follow-up with clear actionable implications when disruptive behavior occurs. Each instance of disruptive behavior should be addressed in a timely manner, rather than delaying interventions until trends become apparent. Competent clinical practice is a basic expectation and cannot be substituted for irresponsible, inappropriate, dysfunctional, or abusive behavior.

COMMON AREAS OF LIABILITY AND PATIENT HARM IN CLINICAL PRACTICE

Following is a summary of the most common foci of professional perinatal liability claims, together with the most current applicable evidence and published standards and guidelines from professional associations and regulatory agencies (Simpson & Knox, 2003a). The purpose of this discussion is to provide a framework for reviewing existing institutional protocols and developing future policies and guidelines that decrease professional liability exposure and minimize the risk of iatrogenic injury to mothers and babies.

Note that most publications about clinical practice from professional organizations include disclaimers that their recommendations are guidelines rather than standards of care. However, when clinical care results in litigation, both the plaintiff and defense frequently offer these professional publications as standards to support their case. Thus, while the intention is to offer guidelines based on the best evidence to date, publications from professional organizations such as ACOG, AAP, ASA, AWHONN, and ACNM do in fact become standards of care for all practical purposes in legal proceedings.

Allegations against nurses, nurse midwives, physicians, and/or institutions often result from a lack of knowledge of or commitment to practice based on current standards, guidelines, and evidence. In other cases, care is based on personal experience and history of practice over a long period during which the care provider has not experienced an adverse outcome. In obstetrics, complications leading to death are rare because mothers and infants are generally healthy to begin with. Even care that would be judged by expert peers to be substandard rarely results in injury or death. Without personal involvement in an adverse outcome, some practitioners tend to continue as they have in the past regardless of their true capabilities and limitations (Chauhan, Magann, McAninch, Gherman, & Morrison, 2003).

Although it is generally thought that practitioners with more experience have accumulated more knowledge and clinical skills and, therefore, provide higher quality care, researchers recently found the opposite to be true (Choudhry, Fletcher, & Soumerai, 2005). Physicians with more experience have less factual knowledge, are less likely to practice based on current science and standards from their professional associations, and are more likely to have a poor patient outcome when compared to physicians with fewer years of experience (Choudhry et al., 2005). Although this study was about physicians, likely the same implications apply to nursing. Admittedly, some of the scientific evidence is counter-intuitive and different from what we all learned years ago. For example, it seems likely that more oxytocin at higher rates will produce a more effective labor process and a clinically significant shorter labor. It also seems that pushing immediately at 10 cm and continued pushing despite a nonreassuring FHR pattern is the best and quickest way to deliver the baby. However, there is a growing body of evidence to the contrary. Given the odds of an adverse outcome for generally healthy patients and a practitioner's years of experience (with practice that may be no longer consistent with current standards, guidelines, and evidence), practitioners are often surprised when the rare adverse outcome does occur (Chauhan et al., 2003). Moving toward a science-based clinical practice environment rather than "the way we've always done it" remains a significant challenge to promoting safe care. It should be noted that many times there is no cause and effect relationship between the allegations and an injury to a mother or baby. However, practices inconsistent with current standards, guidelines, and evidence offer opportunity for the plaintiff to demonstrate "breach of the standard of care," which can be challenging to overcome during a legal proceeding.

Telephone Triage
Common Allegations

- Failure to accurately assess maternal–fetal status over the telephone
- Failure to advise the woman to seek inpatient evaluation and treatment
- Failure to correctly communicate maternal–fetal status to the primary healthcare provider
- Failure of the physician/nurse midwife to come to the hospital to see the patient when requested by the nurse

Standards, Guidelines, and Recommendations

- Telephone advice to pregnant patients from labor and delivery nurses should be limited to two comments: "Call your primary healthcare provider" or "come to the hospital to be evaluated." Ruling out labor and possible maternal–fetal complications cannot be done accurately over the phone. The liability for assessing and diagnosing conditions of pregnancy and labor should remain with the primary care providers rather than being assumed by the institution.

Fetal Heart Rate Pattern Interpretation, Communication, and Documentation

Common Allegations

- Failure to assess accurately maternal–fetal status
- Failure to appreciate a deteriorating fetal condition
- Failure to treat appropriately a nonreassuring FHR
- Failure to correctly communicate the maternal–fetal status to the physician/nurse midwife
- Failure of the physician/nurse midwife to respond appropriately when notified of nonreassuring fetal status
- Failure to institute the chain of command when there is a clinical disagreement between the nurse and responsible physician/nurse midwife

Standards, Guidelines, and Recommendations

- Use the terminology recommended by the National Institute of Child Health and Human Development (NICHD, 1997), ACOG (2005), and AWHONN (2005) to describe FHR patterns in all professional communication and medical record documentation concerning fetal assessment.
- Establish ongoing interdisciplinary fetal monitoring education (JCAHO, 2004). Knowledge and skills in fetal assessment are not discipline-specific. Ensure and document that all care providers are competent to interpret electronic fetal monitoring (EFM) data (Freeman, 2002).
- All members of the team should participate in regularly scheduled case reviews and offer suggestions for future care improvement.
- Include baseline rate, variability, presence or absence of accelerations and decelerations, clinical context, and pattern evolution in communication between team members about nonreassuring FHR patterns (Fox, Kilpatrick, King, & Parer, 2000).
- Establish a clear and agreed-upon definition of fetal well-being (eg, accelerations 15 beats per minute above the baseline rate lasting for 15 seconds for the term fetus; a baseline rate within normal limits; no recurrent late, variable, or prolonged decelerations; and moderate variability) and document fetal well-being on admission, prior to administration of pharmacologic agents for cervical ripening and labor induction, initiation of epidural analgesia, and discharge.
- Consider an initial assessment of fetal status via EFM on admission for women in labor when intermittent auscultation is planned for the primary method of fetal surveillance (Golditch, Ahn, & Phelan, 1998; Sarno, Phelan, & Ahn, 1990).
- Ensure ongoing, timely, and accurate assessment and determination of fetal well-being during labor (Freeman, 2002).
- During absent or minimal baseline FHR variability, use stimulation to evaluate fetal well-being (AAP & ACOG, 2002; Clark, Gimovsky, & Miller, 1984; Freeman, Garite, & Nageotte, 2003).
- Develop common expectations for intrauterine resuscitation, including maternal repositioning, an intravenous fluid bolus of at least 500 mL of lactated Ringer's solution, oxygen administration at 10 L/min via nonrebreather facemask, correction of maternal hypotension, and reduction of uterine activity, based on the FHR pattern (ACOG, 2005; Simpson & James, 2005b).
- Establish agreement among team members concerning which type of FHR patterns require bedside evaluation by the primary care provider and the timeframe involved (Fox et al., 2000).
- If continuous EFM is ordered, monitoring of FHR and uterine activity via EFM should continue until birth.
- Ensure that there are organizational resources and systems to support timely interventions (including emergent cesarean birth) when the FHR is nonreassuring.

Elective Induction of Labor

Common Allegations

- Failure to fully inform the woman of the risks and benefits of elective induction
- Failure to accurately determine gestational age prior to elective induction

- Iatrogenic prematurity as the result of elective induction before 39 completed weeks of pregnancy
- Excessive doses of oxytocin resulting in hyperstimulation of uterine activity (with or without the presence of a nonreassuring FHR pattern)
- Failure to accurately assess maternal–fetal status during labor induction

(See also FHR Pattern Interpretation, Communication, and Documentation; Hyperstimulation of Uterine Activity.)

Standards, Guidelines, and Recommendations

- Obtain informed consent and document it in the medical record (ACOG, 1999; JCAHO, 2006).
- An established gestational age of at least 39 completed weeks by at least one of the following criteria should be documented prior to elective induction: Fetal heart tones have been documented for 20 weeks by nonelectronic fetoscope or for 30 weeks by Doppler; it has been 36 weeks since a positive serum or urine human chorionic gonadotropin pregnancy test was performed by a reliable laboratory; an ultrasound measurement of the crown-rump length, obtained between 6 to 12 weeks supports a gestational age of at least 39 weeks; an ultrasound at 13 to 20 weeks gestation confirms the gestational age of at least 39 weeks; or, alternatively, documentation of fetal lung maturity (ACOG, 1999).
- Adhere to ACOG/AWHONN recommendations for dosages of pharmacologic agents (see misoprostol and oxytocin) (ACOG, 1999; Simpson, 2002).
- Ensure adequate personnel are available to monitor maternal–fetal status (ACOG, 1999).
- Adhere to ACOG/AWHONN recommendations for maternal–fetal assessment: Assess characteristics of uterine activity and the FHR every 15 minutes during the active phase of the first stage of labor and every 5 minutes during the second stage of labor; assess maternal vital signs at least every 4 hours or more often if indicated (AAP & ACOG, 2002).

Misoprostol (Cytotec) for Cervical Ripening/Labor Induction

Common Allegations

- Excessive doses of misoprostol that resulted in hyperstimulation of uterine activity (with or without a nonreassuring FHR pattern)

- Uterine rupture as a result of misoprostol administration
- Use of misoprostol for a woman with a history of a prior cesarean birth or uterine scar
- Failure to accurately assess maternal–fetal status during labor induction

(See also FHR Pattern Interpretation, Communication, and Documentation; Hyperstimulation of Uterine Activity.)

Standards, Guidelines, and Recommendations

- Obtain informed consent and document in the medical record (JCAHO, 2006).
- Have pharmacist prepare the tablets (100-mcg tablets are not scored) (Simpson, 2002).
- Use the lowest possible dose to effect cervical change and labor progress (ACOG, 1999).
- The initial dose should be 25 mcg (1/4 of 100-mcg tablet) inserted into the posterior vaginal fornix. The dose can repeated every 3 to 6 hours, up to six doses in 24 hours as needed. There are lower rates of uterine hyperstimulation with lower dosages (25 mcg) and longer intervals between doses (q 6 hours rather than q 3 hours) (ACOG, 1999).
- Redosing should be withheld if three or more contractions occur within 10 minutes, adequate cervical ripening is achieved with a Bishop score of 8 or more, the cervix is 80% effaced and 3 cm dilated, the patient enters active labor, or the FHR is nonreassuring (ACOG, 1999; Simpson, 2002).
- If oxytocin is needed, it should not be given until at least 4 hours after the last dose (ACOG, 2000b).
- Misprostol should be administered at or near the labor and birth suite, where uterine activity and FHR can be monitored continuously (ACOG, 1999).
- Misoprostol should not be administered to women with a history of prior cesarean birth or uterine scar (ACOG, 1999; 2006a).
- There are not enough data about oral route to recommend oral use at this time (ACOG, 1999).

Oxytocin for Labor Induction/Augmentation

Common Allegations

- Failure to accurately assess maternal–fetal status during labor induction
- Excessive doses of oxytocin resulting in hyperstimulation of uterine activity, with or without a nonreassuring FHR pattern

(See also FHR Pattern Interpretation, Communication, and Documentation; Hyperstimulation of Uterine Activity.)

Standards, Guidelines, and Recommendations

- Administer the lowest possible dose to achieve cervical change and labor progress (ACOG, 1999).
- Starting at 0.05 to 1 mU and increasing by 1 to 2 mU/min no more frequently than every 30 to 40 minutes will result in successful induction of labor for most women (ACOG, 1999). Approximately 90% of women at term will have labor successfully induced with 6 mU/min or less (Arias, 2000).
- Based on physiologic and pharmacokinetic principles, a 30- to 40-minute interval between oxytocin dosage increases is optimal. The full effect of oxytocin on the uterine response to increases in dosage cannot be evaluated until steady-state concentration has been achieved. Increasing the infusion rate before steady-state concentration is achieved results in laboring women receiving higher than necessary doses of oxytocin, which increases risk of side effects such as uterine hyperstimulation and nonreassuring fetal status (Arias, 2000; Crane & Young, 1998; Phaneuf, Rodriguez-Linares, Tambyraja, MacKenzie, & Lopez Bernal, 2000).
- Titrate the dosage to the fetal response and uterine activity/labor progress (ACOG, 1999; Clayworth, 2000; Simpson, 2002).
- Avoid uterine hyperstimulation and treat (decrease or discontinue oxytocin) in a timely manner if it occurs (ACOG, 1999).
- If labor is progressing at 1 cm/hr cervical dilation, there is no need to increase the dosage rate (Crane & Young, 1998; Simpson, 2002).
- If using an active management of labor (AMOL) protocol, follow all aspects of the published protocol rather than just the oxytocin dosages and infusion frequencies. The protocol was designed to be used for nulliparous women in spontaneous active labor. The Dublin AMOL protocol is precisely described and, under these conditions, was found to be safe, although three subsequent studies in the United States (Frigaletto et al., 1995; Lopez-Zeno, Peaceman, Adashek, & Socol, 1992; Rogers, Gilson, Miller, Izquierdo, Curet, & Qualls, 1997) did not find that it led to a decrease in cesarean births: Candidates include only nulliparous women in spontaneous active labor with a singleton pregnancy, cephalic presentation, and no evidence of fetal compromise. To exclude false

and prodromal labor, true labor is specifically defined as contractions with either bloody show, spontaneous rupture of membranes, or complete (100%) cervical effacement. Once labor is diagnosed, the woman receives continuous one-to-one labor support from a birth attendant (midwife). An amniotomy is performed if membranes are not spontaneously ruptured within one hour after labor has been diagnosed. If cervical dilation does not progress at least 1 cm/hr, oxytocin augmentation is initiated beginning at 6 mU/min, increasing by 6 mU/min every 15 minutes until adequate labor is established, to a maximum dose of 40 mU/min. Hyperstimulation of uterine activity is defined as more than seven contractions over 15 minutes (O'Driscoll, Jackson, & Gallagher, 1970).

- To enhance communication among members of the perinatal healthcare team and to avoid confusion, oxytocin administration rates should always be ordered by the physician or certified nurse midwife as mU/min and documented in the medical record as mU/min (ACOG, 1999; Simpson, 2002).

Hyperstimulation of Uterine Activity

Common Allegations

- Failure to appropriately identify and treat uterine hyperstimulation (with and without a nonreassuring FHR pattern)
- Failure to decrease or discontinue the oxytocin infusion or delay the next dose of misoprostol during uterine hyperstimulation
- Physician/nurse midwife orders to continue oxytocin or administer misoprostol despite being notified of uterine hyperstimulation
- Failure to communicate with the physician/nurse midwife when uterine hyperstimulation occurs
- Failure to institute the chain of command when there is a clinical disagreement between the nurse and responsible physician/nurse midwife

(See also FHR Pattern Interpretation, Communication and Documentation; Elective Induction of Labor; Misoprostol for Cervical Ripening/Labor Induction; Oxytocin for Labor Induction/Augmentation [Cytotec].)

Standards, Guidelines, and Recommendations

- A clear definition of hyperstimulation (eg, a series of single contractions lasting two minutes or more, a contraction frequency of six or more in ten minutes, or contractions of normal duration occurring within one minute of each other

[ACOG, 1999, 2003, 2005; Simpson, 2002]) is essential in each institution, because clinical management strategies, policies, and protocols should include expected actions when hyperstimulation is identified.

- All perinatal healthcare providers in each institution should be aware of clinical criteria established for hyperstimulation and the expected actions.
- While hyperstimulation of uterine activity can be the result of endogenous maternal oxytocin and prostaglandins, most hyperstimulation is the result of administration of exogenous pharmacologic agents (Crane, Young, Butt, Bennett, & Hutchens, 2001).
- Treat hyperstimulation by decreasing or discontinuing oxytocin based on the individual clinical situation.
- Hyperstimulation and hyperstimulation accompanied by a nonreassuring FHR pattern are more common during cervical ripening and labor induction when compared with spontaneous labor (Crane et al., 2001).
- Be aware that some practitioners reserve the term "hyperstimulation" for excessive contractions that result in a nonreassuring FHR pattern. Contractions that are excessive without a corresponding nonreassuring FHR are often called "tachysystole" in an unsuccessful attempt to avoid the recognized liability inherent in using the term hyperstimulation. Whatever the term, however, the physiologic implications are similar. From the perspective of maternal–fetal safety, the best approach is to avoid prolonged periods of hyperstimulation (whether designated as such or not) that lead to progressive deterioration in fetal status and subsequent nonreassuring FHR patterns (ACOG & AAP, 2003). Interventions for hyperstimulation should not be delayed until there is evidence of nonreassuring fetal status (Simpson, 2002).
- Empower and encourage all members of the perinatal team to be appropriately assertive in their actions and communications with colleagues to advocate for patient safety if they feel pressured to increase oxytocin rates during uterine hyperstimulation and/or nonreassuring FHR patterns (Simpson et al., 2006).

Pain Relief During Labor and Birth

Common Allegations

- Failure to accurately identify and treat labor pain
- Use of "ability to pay" or insurance status as criteria for treatment of labor pain

Standards, Guidelines, and Recommendations

- Provide adequate pain relief for all women in labor as per their request regardless of ability to pay or whether they sought prenatal care (ACOG, 2006a; JCAHO, 2006).
- Labor results in severe pain for many women. There is no other circumstance under which it is considered acceptable for a person to experience untreated severe pain, amendable to safe intervention, while under a physician's care. In the absence of a medical contraindication, maternal request is a sufficient medical indication for pain relief during labor and birth (ACOG, 2006a).
- The choice of technique, agent, and dosage should be based on patient preference, medical status, and contraindications. Decisions should be closely coordinated among the obstetrician, the anesthesia provider, the patient, and skilled support personnel (ACOG, 2006a).
- There are conflicting data about the effect of epidural analgesia/anesthesia on the risk of cesarean birth; however, based on what is known at present, if the patient desires an epidural during the early stages of labor, there is no reason to deny that request if the denial is related to potential risk of cesarean birth (ACOG, 2006a).

Nurses' Role During Regional Anesthesia

Common Allegations

- Administration of bolus or change in medication rate of epidural anesthesia that resulted in subsequent maternal and/or fetal harm
- Nurses' actions beyond the scope of practice as defined by their professional association (AWHONN, 2001)

Standards, Guidelines, and Recommendations

- Adhere to the AWHONN clinical position statement that describes the role of the nurse during epidural anesthesia. Require that only qualified, credentialed anesthesia providers adjust the dosage for labor epidurals, including boluses, and increases or decreases in rate. Require that only qualified, credentialed anesthesia providers program the epidural pumps during regional anesthesia for labor (AWHONN, 2001).
- Require that the provider who will be administering the narcotics and regional blocking agents sign-out these medications personally from the

medication-dispensing cabinet (including wasted excess dosages) (JCAHO, 2006).

- Acknowledge and support the responsibility of registered nurses to practice within the guidelines of their professional association. Expect that anesthesia providers will acknowledge this right and duty as well.

Fundal Pressure During the Second Stage of Labor
Common Allegations

- Application of fundal pressure during second stage of labor that resulted in shoulder dystocia and/or other maternal–fetal injuries
- Application of fundal pressure during shoulder dystocia that further affected the shoulder and delayed the birth, resulting in maternal–fetal injuries

(See also Shoulder Dystocia.)

Standards, Guidelines, and Recommendations

- Fundal pressure applied during the second stage of labor is associated with risks of adverse outcomes to the mother and the baby (Simpson & Knox, 2001).
- Risks to the baby include inadvertent shoulder dystocia, which in turn places the baby at risk for brachial plexus injuries; fractures of the humerus and clavicles; hypoxemia, asphyxia, and death; an increase in fetal intracranial pressure, resulting in significant decreases in cerebral blood flow and nonreassuring FHR patterns; umbilical cord compression negatively affecting maternal–fetal exchange; functional alterations in the placental intervillious space, which increases the risk of fetal hypoxemia and asphyxia; subgaleal hemorrhage, and spinal cord injuries (ACOG, 2002; Amiel-Tison, Sureau, & Shnider, 1988; Gherman, Ouzounian, & Goodwin, 1998; Hankins, 1998).
- Risks to the mother include perineal injuries such as third- and fourth-degree lacerations, anal sphincter tears, uterine rupture and uterine inversion, pain, hypotension, respiratory distress, abdominal bruising, fractured ribs, and liver rupture (Cosner, 1996; Kline-Kaye & Miller Slade, 1990; Lee, Baggish, & Lashgari, 1978; Rommal, 1996).
- Avoid fundal pressure to shorten an otherwise normal second stage of labor (Simpson & Knox, 2001).
- Avoid fundal pressure during shoulder dystocia (ACOG, 2002b).

- Avoid clinical disagreements about fundal pressures at the bedside in front of the patient by a having an agreed-upon policy.

Shoulder Dystocia
Common Allegations

- Failure to accurately predict risk of shoulder dystocia
- Failure to diagnose labor abnormalities
- Failure to appropriately initiate shoulder dystocia corrective maneuvers
- Failure to perform a cesarean birth
- Application of forceps or vacuum at high station or continued application without evidence of fetal descent resulting in shoulder dystocia
- Application of fundal pressure during shoulder dystocia further affecting the shoulder and delaying birth, thereby resulting in maternal–fetal injuries

(See also Fundal Pressure During the Second Stage of Labor.)

Standards, Guidelines, and Recommendations

- Most cases of shoulder dystocia cannot be predicted or prevented (ACOG, 2002b).
- There is no evidence that any one maneuver is superior in releasing an impacted shoulder; however, the McRoberts maneuver and suprapubic pressure are easily implemented without an associated increase in risk of injury to the baby.
- Excess traction and fundal pressure should be avoided because of increased risk of injuries to the baby (ACOG, 2002b).

Suggestions for Medical Record Documentation (Simpson, 1999)

- Provide emergent nursing care to woman and newborn as a first priority.
- Provide a narrative note that summarizes the series of interventions and clinical events that have taken place, with a focus on a logical step-by-step approach to relieving the affected shoulder and resuscitating the newborn.
- Avoid documenting a minute-by-minute account of the emergency unless it is absolutely certain that the times included are accurate.
- Attempt to closely approximate the time interval between delivery of fetal head and body.
- Review the EFM strip and talk with other providers in attendance to ensure the most accurate details of clinical circumstances are accurately recorded.

- Include fetal assessment data and/or attempts to obtain data about fetal status during the maneuvers.
- List the order of each maneuver used in clear and precise terms.
- Note that nursing assistance with these maneuvers was provided under the direction of the physician or nurse midwife.
- If suprapubic pressure was used, make sure it is noted as such to avoid later allegations of fundal pressure.

Second-Stage Management

Common Allegations

- Iatrogenic nonreassuring FHR patterns as a result of provider-coached pushing efforts
- Failure to appreciate a deteriorating fetal status
- Failure to anticipate resuscitation needs of an infant after a nonreassuring FHR pattern during the second stage of labor
- Injuries to the perineum that resulted in perineal lacerations, loss of pelvic floor integrity, and sexual dysfunction

Standards, Guidelines, and Recommendations

- Follow AWHONN (2000) recommendations for second-stage management.
- Develop common expectations among team members concerning when to begin pushing and how to encourage women to push.
- The active phase of second-stage labor is a period of stress for the fetus; thus, efforts should be made minimize that stress by shortening the active pushing phase and using appropriate pushing techniques (Barnett & Humenick, 1982; Nordstrom, Achanna, Nuka, & Arulkumaran, 2001; Piquard, Schaefer, Hsiung, Dellenbach, & Haberey, 1989; Roberts, 2002).
- Women with epidural anesthesia who do not feel the urge to push at 10 cm cervical dilation should be allowed to rest until the fetus has descended enough to stimulate the urge to push (up to 2 hours for nulliparous women and up to 1 hour for multiparous women) (Fraser, et al., 2000; Roberts, Torvaldsen, Cameron, & Olive, 2004). There is evidence to suggest that for women with epidurals, coached pushing does not significantly decrease the length of the second stage (Fraser, et al., 2000; Hansen, Clark, & Foster, 2002; Mayberry, Hammer, Kelly, True-Driver, & De, 1999). Passive fetal descent will result in about the same length of the second stage for women with epidural analgesia/anesthesia as does the coached pushing approach.

- When the urge to push is noted, women should be encouraged to bear down as long as they can at the peak of the contraction, no more than three times per contraction (Mayberry, Gennaro, Strange, Williams, & De 1999; Roberts, 2002).
- Women should not be told to take a deep breath and hold it while the nurse or physician counts to 10 (Caldeyro-Barcia, 1979; Caldeyro-Barcia et al., 1981; Nordstrom et al., 2001; Sampselle & Hines, 1999; Simpson & James, 2005a). Discourage breath-holding longer than 6 to 8 seconds per pushing effort (Barnett & Humenick, 1982; Roberts, 2002).
- Women should be assisted to appropriate positions for pushing, such as upright, semi-Fowlers, lateral, and squatting (AWHONN, 2000; Mayberry, Strange, Suplee, & Gennaro, 2003; Roberts, Algert, Cameron, & Torvaldsen, 2005). The supine lithotomy position and stirrups should not be used during pushing efforts (AWHONN, 2000; Tubridy & Redmond, 1996).
- The woman's knees should not be forcibly pushed back against her abdomen in positions that stretch the perineum or risk joint or nerve injury; rather, the woman should be allowed to position herself for comfort or keep her feet flat on the bed as desired (Simpson & James, 2005a; Tubridy & Redmond, 1996).
- Repetitive pushing efforts should not be encouraged if the FHR is nonreassuring. Instead, women should be coached to push with every other or every third contraction to maintain a stable baseline FHR and allow the fetus to recover between pushes (Simpson & James, 2005a). If the fetus is not responding well to coached pushing, stop pushing temporarily and let the fetus recover (AWHONN, 2006; PEOPLE, 2003; Simpson & James, 2005b).
- Uterine hyperstimulation should be avoided during the second stage and the same intrauterine resuscitation techniques used during the first stage labor should be used during the second stage (Simpson & James, 2005a).
- As in the first stage of labor, the FHR pattern during the second stage should be used as an indicator of how well the fetus is responding. It is important to recognize nonreassuring FHR patterns and intervene appropriately. It is known that recurrent late and variable decelerations during the second stage are associated with respiratory acidemia at birth (Parer, King, Flanders, Fox, & Kilpatrick, 2006). Some fetuses may develop metabolic acidemia if this type of pattern continues over a long period (Parer et al., 2006). These babies are difficult to resuscitate and may not transition well to extra-uterine life.

Forceps- and Vacuum-Assisted Birth

Common Allegations

- Application of forceps/vacuum at high station that results in maternal–fetal injury
- Inappropriate timing or application of forceps, resulting in fetal injuries such as fractured skull, intracranial bleed, or facial paralysis
- Use of excessive force during a forceps- or vacuum-assisted birth
- Use of a vacuum for rotation of the fetal head
- Use of excessive pressures during a vacuum-assisted birth
- Excessive time of vacuum application

Standards, Guidelines, and Recommendations

- Adhere to ACOG (2000a) indications for operative vaginal birth. No indication for operative vaginal birth is absolute; however, the following indications apply when the fetal head is engaged and the cervix is fully dilated: Prolonged second stage for nulliparous women with lack of continuing progress for 3 hours with regional anesthesia or 2 hours without regional anesthesia, and prolonged second stage for multiparous women with lack of continued progress for 2 hours with regional anesthesia or 1 hour without regional anesthesia; suspicion of immediate or potential fetal compromise; and shortening of the second stage for maternal benefit.
- Operative vaginal birth should only be performed by individuals with privileges for such procedures and in settings in which personnel are readily available to perform a cesarean birth in the event that operative vaginal birth is unsuccessful (ACOG, 2000a).

Forceps-Assisted Vaginal Birth

- Adhere to ACOG (2000a) criteria for types of forceps births:
  - *Outlet forceps:* The fetal scalp is visible at the introitus without separating the labia, the fetal skull has reached the pelvic floor, the sagittal suture is in anterior–posterior diameter or right or left occiput anterior or posterior position, the fetal head is at or on the perineum, and rotation does not exceed 45°.
  - *Low forceps:* The leading point of the fetal skull is at station ≥+2 cm and not on the pelvic floor, rotation is 45° or less (left or right occipute anterior to occiput anterior, or left or right occiput posterior to occiput posterior), and rotation is greater that 45°.
  - *Midforceps:* The station is above +2 cm but fetal head is engaged.
  - *High forceps:* This type is not included in classification and should not be permitted or attempted.

Vacuum-Assisted Vaginal Birth

- Follow the manufacturer's guidelines for the vacuum device being used. Generally, using no more than 600 mmHg pressure and abandoning the procedure after three pop-offs and/or 20 minutes maximum total time of application is consistent with safe care and a decreased risk of fetal injuries (Bofill et al., 1996; Bofill, Martin, & Morrison, 1998).
- The vacuum pressure should not exceed 500 to 600 mm Hg, and the pressure should be released as soon as the contraction ends and the woman stops pushing (Brumfield, Gilstrap, O'Grady, Ross, & Schifrin, 1999).
- As a general guideline, progress in descent should accompany each traction attempt and no more than three pulls should be attempted (ACOG, 2000a; Bofill et al., 1996; Bofill et al., 1998; Brumfield et al., 1999). Traction is only when the woman is actively pushing.
- The vacuum procedure should be timed from the moment of insertion of the cup into the vagina until birth and should not be on the fetal head for longer than 20 to 30 minutes (Bofill et al., 1998; Brumfield et al., 1999).
- When the cup has been applied at maximum pressure for more than 10 minutes, the rate of fetal injuries increases (Brumfield et al., 1999); thus, while total time of cup application can be between 20 to 30 minutes, the time of maximum pressure force should not exceed 10 minutes (Paluska, 1997).
- As with forceps, there should be a willingness to abandon attempts at a vacuum-assisted birth if satisfactory progress is not made. Three pop-offs, evidence of fetal scalp trauma, and/or no descent with appropriate application and traction should warrant abandoning the vacuum procedure (Bofill et al., 1998).
- The FDA (1998) recommendations for vacuum-assisted birth include: rocking movements or torque should not be applied to the device; only steady traction in the line of the birth canal should be used and clinicians caring for the baby should be alerted that a vacuum device has been used so that they can adequately monitor the baby for the signs and symptoms of device-related injuries.
- Vacuum-assisted vaginal birth should not be performed before 34 weeks' gestation (ACOG, 2000a).
- Persistent efforts to achieve a vaginal birth using different instruments may increase the potential for maternal and fetal injury. The incidence of injuries increase with combined methods (forceps and vacuum) of operative vaginal birth (ACOG, 2000a).

30-Minute "Rule"

Common Allegations

- Failure to initiate a cesarean birth in a timely manner (within 30 minutes of the decision to do so)

Standards, Guidelines, and Recommendations

- Have a system in place to ensure that an emergent cesarean birth can be started within 30 minutes of the decision to do so (AAP & ACOG, 2002).
- Acknowledge that some emergencies, such as a prolapsed umbilical cord, a uterine rupture, an abruptio placenta, or a maternal cardiopulmonary arrest, may not result in a positive outcome for the mother or baby even if the cesarean birth is initiated within 30 minutes of the event (AAP & ACOG, 2002).
- Appropriately transfer patients with high-risk conditions to perinatal centers where a surgical team is in house at all times (ACOG & ASA, 2001).
- As applicable, fully inform pregnant women that there is a risk of adverse outcome for the mother and baby when laboring and giving birth at an institution where there is not a surgical team in house at all times (ACOG & ASA, 2001).

Vaginal Birth After Cesarean Birth (VBAC)

Common Allegations

- Failure to fully inform a woman with a history of a prior cesarean birth or uterine scar of risks and benefits of a trial of labor for VBAC
- Use of prostanglandin agents for cervical ripening or labor induction for a woman with a history of a prior cesarean birth or uterine scar that results in uterine rupture
- Use of excessive doses of oxytocin during labor induction or augmentation that results in uterine rupture
- Failure to have a heightened awareness of and identify signs and symptoms of uterine rupture
- Failure to treat uterine rupture in a timely manner
- Failure to have appropriate personnel and equipment during trial of labor for VBAC

Standards, Guidelines, and Recommendations

- Adhere to ACOG (2004c) recommendations for appropriate candidates (eg, one or two prior low-transverse cesarean births, clinically adequate pelvis, no other uterine scars or previous rupture).

- Avoid use of prostaglandin agents for cervical ripening and labor induction (ACOG, 2006b).
- Avoid excessive use of oxytocin and hyperstimulation if labor induction is indicated (ACOG, 2006b).
- Ensure that a full surgical team (obstetrician/surgeon, surgical first assistant, anesthesia provider, scrub technician, circulating nurse, and personnel skilled in neonatal resuscitation) is in-house during a trial of labor for patients attempting a VBAC (ACOG, 2004c).

Multiple Gestation

Common Allegations

- Failure to transfer care of high-risk pregnancy to appropriate healthcare provider or tertiary center
- Failure to diagnosis multiple gestation
- Failure to determine chorionicity of multiple gestation
- Failure to accurately monitor all fetuses during labor and birth
- Failure to have in place appropriate personnel and equipment during birth of multiple gestation

Standards, Guidelines, and Recommendations

- Determine chorionicity during prenatal period using high-resolution ultrasound techniques by practitioners experienced with this technique.
- Confirm fetal lung maturity if elective birth before 38 weeks' gestation is performed.
- Anticipate vaginal birth if both twins are vertex; other presentations and higher-order multiples are usually delivered via cesarean birth.
- Attempt to continuously monitor all fetuses during the first and second stages of labor. This may be challenging with higher-order multiples.
- Have ultrasound equipment immediately available in the labor room to determine fetal presentation during the second stage of labor.
- Have personnel standing by in-house for neonatal resuscitation and anesthesia during the second stage of labor.

Iatrogenic Prematurity

Common Allegations

- Failure to follow the ACOG (1999) recommendations for gestational age for elective induction of labor or repeat cesarean section, resulting in iatrogenic prematurity and subsequent neonatal morbidity, neurological injury, or death

- Failure to accurately determine the gestational age prior to elective repeat cesarean birth or elective induction of labor

Standards, Guidelines, and Recommendations

- Avoid elective induction of labor and elective cesarean birth before 39 weeks of gestation (ACOG, 1999; Wang, Dorer, Fleming, & Catlin, 2004). (See Elective Induction of Labor.)
- Assess fetal lung maturity if there is any question of gestational age before 39 weeks of gestation prior to elective repeat cesarean birth (AAP & ACOG, 2002).

Prevention of Perinatal Group B Streptococcal Disease

Common Allegations

- Failure to adhere to the CDC guidelines for GBS prophylaxis, resulting neonatal infection, and subsequent neonatal neurological damage or death

Standards, Guidelines, and Recommendations

- Universal screening is the preferred recommendation from the CDC for GBS prophylaxis with risk-based screening reserved for those women not previously screened (Schrag, Gorwitz, Fultz-Butts, & Schuchat, 2002). These recommendations are supported by ACOG (2002a, and reaffirmed in 2005).

Current CDC Recommendations (Schrag et al., 2002)

- Universal prenatal culture-based screening for vaginal and rectal GBS colonization of all pregnant women at 35 to 37 weeks' gestation.
- At the time of labor or rupture of membranes, give intrapartum chemoprophylaxis to all pregnant women identified as GBS carriers.
- Penicillin is the first-line agent for intrapartum antibiotic prophylaxis (penicillin G, 5 million units intravenously [IV] as the initial dose, then 2.5 million units IV every 4 hours until birth), with ampicillin an acceptable alternative (2 g IV as the initial dose, then 1 g IV every 4 hours until birth).
- During prenatal screening, all women should be assessed for a history of penicillin allergy and categorized as low risk or high risk for anaphylaxis. Low risk may include a history of rash, especially if the rash-inducing medication was amplicillin. High risk is a history of immediate hypersensitivity to reactions (anaphylaxis, angioedema, uticaria, or

other conditions) that would make anaphylaxis more dangerous. For women who are allergic to penicillin and at low risk for anaphylaxis, the recommended antibiotic is cefazolin. For women determined to be at high risk for anaphylaxis, all GBS specimens sent for culture should be tested for sensitivity to erythromycin and clindamycin. If the isolate is sensitive to either of these medications, they can be used for intrapartum prophylaxis (clindamycin, 900 mg IV every 8 hours until birth or erythromycin, 500 mg IV every 6 hours until birth).
- For penicillin-allergic women at high risk for anaphylaxis and whose isolate is resistant to erythromycin and clindamycin, the recommended antibiotic is vancomycin (vancomycin, 1 g IV every 12 hours until birth). If sensitivity data are unknown at time of labor or ROM and the woman is at high risk for anaphylaxis, vancomycin is recommended for intrapartum prophylaxis (Jolivet, 2002).
- Women whose culture results are unknown at the time of delivery should be managed according to the risk-based approach (risk factors: birth before 37 weeks' gestation, ruptured membranes ≥18 hours, or temperature ≥104°F).
- Women with GBS bacteriuria in any concentration during their current pregnancy or who previously gave birth to an infant with GBS disease should receive intrapartum antimicrobial prophylaxis.
- Women who are undergoing a planned cesarean birth who have not begun labor or had a rupture of membranes should not receive intrapartum antibiotic prophylaxis.
- In the absence of GBS urinary tract infection, antimicrobial agents should not be used before the intrapartum period to treat asymptomatic GBS colonization.
- Routine use of antimicrobial prophylaxis for infants whose mothers received intrapartum chemoprophylaxis for GBS is not recommended. However, therapeutic use of these agents is appropriate for infants with clinically suspected sepsis. If no intrapartum prophylaxis for GBS was administered despite an indication being present, data are insufficient in recommending a single strategy. A full diagnostic workup and empiric therapy is the usual course.

Neonatal Resuscitation at Birth

Common Allegations

- Failure to anticipate resuscitation needs of infant whose mother experienced pregnancy complications and/or after a nonreassuring FHR pattern during labor

- Failure to have appropriate personnel and equipment available for neonatal resuscitation

Standards, Guidelines, and Recommendations

- All members of the perinatal team who are involved in labor and birth should have successfully completed the neonatal resuscitation course sponsored by AAP and the American Heart Association (AHA) (AAP & AHA, 2006).
- There should be one person at every birth whose primary responsibility is the baby and who is capable of initiating resuscitation (AAP & AHA, 2006).
- Either that professional or an alternate who is immediately available should have the skills required to perform a complete resuscitation, including endotracheal intubation and administration of medications (AAP & AHA, 2006).
- When resuscitation is needed, it must be initiated without delay. It is not sufficient to have someone on-call (either at home or in a remote area of the hospital) for newborn resuscitation in the delivery room (AAP & AHA, 2006).
- If the birth is anticipated to be high-risk, and thus may require more advanced resuscitation, at least two persons should be present solely to manage the baby: one with complete resuscitation skills and one or more to assist (AHA & AAP, 2006).

CONFLICT RESOLUTION

No group of individuals can work together in an organization and always share the same expectations, goals, and identical perspectives. Conflict is an inevitable result when reality does not meet with individual expectations. While individual expectations may differ, usually there exists among caregivers a basic commitment to quality and to the best possible outcomes for mothers and babies. Mutual trust and respect and the capacity to engage in agreeable disagreement are the hallmarks of a professional unit. When involved in a clinical or administrative situation that can potentially cause conflict, consider that both parties probably have the best interests of the patient in mind, although there may be different approaches proposed to achieve that goal. At times, clinical practice issues arise when the "way we've always done it" conflicts with a new or an alternate approach.

If the conflict is not related to an emergent patient situation (eg, there is at least some time for discussion), effective communication techniques can enhance the chances of conflict resolution to the satisfaction of both parties, or at least to reach a workable compromise. Taking time to really listen and understand the intent of the other person is a helpful starting point. While

others express their concerns, give visual and verbal feedback to ensure that they know you take them seriously. For example, nod or say, "I see, please go on." or summarize what it is the other person is concerned about by saying, "let me see if I understand you correctly." Then use phrases such as, "I have a different perspective." This usually works better in conflict resolution than, "You are wrong." Other successful strategies include a calm, collected attitude and careful consideration of the goal to be accomplished.

Communication in conflict resolution may not always be so rational and under one's control. This is especially true when dealing with difficult people, particularly those who are hostile or aggressive. These individuals manifest behavior that is abusive, abrupt, intimidating, and overwhelming. Being confronted by this behavior often catches the victim by surprise and generates feelings of helplessness. When being attacked, stand up for yourself and command respect. Calmly wait for the person to stop, then jump in. Use words that express your assertiveness. For example, say, "I am willing to discuss this with you when you are ready to speak to me with respect." This may help stop the verbal attack and allow time for more respectful discussion when the other person is rational.

Selecting the best time and place for interaction is also essential. Ideally the setting will not allow opportunity for patients, family members, or other colleagues to overhear the discussion. The focus of the discussion should remain on the issue, preferably on the potential impact on patient care. If the conversation deteriorates beyond your personal capacity to handle it or the colleague becomes verbally abusive, end the discussion until a later time and inform a third party who has the ability to help or the responsibility to know about the interaction.

An important strategy for promoting positive long-term professional collaboration is the development of interdisciplinary specialty practice opportunities where colleagues can come together to work toward a common goal. This can include developing unit guidelines, learning from a case review or grand rounds, examining quality of research findings, designing unit projects, or discussing conflict resolution. When colleagues come together to identify problems, define objectives, address alternatives, integrate changes, remain patient focused, disagree agreeably, negotiate, demonstrate mutual respect, and recognize and praise positive attributes and actions, it facilitates a professional culture for positive conflict resolution.

Some issues of conflict in the clinical setting cannot be solved at the lowest level and do not allow the luxury of time. If, after careful deliberation, the issue is determined to be a matter of maternal/fetal well-being or there is potential for the clinical situation to deteriorate rapidly, the nurse must initiate an appropriate course of action. One example is failure of the physician to respond to a

CHAIN OF COMMAND

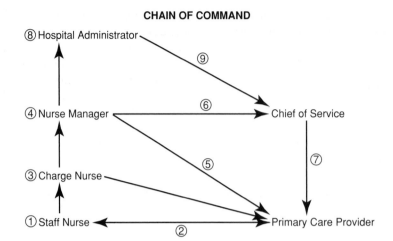

EXAMPLE
1. Conflict exists between judgment of nurse and primary care provider.
2. Direct conversation with primary care provider to verbalize/communicate conflict/concern.
3. Notification of charge nurse, who may confer with provider.
4. Notification of nurse manager.
5. Conversation with primary care provider.
6. Conversation with chief of service.
7. Chief of service confers with primary care provider.
8. Hospital administrator notified.
9. Hospital administrator confirms resolution of conflict.

WHO: Every perinatal nurse
WHAT: A mechanism (usually administrative) to resolve conflict in patient management plans
WHERE: Every patient-care setting
WHEN: Whenever there is a question regarding patient care, patient safety, or the nurse is uncertain about how to proceed in a situation of conflict
HOW: Notification of an administrative line of authority to resolve the conflict

FIGURE 1–1: Each perinatal care setting should have its own administrative chain of command to assist in conflict resolution in the management of patients. Such a chain of command is illustrated here. Adapted from Chez, B. F., Harvey, C. J., & Murray, M. L. (1990). *Critical concepts in fetal heart rate monitoring.* (p. 32). Baltimore: Williams & Wilkins.

nonreassuring FHR pattern or deteriorating maternal condition. Decisive, timely nursing intervention may be necessary to avoid a potentially adverse outcome. Knowledge and the use of the chain of command are ways to attempt to resolve differences of opinion in clinical practice settings. An example of chain of command is presented in Figure 1–1. If discussions with the physician or CNM do not result in care appropriate for the clinical practice situation, the nurse has the responsibility to use the perinatal unit institutional chain of command to avoid harm to the mother and/or baby. Frequently this involves the staff nurse notifying the appropriate, immediately available supervisory nurse (eg, charge nurse, nurse manager, or nursing supervisor) to provide assistance. In selected instances, it may be necessary to go further up the chain of command to resolve the situation. This process may require more time than the situation can accommodate. In other words, invoking the complete use of the chain of command is generally most successful when there is an urgent situation (eg, progressively nonreassuring FHR tracing) rather than an overt emergency (eg, shoulder dystocia).

Institutions have a responsibility to support nurses who use the chain of command. Nurses may be reluc-

tant to invoke this process due to intimidation, sense of personal or professional jeopardy, fear of retribution, or lack of confidence in the institutional lines of authority and responsibility. Medical hierarchy can be a powerful deterrent to speaking up when appropriate and following through on concerns about care that may not be in the best interests of the patient. It is important that nurses and physicians know the institution's policy for chain of command, data about its use be collected and analyzed so that the process can be optimized, and personnel receive positive feedback for its appropriate use. Chain of command should not be the routine method of conflict resolution. Clinical disagreements that result in going up the chain are detrimental to nurse-physician relationships. Soon after a clinical disagreement that results in use of the chain of command, all those involved should meet and calmly discuss what happened and why. Having an objective third party such as the risk manager present during this discussion may facilitate the interaction. Prospective plans should then be developed to avoid this situation in the future. A positive corporate culture that includes selected use of the chain of command recognizes that when personnel are given the resources, support, and guidance that are necessary to carry out the responsibilities of their positions, everyone generally benefits: the institution, its employees, the medical staff, and the patients.

MEDICAL RECORD DOCUMENTATION

Medical record documentation is a vital nursing function. The purpose of the medical record is to communicate patient status to other members of the healthcare team and to provide an accurate, timely description of the course of care and the patient's response. The nurse providing care is in control of the information included in the nursing portions of the medical record; however, documentation has become one of the most time-consuming of nursing activities and, therefore, one that is prone to omissions. Nurses often are concerned that medical record documentation forces them to focus on paper work rather than patient care. Cumbersome documentation systems that require duplicate and triplicate entries of the same data contribute to this real problem. The ongoing challenge is to create a streamlined system for documentation that is cost-effective, easy to use, an efficient use of nursing time, and sufficiently comprehensive for current or subsequent review. There are significant ramifications for inaccuracies and omissions in medical record documentation. Documentation deficiencies may result in decreased communication among team members, denied reimbursement by insurance carriers for care rendered, lost information for statistical or outcome data for quality purposes, and, in the case of litigation, increased difficulty for the defense to prove its case.

Of all strategies to decrease liability, accurate and thorough documentation may be the easiest to accomplish; yet it is the most common missing piece. The medical record is often the single most important document available in the defense of a negligent action. Frequently, in issues of litigation, the nurse cannot recall the specific patient or incident and, therefore, must rely on written or computerized nurses notes completed at the time of patient contact. The time from event to formal legal inquiry may be several years, and the nurse may have limited independent recall without the documentation in the medical record. Without a complete and legible medical record, nurses may be unable to successfully defend themselves against allegations of improper care. Because lack of documentation equals a presumed lack of care, omissions are challenging to defend.

Litigation many times follows clinical events that result in significant adverse outcomes. Therefore, the most complete documentation should focus on the time period surrounding the adverse events. Obviously during emergent situations, medical record documentation occurs retrospectively. The first priority during an emergency is to provide immediate patient care. Then, after the mother or fetus or newborn is stable, documentation is possible. Post-event documentation should focus on reconstructing a summary of all of the assessments, actions, and communication that transpired as accurately and timely as possible. For example, following birth complicated by shoulder dystocia, note the time interval between delivery of the fetal head and the body, fetal assessment data and attempts to obtain data about fetal status during the maneuvers, the order of the maneuvers and interventions, suprapubic pressure (if used) to avoid later allegations of use of fundal pressure, times for calls for assistance and when help arrived, condition of the newborn at birth and the immediate newborn period, any resuscitation efforts (including those who attended the newborn), and a summary of the discussion that occurred between the physician or CNM and the patient and her family about the shoulder dystocia and subsequent condition of the newborn. The neonatal team in attendance must be aware of the difference between suprapubic pressure and fundal pressure to avoid a neonatal note that fundal pressure was used if this is inaccurate.

In the case of a nonreassuring FHR pattern of acute onset resulting in an emergent cesarean birth, summary documentation should include timely recognition of the problem, nursing actions initiated for maternal and/or fetal resuscitation, communication with team members and their responses, time to the surgical suite and incision, and chronologies of interventions performed (and by whom) for newborn resuscitation, followed by a note about the details of the discussion between the physician and the patient and her family. During emergent intrapartum situations, some nurses feel that documentation directly on the FHR strip can assist them in constructing notes after patient stabilization. If this approach is used, ensure that the narrative notes written later coincide with the FHR strip annotations.

The medical record should provide a factual and objective account of care provided, including direct and indirect communication with other members of the healthcare team. Only document clinically relevant information. Address information not related to the patient's care, such as the filing of incident reports, short staffing, or conflicts between nurses and primary care providers, through the appropriate institutional channels rather than in the medical record.

Bedside use of a medical record as the single source of comprehensive data about the maternal–fetal status, nursing interventions, and the events of labor and birth, written or computerized flow sheets facilitate timely and accurate medical record data entry. Well-designed flow sheets are useful tools to prompt appropriate notations and practice consistent with unit guidelines, especially in the labor and birth setting. Ideally this flow sheet is keyed to the NICHD terminology for FHR patterns to facilitate consistent medical record documentation concerning fetal status by all members of the team. Routine assessments and interventions can easily be documented in the flow sheet format. The practice of duplicate documentation of routine care on both the FHR strip and the medical record is outdated (Chez, 1997). Previously, perinatal nurses believed there should be enough documentation on the FHR strip so that the strip could stand alone for subsequent review. However, writing on the strip not only increases the amount of nursing time spent on inpatient care activities, but this practice also contributes to late entries on the medical record and can lead to errors in documentation. If the FHR strips are electronically archived, hand-written notes on the strip do not become part of the permanent medical record.

Use narrative notes to document nonroutine care or events that are not included on the flow sheet. Also use narrative notes to document any nurse-physician communication, ongoing interventions for a nonreassuring FHR that does not resolve with the usual intrauterine resuscitation techniques, significant changes in maternal status, patient concerns or requests, and complete details of emergent situations and the outcome.

Retrospective charting is better than no documentation. However, late entries following an adverse outcome are often areas of controversy in litigation if they are written days after the event. Often these types of late entries have a defensive tone. Ensure that the data entered are accurate and objective. Do not alter the medical record to include data that are not accurate, even if asked to do so by someone in a position of authority. Falsification of the medical record is not only dishonest and unethical, but it can lead to successful claims against the nurse and institution.

One method to promote accurate and timely medical record documentation is to conduct routine medical record audits (see Display 1–1). Ideally this process is coordinated by a committee of perinatal nursing peers who have volunteered to participate. An additional important by-product of medical record audits is the ability to evaluate unit and individual competence in various aspects of clinical care. When the fetal monitoring strip is used to compare FHR pattern interpretation and interventions documented in the medical record, valuable insight can be gained. Based on data collected, strategies can be developed for improvement for unit practice and/or individuals as appropriate.

INCIDENT MANAGEMENT

An incident may be defined as any happening that is not consistent with the routine care of a particular patient. Many adverse perinatal outcomes that result in litigation derive from perinatal incidents that are unexpected or are the result of an emergency occurrence. Emergency occurrences can be categorized as actual, evolving, or perceived. Actual emergencies may include maternal hemorrhage, prolapsed cord, amniotic fluid embolism, shoulder dystocia, or neonatal asphyxia. Evolving emergencies are those that develop gradually and go unrecognized until an acute situation occurs. Examples include progressive deterioration in fetal status evolving to terminal bradycardia, severe preeclampsia converting to overt eclampsia, or an unrecognized malpresentation progressing to precipitous birth without appropriate preparation. Finally, perceived emergencies are the near misses that have the potential to result in adverse outcomes. These may include insufficient resources, inadequate communication, professional knowledge deficits, or ineffective lines of authority and responsibility.

Incident management, therefore, plays an important role not only in reducing institutional liability, but also in promoting a safer care environment. The goal is for members of the interdisciplinary perinatal team to objectively assess what happened (or what might have happened in the case of near misses) so that problem-prone systems or operations can be identified. After identification there may be opportunities for improvement to prevent an adverse event or recurrence of the adverse event. This process requires time, extensive communication, and a systematic framework. Generally, incident management is a retrospective process that includes the examination of all of the events surrounding the incident. Key questions for the review include the following:

- What happened?
- What were the contributing factors?
- Was it preventable?
- How was it handled?
- Were sufficient resources available?
- Was there the opportunity to handle it better?
- Is there a need for remedial action?
- What is the appropriate follow-up?
- What is the required documentation?

Sentinel Events

Some incidents are of such serious nature that they are classified as sentinel events and require specific actions by JCAHO-accredited institutions. A sentinel event is defined by JCAHO (2005b) as an unexpected occurrence involving death or serious physical or psychological injury, or the risk thereof. Serious injury specifically includes loss of limb or function. The phrase "or the risk thereof" includes any process variation for which a recurrence would carry a significant chance of a serious adverse outcome. Such events are called "sentinel" because they signal the need for immediate investigation and response (JCAHO, 2005b).

Sentinel events in perinatal services that are subject to review by JCAHO include any occurrence that meets any of the following criteria (JCAHO, 2005b):

DISPLAY 1-1

Suggested Components of a Medical Record Audit

- Are the times noted on the Admission Assessment, Labor Flow Chart, and initial EFM strip consistent with each other within a reasonable timeframe?
- If elective labor induction, is gestational age of at least 39 weeks confirmed?
- Is it documented that the physician was notified of admission within the timeframe outlined in the policies and procedures?
- Is fetal well-being established on admission?
- Is fetal well-being established prior to ambulation?
- Is fetal well-being established prior to medication administration?
- Does the EFM FHR baseline rate match the FHR baseline documented?
- Does the EFM FHR baseline variability match the FHR baseline variability documented?
- If there is evidence of absent or minimal FHR variability, is it documented?
- If there is evidence of absent or minimal FHR variability, are appropriate interventions documented?
- If there are FHR decelerations on the EFM strip, are they correctly documented?
- Are appropriate interventions documented during nonreassuring FHR patterns?
- Is there documentation of physician notification during nonreassuring FHR patterns?
- If FHR accelerations are documented, are they on the EFM strip?
- Are maternal assessments documented according to policy?
- If there is evidence of a nonreassuring FHR pattern, is oxytocin dosage increased?
- If there is evidence of a nonreassuring FHR pattern, is oxytocin dosage discontinued?
- If there is evidence of uterine hyperstimulation, are appropriate interventions documented?
- If there is evidence of adequate labor, is oxytocin dosage increased?
- If there is evidence of uterine hyperstimulation, is oxytocin dosage increased or decreased?

- Does the frequency of uterine contractions on the EFM strip match what is documented?
- Is the uterine activity monitor (external tocodynamometer or intrauterine pressure catheter [IUPC]) adjusted to maintain an accurate uterine activity baseline?
- Are oxytocin dosage increases charted when there is an inaccurate uterine baseline tracing or an uninterpretable FHR tracing?
- Is the physicians' documentation of fetal status consistent with the nurses' documentation?
- Are automatically generated data from blood pressure and SpO2 devices accurate?
- Does documentation continue during the second stage of labor?
- Are patients in the second stage of labor encouraged to push before they feel the urge to push?
- Are patients in the second stage of labor encouraged to push with contractions when the FHR is nonreassuring (ie, are there variable or late FHR decelerations occurring with each contraction)?
- When the FHR is nonreassuring during the second stage of labor, is pushing discontinued or encouraged with every other or every third contraction to maintain a stable baseline rate and minimize decelerations?
- If the FHR is nonreassuring during the second stage of labor, is oxytocin discontinued?
- Are uterine contractions continuously monitored during the second stage of labor via external tocodynamometer or IUPC?
- Does the time of birth on the medical record match the time of birth at end of the EFM strip?
- If the patient had regional analgesia/anesthesia, is a qualified anesthesia provider involved in the decision to discharge from postanesthesia care unit (PACU) care?
- If the patient had regional analgesia/anesthesia, is the discharge from PACU care scoring evaluation documented?
- Are maternal assessments documented during the immediate postpartum period every 15 minutes for the first hour?
- Are newborn assessments documented during the transition to extrauterine life at least every 30 minutes until the newborn's condition has been stable for 2 hours?

- The event has resulted in an unanticipated death or major permanent loss of function, not related to the natural course of the patient's illness or underlying condition
- The event is one of the following (even if the outcome was not death or major permanent loss of function unrelated to the natural course of the patient's illness or underlying condition):
  - Any individual death, paralysis, coma, or other major permanent loss of function associated with a

medication error. Suicide of any individual receiving care, treatment, or services in an around-the-clock care setting or within 72 hours of discharge.
- Any intrapartum maternal death.
- Any perinatal death unrelated to a congenital condition in an infant having a birth weight greater than 2500 g (eg, unanticipated death of a full-term infant).
- Infant abduction.
- Discharge of an infant to the wrong family.

- Hemolytic transfusion reaction involving administration of blood or blood products having major blood group incompatibilities.
- Surgery on the wrong individual or wrong body part.
- Unintended retention of a foreign object in an individual after surgery or other procedure.
- Severe neonatal hyperbilirubinemia (bilirubin >30 mg/dL).

Accredited organizations are expected to identify and respond appropriately to all sentinel events that occur in the organization or are associated with services that the organization provides, or provides for (JCAHO, 2005b). Appropriate response includes conducting a timely, thorough, and credible root-cause analysis, implementing improvements to reduce risk, and monitoring the effectiveness of those improvements (JCAHO, 2005b). Root-cause analysis is a process for identifying the basic or causal factors that underlie variation in performance, including the occurrence or possible occurrence of a sentinel event (JCAHO, 2005b). A root-cause analysis focuses primarily on systems and processes, not individual performance. It progresses from special causes in clinical processes to common causes in organizational processes and identifies potential improvements in processes or systems that would tend to decrease the likelihood of such events in the future, or determines, after analysis, that no such improvement opportunities exist (JCAHO, 2005b). The product of the root-cause analysis is an action plan that identifies the strategies that the organization intends to implement to reduce the risk of similar events occurring in the future. The plan should address responsibility for implementation, oversight, pilot testing as appropriate, time lines, and strategies for measuring the effectiveness of the actions (JCAHO, 2005b).

Not all sentinel events are the result of errors. For example a maternal death, while unexpected, may be unavoidable if the woman suddenly develops an amniotic fluid embolism or deteriorates as a result of consumptive coagulopathy. A term infant weighing 2,500 g may not survive a complete placental abruption or prolapsed umbilical cord. The key issue is to carefully analyze the event through as interdisciplinary process with the goal of developing strategies to prevent future occurrences. The discussion should avoid blaming individuals and instead focus on systems that may have failed them. Some adverse outcomes in perinatal care are not predictable or avoidable, despite the best efforts of healthcare providers and the availability of sophisticated technology.

METHODS OF MEASURING PATIENT SAFETY

Often the first indication that there are significant gaps in the safety net is the occurrence of a near miss or an adverse outcome. Retrospective review of systems and routine clinical processes reveal areas for improvement, but in some cases they are too late for the patient and healthcare providers involved. Rather than a reactive approach based solely on review of errors and accidents, an ongoing prospective program that includes various measures of safety can be used to develop strategies to minimize risk of patient harm (Simpson, 2006).

Measuring things that do not occur (eg, absence of patient harm as a result of the process of care) is a challenge. Nonetheless, various methods have been proposed as measures of patient safety, each with advantages and limitations. These include mainly structure, process, and outcomes measures. Structure measures cover the organizational context of care, such as the existence of an interdisciplinary practice committee and key clinical protocols for areas of care known to be associated with patient risk (eg, fetal assessment and neonatal resuscitation). Process measures evaluate how care is provided (eg, adherence to science- and standards-based clinical protocols or routinely beginning an emergent cesarean birth within 30 minutes of the decision to do so). Outcome measures for complication rates, morbidity, and mortality such as the Agency for Healthcare Research and Quality (AHRQ, 2003) patient safety indicators (PSIs); JCAHO (2002) core measures; and the National Quality Forum (NQF, 2004) performance measurement set for nursing-sensitive care are the most widely used evaluation method. Qualitative assessment methods also can provide rich actionable data. These include focus groups (Hesse-Biber & Leavy, 2006), story telling (Beyea, Killen, & Knox, 2004) and executive walk rounds (Thomas, Sexton, Neilands, Frankel, & Helmreich, 2005). Other types of measurement tools include safety surveys such as the AHRQ (2004) *Hospital Survey on Patient Safety Culture* and the *Safety Attitude Questionnaire* (Sexton et al., 2003).

Structure Measures

Structure measures are easy to analyze because they are based on concrete objective data. Most can be reported as a simple yes/no or in rates or percentages. Questions include the following: Is there an interdisciplinary practice committee?, Are there standard unit policies for oxytocin, misoprostol, and magnesium sulfate administration?, Are there standard physician order sets; what percentage of the perinatal team holds certification in electronic fetal monitoring?, Is there an anonymous nonpunitive error-reporting system?, etc. Although it may be difficult to determine a direct cause and effect relationship between the existence of certain organizational structures and patient safety, it is generally assumed that they enhance the safe care environment (Leape & Berwick, 2005; Pronovost, Nolan, Zeger, Miller, & Rubin, 2004). (See Table 1–1 for examples of structure measures.)

TABLE 1–1 ■ SELECTED STRUCTURE MEASURES FOR PERINATAL PATIENT SAFETY

Measure	Results
Interdisciplinary perinatal practice committee	Yes/No
Nurse and physician co-chairs of interdisciplinary practice committee	Yes/No
Regularly scheduled interdisciplinary case reviews	Yes/No
Interdisciplinary fetal monitoring education	Yes/No
Medical record documentation forms and electronic systems with cues for use of the NICHD terminology for FHR patterns	Yes/No
Weekly interdisciplinary fetal monitoring strip reviews	Yes/No
Routine medical record audits using fetal monitoring strips as part of the review	Yes/No
Uniform criteria for selecting cases for review	Yes/No
Standard policy for oxytocin administration (start at 1 mU/min and increase by 1 to 2 mU/min based on labor progress and fetal status, no more frequently than every 30 to 40 min; direct bedside physician evaluation required for increases beyond 20 mU/min; IV solution with 30 units in 500 mL for labor induction; IV solution with 20 units in 1000 mL for immediate postpartum; IV solutions prepared by pharmacy)	Yes/No
Standard order set for oxytocin administration based on components of policy listed above	Yes/No
Standard policy for misoprostol administration (25 mcg as the initial dose; every 4 to 6 hours; oxytocin no sooner than 4 hours after last dose; continuous EFM for at least 4 hours after dose)	Yes/No
Standard order set for misoprostol administration based on components of policy listed above	Yes/No
Standard policy for magnesium sulfate administration (IV loading dose administered in 4 g [100 mL] or 6 g [150 mL] solution; maintenance solution 20 g in 500 mL; nurse double-checks for all dosage/pump changes; IV solutions prepared by the pharmacy)	Yes/No
Policy requiring full surgical team in-house during labor of women attempting VBAC	Yes/No
Criteria for prioritizing labor inductions based on medical necessity	Yes/No
Requirement for 39 completed weeks of gestation before elective labor induction and elective cesarean birth	Yes/No
Agree-upon definition of uterine hyperstimulation and expected interventions based on ACOG/AWHONN standards	Yes/No
Clinical algorithm for intrauterine resuscitation during nonreassuring FHR patterns	Yes/No
Protocol for second-stage labor care based on AWHONN guidelines	Yes/No
Policy for prevention of perinatal GBS based on AAP/ACOG/CDC recommendations	Yes/No
Policy for prevention of perinatal transmission of HIV based on ACOG/CDC recommendations	Yes/No
Policy for treatment of neonatal hyperbilirubinemia and kernicterus prevention based on AAP/JCAHO recommendations	Yes/No
Policy requiring analgesia and anesthesia for all circumcision	Yes/No
Criteria for transfer of high-risk mothers and babies	Yes/No
Nurse staffing based on ACOG/AWHONN guidelines	Yes/No
Nurses' role in epidural anesthesia consistent with AWHONN guidelines (ie, no programming epidural pumps, changing doses, giving boluses, or signing out narcotics for anesthesia providers)	Yes/No
Anonymous, nonpunitive error-reporting system	Yes/No
Good citizenship/professional behavior policy	Yes/No
All members of the perinatal leadership team are members of their professional association (ACOG, AAP, ASA, AWHONN, or NANN)	Yes/No
% of physicians who are board-certified	
% of nurses who hold certification in inpatient obstetrics	
% of the perinatal team who hold certification in fetal monitoring	
% of the perinatal team who have attended a fetal monitoring workshop within the past 2 years	
% of the perinatal team who have completed the neonatal resuscitation program course within the past 2 years	

Process Measures

The degree to which institutions and healthcare providers adhere to processes that are supported by scientific evidence or recommended by professional organizations and regulatory agencies can be measured (Pronovost et al., 2004). A process measure should have adequate specificity as defined by NQF (2002) (ie, the process or manner of providing the service should be clearly defined, and its essential components specified, so that one could conduct an audit and readily determine whether the practice is in use). Many healthcare providers are accepting of process measures because they are more in control of and accountable for care processes than patient outcomes, which can be affected by many other variables (Pronovost et al., 2004).

Process evaluation usually requires medical record review, which can be a time-consuming endeavor. Therefore, random samples of cases of each process under investigation are generally used rather than 100% of cases, particularly if the process is common (eg, compliance with appropriate gestational age criteria for elective birth). If the process is rare (eg, care during shoulder dystocia), review of all cases is feasible and should be considered. Although labor-intensive, medical record review as a component of process measurement often uncovers important data concerning clinical care and documentation practices. Some process measures ideally should reveal nearly 100% adherence because there is a cumulative body of evidence or professional standards to support routine use in the absence of emergencies or patient refusal. For example, all baby boys should receive pain relief measures for circumcision (AAP, 1999; AAP & Canadian Paediatric Society, 2000; ACOG, 2001), all pregnant women should be screened for perinatal GBS during their prenatal care and, if positive, treated with chemoprophylaxis during labor (ACOG, 2002a), and all mothers who are HIV-positive should receive antiretroviral prophylaxis during labor (ACOG, 2004b). If the interdisciplinary perinatal practice committee has been empowered to enact policies and require routine adherence, other process measures can also be expected to have a 100% adherence rate. These include physician notification of specific nonreassuring FHR patterns and bedside evaluation of patients with certain maternal–fetal complications within designated timeframes. (See Table 1–2 for examples of process measures.) A reliable and valid tool for measuring fetal safety during labor has been published (Simpson, 2005; 2006). This tool can be used to evaluate the process of care during nonreassuring FHR patterns. Ongoing process evaluation can be a valuable tool for providing continuous feedback and educational reminders to clinicians and to identify gaps in routine care that can potentially be eliminated.

A successful clinical outcome does not mean that the process of care was appropriate or timely. There are not large numbers of maternal or infant deaths in individual hospitals or healthcare systems that allow statistically stable estimates of the death rates or statistical analyses that are usually used with outcome-based patient safety indicators. When evaluating perinatal patient safety, process measurement is likely more useful to practicing clinicians and has more potential to identify errors, omissions, or miscommunication that can help the team develop strategies for improvement (Simpson, 2005). Components of the care processes that are found to consistently work well can be shared with all members of the team and adopted as expectations for routine practice.

Outcome Measures

The AHRQ (2003) recently published a set of PSIs that are intended to measure potentially preventable complications and iatrogenic events for patients treated in hospitals. The PSIs are for use with administrative data sets, particularly those found in hospital discharge abstract data. Many of the AHRQ PSIs exclude obstetric patients from their inclusion criteria. (See Table 1–3 for PSIs that include obstetric patients with information concerning the numerator for each.) The indicators can be risk-adjusted using age, gender, and demographics (Johnson, Handberg, Dobalian, Gurol, & Pearson, 2005). The PSIs are designed to screen for adverse events that patients experience as a result of their exposure to the healthcare system; these events are likely amenable to prevention by changes at the system or provider level. The most useful PSIs measure conditions likely to reflect medical error such as a foreign body accidentally left during a procedure or blood transfusion reaction. Those that measure conditions that conceivably, but not definitely, reflect medical error such as death in low-mortality diagnosis-related groups or postoperative infection require more careful case analysis (AHRQ, 2003).

Reliance on administrative data is both a strength and weakness of the AHRQ PSIs (Johnson et al., 2005). Administrative data sets allow the PSIs to be accessible and low-cost screening tools to help identify potential problems in quality of care and target promising areas for more in-depth review. Conversely, there are known limitations with using administrative data, including the difficulty in perfectly risk-adjusting outcomes and the lack of time relationships with events (Johnson et al., 2005). Reliability of administrative data is based on coding accuracy, timing of entries, and medical record documentation (Romano, Yasmeen, Schembri, Keyzer, & Gilbert, 2005). Errors in any of these areas can significantly obscure potential findings. Additionally, if the outcome is infrequent, it may take some time before providers can receive meaningful feedback in order to make practice changes (Pronovost et al., 2004). In cases of infrequent

TABLE 1–2 ■ SELECTED PROCESS MEASURES

Processes	Denominator	Numerator	Sample
Timely triage and disposition	Patients in sample who present to obstetric triage unit	All patients in denominator cohort who do not have documented decision for treatment or disposition within 2 hours of being seen in triage unit	30 medical records per month randomly selected from triage log who present to the obstetric triage unit
Adherence to unit policy for elective/repeat cesarean birth requiring 39 completed weeks of gestation	Patients in sample who have elective/repeat cesarean birth	All patients in denominator cohort who have cesarean birth before 39 completed weeks of gestation	30 medical records per month randomly selected from unit birth log of women who have elective/repeat cesarean birth
Adherence to unit policy for oxytocin administration for elective labor induction (appropriate gestational age of 39 completed weeks)	Patients in sample who have elective induction of labor	All patients in denominator cohort who are induced before 39 completed weeks of gestation	30 medical records per month randomly selected from unit birth log of women who had elective induction of labor
Adherence to unit policy for oxytocin administration for labor induction/augmentation (start at 1 mU/min and increase by 1 to 2 mU/min based on labor progress and fetal status no more frequently than every 30 to 40 min)	Patients in sample receiving oxytocin for labor induction/augmentation	All patients in denominator cohort who receive oxytocin outside the context of the policy dosage	30 medical records per month randomly selected from unit birth log of women who received oxytocin for labor induction/augmentation
Adherence to unit policy for oxytocin administration for labor induction/augmentation (physician evaluation for dose beyond 20 mU/min)	Patients in sample receiving oxytocin for labor induction/augmentation	All patients in denominator cohort who receive oxytocin dosage higher than 20 mU/min without documentation of bedside evaluation by an attending physician	30 medical records per month randomly selected from unit birth log of women who received oxytocin for labor induction/augmentation
Adherence to unit policy for oxytocin administration for labor induction/augmentation (hyperstimulation)	Patients in sample receiving oxytocin for labor induction/augmentation	All patients in denominator cohort with more than 20 min of unrecognized and untreated hyperstimulation	30 medical records per month randomly selected from unit birth log of women who received oxytocin for labor induction/augmentation (review includes EFM strip)
Adherence to unit policy for intrauterine resuscitation	Patients in sample who have a nonreassuring FHR pattern during labor	All patients in denominator cohort with more than 10 min of unrecognized and untreated nonreassuring FHR pattern	30 medical records per month randomly selected from unit birth log of women who had a nonreassuring FHR pattern during labor (review includes EFM strip)
Pre-epidural IV fluid hydration	Patients in sample who have epidural anesthesia during labor	All patients in denominator cohort who do not receive at least 500 mL of lactated Ringer's solution IV prior to epidural anesthesia during labor	30 medical records per month randomly selected from unit birth log of women who had epidural anesthesia during labor

(continued)

TABLE 1–2 ■ SELECTED PROCESS MEASURES (Continued)

Processes	Denominator	Numerator	Sample
Promoting second stage pushing fetal well-being	Patients in sample who have vaginal birth	All patients in denominator cohort who have unrecognized and untreated nonreassuring FHR during second-stage labor	30 medical records per month randomly selected from unit birth log of women who have vaginal birth
Prophylactic antibiotics prior to cesarean birth based on unit policy	Patients in sample who have cesarean birth	All patients in denominator cohort who do not receive antibiotics prior to cesarean birth	30 medical records per month randomly selected from unit birth log of women who have cesarean birth
Timely cesarean birth	Term patients in sample who have unscheduled cesarean birth after labor with an indication of maternal or fetal compromise	All patients in denominator cohort who do not have incision for cesarean birth within 30 minutes of the documented decision for cesarean birth	30 medical records per month randomly selected from unit birth log of women at term who had an unscheduled cesarean birth after labor with an indication of maternal or fetal compromise

outcomes, process measures may be more valuable. For example, it may take six months to a year to see evidence of decreased rates of iatrogenic preterm birth using outcomes data, whereas improved adherence to 39 completed weeks of gestation as criteria for elective birth (ACOG, 1999) may be seen within one month. Despite limitations, analysis of these inexpensive, readily available indicators may provide a screen for potential errors and a method of monitoring trends in care that put patients at risk.

The JCAHO (2002) pregnancy advisory panel identified interrelated, evidence-based measures that, when used together, can more fully assess the overall quality of care provided for pregnant women and newborns. These include vaginal birth after cesarean birth, inpatient neonatal mortality, and vaginal birth involving third- or fourth-degree perineal lacerations. All three measures in the *Pregnancy and Related Conditions Core Measure Set* can be primarily derived from administrative data and have been field tested in conjunction with the National Perinatal Information Center using its trend database to analyze the measures (JCAHO, 2002). This testing permitted refinement respecting the measures and provided information pertinent to risk adjustment models (JCAHO, 2002). Other measures have been identified for potential future implementation. (See Display 1–2.) According to JCAHO (2005a), the core measures have been developed based on defined attribute criteria, including precise definitions; reliability; validity; interpretable, risk-adjusted or stratified availability of data; the potential to target improve-

ment in the health of populations; usefulness in accreditation process; and under-provider control.

The NQF (2004) has identified 15 National Voluntary Consensus Standards for Nursing-Sensitive Care. They include three categories: patient-centered outcome measures, nursing-centered interventions measures, and system-centered measures. While many of the standards do not apply directly to perinatal care, two of the outcome measures (central line catheter–associated blood stream infection rate and ventilator-associated pneumonia for high-risk nursery patients) and all of the system measures (skill mix, nursing care hours per patient day, practice environment scale, and voluntary turnover) are applicable. The nursing practice environment can be measured using the *Revised Nursing Work Index* (Aiken & Patrician, 2000; Lake, 2002). The value of this set of indicators is that they have been shown to reflect quality of nursing care (NQF, 2004).

Often clinical leaders desire a method that will allow more timely notification of clinical events that may warrant closer scrutiny, rather than waiting for information from administrative data sets. A set of clinical indicators can be developed with requirements for case review. For this process to be successful, all members of the perinatal team must be aware of the indicators and notification procedures. One method that works well is the creation of a form that can be affixed to the front matter of the medical record (but is not a permanent component) with a list of clinical indicators that require notification. (See Display 1–3.)

TABLE 1–3 ■ PERINATAL AND NEONATAL-RELATED AHRQ PATIENT SAFETY INDICATORS AND NUMERATOR DEFINITIONS

Indicator	Numerator Definitions
Complications of anesthesia	Discharges with ICD-9-CM diagnosis codes for anesthesia complications in any secondary diagnosis fields per 1,000 discharges
Death in low-mortality diagnosis-related groups	Discharges with disposition of "diseased" per 1,000 population at risk
Foreign body left during procedure	Discharges with ICD-9-CM codes for foreign body left in during procedure in any secondary field per 1,000 surgical cases
Postoperative hemorrhage or hematoma	Discharges with ICD-9-CM codes for postoperative hemorrhage or postoperative hematoma in any secondary diagnosis field and code for postoperative control of hemorrhage or drainage of hematoma in any secondary procedure code per 1,000 discharges. Procedure code for postoperative control of hemorrhage must occur on the same day or after principal procedure.
Selected infections due to medical care	Discharges with ICD-9-CM code of 9993 or 99662 in any secondary diagnosis field per 1,000 discharges
Transfusion reaction	Discharges with ICD-9-CM code for transfusion reaction in any secondary diagnosis field per 1,000 discharges
Birth trauma: injury to neonate	Discharges with ICD-9-CM code for birth trauma in any diagnosis field per 1,000 live births
Obstetric trauma: cesarean birth	Discharge with ICD-9-CM code for obstetric trauma in any diagnosis or procedure field per 1,000 cesarean births
Obstetric trauma: vaginal birth with instrument	Discharge with ICD-9-CM code for obstetric trauma in any diagnosis or procedure field per 1,000 instrument-assisted vaginal births
Obstetric trauma: vaginal birth without instrument	Discharge with ICD-9-CM code for obstetric trauma in any diagnosis or procedure field per 1,000 vaginal births without instrument assistance

Adapted from Agency for Healthcare Research and Quality. (2003). *Quality indicators: Guide to patient safety indicators.* (AHRQ Publication 03-R203). Rockville, MD: Author.

Safety Attitude and Climate Surveys

Safety culture has been defined as the product of individual and group values, attitudes, perceptions, competence, and patterns of behavior that determine the commitment to, and the style and proficiency of, an organization's health and safety management (Nieva & Sorra, 2003). Over the past several years since the Institute of Medicine (Kohn et al., 1999) recommended changing healthcare organizational characteristics to create a culture of safety, surveys have been developed to measure safety attitudes and cultures. The most commonly known are the *Hospital Survey on Patient Safety Culture* (AHRQ, 2004) and the *Safety Attitude Questionnaire* (SAQ) (Sexton et al., 2003). All use Likert scales to measure individual attitudes. Most cover the five common dimensions of the patient safety climate: leadership, policies and procedures, staffing, communication, and reporting. To date, there are limited data linking a better or improved safety climate score to meaningful patient outcomes. Only the SAQ (Sexton et al., 2003) has been tested to determine whether better scores are associated with improved outcomes; these studies demonstrated a relationship between higher SAQ scores and lower medication error and risk-adjusted mortality rates (Colla, Bracken, Kinney, & Weeks, 2005). Healthcare organizations can use survey tools

DISPLAY 1-2

JCAHO Core Measures of Pregnancy and Related Conditions

INITIAL MEASURES

- Vaginal birth after cesarean birth (VBAC)
- Inpatient neonatal mortality
- Third- or fourth-degree laceration

FUTURE MEASURES

- Presence of prenatal record at time of admission
- Episiotomy rate
- Indications and/or rate of elective labor induction
- Primary cesarean birth rate
- Attempted (unsuccessful) VBAC
- Neonatal transfer to perinatal center
- Maternal transfer to perinatal center

Adapted from Joint Commission on Accreditation of Healthcare Organizations. (2002). *Pregnancy and related conditions core measure set*. Oak Brook, IL: Author.

to better understand their safety culture and identify areas for improvement. The safety culture assessment should be viewed as the starting point from which action planning begins and patient safety changes emerge (Nieva & Sorra, 2003).

Qualitative Methods

Focus groups, executive walk rounds, and story telling are examples of qualitative methods to assess perinatal patient safety. These methods can provide rich data with detailed descriptions of system vulnerabilities that may be otherwise not noted using more traditional types of measurements (Hesse-Biber & Leavy, 2006). Participants often respond favorably to simple questions that ask their opinions and perceptions of safety. Bedside care providers have direct knowledge of how the system actually works and appreciate the opportunity to offer feedback. The potential value is acknowledging their wisdom and engaging them directly in improvement efforts (Thomas et al., 2005). Focus groups using open-ended questions such as "what could be done to improve patient safety on your unit?" or "describe a common situation that you believe puts patients at risk for harm" work well to elicit responses that can be helpful in identifying gaps

DISPLAY 1-3

Sample Form for Request for Review of Clinical Events

CONFIDENTIAL: NOT PART OF MEDICAL RECORD—DO NOT COPY OR RELEASE This report is prepared for quality improvement and/or risk management purposes. The report and the information contained herein are privileged under Peer Review Statute.	Patient Name

DATE: _____

_____ Fetal monitor strip review (ie, Nonreassuring FHR, hyperstimulation, second-stage management)

_____ APGAR score <7 at 5 minutes of life for a term (≥37 weeks) infant

_____ Umbilical artery cord blood <7.10

_____ Infant injury during birth: ___fracture ___laceration ___ hematoma ___ other: _____

_____ Transfer of term (≥37 weeks) infant

_____ Intrapartum fetal death ≥24 weeks (excludes fetal demise known prior to admission)

_____ Emergent "crash" cesarean birth: Time of decision: _____ Time of incision: _____

_____ Placental abruption

_____ Uterine rupture

_____ Shoulder dystocia (circle any maneuver used to disimpact the shoulders: suprapubic pressure, McRoberts maneuver, other: _____.) Time elapsed from birth of fetal head to birth of body: _____ minutes.

_____ Other (eg, amniotic fluid embolism, pulmonary embolism, etc.): _____

_____ Extensive episiotomy/perineal laceration tear and/or repair

_____ Maternal hemorrhage _____ Transfusion _____ Hysterectomy _____ Uterine _____ Artery ligation or embolization

_____ Unplanned maternal return to surgery

_____ Maternal transfer to intensive care unit

_____ Maternal death

_____ RN only present at birth (ie, attending MD not present)

in the safety net. The facilitator can be a member of the leadership team or an external consultant. To be effective, however, participants must be confident that their comments will be confidential and their suggestions for improvement should be acted on as appropriate within a reasonable timeframe.

Executive walk rounds generally involve visits by hospital executives to patient units to discuss patient safety issues with direct care providers. Sample questions for executive walk rounds include Have there been any near misses that almost caused patient harm but didn't?, What aspects of the environment are likely to lead to the next patient harm?, Is there anything we could do to prevent the next adverse event?, and Can you think of a way in which the system or your environment fails you on a consistent basis? The discussions should lead to action followed by feedback to participants (Thomas et al., 2005). Executive walk rounds are visible demonstrations of the executive and the organizational commitment to patient safety. Those who participate in the discussions may develop a more positive attitude about the safety climate in the organization (Thomas et al., 2005).

Patient safety can be enhanced by telling stories about clinical successes and events that did not go as planned. Detailed stories of how situations evolved into adverse events can be more helpful in teaching safety concepts than traditional methods such as lectures and assigned reading (Beyea et al., 2004). Stories help listeners remember facts and details that otherwise might be forgotten. Discussions concerning what worked and what could have been done differently in emergent situations are valuable in planning for future emergencies, particularly in avoiding similar types of errors or miscommunication that may have occurred (Simpson & Knox, 2003b). Story telling opportunities may be provided during unit meetings, interdisciplinary case reviews, grand rounds, or informal teaching sessions.

External Review and Risk Assessment

Often members of the leadership team desire external review to determine the state of perinatal patient safety in an individual hospital or entire healthcare system. Generally this process includes a review of current clinical practices, policies, and protocols; selected medical records; recent sentinel events; and open and closed obstetric professional liability claims. Interviews with key members of the leadership team and individual care providers add qualitative data and confirmation of clinical practices identified during policy and medical record review. Ideally the review team is interdisciplinary, to enhance acceptance of the results and suggestions for improvement by all members of the perinatal team. Based on an objective review process, perinatal patient safety and professional lia-

bility risk can be determined. In some cases, external review is desired to confirm the leadership team's perceptions of quality care, while in other cases, the review follows an adverse outcome, series of adverse outcomes, or significant payout resulting from a successful malpractice claim. Whatever the reason, the process can be useful for identifying gaps in the safety net and planning for improvement.

PERINATAL PATIENT SAFETY NURSES

Some institutions have created a position for an advanced practice nurse whose primary responsibility is to promote safe care for mothers and babies by maintaining a focus on patient safety for all unit operations and clinical practices (Knox et al., 2003; Will, Hennicke, Jacobs, O'Neill, & Raab, 2006). Other responsibilities of the perinatal patient safety nurse include ensuring that all perinatal care providers and unit practices adhere to national professional standards as well as the principles of patient safety; coordinating professional communication education; maintaining professional collaboration and behavior; conducting ongoing objective analysis of practice based on structure, process, and outcome measures; and coordinating fetal monitoring education and certification (Knox et al., 2003; Will et al., 2006). Although the volumes in all hospitals may not support this position on a full-time basis, in some hospitals, a part-time position may be feasible.

SUMMARY

When the focus of care is putting safety of mothers and babies first, practice based on the cumulative body of science and national standards and guidelines is a natural and obvious conclusion. Keeping current is critically important for perinatal nurses to maximize safe care for mothers and babies and to minimize risk of patient injuries and professional liability. Effective leadership and interdisciplinary collaboration are essential. When there is mutual respect and professional behavior among all members of the perinatal team, a safe care environment is enhanced. Practice in a perinatal setting where patient safety is the number-one priority is professionally rewarding and personally fulfilling.

REFERENCES

Agency for Healthcare Research and Quality. (2003). *Quality indicators: Guide to patient safety indicators.* (AHRQ Publication No. 03-R203). Rockville, MD: Author.

Agency for Healthcare Research and Quality: (2004). *Hospital survey on patient safety culture.* Rockville, MD: Author. Retrieved February 7, 2007, from http://www.ahrq.gov/qual/hospculture

Aiken, L. H., & Patrician, P. A. (2000). Measuring organizational traits of hospitals: The revised nursing work index. *Nursing Research, 49*(3), 146–153.

American Academy of Pediatrics. (1999). *Circumcision policy statement.* Washington, DC: Author.

American Academy of Pediatrics & American College of Obstetricians and Gynecologists. (2002). *Guidelines for perinatal care* (5th ed.). Elkgrove Village, IL: Author.

American Academy of Pediatrics & American Heart Association. (2006). *Textbook of neonatal resuscitation* (5th ed.) Chicago, IL: Author.

American Academy of Pediatrics & Canadian Paediatric Society. (2000). *Prevention and management of pain and stress in the neonate.* Washington, DC: Author.

American College of Obstetricians and Gynecologists. (1999). *Induction of labor* (Practice Bulletin No. 10). Washington, DC: Author.

American College of Obstetricians and Gynecologists. (2000a). *Operative vaginal delivery* (Practice Bulletin No. 17). Washington, DC: Author.

American College of Obstetricians and Gynecologists. (2000b). *Response to Searle's drug warning on misoprostol* (Committee Opinion No. 248; Reaffirmed 2003). Washington, DC: Author.

American College of Obstetricians and Gynecologists. (2001). *Circumcision* (Committee Opinion No. 260; Reaffirmed 2004). Washington, DC: Author.

American College of Obstetricians and Gynecologists. (2002a). *Prevention of early-onset group B streptococcal disease in newborns* (Committee Opinion No. 279; Reaffirmed 2005). Washington, DC; Author.

American College of Obstetricians and Gynecologists. (2002b). *Shoulder dystocia* (Practice Bulletin No. 40). Washington, DC: Author.

American College of Obstetricians and Gynecologists. (2003). *Dystocia and augmentation of labor* (Practice Bulletin No. 49).Washington, DC: Author.

American College of Obstetricians and Gynecologists. (2004a). *2003 ACOG survey of professional liability.* Washington, DC: Author.

American College of Obstetricians and Gynecologists. (2004b). *Prenatal and perinatal human immunodeficiency virus testing: Expanded recommendations* (Committee Opinion No. 304). Washington, DC: Author.

American College of Obstetricians and Gynecologists. (2004c). *Vaginal birth after previous cesarean delivery* (Practice Bulletin No. 54). Washington, DC: Author.

American College of Obstetricians and Gynecologists. (2005). *Intrapartum fetal heart rate monitoring* (Practice Bulletin No. 62). Washington, DC: Author.

American College of Obstetricians and Gynecologists. (2006a). *Analgesia and cesarean delivery rates* (Committee Opinion No. 339). Washington, DC: Author.

American College of Obstetricians and Gynecologists (2006b). *Induction of labor for vaginal birth after cesarean delivery* (Committee Opinion No. 342). Washington, DC: Author.

American College of Obstetricians and Gynecologists & American Academy of Pediatrics. (2003). *Neonatal encephalopathy and cerebral palsy: Defining the pathogenesis and pathophysiology.* Washington, DC: Author.

American College of Obstetricians and Gynecologists and American Society of Anesthesiologists. (2001). *Optimal goals for anesthesia care in obstetrics* (Committee Opinion No. 256; Reaffirmed 2004). Washington, DC: Author.

American Nurses Association. (2001). *Code of ethics for nurses.* Washington, DC: Author.

Amiel-Tison, C., Sureau, C., & Shnider, S. M. (1988). Cerebral handicap in full-term neonates related to the mechanical forces of labour. *Baillieres Clinical Obstetrics and Gynaecology, 2*(1), 145–165.

Arias, F. (2000). Pharmacology of oxytocin and prostaglandins. *Clinical Obstetrics and Gynecology, 43*(3), 455–468.

Association of Women's Health, Obstetric and Neonatal Nurses. (2000). *Nursing management of the second stage of labor.* (Evidence-based clinical practice guideline). Washington, DC: Author.

Association of Women's Health, Obstetric and Neonatal Nurses. (2001). *The role of the registered nurse (RN) in the care of pregnant women receiving analgesia/anesthesia by catheter techniques (epidural, intrathecal, spinal, PCEA catheters)* (Clinical Position Statement). Washington, DC: Author.

Association of Women's Health, Obstetric and Neonatal Nurses. (2005). *Fetal heart monitoring principles and practices.* Washington, DC: Author.

Association of Women's Health, Obstetric and Neonatal Nurses (Producer). (2006). *High-touch nursing care during labor: Volume 3: Second stage labor support* [Video series]. Washington, DC: Author.

Barnett, M. M., & Humenick, S. S. (1982). Infant outcome in second stage labor pushing method. *Birth and the Family Journal, 9,* 221–229.

Beyea, S. C., Killen, A., & Knox, G. E. (2004). Learning from stories: A pathway to patient safety. *AORN Journal, 79*(1), 224–226.

Bofill, J. A., Rust, O. A., Schorr, S. J., Brown, R. C., Martin, R. W., Martin, J. N., Jr., et al. (1996). A randomized prospective trial of the obstetric forceps versus the M-cup vacuum extractor. *American Journal of Obstetrics and Gynecology, 175*(5), 1325–1330.

Bofill, J. A., Martin, J. N., Jr., & Morrison, J. C. (1998). The Mississippi operative vaginal delivery trial: Lessons learned. *Contemporary OB/GYN, 43*(10), 60–79.

Brumfield, C., Gilstrap, L. C., O'Grady, J. P., Ross, M. G., & Schifrin, B. S. (1999). Cutting your legal risks with vacuum-assisted deliveries. *OBG Management, 3,* 2–6.

Caldeyro-Barcia, R. (1979). The influence of maternal bearing-down efforts during second stage on fetal wellbeing. *Birth and the Family Journal, 6,* 17–21.

Caldeyro-Barcia, R., Giussi, G., Storch, E., Poseiro, J. J., Kettenhuber, K., & Ballejo, G. (1981). The bearing down efforts and their effects on fetal heart rate, oxygenation, and acid-base balance. *Journal of Perinatal Medicine, 9*(Suppl. 1), 63–67.

Chauhan, S. P., Magann, E. F., McAninch, C. B., Gherman, R. B., & Morrison, J. C. (2003). Application of learning theory to obstetric maloccurrence. *Journal of Maternal-Fetal and Neonatal Medicine, 13*(3), 203–207.

Chez, B. F. (1997). Electronic fetal monitoring: Then and now. *Journal of Perinatal and Neonatal Nursing, 10*(4), 1–4.

Choudhry, N. K., Fletcher, R. H., & Soumerai, S. B. (2005). Systematic review: The relationship between clinical experience and quality of health care. *Annals of Internal Medicine, 142*(4), 260–273.

Clark, S. L., Gimovsky, M. L., & Miller, F. C. (1984). The scalp stimulation test: A clinical alternative to fetal scalp blood sampling. *American Journal of Obstetrics and Gynecology, 148*(3), 274–277.

Clayworth, S. (2000). The nurse's role during oxytocin administration. *MCN American Journal of Maternal Child Nursing, 25*(2), 80–85.

Colla, J. B., Bracken, A. C., Kinney, L. M., & Weeks, W. B. (2005). Measuring patient safety climate: A review of surveys. *Quality and Safety in Healthcare, 14*(5), 364–366.

Cosner, K. R. (1996). Use of fundal pressure during second-stage labor: A pilot study. *Journal of Nurse Midwifery, 41*(4), 334–337.

Crane, J. M., & Young, D. C. (1998). Meta-analysis of low-dose versus high-dose oxytocin for labour induction. *Journal of the Society of Obstetricians and Gynaecologists of Canada, 20,* 1215–1223.

Crane, J. M., Young, D. C., Butt, K. D., Bennett, K. A., & Hutchens, D. (2001). Excessive uterine activity accompanying induced labor. *American Journal of Obstetrics and Gynecology, 97*(6), 926–931.

Food and Drug Administration. (1998). *Need for caution when using vacuum assisted delivery devices.* (FDA Public Health Advisory), Washington, DC: Author.

Fox, M., Kilpatrick, S., King, T., & Parer, J. T. (2000). Fetal heart rate monitoring: Interpretation and collaborative management. *Journal of Midwifery and Women's Health, 45*(6), 498–507.

Fraser, W. D., Marcoux, S., Krauss, I., et al., for the PEOPLE (Pushing Early or Pushing Late with Epidurals) Study Group (2000). Multicenter randomized trial of delayed pushing for nulliparous women in the second stage of labor with continuous epidural analgesia. *American Journal of Obstetrics and Gynecology, 182*(5), 1165–1172.

Freeman, R. K. (2002). Problems with intrapartum fetal heart rate monitoring interpretation, and patient management. *Obstetrics and Gynecology, 100*(4), 813–826.

Freeman, R. K., Garite, T. J., & Nageotte, M. P. (2003). *Fetal heart rate monitoring* (3rd ed.). Philadelphia, PA: Lippincott Williams & Wilkins.

Frigoletto, F. D., Jr., Lieberman, E., Lang, J. M., Cohen, A., Barss, V., Ringer, S., et al. (1995). A clinical trial of active management of labor. *New England Journal of Medicine, 333*(12), 745–750.

Gherman, R. B., Ouzounian, J. G., & Goodwin, T. M. (1998). Obstetric maneuvers for shoulder dystocia and associated fetal morbidity. *American Journal of Obstetrics and Gynecology, 178*(6), 1126–1130.

Golditch, B. D., Ahn, M. O., & Phelan, J. P. (1998). The fetal admission test and intrapartum fetal death. *American Journal of Perinatology, 15*(4), 273–276.

Greenwald, L. M., & Mondor, M. (2003). Malpractice and the perinatal nurse. *Journal of Perinatal and Neonatal Nursing, 17*(2), 101–109.

Hankins, G. D. V. (1998). Lower thoracic spinal cord injury: A severe complication of shoulder dystocia. *American Journal of Perinatology, 15*(7), 443–444.

Hansen, S. L., Clark, S. L., & Foster, J. C. (2002). Active pushing versus passive fetal descent in the second stage of labor: A randomized controlled trial. *Obstetrics and Gynecology, 99*(1), 29–34.

Hesse-Biber, S. N., & Leavy P. (2006). *The practice of qualitative research.* Thousand Oaks, CA: Sage.

Johnson, C. E., Handberg, E., Dobalian, A., Gurol, N., & Pearson, V. (2005). Improving perinatal and neonatal patient safety: The AHRQ patient safety indicators. *Journal of Perinatal and Neonatal Nursing, 19*(1), 15–23.

Joint Commission on Accreditation of Healthcare Organizations. (2002). *Pregnancy and related conditions core measure set.* Oak Brook, IL: Author.

Joint Commission on Accreditation of Healthcare Organizations. (2004). *Preventing infant death and injury during delivery.* (Sentinel Event Alert No. 30.). Oak Brook, IL: Author.

Joint Commission on Accreditation of Healthcare Organizations. (2005a). *Attributes of core performance measures and associated evaluation criteria.* Oak Brook, IL: Author.

Joint Commission on Accreditation of Healthcare Organizations. (2005b). *Sentinel event policy and procedures.* Oak Brook, IL: Author.

Joint Commission on Accreditation of Healthcare Organizations (2006). *Comprehensive accreditation manual for hospitals.* Oak Park, IL: Author.

Jolivet, R. R. (2002). Early-onset neonatal group-B streptococcal infections: 2002 guidelines for prevention. *Journal of Midwifery and Women's Health. 47*(6), 435–446.

Jury Verdict Research. (2004). *Current award trends in personal injury.* Horsham, PA: Author.

Kline-Kaye, V., & Miller-Slade, D. (1990). The use of fundal pressure during the second stage of labor. *Journal of Obstetric, Gynecologic, and Neonatal Nursing, 196*(6), 511–517.

Knox, G. E., Simpson, K. R., & Townsend, K. E. (2003). High reliability perinatal units: Further observations and a suggested plan for action. *Journal of Healthcare Risk Management, 23*(4), 17–21.

Kohn, L. T, Corrigan, J. M., & Donaldson, M. S. (1999). *To err is human: Building a safer health system.* Washington, DC: National Academy Press.

Lake, E. T. (2002). Development of the practice environment scale of the nursing work index. *Research in Nursing and Health, 25*(3), 176–188.

Leape, L. L., & Berwick, D. M. (2005). Five years after to err is human: What have we learned? *Journal of the American Medical Association, 293*(19), 2384–2390.

Lee, W. K., Baggish, M. S., & Lashgari, M. (1978). Acute inversion of the uterus. *Obstetrics and Gynecology, 51*(2), 144–147.

Lopez-Zeno, J. A., Peaceman, A. M., Adashek, J. A., & Socol, M. L. (1992). A controlled trial of a program for the active management of labor. *New England Journal of Medicine, 326*(7), 450–454.

Mayberry, L. J., Gennaro, S., Strange, L., Williams, M., & De, A. (1999). Maternal fatigue: Implications of second stage nursing care. *Journal of Obstetric, Gynecologic and Neonatal Nursing, 28*(2), 175–181.

Mayberry, L. J., Hammer, R., Kelly, C., True-Driver, B., & De, A. (1999). Use of delayed pushing with epidural anesthesia: Findings from a randomized controlled trial. *Journal of Perinatology, 19*(1), 26–30.

Mayberry, L. J., Strange, L. B., Suplee, P. D., & Gennaro, S. (2003). Use of upright positioning with epidural analgesia: Findings from an observational study. *MCN: The American Journal of Maternal Child Nursing, 28*(3), 152–159.

National Institute of Child Health and Human Development Research Planning Workshop (1997). Electronic fetal heart rate monitoring: Research guidelines for interpretation. *American Journal of Obstetrics and Gynecology, 177*(6),1385–1390 and *Journal of Obstetric, Gynecologic and Neonatal Nursing, 26*(6) 635–640.

National Quality Forum. (2002). *Better healthcare through safe practices.* Washington, DC: Author.

National Quality Forum. (2004). *National voluntary consensus standards for nursing-sensitive care: An initial performance measure set.* Washington, DC: Author.

Nieva V. F., & Sorra, J. (2003). Safety culture assessment: A tool for improving patient safety in healthcare organizations. *Quality and Safety in Health Care, 12*(Suppl 2), 17–23.

Nordstrom, L., Achanna, S., Nuka, K., & Arulkumaran, S. (2001). Fetal and maternal lactate increase during active second stage labour. *British Journal of Obstetrics and Gynaecology, 108*(3), 263–268.

O'Driscoll, K., Jackson, R. J., & Gallagher, J. T. (1970). Active management of labor and cephalopelvic disproportion. *Journal of Obstetrics and Gynaecology of the British Commonwealth, 77* (5), 385–389.

Paluska, S. A. (1997). Vacuum-assisted vaginal delivery. *American Family Physician, 55*(6), 2197–2203.

Parer, J. T., King, T., Flanders, S., Fox, M., & Kilpatrick. (2006). Fetal acidemia and electronic fetal heart rate patterns: Is there evidence of an association? *Journal of Maternal-Fetal and Neonatal Medicine. 19*(5), 289–294.

Partnership for Patient Safety. (2002). *First do no harm: Taking the lead.* Chicago, IL: Author.

Piquard, F., Schaefer, A., Hsiung, R., Dellenbach, P., & Haberey, P. (1989). Are there two biological parts in the second stage of labor? *Acta Obstetricia et Gynecologica Scandinavica, 68*(8), 713–718.

Phaneuf, S., Rodriguez-Linares, B., Tambyraja R. L., MacKenzie, I. Z., & Lopez Bernal, A. (2000). Loss of myometrial oxytocin receptors during oxytocin-induced and oxytocin-augmented labour. *Journal of Reproduction and Fertility, 120,* 91–97.

Porto, G., & Lauve, R. (2006). Disruptive clinician behavior: A persistent threat to patient safety. *Patient Safety & Quality Healthcare* (July/August). Retrieved August 31, 2006, from www.psqh.com

Pronovost, P. J., Nolan, T., Zeger, S., Miller, M., & Rubin, H. (2004). How can clinicians measure safety and quality in acute care? *Lancet, 363,* 1061–1067.

Roberts, C. L., Algert, C. S., Cameron, C. A., & Torvaldsen, S. (2005). A meta-analysis of upright positions in the second stage to reduce instrumental deliveries in women with epidural analgesia. *Acta Obstetricia et Gynecologica Scandinavica, 84*(8), 794–798.

Roberts, C. L., Torvaldsen, S., Cameron, C. A., & Olive, E. (2004). Delayed versus early pushing in women with epidural analgesia: A systematic review and meta-analysis. *Journal of Obstetrics and Gynaecology, 111*(12), 1333–1340.

Roberts, J. E. (2002). The "push" for evidence: Management of the second stage. *Journal of Midwifery and Women's Health, 47*(1), 2–15.

Rogers, R., Gilson, G. J., Miller, A. C., Izquierdo, L. E, Curet, L. B., & Qualls, C. R. (1997). Active management of labor: Does it make a difference? *American Journal of Obstetrics and Gynecology, 177*(3), 599–605.

Romano. P. S., Yasmeen, S., Schembri, M. E., Keyzer, J. M., & Gilbert, W. M. (2005). Coding of perineal lacerations and other complications of obstetric care in hospital discharge data. *Obstetrics and Gynecology, 106*(4), 717–725.

Rommal, C. (1996). Risk management issues in the perinatal setting. *Journal of Perinatal and Neonatal Nursing, 10*(3), 1–31.

Rosentein, A. H., & O'Daniel, M. (2005). Disruptive behavior and clinical outcomes: Perceptions of nurses and physicians. *American Journal of Nursing, 105*(1), 54–64.

Ryan, M. J. (2004) Patient safety: A matter of integrity. *Journal of Innovative Management, 9*(1), 11–20.

Sampselle, C., & Hines, S. (1999). Spontaneous pushing during birth. Relationship to perineal outcomes. *Journal of Nurse Midwifery, 44*(1), 36–39.

Sarno, A. P. Jr., Phelan, J. P., & Ahn, M. O. (1990). Relationship of early intrapartum fetal heart rate patterns and fetal outcome. *Journal of Reproductive Medicine. 35*(3), 239–242.

Schrag, S., Gorwitz, R., Fultz-Butts, K., & Schuchat, A. (2002). Prevention of perinatal group B streptococcal disease: Revised guidelines from the CDC. *Morbidity and Mortality Weekly Report, 51*(RR11), 1–22.

Sexton, J. B., Thomas, E. J., Helmreich, R. L., Neilands, T. B., Rowan, K., Vella, K., et al. (2003). *Frontline assessments of healthcare culture: Safety attitudes questionnaire norms and psychometric properties* (Technical Report No. 04-01). The University of Texas Center of Excellence for Patient Safety Research and Practice. Retrieved February 7, 2007, from http://www.utpatientsafety.org

Simpson, K. R. (1999). Shoulder dystocia: Nursing interventions and risk management strategies. *MCN: The American Journal of Maternal Child Nursing, 24*(6), 305–311.

Simpson, K. R. (2002). *Cervical ripening and induction and augmentation of labor* [Practice monograph]. Washington, DC: Association of Women's Health, Obstetric and Neonatal Nurses.

Simpson, K. R. (2004). Second stage labor care. *MCN: The American Journal of Maternal Child Nursing, 29*(6), 416.

Simpson, K. R. (2005). Failure to rescue: Implications for evaluating quality of care during labor and birth. *Journal of Perinatal and Neonatal Nursing, 19*(1), 23–33.

Simpson, K. R., (2006). Measuring perinatal patient safety: Review of current methods. *Journal of Obstetric, Gynecologic and Neonatal Nursing, 35*(3), 432–442.

Simpson, K. R., & James, D. C. (2005a). Effects of immediate versus delayed pushing during second-stage labor on fetal well-being: A randomized clinical trial. *Nursing Research, 54*(3), 149–157.

Simpson, K. R., & James, D. C. (2005b). Efficacy of intrauterine resuscitation techniques in improving fetal oxygen status during labor. *Obstetrics and Gynecology, 105*(6), 1362–1368.

Simpson, K. R., James, D. C., & Knox, G. E. (2006). Nurse-physician communication during labor and birth: Implications for patient safety. *Journal of Obstetric, Gynecologic and Neonatal Nursing, 35*(4), 547–556.

Simpson, K. R., & Knox, G. E. (2001). Fundal pressure during the second stage of labor: Clinical perspectives and risk management issues. *MCN: The American Journal of Maternal Child Nursing, 26*(2), 64–71.

Simpson, K. R., & Knox, G. E. (2003a). Adverse perinatal outcomes: Recognition, understanding and prevention of common types of accidents. *AWHONN Lifelines, 17*(3), 225–236.

Simpson, K. R., & Knox, G. E. (2003b). Common areas of litigation related to care during labor and birth: Recommendations to promote patient safety and decrease risk exposure. *Journal of Perinatal and Neonatal Nursing, 17*(1), 94–109.

Simpson, K. R., & Knox, G. E. (2006). Essential criteria to promote safe care during labor and birth. *AWHONN Lifelines, 9*(6), 478–483.

Thomas, E. J., Sexton, J. B., Neilands, T. B., Frankel, A., & Helmreich, R. L. (2005). The effect of executive walk rounds on nurse safety climate attitudes: A randomized trial of clinical units. *BMC Health Services Research, 5*(1), 28–37.

Tubridy, N., & Redmond, J. M. (1996). Neurological symptoms attributed to epidural analgesia in labour: An observational study of seven cases. *Journal of Obstetrics and Gynaecology, 103*(8), 832–833.

Wang, M. L., Dorer, D. J., Fleming, M. P., & Catlin, E. A. (2004). Clinical outcomes of near-term infants. *Pediatrics, 114*(2), 372–376.

Weber, D. O. (2004). Poll results: Doctors' disruptive behavior disturbs physician leaders. *The Physician Executive, 30*(5), 6–15.

Will, S. B., Hennicke, K. P., Jacobs, L. S., O'Neill, L. M., & Raab, C. A. (2006). The perinatal patient nurse: A new role to promote safe care for mothers and babies. *Journal of Obstetric, Gynecologic and Neonatal Nursing, 35*(3), 417–423.

White, A. A., Pichert, J. W., Bledsoe, S. H., Irwin, C., & Entman, S. S. (2005). Cause and effect analysis of closed claims in obstetrics and gynecology. *Obstetrics and Gynecology, 105*(5, pt 1), 1031–1038.

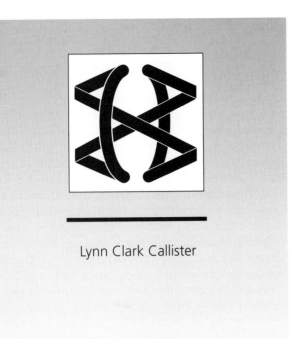

CHAPTER 2

Integrating Cultural Beliefs and Practices When Caring for Childbearing Women and Families

Lynn Clark Callister

MARIA, a Mexican-American woman having her first baby, attended a childbirth education class where the expectant fathers learned labor support techniques. She declined to lie on the floor surrounded by other men while her husband massaged her abdomen.

Inaam, a Muslim Arabic woman experiencing her first labor, was attended by her mother and mother-in-law. As the labor slowly progressed and Inaam began to be more uncomfortable, the two mothers rotated between offering her loving support, chastising her for acting like a child, and praying loudly that mother and baby will be safe from harm.

Nguyet, a Vietnamese immigrant, had been in the United States only a short time when she went into labor for the first time. She arrived at the birthing unit in active labor dilated to 5 cm. Nguyet and the father of the baby, Duc, spoke very limited English. Her labor was difficult, but she did not utter a sound. Duc entered the birthing room only when the nurses asked him to translate for Nguyet. After 20 hours of labor, a cesarean birth was performed. On the mother–baby unit, Nguyet cooperated with the instructions from the nurse to cough and deep breathe, but she became agitated when the nurse set up for a bed bath and began bathing her. When she was encouraged to walk, she shook her head and refused. She also refused the chilled apple juice the nurse brought to her. Because of abdominal distention and dehydration, a nasogastric tube was inserted, and intravenous fluids were restarted. No one could understand why she was so uncooperative.

Because of a nonreassuring fetal heart rate, Koua Khang needed an emergent cesarean birth. The nurse told her she would need to remove a nondescript white string bracelet from her wrist before surgery. Koua became hysterical, gesturing and trying to convey the message that the bracelet would protect her during the birth from evil spirits.

Cynthia, a certified nurse midwife, cared for a Mexican immigrant mother who finally confided in her that during her postpartum hospitalization she went in the shower and turned on the water but was very careful not to get wet. She was following instructions from her nurse while trying to maintain her own cultural beliefs.

Mei Lin, a Chinese woman in graduate school in the United States, promised her mother she would follow traditional Asian practices after her son was born, including "doing the month" and subscribing to the hot/cold theory. Even though this woman was intellectually aware these practices had little scientific basis, she demonstrated her respect for her mother and her culture by honoring her mother's request.

Childbirth is a time of transition and social celebration in all cultures. A Wintu child living in Africa, in deference to his mother, refers to her as, "She whom I made into mother." Culture also influences the experience of perinatal loss, because the meaning of death and rituals surrounding death are culturally bound. Healthcare beliefs and health-seeking behaviors surrounding pregnancy, childbirth, and parenting are deeply rooted in cultural context. Culture is a set of behaviors, beliefs, and practices, a value system that is transmitted from one woman in a cultural group to another (Lauderdale, 2003). It is more than skin color, language, or country of origin. Culture provides a framework within which women think, make decisions, and act. It is the essence of who a woman is. The extent to which a woman adheres to cultural practices, beliefs, and rituals is complex and depends on acculturation and assimilation into the dominant culture within the society, social support, length of time in the United States or Canada, generational ties, and linguistic preference. Even within individual cultural groups, there is tremendous heterogeneity. Although women may share a common birthplace or language, they do not always share the same cultural traditions.

Diversity is a reality in the United States and Canada. Nurses provide care to immigrants, refugees, and women from almost everywhere in the world, many of whom are of childbearing age (Carr & deJoseph, 2001). More than 30% of the US population now consists of individuals from culturally diverse groups other than non-Hispanic whites, whereas only 9% of registered nurses come from racial or ethnic minority backgrounds. It is projected that by the year 2050, minorities will account for more than 50% of the population of the United States. Each year, nearly 1 million immigrants come to the United States, half of whom are immigrant women of childbearing age. One in every 13 US residents is foreign born (http://www.census.gov).

Twenty-seven percent of women living in the United States are women of color. One of the challenges for healthcare in this century is that members of racial and ethnic minorities make up a disproportionately high percentage of persons living in poverty.

Poverty brings many challenges in healthcare delivery (United States Census Bureau [USCB], 2001; United States Department of Health and Human Services, 2000; Office of Minority Health, 2001). Poverty can be considered a culture associated with increased vulnerability in childbearing women. For example, in a recent study of low-income pregnant women (both white and African-American), abuse and depressive symptoms predicted substance use (Jesse, Graham & Swanson, 2006).

Clinical examples in this chapter represent only a fraction of the possible cultural beliefs, practices, and behaviors the perinatal nurse may see in practice (Display 2–1). It is beyond the scope of this chapter to thoroughly discuss in detail each cultural group. Although generalizations are made about cultural groups, a stereotypical approach to the provision of perinatal nursing care is not appropriate. Cultural

---

DISPLAY 2-1

Culture and Birth Traditions

AFRICAN-AMERICAN/BLACK

- Geophagia (ingestion of soil, chalk, or clay) may be present during pregnancy
- Strong extended family support
- Matriarchal society
- Present time orientation
- May engage in folk practices ("granny," "root doctor," voodoo priest, spiritualist) depending on background
- Tend to seek prenatal care after the first trimester

AMERICAN INDIAN AND NATIVE ALASKAN

- Healthcare decision-making by families/tribal leaders
- Often stoic; don't make eye contact, limit touch
- Strong spiritual foundation
- May utilize a medicine man or shaman
- Present time orientation

ASIAN-AMERICAN AND PACIFIC ISLANDER

- Culturally and linguistically hetereogeneous
- Healthcare decision-making by families
- "Hot/cold" theory of illness (pregnancy considered a "hot" condition, except among Chinese women, who consider it a "cold" condition)

- Asians are often stoic
- Strong extended family support
- Asian fathers may choose not to attend the birth
- Chinese postpartum focus on "doing the month"
- AAs have future orientation, PIs have present orientation
- Asians have high respect for others
- Asians may utilize an acupuncturist/acupressurist, herbalist

HISPANIC/LATINO

- Healthcare decision-making by families
- Strong extended family support
- Prenatal care may not be valued because pregnancy is a healthy state
- Enjoy strong extended family support
- Fathers may choose not to attend the birth
- May use folk healers and western medicine concurrently (curandero, espiritualista, yerbero)
- Present time orientation
- Believe in the "evil eye"
- Postpartum maternal/newborn dyad vulnerable or delicate

WHITE/CAUCASIAN

- Often considered a noncultural group
- Value autonomy and personal decision-making
- Eastern European women avoid cutting or coloring hair during pregnancy
- Future time orientation
- Focus on achievement

beliefs and practices are dynamic and evolving, requiring ongoing exploration. In any given culture, each generation of childbearing families perceives pregnancy, childbirth, and parenting differently. Each individual woman should be treated as such—an individual who may or may not espouse specific cultural beliefs, practices, and behaviors.

Cultures are not limited to the obvious traditional ethnic or racial groups. Examples of other "cultures" include refugees and immigrants, poverty-stricken women, women who have experienced ritual circumcision, adolescent childbearing women, and deeply religious women. Perinatal nursing units may also be considered a culture.

CULTURAL FRAMEWORKS AND CULTURAL ASSESSMENT TOOLS

Cultural frameworks and cultural assessment tools have been developed to guide perinatal nursing practice. The Sunrise Model is based on culture care theory (Fig. 2–1) (Leininger & McFarland, 2006). The Transcultural Assessment Model (Giger & Davidhizar, 2005) includes variables such as communication, space, social organization, time, environmental control, and biologic variations (Fig. 2–2). Others have identified the dimensions of culture, including values, worldview, disease etiology, time orientation, personal-space orientation and touch, family organization, and power structure (Moore & Moos, 2003). The Transcultural Nursing Model is illustrated in Figure 2–3 (Andrew & Boyle, 2003). Mattson (2004) has conceptualized specific ethnocultural considerations in caring for childbearing women (Fig. 2–4). Four assumptions define the influence culture has on pregnancy, childbirth, and parenting (Display 2–2). A model has been proposed for those caring for immigrant and minority women that moves beyond the bio-medical, reproductive/ maternal, and cultural models to one focusing on the person, process, environment, and outcomes. This model suggests that "cultural models of care often stereotype women who share the same cultural heritage" (Meleis, 2003).

Cultural Competence

The process of cultural competence in the delivery of healthcare includes cultural awareness, skills, encounters, and knowledge (Fig. 2–5) (Campinha-Bacote, 1994; Andrews, 2003; Purnell & Paulanka, 2003; Suh, 2004). Cultural competence is more than a nicety in healthcare. Cultural competence has become imperative because of increasing health disparities and population diversity; the competitive healthcare market; federal regulations on discrimination; complex legislative, regulatory, and accreditation requirements; and our litigious society (Bazaldua & Sias, 2004; deChesnay, Wharton, & Pamp, 2005).

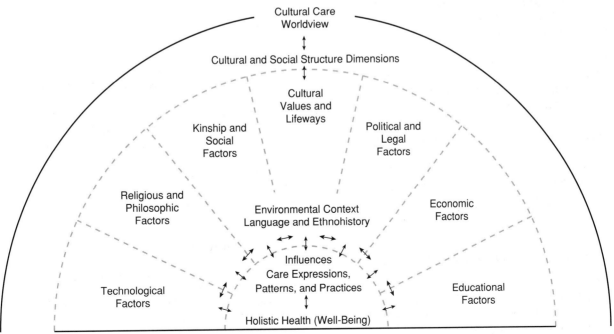

FIGURE 2–1. The sunrise model. (From Leininger, M. & McFarland, M. R. [2006]. *Cultural care diversity and universality* [2nd ed.]. Sudbury, MA: Jones & Bartlett.)

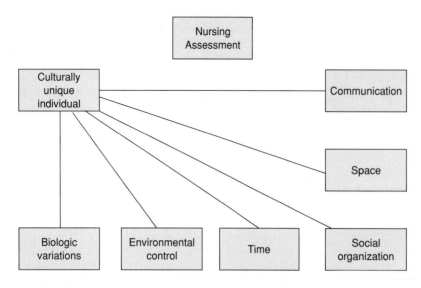

FIGURE 2–2. Giger and Davidhizar's transcultural model. (From Giger, J. N., & Davidhizar, R.E. [2005]. *Transcultural nursing: Assessment and intervention* [pp. 127–161]. St. Louis, MO: Mosby–Year Book.)

Acculturation is a complex variable that is challenging to measure, and current measures need to be refined (Beck, Froman, & Bernal, 2005; Foss, 2001; Zlot, Jackson, & Korenbrot, 2005). Acculturation can be at a cultural or group level and a psychological or individual level (Beck, 2005). The General Acculturation Index scale can be used to assess level of acculturation, and it includes items such as written and spoken language, the country where the childhood was spent, the current circle of friends, and pride in cultural background (Balcazar, Peterson, & Krull, 1997). Other instruments include the Short Acculturation Scale, the Acculturation Rating Scale for Mexican Americans (ARSMA), the ARSMA II, and the Bidimensional Acculturation Scale for Hispanics (Beck, 2005). A framework for acculturation has been identified by Berry (1980). Outcomes include assimilation, the establishment of relationships in the host society made at the expense of the patient's native culture; integration, in which cultural identity is retained and new relationships are established in the host society; rejection, in which one retains cultural identity and rejects the host society; and deculturation, in which one values neither. Nurses will encounter immigrant women who fall into each of these categories of acculturation.

What constitutes a positive and satisfying birth experience varies from one culture to another (Johnson, Callister, Beckstrand, & Freeborn, in press;

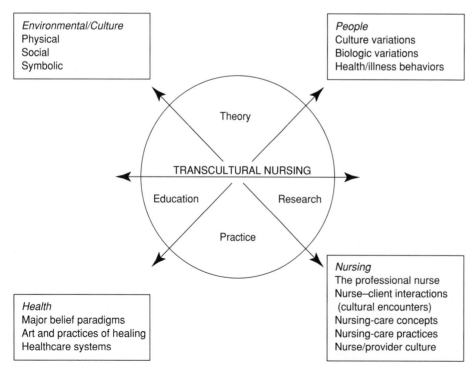

FIGURE 2–3. Transcultural nursing.

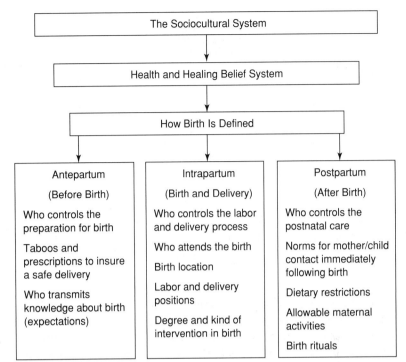

FIGURE 2–4. The sociocultural system, health and healing belief system, and how birth is defined. (From Mattson, S. [1995]. Culturally sensitive perinatal care for Southeast Asians. *Journal of Obstetric, Gynecologic, and Neonatal Nursing, 24*[5], 335–341.)

Melender, 2006). For example, within the Japanese culture, there is the belief in a process called "education of the unborn." A happy mother is thought to ensure joy and good fortune because the unborn child learns, communicates, and responds in utero. The individual personality is formed before birth. Such a belief about the fetus is reflected in many cultures, with concern during pregnancy about evil spirits and birthmarks. Other cultural considerations include fertility rites and beliefs about what determines the gender of the unborn child.

Rich meaning may be created by women espousing traditional religious beliefs (Callister, 2003a, 2005; Callister & Vega, 1998; Callister, Semenic, & Foster, 1999; Khalaf & Callister, 1997; Semenic, Callister, & Feldman, 2004). An Orthodox Jewish mother gives silent thanks in the ancient words of the Psalms following the birth of her first-born son. She believes that by birthing a son she has fulfilled the reason for her creation in

DISPLAY 2-2

Influence of Culture on Pregnancy, Childbirth, and Parenting

- Within the framework of the *moral and value system,* cultural groups have specific *attitudes* toward childbearing and the meaning of the birth experience.
- Within the framework of the *ceremonial and ritual system,* cultural groups have specific *practices* associated with childbearing.
- Within the framework of the *kinship system,* cultural groups prescribe *gender-related roles* for childbearing.
- Within the framework of the *knowledge and belief system,* cultural groups influence *normative behavior* in childbearing and the *pain experience* of childbirth

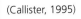
(Callister, 1995)

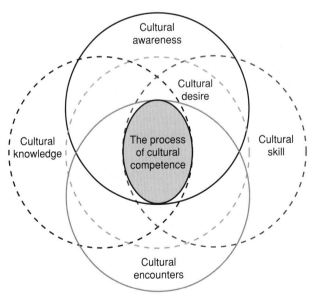

FIGURE 2–5. The process of cultural competence in the delivery of healthcare services. (From Campinha-Bacote, J. [1994]. *The process of cultural competence in healthcare: A culturally competent model of care.* Wyoming, OH: Transcultural CARE Associates.)

obedience to rabbinical law. The creation of life and giving birth represent obedience to religious law and the spiritual dimensions of the human experience.

Giving birth is a significant life event, a reflection of a woman's personal values about childbearing and child rearing and the expression and symbolic actualization of the union of the parents. For Muslim women, giving birth fulfills the scriptural injunctions recorded in the Quran. Muslim women may be asked soon after getting married, "Do you save anything inside your abdomen?" Meaning, "Are you pregnant yet?" Pregnancy in a traditional Asian family is referred to as a woman having "happiness in her body." In Latin America, if you were to ask an expectant mother when her baby is due, the direct translation from Spanish to English is, "when are you going to give light?"

PRACTICES ASSOCIATED WITH CHILDBEARING

There are many diverse cultural rituals, customs, and beliefs associated with childbearing. American Indian mothers believe tying knots or weaving will cause birth complications associated with cord accidents. Navajo expectant mothers do not choose a name or make a cradleboard because doing so may be detrimental to the well-being of the newborn. Arabic Muslim women do not prepare for the baby in advance (eg, no baby showers, layette accumulation, or naming the unborn child) because such planning has the potential for defying the will of Allah regarding pregnancy outcomes. Similarly, Russian women do not make prenatal preparations for the newborn, believing such actions would create bad luck. Filipino women believe that daily bathing and frequent shampoos during pregnancy contribute to having a clean baby. Asian-American women may not disclose their pregnancy until the 120th day, when it is believed the soul enters the fetus. In many cultures, girls are socialized early about childbearing. They may witness childbirth or be present when other women repeat their birth stories, especially extended female family members. In the Sudan, a pregnant woman is honored in a special ceremony, as extended female family members rub her belly with millet porridge, a symbol of regeneration, empowering her to give birth (Davis, 2000). Because of the importance of preserving modesty, Southeast Asian women tie a sheet around their bodies like a sarong during labor and express a preference to squat while giving birth. An Italian maternal grandmother may request permission to give her newborn grandson his first bath. After the bath she dresses him in fine, white silk clothing that she stitched by hand for this momentous occasion. When women in Bali hear the first cries of a newborn, they lavish the new mother with gifts such as dolls, fruit, flowers, or incense to bless, honor, purify, and protect the new child.

The placenta is called "el compañero" in Spanish, translated to mean, "the companion of the child." And there are a variety of cultural rituals associated with the disposal of the placenta, including having it dried, burned, or buried in a specific way. Although disposing of the placenta must meet with standard infection control precautions, individual family preferences should be honored as much as possible.

A variety of cultural practices influence postpartum and newborn care. Laotian women stay home the first postpartum month, near a fire or heater in an effort to "dry up the womb." The traditional postpartum diet for Korean women includes a soup made from beef broth and seaweed that is believed to cleanse the body of lochia and increase breast milk production. In Navaho tradition, a family banquet is prepared following the baby's first laugh because this touches the hearts of all those who surround the baby.

Care of the newborn's umbilical cord includes the use of a binder or belly band, the application of oil, or cord clamping, and then sterile excision. A Southeast Asian woman may fail to bring her newborn to the pediatrician during the first month after birth because this is considered to be a time for confinement and rest.

Postpartum cultural rituals are important for women of different cultures (Kim-Goodwin, 2003). In a study of African-American childbearing women, Amankwaa (2003) concluded that the absence of postpartum cultural rituals increases the likelihood of postpartum depression. Culturally diverse women experience postpartum depression, with an increased risk related to the gender of the child, because in some societies male children are more highly valued (Goldbort, 2005).

GENDER ROLES

Many cultural groups show strong preference for a son. For example, according to Confucian tradition, only a son can perform the crucial rites of ancestor worship. A woman's status is closely tied to her ability to produce a son in many cultures.

A Mexican immigrant woman may prefer that her mother or sister be present during her childbirth, rather than the father of her child. In some cultures, fathers may prefer to remain in the waiting room until after the birth. Vietnamese fathers rarely participate in the birth of their children. Only after the newborn is bathed and dressed may the father see him or her. In cultures in which the husband's presence during birth is not thought to be appropriate, nurses should not assume this denotes lack of paternal involvement and support.

Modesty laws and the law of family purity found in the Torah prohibit the Orthodox Jewish husband from observing his wife when she is immodestly exposed, and from touching her when there is vaginal bleeding. Depending on the specific religious sect, observance of the law varies from the onset of labor or bloody show to complete cervical dilation. Jewish husbands present at birth stand at the head of the birthing bed or behind a curtain in the room and do not observe the birth or touch their wives. In one study, only 37% of Orthodox Jewish husbands attended the birth (Callister et al., 1999). Although cultural factors may limit a husband's ability to physically support or coach his wife during labor and birth, Jewish women still feel supported. Husbands praying, reading Psalms, and consulting with the rabbi represent significant and active support to these women (Callister et al., 1999; Lewis, 2003; Semenic et al., 2004).

DISPLAY 2-3

Culture and Pain Communication

- Assess pain and cultural pain behaviors and practices
- Accept the choices of the woman about pain control after providing available information about pain management
- Demonstrate a willingness to listen to the woman's description of her pain
- Learn about culturally appropriate pain management strategies

(Munoz & Luckmann, 2005)

CHILDBIRTH PAIN AND CULTURE

A major pain experience unique to women is that associated with giving birth. Many cultural differences related to the perception of childbirth pain have been identified (Callister, 2003a; Callister, Khalaf, Semenic, Kartchner, & Vehvilainen-Julkunen, 2003). Some women feel that pain is a natural part of childbirth and that the pain experience provides opportunity for important and powerful growth. Others see childbirth pain as no different from the pain of an illness or injury; that it is inhumane and unnecessary to suffer.

Words used to describe the pain associated with childbirth vary. Labor pain has been described as horrible to excruciating, episiotomy pain described as discomforting and distressing, and postpartum pain described as mild to very uncomfortable. Korean women described pain with words such as "felt like dying" or the "the sky was turning yellow," or the sense of "tearing apart." Mexican-American women view pain as a physical experience, composed of personal, social, and spiritual dimensions. Scandinavian women demonstrate a high level of resilience and hardiness when giving birth. One Finnish woman spoke of her solitary struggle to meet the increasing pain of her contractions, "We were alone, me and my pain. I focused only on the pain and how I could work with the pain" (Callister, Vehvilainen-Julkenen, & Lauri, 2001, p. 30). Women's perceptions of personal control have been found to positively influence their satisfaction with pain management during childbirth (Carlton, Callister, & Stoneman, 2005).

Pain behaviors also are culturally bound. Some Hispanic laboring women may moan in a rhythmic way and rub their thighs or abdomen to manage the pain. During labor, Haitian women are reluctant to accept pain medication and instead use massage, movement, and position changes to increase comfort. Filipino women believe that noise and activity around them during labor increases labor pain. African-American women are more vocally expressive of pain. American Indian women are often stoic, using meditation, self-control, and traditional herbs to manage pain. Puerto Rican women are often emotive in labor, expressing their pain vocally. It has been documented that there is disparity between the estimation of labor pain by caregivers and the pain the women reported they were experiencing (Baker, Ferguson, Roach & Dawson, 2001). Suggestions for communication skills related to pain assessment and management are summarized in Display 2–3.

MAJOR CULTURAL GROUPS

The major cultural groups in the United States include African-American/blacks (AA/B), American Indian/ Alaska Native (AI/AN), Asian-American/Pacific Islander (AA/PI), Hispanic/Latino (H/L), and white/ Caucasian (W/C). Designation in one of these five categories is not equated with within-group homogeneity. The US population by race and ethnic origin is shown in Figure 2–6 (USCB, 2001). The names used to identify these major US cultural groups are those used by the USCB. The following two modifications were made in the year 2000 census data. The AA/PI category was separated into two categories, Asian-American or Native Hawaiian/Pacific Islander; and Latino has been added to the Hispanic category (H/L).

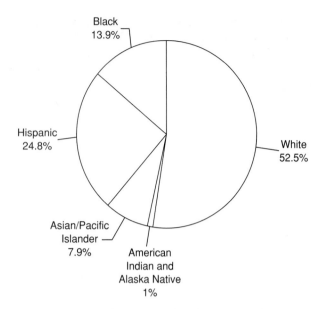

FIGURE 2–6. United States' predicted population by race and ethnic origin, 2050.

African-American or Black

According to 2000 census data, this group constitutes 12.6% of the population in the United States. This heterogeneous group has origins in black racial groups of Africa and the Caribbean Islands, including the West Indies, Dominican Republic, Haiti, and Jamaica. AA/B persons may speak French, Spanish, African dialects, and various forms of English. By 2050, the AA/B population is expected to nearly double its present size to 61 million. A disproportionate percentage of AA/Bs are disadvantaged because of poverty and low educational levels, and they are more likely to have only public insurance. Comparative lifetime pregnancy rates for US women between the ages of 15 and 44 are 2.7 for W/Cs and 4.6 for AA/B and H/L women. Health disparities exist between W/C and AA/B women (Shambley-Ebron & Boyle, 2004). Infant mortality rates for AA/Bs have consistently been twice those of the overall population (HHS, 2000). As a group, AA/Bs have increased risk for diabetes, lupus, HIV/AIDs, sickle cell anemia, hypertension, and cancer of the esophagus and the stomach (St. Hill, 2003; Spector, 2004).

Core Values

AA/B families display resilience and adaptive coping strategies in their struggles with racism and poverty. They have a strong religious commitment, as observed in Southern Baptist, fundamentalist, and black Muslim church communities. Fifty-one percent of AA/B families are headed by women, and more than 55% of all AA/B children younger than three years are born into single-parent families. AA/B families have exten-sive networks of extended families, friends, and neighbors who participate in child rearing with a high level of respect for elders. Children are highly valued, and as a result of extended family networks, the "mothering" a child receives comes from many sources. An example of this is the active role assumed by the maternal grandmother when an adolescent pregnancy occurs. Becoming a mother at a young age is acceptable. AA/Bs are demonstrative; comfortable with touch, physical contact, and emotional sharing; and have an orientation toward the present. AA/B women demonstrate great strength and matriarchal leadership (St. Hill, 2003), even in the face of devastating challenges such as being HIV positive and mothering children who were also HIV positive (Shambley-Ebron & Boyle, 2006). Providing healthcare to this group may be complicated by folk practices, including the belief that all animate and inanimate objects have good or evil spirits. Healers may include family, a "Granny," or a spiritualist. Folk practices may also include pica (ie, ingestion of nonfood items such as starch, clay, ashes, or plaster) and wearing of garlic, amulets, and copper or silver bracelets (Spector, 2004).

Cultural Beliefs and Practices

Some American blacks may resent being called African-Americans because this does not represent their origin (Moore & Moos, 2003). AA/Bs living in poverty may demonstrate a lack of respect or fear of public clinics and hospitals. They tend to seek prenatal care later then other women, usually after the first trimester. The incidence of breast feeding is related to the level of maternal education and social support. AA/B women are more expressive of pain and are usually accompanied during labor and birth by female relatives. Most male newborns are circumcised.

Haitian women are less likely than other groups to seek prenatal care. During pregnancy, they believe they should not swallow their saliva and instead carry a spit cup with them. Fathers are unlikely to be present during birth, believing it is an event only for women. Haitian women are encouraged by their community to breast-feed. However, some inaccurate beliefs, such as thick milk causing skin rashes and thin milk resulting in diarrhea, persist. During the postpartum period, women may believe that a series of three baths aids in their recovery. The first three days, women bathe in a special water infused with herbs. For the next three days, women bathe in water in which leaves have been soaked and warmed by the sun. After four weeks, a cold bath is taken that is believed to tighten muscles and bones loosened during the birth process. Women also believe that wearing a piece of linen or a belt tightly around the waist prevents the entry of gas into their body. Eating white foods such as milk, white lima beans, and lobster are avoided during the postpartum period because they are believed to increase vaginal discharge and hemorrhaging male. Traditionally, Haitian women do not have their newborns circumcised because they believe circumcision decreases sexual satisfaction, but as acculturation occurs, this procedure is becoming more common. West Indian countries of origin are Trinidad, Jamaica, and Barbados. Traditionally, the father of the baby is not present during labor and birth.

Ethiopian woman are considered to be in a delicate state after birth. To be protected from disease and harm, they remain secluded for at least 40 days. A special diet that includes milk and warm foods such as a gruel made of oats and honey is thought to increase breast milk production.

American Indian and Alaskan Native

Descendants of the original peoples of North America (ie, American Indian, Eskimo, and Aleut), this group constitutes 0.9% of the population. There are 500 federally recognized AI nations accessing healthcare from Indian Health Services and/or traditional healers.

AI/ANs have a higher unemployment and poverty rate than the general population. They average 9.6 years of formal education, the lowest rate of any major group in the United States. Urban AI/ANs have a much higher rate of low-birth-weight infants compared with urban W/Cs and rural AI/ANs and a higher rate of infant mortality than urban W/Cs. Urban AI/ANs have a high incidence of risk factors associated with poor birth outcomes, including delayed prenatal care, single marital status, adolescent motherhood, and use of tobacco and alcohol (Dalla & Gamble, 2000). These risk factors resemble the prevalence among AA/ABs except for the higher incidence of alcohol use among AI/ANs. Rural AI/ANs have lower rates of low-birth-weight infants and higher rates of timely prenatal care than their urban counterparts. As a group, AI/ANs have an increased risk for alcoholism, heart disease, cirrhosis of the liver, and diabetes mellitus (Spector, 2004).

Core Values

In general, AI/ANs have a strong spiritual foundation in their lives with a holistic focus on the circular wheel of life. It is important to live in complete harmony with nature. Values include oral traditions passed from generation to generation. Elders play a dominant role in decision-making, and many AI/AN tribes are matrilineal; so involving maternal grandmothers in teaching young mothers is an important and culturally sensitive intervention (Banks, 2003). AI/ANs are present oriented, which may make it difficult to obtain an accurate health history because the past may be perceived as unrelated to current conditions. They believe in harmony. They may avoid eye contact and limit touch. Use of a formal interpreter increases the credibility of the healthcare provider, because listening is highly valued.

Cultural Beliefs and Practices

During pregnancy, women avoid touching their hair. If an infant is born prematurely or expected to die, a family member may request to perform a ceremony that includes ritual washing of the hair. If hair is removed to initiate a scalp intravenous line on a newborn, some families want the hair returned to them. The mother and newborn remain indoors resting for 20 days or until the umbilical cord falls off. The umbilical cord may be saved, because some AI/ANs believe that it has spiritual significance. In a recent study of Cherokee mothers, patterns of infant care include building a care-providing consortium, living spiritually, merging the infant into Indian culture, using noncoercive discipline techniques, and observing the unfolding of the child (Nichols, 2004). Such a community for child rearing is also available for Navajo adolescent mothers (Dalla & Gamble, 2000).

Asian-American and Pacific Islander

AA/PIs are people with origins in the Far East, Southeast Asia, the Indian subcontinent, or the Pacific Islands. AA/PIs constitute 3.6% of the population in the United States, and are projected to make up 8.7% by 2050. There is great diversity in the 28 AA/PI groups designated in the census. Asians comprise 95% of this population and are divided into 17 groups, speaking 32 different primary languages, plus multiple dialects. Major groups of AAs include Chinese, Japanese, Koreans, Filipinos, Vietnamese, Cambodians, and Laotians. The major groups, Chinese and Japanese, are the most long-standing groups of Asian immigrants.

PIs comprise 5% of AA/PIs, with specific groups including Hawaiian, Samoan, Guamanian, Tongan, Tahitian, North Marianas, and Fijian. There are more than 50 subgroups speaking at least 32 different languages. Approximately two-thirds of Asians living in the United States are foreign-born. This group is culturally and linguistically heterogeneous. In the United States, AA/PIs are highly concentrated in the western states and in metropolitan areas.

There is a paucity of data regarding the health status of AA/PIs. Because they are a small minority, AA/PIs are often overlooked in healthcare services planning and research. In relation to healthcare, AA/PIs comprise the most misunderstood, underrepresented, underreported, and understudied ethnic population.

They are often mistakenly referred to as the healthy minority. Their educational attainment has a bi-modal distribution, with 39% having college degrees and 5% assessed as functionally illiterate. Post-traumatic stress syndrome is of concern in AA/PI refugee women, especially Hmong women, who may have suffered atrocities while living in their country of origin. Infant mortality rates are highest in Native Hawaiians (11.4/1,000 live births). As a group, AA/PIs are at increased risk of hypertension, liver cancer, stomach cancer, and lactose intolerance (Spector, 2004).

Core Values

Values embody the philosophical traditions of Buddhism, Hinduism, and Christianity. They believe events are predestined and strive for a degree of spirituality in their lives. Core values include cohesive families, filial piety and respect for the elderly, respect for authority, interdependence and reciprocity (group orientation), interpersonal harmony and avoidance of disagreement and conflict (Willgerodt & Killien, 2004). Pride, fatalism, education/achievement orientation, respect for tradition, and a strong work ethic are also core values. Asians seldom express strong reactions to emotionally arousing events and are taught to suppress feelings to maintain harmonious relationships with others (Yick, Shibusawa, & Agbayani-Siewert, 2003). They avoid public displays of affection, except among family and close friends, and have clearly defined gender roles.

Traditional therapies are often employed concurrently with Western medicine, including acupuncture, herbs, nutrition, and meditation. Asian women may believe Western medicines are too strong and may halve the prescribed dosages. Chinese women avoid oral contraceptives because of a perception that hormones may be harmful. Screening exams such as cervical screening may be avoided because of modesty and discomfort with such intimate procedures (Holdroyd, Twinn, & Adab, 2004).

Cultural Beliefs and Practices

Traditional Asian healthcare beliefs and practices are Chinese in origin, with the exception of Filipino beliefs and practices being based primarily on the Malaysian culture. The yin/yang polarity is a major life force and focuses on the importance of balance for the maintenance of health. Yin represents cold, darkness, and wetness; yang represents heat, brightness, and dryness. For those who subscribe to the hot/cold theory (including Asians and Hispanics), health requires harmony between heat and cold. Balance should be maintained for women to be in harmony with the environment. During pregnancy women eat "cold" foods such

as poultry, fish, fruits, and vegetables. Eating "hot" foods, such as red peppers, spicy soups, red meat, garlic, ginger, onion, coffee, and sweets, at this time is believed to cause abortion or premature labor. A designation of "hot" or "cold" does not necessarily refer to physical temperature but the specific effects the food is believed to have on the body.

Because pregnancy is a "hot" condition, some expectant mothers may be reluctant to take prenatal vitamins, which are considered a "hot" medication. Encouraging the woman to take her prenatal vitamins with fruit juice may resolve the problem. Some pregnant Asian women believe that iron hardens bones and makes birth more difficult, and these women resist taking vitamin preparations containing iron. Many Southeast Asian women believe that exposure of the genital area is inappropriate because this is considered a sacred part of the body. They may be reluctant to have pap smears, wait to seek prenatal care, and communicate poorly about physical changes of pregnancy. Sexual intercourse is avoided during the third trimester because it is thought to thicken amniotic fluid, causing respiratory distress in the newborn.

Vaginal exams and an open hospital gown may be deeply humiliating and unnerving to Southeast Asian women who value humility and modesty. Giving birth is believed to deplete a woman's body of the "hot" element (blood) and inner energy. This places her in a "cold" state for about 40 days after birth, which is assumed to be the period for the womb to heal. Rice, eggs, beef, tea, and chicken soup with garlic and black pepper are foods high in "hotness" and are eaten by postpartum women. During postpartum, pericare and hygiene are considered important, but women are discouraged from showering for several days to two to four weeks. They believe that exposure to water cools the body and interrupts balance, which may cause premature aging. One woman said,

> They make me [take a shower] in the hospital. I have to. The nurse came in and told me. And she would not bring the baby for me. If I don't take a bath, they won't give me the baby to feed . . . So I did, I went in to take a quick shower and then came out. It makes me feel like it's sort of a parent's order. They say to protect the baby from germs [and] all that. I understand, but I have my own beliefs, so when I get home, I do it a different way. I just do what I [am] supposed to do." (Davis, 2001, p. 211)

Most AA/PI women breast-feed for several years. Women in the Hmong community (originally from Laos) may choose to formula feed, inaccurately believing American women do not breast-feed because they do not see this practice in public like they did in their homelands (Riordan, 2004).

Korean mothers may believe that newborns need sleep and little stimulation. They are discouraged from touching the baby. Thus, they may not understand the amazing capabilities of the newborn to see, hear, and interact (Shin, Bozzette, Kenner, & Kim, 2004). Childrearing often occurs within the extended family. A newborn's head is considered sacred, the essence of his being. Touching the newborn's head is distressing to parents and should be avoided. Traditionally, newborns have not been circumcised, but as acculturation occurs, some AA/PIs have adopted this practice.

Cambodian women may avoid certain activities during pregnancy, such as standing in doorways, because they believe this will cause the baby to become stuck in the birth canal. Sexual intercourse is not permitted during the third trimester. It is thought that avoidance of sexual intercourse during pregnancy will produce a more attractive baby. Vernix caseosa is believed to be sperm. Cambodian woman will not be seen cuddling their newborns; instead, the newborn is held down and away from their body. Herbal medications are prepared during the third trimester to be eaten three to four times per day during the postpartum period to restore body heat. Along with eating special foods that are thought to restore lost heat, mothers wear heavy clothing during the postpartum period. Breast-feeding is delayed for several days because colostrum is thought to be harmful for the newborn.

Filipino women are discouraged from remaining in a dependent position late in pregnancy, because sitting or standing may cause retention of fluid. Sexual intercourse is discouraged for the last two months. The women eat eggs, believing that slippery foods help the baby move through the birth canal more easily. Filipino women are accompanied during labor by a woman who has experienced birth herself.

Korean women avoid certain animal foods during pregnancy because they believe these foods can harm the newborn's character or appearance. It is believed that eating duck can cause the newborn to be born with webs between his fingers and that eating eggs causes the child to be born without a spine. Dairy products are not traditionally part of the Korean diet, so care should be taken to ensure women are receiving adequate amounts of calcium during pregnancy. In the Korean culture, the new mother is perceived as being sick and needing care. Postpartum Korean women do not easily participate in self-care activities or care for their newborn. The husband's mother is responsible for caring for the newborn and the recovery of her daughter-in-law. The need to return the hot element to the body after childbirth is accomplished by eating a special seaweed soup made with beef broth and avoiding anything cold, such as ice. The soup is thought to increase breast milk production and rid the body of lochia. Korean women may refuse an ice pack or chemical cold pack for control of perineal edema because of the belief that coldness in any form may cause chronic illness such as arthritis. Women who breast-feed are reluctant to supplement with formula.

Samoan women do not eat octopus or raw fish during pregnancy. Women supporting the laboring woman often gently massage her abdomen to relieve discomfort and determine the position of the baby. Postpartum, the abdomen may be bound and massaged by the midwife. Women do not carry the newborn after dark or stand in front of windows with the newborn at night. Most women choose to breast-feed, and it is customary to abstain from sexual intercourse while breast-feeding. Generally, male infants are circumcised.

Vietnamese women must avoid sexual intercourse and be kept warm during their pregnancy. Special hygiene practices include using salt water to wash their teeth and gums.

Chinese women focus on "doing the month" (*zuo yue zi*), with elaborate and specific restrictions for the first month following giving birth designed to promote the health and well being of both mother and newborn (Holroyd, Twinn, & Yim, 2004; Kartchner & Callister, 2003). Sometimes nurses assume that with acculturation and education, childbearing women will be less likely to practice traditional beliefs, but in a study of professional Chinese childbearing women living in Canada, researchers found that indeed these women still "did the month" and valued other cultural practices (Braithwaite & Williams, 2004).

Hispanic and Latino

H/L women have ethnic origins from countries where Spanish is the primary language, including Mexico, Puerto Rico, Cuba, Spain, and South or Central America. They constitute at least 13% of the population in the United States and are the fastest growing ethnic group (USCB, 2001). Immigration is estimated at one million people per year, and census data does not include the significant number of undocumented H/Ls living and working in the United States. Spanish is the most common second language spoken in the United States. Sixty-seven percent of Hispanics are of Mexican origin (Ramirez & de la Cruz, 2002). Assimilation is minimal, with strongly held cultural beliefs and behaviors. Traditional beliefs, values, and customs govern decision-making behaviors.

Significant increases in the H/L population are related to a natural increase (births over deaths) of 1.8% and a fertility rate 50% higher than W/Cs. Women comprise the largest group among the H/L population in the United States, accounting for an estimated 11 million. Latino women are younger than non-H/L women at the age of first pregnancy. The fertility rate of H/L women is 84% higher than white women and 31% higher than black women. Although H/Ls are the most likely group of women to have children, they are the least likely to initiate early prenatal care (Torres, 2005).

Forty-three percent of H/L births were to unmarried mothers, with adolescents accounting for a large percentage of those births. Two-thirds of H/L births are to Mexican-American mothers. Unintended pregnancies are more common among H/Ls compared with other ethnic groups, especially among women of low socioeconomic status (Erviti, Castro, & Collado, 2004). First generation, or less acculturated, Mexican-American women seem to have a perinatal advantage despite low levels of maternal education, low socioeconomic status, and less than adequate prenatal care. Aspects of their culture that seem to protect them include nutritional intake, lower prevalence of smoking and alcohol consumption, extended family support, and spirituality or a religious lifestyle (Bender, Harbour, Thorp, & Morris, 2001; Callister & Birkhead, 2002; Heilemann, Lee, Stinson, Koshar, & Goss, 2000; Martinez-Schallmoser, MacMullen, & Telleen, 2005).

Immigrants usually favor Depo-Provera or Norplant rather than oral contraceptives for family planning (Brown, Villarruel, Oakley, & Eribes, 2003), and use of the term "well woman visit" is more appropriate than "family planning visit" when scheduling an appointment (Jones, Bond, Gardner, & Hernandez, 2002). Because there may be much distress and embarrassment about touching and inserting fingers into the vagina, diaphragms are not a good choice as a family planning method. H/Ls may not perceive the need for routine checkups such as pap smears (Boyer, Williams, Callister, & Marshall, 2001).

Compared with women born in the United States, foreign-born H/L women are more likely to be economically disadvantaged and uninsured, factors usually associated with poor birth outcomes when adjustments were made for maternal and healthcare factors. Although H/Ls represent only 11.6% of the population under age 65, they make up more than 21% of the uninsured population. With larger families and inadequate sources of income, more than 30% of H/L families have incomes below the poverty level. As a group, H/Ls are at higher risk for diabetes mellitus (twice that of W/Cs—9.8% versus 5%), obesity (especially among adolescents), parasitic disease, and lactose intolerance (Centers for Disease Control and Prevention [CDC], 2004; Gordon-Larsen, Harris, Ward, & Popkin, 2003; Spector, 2004). H/Ls are not a homogenous group, and there are many variations between Puerto Rican, Mexican, Peruvian, Chilean,

and other H/Ls. For example, low birth weight rate is lower among Mexican infants (6%) than among Puerto Rican infants (9.7%) (Gennaro, 2005).

Core Values

In the H/L community, there are strong family ties, large and cohesive kin groups, and a family decision-making process. It is believed that the family has a meditating effect on stress (Callister & Birkhead, in press). Family values include pride and self-reliance, dignity, trust, intimacy, and respect for older family members and authority figures. H/L women usually consult their husbands, significant others, or other important family members such as godparents about major health decisions. *Curanderismo* or folk medicine is frequently used. Mexican-Americans may seek the services of folk healers such as herbalists, bone and muscle therapists, and midwives. These practitioners are more prevalent in border towns and may be used there as an adjunct to the established healthcare systems. An emerging group of healthcare providers are bilingual nurse-*curanderas* (Luna, 2003).

Cultural Beliefs and Practices

Pregnancy is an important family event engendering extensive physical and emotional support from family members (Callister & Birkhead, in press). Motherhood is seen as the most important role a woman can achieve. Most H/L babies are wanted, cherished, and pampered. They are thought to be untouched by sin and evil.

H/Ls have a present orientation. This orientation affects how prenatal care is accessed. Women are frequently late for or miss prenatal appointments and may not understand how high-risk behaviors affect maternal and fetal/neonatal well-being (Torres, 2005). H/Ls have a sense of fatalism, believing that their destiny is controlled by fate or by the will of God. Hispanic women may see early prenatal care as unnecessary because pregnancy outcomes are beyond personal control. This sense of fatalism can also promote a sense of vulnerability and lack of control. They do expect *personalism* and *respecto* from healthcare providers (Tandon, Parillo, & Keefer, 2005; Warda, 2000). During pregnancy, women maintain healthy diets and exercise, and they may take herbs and drink teas recommended by herbalists. Certain folk traditions are thought to prevent birth defects. A safety pin attached to an undergarment helps protect the fetus from a cleft lip or palate. If a pregnant Guatemalan woman sees an eclipse (ie, a "bite" taken out of the moon), her unborn child may have a bite taken out of its mouth, resulting in a cleft lip or palate (Callister & Vega, 1998).

Some H/L women believe that unsatisfied cravings cause defects or injury to the fetus. For example, a strawberry nevus is believed to occur because the pregnant woman had an unsatisfied craving for strawberries during her pregnancy. Vitamins and iron are avoided by some women during pregnancy because they are thought to be harmful. Women believe that walking during labor makes birth occur more quickly and that inactivity decreases the amount of amniotic fluid and causes the fetus to stick to the uterus, delaying the birth. Many Hispanic women prefer not to have epidural analgesia/anesthesia. Cesarean birth is feared and viewed as life threatening for the mother.

Postpartum women are discouraged from taking a shower for several days. Belief in the "evil eye" means that a fixed stare from a person believed to be envious may result in illness. *La manita de azabache*, a black onyx hand, may be placed on or near the newborn to ward off the envious evil eye. An H/L mother may assume that a nurse who overly praises her newborn or is perceived as staring at the child can cause the child to cry excessively and be very restless. H/L women view colostrum as bad or old milk and may delay breast-feeding until several days after the birth (Riordan, 2004; Schlickau & Wilson, 2005). Avoiding foods such as chilies and beans is thought to protect the newborn from illness. In the early postpartum period, the maternal/newborn dyad is considered *muy delicados* (vulnerable or delicate) and stays at home for 7 to 15 days; and for some, up to 40 days postpartum (Spector, 2004). Traditionally, circumcision has not been practiced, but as acculturation occurs, this practice is becoming more acceptable. Some H/L families may want to keep and bury the placenta (Lemmon, 2002a).

White or Caucasian

W/Cs have origins in Europe, North Africa, or the Middle East and constitute 83% of the population of the United States. There are 53 ethnic groups classified as W/C living in the United States. In many ways, W/Cs are perceived as being privileged. For example, there are substantial differences in sources of prenatal care, with 78% of W/C women receiving private care compared with 51% of Mexican-American women, 44% of AA/B women, and 47% of Puerto Rican women.

W/C is generally acknowledged to be the dominant culture. This cultural group seems intent on achieving accomplishments quickly, contributing to a high-energy, high-stress lifestyle, compared with other cultural groups that have more peaceful ways of life. Predominant belief systems accept the Western bio-technologic model of healthcare, including elective inductions, elective cesarean births, and assisted reproductive technology. Women in this group are more likely to embrace such practices, but paradoxically, like women in other cultural groups, most childbearing women want nurturing, supportive, and meaningful care (Callister, 2006a; Callister et al., in press; Callister, Vehvilainen-Julkunen, & Lauri, 2000; Callister et al., 2001; Carlton et al., 2005; Davis-Floyd & Sargent, 1997; Johnson et al., in press; Jordan, 1993; Matthews & Callister, 2004).

Core Values

Core values include individualism, self-reliance, personal achievement and independence, democratic ideals and egalitarianism, work and productivity, materialism, punctuality, and future time orientation, as well as openness, assertiveness, and directness in communication.

Immigrant and Refugee Women

Increasingly, the United States is becoming a global village (Rorie, 2004). Immigrant women are coping with tremendous cultural differences and issues related to making transitions that may be extremely stressful (Barnes & Harrison, 2004; Conrad & Pacquiao, 2005; St. Hill, Lipson, & Meleis, 2003). In addition to multiple challenges, many demonstrate great resiliency and strength (Heilemann, Lee and Kury, 2005; Lindgren & Lipson, 2004; Rutherford & Parker, 2003). Immigrant and refugee women may embrace distinct culture practices and are very heterogeneous (Williams & Hampton, 2005).

Cultural Beliefs and Practices

As first-generation less-acculturated Americans, these women have stronger ties to cultural traditions and customs than second- or third-generation Americans. For instance, they may have given birth previously in their home attended by a traditional midwife and their mother or mother-in-law.

The bio-medical and highly technological environment of birthing units in the United States may be foreign and frightening. There may be a deep sadness for these mothers as they give birth without the assistance of their own mothers. In a recent study, acculturation levels and postpartum depression in Hispanic women were not consistently related, but Puerto Rican ethnicity, cesarean birth, and single marital status were significant predictors of postpartum depression (Beck et al., 2005). Many immigrants and refugees are migrant farm workers, living in unsanitary, unsafe, and crowded conditions. Language, illiteracy, and cultural barriers have a negative impact on access to health-care.

Cultural beliefs, such as the belief among some African immigrants that condoms may lodge in the abdominal cavity and result in obstruction, infection, or cancer, also represent a significant challenge. Another cultural challenge is the resistance of Cambodian refugees to utilize contraception. Other beliefs about gender inequalities and intimate partner violence compromise the health of immigrant childbearing women (Ahmad, Riaz, Barata, & Stewart, 2004; Kasturirangan, Krishnan, & Riger, 2004). Some may be at risk for perinatal depression (Le, Munoz, Soto, Delucchi, & Ippen, 2004). However, one recent study found that arranged marriage and giving birth to a girl were not significantly related to postpartum depression in immigrant Asian Indian women (Goyal, Murphy, & Cohen, 2006).

It is estimated that by 2025, there will be at least 15 million American Muslims, many of whom will be immigrants (Rashidi & Rajaram, 2001). Their beliefs include *shadadah* (monotheism), *salat* (prayer five times daily), *zakat* (purification), *siawm* (fasting during Ramadan), and *hajj* (a pilgrimage to Mecca). Islamic concepts include these five teachings, along with modesty, visiting the ill, and dietary and gender restrictions. The bride's status in the family is uncertain until she has proven fertility with the birth of her first child, and sons are highly valued. Seeking prenatal care is not considered important unless there are complications. Childbirth education classes are considered to be excessive planning that may negatively affect the outcomes of pregnancy (Kridli, 2002).

As conservators of family health, the role of immigrant women in health promotion is critical. Refugees are eligible for special refugee medical assistance during their first 18 months in the United States. After this initial coverage, those who cannot afford private health insurance and are ineligible for Medicaid benefits may become medically indigent. Limitations in literacy and language make it difficult to enter the healthcare system. Feelings of fear and paranoia create circumstances where these women are unwilling to access care. Like other childbearing women, immigrant women appreciate supportive and respectful care, as demonstrated in a study of Vietnamese, Turkish, and Filipino women (Small, Yelland, Lumley, Brown, & Liamputtong, 2002).

Immigrant women may also be more susceptible to helminthic diseases, including tapeworm, roundworm, and hookroom, because these are endemic in Asia. Eighty percent of the five million women of childbearing age who are HIV positive are from Sub-Saharan Africa, with 90% of HIV cases in this area transmitted through heterosexual contact (American Public Health Association [APHA], 2004).

Ritually Circumcised Women

It is estimated that at least 130 million women throughout the world have been ritually circumcised. Immigrants and refugee women from developing countries in Asia (eg, Malaysia, India, Yemen, and Oman) and 28 African countries may have experienced female genital mutilation. Among Somali women, more than 98% of the women have experienced female circumcision/female genital mutilation (APHA, 2004). Genital mutilation may occur at any point between the newborn period and the time a woman gives birth to her first child. These women experience severe pain and complications during childbirth because the inadequate vaginal opening and scarring may prevent cervical dilatation and fetal passage. After giving birth in their native countries, some women experience reinfibulation (ie, suturing together of the labia). Because female circumcision is a culturally bound rite of passage, women may resent Western attitudes about this practice, which has strong social and cultural support (Anuforo, Oyedele, & Pacquiao, 2004; Little, 2003). Perinatal nurses need to create an environment of trust, establish rapport with male family members, ensure privacy, and be sensitive to the stoicism demonstrated toward childbirth pain. Cultural re-patterning may occur with the acceptance of alternatives such as flattening of the clitoris and symbolic cutting of the pubic hair.

Deeply Religious Women

Many religious and spiritual beliefs and practices influence childbearing (Callister, 2002; Lemmon, 2002b). Orthodox Jews have a rich body of traditions associated with childbearing and great reverence for childbearing and child rearing. Some Jewish women feel a moral responsibility to bring at least two children into the world because of the destruction of their progenitors during the Holocaust (Semenic et al., 2004). Circumcision is a Jewish ritual based on a Hebrew covenant in the Old Testament of the Bible (Genesis 17:10–14) performed on all male children by a mohel on the eighth day of life.

For Islamic women, creating an environment that honors traditional practices according to the precepts of Islam is important. Islamic women practice a cleansing process at the end of each menstrual period. Palestinian refugee women feel a strong obligation to bear a significant number of children, especially sons, to continue the generations of the Arabic bloodline (Khalaf & Callister, 1997). A woman espousing the beliefs of the Church of Jesus Christ of Latter-day Saints (Mormon) may request her husband to lay his hands on her head and give her a blessing for strength, comfort, and well-being as she labors and gives birth (Callister, 2003b). Mexican-American women often speak in terms of a person's soul or spirit (*alma* or *espiritu*) when referring to one's inner qualities.

The sacred day of worship varies. Sunday is the Sabbath for most Christians. The Muslim's holy day is sunset Thursday to sunset Friday. Jews and Seventh Day Adventists celebrate the Sabbath from sunset on Friday to sunset on Saturday. For an Orthodox Jewish woman, honoring the Sabbath may mean not raising the head of the bed to breast-feed and not turning on the call light to request assistance, because in the Orthodox culture, these acts would constitute work. Table 2–1 provides common religious dietary prohibitions.

There is a strong relationship between health status and spiritual well-being. Religiosity and a spiritual lifestyle have been found to be the source of powerful strength during childbearing, especially when complications such as fetal or neonatal demise occur (Callister, 2006b). For example, in a study of neonatal loss among Muslim women living in Sweden, one woman said, "We trust in God, it is the will of God" (Lundqvist, Nilstun, & Dykes, 2003, p. 79). Spiritual beliefs and religious affiliations are effective coping mechanisms and sources of support (Khalaf & Callister, 1997; Callister et al., 1999).

TABLE 2–1 ■ RELIGIOUS DIETARY PROHIBITIONS

Religion	Dietary Prohibitions
Hinduism	All meats are prohibited.
Islam	Pork and alcoholic beverages are prohibited.
Judaism	Pork, predatory fowl, shellfish, and blood by ingestion (eg, blood sausage, raw meat) are prohibited. Foods should be kosher (ie, properly prepared). All animals should be ritually slaughtered to be kosher. Mixing dairy and meat dishes at the same meal is prohibited.
Mormonism (Church of Jesus Christ of Latter-day Saints)	Alcohol, tobacco, coffee, and tea are prohibited.
Seventh-Day Adventists	Pork, certain seafood (including shellfish), and fermented beverages are prohibited. A vegetarian diet is encouraged.

HEALTH DIFFERENCES IN POPULATIONS OF CHILDBEARING WOMEN

There is a paucity of research identifying health differences among minority groups and the prevalence of illness among specific populations of childbearing women (Gennaro, 2005). As far as body structure is concerned, AA/PIs typically have small-for-gestational-age neonates. Birth weight is lower in AA/B newborns, but size for size, they are more mature for gestational age. AA/B newborns have a mean nine days' shorter gestation period than other ethnic groups, and there is a slowing of intrauterine growth in black infants after 35 weeks' gestation. Mongolian spots are commonly found in AA/B, AA/PI, AI/AN, and H/L infants.

In addition to physical differences, cultural practices may be misinterpreted during an initial examination. Dermal practices among Southeast Asian refugees may be noticed and assumed to be a sign of physical abuse. An example of a cultural practice that may be misinterpreted is "cupping." In this practice, a cup is heated and placed on the skin, leaving a circular ecchymotic area. Pinching and rubbing may produce bruises or welts. Rubbing the skin with a spoon or coin produces dermal changes. Touching a burning cigarette to the skin may also represent cultural self-care (Spector, 2004).

Chemical substances, including pharmaceuticals, are metabolized differently among groups (Doyle & Faucher, 2002; Munoz & Hilgenberg, 2005). Ethnopharmacologic research is a growing and important specialty. It is essential that as part of a cultural assessment, specific questions are asked about the presence or absence of potentially adverse effects of medication. It may be possible in some instances to reduce dosages in culturally diverse women.

There is an increasing incidence of alcoholism among H/Ls and AA/Bs, while Asians have the lowest alcoholism rate. Most Asians and AI/ANs experience a rapid onset but slow decrease in blood acetaldehyde levels, leaving long periods of exposure to substances that cause alcohol intoxication. Fetal alcohol syndrome, or its effect, is highest among AI/ANs. Caffeine is metabolized and excreted faster by W/Cs than Asians. The incidence of lactose intolerance is 94% in AA/PIs, 90% in AA/Bs, 79% in AI/ANs, 50% in H/Ls, and 17% in W/Cs. This can have a negative effect on breast-feeding, because infants may be lactose intolerant as well.

The Rh negative factor, common in Caucasians, is rare in other groups (especially Asians) and essentially absent in Eskimos. There is a high incidence of diabetes in AI tribes, whereas the disease is rare in Alaskan Eskimos. The prevalence of insulin-dependent diabetes mellitus is highest among AA/Bs. Gestational diabetes mellitus occurs in 20% of pregnant women and is not attributed specifically to race or culture.

Communicable diseases that threaten foreign-born and new immigrants, particularly those from China, Korea, the Philippines, Southeast Asia, and the Pacific, are tuberculosis (TB) and hepatitis B. Among these women, hepatitis B has a prevalence of 8% to 22%, compared with 2% for women living in the United States. Fifty percent of women who give birth to hepatitis B–carrier infants in the United States are foreign-born Asian women. There is a significantly higher incidence of TB in AI/ANs and foreign-born AA/PIs, and the incidence of TB is four times higher among Asians than the overall population. AA/PI and AI/AN women diagnosed with TB tend to be of childbearing age.

There is a higher incidence of hypertension in AA/Bs and H/Ls. The incidence of lupus is four times higher in AA/B women and is twice as prevalent in H/L women when compared to W/C women. Native Hawaiian and Samoan women are reported to have the highest obesity rates in the world, although maternal obesity is increasing at an alarming rate in the developed world in many populations.

Sickle cell anemia occurs predominately in AA/Bs. Tay-Sachs disease is predominately found in Hasidic Jews of Eastern European descent, particularly Ashenazi and Sephardi women. Thalassemia is a genetic blood disorder found in women from the Mediterranean region, the Middle East, and Southeast Asia.

Racial differences have been documented in asthma morbidity during pregnancy, with AA/B childbearing women with asthma more likely to be seen in the emergency department, be hospitalized, or need rescue medications for asthma during their pregnancy (Carroll et al., 2005).

In a retrospective study, Caughey and associates (2005) identified predictors of pregnancy-induced hypertension (PIH), with baseline rates of 5.2% in AA/Bs, 4% in H/Ls, 3.9% in AI/ANs, 3.8% in W/Cs, and 3.5% in Asian women. When the mother and father were of different ethnicities, there was a 13.5% increase in the rates of PIH, except in AI/ANs, whose rates increased to 9.7%.

In recent work supported by the Agency for Healthcare Research and Quality, researchers have also documented racial disparities in complications of pregnancy and childbirth. AA/B women were more likely to have 10 of 11 maternal perinatal complications than W/C women, including preterm labor and premature rupture of membranes (PRM), hypertensive disorders, diabetes, placenta previa (PP) and abruption, infection of the amniotic cavity (IAC), and cesarean birth. H/L women were at a higher risk than white women for diabetes, PP, IAC, and cesarean birth. AA/PIs were more at risk than any other women for diabetes, PP, PRM, IAC, and postpartum hemorrhage (Shen, Tymkow, & MacMullen, 2005). It should be noted that race/ethnicity data are missing in 24% of cases, and this limits these research findings.

Access to care also differs depending on ethnicity and culture. Fifteen percent of the population of the United States as a whole does not have health insurance, compared to 33% of H/Ls, 19% of AA/Bs, and 18% of AA/PIs (USCB, 2002).

BARRIERS TO CULTURALLY COMPETENT CARE

Barriers to culturally competent care include values, beliefs, and customs; communication challenges; and the biomedical healthcare environment (Callister, 2005).

Differences in Values, Beliefs, and Customs

Ethnocentrism is the belief that one's ways are the only way. *Cultural imposition* is the tendency to thrust one's beliefs, values, and patterns of behaviors upon another culture. Characteristics of caregivers that influence their ability to be culturally competent include educational level, multicultural exposure, personal attitudes and values, and professional experiences. Identifying and understanding the childbearing woman's attitudes, behaviors, values, and needs assists the perinatal nurse in identifying interventions that are culturally appropriate; are acceptable to healthcare providers, the women, and their families; have the potential to increase adherence to therapeutic regimens; and will over time result in constructive changes in perinatal healthcare delivery.

Cross and associates (1989) originally developed the cultural competence continuum, which moves incrementally across six stages: destructiveness, incapacity, blindness, pre-competence, competence, and proficiency. This model was later adopted by the National Alliance for Hispanic Health (2001). Nurses demonstrate various levels of commitment when caring for culturally diverse women on a continuum from resistant care to generalist care to impassioned care (Kirkham, 1998). Nurses who are resistant judge behaviors, ignore client needs, and complain. Resistant nurses may ignore or resent culturally diverse women and their families. They may see culture as an inconvenience or problem. Nurses who provide generalist care are respectful and competent but do not differentiate cultural diversities. Culture, to them, is a non-issue.

They may empathize with client experiences but don't feel empowered to bring about substantial change. Racist attitudes of colleagues are tolerated. Nurses who provide impassioned care have a high degree of personal commitment to provide culturally sensitive care. These nurses go beyond accommodation to an appreciation of cultural diversity. They are aware of the complexities of cultural competence and the variability of expressions within cultural groups. Creativity and flexibility are the hallmarks of the care they provide to culturally diverse clients. They feel empowered to make a difference through their clinical practice. Recent work by Braithwaite (2006) found a weak but significant association between fewer years of nursing experience/higher levels of education and increased cultural knowledge/competence.

Display 2–4 provides the characteristics of the culturally competent nurse. Campinha-Bacote (1994)

DISPLAY 2-4

Characteristics of the Culturally Competent Practitioner

- Move from cultural unawareness to an awareness and sensitivity to their own cultural heritage
- Recognize their own values and biases and are aware of how they may affect clients from other cultures
- Demonstrate comfort with cultural differences that exist between herself/himself and clients
- Know specifics about the particular cultural groups they work with
- Understand the significance of historic events and socio-cultural context for specific cultural groups
- Respect and are aware of the unique needs of specific women
- Understand the diversity that exists within and between cultures
- Endeavor to learn more about cultural communities through interactions with diverse women, participation in cultural diversity workshops and community events, readings on cultural dynamics, and consultations with community experts
- Make a continuous effort to understand others points of view
- Demonstrate flexibility and tolerance of ambiguity and is nonjudgmental
- Maintain a sense of humor
- Demonstrate willingness to relinquish control in clinical encounters, to risk failure, and to look within for sources of frustration, anger, and resistance
- Promote cultural practices that are potentially helpful, tolerate cultural practices that are harmless or neutral and works to education women to avoid cultural practices that may be potentially harmful

identified the importance of becoming culturally aware as the nurse becomes sensitive to other cultures. Cultural knowledge involves gaining knowledge of the worldviews of others. Development of assessment skills to understand the values, beliefs, and practices of others, means engaging in cross-cultural interactions rather than avoiding them.

It is essential that the nurse examines his or her own cultural beliefs, biases, attitudes, stereotypes, and prejudice and asks, "Whose birth is it anyway?" The following story is told by Khazoyan and Anderson (1994, p. 226):

> Señor Rojas sat at the bedside of his laboring wife, held her hand, and spoke soft, encouraging words to her. This was the kind of support that she desired during her labor: his presence, his attention, and his affection. Following the birth of their child, Señora Rojas expressed contentment and proudly described the support that her husband had provided. He had met her expectations. The nurses, however, expected more. They had wanted Señor Rojas to participate more actively in his wife's labor by massaging her back and assisting her with breathing techniques.

Communication

Communication barriers include lack of knowledge, fear and distrust, racism, bias and ethnocentrism, stereotyping, nursing rituals, and language barriers (Munoz & Luckmann, 2005). Communication (or lack of communication) between cultures occurs whenever a message produced in one culture must be processed into another culture. A significant barrier to culturally competent care is language and the lack of bilingual personnel and staff with culturally diverse backgrounds. Hospitals frequently enlist nonprofessional employees of the client's ethnic background to act as interpreters. These individuals are often unfamiliar with English medical terminology and may not be able to translate accurately. Interpreters who are members of the client's cultural group may be of a different social class than the client or may be more acculturated and anxious to appear part of the dominant culture. In some cases, interpreters may be disdainful or dismissive of the client's belief system. Using children or other family members to interpret may also lead to problems. Interpretation may be based on the perceptions of the interpreter as to what is best to communicate, and they often may omit important information (Carr & deJoseph, 2001). According to the Office of Minority Health's *National Standards for Culturally and Linguistically Appropriate Services in*

DISPLAY 2-5

Medical Interpreter Code of Ethics

- Confidentiality
- Accuracy: Conveying the content and spirit of what is said
- Completeness: Conveying everything that is said
- Conveying cultural frameworks
- Nonjudgmental attitude about the content to be interpreted
- Client self-determination
- Attitude toward clients
- Acceptance of assignments
- Compensation
- Self-evaluation
- Ethical violations
- Professionalism

(Roat, 1997)

Health Care (2001), using the woman's friends or family members is not recommended. A medical interpreter who follows a specific code of ethics should be provided by the healthcare facility (Display 2–5). The standards for culturally and linguistically appropriate services are described in Display 2–6. Interpreters are visitors to the perinatal unit. They will need the help of the nursing staff to feel comfortable and effectively provide services to the non-English-speaking patient. Guidelines for perinatal nursing staff as they work with a medical interpreter are reviewed in Display 2–7.

Healthcare Environment

This barrier includes bureaucracy (eg, inability of the dietary department to provide culturally appropriate foods), nonsupportive administration, lack of educational opportunities to promote cultural diversity, lack of translators, and rigid policies and protocols that do not support cultural diversity. Consider how difficult it is for the woman who may be living in the United States without the support of extended family (especially female family members), speaking little or no English, having a limited understanding of the dominant culture, having little education, and working in a low-skills-level job without benefits. When this woman arrives at the birthing unit, the unfamiliar environment and procedures serve only to increase her stress. Being hospitalized means entering a new and foreign culture with a high level of technology, the necessity of conforming to unit policies and procedures and unfamiliar schedules, having one's privacy invaded, and behaving as a "patient." This may be very challenging for women. Another issue is our birth language, which may not reflect how women feel about having a baby. For example, use of the term "delivery" versus "birth" "reflects the limited value placed on the woman's role. Phrases such as this devalues the mother's role in the birth process and the cultural and spiritual aspects of birth" (Shilling, 2000, p. 141). The woman is not passively delivered by the omnipotent caregiver; she should be the central figure actively giving birth. Similarly, rather than "cesarean section," the focus should be on the woman giving birth, using the language "cesarean birth." These small but significant linguistic differences are important in the demonstration of respect.

TECHNIQUES TO INTEGRATE CULTURE INTO NURSING CARE

Standards for the Joint Commission for Accreditation of Healthcare Organizations (2000) suggest that understanding the cultural context in which patients live is important to fully appreciate their response to illness and is necessary for planning appropriate nursing and medical interventions. It is essential that culturally competent care be integrated into all standards of practice. Becoming culturally competent is a developmental process. As nurses become more sensitive to the issues surrounding healthcare and the traditional health beliefs of the women they care for, more culturally competent healthcare will be provided (Callister, 2005). Examples of ways that perinatal nursing units might become more culturally competent are described in Display 2–8.

When the cultural expectations of the nurse and the woman conflict, both are left feeling frustrated and misunderstood. The woman's adherence to traditional practices may be seen as strange and backward to the nurse, who responds by trying to "fit" the woman into the bio-technologic Western system. For example, an AI/AN mother may avoid eye contact and fail to ask questions or breast-feed in the presence of the mother–baby nurse. For many women, including Southeast Asian women, there is "loss of face" because they feel responsible for any confusion or cultural conflict with the nurse, who is perceived as a social superior. This experience may discourage them from future contact with healthcare professionals. Moore and Moos (2003) identified assessment information, including place of birth, how long the woman has lived in the United States, ethnic affiliation and the strength of that affiliation, including ethnic communities, personal support systems, language and literacy,

DISPLAY 2-6

Standards for Culturally and Linguistically Appropriate Services (CLAS)

Standard 1. Healthcare organizations should ensure that the patients/consumers receive from all staff members effective, understandable, and respectful care that is provided in a manner compatible with their cultural health beliefs and practices and preferred language.

Standard 2. Healthcare organizations should implement strategies to recruit, retain, and promote at all levels of the organization a diverse staff and leadership that are representative of the demographic characteristics of the service area.

Standard 3. Healthcare organizations should ensure that staff at all levels and across all disciplines provide culturally competent care

Standard 4. Healthcare organizations must offer and provide language assistance services, at no cost, to each patient/consumer with limited English proficiency at all points of contact in a timely manner during all hours of operation.

Standard 5. Healthcare organizations must provide to patients/consumers in their preferred language both verbal offers and written notices informing them of their right to receive language assistance services.

Standard 6. Healthcare organizations must ensure the competence of language assistance provided to limited English proficient patients/consumers by interpreters and bilingual staff. Family and friends should not be used to provide interpretation services (except at the request of the patient/consumer).

Standard 7. Healthcare organizations must make available easily understood patient-related materials and post signage in the language of the commonly encountered group or groups represented in the service area.

Standard 8. Healthcare organizations should develop, implement, and promote a written strategic plan that outlines clear goals, policies, and operational plans and management accountability/oversight mechanisms to provide culturally and linguistically appropriate services.

Standard 9. Healthcare organizations should conduct initial and ongoing organizational self-assessments of CLAS-related activities and are encouraged to integrate cultural and linguistic competence-related measures into their internal audits, performance improvement programs, patient satisfaction assessments, and outcome-based evaluations.

Standard 10. Healthcare organizations should ensure that data on the individual patient's/consumer's race, ethnicity, and spoken and written language are collected in health records, integrated into the organization's management information systems, and periodically updated.

Standard 11. Healthcare organizations should maintain a current demographic, cultural, and epidemiological profile of the community as well as a needs assessment to accurately plan for and implement services that respond to the cultural and linguistic characteristics of the service area.

Standard 12. Healthcare should develop participatory, collaborative partnerships with communities and utilize a variety of formal and informal mechanisms to facilitate community and patient/consumer involvement in designing and implementing CLAS-related activities.

Standard 13. Healthcare organizations should ensure that conflict and grievance resolution processes are culturally and linguistically sensitive and capable of identifying, presenting, and resolving cross-cultural conflict or complaints by patients/consumers.

Standard 14. Healthcare organizations are encouraged to regularly make available to the public information about their progress and successful innovations in implementing the CLAS standards and to provide public notice in their communities about the availability of this information.

(USDHHS Office of Minority Health, 2001)

style of communication, religious practices, dietary practices, and socioeconomic status. Display 2–9 provides the components of a cultural assessment of the childbearing woman.

Enhancing Communication Skills

Display 2–10 contains suggestions for communicating effectively with childbearing women and their families. It is important to remember that effective communication requires a sincere desire to understand the other person's way of behaving and seeing the world. This allows for cultural reciprocity, when a woman feels that she has permission to share her cultural needs, concerns, and feelings. Respect and sensitivity characterize this kind of relationship. A perinatal nurse described the following experience:

> I cared for a Mexican-American woman in maternal/fetal testing. I was able to help her out by being her translator. Modesty was a big issue with her, and she was extremely uncomfortable with undoing her pants and showing her abdomen for the procedure. I felt that there was a unique bond and friendship that was created because of my understanding and sensitivity to her cultural values. It makes all the difference to the woman if she is able to communicate with you and you can convey that you really care.

DISPLAY 2-7

Guidelines for Working with a Medical Interpreter

- Orient the interpreter
- Request a female interpreter the approximate age of the woman
- Be prepared prior to the interpreter coming, and try to communicate with the woman prior to the interpreter arriving
- Ask the interpreter the best way to approach sensitive issues such as sexuality or perinatal loss
- Face the woman and direct your questions to the woman rather than the interpreter
- Ask about one problem at a time, using concise questions and phrases
- Look for nonverbal cues
- After the interaction, review the woman's answers with the interpreter

(Munoz & Luckmann, 2005)

DISPLAY 2-9

Cultural Assessment of the Childbearing Woman

- How is childbearing valued?
- Is childbearing viewed as a normal physiologic process, a wellness experience, a time of vulnerability and risk, or a state of illness?
- Are there dietary, nutritional, pharmacologic, and activity prescribed practices?
- Is birth a private intimate experience or a societal event?
- How is childbirth pain managed, and what maternal and paternal behaviors are appropriate?
- What support is given during pregnancy, childbirth, and beyond, and who appropriately gives that support?
- How is the newborn viewed, what are the patterns regarding care of the infant, and what are the relationships within the nuclear and extended families?
- What maternal precautions or restrictions are necessary during childbearing?
- What does the childbearing experience mean to the woman?

(Callister, 1995)

Be considerate, be polite, and speak softly. Caring behaviors and personal attention from healthcare providers are important to individuals of all cultures. Spend a few minutes talking to the woman and her family as she is admitted to the birthing unit to build rapport. Just a greeting and knowing a few of the social words in the woman's language and use of culturally specific etiquette helps to establish rapport. It is essential to understand cultural communication patterns. For example, Native Americans may maintain silence and not interrupt others. Hispanics appreciate interactions that begin with personal conversation or small talk, which serves to promote trust.

DISPLAY 2-8

Changing Institutional Forces to Facilitate Culturally Competent Care

- Changing birthing room policies and unit protocols to promote individualized and family-centered care
- Lobbying for increased resources such as translation services and cultural mediators
- Designing continuing education opportunities to increase cultural competence
- Hiring a nursing staff reflecting the culture of the community
- Generating a pool of volunteer translators who meet women prenatally and follow them through their births and the postpartum period
- Increasing the availability of language line services
- Developing innovative programs addressing the unique needs of culturally diverse populations and integrating community and acute care services for childbearing women and their families

DISPLAY 2-10

Culturally Competent Communication

- Enhance communication skills (greet respectfully, establish rapport, demonstrate empathy, listen actively, provide appropriate feedback, demonstrate interest)
- Develop linguistic skills
- Determine who the family decision makers are
- Understand that agreement does not indicate comprehension
- Use nonverbal communication
- Use appropriate names and titles
- Use culturally appropriate teaching techniques
- Provide for sufficient time

(Lipson & Dibble, 2005; Munoz & Luckmann, 2005)

Developing Linguistic Skills

Learning a second language is an excellent way to lower cultural barriers. A labor and delivery nurse described her experience caring for a Mexican immigrant woman:

> When I stepped into the room and began to speak in my high-school-level Spanish, her face brightened and she quickly responded in a rapid flow of unintelligible (to me) foreign syllables. Soon, we were able to communicate quite well, and I became comfortable with her. I translated the physician's words and vice versa. I rubbed her leg and stroked her hair when she cried out or moaned. I'd then ask her about the pain and reassured her as much as I could.

Pay attention to changing trends in language and incorporate them into your spoken and written language. Avoid using complex words, medical terms, and jargon that are difficult to understand in any language. Keep instructions simple and repeat as necessary. Saying "I understand" may be patronizing. Speak slowly, speak distinctly, and try to appear unhurried. State your message slowly, sentence by sentence. Find creative ways to convey information. One mother–baby nurse described caring for a woman who spoke no English:

> I was left with hand gestures and body language for communication. It was very difficult for her to understand my actions. Her assessment was especially hard because I was unable to assess her pain, bleeding, and nipple tenderness adequately. I finally found an English to Spanish dictionary, but this was of limited help to me because I was so bad at pronouncing the words that she still had a very difficult time understanding me. Finally, I just let her read the words from the dictionary. This was the most effective way of communicating that I could come up with. I know that she felt somewhat isolated because she had a difficult time communicating her needs to me also.

Determining Who Makes Family Decisions

Ask women whom they wish to include in their birth experience and make sure those persons are present for all discussions and participate in decision-making. Families fulfill several roles for women, including providers of security and support, caregivers, advocates, and liaisons. Families should be treated respectfully with the goal of establishing trust. For some cultural groups, conversation should be directed toward a specific family member. It is important to identify a spokesperson in the family, often the family member most proficient in English. Ask about family roles and respect the preferences of the woman and her family. When a Mexican immigrant woman was asked whether she wanted an epidural, the father of the baby answered, saying it was better for the baby to have an unmedicated labor and birth. The wife complied with this suggestion, and the nurse modeled support for the laboring woman and demonstrated respect for their decision as a couple. Many Mexican women may prefer not to have epidural analgesia/anesthesia.

Understanding the role of different family members in the Korean family system is important because a woman's mother-in-law traditionally cares for her and the newborn during the postpartum period. The nurse needs to recognize that any teaching she does must include the mother-in-law.

Understanding That Agreement May Not Indicate Comprehension or the Ability to Adhere to Healthcare Recommendations

The woman may pretend to understand in an effort to please the nurse and gain acceptance. The woman's smile may mask confusion, and her nod of assent or "uh-huh" may mean only that she hears, not that she understands or agrees. For example, a new mother who did not speak English was admitted to the mother–baby unit during the night shift. When asked if she was voiding sufficient amounts, she responded, "Yes." In the early morning hours, the mother began to complain of intense abdominal pain. She was catheterized and drained of more than 1200 mL of urine. The nurse had incorrectly assumed the woman's understanding.

The story is told of a 14-year-old AN new mother who was instructed to return to the hospital lab within 24 hours to have her newborn's bilirubin level drawn. When the nurse inquired further, she learned that this young mother had only been in the city for two weeks and had never used public transportation and had no money. The nurse was able to assist with community resources to help this young mother, rather than judging her as neglectful for not following discharge instructions (Munoz & Luckmann, 2005).

Using Nonverbal Communication

Use eye contact, friendly facial expressions, and face-to-face positions. Do not assume the woman dislikes you, does not trust you, or is not listening to you because she avoids eye contact. Koreans, Filipinos, and many other Asian groups, as well as AI/ANs, consider direct eye contact rude and confrontational. Islamic women are taught to lower their gaze with members of the opposite sex. Use touch to express caring and comfort. Nonverbal communication makes an important difference. A labor and delivery nurse said,

> I cared for a Korean first-time mother who came to the hospital fully dilated and gave birth to her son unmedicated. She did not speak any English, and her young husband was obviously uncomfortable and had little understanding about what was going on. As she gave birth, I could see the pain in her face, but she was stoic. I felt powerless because of her language and [other] cultural barriers, but I stayed with her and held her hand and encouraged her. Even though she could not understand my words, I hope she understood that I really cared.

Use universally understood language, such as charades (acting out), drawings, and gestures, and repeat the message several times using different common words. Use of simple words that are easily translated serves to improve communication.

Using Names and Titles

Determine how the childbearing woman and her family wish to be addressed. Names and appropriate titles are often complex and confusing. Mexican-American clients appreciate being addressed by their last name. In the Korean culture, family members are addressed in terms of their relationship to the youngest child in the family (eg, "Sung's grandmother"). It is important to learn how the woman wants to be addressed and to record it in the patient record so she won't have to answer the question over and over again.

Teaching Techniques

Use visual aids and demonstrations, and assist with return demonstrations. Do not assume that the woman can read or write. Ensure that teaching or educational materials can be understood by the client and are appropriate for the woman's cultural group and educational level (Freda, 2002). Display 2–11 contains suggestions for beginning the process of developing culturally appropriate patient education material. Appendix 2–A contains a sampling of culturally specific educational resources.

D I S P L A Y   2 - 1 1

Developing Culturally Appropriate Educational Material

- Be aware of your own assumptions and biases
- Develop an understanding of the target culture, including core values
- Work with a multicultural team
- Develop materials in the native language rather than having materials translated
- Have materials reviewed by members of the target cultural group

Accommodating Cultural Practices

Stereotypical generalization involves two dynamics: stereotyping and generalizing. Stereotyping, or believing that something is the same for everyone in a group, should be avoided. Generalizing, however, must be done to understand potential cultural beliefs and practices. The goal of individualizing care is to achieve a balance between what is indigenous to the culture and what may be specific to an individual woman. An experience that made one nurse sensitive to differences among women within the same culture was when she assumed that birth in H/L culture was exclusively a woman's experience, with little involvement by the father of the baby. She said,

> When I helped a Hispanic couple having their first baby, much to my surprise the father was right in there coaching his wife. So I supported his efforts and tried to make the birth experience what they wanted it to be.

If in doubt, ask. A culturally competent labor and delivery nurse described the following experience with a Muslim family:

> I asked the father if there was anything I should know about their customs, and he told me that before anyone could handle the baby [besides the physician], the father had to hold the baby and whisper a prayer into the ear of the baby to protect the baby from evil. I told him that as long as there were no problems with the baby immediately after birth, I would hand him the baby, and if there were problems, he could 'do his thing' while the baby was under the warmer and stabilized. He agreed to that. There were no

problems, and the father got his wishes and I had the opportunity to attend a wonderfully rich cultural birth.

One Muslim husband stayed with his wife 24 hours a day during her hospitalization. The husband observed the tradition of prayers five times each day, which is a religious duty specified in the Holy Quran. It was challenging for the nurse who walked into the room while he was praying on the floor on his prayer mat, but she did all she could to support these religious rituals.

In many cultures, there is a gender preference for male children. For example, a Korean mother gave birth to a healthy baby girl. Her husband was an active, supportive coach during the labor and birth. When he saw the baby girl, however, his demeanor changed, and he shouted at his wife and started to cry. The mother also cried and refused to hold or look at her newborn daughter. The father left the room, and the mother became subdued but still refused to hold the baby. Later, the nurse commented about the beautiful infant, referring to her not as a "baby girl," but as "the baby." The mother asked to hold her newborn. The father came back into the room, and the nurse told him his baby was perfect and beautiful. This reinforcement seemed to appease the father, who then held his infant.

It is important to respect the wisdom of other cultures. Healthcare beliefs and practices can be divided into three categories: potentially beneficial, harmless or neutral, and potentially harmful. Examples in each category are listed in Table 2–2. Preservation of potentially helpful beliefs or practices and harmless or neutral behaviors that respect the natural wisdom of the culture should be encouraged, valued, and celebrated. Beneficial as well as harmless or neutral practices and those of unknown efficacy may increase a woman's connection to her own historical and cultural roots. For example, an East Indian pregnant woman may softly sing songs passed from generation to generation, massaging her abdomen several times a day and continuing that practice with her infant through the first year of life.

Born and Barron (2005) have summarized important facts about the use of herbs and plants during pregnancy. Herbs commonly used include ginger, peppermint, chamomile, cinnamon, and red raspberry leaf for morning sickness; dandelion for constipation; field greens, dandelion, and red raspberry leaf for anemia; cranberry for urinary tract infections; and red raspberry leaf for prevention of preterm labor. Herbs should not be used in the first trimester of pregnancy, and some herbs, including blue or black cohosh, dong quai, ephedra chaste tree, and zinc, should never be used during pregnancy. Some nurse midwives recommend the use of black and blue cohosh for induction of labor in term women.

Focus energy on changing harmful practices. For example, the motivator for a pregnant woman to discontinue a harmful practice, such as the use of certain herbs or smoking, is to appeal to her protective instincts toward her unborn child. It is essential to show genuine interest and appreciation. The culturally competent nurse seeks to understand the woman's unique way of experiencing birth and expressing what birth means. Failure of the nurse to demonstrate interest and caring toward cultural practices she does not understand causes women to lose confidence in the nurse and the larger healthcare system and may

TABLE 2–2 ■ PERINATAL CULTURAL PRACTICES

Potentially Helpful	Harmless or Neutral	Potentially Harmful
Postpartum diet, hygiene practices	Avoidance of sexual activity during menstruation	Avoiding bathing during menstruation
Carrying the infant close in a sling		Avoiding iron supplements during pregnancy or lactation because of the belief that iron causes hardening of the bones and a hard labor
Breast-feeding on demand	Yarn tied around the middle finger to give hope and signify spiritual wholeness	
Spacing of children by long-term breastfeeding		Belief that colostrum is "dirty" or "old" and unfit for the newborn
Remaining active throughout labor	Keeping the mother's head covered at all times with a scarf or wig	Prolonged bed rest after birth
Giving birth in non-recumbent position	Not allowing the newborn to see his image in a mirror	Placing a raisin on the umbilical cord to prevent a hernia
	Garlic charm around the baby's neck to offer protection from the "evil eye"	Use of abdominal binders to prevent umbilical hernia
	Eating garlic to prevent illness	

decrease adherence with suggested health promotion strategies.

Changes are needed in nursing education, healthcare delivery, and in nursing research to increase cultural competence in perinatal nursing practice. The Institute of Medicine (2002) has called for healthcare providers and the healthcare delivery system to confront and overcome their racial and ethnic disparities.

Nursing Education

Most nursing students have little knowledge about any culture other than their own. Changes in basic nursing education programs should begin to increase cultural competence. National nursing education standards require that educational programs prepare nurses to understand the effect cultural, racial, socioeconomic, religious, and lifestyle differences have on health status and responses to health and illness (American Association of Colleges of Nursing, 1998). Graduates should have the knowledge and skills to provide holistic care to culturally diverse women and their families. Nursing education should expose students diversity in a variety of settings; include theoretical and factual information about cultural groups, identify strategies and skills useful in providing nursing care to culturally diverse clients, allow students the opportunity to examine their own personal values and attitudes, and encourage linguistic skills in a second language (Grant & Letzring, 2003; Kleiman, Frederickson, & Lundy, 2004; Sloane, Groves, & Brager, 2004; Wittig, 2004).

Cross-cultural health education materials are available on many Web sites (McCarty, Enslein, Kelley, Choi, & Tripp-Reimer, 2002) and sources are listed in Appendix 2–A.

Healthcare Delivery

Most healthcare systems in the United States exhibit cultural blindness, ignoring differences as if they do not exist. Healthcare in the United States is a culture unto itself, based on the dominant Western biomedical model of health beliefs and practices. In most hospitals, only American food is served, and there is a universal assumption that everyone seeking healthcare understands English. Nurses are in a position to challenge institutional forces that may inhibit culturally sensitive care. Display 2–12 provides examples of institutional changes and strategies that may facilitate culturally competent care. There are ethical issues related to caring for culturally diverse populations who do not speak English, including compromised quality of care, increased risk of adverse events, lack of

DISPLAY 2 - 12

Strategies Fostering Culturally Competent Care on Perinatal Nursing Units

- Educational offerings on ethnic, religious, cultural, and family diversity
- Educational offerings about available community resources
- Literature searches focused on the predominant cultural groups cared for, followed by development of a resource binder available on the unit
- Generating a culture database
- Establishing a task force to create culturally sensitive birth plans for the predominant cultural groups cared for
- Establishing cultural competencies that are part of the yearly staff evaluation
- Making cultural competence part of the interview process
- Supporting each other in frustrating situations
- Nursing grand rounds focusing on cultural issues
- Celebrating successes by peers in providing culturally competent care
- Sharing resources such as books and professional journal articles
- Discouraging negativism and discrimination on the unit
- Creating connections between community and acute care settings

access to health care, and lack of informed consent (Ku & Flores, 2005; McCabe, Morgan, Curley, Begay, & Gohdes, 2005). In addition to diversity in women and their families receiving care, there is also growing diversity within the healthcare work force. Display 2–13 describes how a multicultural health care team might improve communication between members.

Nursing Research

Culturally sensitive scholarship is essential. Many cultures are silent or invisible minorities because of the lack of research on their health needs, status, beliefs, behavior, and family roles. Cross-cultural comparative studies of childbirth demonstrate that much of the information available is medically oriented or narrowly anthropologic in focus. Much of the current literature on how culture influences childbirth is descriptive or focuses on a case study approach (Sperstad & Werner, 2005). There is a need for qualitative approaches to research, with women as participants or co-investigators rather than study subjects.

DISPLAY 2-13

Communication in a Multicultural Healthcare Team

- Assess the personal beliefs of members
- Assess communication variables from a cultural perspective
- Modify communication patterns to enhance communication
- Identify mannerisms that may be threatening and avoid using them
- Understand that respect for others and the needs they communicate is central to positive working relationships
- Use validating techniques when communicating
- Be considerate of a reluctance to talk when the subject might involve culturally taboo topics, such as sexual matters
- Use team members from a different culture as resources, but do not support a dependency by the team on those members
- Support team efforts to plan and adapt care based on communicated needs and cultural backgrounds of individual patients
- Identify potential interpreters for patients whenever necessary in order to improve communication

Shilling (2000, p. 153) suggests the following potential research questions:

1. How do women of different cultures talk about childbearing?
2. What type of concerns do childbearing women have, and how are they similar or different between cultures?
3. How do women of different cultures feel about their bodies during the childbearing year?
4. How have the technologic, political, and social changes influenced childbearing among different cultures?

Qualitative research approaches include focus groups with a bilingual discussion leader or participative research in which results are returned rapidly to participants to improve service. Such approaches are empowering and give legitimacy to healthcare issues of culturally diverse women. The ideal research team includes both members from within the culture being studied as well as nonmembers. Multidisciplinary research teams that include transcultural nurses, nurse anthropologists, sociologists, and others are effective. Cultural issues of specific interest to women have the potential to improve the quality of nursing care provided to women and their quality of life. One understudied area is the measure-

ment of biologic and physiologic differences in cultural, ethnic, and racial groups of women. Studies on the sexual and emotional complications of genital mutilation also are needed. Another important research priority is intervention studies designed to measure the effectiveness of strategies for providing healthcare to vulnerable populations of culturally diverse women.

SUMMARY

The story is told of a Native American childbearing couple who seemed like a typical mainstream American family, but whose grandmother requested to take the placenta home. It would have been helpful if, on admission, the nurse had asked about their heritage and whether there were any cultural traditions that were important to them. The father would have perhaps responded that his mother was traditional and may want to take the placenta home. The nurse then would have had time to explain whether or not the request could be accommodated, demonstrating respect and providing culturally appropriate care (Leininger & McFarland, 2006). Nurses caring for childbearing women and their families should be respectful of women's cultural diversity and the societal context of their lives, balancing professional standards of care with attitudes, knowledge, and skills associated with cultural competence (Callister, 2001; D'Avanzo & Geissler, 2003; Edwards, 2003). Perinatal nurses should seek to create a healthcare encounter with childbearing women and their families that respects the sociocultural and spiritual context of life and moves beyond the superficial to understand the deeper meaning of childbearing (Callister, 2004; Rodriguez, Patel, Jaswal, & de Souza, 2003). Perinatal nurses must never lose sight of the fact that a woman's childbirth experience is not only about making a baby but also about creating a mother—a mother who is strong and competent and who trusts her own capacities because she has been cared for by a culturally competent nurse. Giving birth has the potential to be a rich cultural and spiritual experience facilitated by such a nurse.

REFERENCES

Ahmad, F., Riaz, S., Barata, P., & Steward, D. E. (2004). Patriarchal beliefs and perceptions of abuse among South Asian immigrant women. *Violence Against Women, 10*(3), 262–282.

Amankwaa, L. C. (2003). Postpartum depression, culture, and African-American women. *Journal of Cultural Diversity, 10*(1), 23–29.

American Association of Colleges of Nursing. (1998). *The essentials of baccalaureate education for professional nursing practice.* Washington, DC: Author.

American Public Health Association. (2004). Understanding the health culture of recent immigrants to the United States: A cross-cultural maternal health information catalog. Retrieved February 15, 2006, from http://www.apha.org/pppp/red/summary.htm.

Andrews, M. M. (2003). Culturally competent nursing care. In M. M. Andrew & J. S. Boyle (Eds.), *Transcultural concepts in nursing* (pp. 15–35). Philadelphia: Lippincott Williams & Wilkins.

Andrews, M. M., & Boyle, J. S. (2003). *Transcultural concepts in nursing care*. Philadelphia: J. B. Lippincott.

Anuforo, P. O., Oyedele, L., & Pacquiao, D. F. (2004). Comparative study of meanings, beliefs, and practices of female circumcision among three Nigerian tribes in the United States and Nigeria. *Journal of Transcultural Nursing, 15*(2), 103–113.

Baker, A., Ferguson, S. A., Roach, G. D. & Dawson, D. (2001). Perceptions of labor pain by mothers and their attending midwives. *Journal of Advanced Nursing, 35*(2), 171–179.

Balcazar, H., Peterson, G. W., & Krull, J. L. (1997). Acculturation and family cohesiveness in Mexican American pregnant women: Social and health implications. *Family and Community Health, 20*(3), 16–31.

Banks, J. W. (2003). Ka'nistenhsera Teiakotihsnie's: A native community rekindles the tradition of breastfeeding. *Association of Womens Health, Obstetric, and Neonatal Nursing Lifelines, 7*(4), 340–347.

Barnes, D. M. & Harrison, C. L. (2004). Refugee women's reproductive health in early resettlement. *Journal of Obstetric, Gynecologic, and Neonatal Nursing, 33*(6), 723–728.

Bazaldua, O. V. & Sias, J. (2004). Cultural competence. *Journal of Pharmacy Practice, 17*(3), 160–166.

Beck, C. T. (2005). Acculturation: Implications for perinatal research. *MCN: The American Journal of Maternal Child Nursing, 31*(2), 114–120.

Beck, C. T., Froman, R. D., & Bernal, H. (2005). Acculturation level and postpartum depression in Hispanic mothers. *MCN: The American Journal of Maternal Child Nursing, 30*(5), 299–304.

Bender, D. E., Harbour, C., Thorp, J., & Morris, P. (2001). Tell me what you mean by "si": Perceptions of quality of prenatal care among immigrant Latina women. *Qualitative Health Research, 11*(6), 780–794.

Berry, J. W. (1980). Acculturation as varieties of adaptation. In A. M. Padilla (Ed.), *Acculturation: Theories, models, and some new findings* (pp. 9–25). Boulder, CO: Westview Press.

Born, D., & Barron, M. L. (2005). Herb use in pregnancy: What nurses should know. *MCN: The American Journal of Maternal Child Nursing, 30*(3), 201–206.

Boyer, L. E., Williams, M., Callister, L. C., & Marshall, E. S. (2001). Hispanic women's perceptions regarding cervical cancer screening. *Journal of Obstetric, Gynecologic, and Neonatal Nursing, 30*(2), 240–245.

Braithwaite, A. C., & Williams, C. C. (2004). Childbirth experiences of professional Chinese women. *Journal of Obstetric, Gynecologic, and Neonatal Nursing, 33*(6), 748–755.

Braithwaite, A. C. (2006). Influence of nurse characteristics on the acquisition of cultural competence. *International Journal of Nursing Education Scholarship, 3*(1), Article 3 [Retrieved March 6, 2006 www.bepress.com/IJNES].

Brown, J. S., Villarruel, A. M., Oakley, D., & Eribes, C. (2003). Exploring contraceptive pill taking among Hispanic women in the United States. *Health Education and Behavior, 30*(6), 663–682.

Callister, L. C. (1995). Cultural meanings of childbirth. *Journal of Obstetric, Gynecologic, and Neonatal Nursing, 24*(4), 327–331.

Callister, L. C. (2001). Culturally competent care of women and newborns: Attitudes, knowledge and skills. *Journal of Obstetric, Gynecologic, and Neonatal Nursing, 30*(2), 209–215.

Callister, L. C. (2002). Celebrating life: Spirituality in Judeo-Christian and Muslim childbearing women. *Bridges: The Kennedy Center for International Studies, Spring 2002*. Retrieved June 10, 2002, from http://kennedycenter.byu.edu

Callister, L. C. (2003a). Cultural influences of pain perceptions and behaviors. *Home Health Care Management and Practice, 15*(3), 207–211.

Callister, L. C. (2003b). A perspective from the Church of Jesus Christ of Latter-day Saints. In M. L. Moore & M. K. Moos (Eds.), *Cultural competence in the care of childbearing families* (pp. 68–70). White Plains, NY: March of Dimes.

Callister, L. C. (2004b). Making meaning: Women's birth narratives. *Journal of Obstetric, Gynecologic, and Neonatal Nursing, 33*(4), 508–518.

Callister, L. C. (2005). What has the literature taught us about culturally competent care of women and children? *MCN: The American Journal of Maternal Child Nursing, 30*(6), 380–388.

Callister, L. C. (2006a). Perinatal ethics: State of the science. *Journal of Perinatal and Neonatal Nursing, 20*(1), 37–39.

Callister, L. C. (2006b). Perinatal loss: A family perspective. *Journal of Perinatal and Neonatal Nursing, 20*(3), 227–234.

Callister, L. C., & Birkhead, A. (2002). Acculturation and perinatal outcomes in Mexican immigrant childbearing women. *Journal of Perinatal and Neonatal Nursing, 16*(3), 22–38.

Callister, L. C., Getmanenko, N., Garvrish, N., Eugenevna, M. O., Vladimirova, Z. N., Lassetter, J., et al. (in press). Giving birth: The voices of Russian women. *MCN: The American Journal of Maternal Child Nursing, 32*(1), 18–24.

Callister, L. C., Khalaf, I., Semenic, S., Kartchner, R., & Vehvilainen-Julkunen, K. (2003). The pain of childbirth: Perceptions of culturally diverse women. *Pain Management Nursing, 4*(4), 145–154.

Callister, L. C., Semenic, S., & Foster, J. C. (1999). Cultural and spiritual meanings of childbirth: Orthodox Jewish and Mormon women. *Journal of Holistic Nursing, 17*(3), 280–295.

Callister, L. C., & Vega, R. (1998). Giving birth: Guatemalan women's voices. *Journal of Obstetric, Gynecologic, and Neonatal Nursing, 27*(3), 289–295.

Callister, L. C., Vehvilainen-Julkunen, K., & Lauri, S. (2000). A description of birth in Finland. *MCN: The American Journal of Maternal Child Nursing, 25*(3), 146–150.

Callister, L. C., Vehvilainen-Julkunen, K., & Lauri, S. (2001). Giving birth: Perceptions of Finnish childbearing women. *MCN: The American Journal of Maternal Child Nursing, 26*(1), 28–32.

Campinha-Bacote, J. (1994). *The process of cultural competence in healthcare: A culturally competent model of care*. Wyoming, OH: Transcultural CARE Associates.

Carlton, T., Callister, L. C., & Stoneman, E. (2005). Decision making in laboring women: Ethical issues for perinatal nurses. *Journal of Perinatal and Neonatal Nursing, 19*(2), 145–154.

Carr, C. A., & deJoseph, J. F. (2001). Perinatal care among diverse populations of women. In L. V. Walsch (Ed.), *Midwifery: Community based care during the childbearing year* (pp. 211–218). Philadelphia: Saunders.

Carroll, K. N., Griffin, M. R., Gebretsadik, T., Shintani, A., Mitchel, E., & Hartert, T. V. (2005). Racial differences in asthma morbidity during pregnancy. *Obstetrics & Gynecology, 106*(1), 66–72.

Caughey, A. B., Stotland, N. E., Washington, M. D., & Escobar, G. (2005). Maternal ethnicity, paternal ethnicity, and parental ethnic discordance: Predictors of pre-eclampsia. *Obstetrics and Gynecology, 106*(1), 156–161.

Centers for Disease Control and Prevention. (2004). Prevalence of diabetes among Hispanics. *Morbidity and Mortality Weekly Report, 53*(40), 941–944.

Conrad, M. M., & Pacquiao, D. F. (2005). Manifestation, attribution, and coping with depression among Asian Indians from the perspectives of health care practitioners. *Journal of Transcultural Nursing, 16*(1), 32–40.

Cross, T. F., Brazon, B. J., Dennis, K. W., & Isaacs, M. R. (1989). *Toward a culturally competent system of care*. Washington, DC: Child and Adolescent Service System Program Technical Assistance Center.

Dalla, R. L., & Gamble, W. C. (2000). Mother, daughter, teenager—Who am I? Perceptions of adolescent maternity in a Navajo reservation community. *Journal of Family Issues, 21*(2), 225–245.

D'Avanzo, C. E., & Geissler, E. M. (2003). *Cultural Health Assessment* (3rd ed.). Philadelphia: Mosby.

Davis, E. (2000). The sexuality of pregnancy and birth. In *Women's sexual passages* (pp. 82–120). Alameda, CA: Hunter House.

Davis, R. E. (2001). The postpartum experience of Southeast Asian women in the United States. *MCN: The American Journal of Maternal Child Nursing, 26*(4), 202–207.

Davis-Floyd, R. B., & Sargent, C. F. (1997). *Childbirth and authoritative knowledge*. Berkeley, CA: University of California Press.

deChesnay, M., Wharton, R., & Pamp, C. (2005). Cultural competence, resilience, and advocacy. In M. deChesnay (Ed.), *Caring for the vulnerable* (pp. 31–41). Boston: Jones & Bartlett.

Doyle, E. I., & Faucher, M. A. (2002). Pharmaceutical therapy in midwifery practice: A culturally competent approach. *Journal of Midwifery and Womens Health, 47*(3), 122–129.

Edwards, K. (2003). Increasing cultural competence and decreasing disparities in health. *Journal of Cultural Diversity, 10*(4), 111–112.

Erviti, J., Casro, R., & Callado, A. (2004). Strategies used by low-income Mexican women to deal with miscarriage and "spontaneous" abortion. *Qualitative Health Research, 14*(8), 1058–1076.

Foss, G. F. (2001). Maternal sensitivity, post-traumatic stress, and acculturation in Vietnamese and Hmong mothers. *MCN: The American Journal of Maternal Child Nursing, 26*(5), 257–263.

Freda, M. (2002). *Perinatal patient education*. Philadelphia: Lippincott Williams & Wilkins.

Gennaro, S. (2005). Overview of current state of research on pregnancy outcomes in minority populations. *American Journal of Obstetrics and Gynecology, 192*(Suppl. 5): S3–10.

Giger, J. N., & Davidhizar, R. E. (2005). *Transcultural nursing: Assessment and intervention*. St. Louis, MO: Mosby–Year Book.

Goldbort, J. (2005). Transcultural analysis of postpartum depression. *MCN: The American Journal of Maternal Child Nursing, 31*(2), 121–126.

Gordon-Larsen, P., Harris, K. M., Ward, D. S., & Popkin, B. M. (2003). Acculturation and overweight-related behaviors among Hispanic immigrants to the US: The National Longitudinal Study of Adolescent Health. *Social Science and Medicine, 57*(11), 2023–2034.

Goyal, D., Murphy, S. O., & Cohen, J. (2006). Immigrant Asian Indian women and postpartum depression. *Journal of Obstetric, Gynecologic, and Neonatal Nursing, 35*(1), 98–104.

Grant, L. F., & Letzring, T. D. (2003). Status of cultural competence in nursing education: A literature review. *Journal of Multicultural Nursing and Health, 9*(2), 6–13.

Heilemann, M. S. V., Lee, K. A., & Kury, F. S. (2005). Strength factors among women of Mexican descent. *Western Journal of Nursing Research, 27*(8), 949–965.

Heilemann, M. S. V., Lee, K. A., Stinson, J., Koshar, J. H., & Goss, G. (2000). Acculturation and perinatal health outcomes among women of Mexican descent. *Research in Nursing and Health, 23*(2), 118–125.

Holroyd, E., Twinn, S., & Adab, P. (2004). Socio-cultural influences on Chinese women's attendance for cervical screening. *Journal of Advanced Nursing, 46*(1), 42–52.

Holroyd, E., Twinn, S., & Yim, I. W. (2004). Exploring Chinese women's cultural beliefs and behaviors regarding the practice of "doing the month." *Women's Health, 40*(3), 109–123.

Institute of Medicine. (2002). *Unequal treatment: Confronting racial and ethnic disparities in health care*. Washington, DC: Author.

Jesse, D. E., Graham, M., & Swanson, M. (2006). Psychosocial and spiritual factors associated with smoking and substance use during pregnancy in African American and white low-income women. *Journal of Obstetrics, Gynecologic, and Neonatal Nursing, 35*(1), 68–77.

Johnson, T., Callister, L. C., Beckstrand, R., & Freeborn, D. (in press). Dutch women's perceptions of childbirth in the Netherlands. *MCN: The American Journal of Maternal Child Nursing, 32*(3).

Joint Commission for Accreditation of Healthcare Organizations. (2000). *Comprehensive accreditation manual for hospitals*. Chicago: Author.

Jones, M. E., Bond, M. L., Gardner, S. H., & Hernandez, M. C. (2002). Acculturation levels and family-planning patterns of Hispanic immigrant women. *MCN: The American Journal of Maternal Child Nursing, 27*(1), 26–32.

Jordan, B. (1993). *Birth in four cultures*. Prospect Heights, IL: Waveland Press.

Kartchner, R., & Callister, L. C. (2003). Giving birth: Voices of Chinese women. *Journal of Holistic Nursing, 21*(2), 100–116.

Kasturirangan, A., Krishnan, S., & Roger, S. (2004). The impact of culture and minority status on women's experience of domestic violence. *Trauma, Violence and Abuse, 5*(4), 318–332.

Khalaf, I., & Callister, L. C. (1997). Cultural meanings of childbirth: Muslim women living in Jordan. *Journal of Holistic Nursing, 15*(4), 373–388.

Khazoyan, C. M., & Anderson, N. L. R. (1994). Latinas' expectations of their partners during childbirth. *MCN: The American Journal of Maternal Child Nursing, 19*(4), 226–229.

Kim-Goodwin, Y. S. (2003). Postpartum beliefs and practices among non-Western cultures. *MCN: The American Journal of Maternal Child Nursing, 28*(2), 74–78.

Kirkham, S. R. (1998). Nurses' descriptions of caring for culturally diverse clients. *Clinical Nursing Research, 7*(2), 125–146.

Kleiman, S., Fredrickson, K., & Lundy, T. (2004). Using an eclectic model to educate students about cultural influences on the nurse-patient relationship. *Nursing Education Perspectives, 25*(5), 249–255.

Kridli, S. A. (2002). Health beliefs and practices among Arab women. *MCN: The American Journal of Maternal Child Nursing, 27*(3), 178–182.

Ku, L., & Flores, G. (2005). Pay now or pay later: Providing interpreter services in health care. *Health Affairs, 24*(2), 435–444.

Lauderdale, J. (2003). Transcultural perspectives in childbearing. In M. M. Andrews & J. S. Boyle (Eds.), *Transcultural concepts in nursing care* (4th ed., pp. 95–130). St. Louis, MO: Mosby.

Le, H. N., Munoz, R. F., Soto, J. A., Delucchi, K. L., & Ippen, C. G. (2004). Identifying risk for onset of major depressive episodes in low-income Latinas during pregnancy and postpartum. *Hispanic Journal of Behavioral Sciences, 26*(4), 463–482.

Leininger, M., & McFarland, M. R. (2006). *Cultural care diversity and universality*. Sudbury, MA: Jones and Bartlett.

Lemmon, B. S. (2002a). Exploring Latino rituals in birthing: Understanding the need to bury the placenta. *Association of Women's Health, Obstetric, and Neonatal Nurses, 6*(5), 443–445.

Lemmon, B. S. (2002b). Amish health care beliefs and practices in an obstetrical setting. *The Journal of Multicultural Nursing and Health, 8*(3), 72–77.

Lewis, J. (2003). Jewish perspectives on pregnancy and childbearing. *MCN: The American Journal of Maternal Child Nursing, 28*(5), 306–312.

Lindgren, T., & Lipson, J. G. (2004). Finding a way: Afghan women's experience in community participation. *Journal of Transcultural Nursing, 15*(2), 122–130.

Lipson, J. G., & Dibble, S. L. (2005). *Culture and clinical care.* San Francisco: University of California Nursing Press.

Little, C. (2003). Female genital circumcision: Medical and cultural considerations. *Journal of Holistic Nursing, 10*(1), 30–34.

Luna, E. (2003). Nurse-curanderas: *Las que curan* at the heart of Hispanic culture. *Journal of Holistic Nursing, 21*(4), 326–342.

Lundquist, A., Nilstun, T., & Dykes, A. K. (2003). Neonatal end of life care in Sweden: The views of Muslim women. *Journal of Perinatal and Neonatal Nursing, 17*(2), 77–86.

McCabe, M., Morgan, F., Curley, H., Begay, R., & Gohdes, D. M. (2005). The informed consent process in a cross-cultural setting: Is the process achieving the intended result? *Ethnicity and Disease, 15*(2), 300–304.

McCarty, L. J., Enslein, J. C., Kelley, L. S., Choi, E., & Tripp-Reimer, T. (2002). Cross-cultural health education: Materials on the world wide web. *Journal of Transcultural Nursing, 13*(1), 54–60.

Martinez-Schallmoser, L., MacMullen, N. J., & Telleen, S. (2005). Social support in Mexican American childbearing women. *Journal of Obstetric, Gynecologic, and Neonatal Nursing, 34*(6), 755–760.

Matthews, R., & Callister, L. C. (2004). Child bearing women's perceptions of nursing care that promotes dignity. *Journal of Obstetric, Gynecologic, and Neonatal Nursing, 33*(4), 498–507.

Mattson, S. (2004). Ethnocultural considerations in the childbearing period. In S. Mattson & J. E. Smith (Eds.), *Core curriculum for maternal newborn nursing* (3rd ed.). St Louis, MO: Elsevier & Saunders.

Melender, H. L. (2006). What constitutes a good childbirth? A qualitative study of pregnant Finnish women. *Journal of Midwifery and Womens Health, 51*(5), 331–339.

Meleis, A. (2003). Theoretical considerations of health care for immigrant and minority women. In P. St. Hill, J. G. Lipson, & A. I. Meleis (Eds.), *Caring for women cross-culturally* (pp. 1–10). Philadelphia: F. A. Davis.

Moore, M. L., & Moos, M. K. (2003). *Cultural competence in the care of childbearing families.* New York: March of Dimes.

Munoz, C., & Hilgenberg, C. (2005). Ethnopharmacology. *American Journal of Nursing, 105*(8), 40–49.

Munoz, C., & Luckmann, J. (2005). *Transcultural communication in nursing* (2nd ed.). Clifton Park, NY: Thomson Delmar Learning.

National Alliance for Hispanic Health. (2001). *A primer for cultural proficiency: Toward quality health services for Hispanics.* Washington, DC: Estrella Press.

Nichols, L. A. (2004). The infant caring process among Cherokee mothers. *Journal of Holistic Nursing, 22*(3), 226–253.

Office of Minority Health. (2001). *National standards for culturally and linguistically appropriate service in health care.* Rockville, MD: Government Printing Office. Retrieved February 12, 2006, from http://www.omhrc.gov/clas/finacultural11a.htm

Purnell, L. D., & Paulanka, B. J. (2003). *Transcultural health care* (2nd ed.). Philadelphia: F. A. Davis.

Ramirez, R. R., & de la Cruz, G. P. (2002). *The Hispanic population in the United States.* Washington, DC: U.S. Census Bureau. (Current Population Reports, P20–545)

Rashidi, A., & Rajaram, S. S. (2001). Culture care conflicts among Asian-Islamic immigrant women in United States hospitals. *Holistic Nursing Practice, 16*(1), 55–64.

Riordan, J. (2004). The cultural context of breastfeeding. In J. Riordan & K. G. Auerbach (Eds.), *Breastfeeding and human lactation.* Boston: Jones & Bartlett.

Roat, C. E. (1997). A medical interpreter's code of ethics. In C. E. Roat (Ed.), *Bridging the gap: A basic training for medical inter-preter* (pp. 34–35). Seattle, WA: Cross-Cultural Health Care Program.

Rodriguez, M., Patel, V., Jaswal, S., & de Souza, N. (2003). Listening to mothers: Qualitative studies on motherhood and depression from Goa, India. *Social Science and Medicine, 57*(10), 1797–1806.

Rorie, J. L. (2004). Cultural competence in midwifery practice. In H. Varney, J. M. Kriebs, & C. L. Gego (Eds), *Varney's Midwifery* (5th ed., pp. 49–58). Sudbury, MA: Jones & Bartlett.

Rutherford, M. S., & Parker, K. (2003). Inner strength in Salvadoran women. *Journal of Cultural Diversity, 10*(1), 6–10.

St Hill, P. (2003). African Americans. In P. St Hill, J. G. Lipson, & A. I. Meleis (Eds.), *Caring for Women Cross-culturally* (pp. 11–27). Philadelphia: F. A. Davis.

St Hill, J. G., Lipson, J., & Meleis, A. I. (2003). *Caring for women cross-culturally.* Philadelphia: F. A. Davis.

Schlickau, J. M., & Wilson, M. E. (2005). Breastfeeding: A health-promoting behavior for Hispanic women. *Journal of Advanced Nursing, 52*(2), 200–210.

Semenic, S., Callister, L. C., & Feldman, P. (2004). Giving birth: The voices of Orthodox Jewish women living in Canada. *Journal of Obstetric, Gynecologic, and Neonatal Nursing, 33*(1), 80–87.

Shambley-Ebron, D. Z., & Boyle, J. S. (2004). New paradigms for transcultural nursing: Frameworks for studying African American women. *Journal of Transcultural Nursing, 15*(1), 11–17.

Shambley-Ebron, D. Z., & Boyle, J. S. (2006). Self-care and mothering in African American women with HIV/AIDS. *Western Journal of Nursing Research, 28*(1), 42–60.

Shen, J. J., Tymkow, C., & MacMullen, N. (2005). Disparities in maternal outcomes among four ethnic populations. *Ethnicity and Disease, 15*(3), 492–497.

Shilling, T. (2000). Cultural perspectives on childbearing. In F. H. Nichols & S. S. Humenick (Eds.), *Childbirth education: Practice, research, and theory* (2nd ed., pp. 138–154). Philadelphia: Saunders.

Shin, Y., Bozzette, M., Kenner, C., & Kim, T. I. (2004). Evaluation of Korean newborns with the Brazelton Neonatal Behavioral Assessment Scale. *Journal of Obstetric, Gynecologic, and Neonatal Nursing, 33*(5), 589–596.

Sloane, E., Groves, S., & Brager, R. (2004). Cultural competency education in American nursing programs and the approach of one school of nursing. *International Journal of Nursing Education Scholarship, 1*(1), Article 6. Retrieved March 6, 2006, from http://www.bepress.com/ijnes

Small, R., Yelland, J., Lumley, J., Brown, S., & Liamputtong, P. (2002). Immigrant women's views about care during labor and birth: An Australian study of Vietnamese, Turkish, and Filipino women. *Birth, 29*(4), 266–277.

Spector, R. E. (2004). *Cultural diversity in health and illness* (6th ed.). Upper Saddle River, NJ: Prentice Hall Health.

Sperstad, R. A., & Werner, J. S. (2005). Coming to the cultural "in-between": Nursing insights from a Hmong birth case study. *Journal of Obstetric, Gynecologic, and Neonatal Nursing, 34*(6), 682–688.

Suh, E. E. (2004). The model of cultural competence through an evolutionary concept analysis. *Journal of Transcultural Nursing, 15*(2), 93–102.

Tandon, S. D., Parillo, K. M., & Keefer, M. (2005). Hispanic women's perceptions of patient-centeredness during prenatal care: A mixed-method study. *Birth, 32*(4), 312–317.

Torres, R. (2005). Latina perceptions of prenatal care. *Hispanic Health Care International, 3*(3), 153–160.

United States Census Bureau. (2002). *Health Insurance Coverage.* http://www.census.gov/prod/2002pubs/p60-220.pdf

United States Census Bureau. (2001). *Mapping census 2000: The geography of United States diversity.* http://www.census.gov/main/www/schtool.htm

United States Department of Health and Human Services. (2000). *Healthy people 2010: Understanding and improving health* (2nd ed.). Rockville, MD: Government Printing Office.

Warda, M. R. (2000). Mexican Americans' perceptions of culturally competent care. *Western Journal of Nursing Research, 22*(2), 203–224.

Willgerodt, M. A., & Killien, M. G. (2004). Family nursing research with Asian families. *Journal of Family Nursing, 10*(2), 149–172.

Williams, D. P., & Hampton, A. (2005). Barriers to health services perceived by Marshallese immigrants. *Immigrant Health, 7*(4), 317–326.

Wittig, D. R. (2004). Knowledge, skills and attitudes of nursing students regarding culturally congruent care of Native Americans. *Journal of Transcultural Nursing, 15*(1), 54–61.

Yick, A. G., Shibusawa, T., & Agbayani-Siewert, P. (2003). Partner violence, depression, and practice implications with families of Chinese descent. *Journal of Cultural Diversity, 10*(3), 96–104.

Zlot, A. I., Jackson, D. J., & Korenbrot, C. (2005). Association of acculturation with cesarean section among Latinas. *Maternal and Child Health Journal, 9*(1), 11–20.

APPENDIX **2-A**

Culturally Competent Care Resources

AfricaOnline
http://www.africaonline.com/site/ (African topics such as health, women and education and African countries)

Al-bab.com
http://www.al-bab.com (Arab topics and countries)

Alliance for Hispanic Health
http://www.hispanichealth.org

American Academy of Child and Adolescent Psychiatry
http://www.aacap.org/publications/factsfam/index.htm (Spanish, French, German, Malaysian, Polish, and Icelandic translations available with links from the site, though there is a disclaimer that they have been been reviewed for translation accuracy by the AACAP)

American Diabetes Association
http://www.diabetes.org (English and Spanish)

American Immigration Resources on the Internet
http://www.theodora.com/resource.html (English, Chinese, Russian)

American Public Health Association (Maternal/child health)
http://www.apa.org/ppp/red/index.htm

Ameristat
http://www.ameristat.org (Graphics and text of US population)

Asian and Pacific Islander American Health Forum
http://www.apiahf.org (Focuses on health status of AA/PI communities)

AT&T Language Line
http://www.languageline.com (800) 752-0093
Translation into over 140 languages. Subscribed interpretation (organizations, frequent use); membership interpretation (organizations, predictable need); personal interpreter (individuals, occasional use)

Baylor University Refugee Health Page
http://www.baylor.edu/~Charles_Kemp/refugee_health.htm
Bolane, J. E. (1999). *Labor and birth: Terms, techniques, problem solving.* Waco, TX: Childbirth Graphics. (Pocket glossary of labor and birth terms and interactions. Translated into Spanish, French, Tagalog, Vietnamese, Chinese, and Korean.)

Center for Cross-Cultural Health
http://www.crosshealth.com

Center for Immigration Studies
http://www.cis.org (Immigration issues)

Center for Reproductive Law and Policy
http://www.crlp.org (Global women's rights including reproductive rights)

Centers for Disease Control and Prevention
http://www.cdc.gov/epo/mmwr/international//world.html (Epidemiology International Bulletins)
http://www.cdc.ogh (Office of Global Health)
http://www.cdc.gov/spanish (Spanish website)

Central Intelligence Agency (CIA) *World Factbook*
http://www.cia/gov/cia/publications/factbook

Cross Cultural Health Care Program
http://www.xculture.org

CultureMed
http://www.suny.edu/library/culturemed/

Diversity Rx
http://www.diversityrx.org/htm/divrx.htm

EthnoMed
http://www.ethnomed.org/ (Amharic, Cambodian, Chinese, Eritrean, Ethiopian, Oromo, Somali, Tigrean, Vietnamese)

Georgetown University Child Development Center, National Center for Cultural Competence
http://www.gucdc.georgetown.edu/nccc/index.html

Immigration and Naturalization Service (INS)
http://www.ins.gov

Indian Health Services
http://www.ihs.gov

Indiana University College of Nursing Transcultural Nusing
http://www.lib.iun.indiana.edu/transnurs.htm Lipson, J. G., & Dibble, S. L. (2005). *Culture and clinical care.* San Francisco: University of California at San Francisco Nursing Press. (Not specific to perinatal nursing) Moore, M. L., & Moos, M. K. (2002). *Cultural competence in the care of childbearing families.* New York: March of Dimes. (Includes definitions of culture, cultural competence, cultural profiles)

Multicultural Mental Health Australia
http://www.atmhn.unimelb.edu.au
(Amharic, Arabic, Armenian, Bengali, Bosnian, Burmese, Cambodian, Cantonese, Chinese, Croatian, Czech, Dutch, English, Farsi, Finnish, French, German, Greek, Hebrew, Hindi, Hungarian, Indonesian, Italian, Japanese, Korean, Kurdish, Laotian, Macedonian, Malay, Maltese, Mandarin, Maori, Oromo, Pashto, Polish, Portuguese, Punjabi, Romanian, Russian, Samoan, Serbian, Serbo-Croatian, Singhalese, Slovak, Somali, Spanish, Tagalog, Tamil, Thai, Tigrinya, Tongan, Turkish, Ukrainian, Urdu, Vietnamese)

National Asian Women's Health Organization
http://www.nawho.org

National Center for Cultural Competence
http://www.guccdc.georgetown.edu/nccc/

National Institutes of Health Office of Research on Minority Health
http://www.od.nih.gov/ormh

NOAH: New York Online Access to Health
http://ww.noah-health.org (English and Spanish)

Oregon Health Sciences University Patient Education Resources for Clinicians
http://www.ohsu.edu/library

Pan American Health Organization (PAHO)
http://www.paho.org

Population Reference Bureau (PRB)
http://www.prb.org (US and international population trends)

Princeton University Office of Population Research
http://www.opr.princeton.edu/archive

RAINBO—Research, Action, and Information Network for Bodily Integrity of Women Task Force on Caring for Circumcised Women
http://www.rainbo.org

Reproductive Health Outlook
http://www.rho.org (Transcultural issues)

Safe Motherhood Initiative
http://www.safemotherhood.org

Transcultural C.A.R.E. Associates
http://www.transculturalcare.net

Transcultural Nursing Society
http://www.tcns.org/

UNICEF Statistical Data
http://www.unicef.org/statis

United States Census Bureau, International Statistical Agencies
http://www.census.gov/main/www/stat_int.html

United States Department of Health and Human Services
http://www.raceandhealth.hhs.gov

United States Department of Health and Human Services, Office of Minority Health
http://www.omhrc.gov

Utah Department of Health, Office of Ethnic Health
http://www.health.state.ut.us

World Health Organization
http://www.who.int/

World Wide Web Virtual Library Migration and Ethnic Relations
http://www.ercomer.org/wwwvl/

Journals
Cross Cultural Issues
Hispanic Health Care International
Hmong Studies Journal
Journal of Cultural Diversity
Journal of Multi-cultural Nursing
Journal of Transcultural Nursing
Western Journal of Medicine

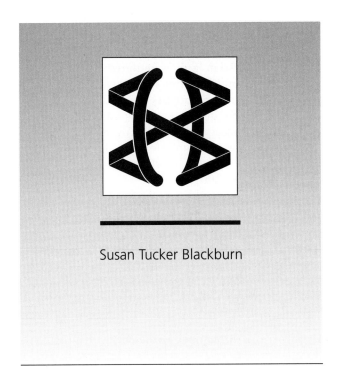

Susan Tucker Blackburn

CHAPTER **3**

Physiologic Changes of Pregnancy

THE pregnant woman experiences dramatic physiologic changes to meet the demands of the developing fetus, maintain homeostasis, and prepare for birth and lactation. Maternal adaptations during pregnancy result from the interplay of multiple factors, including the influences of reproductive and other hormones, growth factors, cytokines, and other signaling proteins, as well as mechanical pressures exerted by the growing fetus and enlarging uterus. An understanding of the normal physiologic changes of pregnancy is essential for discriminating between normal and abnormal states. Laboratory values and physical findings considered normal in the nonpregnant woman may not be normal for women during pregnancy. This chapter reviews physiologic changes during pregnancy to provide baseline information to guide the perinatal nurse in conducting an accurate and thorough assessment of the pregnant woman.

HORMONES AND OTHER MEDIATORS

Many of the physiologic changes during pregnancy are mediated by hormones. Hormones are responsible for maintaining homeostasis, regulation of growth, and development and cellular communication. They are transported by the blood from the site of production to their target cells throughout the pregnant woman's body, and are responsible for many physiologic adaptations to pregnancy. During pregnancy, the placenta serves as an endocrine gland, secreting many hormones, growth factors, and other substances. The major hormones produced by the placenta are human chorionic gonadotropin, human placental lactogen, estrogen, and progesterone. However, the placental also produces pituitary-like and gonad-like hormones (ie, placental corticotrophin, human chorionic thyrotropin, placental growth hormone), hypothalamus-like releasing hormones (ie, human chorionic somatostatin, corticotrophin-releasing hormone), gastrointestinal-like hormones (ie, gastrin, vasoactive intestinal peptide), and parathyroid hormone–related protein (PTHrP) (Blackburn, 2003). The placental hormones are critical for many of the metabolic and endocrine changes during pregnancy. For example, PTHrP mediates placental calcium transport and fetal bone growth; corticotropin-releasing hormone stimulates release of prostaglandins and has a major role in initiation of myometrial contractility and labor onset.

The placenta, membranes, and fetus also synthesize peptide growth factors such as epidermal growth factor, nerve growth factor, platelet-derived growth factor, transforming growth factor-β (TGF-β), skeletal growth factor, and insulin-like growth factor-I (IGF-I) and II (IGF-II) (Liu, 2004). These growth factors stimulate localized hormone release, regulate cell growth and differentiation, and enhance metabolic processes during pregnancy (Blackburn, 2003). For example, IGF-I and IGF-II enhance amino acid and glucose uptake and prevent protein breakdown, thus helping to regulate cell proliferation and differentiation to maintain fetal growth. TGF-β stimulates cell differentiation and is important in embryogenesis and neural migration and differentiation (Liu, 2004).

Human Chorionic Gonadotropin

Human chorionic gonadotropin (hCG) is secreted by the blastocyst (pre-embryo) and the placenta. The major function of hCG is to maintain progesterone and estrogen production by the corpus luteum until the placental function is adequate (about 10 weeks post-conception). hCG is also thought to have a role in fetal testosterone and corticosteroid production as well as immune function during pregnancy (Keay, Vatish, Karteris, Hillhouse, & Randeva, 2004). hCG is found in the blastocyst prior to implantation and is detected in maternal serum and urine around the time of implantation (7 to 8 days after ovulation) (Liu, 2004). hCG levels increase to peak about 60 to 90 days after conception, then decrease rapidly after 10 to 12 weeks (when the placental becomes the main producer of estrogens and progesterone and the corpus luteum is no longer needed) to a nadir at 100 to 130 days (Keay et al., 2004). Maternal urine pregnancy testing reads hCG levels and can declare a positive result 3 weeks after conception (about 5 weeks after the last normal menstrual period) (Moore & Persaud, 2003). hCG levels are elevated in multiple and molar pregnancies and low with ectopic pregnancy or abnormal placentation (Liu, 2004).

Human Placental Lactogen

Human placental lactogen (hPL), also known as human chorionic somatomammotropin, is produced by the syncytiotrophoblast tissues of the placenta. Maternal serum hPL levels increase parallel to placental growth and peak near term. hPL is critical to fetal growth because it alters maternal protein, carbohydrate, and fat metabolism and acts as an insulin antagonist (Liu, 2004). This hormone increases free fatty acid availability for maternal metabolic needs and decreases maternal glucose uptake and use. Thus, glucose (the major fetal energy substrate) is reserved for fetal use, and free fatty acids are used preferentially by the mother (Blackburn, 2003). This preferred breakdown of free fatty acids increases levels of ketones and the risk of ketosis with significant decreased maternal food intake.

Estrogens

Estrogens (estrone, estradiol, and estriol) are steroid hormones secreted by the ovaries during early pregnancy and the placenta for most of pregnancy. Estrogen prevents further ovarian follicular development during pregnancy. Both luteinizing hormone (LH) and follicle-stimulating hormone (FSH) are inhibited by high concentrations of progesterone in the presence of estrogen. Estrogen affects the renin-angiotensin-aldosterone system and stimulates production of hormone-binding globulins in the liver during pregnancy. It prepares the breasts for lactation, increases blood flow to the uterus, and may be involved in the timing of the onset of labor. Estrogen stimulates the growth of the uterine muscle mass. It also plays an important role in fetal development (Cunningham, Gant, & Leveno, 2001).

Estriol is the primary estrogen produced by the placenta during pregnancy. Production of estriol involves interaction of the mother, fetus, and placenta. The mother provides cholesterol and other precursors, which are metabolized by placenta. These metabolites are sent to the fetus for further processing by the fetal liver and adrenal gland to produce dehydroepiandrosterone sulfate, which is sent back to the placenta to produce estriol. Maternal serum and urinary estriol levels increase throughout pregnancy, with a rapid rise during the last 6 weeks. This late increase in estriol alters the local (uteroplacental area) ratio of estrogens to progesterone, which is a factor in the onset of labor (Cunningham et al., 2001; Challis & Lye, 2004). Maternal estriol levels were historically used as an index of fetal and placental function; however, numerous problems with interpretation have limited their usefulness.

Progesterone

Progesterone is initially produced by the corpus luteum in early pregnancy and later primarily by the placenta. Progesterone maintains decidual secretory activities required for implantation and helps to maintain myometrial relaxation by acting on uterine smooth muscle to inhibit prostaglandin production (Bagchi & Kumar, 1999). Progesterone acts on smooth muscle in other areas of the body as well, especially in the gastrointestinal and renal system; relaxes venous walls to accommodate the increase in blood volume; alters respiratory center sensitivity to carbon dioxide and aids in the development of acini and lobules of the breasts in preparation for lactation (Cunningham et al., 2001). Progesterone also mediates changes in immune function during pregnancy, which helps prevent rejection by the mother of the fetus and placenta as foreign antigens (Druckmann & Druckmann, 2005).

Relaxin

Relaxin is secreted by the corpus luteum and in small amounts by the myometrium, decidua, and placenta. Relaxin interacts with other mediators to inhibit uterine activity, thereby maintaining myometrial quiescence during pregnancy and diminishing the strength of uterine contractions. Relaxin also plays a role in cervical ripening and may help suppress oxytocin release during pregnancy (Monga & Sanborn, 2004).

Prostaglandins

Prostaglandins (PGs) are found in high concentrations in the female reproductive tract and in the decidua and fetal membranes during pregnancy. Prostaglandins are part of a family of substances called eicosanoids that are synthesized from arachidonic acid, which is present in plasma membrane phospholipids. This family includes prostaglandins, prostacyclins, thromboxanes, and leukotrienes. Eicosanoids are released quickly with plasma membrane stimulation and act near the site of release. Prostaglandins affect smooth muscle contractility. The interplay between thromboxanes and prostacyclin (PGI2) is believed to contribute to hypertensive disorders in pregnancy. PGI2 release is mediated by nitric oxide, which regulates vascular tone and is an important mediator of reduced vascular resistance and myometrial relaxation during pregnancy (Blackburn, 2003).

PGs mediate the onset of labor, myometrial contractility, and cervical ripening. Throughout most of pregnancy, myometrial PG receptors are down regulated (Lockwood, 2004). Changes in receptor responsivity and increases in PG receptors and levels of stimulatory PG near the end of pregnancy are mediated by corticotropin-releasing hormone (CRH), fetal cortisol, and uterine stretch (Hertelendy & Zakar, 2004). PGs play a critical role in labor onset via a variety of mechanisms, including formation of gap junctions (needed to transmit action potentials) and oxytocin receptors in the myometrium, increasing frequency of action potentials, stimulating myometrial contractility, and enhancing calcium availability (calcium is essential for smooth muscle contraction) (Mohan, Loudon, & Bennett, 2004). The physiologic roles of endogenous PGs have led to the use of various PGs for cervical ripening and induction of labor (Stitely & Satin, 2002).

Prolactin

Prolactin is released from the anterior pituitary. This hormone is responsible for the increase in and maturation of ducts and alveoli in the breasts and for initiation of lactation after birth. During pregnancy, there is a marked increase of prolactin secondary to the effects of angiotensin II, gonadotropin-releasing hormone, and arginine vasopressin on the pituitary. However, the high estrogen levels throughout pregnancy inhibit initiation of lactation. After birth, this inhibition quickly disappears with removal of the placenta, the major source of estrogen during pregnancy. The anterior pituitary begins to produce larger amounts of

prolactin, which stimulate the breast to begin lactation. The serum prolactin concentration begins to rise in the first trimester and by term may reach 10 times the nonpregnant concentration (Lu, 2004). After birth, prolactin levels rise rapidly, returning to prepregnancy levels by 7 to 14 days in non–breast-feeding mothers (Molitch, 2004). In lactating women, baseline prolactin levels are elevated further during sucking; the baseline decreases over the first months of lactation.

CARDIOVASCULAR SYSTEM

The cardiovascular system undergoes numerous and profound adaptations during pregnancy (Table 3–1). Cardiovascular anatomy, blood volume, cardiac output, and vascular resistance are altered to accommodate the additional maternal and fetal circulatory requirements. Increased ventricular wall muscle mass, an increased heart rate, cardiac murmurs, and dependent peripheral edema are evidence of these anatomic and functional changes. Physical symptoms may occur during pregnancy in response to normal cardiovascular changes. Some women report palpitations, lightheadedness, or decreased tolerance for activity. Cardiovascular adaptations have a significant impact on all organ systems. Women with normal cardiovascular function are generally able to accommodate the dramatic cardiovascular changes associated with pregnancy. Women with cardiovascular disease are at increased risk for complications during pregnancy, labor, or the immediate postpartum period, in part because of alterations in blood and plasma volume and cardiac output.

TABLE 3–1 ■ CARDIOVASCULAR CHANGES DURING PREGNANCY

Parameter	Change
Heart rate	Increases 15% (10–20 bpm)
Blood volume	Increases 30%–50% (1,450–1,750 mL)
Plasma volume	Increases 40%-60% (1,200–1,600 mL)
Red cell mass	Increases 20%–30% (250–450 mL)
Cardiac output	Increases 30%–50% (average 40%–45%)
Stroke volume	Increases 30%
Systemic vascular resistance	Decreases 20%
Colloid oncotic pressure	Decreases 20% (23 mm Hg)
Diastolic blood pressure	Decreases 10–15 mm Hg by 24–32 weeks

Heart

The position, appearance, and function of the heart change during pregnancy. As the growing uterus exerts pressure on the diaphragm, the heart is displaced upward, forward, and to the left, to lie in a more horizontal position. The first-trimester increase in ventricular muscle mass and the second- and early third-trimester increase in end-diastolic volume cause the heart to undergo a physiologic dilation (Gei & Hankins, 2001; Monga, 2004). The point of maximal impulse is deviated to the left at the fourth intercostal space. During the first few days postpartum, the left atrium also appears to be enlarged because of the increased blood volume that occurs with removal of the placenta.

Maternal heart rate begins to increase at 4 to 5 weeks' gestation and peaks at about 32 weeks to 10 to 20 beats/min above baseline (Caulin-Glaser & Setaro, 2004; Monga, 2004). In twin pregnancies, the maternal heart rate at term increases as much as 40% above nonpregnant rates (Cunningham et al., 2001). Heart rate and atrial size return to normal prepregnancy values in the first 10 days postpartum, whereas left ventricular size normalizes after 4 to 6 months (Cunningham et al., 2001; Monga, 2004).

Between 12 and 20 weeks, a change in heart sounds and a systolic murmur is heard in approximately 90% to 95% of pregnant women because of the increased cardiovascular load (Blanchard & Shabetal, 2004). Ninety percent of pregnant women have a wider split in the first heart sound (which also becomes louder) and an audible third heart sound. Around 30 weeks' gestation, the second heart sound also demonstrates an audible splitting. About 5% of pregnant women also have an audible fourth heart sound. Systolic murmurs are auscultated in more than 95% of pregnant women during the last two trimesters. However, systolic murmurs greater than grade 2/4 and any type of diastolic murmur are considered abnormal (Monga, 2004). Systolic murmurs can be best auscultated along the left sternal border and result from aortic and pulmonary artery blood flow (Gei & Hankins, 2001).

Blood Volume

Blood volume increases approximately 30% to 50% beginning as early as 6 weeks and peaking at 28 to 34 weeks (Monga, 2004). Blood volume then plateaus or decreases slightly to term, returning to prepregnant values by 6 to 8 weeks postpartum or sooner (Bridges, Womble, Wallace, & McCartney, 2003). The increased blood volume is necessary to provide adequate blood flow to the uterus, fetus, and maternal tissues; to maintain blood pressure; to assist with temperature regulation by increasing cutaneous blood flow; and to accommodate blood loss at birth (Blackburn, 2003). Failure of blood volume to increase is associated with altered fetal and placental growth. Blood volume is greater in multiple gestations and increases proportionally according to the number of fetuses (Monga, 2004).

Changes in blood volume are due to increases in both plasma volume and red blood cell (RBC) mass. Plasma volume increases approximately 50% (range, 40% to 60% or about 1200 to 1600 mL) by term, and red cell mass increases 20% to 30% (250 to 450 mL) (Monga, 2004). The rapid increase in plasma volume and later rise in RBC volume results in relative hemodilution. Even with increased RBC production, there is a decrease in both hemoglobin (12 to 16 g/dL) and hematocrit (37% to 47%) values during pregnancy. This decrease is more obvious during the second trimester, as blood volume peaks.

One proposed mechanism for expansion of blood volume is hormonal stimulation of plasma renin activity and aldosterone levels. Increases in the renin-angiotensin-aldosterone system stimulate renal tubular reabsorption of sodium and a subsequent increase of 6 to 8 L in total body water (extracellular and plasma fluid volume) (Blackburn, 2003). Changes in systemic vascular resistance decrease venous tone and increase the capacity of the blood vessels to accommodate the extra blood volume without overloading the maternal system.

The extra blood volume helps protect the woman from shock with the normal blood loss at birth. To prevent hemorrhage immediately after childbirth, the uterus contracts, shunting blood from uterine vessels into the systemic circulation, and causing an autotransfusion of approximately 1,000 mL. Although up to 500 mL (10%) of blood may be lost with a vaginal birth and 1,000 mL (15% to 30%) with a cesarean birth, average loss is usually less. These changes are accompanied by a postpartum diuresis that further reduces the plasma volume during the first several days postpartum. Plasma volume returns to prepregnancy levels by 6 to 8 weeks and perhaps as early as 2 to 3 weeks postpartum (Blackburn, 2003).

Cardiac Output

Cardiac output is the product of heart rate times stroke volume, both of which increase during pregnancy. Cardiac output is also influenced by blood volume, cardiac contractility, vascular resistance, and maternal position. Cardiac output increases 30% to 50% during pregnancy when measured in the left lateral recumbent position (Monga, 2004). It begins early, with approximately half of the increase occurring by 8 weeks' gestation, peaks in the second trimester, and then plateaus until term (Blanchard & Shabetal, 2004;

Bridges et al., 2003). In early pregnancy, the increase in cardiac output primarily results from an increase in stroke volume. Stroke volume increases by as early as 8 weeks, peaks at 16 to 24 weeks, and then declines to term. The increase in cardiac output results initially from the increase in both heart rate and stroke volume, but by late pregnancy is due primarily to the changes in heart rate, which continues increasing to term (Monga, 2004). Cardiac output increases are greater in multiple pregnancies, especially after 20 weeks' gestation (Blackburn, 2003).

Maternal position can greatly influence cardiac output, most dramatically during the third trimester. Cardiac output is optimized in the lateral position, somewhat decreased in the sitting position, and markedly decreased in the supine position (Tsen, Gerard, & Ostheimer, 2005). In the supine position, pressure exerted on the inferior vena cava from the gravid uterus decreases venous return and results in decreased cardiac output. This position may lead to supine hypotension with diaphoresis and possible syncope.

Cardiac output rises progressively during labor (Abbas, Lester, & Connolly, 2005). Changes in cardiac output during the intrapartum period depend on maternal position, type of anesthesia, and method of birth. During the first stage of labor, approximately 300 to 500 mL of blood are shunted from the uterus into the systemic circulation with each contraction. This results in a progressive and cumulative rise in cardiac output during the first and second stages (Abbas et al., 2005). Average increases during labor are summarized in Table 3–2. Epidural anesthesia causes a sympathectomy and a marked decrease in peripheral vascular resistance that may cause a decrease in venous return, resulting in decreased cardiac output. An intravenous fluid bolus before epidural placement may mitigate these effects.

Immediately after birth, cardiac output is 60% to 80% higher than during prelabor levels, declining rapidly after 10 to 15 minutes to stabilize at prelabor values after 1 hour (Monga, 2004). As a result of these hemodynamic changes, the intrapartum and immediate postpartum periods are times of increased vulnerability in women with cardiovascular disease. Cardiac output remains high for 24 to 48 hours after birth, and then progressively decreases and returns to nonpregnant levels by 6 to 12 weeks postpartum in most women (Resnick, 2004).

Distribution of Blood Flow

Most of the increase in blood volume during pregnancy is distributed to the uterus, kidneys, breasts, and skin. The uterus accommodates one-third of the additional blood volume at term. The kidneys receive approximately 400 mL/min. Glandular growth, distended veins, and tissue engorgement reflect the increased blood flow to the breasts, which may lead to a sensation of heat and tingling. Hyperemia of the cervix and vagina is also evident. Blood flow to the maternal skin increases to compensate for the heat loss created by fetal and placental metabolism as well as increases in maternal metabolic rate. This increased blood flow can result in alterations in nail and hair growth, increased nasal congestion, rhinitis, increased risk of nose bleeds, and sensations of warm hands and feet (Blackburn, 2003).

Blood Pressure

Maternal position during blood pressure (BP) measurement significantly affects BP values. Sitting or standing BP measurement shows minimal change in systolic blood pressure (SBP) throughout pregnancy. Diastolic blood pressure (DBP), measured while in the sitting or standing positions, gradually decreases by approximately 10 to 15 mm Hg over the first-trimester values, with lowest values seen at 24 to 32 weeks followed by a gradual increase toward nonpregnant baseline values by term (Monga, 2004). DBP measurements can vary as by much as 15 mm Hg depending on the measurement method: a mercury cuff with Korotkoff sounds assessed with a stethoscope, intraarterial catheters, or automated BP devices (Blackburn, 2003). Accurate comparison of BP values depends on consistent techniques of measurement and consistent maternal positioning. Changes in BP are thought to be related to the vasodilatory effects of nitric oxide, prostacyclin, and relaxin that mediate a decrease in systemic vascular resistance (Monga).

Systemic Vascular Resistance

Systemic vascular resistance (SVR) decreases by about 20%. Changes in SVR are related to the increased capacity of the uteroplacental blood vessels, progesterone, nitric oxide, and prostacyclin. The uteroplacental vascular system is a low-resistance network that accommodates a large percentage of maternal cardiac output. Progesterone and PGs relax smooth muscle

TABLE 3–2 ■ INCREASES IN OUTPUT DURING LABOR AND BIRTH

Labor Phase or Stage	Increase Above Prelabor Values
Latent phase	15%
Active phase	30%
Second stage	45%
Immediately after birth	65%

and produce vasodilation. Uterine vascular resistance also decreases during pregnancy and enhances uterine blood flow. SVR decreases by 5 weeks' gestation, is lowest at 16 to 34 weeks' gestation, and gradually increases by term, when the mean SVR may approximate nonpregnant values (Bridges et al., 2003; Monga, 2004).

HEMATOLOGIC CHANGES

To meet additional oxygen requirements of pregnancy, RBC volume increases approximately 17% to 33% (Duffy, 2004). However because plasma volume increases to a greater degree than the erythrocyte volume, the hematocrit decreases approximately 3% to 5%. This decrease is most obvious during the second trimester, after blood volume peaks.

Hemoglobin levels during pregnancy are between 12 and 16 g/dL. With the increase in the number of RBCs, the need for iron for the production of hemoglobin also increases. Serum ferritin levels decrease, with the greatest decline seen at 12 to 25 weeks (Allen, 2000). Approximately 500 mg of iron is needed for the increases in maternal RBCs, 270 mg by the fetus and 90 mg by the placenta. Total iron needs during pregnancy, including replacement of losses are estimated at 1 g (Lynch, 2000). Iron needs increases from 0.8 g/day in early pregnancy to 7.5 mg/day by term (Milman, Bergholt, Byg, Eriksen, & Graudal, 1999).

Gastrointestinal absorption of iron is increased during pregnancy, but additional iron supplementation is nonetheless necessary for most women to maintain maternal iron stores. If iron stores are initially low and supplemental iron is not added to enhance the diet, iron deficiency anemia may result (Allen, 2000, Milman et al., 1999). There is controversy surrounding the efficacy and benefit of prophylactic oral iron supplementation during pregnancy (Beard, 2000; Milman et al., 1999). Thus, supplementation may not be needed to prevent iron deficiency anemia in a woman who has good iron stores prior to pregnancy and a diet during pregnancy that is high in bioavailable iron. However, the majority of women of childbearing age have marginal iron stores (an average of 300 mg of stored iron estimated in most women in the United States at the beginning of pregnancy) (Lynch, 2000). Iron supplementation does not prevent the normal fall in hemoglobin (due to hemodilution), but can prevent depletion of stores and onset of iron-deficiency anemia (Institute of Medicine, 1990).

Leukocyte (especially neutrophil) production also increases in pregnancy. The average white blood cell (WBC) count in the third trimester is 5,000 to 12,000/mm^3 (Kilpatrick & Laros, 2004). Labor and early postpartum levels may reach 20,000 to 30,000/mm^3 without an infection. The increase in WBC count begins during the second month, and the level returns to the normal range for nonpregnant women by 6 days postpartum. Slight increases in eosinophil levels and slight decreases in basophil levels have also been reported (Kilpatrick & Laros, 1999). Platelet counts range between 150,000/mm^3 and 400,000/mm^3, with perhaps a slight decrease in the third trimester (Bremme, 2003).

Plasma proteins and other components are also altered during pregnancy. Serum electrolytes and osmolality decrease. Serum lipids, especially cholesterol (needed for steroid hormone synthesis) and phospholipids (needed for cell membranes) increase 40% to 60%. Total plasma protein decreases 10% to 14% due primarily to hemodilution, but with both absolute and relative decreases in serum albumin. This leads to decreased serum oncotic pressure that contributes to the dependent edema seen in many pregnant women. The decrease in albumin also results in less bound and increases in the free fraction of substances such as calcium and some drugs (Blackburn, 2003).

Coagulation and fibrinolytic systems undergo significant changes during pregnancy. Pregnancy is considered a hypercoagulable state because of increased levels of many coagulation factors and a decrease in factors such as protein S that inhibit coagulation. The most marked increases occur in factors I (fibrinogen), VII, VIII, X, and von Willebrand factor (vWF) antigen (Bremme, 2003; Hellgren, 2003). These changes are partially balanced by alterations in the plasminogen system that enhances clot lysis. Prothrombin time (PT) and activated partial thromboplastin time (aPTT) decrease slightly as the pregnancy comes to term; however, bleeding time and clotting time remain unchanged despite the increase in clotting factors (Bremme, 2003). Table 3–3 summarizes the changes in clotting factors during pregnancy. The net effect of these alterations places pregnant women at increased risk for thrombus formation and consumptive coagulopathies. After birth, coagulation is initiated to prevent hemorrhage at the placental site. Fibrinogen and platelet counts decrease as platelet plugs and fibrin clots form to provide hemostasis.

RESPIRATORY SYSTEM

Changes in the respiratory system are essential to accommodate increased maternal–fetal requirements and to ensure adequate gas exchange to meet maternal and fetal metabolic needs. The respiratory system must provide an increased amount of oxygen and efficiently remove carbon dioxide. Changes in the respiratory system are due to primarily to a combination of mechanical forces (eg, the enlarging uterus) and biochemical

TABLE 3–3 ■ CLOTTING FACTORS DURING PREGNANCY	
Parameter	Change
Fibrin	Increases 40% at term
Plasma fibrinogen	Increases 50%, 300–600 mg/dL
Coagulation factors I, VII, VIII, X, XII	Increases markedly
von Willebrand factor antigen	Increased markedly
Coagulation factor XI	Decreases 60%–70%
Coagulation XIII	Decreases slightly
Coagulation factors II, V	Increased slightly or unchanged
Protein S (anticoagulant) activity	Decreased
Clotting and bleeding time	Unchanged
Prothrombin time	Increases slightly or unchanged
Partial plasma thromboplastin time	Increases slightly or unchanged
Fibrin degradation products	Increased (D-Dimer increased)
Platelets	Unchanged, 150,000–500,000/mm^3

TABLE 3–4 ■ RESPIRATORY CHANGES DURING PREGNANCY	
Parameter	Change
Tidal volume	Increases 30%–40% (500–700 mL)
Vital capacity	Unchanged
Inspiratory reserve volume	Unchanged
Expiratory reserve volume	Decreases 20%
Respiratory rate	Unchanged or slight increase
Functional residual capacity	Decreases 18%–20%
Total lung volume	Decreases 5%
Residual volume	Decreases 20%
Minute ventilation	Increases 40%
pH	Slight increase to 7.40–7.45
PaO2 (first trimester)	106–108 mm Hg
PaO2 (by term)	101–104 mm Hg
PaCO2	27–32 mm Hg
Bicarbonate	18–21 mEq/L (base deficit of −3 to −4 mEq/L)

effects, especially the effects of progesterone and prostaglandins on the respiratory center and bronchial smooth muscle. Table 3–4 summarizes the changes in respiratory function during pregnancy.

Structural Changes

Pressure from the uterus shifts the diaphragm upward approximately 4 cm, decreasing the length of the lungs. To adjust to this decreased length, the anterioposterior diameter of the chest enlarges by 2 cm. Increased pressure from the uterus widens the substernal angle 50%, from 68 to 103 degrees, and causes the ribs to flare out slightly (Whitty & Dombrowsky, 2004). The circumference of the thoracic cage may increase 5 to 7 cm, compensating for the decreased lung length (Harvey, 1999). Many of these changes are probably caused by hormonal influence, because they occur before pressure is exerted from the growing uterus. Despite the mechanical elevation of the diaphragm in pregnancy, most of the work of breathing remains diaphragmatic.

Lung Volume

Lung volumes are altered during pregnancy. Total lung volume (ie, the amount of air in lungs at maximal inspiration) decreases slightly (5%). Residual volume (ie, the amount of air in lungs after maximum expira-

tion), expiratory reserve volume (ie, the maximal amount of air that can be expired from the resting expiratory level), and functional residual capacity (ie, the amount of air remaining in the lungs at resting expiratory level, permitting air for gas exchange between breaths) fall by about 18% to 20% (Whitty & Dombrowsky, 2004). Tidal volume (ie, the amount of air inspired and expired with normal breath), increases 30% to 40% (500 to 700 mL/min) during pregnancy and compensates for decreases in expiratory reserve volume and residual volume. Vital capacity (ie, the maximum amount of air that can be forcibly expired after maximum inspiration) and inspiratory reserve volume (ie, the maximum amount of air that can be inspired at end of normal inspiration) remain unchanged (Blackburn, 2003). The net effect of these lung volume changes is that there is no change in maximum breathing capacity during pregnancy. Spirometric measurements used for the diagnosis of respiratory problems do not change and remain useful evaluation tools.

Ventilation

Alveolar ventilation increases by 50% to 70% (Mandel & Weinberger, 2004). Minute ventilation (ie, amount of air inspired in 1 minute) increases during the first trimester and reaches 6.5 to 10 L/min at term. Minute ventilation is the product of the respiratory rate and the tidal volume. The increase in minute ventilation is caused by an increase in tidal volume, because the respiratory rate remains unchanged or increases only slightly (Blackburn, 2003). Progesterone stimulates ventilation by lowering the carbon dioxide threshold of the respiratory center and may also act as a primary stimulant to the respiratory center, independent of carbon dioxide sensitivity and threshold. For example, in the nonpregnant woman, an increase of 1 mm Hg in $PaCO_2$ increases minute ventilation by 1.5 L/min, whereas in pregnancy this same change in $PaCO_2$ results in a 6 L/min change in minute ventilation (Whitty & Dombrowsky, 2004).

Oxygen and Carbon Dioxide Exchange

Oxygen consumption increases to approximately 50 mL/min at term to meet increasing oxygen demand in maternal, placental, and fetal tissues. Further increases of 40% to 60% occur during labor (Whitty & Dombrowsky, 2004). The increased oxygen demand during pregnancy is met by the increases in minute ventilation and cardiac output. Increased minute ventilation increases arterial partial pressures of oxygen (PaO_2) and decreases alveolar carbon dioxide tension.

The PaO_2 during pregnancy is mildly elevated to between 106 to 108 mm Hg during the first trimester and 101 to 104 mm Hg at term (Mandel & Weinberger, 2004). $PaCO_2$ is decreased to between 27 and 32 mm Hg (Thornberg, Jacobson, Giraud, & Morton, 2000). The decrease in $PaCO_2$ is accompanied by a fall in plasma bicarbonate concentration to 18 to 21 mEq/L (base deficit of -3 to -4 mEq/L). Decreased carbon dioxide levels in the blood lead to higher pH values that are compensated for by renal excretion of bicarbonate, and the woman maintains a normal pH in the range of 7.40 to 7.45. The result of these changes is mildly elevated PaO_2 and decreased $PaCO_2$ and serum bicarbonate levels compared with normal values for nonpregnant women (Blackburn, 2003). Thus, the acid-base status during pregnancy is that of a compensated respiratory alkalosis.

Up to 60% to 70% of pregnant women experience dyspnea (Mandel & Weinberger, 2004). The exact cause of this dyspnea is unclear, but it may be due to the woman's sensation of hyperventilation, effects of progesterone, increased oxygen consumption, and decreased $PaCO_2$ levels. Mechanical forces from pressure of the uterus on the diaphragm may increase the sensation of dyspnea, but these forces are not the primary cause, because dyspnea usually begins during the first or second trimester. Symptoms of nasal stuffiness, rhinitis, and nose bleeds are also more common for pregnant women and are related to vascular congestion resulting from increased levels of estrogen (Blackburn, 2003). The respiratory system rapidly returns to the prepregnant status within 1 to 3 weeks after birth.

RENAL SYSTEM

The renal system undergoes structural and functional changes during pregnancy. Changes in renal function accommodate the increased metabolic and circulatory requirements of pregnancy. The renal system excretes maternal and fetal waste products. Pressure placed on the renal system and the relaxant effects of progesterone on vascular tissue enhance the ability of the renal system to accommodate the cardiovascular changes of pregnancy.

Structural Changes

Increased renal blood flow, interstitial volumes, and hormonal influences increase renal volume by 30% and lengthen the kidneys by 1 to 1.5 cm (Chaliha & Stanton, 2002). The relaxing effects of progesterone on smooth muscle are probably primarily responsible for the dilation of the renal calyces, pelvis, and ureters (Blackburn, 2003). This muscular relaxation, coupled with increased urine volume and stasis, is associated with an increased risk of urinary tract infection.

During late gestation, the growing uterus and the dilated ovarian vein plexus place pressure on and displace the ureters and bladder. The ureters become dilated, elongated, and more tortuous, primarily in portions above the pelvic rim. The urethra also lengthens. Dilation of the ureters on the right side is more pronounced than that on the left because of the cushioning that occurs on the left side and dextrarotation of the uterus by the sigmoid colon. The right ovarian vein crosses the pelvic brim, and therefore experiences greater compression by the growing uterus than the left ovarian vein, which parallels the brim. About 80% of pregnant women experience physiologic hydronephrosis and hydroureter of pregnancy (Monga, 2004).

During the second trimester, hyperemia of pelvic organs, hyperplasia of all muscles and connective tissues, and the gravid uterus elevate the bladder trigone and cause thickening of the interuretic margin (Chaliha & Stanton, 2002). The bladder is displaced forward and upward in late pregnancy. Mechanical pressure placed on the bladder by the gravid uterus changes it from a convex to a concave organ. Urine output is increased primarily due to changes in sodium excretion. Urinary frequency (>7 daytime voidings) is reported in about 60% of pregnant women, with an increased incidence of stress and urge incontinence (Chaliha & Stanton, 2002; Thorp, Norton, Wall, Kuller, Eucker, & Wells, 1999). These changes regress after birth in most women. Nocturia is due to increased sodium and therefore water excretion, mediated by the effects of the lateral position, which decrease stasis and increase venous return renal blood flow and glomerular filtration rate (Blackburn, 2003).

Pressure on the renal system can impair drainage of blood and lymph and impede urine flow, which increases risk of infection and trauma during pregnancy. Renal volumes normalize with the first week after birth. However, hydronephrosis and hydroureter may take 3 to 4 months to return to normal (Monga, 2004).

Renal Blood Flow, Glomerular Filtration, and Tubular Function

Renal plasma flow (RPF) increases 60% to 80% by the end of the first trimester because of increased blood volume and cardiac output and the lowered systemic vascular resistance caused by progesterone. RPF then progressively decreases by term to a level 50% greater than nonpregnant values (Monga, 2004). Women lying in the supine position can have decreased RPF in late pregnancy, compared with values obtained while in lateral positions. The glomerular filtration rate (GFR) begins to rise after 6 weeks of gestation and peaks by the end of the first trimester, at 40% to 50% greater than nonpregnant levels or at an average of 110 to 180 mL/min (Thornberg et al., 2000). This rise in GFR probably results from vasodilation of preglomerular and postglomerular resistance vessels without any alteration in glomerular capillary pressure (Monga, 2004).

The filtered load of many substances exceeds the tubular reabsorptive capacity. As a result, renal clearance of many substances is elevated during pregnancy, with increased excretion and a related decrease in serum levels of some substances (Table 3–5). Amino acids, glucose, many electrolytes, and water-soluble vitamins are excreted in amounts higher than in nonpregnant women. Calcium excretion increases, but is balanced by increased intestinal absorption. Serum potassium values are influenced by both elevated plasma aldosterone levels, which promotes potassium excretion, and by progesterone, which promotes potassium retention (Monga, 2004). The net change favors potassium retention, with a net retention of 300 to 350 mEq/L. Because the extra potassium is used by maternal and fetal tissues, serum potassium is only slightly changed.

Serum urea and creatinine levels decline because of increased GFR. Blood urea nitrogen levels fall 25%. Serum uric acid levels decrease in early pregnancy and rise after 24 weeks. As a result, normal lab values during pregnancy and critical values indicating abnormality may be altered (Table 3–5). Examples of critical values indicative of abnormal renal function during pregnancy include plasma creatinine >0.8 mg/dL, blood urea nitrogen >14 mg/dL, and urinary protein >300 mg/dl (Blackburn, 2003).

Fluid and Electrolyte Balance

The kidneys play a significant role in the regulation of body sodium and water content. Renal sodium is the primary determinant of volume homeostasis. The filtered load of sodium increases from nonpregnant levels of 20,000 mEq/day to approximately 30,000 mEq/day during pregnancy (Monga, 2004). Sodium balance is mediated by factors that promote sodium

TABLE 3–5 ■ LABORATORY MEAN VALUES DURING PREGNANCY: RENAL FUNCTION

	Nonpregnant	Pregnant
Blood		
Serum creatinine	0.6–1.2 mg/dL	Decreases to: First trimester—0.73 mg/dL Second trimester—0.58 mg/dL Third trimester—0.53 mg/dL
Blood urea nitrogen	8–20 mg/dL	Decreases to: First trimester—11 mg/dL Second trimester—9 mg/dL Third trimester—10 mg/dL
Uric acid	4.5–5.8 mg/dL	Decreases to: First trimester—3.1 mg/dL Second trimester—2.0–3.0 mg/dL Increases to: Term—4.5–5.8 mg/dL
Urine		
Creatinine clearance	90–130 mL/min/1.73 m^2	Increases to 150–200 mL/min/1.73 m^2
Urea		Increases
Uric acid	250–750 mg/24 hr	Increases
Glucose	60–115 mg/dL	Increases

excretion versus those that promote sodium retention. Factors promoting sodium excretion during pregnancy include increased GFR, increased atrial natriuretic factor, decreased plasma albumin, elevated progesterone and prostaglandin levels, and decreased vascular resistance. The physiologic changes that cause excretion of sodium are accompanied by increases in tubular reabsorption of sodium to avoid sodium depletion. Increases in aldosterone, estrogen, and cortisol all contribute to sodium reabsorption (Blackburn, 2003). The end result favors sodium retention, with a net retention of 950 mg of sodium or an additional 2 to 6 mEq of sodium reabsorbed each day for fetal and maternal stores.

Sodium retention (and thus water retention, because as sodium is reabsorbed from the tubule back into the blood, it pulls water with it) is mediated by the changes in the renin-angiotensin-aldosterone system. Aldosterone acts on the distal tubule and cortical collecting ducts to enhance sodium reabsorption. Aldosterone release is controlled by a specialized region of the kidney, which secretes the peptide hormone renin in response to decreases in blood pressure, or sodium contents of the renal tubules, and stimulation of the sympathetic nervous system. Renin converts angiotensinogen to angiotensin I. Angiotensin I is cleaved in the lungs by angiotensin-converting enzyme (ACE) to form angiotensin II. Angiotensin II is a potent stimulator of aldosterone secretion and a potent vasopressor. Angiotensinogen, plasma renin activity, plasma renin, angiotensin II, and aldosterone levels are all increased in pregnancy (Shah, 2005).

During pregnancy, renin is produced by the uterus, placenta, and fetus as well as the kidney. Release is stimulated by estrogen, changes in blood pressure, prostaglandins, and progesterone (an aldosterone antagonist). Increased plasma levels of aldosterone promote water and sodium retention, which results in the natural volume-overload state of pregnancy. Despite the elevated levels of angiotensin II, blood pressure is not elevated in normal pregnancy due to a 60% decrease in sensitivity of the blood vessels to the vasoconstrictor effects of angiotensin II. This decreased sensitivity is thought to be due to decreased responsiveness of angiotensin II receptors and the relaxant effects of vasodilatory prostaglandins and endothelial factors such as nitric oxide. Women with preeclampsia do not maintain this reduced sensitivity to angiotensin II, and blood pressure rises (Shah, 2005). In healthy pregnant women, the net effect of these changes is the establishment of a new equilibrium that the women sense as normal. From this new baseline, she responds to changes in fluid and electrolytes in a manner similar to a nonpregnant woman (Blackburn, 2003).

Glycosuria

During pregnancy, the amount of glucose that is filtered by the kidneys increases 10- to 100-fold due to the increased RPF and GFR. The renal tubules increase reabsorption of glucose from the tubules back into the blood, but are unable to match the dramatic increase in filtered glucose. The glucose that cannot be absorbed is lost in the urine; therefore, glycosuria is common. The glucose tolerance test is normal with most pregnant women with glycosuria, suggesting that this glycosuria is secondary to altered renal function and not abnormal carbohydrate metabolism (Blackburn, 2003). Clinical management of the woman with diabetes requires serum glucose evaluation rather than urine glucose evaluation during pregnancy.

Proteinuria

Protein excretion is also increased during pregnancy because the increased filtered load of protein exceeds the tubular reabsorptive capacity. Thus, urinary protein measurements should not be considered abnormal until 24-hour urine values greater than 300 mg are reached. Levels higher than 300 mg/24 hours may indicate renal disease, preeclampsia, or urinary tract infection (Monga, 2004).

GASTROINTESTINAL SYSTEM

Nutritional requirements during pregnancy increase, and changes in the gastrointestinal (GI) system meet these demands. The GI tract is altered physiologically and anatomically during pregnancy. Many of the common discomforts of pregnancy (eg, heartburn, gingivitis, constipation, nausea, and vomiting) can be attributed to the GI system. Pregnancy is associated with increased appetite and consumption of food. Many women experience food cravings and avoidances, sometimes mediated by alterations in sensitivity to taste and smell.

Mouth and Esophagus

Thirty percent to 80% of pregnant women experience gingival edema and hyperemia (Muallem & Rubeiz, 2006). This usually begins in the second month and peaks in the third trimester. Gingival changers are probably related to increased vascularity and blood flow, changes in connective tissue, and the release of inflammatory mediators. Tooth enamel is not altered, but increases in dental plaques and calculus have been reported (Barak, Oettinger-Barak, Oettinger, Machtei, Peled, & Ohel, 2003). Existing periodontal disease may be exacerbated by pregnancy, and associations between periodontal disease and preterm birth and low birth weight have been reported in some studies (Xiong, Buekens, Fraser, Beck, & Offenbacher, 2006). Three percent to 5% of women develop an angiogranuloma (epulis) between their upper, anterior maxillary teeth. Epulis regresses postpartum, but may recur with subsequent pregnancies (Barak et al., 2003; Laine, 2002).

Lower esophageal sphincter (LES) muscle tone and pressure decrease due to the effects of progesterone. LES function is further altered after the uterus is large enough to change the positioning of the stomach and intestines and to move the LES into the thorax (Richter, 2005). These changes increase the risk of reflux and heartburn.

Nausea and Vomiting

Nausea and vomiting of pregnancy (NVP) affect 70% to 80% of pregnant women in Western cultures. The exact mechanism for NVP is unclear. "Many theories have been proposed, focusing on mechanical, endocrinologic, allergic, metabolic, genetic, and psychosomatic etiologies, but none have substantial research support" (Blackburn, 2003). The most frequent hormones linked with NVP are estrogens and especially hCG, whose secretion patterns parallel the appearance and disappearance of NVP in most women. Many studies have examined this link; however, data are inconsistent and inconclusive (Goodwin, 2002). NVP usually begins between 4 and 6 weeks and peaks at 8 to 12 weeks, but may begin earlier or last longer in some women (Bryer, 2005). Treatment is supportive and involves suggesting that the woman avoid foods that trigger nausea and to eat frequent, small meals. Ginger has been reported to be effective in reducing nausea (Bryer, 2005). Hyperemesis gravidarum is a more severe and persistent form of nausea and vomiting and is associated with weight loss, electrolyte imbalance, ketosis, and dehydration. Any underlying illness should be excluded; hospitalization for fluid and electrolyte replacement may be necessary.

Stomach

Progesterone decreases stomach gastric smooth muscle tone and motility, while the gravid uterus displaces the stomach. Gastric emptying is probably unchanged in early pregnancy, but may be delayed with a tendency toward reverse peristalsis later in gestation. Relaxation of the lower esophageal sphincter permits reflux of gastric contents into the esophagus, causing heartburn. Gastric reflux is more common later in pregnancy. A decrease in hydrochloric acid production during the first two trimesters reduces symptoms in women with peptic ulcer (Cunningham, 1998).

Small and Large Intestines

The intestines are pushed upward and laterally. The appendix is displaced superiorly, reaching the right costal margin by term, which, along with milder guarding and rebound tenderness due to cushioning by the uterus, may delay diagnosis of appendicitis during pregnancy. Increased progesterone levels relax gastrointestinal tract tone and decrease intestinal motility, allowing time for increased absorption from the colon. Increased height of the duodenal villi and activity of brush border enzymes also increase nutrient absorptive capacity (Scott, 2004). As a result, absorption of substances such as calcium, amino acids, iron, glucose, sodium, chloride, and water are increased. Reduced motility, mechanical obstruction by the uterus, and increased water absorption from the colon increase the risk of constipation. Hemorrhoids may develop when there is straining during bowel movements related to constipation, and from the increased pressure exerted on the vessels below the level of the uterus.

Liver

Liver size and morphology do not significantly change during pregnancy, but liver production of many proteins is altered due to the effects of estrogen. Hepatic blood flow increases during pregnancy, but the percentage of circulating blood volume reaching the liver remains unchanged. Some tests of liver function during pregnancy produce values that would suggest hepatic disease in nonpregnant women. For example, fibrinogen levels increase by 50% by the end of the second trimester. Plasma albumin concentration decreases, which in nonpregnant patients could indicate liver disease. Serum alkaline phosphatase activity and serum cholesterol concentration can be twice the normal range or even higher in multiple gestations (Blackburn, 2003). On the other hand, serum bilirubin, aspartate aminotransferase (AST), and alanine aminotransferase (ALT) are unchanged in normal pregnancy and therefore can be used to evaluate liver function during pregnancy (Table 3–6).

Gallbladder

Gallbladder size and function are altered during pregnancy. Elevated progesterone levels cause the gallbladder to be hypotonic and distended. Gallbladder smooth muscle contraction is impaired and may lead to stasis. Emptying time is slow after 14 weeks' gestation. In the second and third trimesters, fasting and residual volumes are twice as large as in the nonpregnant woman. As a result of these changes, cholesterol may be sequestered in the gall bladder, increasing the risk of gall stones (Blackburn, 2003).

TABLE 3–6 ■ LIVER FUNCTION DURING PREGNANCY

Parameter	Normal Range	Change
Increased		
Alkaline phosphate		Progressive to 2 to 4 times greater by term
Fibrinogen		50% by second trimester
		Progressive to term
Globulins, alpha and beta		Progressive to term
Lipids		Progressive to term
Decreased		
Albumin		20% during first trimester
Globulins, gamma		Minor or unchanged
Unchanged		
Bilirubin	0.1–1.2 mg/dL	
Aspartate aminotransferase (ASAT [SGOT])	0–35 U/L	No change; may be lower than nonpregnant reference levels
Alanine aminotransferase (ALT [SGPT])	0–35 U/L	No change; may be lower than nonpregnant reference levels
5-Nucleotidase		
Prothrombin time	11–15 seconds	Unchanged or slight increase

Weight Gain

Prenatal care, socioeconomic factors, and adequate nutrition influence pregnancy outcome. Women who are underweight before conception and women who have inadequate weight gain during pregnancy are at greater risk for having a low-birth-weight infant. The risk is greatest for women with both factors (Abrams, Minassian, & Pickett, 1999). Maternal obesity and excessive weight gain during pregnancy have been associated with fetal macrosomia (Abrams et al., 2004). A nutritional assessment should be made at the initial prenatal visit, with referral to a registered dietitian as needed. Table 3–7 summarizes the approximate weight gain distribution that occurs during pregnancy.

The woman's prepregnancy height and weight determine her actual caloric intake needs. On average, the increased demands of pregnancy require an additional 300 kcal each day. Women who are pregnant with twins or higher-order multiples need an additional 300 kcal per fetus each day. There are differences in suggested weight gain based on prepregnancy weight and body mass index. Women who are underweight before pregnancy are encouraged to gain more weight than women who are overweight before conception. Recommended weight gain is 28 to 40 pounds for underweight women, 25 to 35 pounds for normal-weight women, and 15 to 25 pounds for overweight women (Institute of Medicine, 1990).

METABOLIC CHANGES

Profound metabolic changes occur throughout pregnancy to provide for the development and growth of the fetus. Adequate maternal weight gain and changes in maternal glucose, protein, and fat metabolism are important factors in normal fetal growth and development. During the course of pregnancy, approximately 3.5 kg of fat is deposited, approximately 30,000 kcal of energy is stored, and 900 g of new protein is synthesized to meet maternal and fetal needs (Blackburn, 2003). Estrogens, progesterone, and hPL influence metabolic processes during pregnancy by altering glucose utilization, fat metabolism and use, protein homeostasis, and insulin action. These changes meet fetal growth needs by increasing the availability of glucose and amino acid for transfer to the fetus, while providing increased availability of fatty acids as an

TABLE 3–7 ■ WEIGHT INCREASE DISTRIBUTION DURING PREGNANCY

Source	Pounds
Fetus, placenta, amniotic fluid	11
Uterus, breasts	2
Blood volume	4
Maternal stores	5
Tissue, fluid	3

alternative energy substrate to meet maternal needs and maintain homeostasis (Blackburn, 2003). "The changes in carbohydrate and lipid metabolism parallel the energy needs of the mother and fetus, whereas the changes in maternal nitrogen and protein metabolism occur early in pregnancy, before fetal demand" (Blackburn, 2003). Pregnancy can be divided into two metabolic phases: an initial anabolism dominant phase and a later catabolism predominant phase.

During the first part of pregnancy, anabolism is prominent with nutrient uptake, energy stored as fat, and maternal weight gain. Estrogen stimulates pancreatic beta cell hypertrophy and hyperplasia with increased insulin production. During this phase, insulin sensitivity is not significantly affected, and insulin increases in response to the influx of glucose from the GI track after a meal (Kenshole, 2004). The increased insulin promotes storage of glucose as glycogen increased fat synthesis, storage of triglycerides and fat, fat cell hypertrophy, and inhibition of lipolysis. Both low-density and high-density lipoproteins increase (Herrera, 2000). Maternal protein storage increases, with a net retention of 1.3 g/day of nitrogen for use both by the mother and the fetus (King, 2000).

As pregnancy progresses, the maternal metabolic status becomes more catabolic, and maternal weight gain is due primarily to fetal growth. Adipose tissue lipolytic activity is enhanced, and plasma free fatty acids, glycerol, and ketones increase (Herrera, 2000). These provide alternate energy sources for maternal needs, conserving glucose for transfer to the fetus (the fetus is an obligatory glucose user whose enzyme systems promote fat storage, and who cannot readily breakdown fat to use for energy). During this phase, maternal urinary nitrogen excretion decreases, conserving protein for fetal transfer. Maternal hyperinsulinemia increases as insulin resistance in the peripheral tissues becomes prominent (Blackburn, 2003).

Insulin antagonism is caused by hPL and other placental hormones (ie, progesterone, estrogen, cortisol, and prolactin) that oppose the action of insulin and promote maternal lipolysis (Butte, 2000). Insulin normally helps to clear glucose from the blood and promotes glycogen and fat storage. Insulin resistance (mean insulin sensitivity decreases 50% to 70%) means that maternal glucose levels remain higher for a longer period of time after a meal to promote fetal transfer (Kenshole, 2004). Thus, decreased sensitivity to insulin in the liver and peripheral tissues leads to a persistent relative hyperglycemia after meals. This relative hyperinsulinemia and hyperglycemia of pregnancy has been referred to as a diabetogenic state.

Maternal metabolic responses alter responses on glucose tolerance tests so that these tests need to be interpreted using pregnancy-specific norms. These changes, in comparison to a nonpregnant individual, include (1) a lower initial fasting blood glucose value (due to decreased glucose utilization and increased fat utilization enhancing glucose availability for the fetus) and (2) elevated blood glucose for a longer period of time after ingestion of carbohydrates (due to insulin antagonism and decreased insulin sensitivity) (Kenshole, 2004; Moore, 2004).

ENDOCRINE SYSTEM

Thyroid Gland

The production, circulation, and disposal of thyroid hormone are altered in pregnancy to support maternal metabolic changes and fetal growth and development. Increased vascularity and hyperplasia of the thyroid gland result in increased hormone production and an increase in thyroid size, although not in the form of a goiter in populations with adequate iodine intake (Lazarus, 2005). Most of the changes in the thyroid gland occur during the first half of pregnancy and lead to a state of "euthyroid hyperthyroxinemia," in which levels of thyroxine (T4) are elevated. These changes are due to estrogen (increasing thyroxine-binding globulin [TBG] production by the liver), hCG, and increased urinary iodide excretion (Golden & Burrow, 2004). Human chorionic gonadotropin, which has mild thyroid-stimulating-like activity, stimulates production of T4 and triiodothyronine (T3).

Total T4 and T3 increase and peak by 10 to 15 weeks and remain 40% to 100% higher to term (Fantz, Dagogo-Jack, Ladenson, & Gronowski, 1999). Free T4 and T3 increase during the first trimester, but decrease during the second and third trimesters as levels of thyroxine binding globulin increase. Thus, more T3 andT4 are produced (increased total), but because much of the extra thyroid hormone is bound to TBG, the amount of free hormone is reduced. Serum protein-bound iodine increases. Increased production of thyroid hormone increases thyroid iodine uptake. At the same time, urinary iodide excretion increases and iodide is sent to the fetus, leading to a smaller iodine pool. These changes are partially compensated for by increased thyroid clearance and recycling of iodide; however, maternal iodide needs increase during pregnancy (Glinoer, 2004).

Maternal thyroid hormone is critical for fetal central nervous system (CNS) development, especially in early pregnancy, when the CNS undergoes critical development prior to the time the fetus is able to produce T4 (Morreale-de-Escobar, Obregon, & Escobar del Rey, 2004). Untreated maternal hypothyroidism increases the risk of pregnancy loss and altered fetal brain development and later mental retardation.

Iodine supplementation has been found to decrease the incidence of these complications in populations with high endemic levels of hypothyroidism (Mahomed & Gulmezoglu, 2000).

Transient hyperthyroidism is seen during the first trimester in about 15% of healthy pregnant women (Fantz et al., 1999). The incidence of chronic hyperthyroidism in pregnant women is 0.1% to 0.4%. Diagnosis of hyperthyroidism during pregnancy is challenging because normal signs of symptoms of pregnancy, including heat intolerance, tachycardia, wide pulse pressure, and vomiting, mimic hyperthyroidism (LeBeau & Mandel, 2006). Poor control during pregnancy can result in preterm labor, fetal loss, or thyroid crisis in these women. Diagnosis of abnormal thyroid function in the pregnant woman requires an understanding of the normal changes in thyroid function during pregnancy in order to appropriately interpret results of laboratory tests.

Transient postpartum thyroid disorder (PPTD) is seen in 6% to 9% of postpartum women and is thought to have an autoimmune basis. PPTD is usually characterized by a period (average, 2 to 4 months) of mild hyperthyroidism, followed by a period of hypothyroidism, with a return to normal thyroid function in most women by 12 months postpartum. Some women only experience one of these phases. Up to one-fourth of these women develop permanent hypothyroidism within 5 to 15 years (Stagnaro-Green, 2004).

Pituitary Gland

The anterior pituitary enlarges, with a 30% increase in weight and 2-fold increase in volume, and becomes more convex and dome-shaped (Foyouzi, Frisbaek, & Norwitz, 2004). These changes are primarily due to an increase in the group of cells that produce prolactin. Adrenocoricotropin (ACTH) secretion and serum levels increase, peaking during the intrapartum period (Foyouzi et al., 2004). This increase is probably due primarily to stimulation by increased placental, rather than hypothalamic CRH. Pituitary growth hormone secretion is suppressed by placental growth hormone, which increases from 15 to 20 weeks to term (Molitch, 2006). FSH (stimulates ovum follicle growth) and LH (needed for ovulation) are both inhibited during pregnancy.

The posterior pituitary hormones are oxytocin and arginine vasopressin (AVP). Oxytocin influences contractility of the uterus, and after birth, it stimulates milk ejection from the breasts. Secretion increases during the intrapartum and postpartum periods. AVP, also called antidiuretic hormone, causes vasoconstriction when released in large amounts, which increases blood pressure. The major role of AVP is its antidiuretic action in the regulation of water balance. Secretion of AVP is controlled by changes in plasma osmolarity and blood volume. Plasma levels of AVP do not change during pregnancy, despite the changes in blood volume, indicating that AVP is secreted at a lower plasma osmolality in pregnancy (Blackburn, 2003).

Adrenal Glands

The elevated ACTH stimulates increased cortisol production by the adrenal glands during pregnancy. The adrenal gland undergoes hypertrophy with increases in the zona fascullta (the portion of the adrenal that produces glucocorticoids such as cortisol) (Garner & Burrow, 2004). Plasma levels of CRH progressively increase during the second and third trimesters of pregnancy. Circulating cortisol levels regulate carbohydrate and protein metabolism. Total and free cortisol increase 2- to 8-fold (Rainey, Rehman, & Carr, 2004). Thus, pregnancy is characterized by a transient hypercortisolemia (Mastorakas & Ilias, 2000). Normally increased cortisol would turn off ACTH release. Therefore, the increased ACTH with increased cortisol during pregnancy suggests changes in the set point for cortisol release. Thus, in spite of the elevated cortisol and ACTH, physiologic responses to stress (such as blood pressure, heart rate, and cortisol reactivity) are maintained during pregnancy, although they may be somewhat blunted, with wide individual differences reported (Blackburn, 2003).

Other adrenal cortex hormones, aldosterone (see section on changes in the renal system) and steroid hormones also increase. Total testosterone levels also increase in pregnancy because of an increase in sex hormone–binding globulin. Free testosterone levels are low normal before 28 weeks' gestation.

Parathyroid Glands

Immunoradiometric assays demonstrate a decrease in parathyroid hormone (PTH) during pregnancy that is balanced by increased PTHrp production by the fetus and placenta (Seki, Wada, Nagata, & Hagata, 1994). Regulation of calcium is closely related to magnesium, phosphate, PTH, vitamin D, and calcitonin levels. Any alteration in one is likely to alter the others. Increases in serum-ionized calcium or magnesium suppress PTH levels, whereas decreases in serum-ionized calcium or magnesium stimulate the release of PTH (Hosking, 1996).

Maternal calcium homeostasis changes during pregnancy. Total serum calcium falls, primarily related to the fall in albumin, reaching its lowest at 28–32 weeks, then plateaus or increases slightly to term (Blackburn, 2003). There is no significant change in mean serum-ionized calcium. Daily maternal intestinal calcium absorption increases and doubles by the third trimester, due to increased calciferol (active form of vitamin D) and its binding proteins (Kovacs & Kronberg, 1997). This change begins in the first trimester, before fetal demand, so that maternal bone stores of calcium are increased during early pregnancy. These stores are used to meet the increased fetal demand in late pregnancy. Overall significant maternal bone mass is not lost during pregnancy.

NEUROMUSCULAR, SENSORY, AND INTEGUMENTARY SYSTEMS

In general, there are no major CNS changes during pregnancy, although several discomforts reported by pregnant women are associated with the nervous system. Mild frontal headaches may occur in the first and second trimesters and may be caused by tension or may be related to hormonal changes. Severe headache, especially after 20 weeks' gestation, may be associated with preeclampsia. This type of headache is a result of cerebral edema from vasoconstriction. Dizziness may result from vasomotor instability, postural hypotension, or hypoglycemia, especially after prolonged periods of sitting or standing. Paresthesia of the lower extremities can occur because of pressure from the gravid uterus, interfering with circulation. Excessive hyperventilation, resulting in lower PaCO2 levels, creates a tingling sensation in the hands (Harvey, 1999).

Sleep patterns change during pregnancy, mediated by hormonal changes and mechanical forces. Changes include a increases in total sleep time, insomnia, night awakenings, and daytime sleepiness and decreased stage 3 and 4 non–rapid eye movement sleep (Santiago, Nolledo, Kinzler, & Santiago, 2001). Night awakenings are often related to nocturia, fetal activity, backache, dyspnea, and heartburn. Sleep is also altered in the postpartum period, especially in the first 2 weeks.

The pregnant woman may experience ocular and otolaryngeal changes. Intraocular pressure tends to drop during the second half of gestation. The cornea becomes thicker, and mild corneal edema may be present. These changes can slightly alter refractory power and may lead to mild discomforts in women who wear contact lenses. Otolaryngeal changes are due to altered fluid dynamics, increased vascular permeability, vasomotor changes, increased vascularization, and the effects of estrogen. These changes can lead to an increase in ear and nasal stuffiness, hoarseness, and snoring (Blackburn, 2003).

Skin changes induced by pregnancy include vascular alterations, variations in nail and hair growth, connective tissue changes, and altered pigmentation (Rapini, 2004; Rosen, 2004). Blood flow to the skin increases three to four times above prepregnant levels. Vascular

spider nevi appear on the face, neck, chest, arms, and legs. These are small, bright red elevations of the skin radiating from a central body. Spider nevi are related to increased subcutaneous blood flow and potentially to increased estrogen levels in the tissue. Palmar erythema is a normal vascular change during pregnancy, but it has also been associated with liver and collagen vascular diseases.

During early pregnancy, the number of hairs in the growth phase remains stable. In the later stages of pregnancy, however, hormonal levels apparently increase the number of hairs in the growth phase and decrease the number of hairs in the resting phase. After birth, the proportion of hairs that enters the resting phase doubles, and women may experience an increase in hair loss 2 to 4 months postpartum. Occasionally, nail growth may be affected, and nail changes include transverse grooving, softening, and increased brittleness (Rapini, 2004).

Striae gravidarum (ie, stretch marks) may occur on the skin of the breasts, hips, and upper thighs and are usually most pronounced on the abdomen. Striae, which result from the normal stretching of the skin and softening and relaxing of the dermal collagenous and elastic tissues during the last months of pregnancy, occur in about 50% of pregnant women (Blackburn, 2003).

Increases in estrogen and progesterone may cause an increase in melanocyte-stimulating hormone, causing hyperpigmentation in the integumentary system. Darkening of the nipples, areolae, and perianal and genital areas occurs. The linea alba becomes the linea nigra and divides the abdomen longitudinally from the sternum to the symphysis. Melasma (ie, the "mask of pregnancy," previously referred to as chloasma) appears as irregularly shaped brown blotches on the face, with a mask-like distribution on the cheekbones and forehead and around the eyes. Chloasma is thought to result from elevated serum levels of estrogen and progesterone, which also stimulate melanin deposits. Chloasma disappears after pregnancy, but may reappear with excessive sun exposure or with oral contraceptive use (Rapini, 2004; Rosen, 2004).

Early in pregnancy, the ligaments of the pregnant woman soften from the effects of progesterone and relaxin. This softening, especially evident in the sacroiliac, sacrococcygeal, and pubic joints of the pelvis, facilitates birth. The center of gravity changes with advancing pregnancy because of the increase in weight gain, fluid retention, lordosis, and mobilization of ligaments. To accommodate the increased weight of the uterus, the lumbodorsal spinal curve is accentuated, and the woman's posture changes. The rectus abdominis muscle may separate because of the pressure exerted by the growing uterus, producing diastasis recti.

REPRODUCTIVE ORGANS

Uterus

Before pregnancy, the uterus is a small, semisolid, pear-shaped organ that weighs 50 to 70 g. During pregnancy, the uterus becomes globular and increases in length. At term, the uterus weighs approximately 800 to 1,200 g, due to hypertrophy of the myometrial cells (Monga & Sanborn, 2004). Ten percent to 20% of the maternal cardiac output flows through the vascular system of the uterus. During the first few months of pregnancy, the wall of the uterus thickens due to hyperplasia and hypertrophy in response to elevated estrogen and progesterone levels. After this time, the muscle wall thins, allowing easier palpation of the fetus. The size and number of blood and lymphatic vessels increase.

The uterus remains relatively quiescent during most of pregnancy. Even in nonpregnant women, the myometrium has periodic low-frequency, low-amplitude activity. This baseline activity increases during pregnancy and becomes more apparent to the women as gestation progresses. Near the end of pregnancy the myometrium goes through a preparatory stage involving activation of uterine contractility, cervical ripening, and activation of fetal membranes. Activation is thought to be stimulated by uterotrophins such as such as estrogen and by increased formation of gap junctions (needed for transmission of the action potential between muscle cells), oxytocin receptors, prostaglandin receptor activation, and ion channels to enhance movement of calcium (essential for muscle contraction) into the myocytes (Challis & Lye, 2004). Chapter 7 provides a comprehensive discussion of the initiation of labor.

Uteroplacental blood flow is essential for adequate fetal growth and survival. By term, the blood flow from the uterine and ovarian arteries to the uterus is approximately 500 to 600 mL/min, 80% of which is directed to the placental bed (Monga, 2004). Maternal position, maternal arterial pressure, and uterine contractility influence uterine blood flow. The uterine spiral arteries are altered by the fetal trophoblast, which migrates out of the placenta and remodels the elastic and muscle elements of the maternal spiral arteries underlying the site of placental implantation. As a result of these changes, the spiral arteries (called uteroplacental arteries during pregnancy) are greatly increased in diameter and can accommodate the vast supply of blood needed to supply the placenta.

Cervix

The cervix undergoes changes characterized by increased vascularity and water content, softening, and dilation (Leppert, 1995). Estrogen stimulates glandular tissue of the cervix, which increases the number of cells. Early in pregnancy, increased vascularity causes a softening and a bluish discoloration of the cervix known as Chadwick's sign. Endocervical glands, which occupy one-half of the mass of the cervix at term, secrete a thick, tenacious mucus that forms the mucous plug and prevents bacteria and other substances from entering the uterus. This mucous plug is expelled before the onset of labor and may be associated with a bloody show. Hyperactive glandular tissue also causes an increase in the normal mucus production during pregnancy.

Ovaries

Ovulation ceases during pregnancy. Cells that line the follicles, known as thecal cells, become active in hormone production and serve as the interstitial glands of pregnancy. The corpus luteum persists and secretes progesterone until the 10th to 12th week, which maintains the endometrium until adequate progesterone is secreted by the placenta.

Vagina

Vaginal epithelium and muscle layers undergo hypertrophy, increased vascularization, and hyperplasia during pregnancy in response to estrogen levels. Loosening of the connective tissue and thickening of the mucosa increase vaginal secretions. These secretions are thick, white, and acidic and play a role in preventing infection. By the end of pregnancy, the vaginal wall and perineal body become relaxed enough to permit stretching of the tissues to accommodate the birth of the infant.

Breasts

Breasts increase in size and nodularity to prepare for lactation. Nipples become more easily erectile, and veins are more prominent. Areolar pigmentation increases. Montgomery's follicles, the sebaceous glands located in the areola, hypertrophy. Striae may develop as the breasts enlarge. Colostrum, a yellow secretion rich in antibodies, may leak from the nipples during the last trimester of pregnancy. Feelings of fullness, tingling, and increased sensitivity begin in the first few weeks of gestation.

IMMUNE SYSTEM

One mystery in pregnancy is the process by which the mother's immune system remains tolerant of the foreign paternal antigens on fetal tissues and yet maintains adequate immune competence against microorganisms. Protection of the fetus from rejection is a multifactorial, complex process that seems to be predominately a localized uterine response, although there are also systemic responses mediated primarily by endocrine factors.

The mother initially has a weak immune response to the fetus/placenta that leads to an activation (facilitation) reaction rather than rejection. These initial responses, thought to help the mother recognize and protect the fetus, are mediated by Th2 cytokines (interleukins) and growth factors. Trophoblast cells fail to express major histocompatibility complex class (MHC) I or II molecules, and this may be the major reason the fetus is not targeted by the maternal immune system. The absence of the usual MHC class I and II molecules prevents maternal T-cell activation and cytotoxic T-cell destruction (Vince & Johnson, 2000). Factors that may have a role in maternal tolerance of the fetus include histocompatibility antigen, class 1, G (HLA-G) (MHC class I molecule found only on the trophoblast), progesterone, blocking factors induced by progesterone, natural killer (NK) cell function at the fetal–maternal interface, changes in the Th1–Th2 cytokine balance and inodoleamine 2,3 dehydrogenase, suppressor macrophages, annexin II, and changes in the maternal immune system (Blackburn, 2003). Cytokines, prostaglandin E2, steroid hormones, estrogen, hCG, and various pregnancy-specific proteins exert immunosuppressive effects during pregnancy.

Immune responses include innate responses and adaptive responses. Both types of responses are altered during pregnancy. Innate responses include initial actions to the entry of pathogens and inflammatory reactions. Circulating WBCs (especially neutrophils and monocytes) are increased. However, decreased neutrophil chemotaxis (organized movement of neutrophils toward the site of pathogen entry) may delay initial responses to infection (Silver, Peltier, & Branch, 2004). NK cell cytotoxic activity is down regulated by progesterone especially in the second and third trimesters (Druckmann & Druckmann, 2005). Enhanced monocyte and neutrophil activity may enhance phagocytosis. Complement levels and activity are normal to increased, but may be delayed (Richani, Soto, Romero, Espinoza, Chaiworapongsa, Nien, et al., 2005). Inflammatory responses are suppressed at the fetal–maternal border by a pregnancy zone protein.

Adapt responses include antibody-mediated (B lymphocyte) and cell-mediated (T-lymphocyte) responses. Pregnancy is characterized by a switch in the balance of Th1 to Th2 cytokines (Formby, 1995). Th2 type cytokines are increased, enhancing antibody-mediated immunity; while Th1 cytokines are decreased, reducing cell-mediated responses. This may increase the susceptibility to viral infection. B-lymphocyte function (antibody-mediated immunity) is not significantly altered and may be enhanced by the increase in Th2 cytokines. The slight decrease in immunoglobulin G (IgG) may increase the risk of bacterial colonization. Cell-mediated (T lymphocyte) immunity is somewhat suppressed during pregnancy, which may help prevent maternal rejection of the fetus. This suppression is mediated by cortisol, hCG, progesterone, and alpha fetoprotein (Blackburn, 2003). T-cell total numbers and subpopulations are probably unchanged and systemic T-cell function maintained. However, selective localized (reproductive) immunosuppression may occur that may increase the risk of viral and mycotic infections (Blackburn, 2003).

SUMMARY

Significant physical, metabolic, and structural changes occur from conception until weeks into the postpartum period. A thorough understanding of these changes facilitates assessment of normal pregnancy progression. Recognition of variations from normal may result in early identification of risk factors and potential complications. Prompt management can be initiated to help ensure optimal outcomes for both mother and fetus.

REFERENCES

Abbas, A. E., Lester, S. J., & Connolly, H. (2005). Pregnancy and the cardiovascular system. *International Journal of Cardiology, 98,* 179.

Abrams, B., Minassian, D., & Pickett, K. E. (1999). Maternal nutrition. In R. K. Creasy, R. Resnik, & J. D. Iams (Eds.), *Maternal-fetal medicine* (5th ed). Philadelphia: Saunders.

Allen, L. H. (2000). Anemia and iron deficiency: Effects on pregnancy outcome. *American Journal of Clinical Nutrition, 71*(Suppl.), 1280S.

Barak, S., Oettinger-Barak, O., Oettinger, M., Machtei, E. E., Peled, M., & Ohel G. (2003). Common oral manifestations during pregnancy: A review. *Obstetrical and Gynecological Survey, 58,* 624.

Bagchi, I. C., & Kumar, S. (1999). Steroid-regulated molecular markers of implantation. *Seminars in Reproductive Endocrinology, 17,* 235.

Beard, J. L. (2000). Effectiveness and strategies of iron supplementation during pregnancy. *American Journal of Clinical Nutrition, 71*(Suppl. 5), 1288S.

Blackburn, S. T. (2003). *Maternal, fetal and neonatal physiology: A clinical perspective* (2nd ed.). Philadelphia: Saunders.

Blanchard, D. G., & Shabetal, R. (2004). Cardiac disease. In R. K. Creasy, R. Resnik & J. D. Iams (Eds.), *Maternal-fetal medicine* (5th ed.). Philadelphia: Saunders.

Bremme, K. A. (2003). Haemostatic changes in pregnancy. *Best Practice & Research Clinical Haematology, 16,* 153.

Bridges, E. J., Womble, S., Wallace, M., & McCartney, J. (2003). Hemodynamic monitoring in high-risk obstetrics patients, I. Expected hemodynamic changes in pregnancy. *Critical Care Nurse, 23,* 53.

Bryer E. (2005). A literature review of the effectiveness of ginger in alleviating mild-to-moderate nausea and vomiting of pregnancy. *Journal of Midwifery and Womens Health, 50,* e13.

Butte, N. F. (2000). Carbohydrate and lipid metabolism in pregnancy: Normal compared with gestational diabetes mellitus. *American Journal of Clinical Nutrition, 71*(Suppl.), 1256S.

Caulin-Glaser, T., & Setaro, J. F. (2004). Pregnancy and cardiovascular disease. In G. N. Burrow, T. F. Ferris & J. A. Copel (Eds.) *Medical complications during pregnancy* (6th ed.). Philadelphia: Saunders.

Chaliha C., & Stanton S. L. (2002). Urological problems in pregnancy. *British Journal of Urology International, 89,* 469.

Challis, J. R., & Lye, S. J. (2004). Characteristics of parturition. In R. K. Creasy, R. Resnik, & J. D. Iams (Eds.), *Maternal-fetal medicine* (5th ed.). Philadelphia: Saunders.

Cunningham, F. G., Gant, N. F., & Leveno, K. J. (2001). *Williams obstetrics* (21st ed.). New York: McGraw-Hill.

Cunningham, J. T. (1998). Upper gastrointestinal tract disease. Small and large bowel disease. In N. Gleicher (Ed.), *Principles and practice of medical therapy in pregnancy* (3rd ed.). Stamford, CT: Appleton & Lange.

Druckmann, R., & Druckmann, M. A. (2005). Progesterone and the immunology of pregnancy. *Journal of Steroid Biochemistry and Molecular Biology, 97,* 389.

Duffy, T. P. (2004). Hematologic aspects of pregnancy. In G. N. Burrows, T. P. Duffy & J. A. Copel. (Eds.), *Medical complications during pregnancy* (6th ed.). Philadelphia: Saunders.

Fantz, C. R., Dagogo-Jack, S., Ladenson, J. H., & Gronowski, A. M. (1999). Thyroid function during pregnancy. *Clinical Chemistry Outlook, 45,* 2250.

Formby, B. (1995). Immunologic response in pregnancy. Its role in endocrine disorders of pregnancy and influence on the course of maternal autoimmune diseases. *Endocrinology and Metabolism Clinics of North America, 24,* 187.

Foyouzi, N., Frisbaek, Y., & Norwitz, E. R. (2004). Pituitary gland and pregnancy. *Obstetrics and Gynecology Clinics of North America,, 31,* 873.

Garner, P. R., & Burrow, G. N. (2004). Adrenal and pituitary disorders. In G. N. Burrow, T. P. Duffy, & J.A. Copel (Eds.), *Medical complications during pregnancy* (6th ed.). Philadelphia: Saunders.

Gei, A. F., & Hankins, G. D. (2001). Cardiac disease and pregnancy. *Obstetrics and Gynecology Clinics of North America, 28,* 465.

Glinoer, D. (2004). The regulation of thyroid function during normal pregnancy: Importance of the iodine nutrition status. *Best Practice & Research Clinical Endocrinology & Metabolism, 18,* 133.

Golden, L. H., & Burrow, G. N. (2004). Thyroid diseases. In G. N. Burrow, T. P. Duffy, & J. A. Copel (Eds.), *Medical complications during pregnancy* (6th ed.). Philadelphia: Saunders

Goodwin T. (2002). Nausea and vomiting of pregnancy: An obstetric syndrome. *American Journal of Obstetrics and Gynecology,. 186,* S184–S189.

Harvey, M. (1999). Physiologic changes during pregnancy. In L. K. Mandeville & N. H. Troiano (Eds.), *AWHONN's high risk and critical care intrapartum nursing.* Philadelphia: Lippincott Williams & Wilkins.

Hellgren, M. (2003). Hemostasis during normal pregnancy and puerperium. *Seminars in Thrombosis and Hemostasis, 29,* 125.

Herrera, E. (2000). Metabolic adaptations in pregnancy and their implications for the availability of substrates to the fetus. *European Journal of Clinical Nutrition, 54,* S47.

Hertelendy, F., & Zakar, T. (2004). Prostaglandins and the myometrium and cervix. *Prostaglandins, Leukotrienes, and Essential Fatty Acids, 70,* 207.

Hosking, D. J. (1996). Calcium homeostasis in pregnancy. *Clinical Endocrinology, 45*(1), 1.

Institute of Medicine. (1990). *Nutrition during pregnancy: Weight gain and nutrient supplements.* Washington, DC: National Academy Press.

Keay, S. D., Vatish, M., Karteris, E., Hillhouse, E. W., & Randeva, H. S. (2004). The role of hCG in reproductive medicine. *British Journal of Obstetrics and Gynaecology, 111,* 1218.

Kenshole, A. B. (2004). Diabetes and pregnancy. In G. N. Burrow, T. P. Duffy & J. A. Copel (Eds.), *Medical complications during pregnancy* (6th ed.). Philadelphia: Saunders.

Kilpatrick, S. J., & Laros, R. K. (2004). Maternal hematologic disorders. In R. K. Creasy, R. Resnik & J. D. Iams (Eds.), *Maternal-fetal medicine* (5th ed.). Philadelphia: Saunders.

King, J. C. (2000). Physiology of pregnancy and nutrient metabolism. *American Journal of Clinical Nutrition, 71*(Suppl.), 1218S.

Kovacs, C. S., & Kronberg, H. M. (1997). Maternal-fetal calcium and bone metabolism during pregnancy, puerperium and lactation. *Endocrine Reviews, 18,* 832.

Laine, M. A. (2002). Effect of pregnancy on periodontal and dental health. *Acta Odontologica Scandinavica, 60,* 257.

Lazarus, J. H. (2005). Thyroid disorders associated with pregnancy: Etiology, diagnosis, and management. *Treatments in Endocrinology, 4,* 31.

LeBeau, S. O., & Mandel, S. J. (2006). Thyroid disorders during pregnancy. *Endocrinology and Metabolism Clinics of North America, 35,* 117.

Leppert, P. C. (1995). Anatomy and physiology of cervical ripening. *Clinical Obstetrics and Gynecology, 38,* 267.

Liu, J. H. (2004). Endocrinology of pregnancy. In R. K. Creasy, R. Resnik & J. D. Iams. (Eds.), *Maternal-fetal medicine* (5th ed.). Philadelphia: Saunders.

Lockwood, C. J. (2004). The initiation of parturition at term. *Obstetrics and Gynecology Clinics of North America, 31,* 935.

Lynch, S. R. (2000). The potential impact of iron supplementation during adolescence on iron status in pregnancy. *Journal of Nutrition, 120*(Suppl.), 448S.

Mahomed, K., & Gulmezoglu, A. M. (2000). Maternal iodine supplements in areas of deficiency (Cochrane Review). *Cochrane Library, 2.*

Mandel, J., & Weinberger, S. E. (2004). Pulmonary disease. In G. N. Burrows, T. P. Duffy & J. A. Copel. (Eds.), *Medical complications during pregnancy* (6th ed.). Philadelphia: Saunders.

Mastorakos, G., & Ilias, I. (2000). Maternal hypothalamic-adrenal axis in pregnancy and the postpartum period. Postpartum-related disorders. *Annals of the New York Academy of Sciences, 900,* 95.

Milman, N., Bergholt, T., Byg, K. E., Eriksen, L., & Graudal, N. (1999). Iron status and iron balance during pregnancy. A critical reappraisal of iron supplementation. *Acta Obstetricia et Gynecologica Scandinavica, 78,* 749.

Mohan, A. R., Loudon, J. A., & Bennett, P. R. (2004). Molecular and biochemical mechanisms of preterm labour. *Seminars in Fetal & Neonatal Medicine, 9,* 437.

Molitch, M. E. (2004). Prolactin in human reproduction. In J. F. Strauss & R. L. Barbieri (Eds.), *Yen & Jaffe's Reproductive Endocrinology* (5th ed.) Philadelphia: Saunders.

Molitch, M. E. (2006). Pituitary disorders during pregnancy. *Endocrinology and Metabolism Clinics of North America, 35,* 99.

Monga, M. (2004). Maternal cardiovascular and renal adaptations to pregnancy. In R. K. Creasy, R. Resnik & J. D. Iams (Eds.), *Maternal-fetal medicine* (3rd ed.). Philadelphia: Saunders.

Monga, M., & Sanborn, B. M. (2004). Biology and physiology of the reproductive tract and control of myometrial contraction, In R. K. Creasy, R. Resnik & J. D. Iams (Eds.), *Maternal-fetal medicine* (5th ed.). Philadelphia: Saunders.

Moore, K. L., & Persaud, T. V. N. (2003). *The developing human: Clinically oriented embryology* (7th ed.). Philadelphia: Saunders.

Moore, T. R. (2004). Diabetes and pregnancy. In R. K. Creasy, R. Resnik & J. D. Iams (Eds.), *Maternal-fetal medicine: Principles and practice* (5th ed.). Philadelphia: Saunders.

Morreale-de-Escobar, G., Obregon, M. J., & Escobar del Rey, F. (2004). Maternal thyroid hormones early in pregnancy and fetal brain development. *Best Practice & Research Clinical Endocrinology & Metabolism, 18*, 225.

Muallem, M. M., & Rubeiz, N. G. (2006). Physiological and biological skin changes in pregnancy. *American Journal of Clinical Dermatology, 24*, 80.

Rainey, W. E., Rehman, K. S., & Carr, B. R. (2004). Fetal and maternal adrenals in human pregnancy. *Obstetrics and Gynecology Clinics of North America, 31*, 817.

Rapini, R. P. (2004). The skin and pregnancy. In R. K. Creasy, R. Resnik & J. D. Iams (Eds.), *Maternal-fetal medicine* (5th ed.). Philadelphia: Saunders.

Resnik, R. (2004). The puerperium. In R. K. Creasy, R. Resnik & J. D. Iams (Eds.), *Maternal-fetal medicine* (5th ed.). Philadelphia: Saunders.

Richani, K., Soto, E., Romero, R., Espinoza, J., Chaiworapongsa, T., Nien, J. K., et al. (2005). Normal pregnancy is characterized by systemic activation of the complement system. *Journal of Maternal-Fetal Medicine, 17*, 239.

Richter, J. E. (2005) Review article: The management of heartburn in pregnancy. *Alimentary Pharmacology & Therapeutics, . 22*(9), 749–757.

Rosen, C. F. (2004). The skin in pregnancy. In G. N. Burrow, T. P. Duffy & J. A. Copel (Eds.), *Medical complications during pregnancy* (6th ed.). Philadelphia: Saunders.

Santiago, J. R., Nolledo, M. S., Kinzler, W., & Santiago, T. V. (2001). Sleep and sleep disorders in pregnancy. *Annals of Internal Medicine, 134*, 396.

Scott, L. D. (2004). Gastrointestinal disease in pregnancy. In R. K. Creasy, R. Resnik & J. D. Iams (Eds.), *Maternal-fetal medicine* (5th ed.). Philadelphia: Saunders.

Seki, K., Wada, S., Nagata, N., & Nagata, I. (1994). Parathyroid hormone-related protein during pregnancy and the perinatal period. *Gynecologic and Obstetric Investigation, 37*, 83.

Shah, D. M. (2005). Role of the renin-angiotensin system in the pathogenesis of preeclampsia. *American Journal of Physiology. Renal Physiology, 288*, F614.

Silver, R. M., Peltier, M. R., & Branch D. W. (2004). The immunology of pregnancy. In R. K. Creasy, R. Resnik, & J. D. Iams (Eds.), *Maternal-fetal medicine* (5th ed., pp. 89–109). Philadelphia: Saunders.

Stagnaro-Green, A. (2004). Postpartum thyroiditis. *Best Practice & Research. Clinical Endocrinology & Metabolism, 18*, 303.

Stitely, M. L., & Satin, A. J. (2002). Cervical ripening agents and uterine stimulants. *Clinical Obstetrics and Gynecology, 45*, 114.

Thornberg, K. L., Jacobson, S. L., Giraud, G. D., & Morton, M. J. (2000). Hemodynamic changes in pregnancy. *Seminars in Perinatology, 24*, 11.

Thorp, J. M., Norton, P. A., Wall, L. L., Kuller, J. A., Eucker, B. & Wells, E. (1999). Urinary incontinence in pregnancy and the puerperium: A prospective study. *American Journal of Obstetrics and Gynecology, 181*, 266.

Tsen, L. C., Gerard, W., & Ostheimer. (2005). What's New in Obstetric Anesthesia (Lecture). *Anesthesiology, 102*, 672.

Vince, G. S., & Johnson, P. M. (2000). Leukocyte populations and cytokine regulation in human uteroplacental tissues. *Biochemical Society Transactions, 28*, 191.

Whitty, J. E., & Dombrowsky, M. N. (2004). Respiratory diseases in pregnancy. In R. K. Creasy, R. Resnik & J. D. Iams (Eds.), *Maternal-fetal medicine* (3rd ed.). Philadelphia: Saunders.

Xiong, X., Buekens, P., Fraser, W. D., Beck, J., & Offenbacher, S. (2006). Periodontal disease and adverse pregnancy outcomes: a systematic review. *British Journal of Obstetrics and Gynaecology, 113*, 135.

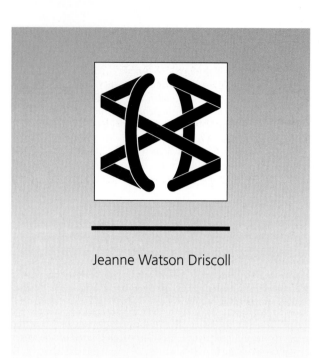

Jeanne Watson Driscoll

CHAPTER **4**

Psychosocial Adaptation to Pregnancy and Postpartum

THE goal of psychosocial care is the integration and normalization of the pregnancy and postpartum experience. It is hoped that, with caring concern, the emotional development of the new family will be encouraged, supported, and valued.

Many changes occur during pregnancy and postpartum. The woman experiences changes in physiology, body size, body shape, relationships, roles, and responsibilities. The partner also undergoes changes, in the manner of roles, relationships, responsibilities, and coping strategies. Pregnancy, childbirth, and the postpartum experience are life events. The way in which they are experienced is influenced by past events in women's lives, and will continue to influence future life experiences (Clement, 1998).

Although family development is an ongoing process that occurs during pregnancy and postpartum, it is not the focus of this chapter; this chapter focuses on the psychosocial aspects of the woman as she progresses through the normal process of pregnancy and postpartum. The purpose here is to provide the perinatal nurse with an overview of these normal psychosocial experiences so that she or he can provide comprehensive care to the woman and her family. It is by knowledge of normal experiences that the nurse is able to recognize deviations that may require referrals to multidisciplinary colleagues for collaborative, quality, holistic care.

As the woman moves through her pregnancy, the perinatal nurse provides anticipatory education and guidance regarding the physiologic, psychological, and spiritual journey. One cannot stress enough the significance of the role the nurse plays as confidant, information provider, and supporter.

And each woman is unique. To her pregnancy she brings experiences, relationships, and realities as she perceives them. It is this unique experiential history that makes her who she is. It is this identity of self that forms the foundation for her development of the maternal self and adaptation to the maternal role.

PSYCHOSOCIAL NURSING CARE

Psychosocial Assessment

The perinatal nurse plays an important role in the woman's psychosocial adaptation. A psychosocial relationship develops based on trust, mutuality, security, validation, and support. The nurse's knowledge of normal developmental and psychosocial processes allows for rapid identification of problems or alterations in the experience. Critical to the adaptation process are the concepts of care and communication. It is important for the woman to feel she is heard and validated. The perinatal nurse needs to be actively involved in the interaction, clarifying communications frequently and avoiding assumptive thinking. For instance, people commonly ask, "You know what I mean?" If the nurse does not understand what the woman is saying, her response should be, "No, I don't know what you mean. Help me understand what you are saying or feeling." This communication strategy places the responsibility onto the woman to describe her experience in her words and her reality.

The nurse needs to establish an atmosphere in which the woman can freely ask questions and engage in discussions about things that concern her. The most difficult aspect of the interaction may be that the nurse will, at times, have to sit with the woman as she bares her soul, all the while knowing there is no magic to make the woman feel better. It is important to validate the woman's uncertainties without paternalism, indifference, or judgment. Nursing actions should be directed at supporting, facilitating, and encouraging the woman's personal exploration and understanding of the experience so that she can integrate this significant life event into her reality.

Because there are transference issues in any relationship, the nurse's self-awareness is a necessity. If the nurse is unaware of his or her own issues, those issues may be projected onto the woman. Such projections can lead to misinformation, lack of concern, validity, and disconnected relationships, resulting in the woman not feeling safe. If the nurse finds that she or he is reacting to something that has been said, it is imperative that the reactions be processed through self-inquiry or with consultation. For example, the fact that a nurse has been pregnant does not mean that she knows how every pregnant woman feels. It merely means that the nurse knows what she personally felt. An example of potential projection is during the admission of a 16-year-old primipara, when the admitting nurse has a daughter of the same age. Self-awareness is especially important in cases like this, because many healthcare providers are the same age as their patients and at similar stages in development. But healthy, clear boundaries are necessary for the development of a therapeutic relationship.

Emphasis of the psychosocial assessment is on normalcy, health, universality, strengths, and developmental concepts, rather than on the formulation of a psychiatric diagnosis. The physiologic aspects of pregnancy often get more attention than the psychosocial aspects, but pregnancy and postpartum are holistic experiences. The mind, body, and soul are affected by these major changes and transitions. The perinatal nurse can use the holistic model to provide total care for this woman.

Psychosocial assessment is dynamic and ongoing. The process includes the pregnant woman, her family, and the nurse. The focus of the assessment is to gather biopsychosocial-spiritual and cultural data. It is from these data that nursing diagnoses can be identified; care plans developed in collaboration with the woman and her family; and strategies developed, implemented, and evaluated (Beck & Driscoll, 2006). Because the psychosocial assessment is an ongoing process, assessment is made during every visit. Key elements to be included in a psychosocial assessment are listed in Display 4–1.

The style of obtaining information is derived from the interviewing skills of the clinician. It may be helpful to use permission-giving statements such as, "Many women have told me they have some periods when they cry. Has this happened to you?" This allows the woman to hear that the nurse is open to her

DISPLAY 4-1

Elements of a Psychosocial Assessment

- Family and social history
- Psychiatric history (mood or anxiety disorders)
- Mental status
- Self-concept or self-esteem
- Support systems
- Stressors: personal and occupational
- Coping strategies
- Spirituality: faith and beliefs
- Cultural history
- Neurovegetative signs:
  Sleep patterns
  Appetite
  Energy or motivation
  Mood or anxiety state
  Sexual desires
- Knowledge of pregnancy experience

worries and concerns and that she does not have to feel "fine." The timing and location of the interview are also important. If there is limited time for interaction and more time is necessary for disclosure and discussion, make another appointment. This strategy validates the woman's issues and demonstrates the nurses' caring and concern.

Collaborative Care and Referral

A critical aspect of holistic care planning is the coordination of the multidisciplinary team to provide care for this woman and her family. Often, women present with issues, needs, or concerns that are beyond the realm of the perinatal nurse. These issues may require collaboration with the members of the psychiatric or mental health specialties, nutrition services, social services, or community agencies.

There is a strong correlation between the onset of mood and anxiety disorders before pregnancy and their exacerbation in the postpartum period (Beck & Driscoll, 2006; Sichel & Driscoll, 1999). All too often, when women talk about mood swings and increased anxiety during pregnancy, the reports of these uncomfortable symptoms are devalued with statements such as, "It's just because of your hormones. It will go away after you have the baby." This type of paternalistic remark denigrates the importance of the woman's feelings and may silence her. It is important for perinatal healthcare providers to be aware that a woman with previous mood and anxiety disorders is at high risk for recurrence of these disorders during pregnancy and postpartum (Beck & Driscoll, 2006; Sichel & Driscoll,

1999). A history of mood and anxiety disorders mandates coordination of the woman's care in a holistic manner that involves the mind, body, and soul. If the perinatal nurse is vigilant about the adaptation and attainment processes during pregnancy, referrals to multidisciplinary colleagues can be made as appropriate to facilitate this woman's journey to motherhood.

The perinatal nurse should be aware of community mental health resources. This may require developing a resource list, talking with providers, and developing referral relationships.

In the following sections, the psychosocial aspects of pregnancy are presented. Ongoing assessment of mood and anxiety levels in addition to the need for information and support is mandatory. Offering anticipatory guidance about physiologic and psychological changes during pregnancy supports the woman as she moves through a period of transition between two lifestyles and two states of being: the woman without child and the woman with child (Lederman, 1996).

Reva Rubin, in her classic work (1984), described tasks that a woman needs to accomplish during her pregnancy. These tasks include ensuring a safe passage for herself and her child, ensuring social acceptance of the child by significant others, increasing affinity ties in the construction of the image and identity of the "I" and the "you," and exploring the meaning of the transitive act of giving and receiving. Regina Lederman (1996) described seven psychosocial variables that are relevant to a woman's transition into self during pregnancy. These include acceptance of pregnancy, identification with a motherhood role, relationship with the woman's mother and partner or husband, preparation for labor, and prenatal fears of loss of control and self-esteem in labor. The perinatal nurse plays a significant role in the facilitation of a woman's attainment of these tasks and as well as helping her to navigate the psychosocial transitions. It is through the establishment of a strong professional relationship of care and concern that this relationship develops and grows.

ADAPTATIONS DURING PREGNANCY

First Trimester

Experience of the Mother

Myriad physiologic symptoms occur during the first trimester, and it is a time of strange feelings and secrets. The woman may know that she is pregnant as a result of a home pregnancy test, or she may deny the possibility until she requests a pregnancy test. Often, the nurse calls the woman to tell her the test result is positive. Psychosocial assessment begins at this initial nurse–patient contact. What was her response to the

DISPLAY 4 - 2

Assessment Issues in the First Trimester

- Mood and anxiety changes
- Meaning of the pregnancy (personal)
- Physical concerns or issues
- Partner or significant other's response
- Sexuality: issues or concerns
- Concerns regarding pregnancy or postpartum experience
- Relationship with family
- Support system
- Coping strategies
- Neurovegetative signs:
  Sleep patterns
  Appetite
  Energy or motivation
- Spirituality: beliefs and values

news that she is pregnant: shock, disbelief, joy, anticipation, denial, or fear? Major areas of assessment are listed in Display 4–2.

"The task of the first trimester is progressive movement of the woman from a state of conflict and ambivalence to one of acceptance of the pregnancy, the child, and the motherhood role" (Lederman, 1990). The nurse promotes this transition through concern, care, and support. Many women share that they are not sure what to feel. Moods can range from high to low, calm to panic, happy to sad, and acceptance to denial. She may feel a bit detached, emotionally labile, nauseated, fatigued, anxious, and concerned.

Often, women describe the feelings of the first trimester as akin to riding a roller coaster. Ambivalence is high during this time, and women may wonder, "This is what I thought I wanted; why do I feel so confused and sick?" Anticipatory guidance helps the woman resolve some of these feelings. If this is her first pregnancy, she needs consistent information and support. If she is a multiparous woman, how did she experience her other pregnancies? Has she had any abortions? Were they spontaneous or elective? What was her response at that time? Does she have live children? Has she had a stillborn infant? The woman's history affects this pregnancy experience.

Today, with regular use of amniocentesis, the woman may delay attachment to the pregnancy until results of an amniocentesis are available, usually at about 20 weeks of pregnancy. So for almost 20 weeks, she may remain disconnected from her feelings and emotions in an effort to protect herself from potential pain and disappointment. If she has a history of miscarriage, she may be afraid to become attached to the pregnancy until she passes the "critical week" when she lost the other pregnancy. It is not uncommon for women with histories of loss to delay attachment until they see a live baby at birth.

Developing a therapeutic relationship with the woman takes work. Key aspects of this relationship include the development of trust, confidence, mutuality, active listening, and empowerment. Pregnancy is a time of emotional changes, and she needs a "safe place" to share her thoughts and concerns. Suggest that she begin a journal of her pregnancy experiences as a place to share personal thoughts. What about the woman's partner? What are his or her thoughts? How does she think the partner is doing with this new information? Meeting with the woman's partner or significant other provides additional information to help the nurse with the complete family assessment. Ascertain any misconceptions, needs for information, and feelings about the pregnancy. What is the partner's availability? What about other support people? Does the woman have a best friend or confidant, or can she talk with other women who have experienced pregnancy and birth? What about her concepts of spirituality; is her faith or belief system helpful to her?

The pregnant woman needs validation and support. A major nursing role is to listen to the woman's experience. What does it feel like for her? All too often, she feels as though the people in the physician's office care only about her urine samples, vital signs, and weight status. She is nervous and will do well with anticipatory information, support, and permission to feel as she moves through this first trimester.

Role of the Nurse

The role of the nurse during the first trimester includes the following tasks:

- Begin psychosocial assessment at initial contact; assess the woman's response to pregnancy.
- Promote the woman's accomplishment of the first task of pregnancy by showing concern and providing care and support.
- Give anticipatory guidance related to the experiences of the first trimester.
- Continue to make assessments by interviewing the partner or significant other.
- Validate the woman's concerns and support her emotional state.

Second Trimester

Experience of the Mother

As she moves into the second trimester, the pregnant woman begins to feel fetal activity. She may have previously seen an image of the fetus by ultrasound, but now she feels the baby move. "Fantasies during pregnancy, expressed as descriptions of the unborn child, are believed to be a key component in maternal–child relational and concomitant maternal role formation" (Sorenson & Schuelke, 1999). This is a good time to engage the woman in questions: What are her fantasies? Who does she imagine her baby looks like? What does she think it will be like to have a baby? It is by asking these types of questions that role development may be facilitated. Building on prior assessments, Display 4–3 contains issues critical to the second trimester.

During the second trimester, the woman deals with issues related to body changes. She begins to wear maternity clothes and people ask her about her pregnancy; it is no longer a secret. She may need to talk and grieve about the loss of her body shape and size. The perinatal nurse must exercise caution and not project personal feelings onto the woman. For example, the perinatal nurse may say, "You must be excited about feeling the baby move." However, the woman may feel as though there is an alien inside; it is more frightening than exciting. Now she knows that the nurse thinks that she should be excited, so she better not reveal how she really feels. She is afraid the nurse may think something is wrong with her if she is not excited. She is vulnerable and needs to feel safe and confident that her feelings are heard in a nonjudgmental way.

Pregnant women have increased vulnerability to emotional nuances in relationships. They perceive from the nurse's looks, innuendos, and responses whether they are being valued. Women have been socialized to be other-centered, so she may need help redirecting and focusing on her own needs, wants, and

DISPLAY 4-3

Assessment Issues in the Second Trimester

- Mood and anxiety changes
- Feelings and perceptions about fetal movements
- Feelings about body changes and body image
- Attachment to fetus
- Neurovegetative signs:
  Sleep patterns
  Appetite
  Energy or motivation
- Relationship with partner or significant other
- Sexuality: issues and concerns
- Relationship with work and family
- Knowledge about the pregnancy experience
- Spirituality: faith and beliefs

concerns (Miller, 1986). It is difficult to share feelings that may not seem nice. If the nurse reacts negatively to the woman's feelings, it will close the door to the woman's development of trust, mutuality, and confidence in her own feelings as valid and real. Permission-giving statements should be used, such as, "In my clinical practice, women have shared with me that they are not too excited about the changes in their body. How do you feel about this?" This allows her to know that you have heard negative things from other women and that perhaps it is safe for her to disclose her real feelings, contrary to what she has been told she should feel.

Although the second trimester is often thought to be a time of tranquility and quiescence, a pregnant woman may experience increased anxiety as the baby makes his or her presence known. She begins to feel better physiologically, and her focus may shift from self-concern to baby-concern. She may begin to experience fears or phobias that something bad may happen. If the nurse feels that the woman's anxieties and concerns are getting in the way of her healthy day to day functioning, a referral to a psychiatric or mental healthcare provider may be necessary. This lets the woman know that her concerns and fears are valued and that the goal is to provide holistic care.

A pregnant woman may tell you that she is having weird, sometimes frightening, dreams about strangers entering her life. When one stops to think about it, there is a stranger in her life. A woman's perception of her unborn child develops through watching images during ultrasound examinations or the personal characteristics the woman imagines in response to fetal movements. For example, many women describe in detail the attributes of their baby based on ultrasound images or cycles of fetal activity. If fetal sex is known as a result of ultrasonography or genetic testing, more gender-specific traits can be imagined. It is not unusual for women to report, "He's a wild one," or "She likes to keep me up at night." Encourage her to share her perceptions and dreams with her partner or another significant person in her life. Tell the woman that it often helps to just talk about them. Let her know that some women find it worthwhile to write about their dreams and feelings in a journal during pregnancy. Benefits of keeping a journal are not only instantly therapeutic, but also provide the woman the opportunity to review entries at a later date and analyze the development of her impressions as the pregnancy progressed.

Anticipatory information and education about the childbirth experience begin to be of importance during the second trimester. It is time to register for prepared childbirth classes. Attending these classes appeals to the cognitive side of the process, because she is becoming informed about her body and the upcoming labor and birth. And childbirth classes could mean the development of new friendships among the participants based on shared experiences. These relationships often carry over into the postpartum period and beyond.

Role of the Nurse

The role of the nurse during the second trimester includes the following tasks:

- Continue ongoing psychosocial assessments of the woman and her partner or significant other.
- Encourage verbalization regarding the grief process (eg, body image).
- Maintain a nonjudgmental attitude.
- Refer to a psychiatric care provider if anxieties seem greater than normal.
- Encourage the woman to share dreams, thoughts, and feelings with a close friend or her partner or to keep a personal journal.
- Provide anticipatory guidance regarding normal changes and concerns.
- Provide information regarding childbirth classes for the woman and her partner.

Third Trimester

Experience of the Mother

During the third trimester, frequency of visits to healthcare providers increases. The woman may begin to ask more questions and verbalize increased concerns about what will happen during labor and birth. The major issues during the third trimester are birth preparation and the baby's well-being. The mother may begin to experience an approach-avoidance conflict related to childbirth and the possible consequences that may evolve, such as pain and loss of control (Rofe, Blittner, & Lewin, 1993). Display 4–4 describes assessment issues pertinent to this trimester.

During this trimester, some women experience physical discomforts because of body size and physiologic changes. They worry about what will happen when they go into labor. Role responsibilities are changing. The woman may leave work to begin maternity leave, a role change that may affect daily interaction with adults and potentially her identity. She may begin to talk about her fear of losing control during labor and birth and ask many questions: "What if I scream?" "How will I know when I am in labor?" "What if my water breaks in the mall?" Her anxieties begin to rise. Ongoing assessment of her anxiety level is necessary. It is important to validate her concerns and support her normalcy.

Attention to the mental health aspects of the woman's care becomes crucial, in that depression that occurs or exacerbates during the pregnancy is a precursor for the onset of a postpartum mood and/or anxiety disorder (Beck & Driscoll, 2006). Jesse and Grajam (2005) published a study that showed that asking two-item screening questions of women in pregnancy related to symptoms of depression could be an essential first step in identification and referral. The two-item depression screening measure questions are: "Are you often sad and depressed?" and "Have you had a loss of pleasurable activities?" These questions may help the nurse assess the woman's emotional state; if the nurse feels that the woman's mood is more intense than usual, referral may be necessary for evaluation by the psychiatric or mental health team. It cannot be stressed enough that if the woman does have a history of mood and anxiety disorders, whether occurring prior to pregnancy, during a previous pregnancy or postpartum, this is a good time to have her meet with the psychiatric treatment team so that a her care plan could be developed for prophylaxis postpartum (Beck & Driscoll, 2006).

Her dreams may begin to include fears of being stuck or trapped, fears of some harm happening to her or the baby, and concerns for survival. It is not uncommon at this time for the woman to experience increased anxiety secondary to hearing other women's stories of their birth experiences. She worries about her performance and about the "awful" things that might happen. She needs to have a safe place to share her concerns and worries.

It is important to discuss and plan for the postpartum experience. What about support? Who is going to help her? What are her expectations of the experience? If there are other children, who will take care of them and help her after she gets home with the new baby? Assist the woman to develop lists of things to do and

people she needs to contact and enlist support from before the birth. If she will be breast-feeding, encourage her to attend breast-feeding support groups before birth to promote relationship and resource development.

Role of the Nurse

The role of the perinatal nurse continues to be one of assessment, information, and support. The nurse's role in the third trimester includes the following tasks:

- Continue ongoing psychosocial assessment of the woman and her partner or significant other.
- Support and reinforce information obtained during childbirth education classes.
- Facilitate verbalization of concerns related to employment status and role changes.
- Encourage sharing of feelings and concerns with her partner or significant other.
- Provide anticipatory education regarding the postpartum experience.
- Facilitate planning for help at home after the birth.
- Encourage her to obtain information about new mothers' support groups and breast-feeding support groups.

ADAPTATIONS DURING LABOR AND BIRTH

Labor and Birth

Experience of the Mother

The labor and birth experience is a critical turning point. The mother makes the major physical and psychological transition during birth. The onset of labor can be a scary experience, especially when she realizes that there is no way back. Often, she calls with the first twinges and asks, "What should I do?" She needs a lot of support and gentle guidance. She is concerned about her well-being, that of her baby, and of her partner. She is afraid that she will lose control, and she wants to "be a good patient." Her sense of reality is intense.

If she is having her baby in the hospital or birth center, it is important that the perinatal nurse orient the woman and her partner to the unit and talk with them about their hopes and desires for this birth experience. The establishment of an empathic, therapeutic relationship is necessary to provide the woman with the connection and concern that she needs to proceed in the labor experience. Anticipatory guidance and information sharing need to be ongoing, as she may lose her sense of time because of the crisis of labor. Continual assessment of her psychosocial ability to stay focused and connected to the experience is important. Pay close attention to the interaction between the laboring woman and her support person so that you will be available as needed to support them both. In Beck's phenomenological study of birth trauma, it was shown that the mother's perceptions of the birth trauma can be based not only on the birth event, but also the unmet expectations of the woman during the birth (Beck, 2004). Nurses can play a proactive role in preventing birth trauma by enhancing a woman's sense of control over the birth and being with the woman during the experience.

Each woman will labor and birth in a unique way, and nursing care should be individualized rather than routine. Similarly, there is no behavior or response that one would expect to see after the birth. Some women will be jubilant and excited, want to hold their baby, count fingers and toes, and breast-feed. Other women need to go into themselves to regroup on an intrapersonal level. There is no one right way to act. One woman, after a precipitous birth experience, when asked if she wanted to hold her new baby, said, "Not yet; give me some time to get myself together. I can't believe this is over." With all the pressure about bonding, it is important for the nurse to support the new mother's request at this time. This is the beginning of the conflicts of new motherhood: do I take care of myself, or do I put the baby first? Klaus, Kennell, and Klaus (1995) found that the care the woman receives during this phase appears to affect her attitudes, feelings, and responses to her family, herself, and especially her new baby to a remarkable degree. The psychosocial assessment issues of this experience are listed in Display 4–5.

Role of the Nurse

The role of the nurse during adaptation to the labor and birth experience is intense and critical. The woman may be scared, vulnerable, or excited. She may even regress in response to the stress of the situation. The role of the nurse during labor and birth includes the following tasks:

- Establish an empathic relationship based on trust.
- Orient the laboring woman and her support person to the unit or birth center.
- Facilitate the interaction between the woman and her labor support person.
- Provide ongoing psychosocial assessment.
- Provide anticipatory guidance regarding the labor experience.
- Encourage attachment to the baby after it is born, in relation to the new mother's needs.

ADAPTATIONS IN THE POSTPARTUM PERIOD

Postpartum Period

Experience of the Mother

The birth occurs. The family has a new member. The new mother begins her physiologic recovery, relationship development with the "real" baby, and psychological transition to motherhood.

During this early postpartum period, it is important for the perinatal nurse to observe the maternal–newborn attachment process and identify behavior patterns that may indicate the need for further follow-up care. It is critical to differentiate behaviors related to maternal exhaustion or discomfort from real problems with attachment. For example, the woman who asks that her baby spend the night in the nursery so she can get some rest is probably physically exhausted from the labor and birth, and the woman who does not want to hold her baby after a cesarean birth may be having significant incisional pain. Each woman is unique and responds to her newborn in her own way. A series of interactions are necessary for accurate assessment of maternal–newborn attachment. Nursing assessment should also focus on maternal confidence in basic newborn care skills, such as comforting strategies, formula or breast-feeding, bathing, and diapering. Encouragement and reinforcement may be necessary as the new mother tries to learn all she needs to know about newborn care in the very short time she is hospitalized.

The new mother needs time to share her labor and birth experience (Rubin, 1984). This is often done by calling all of her friends on the phone or by meeting other new mothers in the perinatal unit and chatting. She is putting meaning into the experience by verbalizing her reality. This integration of the childbirth experience into her self-system is a major issue of the early postpartum experience (Rubin, 1984). There is the need to talk about and process reality versus fantasy.

DISPLAY 4-5

Assessment Issues During Labor and Birth

- Mood and anxiety changes
- Coping strategies
- Adjustment to the environment
- Relationship with partner or significant other
- Assess ability to focus and work with the labor process
- Cultural aspects of childbirth
- Spirituality: faith and beliefs

There is an element of loss as she begins to mourn the imagined childbirth experience (Driscoll, 1990; Nicolson, 1999). The perinatal nurse plays a significant role in the validation and clarification of the experience for this woman by listening and supporting her evolving maternicity.

Today, with the reality of shortened postpartum lengths of stay, the new mother has to move quickly from self-concern to other-concern, focusing now on her newborn. It is important that the new mother's physical and psychological needs be met so that she will be better able to focus on her newborn's care. She may become intensely focused on the cognitive learning needs related to newborn feeding and physical care, and she may verbalize anxiety and concern. If so, she needs to be heard and her concerns must be validated. The newly evolving relationship with the newborn is based on connection and care. If she has difficulty with these beginning skills, it may alter her self-esteem and maternal development (Driscoll, 1993). The woman brings with her many performance expectations that need to be discussed and clarified. Mercer (1986) described maternal role attainment as a process that takes a period of about 10 months to develop. In 2004, Mercer presented evidence for replacing the term "maternal role attainment" (MRA) with the term "becoming a mother" (BAM). She stated that the term BAM "more accurately encompasses the dynamic transformation and evolution of a woman's persona than does MRA, and the term MRA should be discontinued" (p. 226) This seems to be more contextually accurate in that the process of becoming a mother is a transition that changes throughout the maternal–child relationship.

During this postpartum phase, the new mother attaches to her newborn, gains competence as a mother, and expresses gratification in the mother–infant interaction. This transition can be delayed or altered if the woman's health and mental status is less than optimal. The reality of the current healthcare delivery system is that much of the work of the postpartum maternal adjustment and becoming a mother is done after discharge. Referral to community resources and discharge planning are imperative in the total care plan.

Emotionally, these early days can be disconcerting. It is supposed to be such an exciting time, but she may be experiencing irritability, anxiety, headaches, confusion, forgetfulness, depersonalization, fatigue, and alternating periods of tears and joy. She may have the "baby blues." Between 70% and 80% of new mothers may experience this transitory mood disorder. Unfortunately, this phenomenon occurs so frequently that it is often considered normal and therefore does not get the attention that it deserves. It is felt that this disorder is related to the normal phys-

DISPLAY 4-6

Assessment Issues During the Postpartum Period

- Mood and anxiety states
- Perceptions of the birth experience
- Maternal–newborn attachment
- Relationship with partner or significant other
- Neurovegetative signs:
  Sleep patterns
  Energy or motivation
  Pain levels
- Coping strategies
- Support systems
- Cultural aspects of childbearing
- Knowledge about postpartum process after discharge
- Spirituality: faith and beliefs

iologic and psychosocial changes that occur in the process of becoming a new mother. There is a rapid drop in pregnancy hormones after delivery of the placenta, which may alter biochemical neurotransmitters in the brain (Sichel & Driscoll, 1999). This transitory mood disorder can greatly affect the new mother and her family, especially if they are unaware of the possibility or what to do about it. Assessment issues relevant to the postpartum experience are listed in Display 4–6.

Women and their families need information about normal mood changes after childbirth. They should be aware that with much support, reassurance, rest, and good nutrition, these labile moods usually balance out, and the woman will begin to feel better and more organized and confident. However, if the moods do not stabilize by about the 21st day, referral should be made to the psychiatric or mental health team specialists in postpartum mood and anxiety disorders (Beck & Driscoll, 2006).

A study of first-time mothers surveyed during the postpartum period revealed a 63% incidence of depressive disorders of early onset and lengthy duration (McIntosh, 1993). Most affected women reported that they did not seek help because they felt their depression was caused by the stress of becoming a mother; they thought it was a normal reaction. An additional reason women cited for not talking to a professional healthcare provider about their feelings was the fear that they would be labeled mentally ill and considered unfit mothers (McIntosh, 1993). Perinatal nurses must be proactive in identifying women with mood or anxiety disorders during the postpartum period to facilitate early intervention and referral to psychiatric or mental health specialists.

Postpartum Depression

Postpartum depression is a mood disorder that is estimated to affect 3% to 30% of women (Beck & Driscoll, 2006). Symptoms of postpartum depression may include anxiety, irritability, fatigue, a demoralizing sense of failure, feelings of guilt, sleep disorders, appetite changes, suicide ideation, and excessive concerns about the baby. Treatment for postpartum depression and related mood and anxiety disorders may include antidepressant agents, antianxiety agents, psychotherapy, counseling, and support groups. With appropriate intervention, prospects for recovery are excellent.

Postpartum Psychosis

The most serious psychiatric disorder that can occur after the birth of a baby is postpartum psychosis. This is an organic psychosis that affects 1 or 2 women per 1,000 births. This disorder is a psychiatric emergency. The woman can demonstrate symptoms of psychosis within 1 to 2 days after the birth of her baby. The signs and symptoms of psychosis are sleep disturbances, confusion, agitation, irritability, hallucinations, delusions, and potential for suicide or infanticide. Hospitalization is mandatory. With aggressive treatment, most women recover from this disorder (Beck & Driscoll, 2006).

Postpartum Anxiety Disorders

Anxiety disorders may present as a panic disorder or obsessive compulsive disorder (OCD). Often, women with a history of panic disorder experience exacerbations postpartum. The symptoms include palpitations, pounding heart, rapid heart rate, sweating, trembling, sensations of smothering, shortness of breath, feeling of choking, chest pain or tightness, nausea, dizziness, lightheadedness, feeling detached, fear of dying or of going crazy, numbness in fingers, and chills or hot flashes. These episodes begin to occur regularly, out of the blue, and interfere with the woman's everyday living. Treatment includes antianxiety medications, antidepressant medications, and cognitive-behavioral strategies (Beck and Driscoll, 2006).

OCD is typified by repetitive thoughts and behaviors that have no particular meaning and over which sufferers have little or no control. Postpartum onset of OCD often presents during the postpartum period. The woman describes the onset of ego-alien thoughts that something harmful might happen to the baby. She cannot get the thought out of her mind, and she begins to imagine that she could be capable of doing the baby harm, which increases her anxiety. In response to these thoughts, women develop avoidance behaviors to ensure they will not act on their thoughts. Anxiety symptoms surge, and depression can occur. This is not a psychotic disorder; the woman knows that these thoughts are bizarre. The cause of this disorder is not clear, but there may be some correlation between the rapid decrease in estrogen and oxytocin levels in the brain (Beck and Driscoll, 2006). Treatment includes antidepressants, antianxiety agents, and cognitive-behavioral strategies.

Posttraumatic Stress Disorder (PTSD) Secondary to Birth Trauma

The reported prevalence of diagnosed PTSD caused by childbirth is between 1.5% and 6% (Beck and Driscoll, 2006). Women present with symptoms of nightmares, hypervigilant anxiety, and sometimes depression. It is imperative that perinatal nurses who are aware that a woman has experienced a traumatic birth encourage her to talk about her experience. Nurses need to provide acceptance and validation of the woman's feelings and concerns and, if necessary, to refer to mental health colleagues.

It cannot be stressed enough that women and their families need anticipatory information about postpartum mood disorders so that prompt identification and early treatment can be initiated. A heightened awareness among perinatal healthcare providers regarding the incidence of postpartum mood and anxiety disorders, knowledge of common signs and symptoms, and the prospects for recovery can contribute to successful outcomes for affected women and their families.

Discharge planning has become a critical issue in this time of shortened length of stay. Before discharge from the hospital, give the woman a list of telephone numbers of her care providers as well as any emergency services that she may need. Discuss the key support people with the new mother and her partner during discharge teaching.

Role of the Nurse

The role of the perinatal nurse during the postpartum experience is changing continually in response to current lengths of stay. Hospitals are developing home-discharge programs, private home health agencies are being established, and most postpartum care occurs in the community. The nurse has several tasks during the postpartum period:

- Continue ongoing psychosocial assessment of woman and her partner or significant other.
- Assess and facilitate maternal attachment.
- Encourage verbalization of birth experience to promote integration.

- Assess and facilitate family development.
- Assess support systems and networks in the family and community.
- Provide education about normal postpartum emotional adjustments and provide anticipatory guidance regarding postpartum mood and anxiety disorders.
- Make referrals to psychiatric or mental healthcare providers who specialize in perinatal psychiatric care if needed.

SUMMARY

Psychosocial adaptation to pregnancy and postpartum is a dynamic process. The nurse plays a significant role in the promotion and facilitation of this experience in a healthy way. It is a time when the woman is open to great psychological growth and relies on the healthcare team for information and support. The nurse needs to be aware of the normal process to better identify any process that is not. It is helpful in the assessment of mood, anxiety, and emotional states to remember three words: frequency, duration, and intensity. If the woman says she is having difficulty functioning in her activities of daily living and having a tough time coping because of emotional, mood, or anxiety changes, referral is necessary. The referral process needs to be managed in an empowering, supportive way. Letting her know that she is valued and that her concerns and feelings are important is a way for the perinatal nurse to give the woman the message that she deserves good care. Appropriate healthcare provider attitudes support the referral process.

Because of the rapid changes in the healthcare delivery system and decreasing lengths of stay, it is imperative for the perinatal nurse to actively pursue, nurture, and promote collaborative relationships with colleagues in the community. This active communication and relational approach to the care of this new mother and her family promotes, facilitates, and encourages healthy maternal and paternal psychosocial transition and adjustment.

REFERENCES

Beck, C. T. (2004). Birth trauma: In the eye of the beholder. *Nursing Research, 53*(1), 28–35.

Beck, C. T., & Driscoll, J. W. (2006). *Postpartum mood and anxiety disorders: A clinician's guide.* Sudbury, MA: Jones and Bartlett Publishers.

Clement, S. (1998). *Psychological perspectives on pregnancy and childbirth.* New York: Churchill Livingstone.

Driscoll, J. W. (1990). Maternal parenthood and the grief process. *Journal of Perinatal and Neonatal Nursing, 4*(2), 1–10.

Driscoll, J. W. (1993). The transition to parenthood. In C. S. Fawcett (Ed.), *Family psychiatric nursing* (pp. 97–108). St. Louis, MO: C. V. Mosby.

Driscoll, J. W. (2005). Recognizing women's common mental health problems: The Earthquake Assessment Model. *Journal of Obstetric, Gynecologic and Neonatal Nursing, 34*(2), 246–254.

Jesse, D. E., & Graham, M. (2005). Are you often sad and depressed? Brief measures to identify women at risk for depression in pregnancy. *MCH American Journal of Maternal Child Nursing, 30*(1), 40–45.

Lederman, R. P. (1990). Anxiety and stress in pregnancy: Significance and nursing assessment. *NAACOG's Clinical Issues in Perinatal and Women's Health Nursing, 1*(3), 279–288.

Lederman, R. P. (1996). *Psychosocial adaptation in pregnancy.* (2nd ed.). New York: Springer Publishing.

Klaus, M. H., Kennell, J. H., & Klaus, P. H. (1995). *Bonding: Building foundations of secure attachment and independence.* Reading, MA: Addison-Wesley Publishing.

McIntosh, J. (1993). Postpartum depression: Women's help seeking behavior and perceptions of cause. *Journal of Advanced Nursing, 18*(2), 178–184.

Mercer, R. T. (1986). *First-time motherhood: Experiences from teens to forties.* New York: Springer-Verlag.

Mercer, R. T. (2004). Becoming a mother versus maternal role attainment. *Journal of Nursing Scholarship, 36*(3), 226–232.

Miller, J. B. (1986). *Toward a new psychology of women* (2nd ed.). Boston: Beacon.

Nicolson, P. (1999). *Post-natal depression: Psychology, science, and the transition to motherhood.* New York: Routledge.

Rofe, Y., Blittner, M., & Lewin, I. (1993). Emotional experiences during the three trimesters of pregnancy. *Journal of Clinical Psychology, 49*(1), 3–12.

Rubin, R. (1984). *Maternal identity and the maternal experience.* New York: Springer-Verlag.

Sichel, D., & Driscoll, J. W. (1999). *Women's moods.* New York: William Morrow.

Sorenson, D. S., & Schuelke, P. (1999). Fantasies of the unborn among pregnant women. *Maternal Child Nursing, 24*(2), 92–97.

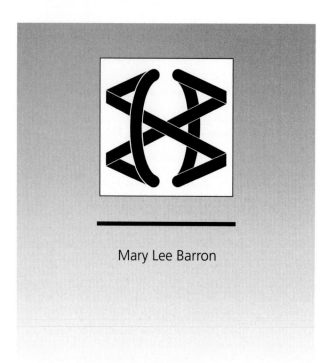

CHAPTER **5**

Antenatal Care

Mary Lee Barron

CARE of the pregnant woman in the antenatal setting is multifaceted, requiring knowledge of the normal and abnormal pregnancy, risk factors affecting pregnancy outcome, screening tests, common pregnancy discomforts and treatments, and psychosocial tasks and issues surrounding the childbearing continuum and appropriate nursing interventions. The purpose of this chapter is to present an overview of essential aspects of prenatal care for perinatal nurse caring for women during the childbearing process. It is beyond the scope of this chapter to present a comprehensive description of antenatal nursing interventions. Preterm labor assessment, hypertensive disorders of pregnancy, and childbirth education are specific topics that are discussed in depth in Chapters 6 and 10.

PRECONCEPTION CARE

Prenatal care begins with preconception healthcare. The purpose of preconception care is to deliver risk screening, health promotion, and effective interventions as a part of routine healthcare (Centers for Disease Control and Prevention [CDC], 2006). Preconception healthcare is critical because the behaviors and exposures that occur before prenatal care is initiated may affect fetal development and subsequent maternal and perinatal outcomes. Recently, the CDC (2006) developed ten recommendations for improving preconception care as part of a strategic plan to improve the health of women, their children, and their families (see Display 5–1). These recommendations, based on existing knowledge and evidence-based practice, were developed for improving preconception health through changes in consumer knowledge, clinical practice, public health programs, healthcare financing, and data and research activities. Each recommendation has specific action steps. If each action step is implemented, benefits might be observed within 2 to 5 years, which would help achieve the *Healthy People 2010* objectives to improve maternal and child health outcomes. The recommendations are aimed at achieving four goals, based on personal health outcomes.

Goal 1. Improve the knowledge and attitudes and behaviors of men and women related to preconception health.
Goal 2. Ensure that all women of childbearing age in the United States receive preconception care services (ie, evidence-based risk screening, health promotion, and interventions) that will enable them to enter pregnancy in optimal health.
Goal 3. Reduce risks indicated by a previous adverse pregnancy outcome through interventions during the interconception period.
Goal 4. Reduce the disparities in adverse pregnancy outcomes.

Preconception care should be tailored to meet the needs of the individual woman. Because preconception care needs to be provided across the life span and not during only one visit, certain recommendations will be more relevant to women at different life stages and with varying levels of risk. Health promotion, risk screening, and interventions are different for a young woman who has never experienced pregnancy than for a woman aged 35 years who has had three children. Women who present with chronic diseases, previous pregnancy

DISPLAY 5-1

Recommendations to Improve Preconception Health

Recommendation 1. Individual Responsibility Across the Life Span. Each woman, man, and couple should be encouraged to have a reproductive life plan.

Recommendation 2. Consumer Awareness. Increase public awareness of the importance of preconception health behaviors and preconception care services by using information and tools appropriate across various ages; literacy, including health literacy; and cultural/linguistic contexts.

Recommendation 3. Preventive Visits. As a part of primary care visits, provide risk assessment and educational and health promotion counseling to all women of childbearing age to reduce reproductive risks and improve pregnancy outcomes.

Recommendation 4. Interventions for Identified Risks. Increase the proportion of women who receive interventions as follow-up to preconception risk screening, focusing on high-priority interventions (ie, those with evidence of effectiveness and greatest potential impact).

Recommendation 5. Interconception Care. Use the interconception period to provide additional intensive interventions to women who have had a previous pregnancy that ended in an adverse outcome (eg, infant death, fetal loss, birth defects, low birth weight, or preterm birth).

Recommendation 6. Prepregnancy Checkup. Offer, as a component of maternity care, one prepregnancy visit for couples and persons planning pregnancy.

Recommendation 7. Health Insurance Coverage for Women with Low Incomes. Increase public and private health insurance coverage for women with low incomes to improve access to preventive women's health and preconception and interconception care.

Recommendation 8. Public Health Programs and Strategies. Integrate components of preconception health into existing local public health and related programs, including emphasis on interconception interventions for women with previous adverse outcomes.

Recommendation 9. Research. Increase the evidence base and promote the use of the evidence to improve preconception health.

Recommendation 10. Monitoring Improvements. Maximize public health surveillance and related research mechanisms to monitor preconception health.

CDC. (2006) Recommendations to improve preconception health and health care—United States: A report of the CDC/ATSDR preconception care work group and the select panel on preconception care. *Morbidity and Mortality Weekly Report Recommendations and Reports, 55*(RR 06), 1–12.

---

complications, or behavioral risk factors might need more intensive interventions. Social determinants of women's health also play a role in birth outcome. An example would be the correlation between women with low incomes and the risk of preterm labor (Haas, Meneses, & McCormick, 1999). Identified modifiable risk factors include isotretinoins (Accutane) use, alcohol misuse, anti-epileptic drug use, diabetes (preconception), folic acid deficiency, hepatitis B, HIV/AIDS, hypothyroidism, maternal phenylketonuria, rubella seronegativity, obesity, oral anticoagulant use, sexually transmitted disease, and smoking (CDC, 2006). Implementation of the CDC recommendations is targeted to (a) women and men of childbearing age having high reproductive awareness (ie, they understand risk factors related to childbearing); (b) women and men have a reproductive life plan; (c) pregnancies are intended and planned; (d) women and men of childbearing age have healthcare coverage; (e) women of childbearing age are screened before pregnancy for risks that could affect the pregnancy; and (f) women with previous adverse pregnancy outcomes (eg, infant death, very low birth weight, or preterm birth) have access to interconception care aimed at reducing their risks. The reader is referred to http://www.cdc.gov/mmwr/preview/mmwrhtml/rr5506a1.htm for complete recommendations.

PRENATAL CARE

Adequate prenatal care is a comprehensive process in which problems associated with pregnancy are identified and treated. Three basic components of adequate prenatal care have been identified: early and continuing risk assessments, health promotion, and medical and psychosocial interventions with follow-up (United States Department of Health and Human Services [VSDHHS] Expert Panel on the Content of Prenatal Care, 1989). Quality prenatal care includes education and support for the pregnant woman, ongoing maternal–fetal assessment, preparation for parenting, and promotion of a positive physical and emotional family experience. Prenatal care has several goals:

- Maintenance of maternal–fetal health
- Accurate determination of gestational age
- Ongoing risk assessment and risk-appropriate intervention
- Woman and family education about pregnancy, birth, and parenting
- Rapport with the childbearing family
- Referral to appropriate resources

Comprehensive services include health education; nutrition education; the Women, Infants, and Children's (WIC) program; social services assessment; medical risk assessment; and referral as appropriate. To provide optimal, individualized care, nurses must recognize the effect of pregnancy on a woman's life span. Although a woman's preconceptional health has an impact on pregnancy, it is also true that childbearing is an event that may affect her long-term health. It is important to consider pregnancy within the larger context of women's health.

Early, adequate prenatal care has long been associated with improved pregnancy outcomes. Continued contact with the pregnant woman through comprehensive prenatal care provides an ideal opportunity for the healthcare provider to assess for and identify potential problems that may place the woman and fetus at risk. Risk-appropriate prenatal care further enhances the possibility of a positive pregnancy outcome among women who are at increased medical or social risk. The nurse should view those women with risk factors to be at higher risk than those without, but should avoid concentrating efforts on only those in a high-risk category.

Prenatal care has been based on tradition and expert opinion rather than on evidence. The VSDHHS Expert Panel on Prenatal Care (1989) recommended that healthy, pregnant women who are at low risk for pregnancy complications could attend fewer visits without negative consequences. For nulliparous women, nine visits were recommended; for multiparous women, seven visits were recommended. Villar and colleagues (2001) found that fewer visits did not result in negative outcomes. However, adoption of the VSDHHS 1989 recommendation has been very slow. Another emerging model of group prenatal care, CenteringPregnancy, integrates group support with prenatal care and is in use in at least 50 sites in the United States (Walker & Rising, 2004). CenteringPregnancy is care given in a group setting that uses the essential components of prenatal care: risk assessment, health promotion, medical and psychosocial interventions, and follow-up. The program is based on the idea that women should be equal partners in care and work actively with care providers to reach their goals (Walker & Rising, 2004). This model involves ten 90- to 120-minute sessions that begin at 16 weeks' gestation and conclude with a postpartum meeting (Rising, 1998). The initial prenatal visit is an individual appointment. Each woman is invited to join a group of 8 to 12 other women with similar estimated dates of birth. Sessions allow for individual time with the care provider and group sharing and education. Groups are led by advanced practice nurses or other healthcare professionals with expertise in group process. Nurses must be aware of these developing models in order to offer the highest quality evidence-based care to pregnant women.

PRENATAL RISK ASSESSMENT

The goal of risk assessment is to identify women and fetuses at risk for developing antepartum, intrapartum, postpartum, or neonatal complications to promote risk-appropriate care that will enhance the perinatal outcome. The underlying causes of preterm labor and intrauterine growth restriction are not fully understood. However, a large body of knowledge regarding risk factors associated with prematurity and low birth weight has developed. These factors include demographic, medical, obstetric, sociocultural, lifestyle, and environmental risks. It is important to note that many risk factors have been identified in studies of women who develop complications of pregnancy or deliver preterm; however, no firm cause and effect relationship between some of the commonly associated risk factors and poor outcome has been established. For example, being an adolescent does not cause poor pregnancy outcomes; however, many teens who live in poverty do experience complications of pregnancy (Cunningham et al., 2005; Markovitz, Cook, Flick, & Leet, 2005). Risk-assessment tools may be helpful in distinguishing between women at high and low risk (see Display 5–2 for a list of assessment factors). Unfortunately, the predictive value of these tools is limited. Enthusiasm for risk assessment must be tempered with reality. Identification of real or potential problems should be a shared process in which the nurse assesses the woman's individual perception of risk. However, note that labeling may actually result in a heightened personal perception of risk (Gupton, Heaman, & Cheung, 2001). Approximately one-third of the potential complications of pregnancy occur during the intrapartum period and are not predictable by current risk-assessment systems (American Academy of Pediatrics [AAP] & American College of Obstetricians and Gynecologists [ACOG], 2002). However, risk assessment directs the provider toward areas in which intervention can have a positive impact on perinatal outcomes. The nurse's knowledge of prenatal risk assessment allows for anticipatory planning, individualized education, and appropriate referral. Outcomes of risk assessment provide guidelines by which the effectiveness of the care can be evaluated. The nurse's role in prenatal care is discussed within these parameters.

Initial Prenatal Visit

Antepartum assessment begins with the first prenatal visit. Generally, a woman with an uncomplicated

D I S P L A Y   5 – 2

Risk Assessment

OBSTETRIC HISTORY

History of infertility
Grand multiparity
Previous stillborn/neonatal death
Incompetent cervix
Previous multiple gestation
Uterine or cervical anomaly
Previous prolonged labor
Previous preterm labor or preterm birth
Previous low-birth-weight infant
Previous cesarean birth
Previous midforceps delivery
Previous macrosomic infant
Previous pregnancy loss (spontaneous or induced)
Last delivery <1 year before present conception
Previous hydatidiform mole or choriocarcinoma
Previous infant with neurologic deficit, birth injury, or congenital anomaly

MEDICAL HISTORY

Cardiac disease
Metabolic disease
Gastrointestinal disorders
Seizure disorders
Malignancy
Reproductive tract anomalies
Renal disease, repeat urinary tract infections, bacteriuria
Emotional disorders, mental retardation
Family history of severe inherited disorders

History of abnormal Pap smear
Previous surgeries, particularly involving the reproductive organs
Pulmonary disease
Chronic hypertension
Endocrine disorders
Hemoglobinopathies
Sexually transmitted diseases
Surgery during pregnancy

CURRENT OBSTETRIC STATUS

Inadequate prenatal care
Intrauterine growth-restricted fetus

Rh sensitization
Preterm labor

Polyhydramnios
Large for gestational age fetus
Placenta previa
Abnormal presentation
Maternal anemia
Weight gain < 10 lb
Weight loss > 5 lb
Sexually transmitted diseases
Pregnancy-induced hypertension, preeclampsia
Premature rupture of membranes

Overweight or underweight
Immunization status
Fetal or placental malformations
Abnormal fetal surveillance tests
Abruptio placentae
Multiple gestation
Postdatism
Fibroids
Fetal manipulation
Cervical cerclage
Maternal infection

PSYCHOSOCIAL FACTORS

Inadequate finances
Poor housing
Social problems
Unwed, father of baby uninvolved or unsupportive
Adolescent
Minority status
Poor nutrition
Parental occupation
More than two children at home, no help
Inadequate support systems
Unacceptance of pregnancy
Dysfunctional grieving
Psychiatric history
Attempt or ideation of suicide
Domestic violence
Demographic Factors
   Maternal age <16 or >35 years
   Education <11 years
Lifestyle
   Smokes >10 cigarettes/day
   Alcohol intake
   Substance abuse
   Heavy lifting, long periods of standing
   Long commute
   Unusual stress

---

pregnancy is examined approximately every 4 weeks for the first 28 weeks of pregnancy, every 2 to 3 weeks until 36 weeks' gestation, and weekly thereafter. Women with medical or obstetric problems may require closer surveillance. Intervals between visits are determined by the nature and severity of the problem (AAP & ACOG, 2002).

The initial prenatal visit is of vital importance and requires careful attention to detail. The nurse is obligated to practice within the framework of professional standards, such as the Association of Women's Health, Obstetric and Neonatal Nurses' (AWHONN) *Standards*

and Guidelines (2003) and *Guidelines for Perinatal Care* (AAP & ACOG, 2002), which provide guidelines for practice in the ambulatory care setting. During the first prenatal visit, baseline health data are obtained and assessed, a patient-centered relationship is established, and the plan of care is initiated. Risk assessment during the initial prenatal visit should include the following:

- A careful family medical history, individual medical history, and reproductive health history
- A comprehensive physical examination designed to evaluate potential risk factors

- Appropriate prenatal laboratory screening
- Individualized, risk-appropriate laboratory evaluation
- Fetal assessment, as developmentally appropriate (eg, fetal heart rate [FHR], fetal activity, kick counts) and individualized fetal surveillance, as indicated (eg, ultrasonography, biophysical profile [BPP])

Maternal Age

The association between Down syndrome and advanced maternal age has been long documented (Hook, 1981). Maternal age of 35 years and older is associated with an increased risk of fetal death (Silver, 2007), whereas children born to mothers younger than 19 or older than 35 years of age have an increased risk of prematurity, congenital anomalies, and risks from other complications of pregnancy (March of Dimes, 2006). However, researchers recently reported that pregnancy outcomes previously linked to maternal age are mitigated by poverty (Cunningham et al., 2005; Markovitz et al., 2005). With poor socioeconomic status, the risk of perinatal morbidity increases after the age of 35, but with adequate income and healthcare, women in that age group experienced only a slight increase in gestational diabetes, pregnancy-induced hypertension, placenta previa or abruption, and cesarean birth (Cunningham et al., 2005). Complications common in pregnant adolescents include low birth weight, preeclampsia and pregnancy-induced hypertension, intrauterine growth restriction (IUGR), and preterm labor. In younger mothers, socioeconomic factors largely explain increased neonatal mortality risk (Markovitz et al., 2005). Knowledge of these risks serves as a guide for counseling women for whom age is a risk factor.

Medical and Obstetric History

Assessment of health factors that may influence pregnancy outcome includes careful evaluation of the woman's individual medical, gynecologic, obstetric, psychosocial, and environmental history. Pertinent family history of the woman and her partner is necessary for complete evaluation. Maternal–family reproductive health history (eg, preeclampsia, hypertension, preterm birth) may be particularly significant. The additional physiologic stress of pregnancy affects chronic conditions (eg, diabetes, hypertension, or cardiac disease). Likewise, factors such as a recent history of sexually transmitted diseases (STDs) or chemical dependency may be indicative of lifestyle behaviors that threaten maternal–fetal well-being.

Obstetric history, such as length of previous labors, cesarean birth, birth weight, gestational age, history of

preterm labor or preterm birth, grand multiparity, elective or spontaneous abortion, instrument-assisted birth, previous stillbirth, or uterine or cervical anomaly may indicate potential risks for the current pregnancy (see Display 5–3). Apply these risk factors within the context of the gestational age. For example, a history of preterm birth would be a pertinent risk to a woman who is presently at 20 weeks' gestation, but is not relevant when the woman is at 37 weeks' gestation. Note familial history, including cardiac disease, diabetes, and bleeding disorders. The woman may also be affected by her mother's obstetric history. There is a familial predisposition to develop preeclampsia. The medical and genetic history of the birth parents serves to guide counseling and testing for predisposed genetic complications. The family history is the most important source of genetic information. The ideal time for genetic screening is before attempting pregnancy. Although general population screening is not considered appropriate, Williams and Lea (2003) recommend

DISPLAY 5-3

Spotlight on Thrombophilias

Thrombophilia is a genetic disorder common in women with unexplained recurrent pregnancy loss and possibly other serious complications, although the precise risk is unknown (Robertson, Wu, & Greer, 2004). The prevalence is as high as 65% in selected populations. The available evidence suggests an increased risk throughout pregnancy, although the risk may be higher during the second and third trimesters. The ACOG guidelines state that Protein C, protein S, AT III, FVL, PT gene mutation, and MTHFR gene mutation have been associated with severe early preeclampsia, unexplained fetal loss or stillbirth, and placental abruption (ACOG, 2000). Thrombophilic disorders are found in up to 20% of women with normal pregnancies, suggesting additional risk factors are required for the development of complications (Robertson et al., 2004). Because the probability of a successful pregnancy outcome is still high, *routine* screening of all pregnant women is **not** recommended. There is currently no consensus on the indications for screening. The ACOG practice guidelines suggest that women with recurrent fetal loss, early or severe preeclampsia, or severe unexplained intrauterine growth restriction be offered screening for antiphospholipid antibodies because prophylactic anticoagulation use in these patients has been shown to improve pregnancy outcome (ACOG, 2000). The most recent data would suggest that screening for genetic thrombophilia is not required for patients with a history of recurrent early (less than 10 weeks) losses (Lockwood, 2002).

that persons with the following conditions be offered genetic screening:

- Developmental disability of unknown etiology, including women with developmental disabilities who present for preconception or prenatal care
- Autism
- Unexplained mental retardation or developmental delay, particularly if the member of the family is related to the patient through females
- Family history of fragile X syndrome
- Family history that suggests increased risk for specific autosomal recessive disease

Probably the most common indications for genetic counseling and prenatal diagnosis are maternal age and abnormal maternal serum screening. If the initial prenatal risk assessment reveals factors that carry risk for the baby (eg, Tay-Sachs, sickle cell disease/trait, thalassemia, and cystic fibrosis), the woman (and her partner) should be offered genetic counseling and additional testing if the woman so desires.

Genetic counseling has grown into a well-recognized specialty. Our understanding of genetics and genomics in healthcare has changed in recent years, however. Genetic conditions inherited in families are caused by gene mutations present on one or both chromosomes of a pair. The three main patterns of Mendelian inheritance are autosomal dominant, autosomal recessive, and X-linked (see Fig. 5–1). The term "genomics" refers to the study of all the genes in the human genome together, including their interactions with each other and the environment (Feetham, Thomson, & Hinshaw, 2005). Genes can cause diseases, and they also may affect disease susceptibility and resistance, prognosis and progression, and responses to illnesses and their treatments. For example, a genetic test for cystic fibrosis (CF) mutations has been developed and is beginning to be widely used for preconception, prenatal, and postnatal diagnostic testing. In 1989, the gene associated

with CF was identified on chromosome number 7. At the time, a single mutation, a three base-pair deletion, was found to account for about half of the people in the United States with CF. As a more diverse population has been tested, more than a thousand mutations have been described in the CF gene, accounting for 90% of classical CF. The findings conclude that (a) not all people with "classical CF" have been found to have mutations in cystic fibrosis transmembrane conductance regulator (CFTR); (b) people with the same CFTR mutations can have quite different courses of disease even when they are from the same family; (c) not all people who have two mutations in their CFTR gene have "classical CF"; and (d) the frequency of CF mutations varies from one population group to another(eg, Ashkenazi Jewish, 1 in 29; European Caucasian, 1 in 29; Hispanic-American, 1 in 46; African-American, 1 in 65; Asian-American, 1 in 90 [ACOG, 2005a]). This range results in variable testing sensitivity, specificity, and predictive value of the genetic test (Feetham, Thomson, & Hinshaw, 2005).

As knowledge of the behavioral, environmental, and genetic mechanisms of disease increases, individuals and families will need to reframe their concepts and experiences with diagnosis, treatment, and prevention (Feetham, Thomson, & Hinshaw, 2005). Therefore, individualized education, planning, and support are vital to the process of genetic counseling. Genetic counseling and fetal surveillance techniques forces a woman (and her partner) to consider the amount and kind of information desired, subsequent decisions related to that information, and what those decisions may reflect about their self-image and personal values. Nurses are knowledgeable, nonthreatening confidants as the woman and her partner sort through the information and decision-making. Nurses, therefore, need to be cognizant of the benefits, limitations, and social implications of the counseling and testing process.

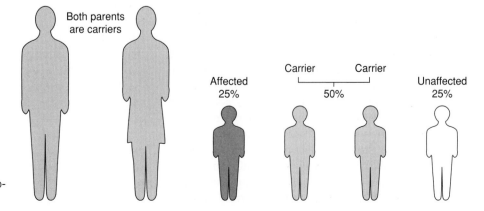

FIGURE 5–1. The inheritance pattern of offspring when both parents are carriers of an autosomal recessive gene.

Lifestyle Factors

Lifestyle or behavioral factors significantly affect women's health in general and perinatal health specifically. Living conditions, marital status, occupation, nutrition, and use of tobacco, alcohol, and illicit substances can all affect pregnancy outcome. Socioeconomic factors may influence gestational age at entry to prenatal care, nutritional status, and availability of support systems. Number of years of completed maternal education has been correlated with birth weight, perinatal mortality and morbidity, and neonatal neurologic sequelae. In general, as years of maternal education increase, incidence of perinatal mortality and morbidity decrease. Not surprising, adolescents are more likely to begin prenatal care later than adults (March of Dimes, 2006). Pregnant women who have more education are more likely to start prenatal care early and have more visits. Between 1989 and 1997, the percentage of women with delayed prenatal care or no prenatal care decreased from 25% to 18%, with improvement in both delayed prenatal care (from 22% to 16%) and in no prenatal care (from 2% to 1%). Groups more likely to have delayed or no prenatal care between 1989 and 1997 included non-Hispanic blacks, Hispanics, women aged <20 years, women with <12 years of education, and multiparous women (CDC, 2000). This association may be a reflection of education as an indicator of socioeconomic status. Women in lower socioeconomic groups tend to initiate prenatal care later than their middle socioeconomic group counterparts. The three most common reasons for late entry into care are (a) no knowledge that she was pregnant; (b) financial barriers; and (c) inability to get an appointment (CDC, 2000).

The marital status of the mother and the presence of the father as related to perinatal outcome are complex social phenomenons. Findings of older studies demonstrated an increase in perinatal morbidity and mortality associated with single motherhood (Bennett, Braveman, Egerter, & Kiely, 1994; Cooperstock, Bakewell, Herman, & Schramm, 1998; Hein, Burmeister, & Papke, 1990; Luo, Wilkins, & Kramer, 2004; Mathews, MacDorman, & Menacker, 2002). That unmarried mothers often are younger, are less well educated, and have a lower socioeconomic status than married mothers was controlled for in the older studies. More recently, births to women who live in an intimate relationship with a partner but without legal marriage have become increasingly common and widely accepted in many Western societies. However, pregnancy outcomes are worse among mothers in common-law unions versus traditional marriage relationships. Raatikainen, Heiskanen, and Heinonen (2005) found an overall 20% increase of adverse outcomes in unmarried, cohabiting mothers, and that free maternity care did not overcome the difference. The highest incidence of perinatal morbidity and loss occurs in families where the father is not present (Luo et al., 2004).

Teratogen Exposure

The cause of congenital malformations can be divided into three categories: unknown, genetic, and environmental. The cause of a majority of human malformations is unknown. More than 50 teratogenic environmental drugs, chemicals, and physical agents have been described using modern epidemiologic tools and clinical dysmorphology (see Appendices 5–A and 5–B). Severe congenital malformations occur in 3% of births. According to the CDC (Martin et al., 2006), severe congenital malformations include birth defects that cause death, hospitalization, mental retardation; necessitate significant or repeated surgical procedures; are disfiguring; or interfere with physical performance. Each year in the United States, 120,000 newborns are born with severe birth defects. Genetic diseases occur in approximately 11% of births (Brent, 2004). Careful assessment of the woman's daily routine provides valuable information about potential teratogen exposure.

Counseling regarding possible teratogenic influences should be performed in a factual yet sympathetic and supportive way so the woman is not unduly alarmed or burdened with guilt (ACOG, 1997). Nurses should also be cognizant of the common potential teratogens in the population for which they provide care. For example, if the majority of the women come from an urban setting in which it is known that lead exposure is problematic, the history should include special attention to the risk. Maternal blood lead levels of approximately 10 mcg/dL have been linked to increased risks of pregnancy hypertension, spontaneous abortion, and reduced neurobehavioral development in the child. Some studies suggest that higher maternal lead levels are linked to reduced fetal growth and a link between increased parental lead exposure and congenital malformations, although uncertainty remains regarding the specific malformations and the dose–response relationships (Bellinger, 2005).

Teratogen exposure may be associated with an occupation (eg, x-rays, chemicals, viruses) or a lifestyle. Alcohol is a potent teratogen in humans, and prenatal alcohol exposure is a leading preventable cause of birth defects and developmental disabilities. Substance use and abuse may have disastrous effects in pregnancy, affecting all body systems and causing cardiac, pulmonary, gastrointestinal, and psychiatric complications. Illicit drug use is highest among women during their peak childbearing years (Misra, 2001). Screening for alcohol and substance use and abuse is discussed in more detail later in this chapter.

Assess use of prescription or over-the-counter medications and use of complementary and alternative therapies such as herbs, homeopathy, and folk remedies. This provides nurses with a more complete picture of the woman's approach to heathcare and allows them to identify potentially harmful practices. If there is a potential substance or practice about which there is a question of teratogenicity, nurses can contact the Organization of Teratology Information Services at its toll-free number ([866] 626-OTIS or [866] 626-6847) or visit www.otispregnancy.org for more information. This organization is a national service that can answers questions or refer pregnant women or nurses to local resources.

Nutrition

The impact of nutrition on maternal and fetal well-being cannot be underestimated. The special physiology of a woman creates variable nutrient requirements during different stages of the life cycle. Nutritional practices influence every pregnancy, as well as a woman's risk for diabetes mellitus, cardiovascular disease, osteoporosis, and several types of cancer. Specific complications of pregnancy, such as pre-eclampsia, preterm birth, intrauterine growth retardation, and low-birth-weight infants with associated detrimental outcomes, can be correlated to nutritional status. A healthy, well-nourished woman has a surplus of all nutrients. Many women in the United States do not consume the recommended daily allowance (LeMone, 1999). For example, preconception deficiencies in folic acid may have devastating effects in the formation of neural tube defects in the baby (March of Dimes, 1999). Folic acid requirements, essential for red blood cell production, are increased to 5 to 10 times normal during pregnancy, and dietary intake may not meet these requirements. A surplus of nutrients can be crucial during the first trimester of pregnancy, when the ability to eat is impaired by hormonal shifts and the tissues and organs of the embryo are being differentiated.

In 1990, the Institute of Medicine (IOM) issued guidelines that recommend an optimal weight gain range for women based on their prepregnancy body-mass index (BMI) [see Table 5–1]. Normal-weighted women (BMI=19.8–25) who gain the recommended weight during pregnancy have the lowest risk for pregnancy–birth complications (Thorsdottir, Torfadottir, Birgisdottir, et al., 2002). Women gaining either above or below IOM guidelines have higher risks of adverse outcomes. Stotland et al. (2005) found that prepregnancy BMI was the strongest predictor of maternal target weight gain outside the IOM guidelines. Observational studies have found that prenatal weight gains below the recommended range are associated with low birth weight and preterm birth. Weight gains above the recommended range are associated with increased risk of macrosomia, cesarean birth, and postpartum weight retention (Abrams, Altman, & Pickett, 2000). Women with low BMIs are more likely to gain below the guidelines. Conversely, women with high BMIs had the highest risk for excessive weight gain (see Display 5–4 for more information about obesity and pregnancy). However, a woman should be evaluated for what factors may be causing her to have excessively high or low gain (eg, lack of money to buy food, stress, presence of infection, or other medical problems) in order to determine a meaningful, personalized recommendation.

Nurses should pay special attention to women with lower educational status with regard to weight gain and nutritional counseling. People with poor health literacy have lower health knowledge, health status, and use of health services. Less-educated women or those who reported *provider advice to gain less than the guidelines* were significantly more likely to have a target weight gain below the IOM guidelines (Stotland et al., 2005). Researchers also found that African-American and Latina women were more likely than white women to report a target weight gain below the IOM guidelines, even when controlling for educational status (Stotland et al., 2005).

The IOM (1990), supported by AAP and ACOG (2002), recommends a weight gain for women that is based on their prepregnant weights and single births (Table 5–1). A weight gain of 35 to 45 pounds

TABLE 5–1 ■ RECOMMENDATIONS FOR WEIGHT GAIN DURING PREGNANCY

Prepregnant Status	BMI	Weight Gain (Pounds/Kilograms)
Underweight	<19.8	28–40 lb (12.7–18.2 kg) (body weight +25 lbs)
Average weight	19.8–25	25–35 lb (11.4–15.9 kg)
Overweight	25–29	15–25 lb (6.8–11.4 kg)
Obese	>29	15 lb (6.8 kg)
Twin gestation	—	35–45 lb (15.9–20.4 kg)

From Institute of Medicine. (1990). *Nutrition during pregnancy.* Washington, DC: National Academy Press; and from American College of Obstetricians and Gynecologists. (1993). *Nutrition during pregnancy* (Technical Bulletin No. 179). Washington, DC: Author.

DISPLAY 5-4

Spotlight on Obesity in Pregnancy

Obesity in pregnancy has garnered more attention as American obesity rates have risen. Obesity is a chronic multifactorial disease that affects 61% of the American population. The definition of overweight is a BMI: 25 kg/m²–29.9 kg/m², and the definition of obese is a BMI of ≥30 kg/m². Specific risks associated with obesity and pregnancy are summarized as follows (Gray, Power, Zinberg, & Schulkin, 2006; Hall & Neubert, 2005):

1. Increased rates of gestational diabetes, gestational hypertension and preeclampsia, antepartum venous thromboembolism, and excessive weight gain
2. Higher likelihood of requiring labor induction and cesarean delivery
3. Fetuses that are large for gestational age and macrosomic, increasing the risk of shoulder dystocia during the second stage of labor
4. Increased term antepartum stillbirth (Silver, 2007; Stephansson, Dickman, Johansson, & Cnattingius, 2001)

5. Postpartum hemorrhage, wound infections, and longer hospital stays
6. More difficulty losing weight after delivery, contributing to increased overweight and obesity postpartum
7. Increased risk of gestational diabetes during a second pregnancy
8. Babies who have an increased risk of neural tube defects and central nervous system defects
9. Delayed lactogenesis

Obesity may also be an independent risk factor in infant mortality. Comorbidities that may be life-threatening include coronary artery disease, type 2 diabetes, and sleep apnea. Comorbidities that may increase risk during pregnancy but are not life-threatening include osteoarthritis, gallstones, stress incontinence, and gynecologic abnormalities.

Obese women should be encouraged to lose weight prior to pregnancy and should not attempt to lose weight while pregnant. Current approaches during pregnancy include giving information on maternal and fetal risks, perform a transumbilical ultrasound to visualize fetal anatomy as necessary, conduct an early screening for gestational diabetes, encourage more frequent visits to detect preeclampsia, schedule an anesthesia consult in early labor, and explain antithrombotic precautions.

Gray, A. D., Power, M. L., Zinberg, S., & Schulkin, J. (2006). Assessment and management of obesity. *Obstetrical and Gynecological Survey, 61*(11), 742–748.
Hall, L., & Neubert, A. G. (2005). Obesity and pregnancy. *Obstetrical and Gynecological Survey, 60*(4), 253–260.

is recommended for women with twins (IOM, 1990). Weight gain should be carefully monitored during each prenatal visit. Weight gain or loss may be indicative of maternal nutritional status or development of complications. Excessive weight gain, excessive weight loss, or inadequate weight gain indicates a need for consultation with a nutritionist. The *pattern* of weight gain is as important as the *total amount*. Early studies indicated that second-trimester weight gain was more predictive of infant birth weight than total maternal weight gain (Abrams et al., 2000; Hickey, Cliver, McNeal, Hoffman, & Goldenberg, 1996; Li, Haas, & Habicht, 1998; Strauss & Dietz, 1999). These studies relied on maternal recall to determine pregravid weight. However, when prepregnancy weight was prospectively measured, maternal weight change during the first trimester more strongly influences newborn size than does weight change during the second or third trimester (Brown, Murtaugh, Jacobs, & Margellos, 2002).

Nutritional care during the antepartum period should include assessment of nutritional risk factors, nutritional assessment, nutritional knowledge, and nutrient supplements, as appropriate. Some risk factors for nutritional problems include adolescence, low income, cigarette smoking, substance use or abuse, history of frequent dieting, vegan diet, pica, high parity, physical or mental illness (including depression), use of certain medications such as phenytoin, mental retardation, chronic diseases, and disordered eating.

The nutrition assessment includes diet intake information (3-day recall), monitoring weight gain, and hematologic assessment. Assessment of usual dietary patterns provides a basis for understanding nutritional health. Variations from the normal dietary routine, such as eating disorders, food shortages, and metabolic disorders such as diabetes, warrant additional interventions. Women who have eating disorders may be reticent to reveal this information. This assessment may require a number of prenatal visits and a building of a trusting relationship between the nurse and the woman. After an eating disorder is revealed, the nurse should ask the woman how she manages eating food and meals, as well as what her attitude is toward eating (eg, preoccupation with food, feeling guilty after eating, engaging in dieting, enjoyment of food).

The current dietary recommendations developed by the IOM include (a) increased intake of protein from 60 to 80 g/day; (b) 300 additional calories per day; (c) increased iron intake from 18 to 27 g/day; and (d) increased folate consumption from 400 to 600 mcg/day (1992). The recommended amount of calcium for women ages 19 to 50, pregnant or not, is

1,000 mg/day; for adolescents up to age 18, it is 1,300 mg daily. Nurses should encourage women to consume a variety of foods, eat at regular intervals (three meals a day and snacks), drink milk two to three times per day, reduce caffeine, and avoid alcohol. Common discomforts (eg, nausea and vomiting of pregnancy, heartburn, and varied reactions to taste or smell of food) can prove challenging to the woman who is trying to follow pregnancy dietary recommendations. Knowledge of safe remedies is the basis for advice when helping women with these discomforts. For example, acupressure wristbands and small, frequent feedings can be of help to some women to decrease nausea.

Another aspect of the nutritional assessment is the use of vitamins and herbs. Because herbs and vitamins are considered dietary supplements, these products are not regulated in the same manner that prescription and over-the-counter medications are. Often the products are labeled as "natural," and the woman may conclude that the product is therefore not harmful. Excesses of one nutrient can alter the need for, absorption of, or use of other nutrients. Supernutrient regimens or megadoses of vitamins (especially those that are fat soluble) may be harmful and cannot ensure a healthy pregnancy.

Many pregnant women experience pica or olfactory cravings during pregnancy. Some women are embarrassed to tell the nurse about these cravings, yet they may significantly interfere with dietary intake of proper nutrients during pregnancy. Pica and olfactory cravings are not limited to any one group, educational level, race, ethnic group, income level, or religious belief (Cooksey, 1995; Corbett, Ryan, & Weinrich, 2003); however, the type of substance ingested does seem to be culturally influenced (Simpson, Mull, & East, 2000). Pagophagia (eating ice) seems to be common among those with pica. The exact mechanism is unknown, but pagophagia is frequently associated with disordered eating and anemia (Parry-Jones, 1992). In the United States, the practice of pica during pregnancy is linked to lower-income women, African-American heritage, family or personal history of pica during childhood or before pregnancy, strong cravings during pregnancy, and cultural groups that endorse pica during pregnancy as important for fertility and femininity (Corbett et al., 2003). As a part of nutrition assessment, nurses should question (in a nonjudgmental style) patients at each prenatal visit regarding pica practice. Pica may be practiced for cultural or other reasons unknown to nurses. Working with patients to discover what they are eating, and helping them to substitute foods with nutritional value, can be a part of a nursing care plan that results in a positive pregnancy outcome (Corbett et al., 2003).

Occupation

Women in low-income positions or employed as unskilled laborers are at increased risk for preterm labor. A meta-analysis of working conditions and pregnancy outcome showed a significant positive association between preterm birth and physically demanding work, shift work, standing for longer than 3 hours/day or standing as the predominant occupational posture, and a high cumulative work fatigue score. Additionally, physically demanding work is positively associated with small for gestational age babies, hypertension, and/or preeclampsia. Working long hours was not associated with an adverse pregnancy outcome (Mozurkewich, Luke, Avni, & Wolf, 2000). However, decreasing or eliminating work during pregnancy may place the woman at greater socioeconomic risk by threatening her livelihood. Activities that cause excessive fatigue, such as heavy work; job-related stress; or daily automobile, train, or bus commutes, may stimulate uterine contractions and increase the risk of perinatal complication (Papiernik, 1993). Areas to ask about in the nature of the woman's job include whether she sits or stands continuously, lifts heavy objects, perceives problems with ventilation, and is exposed to toxic chemicals or radiation. Hobbies and the home environment should be assessed also. Household tasks may be a source of fatigue equal to or greater than job-related fatigue.

Psychosocial Screening

Psychosocial screening of every woman presenting for prenatal care is an important step toward improving the woman's health and the birth outcome. In this way, the nurse can identify areas of concern, validate major issues, and make suggestions for possible changes. Depending on the nature of the identified problem, a referral may be made to an appropriate member of the healthcare team. A woman may be reluctant to share information until a trusting relationship has been formed. Questions asked at the first prenatal visit bear repeating with ongoing prenatal care. The woman may need reassurance as to the confidentiality of the information. For example, if she reveals she uses cocaine, would she be turned over to the judicial system and possibly jailed? Nurses are obligated to know how to answer the woman when these issues arise.

Pregnancy affects the entire family, and, therefore, assessment and intervention must be considered in a family-centered perspective. Stress has been suggested as a potential contributor to preterm birth and physical complications during pregnancy and birth, including prolonged labor, increased use of intrapartum analgesics and barbiturates, and other complications. Unusual stressful events, such as the death of a significant family member or friend, job loss, or a problematic relationship with the baby's father may increase risk of poor pregnancy outcome. Home conditions (eg, private or government housing), quality of comfort (eg, heat, water), housekeeping burden, and number and age of previous children influence stress levels. Nurses should be aware that many women continue to work under hazardous or stressful conditions out of economic necessity, but that they will attempt to minimize any known risk factors as much as possible. Additionally, nurses should assess how the woman appraises her situation (eg, what one woman finds stressful, another may not). Nurses should identify resources available to the pregnant woman (eg, support groups, social worker, counselor, etc.).

Symptoms of dysfunctional family relationships, such as violence toward the pregnant woman, child abuse, or psychosomatic illnesses, are also indicative of risk and warrant investigation. Intimate partner violence is a serious problem in the United States. It is estimated that approximately 4.4 million women are battered each year; more than one-third of adult women's emergency room visits are related to injuries from a current or former spouse or intimate partner (AWHONN, 2004). Domestic violence against women covers a broad spectrum of behaviors, including actual or threatened physical, sexual, or psychological abuse between family members or intimate partners.

In a study of pregnant adolescents, those who had suffered from abuse gave birth to infants with significantly lower birth weights than those who were not abused (Renker, 1999). They also had significantly more miscarriages, substance use, and triage visits during pregnancy. Identification of adolescents dealing with abuse and their social resources during pregnancy may enhance prediction of infants at high risk as well as provide opportunities for intervention.

Abused women frequently state that they are concerned that their healthcare providers will report their abuse to the police and that this inhibits them from disclosing abuse when asked (Geilen et al., 2000, Renker, 2003). Consequently, true numbers for abuse during pregnancy are difficult to determine. However, prevalence studies indicate that the rate ranges between 4% and 8%. Some of the presenting patterns include the following:

- Unwanted pregnancy
- Late entry into prenatal care, missed appointments
- Substance use or abuse
- Poor weight gain and nutrition
- Multiple, repeated somatic complaints (AAP & ACOG, 2002)

Yost and colleagues (2005) surveyed 16,041 women presenting to a labor and delivery unit. Researchers found that when compared with women denying domestic violence, women ($n = 949$) reporting verbal abuse had an increased rate of low-birth-weight infants, and neonatal deaths were significantly increased in women experiencing physical abuse. Second, women who declined to participate ($n = 94$) in their survey were found to have significantly increased rates of a variety of pregnancy complications that adversely affected their infants' outcomes (Yost, Bloom, McIntire, & Leveno, 2005).

AWHONN (2004) strongly urges nurses to take the time to ask their patients whether they are safe in their homes, particularly if patients present with injuries. Integrating a standardized screening protocol into routine history-taking procedures increases identification, documentation, and referral for intimate partner violence. The following standardized screening questions have a sensitivity of 65% to 70% and a specificity of 80% to 85%: (a) Have you been hit, kicked, or otherwise hurt by someone within the past year?; (b) Do you feel safe in your current relationship?; and (c) Is there a partner from a previous relationship who is making you feel unsafe now? (Feldhaus et al., 1997; McFarlane, Parker, Soeken, & Bullock, 1992). There is no single profile of the woman who suffers abuse, and the abuse is likely to continue or escalate during pregnancy (AAP & ACOG, 2002).

Assessing for abuse carries the responsibility of intervention if abuse is identified or suspected. At minimum, nurses should have referral sources readily available. Nurses should document the frequency and severity of present and past abuse (using patient quotes as much as possible), location and extent of injuries, treatments, interventions, escape plan, and educational materials (including phone numbers to a shelter and the police). Discuss a plan of escape and document whether shelter assistance was declined or accepted by the woman. For more information on this important topic and a Domestic Violence and Abuse Assessment Screening tool (The Nursing Network on Violence Against Women, International [NNVAWI], 2003), the reader is directed to www.nnvawi.org/assessment.htm.

Addressing psychosocial issues during pregnancy has the potential to reduce costs to the individual and to society (ACOG, 2006; AWHONN, 2004). A simple screening system was developed by the Healthy Start Program of the Florida Department of Health and has been refined and in use since 1992. This tool is a concise (nine questions) way to open the questioning about perinatal psychosocial risk factors (Display 5–5). If the patient answers in a way indicative of risk to any of the questions, the nurse can further explore the topic with the woman.

Major depression is one of the most frequently encountered medical complications in pregnancy, and the risk for depression increases even more during the

DISPLAY 5-5

Psychosocial Screening Tool

1. Yes   No   Do you have any problems (job, transportation, etc.) that prevent you from keeping your healthcare appointments?

2. Yes   No   Do you feel unsafe where you live?

3. Yes   No   In the past 2 months, have you used any form of tobacco?

4. Yes   No   In the past 2 months, have you used drugs or alcohol (including beer, wine, or mixed drinks)?

5. Yes   No   In the past year, have you been threatened, hit, slapped, or kicked by anyone you know?

6. Yes   No   Has anyone forced you to perform any sexual act that you did not want to do?

7. On a 1 to 5 scale, how do you rate your current stress level?

1	2	3	4	5
Low				High

8. How many times have you moved in the past 12 months? _____

9. If you could change the timing of this pregnancy, would you want it
   earlier
   later
   not at all
   no change

American College of Obstetricians and Gynecologists. (2006). *Psychosocial risk factors: Perinatal screening and intervention* (Committee Opinion No. 343) Washington, DC: Author.

---

postpartum period (Robertson, Grace, Wallington, & Stewart, 2004). Clinical depression is defined as any period of unremitting sadness, unhappiness, or loss of pleasure in once pleasurable activities that has lasted for two weeks or more and impairs the ability to function (Misra & Kostaras, 2001). Women suffer from depression at twice the rate of men (Altshuler et al., 2001). Depression in pregnancy is associated with greater maternal lifestyle risks, increased incidence of postpartum depression, suicide, and adverse birth outcomes (Beck, 2002; DaCosta, Larouche, Dritsa, & Brender, 2000; Misra & Kostaras, 2001; Orr, James, & Prince, 2002). The impact of depression during pregnancy is significant for the mother and to her baby. Researchers during the past decade have identified that untreated maternal depression that extends into the postpartum period has a negative effect on the emotional, cognitive, and developmental growth of young infants

(Misra & Kostaras, 2001). While it is unclear as to why pregnancy and childbirth represent a time of increased vulnerability for the onset or exacerbation of depression, it may be that it is the combination of hormonal shifts, neuroendocrine changes, and psychosocial adjustments (Misra & Kostaras, 2001).

The prevalence of depression in pregnancy ranges from 6.9% to 20% (Mian, 2005). In spite of the high risk for depression during pregnancy, many clinicians are limited in their ability to recognize, diagnose, and offer appropriate treatment. Kelly, Zatzick, and Anders (2001) found that only one in five women being seen in obstetrical practices who screened positive for a psychiatric disorder or substance use had any evidence of treatment in their charts.

Brief screens for symptoms of depression in pregnancy during the initial interview assist clinicians in identifying pregnant women who have symptoms of depression. Effective identification of depression in obstetrical practice meets Healthy People 2010's (HHS, 2000) recommendation for additional research to discover health indicators that place women at risk in pregnancy. The U.S. Preventive Task Force (Pignone et al., 2002) recommended that the following two questions be part of the basic repertoire of every adult patient visit:

- "Over the past 2 weeks have you felt down, depressed, or hopeless?"
- "Over the past 2 weeks, have you felt little interest in doing things?"

Jesse and Graham (2005) validated the use of these two questions in pregnancy; sensitivity was 91%, and specificity was 52%. If the responses are positive, nurses must assess the patient's safety (ie, risk of suicide). These questions can be the first step in determining which women should be referred for a clinical diagnostic evaluation by a psychiatric nurse practitioner, social worker, psychologist, or a psychiatrist. For some women, a pregnancy support group may be helpful. Women who are diagnosed with depression during pregnancy should be followed carefully for postpartum depression. Predisposing risk factors for the development of postpartum depression have been identified (Display 5–6).

It is possible to identify prenatally women who are at risk for experiencing parenting difficulties. Asking the woman how she thinks her pregnancy is progressing and questions about her preparations for the care of the baby opens up areas of discussion that may provide insight into positive or negative reactions to the experience of pregnancy and preparation for parenthood. The woman is given the opportunity to verbalize thoughts about the changes she is experiencing, fantasies about the baby, and acceptance of pregnancy and the child by the family.

DISPLAY 5-6

Predisposing Factors for Postpartum Depression

Depression during pregnancy
Not being married or cohabiting with partner
Poor social support
Low socioeconomic status
Birth complications
Smoking
Multiparity
BMI >30
Stressful life event during pregnancy and/or puerperium

- Loss of loved one (fetus, newborn, partner, or other child)
- Illness of partner, parent, or child
- Financial difficulties
- Job loss
- Move of household

Nausea, vomiting, fatigue in early pregnancy (unclear as to whether depression results or precedes these symptoms)

Adapted from: Andersson L., Sundstrom-Poromaa, I., Wulff, M., Astrom, M., & Bixo, M. (2004). Implications of antenatal depression and anxiety for obstetric outcome. *Obstetrics and Gynecology, 104*(3), 467–476; and Johnstone, S. J., Boyce, P. M., Hickey, A. R., Morris-Yates, A. D., & Harris, M. G. (2001). Obstetric risk factors for postnatal depression in urban and rural community samples. *Australian & New Zealand Journal of Psychiatry, 35*(1), 69–74.

Substance Abuse

Alcohol use has been identified as the leading preventable cause of birth defects (Sidhu, 2005). The National Institute on Drug Abuse suggest that more than 1 million children per year are exposed to alcohol and illicit drugs during gestation (VSDHHS, 2005). At least one in ten women will continue to consume alcohol during pregnancy, putting her fetus at risk for the effects of alcohol exposure (HHS, 2005). Fetal alcohol syndrome (FAS) has four criteria: maternal drinking during pregnancy, a characteristic pattern of facial abnormalities, growth retardation, and brain damage (often manifested by intellectual difficulties or behavioral problems). As surveillance and research have progressed, it has become clear that FAS is a rare example of a wide array of defects that can occur from fetal exposure to alcohol (Krulewitch, 2005).

Illicit drug use is highest among women during their peak childbearing years (Misra, 2001). Substance abuse or chemical dependency affects all body systems and can cause cardiac, pulmonary, gastrointestinal, and psychiatric complications. Use of unsterile drug paraphernalia contributes to infection and disease transmission. Substance abusers rarely abuse a single substance (Chasnoff, Neuman, Thornton, & Callaghan, 2001). The woman's lifestyle when using drugs, which may include alcohol abuse, cigarette smoking, poor nutrition, and sexual promiscuity, further complicates the pregnancy.

Using a diverse sample, Chasnoff and colleagues (2005) developed a five-item brief screening instrument, 4Ps Plus©, to identify pregnant women at highest risk for substance use receiving prenatal care. The questions are easily integrated into prenatal care. The four screening questions are aimed at the following:

1. Parents: Did either of your parents ever have a problem with alcohol or drugs?
2. Partner: Does your partner have a problem with alcohol or drugs?
3. Past: Have you ever drunk beer, wine, or liquor?
4. Pregnancy: In the month before you knew you were pregnant, how many cigarettes did you smoke? In the month before you knew you were pregnant, how many beers/how much wine/how much liquor did you drink?

The women fall into low-, average-, and high-risk categories based on these questions. High-risk are those women who used any alcohol or smoked three or more cigarettes in the month before pregnancy: 34% of women in the high-risk group were found to be using either illicit drugs or alcohol or both during the time they were pregnant. The rate of use for cocaine, heroin, and methamphetamine was 1% after awareness of pregnancy and of women continuing to consume alcohol; the majority drank less than 2 days per week. Because substance abuse or chemical dependency can adversely affect the health of the woman and the fetus, it is essential to include drug use assessment and education strategies in prenatal and women's healthcare encounters (see Display 5–7).

Cigarette Smoking

Cigarette smoking has been linked to an increased incidence of low birth weight and prematurity (ACOG, 2001b; 2005b). In the United States, among women age 15 to 44, combined data for 2003 and 2004 indicated that 18% of those who were pregnant smoked cigarettes in the past month compared with 30% of those who were not pregnant. Rates of past-month cigarette smoking were lower for pregnant than for non-pregnant women among those age 26 to 44 (11.7% vs. 29.1%) and among those age 18 to 25 (28% vs. 36.3%). However, among those age 15 to 17, the rate of cigarette smoking for pregnant women was higher than for non-pregnant women (26% vs. 19.6%), although the difference was not significant (HHS, 2005).

DISPLAY 5-7

Spotlight on Methamphetamine Use in Pregnancy

Methamphetamine is a powerfully addictive stimulant with a high potential for abuse. It stimulates the central nervous system, producing increasing alertness, sleeplessness, euphoria, and exhilaration. It has become popular because it is easy to make and use. Methamphetamines metabolize slowly; a methamphetamine high lasts 8 to 24 hours, whereas the effects of cocaine last only 20 to 30 minutes. Maternal methamphetamine use is associated with risk factors such as poverty, chaotic and dangerous lifestyles, symptoms of psychopathology, history of childhood sexual abuse, and involvement in difficult or abusive relationships with male partners (Wouldes, LaGasse,

Sheridan, & Lester, 2004). Pregnant women who use methamphetamines tend to be young, single, and report psychological morbidity, and have a clustering of risk factors that may compromise the pregnancy and fetus. Smoking, heavy alcohol intake, and polydrug use, combined with a higher than expected rate of unplanned pregnancies, increases the risk of fetal exposure to potentially harmful substances (Ho, Karimi-Tabesh, & Koren, 2001). Methamphetamine use during pregnancy has been associated with decreased growth in infants exposed only for the first two trimesters. Exposed newborns were found to be significantly smaller for gestational age compared with the unexposed group; 4% required pharmacologic intervention for withdrawal from methamphetamine. Tobacco exposure combined with methamphetamine resulted in a decreased growth relative to infants exposed to methamphetamine alone (Smith et al., 2003). Additionally, clefting, cardiac anomalies, and fetal growth reduction deficits have been seen in infants exposed to amphetamines during pregnancy (Marwick, 2000).

From a preventive perspective, it is not enough to discourage smoking in pregnant women. The focus must be on discouraging smoking in any woman of childbearing age who may potentially become pregnant. Smoking during pregnancy presents major, avoidable health risks to the fetus. Smoking has been linked to increased risk of miscarriage, intrauterine growth restriction, low birth weight and very low birth weight, preterm labor and premature birth, placenta previa, placental abruption, perinatal loss, and Sudden Infant Death Syndrome. Infants and young children are affected by environmental tobacco smoke, which has been linked with an increased risk of lower respiratory infections in children, fluid in the middle ear, symptoms of upper respiratory tract irritation, reduced lung function, and additional episodes and increased severity of asthma in children (AWHONN, 2000).

The risk of fetal death is typically 1.5-fold over non-smokers; the risk decreases to that of non-smokers in women who stop smoking after the first trimester (Silver, 2007). Infants who live with a smoker face an increased risk of sudden infant death syndrome. During pregnancy, many women are more highly motivated to stop or decrease their smoking; however, simply providing information may not be enough for the pregnant woman with a long history of smoking. Healthcare professionals should routinely screen pregnant clients and women of childbearing age for tobacco use and should implement evidence-based smoking-cessation strategies appropriate for pregnant women and women who may become pregnant. Counseling interventions of at

least 10 minutes have been shown to increase quit rates (AWHONN, 2000). One evidence-based approach is the "5 A's." In practices that have used the 5 A's approach, quit rates among pregnant women have risen by 30% or more (Martin et al., 2006). This approach to smoking cessation is easily integrated into prenatal care.

- *Ask:* ask the patient to choose a statement that best describes her smoking status
- *Advise:* ask permission to share the health message about smoking during pregnancy
- *Assess:* readiness to change
- *Assist:* briefly explore problem-solving methods and skills for smoking cessation
- *Arrange:* let the woman know that you will be following up on each visit; assess smoking status at subsequent prenatal visits; affirm efforts to quit

This 5 to 15 minute intervention is most effective with pregnant women who smoke fewer than 20 cigarettes per day. The nurse can give pregnant smokers personalized messages about the health risks that smoking poses and self-help materials developed specifically for pregnant smokers. Each step has detailed information to guide use (Washington State Department of Health, 2002). The program is described and available to the reader at: www.doh.wa.gov/CFH/mch/documents/CessationFinal_122.pdf

Physical Activity

Despite the fact that pregnancy is associated with profound anatomical and physiological changes, exercise

DISPLAY 5 - 8

Exercise During Pregnancy

ABSOLUTE CONTRAINDICATIONS TO AEROBIC EXERCISE DURING PREGNANCY

- Hemodynamically significant heart disease
- Restrictive lung disease
- Incompetent cervix/cerclage
- Multiple gestation at risk for premature labor
- Persistent second- or third-trimester bleeding
- Placenta previa after 26 weeks' gestation
- Premature labor during the current pregnancy
- Ruptured membranes
- Preeclampsia/pregnancy-induced hyertension

RELATIVE CONTRAINDICATIONS TO AEROBIC EXERCISE DURING PREGNANCY

- Severe anemia
- Unevaluated maternal cardiac arrhythmia
- Chronic bronchitis

- Poorly controlled type 1 diabetes
- Extreme morbid obesity
- Extreme underweight (BMI <12)
- History of extremely sedentary lifestyle
- Intrauterine growth restriction in current pregnancy
- Poorly controlled hypertension
- Orthopedic limitations
- Poorly controlled seizure disorder
- Poorly controlled hyperthyroidism
- Heavy smoker

WARNING SIGNS TO TERMINATE EXERCISE WHILE PREGNANT

- Vaginal bleeding
- Dyspnea prior to exertion
- Dizziness
- Headache
- Chest pain
- Muscle weakness
- Calf pain or swelling (need to rule out thrombophlebitis)
- Preterm labor
- Decreased fetal movement
- Amniotic fluid leakage

From American College of Obstetricians and Gynecologists. (2002b). *Exercise during pregnancy and the postpartum period* (Committee Opinion No. 267). Washington, DC: Author.

---

has confirmed benefits and minimal risks for most women (Artal & O'Toole, 2003).

A woman's overall health, including obstetric and medical risks, should be assessed before initiating an exercise program (see Display 5–8). Generally, participation in a wide range of recreational activities appears to be safe during pregnancy; however, each sport should be reviewed individually for its potential risk, and activities with a high risk of falling or those with a high risk of abdominal trauma should be avoided during pregnancy. Scuba diving also should be avoided throughout pregnancy because the fetus is at an increased risk for decompression sickness during this activity. In the absence of either medical or obstetric complications, 30 minutes or more of moderate exercise a day on most, if not all, days of the week is recommended for pregnant women (ACOG, 2002b).

Many women are committed to exercising regularly and wish to continue throughout the pregnancy. Pregnant women who have been sedentary before pregnancy should gradually progress up to 30 minutes a day (Artal & O'Toole, 2003). Overall exercise benefits the woman psychologically and physically. Recreational and competitive athletes with uncomplicated pregnancies may remain active during pregnancy and modify their usual exercise routines to refrain from contact sports or other activities that might possibly cause abdominal distress. Particular attention should be paid to maintaining proper hydration during these exercise sessions. Pregnant women with diabetes, morbid obesity, or chronic hypertension should have individualized exercise prescription. Epidemiological data suggest that exercise may even be beneficial in the primary prevention of gestational diabetes, particularly in morbidly obese women (BMI >33), but not in women of normal weight (Dye, Knox, Artal, Aubry, & Wojtowycz, 1997). Women with medical or obstetric complications should be carefully evaluated before recommendations on physical activity participation during pregnancy are made.

Maternal Infections

Maternal infections have long been recognized as risk factors for adverse pregnancy outcomes. Infections have been reported to account for 10% to 25% of fetal deaths in developed countries (Silver, 2007). The mechanism likely involves both maternal and fetal inflammatory responses, but is unknown. There is epidemiological, microbiological, and clinical evidence of an association between infection and preterm birth. Spontaneous preterm birth epidemiological studies reveal that births at less than 34 weeks' gestation are much more frequently accompanied by clinical or subclinical infection than those at more than 34 weeks. Both maternal and neonatal infections are more common after preterm than term birth. The earlier the birth the more risk there is of an associated infection (Boggess, 2005).

The proportion of fetal deaths due to viral infections is uncertain because there is no way to systematically evaluate by cultures. Parvovirus B19 is perhaps the most common viral infection to cause pregnancy loss (Silver, 2007). The mechanism is thought to be fetal anemia leading to fetal hydrops. The most common viral infection is cytomegalovirus, occurring in 1% of U.S. women. Coxsackie virus has also been reported to cause fetal death as well as other sporadically occurring viruses (eg, echoviruses, enteroviruses, chickenpox, measles, mumps, and rubella). Herpes is rarely transmitted in utero. HIV-positive women may have other risk factors that contribute to fetal death (Silver, 2007).

Maternal genitourinary and reproductive tract infections have been implicated as a main risk factor in 15% to 25% of preterm deliveries. Bacterial vaginosis is a gram-negative, anaerobic infection of the vagina that occurs in up to 20% of all pregnancies. Chlamydia and bacterial vaginosis are both important agents in infections associated with preterm birth (Boggess, 2005).

Dental care during pregnancy has received more attention lately, as there has been evidence to support an association between gingivitis and preterm birth, low birth weight, and preeclampsia (Boggess et al., 2003; Lopez, Smith, & Gutierrez, 2002). Gingivitis occurs in 60% to 75% of pregnant women, and it surfaces most frequently during the second trimester (Barak et al., 2003; Khader & Ta'ani, 2005). Symptoms include swollen red gums and bleeding with brushing the teeth. Elevated levels of estrogen and progesterone cause the gums to react differently to the bacteria found in plaque. Gums infected with periodontal disease become toxic reservoirs of bacteria resulting in increased prostaglandin production (Barak et al., 2003). Although it is important to promote good oral hygiene during routine prenatal visits, there is no definitive evidence that treatment of periodontal disease will reduce the risk of preterm birth (Khader & Ta'ani, 2005).

Culture

Cultural assessment is an important part of prenatal care. A comprehensive discussion of culture as it relates to pregnancy and childbirth practices is presented in Chapter 2. Cultural beliefs and practices can affect the health status of the woman by influencing her use of healthcare services, confidence in and acceptance of recommended prevention and treatment strategies, and global beliefs regarding her body, illness, religion, and so forth (Seidel, Ball, Dains, & Benedict, 2006). Principal beliefs, values, and behaviors that relate to pregnancy and childbirth should be identified, taking care to avoid sweeping generalizations about cultural characteristics or cultural values. Not every individual in a culture may display certain characteristics, as there are variations among cultures and within cultures. Planning culturally specific care requires information about ethnicity, degree of affiliation with the ethnic group, religion, patterns of decision-making, language, style of communication, norms of etiquette, and expectations about the healthcare system (Seidel et al., 2006). Nutritional practices and beliefs about medication are particularly significant during pregnancy. Certain behavioral differences can be expected if a culture views pregnancy as an illness, as opposed to a natural occurrence; for example, seeking prenatal care may or may not be important if pregnancy is viewed as a natural occurrence. Healthcare practices during pregnancy are influenced by numerous factors, such as the prevalence of folk remedies, the prevalence of indigenous healers, and the influence of professional healthcare workers. Socioeconomic status and living in an urban or rural setting affect patterns of use of home remedies and use of the healthcare system.

Without cultural awareness, nurses and other healthcare providers tend to project their own cultural responses onto women and families from different socioeconomic, religious, or educational groups. This leads caregivers to assume patients are demonstrating a certain type of behavior for the same reason that they themselves would. Additionally, some nurses may fail to recognize that healthcare has its own culture, which has been dominated historically by traditional middle-class values and beliefs. In an ethnocentric approach, caregivers sometimes believe that if members of other cultures do not share Western values, they should adopt them. An example of this is a nurse who values equality of the sexes dealing with an Asian woman who defers to the husband to make the decisions. Pressuring the woman to defy cultural values and beliefs can prove stressful for the woman and significantly interfere with a therapeutic relationship.

When a language barrier exists, the woman may be reluctant to provide information if the interpreter is male, a relative, or a child of the pregnant woman. Reviewing the goals and purposes of the interview with the interpreter in advance generally enhances the interaction with the woman (Wheeler, 2002). Gender is an important factor in health beliefs. In many cultures, a male physician would not be allowed to examine a woman, much less deliver her baby.

Nurses cannot expect to be culturally competent for every woman they care for. However, culturally sensitive behaviors can enhance prenatal care. If a particular ethnic group dominates the local population, it is a professional responsibility to learn as much about that culture so as to provide optimal care. A cultural assessment should include the following points (adapted from Seidel et al., 2006):

- *Health beliefs and practices*: assessment of methods used to maintain health (ie, hygiene and self-care practices), treatment of illness, attitude toward necessity of prenatal care, family member responsible for healthcare decisions, and healthcare topics that are taboo for discussion
- *Religious influences and special rituals*: assessment of religious preference, significant persons she looks to for guidance, any special practices with regard to birth (eg, baptism for a dying baby), religious view of pregnancy when not married
- *Language and communication*: assessment of oral and written language spoken in the home and elsewhere, appropriate nonverbal communication such as touch and eye contact and its meaning, and culturally appropriate ways to enter and leave situations
- *Parenting styles and role of the family*: assessment of who is making the decisions in the family, composition of the family, attitude toward marriage and divorce, role and attitude toward children, and special beliefs toward conception, pregnancy, childbirth, lactation, and child rearing
- *Source of support beyond the family*: assessment of the woman's social network that influences her perception of health and illness, including the process of childbearing; woman's need of relationships with others
- *Dietary practices*: assessment of food preferences, person responsible for food preparation, forbidden foods by culture or religion, required foods for special rite or custom, method used to prepare food, specific beliefs concerning food's role in causing or curing illness

Current Pregnancy Status

Assessment of current pregnancy status includes analysis of current pregnancy history, psychosocial factors, nutritional status, and laboratory data; a review of symptoms guided by the gestational age and that may reflect medical or pregnancy complications; assessment of the pregnant woman's concerns; and a complete physical examination. Symptom review includes questions about nausea and vomiting, headache, abdominal or epigastric pain, visual changes, fever, viral illness, vaginal bleeding, dysuria, cramping, and other concerns. This screening process incorporates assessment of historical and social factors with current health status. Evaluation of current pregnancy status provides baseline data that guides planning for future evaluation and health promotion activities.

The physical examination is comprehensive and covers a review of the cardiovascular, respiratory, neurologic, endocrine, gastrointestinal, reproductive, and genitourinary systems. Particular attention should be directed to the anthropometric assessment, including the woman's height, weight, and pelvimetry data because these physical characteristics can influence the pregnancy course and birth (Cunningham et al., 2005). Pelvic examination includes measurement of cervical length, a Pap smear, and assessment for STDs. The abdominal examination compares data from the woman's report of her last menstrual period with physical findings. Depending on weeks of gestation, the FHR may be auscultated.

Selected laboratory data are valuable to the assessment process. Biochemical information provides information about current prenatal health, as well as general wellness status. Evaluation of specific laboratory data is discussed later in this chapter.

ONGOING PRENATAL CARE

Nurses who interact with the childbearing family in the prenatal period assess the well-being of the woman and the growth and well-being of the fetus. Nursing intervention is directed by the data obtained from ongoing comprehensive maternal–fetal assessments. Evaluation of the growth and development of the fetus can be shared with the parents to promote prenatal parent–infant attachment (see Display 5–9 for normal fetal developmental events).

Risk status in pregnancy is a dynamic process that affects clinical and nonclinical parameters. Psychosocial factors, socioeconomic factors, and lifestyle patterns also require ongoing evaluation. Employment status, family economic status, and relationship status could change from visit to visit. These changes affect the woman's psychosocial stress level, potentiating existing risk factors. In general, factors with potential to affect the pregnancy are in a constant state of fluctuation and require continued surveillance.

Subsequent prenatal visits should be structured to promote continuous, rather than episodic, risk assessment. Each prenatal visit should include a maternal–fetal physical assessment, including vital signs, weight, fundal height, FHR, and fetal movement (Display 5–10), as well as a review of pertinent laboratory data, dating data, the problem list, and the woman's response to recommended interventions (eg, smoking cessa-

DISPLAY 5-9

Major Normal Events of the Fetal Period (9th to 40th Week)

WEEKS 9 TO 12

- Crown-rump length doubles between 9 and 12 weeks.
- Upper limbs develop to normal proportions, while lower limbs remain less developed.
- Male and female genitalia are recognizable by 12 weeks.
- Production of red blood cells transfers from the liver to the spleen at 12 weeks.

WEEKS 13 TO 16

- Rapid fetal growth occurs.
- Fetus doubles in size.
- Lanugo begins to grow.
- Fingernails are formed.
- Kidneys begin to secrete urine.
- Fetus begins to swallow amniotic fluid.
- Fetus appears human.
- Placenta is fully formed.

WEEKS 17 TO 23

- Fetal growth slows.
- Lower limbs are fully formed.

- Fetal body is covered with lanugo.
- Vernix caseosa covers the body to protect the skin from amniotic fluid.
- Brown fat forms.

WEEKS 24 TO 27

- Skin growth is rapid, and skin appears red and wrinkled.
- The eyes open, and eyelashes and eyebrows are formed.
- The fetus becomes viable at 26 to 27 weeks.

WEEKS 28 TO 31

- Subcutaneous fat is deposited.
- If the fetus is born at this time with immature lungs, respiratory distress syndrome may occur.

WEEKS 32 TO 36

- Lanugo has disappeared from the body but remains on the head.
- Weight gain is steady.
- Fingernails are growing.
- The fetus has a good chance of surviving if born.

WEEKS 37 TO 40

- Subcutaneous fat builds, and fetal contours appear round.
- Both testes have descended in the male.
- The skull is fully developed.

---

tion). At return prenatal visits, risk factors must be analyzed to evaluate their relevance to the gestational age. For example, if a woman has a history of preterm labor and is at 37 weeks' gestation in the current pregnancy, this risk factor would no longer be relevant. Conversely, new risk factors may develop during the pregnancy, such as preeclampsia or gestational diabetes. Ongoing prenatal care is a dynamic process in which risk factors may change from month to month. Achieving healthy pregnancy outcomes is a multifaceted and sometimes complex process. Nurses can be credible sources of information, offering support as the woman and her partner or family sort through information and decision-making during pregnancy.

Particular attention should be given to evaluation of blood pressure trends (see Chapter 6 for a complete discussion of hypertensive disease during pregnancy). During pregnancy, blood pressure values decrease slightly during the second trimester but return to early pregnancy values by the third trimester. Ideally, during preconception care or early prenatal care, a baseline blood pressure is noted. It is important to evaluate and document blood pressure measurements in the same

arm with the woman in the same position (eg, sitting or semi-Fowler's) with the blood pressure cuff at the level of the heart. Use of the same device for assessing blood pressure is also critical to accuracy. Consistency in blood pressure monitoring allows for more accurate assessment and comparison across prenatal visits. Traditionally, an elevation of systolic blood pressure of 30 mm Hg or an elevation of 15 mm Hg for diastolic blood pressure over prepregnancy or first-trimester measurements was thought to be predictive of the development of preeclampsia, but these criteria may be of questionable value for diagnosis. Newer guidelines simplify this to a blood pressure reading of >140/90 (ACOG, 2002a). Other clinical data are important to assess as blood pressure change is not usually a lone sign of complications. When there is a change in blood pressure, the woman should be assessed for the concurrent development of proteinuria, headaches, dizziness, visual disturbances, epigastric pain, or edema.

Basic fetal surveillance includes assessment of fundal height, FHR, and fetal activity. Fundal height is the measurement of the uterus from the symphysis pubis to the top of the fundus. The measurement of the fundal height in centimeters (± 2 cm) should correlate with gestational

DISPLAY 5-10

Schedule of Prenatal Care

INITIAL PRENATAL VISIT

Intake assessment
Comprehensive medical and reproductive health
  history
Comprehensive family history
History of current pregnancy
Psychosocial assessment
Nutrition assessment
Comprehensive physical examination
Complete blood count (CBC)
Blood type and Rh, antibody screen
PAP smear
Gonorrhea culture or test
Chlamydia test
Serology (RPR, VDRL)
Rubella
Hepatitis B surface antigen (HBsAg)
Urine culture and sensitivity
Sickle cell screen (for women of African, Asian, or
  Middle Eastern descent)
Genetic screening (for women at risk of genetic
  disease)
Glucose challenge test (GCT) if woman is at risk
HIV testing
PPD (tuberculin screen)
Obtain if indicated:
  TORCH titers
  Group B *Streptococcus* culture
  Ultrasound examination

SUBSEQUENT VISITS

Assessment (each visit)
  Vital signs

Urine dipstick for glucose, albumin, and ketones
Weight
Fundal height
Fetal heart rate (FHR)
Fetal movement
Leopold's maneuvers to evaluate fetal lie/presentation
Assess presence or absence of edema
15 to 20 weeks
  Maternal serum screening
  Begin preterm birth prevention education
  One-hour glucose challenge test (GCT) as indicated
    by risk
20 to 24 weeks
  Preterm birth prevention education
24 to 28 weeks
  Cervical examination at 28 weeks as indicated by risk
    status
  1-hour 50 g GCT
  Ongoing education about preterm birth prevention
    and warning signs of pregnancy complications
28 to 36 weeks
  CBC at 28 weeks for selected at-risk women
  Blood group antibody screen at 28 weeks if Rh
    negative; RhoGAM if indirect Coombs negative
  Initiate education regarding family planning
  Group B strep culture
  Cervical examination at 32 weeks, as indicated by risk
    status
  Follow-up visit with dietition/nutritionist
  Breast assessment/educational preparation for breast-
    feeding
  Ongoing education about preterm birth prevention
    and warning signs of pregnancy complications
  Initiate parenting education
36 to 40 weeks
  CBC if Hbg <11g/dL or Hct <33% at 28 weeks
  Repeat GC, Chlamydia, RPR, HIV, HBsAg, if indicated
  Initiate education about signs of labor, preparation for
    birth
  Postpartum anticipatory guidance

Adapted from American Academy of Pediatrics & American College of Obstetricians and Gynecologists. (2002). *Guidelines for perinatal care* (5th. ed.). Elk Grove Village, IL: Author.

---

age between 22 and 34 weeks. Fundal height less than gestational age may be indicative of IUGR. Fundal height greater than gestational age may indicate multiple gestation, polyhydramnios, fibroids, or other conditions that cause uterine distension. Fetal activity is an indirect measure of central nervous system function and is predictive of fetal well-being. Fetal movement counting (ie, "kick counts") is discussed later in this chapter.

Preterm Labor and Birth

Preterm birth before 37 weeks' gestation is a common problem in obstetric care, with a preterm birth rate of 12.7% in the United States (Hamilton, Martin & Ven-

tura, 2006). Preterm and low-birthweight births are related to more than two-thirds of infant deaths in the United States (Martin et al., 2006). Therefore, these problems are considered by many to be the most urgent problem in the care of pregnant women. Because this is such an important issue in prenatal care, the reader is referred to Chapter 6 for an in-depth discussion of this topic.

Biochemical Screening and Laboratory Assessment

Selected biochemical screens may be repeated at specific intervals during pregnancy (Table 5–2). Subse-

TABLE 5–2 ■ COMMON PRENATAL LABORATORY TESTS

Test	Timing	Significant Values
Complete blood count		
Hematocrit	Initial visit, 28, 36 weeks	<32%
Hemoglobin	Initial visit, 28, 36 weeks	<11 g/dL
White blood cell count	Initial visit, 28, 36 weeks	>15,000/mm^3
Type and Rh	Initial visit	Mother Rh negative, Father Rh positive
Antibody screen	Initial visit, 36 weeks	Positive
Serology	Initial visit, 36 weeks	Positive
Rubella	Initial visit	1:8; significant rise
50 g 1-hr glucose challenge test	24 to 28 weeks	>140 g/dl
HBsAg	Initial visit, as indicated	Positive
Urinalysis	Initial visit	Positive
Urine culture and sensitivity	Initial visit	Positive
Glucose/protein	Each visit	>2+, + ketones
Pap smear	Initial visit	Abnormal cervical cytology
Group B Strep culture	36 weeks	Positive
GC/Chlamydia probe	Initial visit, 36 weeks	Positive
Rh antibody	Initial visit, 28 weeks	Negative
HIV	Initial visit, 36 weeks	Positive
Maternal serum screening (double, triple, quadruple screen)	15 to 20 weeks	Risk indicated by report
Sickle cell screen, Hgb electrophoresis	Initial visit	Positive for trait/anemia
Tay-Sachs screen	Initial visit	Carrier
PPD (tuberculin screen)	Initial visit	Positive

Adapted from Barron, M. L. (1998). *Nursing assessment of the pregnant woman: Antepartum screening and laboratory evaluation* (Nursing Module). White Plains, NY: March of Dimes Birth Defects Foundation.

quent prenatal visits usually include urinalysis by dipstick for evidence of proteinuria, glucosuria, and ketonuria. Although it is common practice, there is little evidence to suggest routine urinalysis by means of dipstick provides useful clinical information or is predictive of women who will develop complications of pregnancy (Murray et al., 2002; Waugh et al., 2004). Dipstick urinalysis does not detect proteinuria reliably in patients with early preeclampsia; measurement of 24-hour urinary protein excretion is the gold standard but is not always practical. Trace glycosuria also is unreliable, although higher concentrations may be useful (Kirkham, Harris, & Grzybowski, 2005).

After a baseline complete blood cell count (CBC) is obtained, periodic assessment of hematocrit and hemoglobin values may be indicated for certain at-risk populations.

Based on medical and obstetric history, clinical symptoms, and assessment information, more extensive laboratory data may be indicated, including screening for STDs (eg, gonorrhea, chlamydia, hepatitis B, syphilis, and HIV) (AAP & ACOG, 2002). Data indicate risk of maternal–fetal transmis-

sion of HIV can be reduced by prophylactic administration of antiretroviral medications during the antepartum and intrapartum periods to pregnant women who are HIV seropositive and to their infants (CDC, 2001). All pregnant women should tested for HIV as a part of a routine battery of tests in order to initiate timely treatment (ACOG, 2004; CDC, 2006). Appropriate counseling and referral services should be available for women with positive test results.

Screening for gestational diabetes (GDM) is generally carried out at 24 to 28 weeks' gestation using a 1-hour, 50-gram glucose challenge test (ACOG, 2001a). Serum glucose evaluation before 24 to 28 weeks' gestation may be indicated based on family history or maternal factors such as glucosuria, advanced maternal age, marked obesity, family history of diabetes mellitus, personal history of GDM, previous macrosomic infant, or previous unexplained fetal loss. The woman does not need to be fasting for the screening test. One hour after ingesting a glucose load (Glucola), the serum glucose level should be is less than 140 mg/dL. If the screening result is greater than or equal to 140 mg/dL, a 3-hour 100-g oral glucose tolerance test (OGTT) is recommended. Non-fasting plasma glucose over 200 mg/dL on screening or a fasting greater than 105 mg/dL is indicative of diabetes mellitus and no OGTT is necessary for diagnosis.

The diagnostic test for GDM is administered after a fast of at least 8 hours, but with the patient consuming her usual unrestricted daily diet in the days preceding the test. On the day of the test, only water may be consumed, and cigarette smoking should be avoided. Diagnosis of GDM is based on two or more abnormally elevated venous plasma glucose values (ACOG, 2001a). Women diagnosed with GDM require education about appropriate nutrition, self-management, and self-glucose monitoring and referral for appropriate medical care and counseling. The diagnosis of gestational diabetes is made when two or more of the values at the 3-hour OGTT are elevated above the following values (in plasma mg/dL):

Fasting: 105
1 hour: 190
2 hour: 165
3 hour: 145

If only one level is elevated, repeat testing at a later gestation may be ordered or dietary restriction recommended. Approximately 15% to 20% of those with GDM will develop overt diabetes mellitus.

Laboratory data such as CBC, urinalysis, blood type & Rhesus factor (Rh), antibody screen, rubella titer, rapid plasma reagin test, hepatitis B surface antigen, gonorrhea and Chlamydia testing, and cervical cytology should be obtained from all pregnant women. Additional laboratory tests (eg, STD screens, group B streptococci, fetal fibronectin, TORCH titers, tuberculin testing, toxicology screens, and genetic screens) should be performed as indicated, based on historical indicators or clinical findings (AAP & ACOG, 2002).

Maternal serum alpha-fetoprotein (MSAFP) screening should be offered to all pregnant women between 15 and 20 weeks' gestation (AAP & ACOG, 2002; ACOG, 2007). The goal of MSAFP is to identify women who have an increased risk of neural tube defects (NTD), Down syndrome, or trisomy 21. Screening should be voluntary, and the woman should be counseled about its limitations and benefits (ACOG, 2007).

Alpha-fetoprotein (AFP) is a protein that is produced in the fetal yolk sac during the first trimester and in the fetal liver during later gestation. The concentration of AFP in maternal serum is altered by factors that include inaccurate dating of gestational age, maternal weight and race, multiple gestation, and maternal diabetes. Most screening programs establish a cut-off of 2–2.5 times the median values (2–2.5 MoM) to be designated as a positive result for NTD

(AAP & ACOG, 2002). In contrast to the absolute cutoff of 2–2.5 MoM used in NTD screening, Down syndrome screening uses a series of age-specific cutoff levels for each MSAFP level. There is a direct relationship between the age of the patient and the chance of her result being designated as positive.

Abnormally elevated MSAFP levels have been associated with birth defects and chromosomal anomalies, such as open NTDs, open abdominal defects, and congenital nephrosis (AAP & ACOG, 2002). High MSAFP levels also may result from multiple gestations. Low MSAFP levels have been associated with Down syndrome and other chromosomal anomalies (AAP & ACOG, 2002). Double-marker screening (ie, AFP and human chorionic gonadotropin [hCG]), triple-marker screening (ie, AFP, hCG, and estriol) and quadruple (AFP, hCG, estriol, and inhibin A) are also available to screen for trisomy 18, trisomy 21, and NTDs. Average hCG levels are higher and unconjugated estriol levels are lower in Down syndrome pregnancies. The hCG and estriol levels are lower in trisomy 18 pregnancies. When more parameters are evaluated, there is an increased accuracy in diagnosis. Although maternal serum screening with the use of double and triple markers is superior to the use of MSAFP alone when screening for fetal Down syndrome, this method still fails to detect Down syndrome in women less than 35 years of age (AAP & ACOG, 2002). The quadruple is the most effective multiple-marker screening test for Down syndrome in the second trimester. This approach yields an 81% detection rate and a false-positive rate of 5% (Dugoff et al., 2005). New testing techniques, such as nuchal translucency (NT) or the combined test (NT and two serum markers, free beta hCG and pregnancy-associated plasma protein-A), in the first trimester may enhance detection rates and provide earlier risk assessment of Down syndrome.

Women should be counseled that maternal serum screening tests are optional, about the limited sensitivity and specificity of maternal screening tests, and the psychological implications of a positive test prior to the performance of the tests. Any abnormal finding warrants additional testing; however, screening protocols vary. If the initial ultrasound examination does not provide an explanation for the MSAFP elevation (such as inaccurate dating, multiple gestation, or fetal demise) a comprehensive (Level II) ultrasound examination is performed to evaluate the fetus for malformations. Genetic counseling and amniocentesis may be offered in some centers as a follow-up to abnormal findings as well. Hemoglobin electrophoresis is used to detect genetic hemoglobin disorders, including sickle cell anemia, sickle cell disease, and thalassemia. These recessive inherited conditions occur in the United

DISPLAY 5-11

Patient Teaching Tool for Genetic Transfer of Sickle Cell Disease/Trait

1. Two parents affected with sickle cell trait:
SA+SA = 25% of children will have sickle cell disease
50% of children will have sickle cell trait
25% of children will not be affected by the trait or disease
2. One parent affected with sickle cell trait, one parent affected with sickle cell disease:
SA+SS = 50% of children will have sickle cell disease
50% of children will have sickle cell trait
0 children will not be affected by the trait or disease

3. Two parents affected by sickle cell disease:
SS+SS = 100% of children will have sickle cell disease
0 children will have sickle cell trait
0 children will not be affected by the disease
4. One parent affected by sickle cell disease, one parent unaffected:
SS+AA = 100% of children will have sickle cell trait
0 children will have sickle cell disease
0 children will not be affected by trait
5. One parent affected by sickle cell trait, one parent unaffected:
SA+AA = 50% of children will have sickle cell trait
50% of children will not be affected by the trait
0 children will not be affected by sickle cell disease

SA = sickle cell trait; SS = sickle cell disease; AA = unaffected.

From Larrabee, K., & Cowan, M. (1995). Clinical nursing management of sickle cell disease and trait during pregnancy. *Journal of Perinatal and Neonatal Nursing, 9*(2), 29–41.

States primarily in families of African descent, but can also be found in families of Asian, Middle Eastern, or Mediterranean descent (Larrabee & Cowan, 1995). Women of African descent are routinely screened for these disorders. Although prevalence of sickle cell trait is common among African-Americans (8% to 12%), information related to inheritance patterns is not well known to those at risk. Figure 5–1 and Display 5–11 provide teaching tools that may be helpful in explaining the genetic transfer of sickle cell trait and sickle cell disease to women and their partners.

Prenatal Diagnosis

Prenatal diagnostic evaluation should be offered to families with any of the following: maternal age of 35 years or more, maternal age of 32 or more and pregnant with twins, women carrying a fetus with an ultrasonographically identified structural anomaly, women with ultrasound markers of aneuploidy (including increased nucchal thickness), women with a known positive serum screen, a family history of chromosomal anomalies, parental balanced translocation carrier, the mother a known or at-risk carrier for X-linked disorder, parents who are carriers of an autosomal recessive disorder detectable in utero, a parent affected with an autosomal dominant disorder detectable in utero, a family history of neural tube defects (Kirkham et al., 2005) [see Table 5–3]. Some women "may benefit from a more extensive discussion with a genetics professional or a maternal–fetal medicine specialist, especially if there is a family history of a chromosome abnormality, genetic disorder, or a congenital malformation" (ACOG, 2007).

Chorionic Villus Sampling

Chorionic villus sampling (CVS) involves the removal of a small sample of chorionic (placental) tissue through a catheter inserted through the cervix. The villi are harvested and cultured for chromosomal analysis and processed for DNA and enzymatic analysis as indicated. Results are available in 4 days. CVS is ideally performed between 10 and 11.5 weeks' gestation. The risk of fetal loss is approximately 1%. As with amniocentesis, information about benefits and risks must be provided before the procedure (Cunningham et al., 2005).

Ultrasonography

Ultrasonography (ie, fetal imaging by intermittent, high-frequency sound waves) is the most commonly used prenatal diagnostic procedure. Indications vary widely and depend on gestational age and type of diagnostic information sought. During early pregnancy, ultrasound is frequently used to determine presence of an intrauterine gestational sac, fetal number, and cardiac activity and to measure crown-rump length. Early ultrasonography (ie, before 14 weeks' gestation) accurately determines gestational age (± 1 week), decreases the need for labor induction after 41 weeks' gestation, and detects multiple pregnancies

TABLE 5–3 ■ CURRENT PRENATAL SCREENING TESTS

Preconception	0 to 12 weeks	12 to 24 weeks	24 to 40+ weeks
Carrier Screening Cystic Fibrosis, fragile X, Tay-Sachs, hemoglobinopathies	Early amniocentesis Chorionic villus sampling Ultrasound	Ultrasound Amniocentesis Serum screening: AFP, HCG, estriol, Inhibin-A	Ultrasound Percutaneous umbilical blood sample Fetal fibronectin Group B strep culture

Test	Indication	Risk	Accuracy	Limitations
CVS	Fetal karyotype, diagnosis of X-linked or enzymatic disorders	0.5% to 2% risk of fetal loss; maternal Rh immunization; infection, possible limb abnormalities	99.5%; chance of doubtful results due to mosaicism	Does not supply AFP or AChE for analysis
Amnio-centesis	To obtain fetal karyotype, to screen for NTDs using AFP levels; to diagnose infections	1% risk of spontaneous abortion, maternal Rh iso-immunization; infection	99% accurate	Does not detect birth defects caused by teratogens
PUBS	Fetal karyotype; infection, isoimmunization; enzyme analysis; evaluation of fetal hypoxia; hemoglobinopathy; fetal therapy	Fetal loss rate 2% due to infection, membrane rupture, and fetal bradycardia		Anomalous or growth retarded fetus not as "tolerant" of procedure as normal fetus
AFP	To screen for NTDs, midline ventral fusion defects, fetal Down syndrome	Negligible	MSAFP detects 70% to 80% of open NTDs. Detects 40% of DS.	Correct dating essential. Does not detect closed NTDs. At 16–18 weeks for greatest sensitivity. Must have accurate dating for correct interpretation. Inevitable false-positive and false-negative.
Double screen	To screen for Down syndrome and trisomy 18	Negligible	Detects two-thirds of Down syndrome cases, 90% of open NTDs	Provides calculated risk; need amniocentesis for diagnosis
Triple screen	To screen for Down syndrome and trisomy 18	Negligible	57% to 67% detection rate of Down syndrome; false-positive rate of 5%	Provides calculated risk; need amniocentesis for diagnosis
Quad-ruple screen	To screen for Down syndrome and trisomy 18	Negligible	81% detection rate; false-positive rate of 5% for Down syndrome	Provides calculated risk; need amniocentesis for diagnosis

(ACOG, 2001b). Components of the basic ultrasound examination include the following:

- Presence of gestational sac and an evaluation of uterus and adnexa when performed during the first trimester
- Estimated gestational age
- Number of fetuses
- Viability
- Location of placenta
- Volume of amniotic fluid
- Fetal presentation and anatomical survey when performed during the second and third trimesters

Ultrasound during the second and third trimesters can be useful when there is a discrepancy between the woman's last menstrual period and uterine size, to detect fetal anatomic defects, and for placental localization and amniotic fluid volume estimates. When maternal or fetal complications are suspected or identified, ultrasonography serves as a valuable tool to confirm the diagnosis and follow-up on fetal status. Ultrasonography is also used to guide the obstetrician during other diagnostic procedures, such as CVS, amniocentesis, and fetal blood sampling. In women for whom preterm birth is a concern, cervical length can be measured via ultrasound. However, the value of doing this test lies in its negative predictive value. That is, the test is more useful for those women who are not likely to experience preterm labor than for predicting preterm labor (ACOG, 2001b).

Controversy exists over the benefits of routine ultrasound examination for all pregnant women. Advocates suggest routine screening can decrease incidence of labor induction for suspected postdate pregnancies and avoid undiagnosed fetal anomalies and twin gestations. However, no evidence directly links improved fetal outcomes with routine ultrasound screening (Kirkham et al., 2005).

Amniocentesis

Amniocentesis is the collection of a sample of amniotic fluid from the amniotic sac for identification of genetic diseases, selected birth defects, and fetal lung maturity; therapy for polyhydramnios; and progressive evaluation of isoimmunized pregnancies. Amniocentesis for genetic evaluation may be performed between 15 and 20 weeks' gestation. Genetic amniocentesis allows for detection of chromosomal anomalies, biochemical disorders, NTDs, some ventral wall defects, and DNA analysis for a number of single gene disorders. Early amniocentesis, between 11 and 14 weeks' gestation, is offered at some centers with outcomes similar to mid-trimester amniocentesis (Cunningham et al., 2005). Before testing, families should be given information about indications for amniocentesis, how the procedure is done, risks involved, and ramifications of findings.

Fetal Blood Sampling

Fetal blood sampling, also known as percutaneous umbilical blood sampling (PUBS) or cordocentesis, allows direct evaluation of fetal blood obtained from the umbilical cord. Using ultrasonography to guide placement, a needle is inserted into one of the umbilical vessels (usually the vein), and a small amount of blood is withdrawn. Valuable information can be gained from analysis of fetal blood, including prenatal diagnosis of fetal blood disorders, isoimmunization, metabolic disorders, infections, and karyotyping (Cunningham et al., 2005). Cordocentesis can also be used for fetal therapies such as red blood cell and platelet transfusions.

Biochemical Markers

Fetal fibronectin (fFN), a protein secreted by the trophoblast, can be detected by use of a monoclonal antibody: FDC-6. The exact function is unknown, but this protein is thought to play a role in mediating placental–uterine attachment. fFN is normally present in the cervical or vaginal fluid before 20 weeks' gestation. However, after 20 weeks, the presence of fFN may indicate a disruption of the attachment of the fetal membranes, and therefore it has been investigated as an early marker for preterm birth.

Birth before 37 weeks' gestation complicates >12.7% of all pregnancies in the United States (Hamilton, et al., 2006). Predicting women truly at risk for preterm birth and those destined to deliver at term may result in the ability to initiate interventions to prolong pregnancy and avoid preterm birth (see Chapter 6). fFN is a glycoprotein found in high concentrations in the amniotic fluid. It is normally found in the cervical and vaginal secretions before 16 to 20 weeks' gestation, but its presence in the cervicovaginal secretion after 20 weeks' gestation is abnormal, except as a marker of the imminent onset of labor at term (ACOG, 2001b). Elevation of fFN levels is hypothesized to reflect mechanical or inflammatory damage to the membranes or placenta. The fFN cutoff for a positive test is $>/=50$ ng/mL (Fischbach & Dunning, 2004).

The fFN test is a better predictor of women who will not go into preterm labor than those who will, however (Honest, Bachmann, Gupta, Kleijnen, & Khan, 2002). Among all women, the sensitivity of fFN testing was highest for birth within 7 to 14 days (67% to 71%). However, negative predictive value was more specific (96% to 97%) for asymptomatic women than for women with symptoms of preterm labor (85% to 90%). fFN appears to be an especially strong marker for preterm births associated with infection (Honest et al., 2002).

To collect a specimen for fFN testing, a Dacron swab is placed in the posterior fornix of the vagina and rotated for 10 seconds. Sexual activity within 24 hours of sample collection, recent cervical examination, and vaginal bleeding may result in false-positive tests (Adeza Biomedical, 2005) For this reason, a specimen should not be collected if the patient has had intercourse within 24 hours, and the specimen should be collected before performance of a digital cervical exam, measurement of transvaginal cervical length, or performance of Pap smear or cervical cultures. fFN testing should be limited to women with intact amniotic membranes and cervical dilatation <3 cm. Sampling should be carried out no earlier than 24 weeks and no later than 34 weeks and 6 days (ACOG, 2001b). This provides the nurse with the opportunity to review signs and symptoms of preterm labor and to address any fears or anxieties the woman or family may have regarding preterm birth. Ultrasonography to determine cervical length, fFN, or a combination of both may be useful in identifying women at high risk for preterm labor. (Tekesin, Marek, Hellmeyer, Reitz, & Schmidt, 2005; Schmitz, et al., 2006).

FETAL SURVEILLANCE

Fetal assessment is an integral component of prenatal care. Careful assessment of fetal well-being enhances perinatal outcome through early identification and intervention for fetal compromise. The goal of antepartum fetal surveillance is to prevent fetal death. Display 5–12 provides the indications for antepartum fetal surveillance. Techniques based on FHR patterns have been in use for almost 3 decades (ACOG, 1999). Ultrasonography may be used as indicated throughout the pregnancy to assess fetal growth and development.

DISPLAY 5-12

Indications for Antepartum Fetal Surveillance

MATERNAL CONDITIONS

- Antiphospholipid syndrome
- Hyperthyroidism (poorly controlled)
- Hemoglobinopathies (hemoglobin SS, SC, or S-thalassemia)
- Cyanotic heart disease
- Systemic lupus erythematosus
- Chronic renal disease
- Type 1 diabetes mellitus
- Hypertensive disorders

PREGNANCY-RELATED CONDITIONS

- Pregnancy-related hypertension
- Decreased fetal movement
- Oligohydramnios
- Polyhydramnios
- Intrauterine growth restriction
- Postterm pregnancy
- Isoimmunization
- Previous fetal demise (unexplained or recurrent risk)
- Multiple gestation (with significant growth discrepancy)

From American College of Obstetricians and Gynecologists. (1999). *Antepartum fetal surveillance* (Practice Bulletin No. 9). Washington, DC: Author.

Doppler ultrasound may be used during the second half of pregnancy to assess blood flow changes in the fetal heart, aorta, cerebrum, and the uterine and umbilical arteries and is useful in assessing intrauterine growth restriction associated with postterm gestation, diabetes mellitus, systemic lupus erythematosus, or antiphospholipid syndrome (ACOG, 1999).

Assessment of Fetal Activity

Fetal movement counting (ie, "kick counts") has been proposed as a primary method of fetal surveillance for all pregnancies. Cessation of fetal movement is correlated with fetal death. The mother's observation of fetal movement has been validated through an 80% to 90% correlation of maternal perception of movement with movement detected on real-time ultrasonography (Moore & Piacquadio, 1989).

Several methods of fetal movement counting have been proposed; however, neither the ideal number of kicks nor the ideal duration for movement counting has been defined (ACOG, 1999). Perception of 10 distinct movements in a period of up to 2 hours is considered reassuring. After 10 movements have been perceived, the count may be discontinued. Another approach is to instruct women to count fetal movements for 1 hour three times per week. The count is considered reassuring if it equals or exceeds the woman's established baseline count (ACOG, 1999). Monitoring of fetal movement is recommended for pregnant women at high risk for antepartum fetal death beginning as early as 26 to 28 weeks' gestation. For most at-risk patients, however, initiating testing at 32 to 34 weeks is appropriate (ACOG, 1999). Because fetal movement counting is inexpensive, reassuring, and a relatively easily taught skill, all women could benefit from instruction on fetal activity assessment.

Although fetal activity is a reassuring sign, decreased fetal movement is not necessarily ominous. A healthy fetus usually has perceivable movements within 10 to 60 minutes (Harman, 2004). However, perception of fetal movement can be influenced by many factors, including time of day, gestational age, placental location, glucose loading, maternal smoking, maternal medications, and decreased uterine space as gestation increases. Decreased fetal movement may also reflect the fetal sleep state. Early identification of conditions that can affect pregnancy outcome can minimize perinatal morbidity by allowing for the establishment of an appropriate treatment plan and referrals (AAP & ACOG, 2002). Report of decreased fetal movement is an indication for further assessment. The woman should be instructed to have something to eat and drink, rest, and focus on fetal movement for 1 hour. Four movements in 1 hour are considered reassuring. If fewer than four movements are perceived in 2 hours, the woman should call her primary healthcare provider immediately.

Nonstress Test

The nonstress test (NST) is one of the most common methods of prenatal screening and involves electronic FHR monitoring for approximately 20 minutes. The NST is based on the premise that the normal fetus moves at various intervals and that the central nervous system and myocardium responds to movement with acceleration of the FHR. Acceleration of the FHR during fetal activity is a sign of fetal well-being (ACOG, 1999). Various definitions of reactivity have been used. Using the most common definition, the NST is considered to be reactive when two or more FHR accelerations of 15 beats per minute above baseline and lasting at least 15 seconds occur within a 20-minute time frame with or without perception of fetal movement by the woman (ACOG, 1999). These accelerations should occur within 40 minutes of testing. An NST that does not meet these criteria is nonreactive. A reactive NST is reassuring, indicating less than a 1% chance of fetal death within 1 week of a reactive NST. Most deaths within 1 week of a reactive NST fall into nonpreventable categories, such as abruptio placentae, sepsis, and cord accidents. However, a nonreactive NST is not necessarily an ominous sign. Rather, the nonreactive NST indicates a need for further testing and should be followed by a contraction stress test or BPP (Harman, 2004). The NST of the noncompromised preterm fetus (24 to 28 weeks' gestation) is frequently nonreactive, and up to 50% of NSTs may not be reactive from 28 to 32 weeks' gestation (ACOG, 1999).

Biophysical Profile

The BPP combines electronic FHR monitoring with ultrasonography to evaluate fetal well-being based on multiple biophysical variables. Five parameters are assessed: fetal muscle tone, fetal movement, fetal breathing movements, amniotic fluid volume, and FHR reactivity as demonstrated by NST. Each item has a maximum score of 2, with a summed score of 8 to 10 indicating fetal well-being (ie, reassuring). A score of 6 is considered "equivocal," and the test should be repeated the next day in a preterm fetus. A term fetus should be delivered. A score of 4 usually indicates that birth is warranted, although for extremely premature pregnancies, management is individualized. Scores of 0 to 3 are "abnormal," with expeditious birth considered (ACOG, 1999). Indications for BPP are those listed for antepartum fetal surveillance with weekly testing usually recommended. A BPP may also be indicated to follow-up on a nonreactive NST (Harman, 2004).

Modified Biophysical Profile

The modified BPP combines the use of a NST as a short-term indicator of fetal well-being with the assessment of amniotic fluid index as an indicator of long-term placental function. The amniotic fluid index (AFI) is the sum of the measurements of the deepest cord-free amniotic fluid pocket in each of the four abdominal quadrants. An AFI value greater than 5 cm generally is considered to represent an adequate volume of fluid. A modified BPP is considered reassuring if the NST is reactive and the AFI is greater than 5 but abnormal if the NST is nonreactive or the AFI is 5 or less (ACOG, 1999). The modified BPP is less cumbersome and appears to be as predictive of fetal status as other approaches of biophysical fetal surveillance (AAP & ACOG, 2002; ACOG, 1999).

NURSING ASSESSMENT AND INTERVENTIONS

Nursing interventions are based on a collaborative approach to the identification of strengths and conditions with potential to increase risk of complications. Together, the nurse and woman set goals and strategize ways to implement a plan of care to meet these goals. During the antepartum period, nursing care typically includes comfort promotion (ie, measures to relieve discomforts caused by the physiologic changes of pregnancy), counseling for family adaptation in planning the addition of a new member, and encouraging behaviors to enhance maternal and fetal well-being. Providing education, especially for the woman experiencing a first–time pregnancy, is an important aspect of antepartum care. The nurse has the opportunity and the responsibility to teach the woman and her family about beneficial and detrimental lifestyle practices, potential risks, and care required to promote maternal and fetal well-being. The nurse in ambulatory care provides anticipatory planning, assesses all available data, and structures education and nursing interventions accordingly. Inherent in competent antenatal nursing practice is the ability to differentiate between normal pregnancy variations and high-risk complications, and the initiation of appropriate nursing interventions.

Total care management of the childbearing family requires cooperation, collaboration, and communication across disciplines. Risk factors must be evaluated in terms of individual risk versus benefit to be effective. Healthcare providers are charged with the task of finding the goodness of fit between the recommended healthcare regimen and the individual's reality to optimize outcome. Case management allows for a single healthcare professional to coordinate healthcare management in collaboration with the pregnant woman.

Case Management

The childbearing woman and her family are the core of the perinatal healthcare team. Family-centered perinatal care is a model of care based on the philosophy that the physical, social, spiritual, and economic needs of the total family unit should be integrated and considered collectively (AWHONN, 2003). The nurse's role as case manager, advocate, and educator is of primary importance in facilitating a family-friendly system that validates the woman's own knowledge and promotes empowered healthcare decision-making.

Nutrition

Nutrition assessment and counseling is a vital component of prenatal care. The woman may benefit from regularly scheduled appointments with the nutritionist during an early prenatal visit and again at 28 weeks' gestation. Additional visits with the nutritionist should be scheduled as indicated (eg, for inadequate or excessive weight gain, anemia, metabolic disorders such as GDM). Weight-gain charts; 24-hour diet recall; or simple, self-report dietary assessment tools are valuable education resources.

Nutritional status may change because of availability of appropriate foods and financial resources for groceries. The most significant food shortages for low-income women occur at the end of the month, when federal and local resources are depleted or when food is shared among a disproportionate number of household members. Likewise, religious practices may dictate fasting during specific times of the year (eg, Lent or Ramadan), limiting the woman's food intake. Awareness and ongoing assessment of these factors allows for timely interventions and appropriate referral to nutrition counseling, social work, and community support services. Referrals to food and nutrition supplement programs may be warranted. Women in the United States should be referred to the Special Supplemental Feeding Program for WIC. Other supplemental food and nutrition programs are available to childbearing families on a regional or local basis. The prenatal healthcare team must be knowledgeable about such resources in their area.

Social Services

The emphasis on individualized, holistic prenatal care, encompassing physiologic and psychosocial needs, promotes a prevention-oriented model of care. Today's families may face unemployment, homelessness, chemical dependency, increased family and neighborhood violence, and lack of support systems that may precipitate crises and affect perinatal outcome. Early recognition of potential risk allows for prompt intervention

and referral. The role of the perinatal social worker is critical in providing interventions that relieve stress, providing for woman's basic needs, following crisis situations, and facilitating healthcare decision-making. Social work referrals are appropriate for pregnant women experiencing medical, psychological, or socioeconomic crises. Psychosocial and socioeconomic factors are evaluated on a continuing basis, with referral to social services as needed. Chapter 4 provides a more extensive discussion of psychological factors related to pregnancy.

From a practical point of view, pregnant women have much to benefit from a team approach. The woman has access to health professionals offering expertise in a specific area, and the perinatal team may be more likely to thoroughly assess and plan for a woman's individual needs. A pregnant woman may communicate about some concern to a nutritionist or social worker regarding a problem area that she did not reveal to the physician or nurse. With professional collaboration and communication among team members, problems can be better identified and addressed.

Education and Counseling

Educational and health promotional activities that include the father (depending on his relationship with the pregnant woman) can be integrated into prenatal care. Prenatal education should focus not only on a positive labor and birth experience but, more important, on laying the groundwork for a successful pregnancy outcome and family experience (AWHONN, 2003). Education regarding nutrition, sexuality, stress reduction, lifestyle behaviors, and hazards in the work place is appropriate to include in prenatal education (Display 5–13). Chapter 10 provides a more comprehensive review of childbirth education.

Early identification of conditions that can affect pregnancy outcome can minimize perinatal morbidity by allowing for the establishment of an appropriate treatment plan and referrals (AAP & ACOG, 2002). Women must receive information regarding risk factors, warning signs, and criteria for provider notification. Routine prenatal care should include education to enhance recognition of warning signs of preterm labor and preeclampsia (see Chapter 6), fever, rupture of membranes or leaking of fluid, decreased fetal movement, vaginal bleeding, persistent nausea and vomiting, and signs and symptoms of viral or bacterial infection.

With current postpartum lengths of stay, it is increasingly difficult to teach the woman and family all they need to know about maternal–newborn care during hospitalization. The last trimester of pregnancy may be a potentially effective time to introduce maternal–newborn care content, including parenting issues and

D I S P L A Y   5 - 1 3

Prenatal Education Topics

FIRST TRIMESTER

Healthy lifestyle
Nutrition
Smoking cessation
Teratogen avoidance
Alcohol avoidance
Illicit drug avoidance
Seat belt use
Sexuality
Work and rest patterns
Physiologic changes of pregnancy
Emotional changes of pregnancy
Discomforts of pregnancy
Screening, diagnostic tests
What to expect during prenatal care
Nipple assessment, breast-feeding promotion
Warning signs of pregnancy complications
Criteria and mechanism for notification of health care
    provider
(Information may be given at individual prenatal care visit
    or early pregnancy class)

SECOND TRIMESTER

Nutrition
Smoking cessation
Teratogen avoidance

Alcohol avoidance
Illicit drug avoidance
Prenatal laboratory tests
Physiologic changes of pregnancy
Emotional changes of pregnancy
Healthy lifestyle
Discomforts of pregnancy
Sexuality
Family roles
Fetal growth and development
Breast-feeding promotion
Childbirth education
Perineal exercises
Clothing choices/shoes
Body mechanics
Preterm birth prevention
Preeclampsia precautions/warning signs of pregnancy
    complications

THIRD TRIMESTER

Reproductive health
Discomforts of pregnancy
Where to go/whom to call
Warning signs of pregnancy complications
Fetal growth and development
Newborn care
Infant car seat use
Discussion of planned infant feeding
Childbirth education
Postpartum self-care choices
Postpartum emotional changes
Preparation for childbirth

Adapted from United States Department of Health and Human Services Expert Panel on the Content of Prenatal Care. (1989). *Caring for our future: The content of prenatal care.* Washington, DC: United States Public Health Service.

family planning information. Because there is no accurate way to predict which women will develop postpartum emotional disorders, all childbearing women and family members should be provided information about postpartum depression and where to seek help.

Confidence-building strategies that promote breast-feeding are an important component of prenatal nutrition education. Providing information about breast-feeding convenience, infant benefits, and potential formula cost savings can enhance maternal motivation. Acknowledging that some women may feel embarrassed or uncomfortable about breast-feeding and providing tips for discreet breast-feeding techniques are also helpful approaches.

Maternal breastfeeding self-efficacy is a significant predictor of breastfeeding duration and level. Therefore, Blyth and others (2002) recommend integrating self-efficacy enhancing strategies to increase a new mother's confidence in her ability to breastfeed, and to

persevere if she does encounter difficulties. Chezem, Friesen, and Boettcher (2003) studied infant feeding plans and breastfeeding confidence to explore their effect on actual practices. Breastfeeding knowledge was strongly correlated with breastfeeding confidence and actual lactation duration. Expectations and the actual breastfeeding experience differed among women planning to combination feed and those planning to exclusively breastfeed. Whether a cause or consequence, daily human milk substitute feeding was associated with negative breastfeeding outcomes (Chezem et al., 2003). De Oliveira, Camacho, and Tedstone (2001) found that during prenatal care, group education was the only effective strategy to extend the duration of breastfeeding. Class information commonly given to pregnant mothers includes benefits of breastfeeding, early initiation, how breast milk is produced, hazards of bottle feeding, breastfeeding on demand, prolonged breastfeeding, family planning and the lactational amenorrhea method. A session with the nutritionist, focusing on nutrition during lactation, may be helpful in encouraging initiation of breast-feeding and a successful breast-feeding experience. Chapter 13 provides an in-depth discussion about breast-feeding.

The childbearing continuum is a transition involving each family member. Childbirth education provides the opportunity for enhancement of family systems and facilitation of empowered behaviors that may last a lifetime. Forty years ago, the first childbirth education classes began as a means to provide information for women wishing to be awake, active participants in the birth of their child. Since then, childbirth education focusing on coping strategies for labor has been shown to decrease use of anesthesia in labor and enhance maternal confidence and satisfaction. Today, childbirth education goes well beyond basics to include information about birth as a natural process; environments that enhance the woman's ability to give birth; care options; and, most important, the tools necessary to make informed healthcare decisions that are appropriate for individual families. Childbirth education has expanded in some centers to meet consumers' need for information concerning preconception wellness, care provider and birthing options, and maternal–newborn care during the postpartum period. Current, accurate information; effective coping skills; and intact support systems fostered by childbirth education provide families with the skills to explore alternatives and make informed decisions that are congruent with their personal goals. It is important that childbirth education is available to all women. Perinatal nurses are challenged to move childbirth education from traditional services to time frames and locations that meet consumer needs.

Health Promotion

Preconception health promotion is increasingly recognized as an important factor influencing perinatal outcome. The addition of a prepregnancy visit and the recommended prenatal and postpartum visits has been identified as an essential step toward improving pregnancy outcomes, particularly for those planning pregnancy (CDC, 2006). If women have not been exposed to this information before pregnancy, healthcare professionals should seize the opportunity to provide information and experiences that promote these activities during prenatal care. Awareness of reproductive risk, healthy lifestyle behaviors, and reproductive options is essential in improving pregnancy outcome. Additionally, use the interconception period to provide additional intensive interventions to women who have had a previous pregnancy that ended in an adverse outcome (eg, infant death, fetal loss, birth defects, low birth weight, or preterm birth). Experiencing an adverse outcome in a previous pregnancy is an important predictor of future reproductive

risk. However, many women with adverse pregnancy outcomes do not receive targeted interventions to reduce risks during future pregnancies (CDC, 2006). Whereas a preterm birth is identified on birth certificates and a woman's primary care provider typically knows this information, professional guidelines do not include systematic follow-up and intervention for women with this critical predictor of risk.

SUMMARY

Prenatal care provides numerous opportunities for increasing reproductive awareness from a woman's health perspective. Aside from providing valuable information regarding the current pregnancy, laboratory evaluation also provides indicators of general health status and opportunities for health promotion. Screening tests that allow for health promotion are also offered during pregnancy. Nursing care during the prenatal period is multifaceted, requiring knowledge of the psychosocial tasks and issues surrounding the childbearing continuum, as well as knowledge of normal physiologic processes and potential risks. Anticipatory guidance during the prenatal period can have a significant impact on perinatal outcome. Education based on individual assessment empowers women and underscores their partnership in healthcare decision-making. The goal of prenatal care must go a step farther than targeting a positive physical outcome. Rather, we must work toward providing care and education that facilitates holistic family wellness and the best possible outcomes for mothers and babies.

REFERENCES

Abrams, B., Altman, S. L., Pickett, K. E. (2000). Pregnancy weight gain: Still controversial. *American Journal of Clinical Nutrition, 71*(Suppl. 5), 1233S–1241S.

Adeza Biomedical. (2005). *Fetal fibronectin enzyme immunoassay and rapid fFN for the TLi™ system: Information for health care providers.* Sunnyvale, CA: Author.

Altshuler, L. L., Cohen, L. S., Moline, M. L., Kahn, D. A., Carpenter, D., & Docherty, J. B. for the Expert Consensus Panel on Depression in Women. (2001). *The expert consensus guideline series: Treatment of depression in women.* (A Postgraduate Medicine Special report) pp. 1–107.

American Academy of Pediatrics & American College of Obstetricians and Gynecologists. (2002). *Guidelines for perinatal care* (5th ed.). Elk Grove Village, IL: Author.

American College of Obstetricians and Gynecologists. (1993). *Nutrition during pregnancy* (Technical Bulletin No. 179). Washington, DC: Author.

American College of Obstetricians and Gynecologists. (1997). *Teratology* (Educational Bulletin No. 236). Washington, DC: Author.

American College of Obstetricians and Gynecologists. (1999). *Antepartum fetal surveillance* (Practice Bulletin No. 9). Washington, DC: Author.

American College of Obstetricians and Gynecologists. (2000). *Thromboembolism in pregnancy* (Practice Bulletin No. 19). Washington, DC: Author.

American College of Obstetricians and Gynecologists. (2001a). *Gestational diabetes* (Practice Bulletin No. 30). Washington, DC: Author.

American College of Obstetricians and Gynecologists (2001b). *Assessment of risk factors for preterm birth* (Practice Bulletin No. 31). Washington, DC: Author.

American College of Obstetricians and Gynecologists. (2002a). *Diagnosis and management of preeclampsia and eclampsia* (Practice Bulletin No. 33). Washington, DC: Author.

American College of Obstetricians and Gynecologists. (2002b). *Exercise during pregnancy and the postpartum period* (Committee Opinion No. 267). Washington, DC: Author.

American College of Obstetricians and Gynecologists. (2003). *Immunization during Pregnancy* (Committee Opinion No. 282). Washington, DC: Author.

American College of Obstetricians and Gynecologists. (2004). *Prenatal and perinatal human immunodeficiency virus testing: Expanded recommendations* (Committee Opinion No. 304). Washington, DC: Author.

American College of Obstetricians and Gynecologists. (2005a). *Update on carrier screening for cystic fibrosis* (Committee Opinion No. 325). Washington, DC: Author.

American College of Obstetricians and Gynecologists. (2005b). *Smoking cessation during pregnancy* (Committee Opinion No. 316). Washington, DC: Author.

American College of Obstetricians and Gynecologists. (2006). *Psychosocial risk factors: Perinatal screening and intervention* (Committee Opinion No. 343). Washington, DC: Author.

American College of Obstetricians and Gynecologists. (2007). *Screening for fetal chromosomal abnormalities* (Practice Bulletin No. 77). Washington, DC: Author.

Artal, R., & O'Toole M. (2003). Guidelines of the American College of Obstetricians and Gynecologists for exercise during pregnancy and the postpartum period. *British Journal of Sports Medicine, 37*(1), 6–12.

Association of Women's Health, Obstetric and Neonatal Nurses. (2000). *Smoking and childbearing* (Clinical Position Statement). Washington, DC: Author.

Association of Women's Health, Obstetric and Neonatal Nurses. (2003) *Standards and guidelines for professional nursing practice in the care of women and newborns* (6th ed.). Washington, DC: Author.

Association of Women's Health, Obstetric and Neonatal Nurses. (2004). *Response to the U.S. Preventive Services Task Force Report on Screening for Family and Intimate Partner Violence published in the March 2 Annals of Internal Medicine.* Washington, DC: Author.

Andersson, L., Sundstrom-Poromaa, I., Wulff, M., Astrom, M., & Bixo, M. (2004). Implications of antenatal depression and anxiety for obstetric outcome. *Obstetrics and Gynecology, 104*(3), 467–476.

Barron, M. L. (1998). *Nursing assessment of the pregnant woman: Antepartal screening and laboratory evaluation* (Nursing Module). White Plains, NY: March of Dimes Birth Defects Foundation.

Barak S., Oettinger-Barak, O., Oettinger, M., Machtei, E. E., Peled, M., & Ohel, G. (2003). Common oral manifestations during pregnancy: A review. *Obstetrical and Gynecological Survey. 58*(9), 624–628.

Beck, C. T. (2002). Revision of the postpartum depression predictors inventory. *Journal of Obstetric, Gynecologic, and Neonatal Nursing, 31*(4), 394–402.

Bellinger, D. C. (2005). Teratogen update: Lead and pregnancy. *Birth Defects Research, 73*(6), 409–420.

Bennett, T., Braveman P., Egerter, S., & Kiely, J. L. (1994). Maternal marital status as a risk factor for infant mortality. *Family Planning Perspectives, 26*(6), 252–256, 271.

Blyth, R., Creedy, D., Dennis, C., Moyle, W., Pratt, J., & De Vries, S. (2002). Effect of maternal confidence on breastfeeding duration: an application of breastfeeding self-efficacy theory. *Birth, 29*(4), 278–284.

Boggess K. A. (2005). Pathophysiology of preterm birth: Emerging concepts of maternal infection. *Clinics in Perinatology, 32*(3), 561–569.

Boggess, K. A., Lief, S., Murtha, A. P., Moss, K., Beck, J., & Offenbacher S. (2003). Maternal periodontal disease is associated with an increased risk for preeclampsia. *Obstetrics and Gynecology, 101*(2), 227–231.

Brent, R. L. (2004). Environmental causes of human congenital malformations: the pediatrician's role in dealing with these complex clinical problems caused by a multiplicity of environmental and genetic factors. *Pediatrics, 113*(Suppl. 4), 957–968.

Brown, J. E., Murtaugh, M. A., Jacobs, D. R., & Margellos, H. C. (2002). Variation in newborn size according to prepregnancy weight change by trimester. *American Journal of Clinical Nutrition, 76*(1), 205–209.

Centers for Disease Control and Prevention. (2000). Entry into prenatal care–United States, 1989–1997. *Morbidity and Mortality Weekly Report, 49*(18), 393–398.

Centers for Disease Control and Prevention. (2001). HIV screening of pregnant women, *Morbidity and Mortality Weekly Report, 50*(RR 19), 59–86.

Centers for Disease Control and Prevention. (2006). Recommendations to improve preconception health and health care—United States: A report of the CDC/ATSDR preconception care work group and the select panel on preconception care. *Morbidity and Mortality Weekly Report Recommendations and Reports, 55*(RR 06), 1–23.

Chasnoff, I. J., Neuman, K., Thornton, C., & Callaghan, M. A. (2001). Screening for substance use in pregnancy: A practical approach for the primary care physician. *American Journal of Obstetrics and Gynecology, 184*(4), 752–758.

Chasnoff, I. J., McGourty, R. F., Bailey, G. W., Hutchins, E., Lightfoot, S. O., Pawson, L. L., et al. (2005). The 4Ps Plus*(c)* screen for substance use in pregnancy: Clinical application and outcomes. *Journal of Perinatalogy, 25*(6), 368–374.

Chezem, J., Friesen, C., & Boettcher, J. (2003). Breastfeeding knowledge, breastfeeding confidence, and infant feeding plans: Effects on actual feeding practices. *Journal of Obstetric, Gynecologic, and Neonatal Nursing, 32*(1), 40–47.

Cooksey, N. (1995). Pica and olfactory cravings of pregnancy: How deep are the secrets? *Birth: Issues in Perinatal Care, 22*(3), 129–137.

Cooperstock, M. S., Bakewell, J,. Herman, A., & Schramm, W. F. (1998). Effects of fetal sex and race on risk of very preterm birth in twins. *American Journal of Obstetrics & Gynecology. 179*(3 Pt 1), 762–765.

Corbett, R. W., Ryan, C., & Weinrich, S. P. (2003). Pica in pregnancy: Does it affect pregnancy outcomes? *MCN: The American Journal of Maternal Child Nursing, 28*(3), 183–191.

Cunningham, F. G., Leveno, K. J., Bloom, S. L., Hauth, J. C., Gilstrap, L. C., & Wendstrom, K. D. (2005). *William's Obstetrics* (22nd ed.). New York: McGraw-Hill.

DaCosta, D., Larouche, J., Dritsa, M., & Brender, W. (2000). Psychological correlates of prepartum and postpartum depressed mood. *Journal of Affective Disorders, 59*(4), 31–40.

de Oliveira, M. I., Camacho, L. A., & Tedstone, A. E. (2001). Extending breastfeeding duration through primary care: A systematic review of prenatal and postnatal interventions. *Journal of Human Lactation, 17*(4), 326–343.

Dugoff, L., Hobbins, J. C., Malone, F. D., Vidaver, J., Sullivan, L., Canick, J. A., et al. (2005). FASTER Trial Research Consortium. Quad screen as a predictor of adverse pregnancy outcome. *Obstetrics and Gynecology, 106*(2), 260–267.

Dye, T. D., Knox, K. L., Artal, R., Aubry, R. H., & Wojtowycz, M. A. (1997). Physical activity, obesity, and diabetes in pregnancy. *American Journal of Epidemiology, 146*(11), 961–965.

Feetham, S., Thomson, E. J., & Hinshaw, A. S. (2005). Nursing leadership in genomics for health and society. *Journal of Nursing Scholarship, 37*(2), 102–110.

Feldhaus, K. M., Koziol-McLain, J., Amsbury, H. L., Norton, I. M., Lowenstein, S. R., & Abbott, J. T. (1997). Accuracy of 3 brief screening questions for detecting partner violence in the emergency department. *Journal of the American Medical Association, 277*(17), 1357–1361.

Fischbach, F., & Dunning, M. (2004) *A Manual of Laboratory and Diagnostic Tests.* (7th ed.) Philadelphia: Lippincott Williams & Wilkins.

Gielen, A. C., O'Campo, P. J., Campbell, J. C., Schollenberger, J., Woods, A. B., Jones, A. S., et al. (2000). Women's opinions about domestic violence screening and mandatory reporting. *American Journal of Preventive Medicine, 19*(4), 279–285.

Gray, A. D., Power, M. L., Zinberg, S., & Schulkin, J. (2006). Assessment and management of obesity. *Obstetrical and Gynecological Survey, 61*(11), 742–748.

Gupton, A., Heaman, M., & Cheung, L. (2001). Complicated and Uncomplicated pregnancies: Women's perception of risk. *Journal of Obstetric, Gynecologic, and Neonatal Nursing, 30*(2), 192–201.

Haas, J. S., Meneses, V., & McCormick, M. C. (1999). Outcomes and health status of socially disadvantaged women during pregnancy. *Journal of Women's Health and Gender Based Medicine, 8*(4), 547–553.

Hall, L., & Neubert, A. G. (2005). Obesity and pregnancy. *Obstetrical and Gynecological Survey, 60*(4), 253–260.

Hamilton B. E., Martin J. A., & Ventura, S. J. (2006). Births: Preliminary Data for 2005. Retrieved from the world wide web retrieved 1-2-07 www.cdc.gov/nchs.

Harman, F. (2004). Assessment of fetal health. In R. Creasy, R. Resnick, & J. Iams (Eds.), *Maternal–fetal medicine: Principles and practice* (5th ed., pp. 357–402). Philadelphia: WB Saunders.

Hein, H. A., Burmeister, L. F., & Papke, K. R. (1990). The relationship of unwed status to infant mortality. *Obstetrics & Gynecology, 76*(5 Pt l), 763–768.

Hickey, C. A., Cliver, S. P., McNeal, S. F., Hoffman, H. J., & Goldenberg, R. L. (1996). Prenatal weight gain patterns and birth weight among nonobese black and white women. *Obstetrics and Gynecology, 88*(4, Pt.1), 490–496.

Ho, E., Karimi-Tabesh, L., & Koren G. (2001). Characteristics of pregnant women who use ecstasy (3, 4-methylenedioxymethamphetamine). *Neurotoxicology and Teratology, 23*(6), 561–567.

Honest, H., Bachmann, L. M., Gupta, J. K., Kleijnen, J., & Khan, K. S. (2002). Accuracy of cervicovaginal fetal fibronectin test in predicting risk of spontaneous preterm birth: Systematic review. *British Medical Journal, 325*(7359), 301–313.

Hook, E. B. (1981). Rates of chromosome abnormalities at different maternal ages. *Obstetrics and Gynecology, 58*(3), 282–285.

Institute of Medicine. (1990). *Nutrition during pregnancy.* Washington, DC: National Academy Press.

Jesse, D. E., & Graham, M. (2005). Are you often sad and depressed? Brief measures to identify women at risk for depression in pregnancy. *MCN: The American Journal of Maternal Child Nursing, 30*(1), 40–45.

Johnstone, S. J., Boyce, P. M., Hickey, A. R., Morris-Yates, A. D., & Harris, M. G. (2001). Obstetric risk factors for postnatal depression in urban and rural community samples. *Australian & New Zealand Journal of Psychiatry, 35*(1), 69–74.

Kelly, R., Zatzick, D., & Anders, T. (2001). The detection and treatment of psychiatric disorders and substance use among pregnant women cared for in obstetrics. *American Journal of Psychiatry, 158*(2), 213–219.

Khader, Y. S., & Ta'ani, Q. (2005). Periodontal diseases and the risk of preterm birth and low birth weight: A meta-analysis. *Journal of Periodontology, 76*(2), 161–165.

Kirkham, C., Harris, S., & Grzybowski, J. (2005). Evidence based prenatal care: Part I. General prenatal care and counseling issues. *American Family Physician, 71*(7), 1307–1316.

Krulewitch, C. J. (2005). Alcohol consumption during pregnancy. *Annual Review of Nursing Research, 23*, 101–134.

Larrabee, K., & Cowan, M. (1995). Clinical nursing management of sickle cell disease and trait during pregnancy. *Journal of Perinatal and Neonatal Nursing, 9*(2), 29–41.

LeMone P. (1999). Vitamins and minerals. *Journal of Obstetric, Gynecologic, and Neonatal Nursing, 28*(5), 520–533.

Li, R., Haas, J. D., & Habicht, J. P. (1998). Timing of the influence of maternal nutritional status during pregnancy on fetal growth. *American Journal of Human Biology, 10*, 529–539.

Lockwood, C. J. (2002). Inherited thrombophilias in pregnant patients: Detection and treatment paradigm. *Obstetrics and Gynecology, 99*(2), 333–341.

Lopez, N. J., Smith, P. C., & Gutierrez J. (2002). Higher risk of preterm birth and low birth weight in women with periodontal disease. *Journal of Dental Research, 81*(1), 58–63.

Luo, Z. C., Wilkins, R., & Kramer, M. S. (2004). Disparities in pregnancy outcomes according to marital and cohabitation status. *Obstetrics and Gynecology, 103*(6), 1300–1307.

March of Dimes. (1999). *Folic acid fact sheet.* White Plains, NY: March of Dimes Birth Defects Foundation.

March of Dimes. (2006). *Peristats.* White Plains, NY: March of Dimes Birth Defects Foundation.

Markovitz, B. P., Cook, R., Flick, L. H., & Leet, T. L. (2005). Socioeconomic factors and adolescent pregnancy outcomes: Distinctions between neonatal and post-neonatal deaths? *BMC Public Health, 5*, 79.

Martin, J. A., Hamilton, B. E., Sutton, P. D., Ventura, S. J., Menacker, F., & Kirmeyer, S. (2006). Births: Final data for 2004. *National Vital Statistics Reports, 55*(1), 1–102.

Marwick C. (2000). NIDA seeking data on effect of fetal exposure to methamphetamine. *Journal of the American Medical Association, 283*(17), 2225–2226.

Mathews, T. J., MacDorman, M. F., & Menacker, F. (2002). Infant mortality statistics from the 1999 period linked birth/infant death data set. *National Vital Statistics Reports. 50*(4), 1–28.

McFarlane, J., Parker, B., Soeken, K., & Bullock, L. (1992). Assessing for abuse during pregnancy. Severity and frequency of injuries and associated entry into prenatal care. *Journal of the American Medical Association, 267*(23), 3176–3178.

Mian, A. I. (2005). Depression in pregnancy and the postpartum period: Balancing adverse effects of untreated illness with treatment risks. *Journal of Psychiatric Practice, 11*(6), 389–396.

Misra, D. (2001). *The Women's Health Data Book.* (3rd ed.). Jacobs Institute of Women's Health. Elsevier Science.

Misra, S., & Kostaras, X. (2001). Depression during pregnancy: 1st world congress on women's mental health. Retrieved October 31, 2005, from http://www.medscape.com/viewarticle/420029

Moore, T. R., & Piacquadio, K. (1989). A prospective evaluation of fetal movement screening to reduce the incidence of antepartum fetal death. *American Journal of Obstetrics and Gynecology, 160*(5, Pt. 1), 1075–1080.

Mozurkewich, E. L., Luke, B., Avni, M., & Wolf, F. M. (2000). Working conditions and adverse pregnancy outcome: A meta-analysis. *Obstetrics and Gynecology, 95*(4), 623–635.

Murray, N., Homer, C. S., Davis, G. K., Curtis, J., Mangos, G., & Brown, M. A. (2002). The clinical utility of routine urinalysis in pregnancy: A prospective study. *Medical Journal of Australia, 177*(9), 477–480.

Nursing Network on Violence Against Women, International. (2003). *Abuse Assessment Screen.* Retrieved January 1, 2007, from http://www.nnvawi.org/assessment.htm

Orr, S. T., James, S. A., & Prince, C. B. (2002). Maternal prenatal depressive symptoms and spontaneous preterm births among African-American women in Baltimore, Maryland. *American Journal of Epidemiology, 156*(9), 797–802.

Papiernik, E. (1993). Prevention of preterm labor and delivery. *Balliere's Clinical Obstetrics and Gynecology, 7*(3), 499–521.

Parry-Jones, B. (1992). Pagophagia, or compulsive ice consumption: A historical perspective. *Psychological Medicine, 22*(3), 561–571.

Pignone, M. P., Gaynes, B. N., Rushton, J. L., Burchell, C. M., Orleans, C. T., Mulrow, C. D., et al. (2002). Screening for depression in adults: A summary of the evidence for the U.S. Preventive Services Task Force. *Annals of Internal Medicine, 136*(10), 765–776, I56.

Raatikainen, K., Heiskanen, N., & Heinonen, S. (2005). Marriage still protects pregnancy. *British Journal of Obstetrics and Gynaecology, 112*(10), 1411–1416.

Renker, P. R. (1999). Physical abuse, social support, self-care, and pregnancy outcomes of older adolescents. *Journal of Obstetric, Gynecologic, and Neonatal Nursing, 28*(4), 377–387.

Renker, P. R. (2003). Keeping safe: Teens' strategies for dealing with perinatal violence. *Journal of Obstetric, Gynecologic, and Neonatal Nursing, 32*(1), 58–67.

Rising, S. S. (1998). Centering pregnancy. An interdisciplinary model of empowerment. *Journal of Nurse Midwifery, 43*(1), 46–54.

Robertson, E., Grace, S., Wallington, T., & Stewart, D. E. (2004). Antenatal risk factors for postpartum depression: A synthesis of recent literature. *General Hospital Psychiatry, 26*(4), 289–295.

Robertson, L. Wu, O., & Greer I. (2004). Thrombophilia and adverse pregnancy outcome. *Current Opinion in Obstetrics & Gynecology, 16*(6), 453–458.

Schmitz, T., Maillard, F., Bessard-Bacquaert, S., Kayem, G., Fulla, Y., Cabrol, D., & Gofiet, F. (2006). Selective use of fetal fibronectin detection after cervical length measurement to predict spontaneous preterm delivery in women with preterm labor. *American Journal of Obstetrics and Gynecology. 194*(l), 138–143.

Seidel, H. M., Ball, J. W., Dains, J. E., & Benedict, G. W. (2006). *Mosby's Guide to Physical Examination* (6th ed.). CV Mosby: Philadelphia.

Sidhu, J. S. (2005). Alcohol Use Among Women of Childbearing Age: United States, 1991–1999. *Morbidity and Mortality Weekly Report, 51*(13), 273–276.

Silver, R. M. (2007). Fetal death. *Obstetrics and Gynecology, 109*(1), 153–167.

Simpson, E., Mull, J. D., & East, J. (2000). Pica during pregnancy in low-income women born in Mexico. *Western Journal of Medicine, 173*(1), 20–24.

Smith, L., Yonekura, M. L., Wallace, T., Berman, N., Kuo, J., & Berkowitz, C. (2003). Effects of prenatal methamphetamine exposure on fetal growth and drug withdrawal symptoms in infants born at term. *Journal of Developmental and Behavioral Pediatrics, 24*(1), 17–23.

Stephansson, O., Dickman, P. W., Johansson, A., & Cnattingius S. (2001). Maternal weight, pregnancy weight gain and the risk of antepartum stillbirth. *American Journal of Obstetrics and Gynecology, 184*(3), 463–469.

Stotland, N. E., Haas, J. S., Brawarsky, P., Jackson, R. A., Fuentes-Afflick, E., & Escobar, G. J. (2005). Body mass index, provider advice, and target gestational weight gain. *Obstetrics and Gynecology, 105*(3), 633–638.

Strauss, R. S., & Dietz, W. H. (1999). Low maternal weight gain in the second or third trimester increases the risk for intrauterine growth retardation. *Journal of Nutrition, 129*(5), 988–993.

Tekesin, I., Marek, S., Hellmeyer, L., Reitz, D., & Schmidt, S. (2005). Assessment of rapid fetal fibronectin in predicting preterm delivery. *Obstetrics and Gynecology, 105*(2), 280–284.

Thorsdottir, I., Torfadottir, J. E., Birgisdottir, B. E., & Gerisson, R. T. (2002). Weight gain in women of normal weight before pregnancy: Complications in pregnancy or delivery and birth outcome. *Obstetrics and Gynecology, 99*(5, Pt 1), 799–806.

United States Department of Health and Human Services. (2000). *Health People 2010.* Washington, DC: Author. Retrieved January 1, 2007, from http://www.healthypeople.gov/

United States Department of Health and Human Services. (2005). *The NSDUH report: Substance use during pregnancy: 2002 and 2003 update.* Washington, DC: Author. Retrieved January 1, 2007, from http://www.oas.samhsa.gov/2k5/pregnancy/pregnancy.cfm

United States Department of Health and Human Services Expert Panel on the Content of Prenatal Care. (1989). *Caring for our future: The content of prenatal care.* Washington, DC: United States Public Health Service.

Villar, J., Carroli, G., Khan-Neelofur, D., Piaggio, G., & Gulmezoglu, M. (2001). Patterns of routine antenatal care for low-risk pregnancy. *Cochrane Database of Systematic Reviews, 4,* CD000934.

Walker, D. S., & Rising, S. S. (2004). Revolutionizing prenatal care: New evidence-based prenatal care delivery models. *Journal of the New York State Nurses Association, 35,* 18–21.

Washington State Department of Health. (2002). *Smoking cessation during pregnancy: Guidelines for intervention.* Spokane, WA: Author. Retrieved January 1, 2007, from www.doh.wa.gov/CFH/mch/documents/CessationFinal_122.pdf

Waugh, J. J., Clark, T. J., Divarkaran, T. G., Khan, K. S., & Kilby, M. D. (2004). Accuracy of urinalysis dipstick techniques in predicting significant proteinuria in pregnancy. *Obstetrics and Gynecology, 103*(4), 769–777.

Williams, J. K., & Lea, D. H. (2003). *Genetic Issues for Perinatal Nurses* (Nursing Module 2nd ed.). White Plains, NY: March of Dimes Birth Defects Foundation.

Wheeler, L. (2002). *Nurse-midwifery handbook: A practical guide to prenatal and postpartum care.* (2nd ed.) Philadelphia: Lippincott Williams & Wilkins.

Wouldes, T., LaGasse, L., Sheridan, J., & Lester, B. (2004). Maternal methamphetamine use during pregnancy and child outcome: What do we know? *New Zealand Medical Journal, 117*(1206), 1–10.

Yost, N. P., Bloom, S. L., McIntire, D. D., & Leveno, K. J. (2005). A prospective observational study of domestic violence during pregnancy. *Obstetrics and Gynecology, 106*(1), 61–65.

APPENDIX **5-A**

Teratogenic Agents

Agent	Effects	Comments
Drugs and chemicals		
Alcohol	Growth restriction before and after birth, mental retardation, microcephaly, midfacial hypoplasia producing atypical facial appearance, renal and cardiac defects, various other major and minor malformations	Nutritional deficiency, smoking, and multiple drug use confound data. Risk from ingestion of one to two drinks per day is not well defined but may cause a small reduction in average birth weight. Fetuses of women who ingest six drinks per day have a 40% risk of developing some features of the fetal alcohol syndrome.
Androgens and testosterone derivatives (eg, danazol)	Virilization of female, advanced genital development in males	Effects are dose dependent and related to the stage of embryonic development at the time of exposure. Given before 9 weeks of gestation, labioscrotal fusion can be produced; clitoromegaly can occur with exposure at any gestational age. Risk related to incidental brief androgenic exposure is minimal.
Angiotensin-converting enzyme (ACE) inhibitors (eg, enalapril, captopril)	Fetal renal tubular dysplasia, oligohydramnios, neonatal renal failure, lack of cranial ossification, intrauterine growth restriction	Incidence of fetal morbidity is 30%. The risk increases with second- and third-trimester use, leading to in utero fetal hypotension, decreased renal blood flow, and renal failure.
Coumarin derivatives (eg, warfarin)	Nasal hypoplasia and stippled bone epiphyses are most common; other effects include broad, short, hands with shortened phalanges, ophthalmologic abnormalities, intrauterine growth restriction, developmental delay, anomalies of neck and central nervous system	Risk for a seriously affected child is considered to be 15–25% when anticoagulants that inhibit vitamin K are used in the first trimester, especially during 6–9 weeks of gestation. Later drug exposure may be associated with spontaneous abortion, stillbirths, central nervous system abnormalities, abruptio placentae, and fetal or neonatal hemorrhage.
Carbamazepine	Neutral tube defects, minor craniofacial defects, fingernail hypoplasia, microcephaly, developmental delay, intrauterine growth restriction	Risk of neural tube defect, mostly lumbosacral, is 1–2% when used alone during first trimester and increased when used with other antiepileptic agents.
Folic acid antagonists (methotrexate and aminopterin)	Increased risk for spontaneous abortions, various anomalies	These drugs are contraindicated for the treatment of psoriasis in pregnancy and must be used with extreme caution in the treatment of malignancy. Cytotoxic drugs are potentially teratogenic. Effects of aminopterin are well documented. Folic acid antagonists used during the first trimester produce a malformation rate of up to 30% in fetuses that survive.

Cocaine	Bowel atresias; congenital malformations of the heart, limbs, face, and genitourinary tract; microcephaly; intrauterine growth restriction; cerebral infarctions	Risks may be affected by other factors and concurrent abuse of multiple substances. Maternal and pregnancy complications include sudden death and placental abruption.
Diethylstilbestrol	Clear cell adenocarcinoma of the vagina or cervix, vaginal adenosis, abnormalities of cervix and uterus, possible infertility in males and females	Vaginal adenosis is detected in more than 50% of women whose mothers took these drugs before 9 weeks of gestation. Risk for vaginal adenocarcinoma is low. Males exposed in utero may have a 25% incidence of epididymal cysts, hypotrophic testes, abnormal spermatozoa, and induration of the testes.
Lead	Increases abortion rate, stillbirths	Fetal central nervous system development may be adversely affected. Determining preconceptional lead levels for those at risk may be useful.
Lithium	Congenital heart disease, particularly Ebstein anomaly	Risk of heart malformations due to first-trimester exposure is low. The effect is not as significant as reported in earlier studies. Exposure in the last month of gestation may produce toxic effects on the thyroid, kidneys, and neuromuscular systems.
Organic mercury	Cerberal atrophy, microcephaly, mental retardation, spasticity, seizures, blindness	Cerebral palsy can occur even when exposure is in the third trimester. Exposed individuals include consumers of fish and grain contaminated with methyl mercury.
Phenytoin	Intrauterine growth restriction, mental retardation, microcephaly, dysmorphic craniofacial features, cardiac defects, hypoplastic nails and distal phalanges	The full syndrome is seen in less than 10% of children exposed in utero, but up to 30% have some manifestations. Mild to moderate mental retardation is found in some children who have severe physical stigmata. The effect may depend on whether the fetus inherits a mutant gene that decreases production of epoxide hydrolase, an enzyme necessary to decrease the teratogen phenytoin epoxide.
Streptomycin and kanamycin	Hearing loss, eighth-nerve damage	No ototoxicity in the fetus has been reported from use of gentamicin or vancomycin.
Tetracycline	Hypoplasia of tooth enamel, incorporation of tetracycline into bones and teeth, permanent yellow-brown discoloration of deciduous teeth	Drug has no known effect unless exposure occurs in second or third trimester.

(continued)

Teratogenic Agents (*Continued*)

Agent	Effects	Comments
Drugs and chemicals (*Continued*)		
Thalidomide	Bilateral limb deficiencies, anotia and microtia, cardiac and gastrointestinal anomalies	Of children whose mothers used thalidomide between 35 and 50 days of gestation, 20% show the effect.
Trimethadione and paramethadione	Cleft lip or cleft palate; cardiac defects; growth deficiency; microcephaly; mental retardation; characteristic facial appearance; ophthalmologic, limb, and genitourinary tract abnormalities	Risk for defects or spontaneous abortion is 60–80% with first-trimester exposure. A syndrome, including V-shaped eyebrows, low-set ears, high arched palate, and irregular dentition, has been identified. These drugs are no longer used during pregnancy due to the availability of more effective, less toxic agents.
Valproic acid	Neural tube defects, especially spina bifida; minor facial defects	Exposure must occur before normal closure of neural tube during first trimester to produce open defect (incidence of approximately 1%).
Vitamin A and its derivatives (eg, isotretinoin, etretinate, and retinoids)	Increased abortion rate, microtia, central nervous system defects, thymic agenesis, cardiovascular effects, craniofacial dysmorphism, microphthalmia, cleft lip and palate, mental retardation	Isotretinoin exposure before pregnancy is not a risk because the drug is not stored in tissue. Etretinate has a long half-life, and effects occur long after drug is discontinued. Topical application does not have a known risk.
Infections		
Cytomegalovirus	Hydrocephaly, microcephaly, chorioretinitis, cerebral calcifications, symmetric intrauterine growth restriction, microphthalmos, brain damage, mental retardation, hearing loss	Most common congenital infection. Congenital infection rate is 40% after primary infection and 14% after recurrent infection. Of infected infants , physical effects as listed are present in 20% after primary infection and 8% after secondary infection. No effective therapy exists.
Rubella	Microcephaly, mental retardation, cataracts, deafness, congenital heart disease; all organs may be affected	Malformation rate is 50% if the mother is infected during first trimester. Rate of severe permanent organ damage decreases to 6% by midpregnancy. Immunization of children and nonpregnant adults is necessary for prevention. Immunization I not recommended during pregnancy, but the live attenuated vaccine virus has not been shown to cause the malformations of congenital rubella syndrome.
Syphilis	If severe infection, fetal demise with hydrops; if mild, detectable abnormalities of skin, teeth, and bones	Penicillin treatment is effective for *Treponema pallidum* eradication to prevent progression of damage. Severity of fetal damage depends on duration of fetal infection; damage is worse if infection is greater than 20 weeks. Prevalence is increasing; need to rule out other sexually transmitted diseases.

Toxoplasmosis	Possible effects on all systems but particularly central nervous system: microcephaly, hydrocephaly, cerebral calcifications. Chorioretinitis is most common. Severity of manifestations depends on duration of disease.	Low prevalence during pregnancy (0.1–0.5%); initial maternal infection must occur during pregnancy to place fetus at risk. *Toxoplasma gondii* is transmitted to humans by raw meat or exposure to infected cat feces. In the first trimester, the incidence of fetal infection is as low as 9% and increases to approximately 59% in the third trimester. The severity of congenital infection is greater in the first trimester than at the end of gestation. Treat with pyrimethamine, sulfadiazine, or spiramycin.
Varicella	Possible effects on all organs, inluding skin scarring, chorioretinitis, cataracts, microcephaly, hypoplasia of the hands and feet, and muscle atrophy	Risk of congenital varicella is low, approximately 2–3%, and occurs between 7 and 21 weeks of gestation. Varicella-zoster immune globulin is available regionally for newborns exposed in utero during last 4–7 days of gestation. No effect from herpes zoster.
Radiation	Microcephaly, mental retardation	Medical diagnostic radiation delivering less than 0.05 Gy* to the fetus has no teratogenic risk. Estimated fetal exposure of common radiologic procedures is 0.01 Gy or less (eg, intravenous pyelography, 0.0041 Gy).

*1 gray (Gy) = 100 rad.

From American College of Obstetricians and Gynecologists. (1997). *Teratology* (Educational bulletin no. 236). Washington, DC: Author.

Vaccine and Immune Globulin During Pregnancy

RECOMMENDED VACCINE DURING PREGNANCY

Influenza

Recommended for all women in second and third trimester during flu season (October–March) and women at high risk for pulmonary complications regardless of trimester.

CONTRAINDICATED/NOT RECOMMENDED VACCINES IN PREGNANCY

Anthrax	Measles	Yellow Fever
Mumps	Rubella	

RISK VS. BENEFIT: NOT ROUTINELY RECOMMENDED EXCEPT IN PERSONS AT INCREASED RISK OF EXPOSURE

Polio	Plague	Typhoid

CONTRAINDICATED BUT NO ADVERSE OUTCOMES REPORTED IF GIVEN IN PREGNANCY

Varicella

INDICATIONS FOR VACCINE THAT ARE NOT ALTERED BY PREGNANCY

Cholera	Pneumococcus
Hepatitis A	Rabies
Hepatitis B	Tetanus-diphtheria
Meningococcus	

INDICATED FOR IMMUNE GLOBULINS AS POST-EXPOSURE PROPHYLAXIS

Hepatitis A	Rabies
Hepatitis B	Tetanus
Measles	Varicella

Adapted from ACOG. (2003). *Immunization during Pregnancy* (Committee Opinion No. 282). Washington, DC: Author. More complete information may be found at http://www.acog.org/from_home/publications/misc/bco282.pdf (last accessed January, 2007)

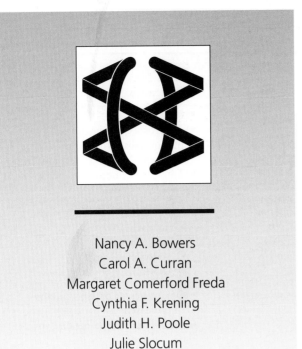

High-Risk Pregnancy

Nancy A. Bowers
Carol A. Curran
Margaret Comerford Freda
Cynthia F. Krening
Judith H. Poole
Julie Slocum
Mary Ellen Burke Sosa

ALTHOUGH the majority of pregnant women have a normal healthy pregnancy, labor, and birth, some women experience complications. These complications may be the result of preexisting conditions or develop as a result of the pregnancy. In some cases, complications arise unexpectedly in a previously healthy pregnancy. The status of the mother or fetus may be in jeopardy. Perinatal nurses need to be aware of signs and symptoms of common complications of pregnancy and be ready to intervene based on the latest science, standards, and guidelines. Providing safe and effective perinatal care requires an interdisciplinary effort by all members of the perinatal team. Because perinatal nurses are the clinicians who provide the majority of direct bedside care, they are often the first members of the healthcare team to recognize when the clinical condition of the mother and baby has changed from the expected normal course to a situation that involves risk of perinatal harm. The expert-nurse authors of this chapter present a review of selected complications and clinical conditions of pregnancy, labor, birth, and the postpartum period including hypertensive disorders, bleeding, preterm labor and birth, diabetes, cardiac disease, pulmonary disease, and multiple gestations.

HYPERTENSIVE DISORDERS

Definitions

Terminology used to describe the hypertensive disorders of pregnancy has suffered from imprecise usage, causing confusion for healthcare providers caring for women with hypertensive complications during pregnancy, childbirth, and postpartum. *The National High Blood Pressure Education Program Working Group Report on High Blood Pressure in Pregnancy*, published through the National Institutes of Health, National Heart, Lung, and Blood Institute, outlines current accepted terminology for the hypertensive disorders of pregnancy (Gifford et al., 2000; National High Blood Pressure Education Program Working Group on High Blood Pressure in Pregnancy [Working Group], 2000; National High Blood Pressure Education Program [NHBPEP], 2000). See Table 6–1 for the current classification of hypertension in pregnancy. The American College of Obstetricians and Gynecologists (ACOG) published a revised Practice Bulletin in 2002 on the diagnosis and management of preeclampsia and reinforced the new classification scheme. Clinically, there are two basic types of hypertension during pregnancy, chronic hypertension and gestational hypertension, with the distinction based on the onset of hypertension in relation to the pregnancy.

Chronic Hypertension

Chronic hypertension is hypertension present and observable before the pregnancy, diagnosed before 20 weeks gestation, or hypertension continuing beyond the 42nd day postpartum (Gifford et al., 2000; NHBPEP, 2000; Working Group, 2000). Hypertension is defined as a systolic blood pressure equal to or greater than 140 mm Hg or a diastolic blood pressure equal to or greater than 90 mm Hg (Gifford et al.; NHBPEP; Working Group). Hypertension is diagnosed

TABLE 6–1 ■ CLASSIFICATION OF HYPERTENSIVE DISORDERS OF PREGNANCY

Type of Hypertension	Diagnostic Criteria	Significance

Gestational hypertension	• New onset of hypertension, generally after 20 weeks of gestation
	• Hypertension defined as:
	  • SBP ≥140 mm Hg, *OR*
	  • DBP ≥90 mm Hg
		• Replaces PIH
		• A retrospective diagnosis
		• BP normalizes to prepregnancy values by 12 weeks' postpartum
		• Think oxygenation and perfusion

Preeclampsia	• Gestational hypertensive plus gestational proteinuria in a previously normotensive woman
	• Gestational proteinuria defined as
	  • >300 mg on random specimen
	  • ≥1+ on dipstick
		• In absence of proteinuria, suspect if any of the following are present:
		  • Headache
		  • Blurred vision
		  • Abdominal pain
		  • Abnormal laboratory tests

Severe	• Diagnosis of preeclampsia plus at least one of the following:
	  • SBP ≥160 mm Hg
	  • DBP ≥110 mm Hg
	  • Proteinuria >2 g/24 hr
	  • Serum creatinine >1.2 mg/dL
	  • Platelets <100,000
	  • ↑ LD (hemolysis)
	  • ↑ ALT or AST
	  • Persistent HA, cerebral/visual disturbances
	  • Persistent epigastric pain
		• One of sickest patients on unit
		• At increased risk for complications
		• Additional criteria for diagnosis may include:
		  • Oliguria defined as <500 mL/24 hr
		  • Pulmonary edema
		  • Impaired liver function of unclear etiology
		  • IUGR
		  • Oligohydramnios
		  • Grand mal seizures (eclampsia)

HELLP syndrome	• Diagnosis based on presence of:
	  • Hemolysis
	  • Elevated Liver Enzymes
	  • Low Platelets
	• Hemolysis
	  • Abnormal peripheral smear
	  • Lactate dehydrogenase (LD) >600 Units/L
	  • Total bilirubin ≥1.2 mg/dL
	• Elevated Liver Enzymes
	  • Serum aspartate aminotransferase >70 U/L
	  • LD >600 U/L
	• Low Platelets <150,000
		• Form of severe preeclampsia
		• Laboratory diagnosis
		• Impairs oxygenation and perfusion
		• Severity of disease, morbidity/mortality, and recovery related to platelet levels
		  • <150,000 BUT >100,000
		  • <100,000 BUT >50,000
		  • <50,000

Eclampsia	• Diagnosis of preeclampsia
	• Occurrence of seizures
	• No other possible etiology for seizure
		• Critically ill patient
		• At risk for cerebral hemorrhage and aspiration
		• Foley's Rule of 13:
		  • 13% Mortality
		  • 13% Abruption
		  • 13% Seize after MgSO$_4$ therapy
		  • 13% Seize >48 hr postpartum

Chronic hypertension	• Hypertension defined as:
	  • SBP ≥140 mm Hg, *OR*
	  • DBP ≥90 mm Hg
	• Hypertension
	  • Present and observable before pregnancy
	  • Diagnosed before 20 weeks' gestation
	  • Persist beyond 12 weeks' postpartum
		• Diagnosis may not be known prior to pregnancy
		• Places pregnancy at increased risk for abruption

TABLE 6–1 ■ CLASSIFICATION OF HYPERTENSIVE DISORDERS OF PREGNANCY (Continued)

Type of Hypertension	Diagnostic Criteria	Significance

Superimposed preeclampsia	• Diagnosis based on presence of 1 or more of the following in the woman with chronic hypertension:
	  • New onset of proteinuria
	  • Hypertension and proteinuria before 20th week of gestation
	  • Sudden ↑ in proteinuria
	  • Sudden ↑ BP (previously well controlled)
	  • ↑ ALT or AST to abnormal levels
	  • Thrombocytopenia
		• Prognosis worse for woman and fetus
		• Mandates close observation
		• Timing of birth indicated by overall assessment of maternal–fetal well-being rather than fixed end point

Adapted from American College of Obstetricians and Gynecologists, 2002; August, 2004; Gifford et al., 2000; National High Blood Pressure Education Program Working Group on High Blood Pressure in Pregnancy, 2000; National High Blood Pressure Education Program, 2000).

when either value is above the defined values; elevation of both systolic and diastolic pressures is not necessary for the diagnosis. The severity of hypertension is determined by the higher value, even if the other value is within normal parameters.

Gestational Hypertension

Gestational hypertension is the onset of hypertension, generally after the 20th week of pregnancy, appearing as a marker of a pregnancy-specific vasospastic condition (Roberts, 2004). Gestational hypertension in clinical practice is a retrospective diagnosis. If hypertension is first diagnosed during pregnancy, is transient, does not progress into preeclampsia, and the woman is normotensive by 12 weeks postpartum, the diagnosis is gestational hypertension; if the blood pressure elevation persists then the diagnosis is chronic hypertension (Gifford et al., 2000; NHBPEP, 2000; Working Group, 2000). These two types of hypertension (chronic hypertension and gestational) may occur independently or simultaneously.

Once gestational hypertension is present, hypertension is further classified according to the maternal organ systems affected. The practitioner must keep in mind that hypertension during pregnancy represents a continuum of disease processes. Hypertension may be the first sign, but the underlying pathophysiology can involve all major organ systems.

Preeclampsia

Preeclampsia is characterized by renal involvement, as evidenced by the onset of proteinuria. It must be remembered that preeclampsia is a pregnancy-specific syndrome of reduced organ perfusion, including the utero–placental–fetal unit, secondary to cyclic vasospasms, and activation of the coagulation cascade (Gifford et al., 2000; NHBPEP, 2000; Working Group, 2000). The disease process is said to be mild or severe on the basis of maternal or fetal findings. If signs and symptoms of preeclampsia or eclampsia occur in women with chronic hypertension, the diagnosis of superimposed preeclampsia or eclampsia is made.

HELLP Syndrome

HELLP syndrome is a clinical and laboratory diagnosis characterized by hepatic involvement as evidenced by Hemolysis, Elevated Liver enzymes, and Low Platelet count. HELLP syndrome is not part of the current classification system but is a reflection of disease progression to severe preeclampsia.

Eclampsia

Eclampsia is characterized by the onset of seizure activity or coma in the woman diagnosed with preeclampsia, with no history of preexisting neurologic pathology (Gifford et al., 2000; NHBPEP, 2000; Working Group, 2000).

Significance and Incidence

Hypertensive disorders of pregnancy are the most common medical complications during pregnancy, labor, birth, and the postpartum period. A diagnosis of hypertension complicating pregnancy challenges the care provider, who must weigh the risk, benefits, and alternatives of treatment related to maternal, fetal, and neonatal well-being. Everyone caring for the woman during her pregnancy must be aware of the significance of the disease process, current diagnostic criteria, and management recommendations. Prompt recognition of the disease process and monitoring for potential complications decreases the risk of significant morbidity for the woman and her baby.

Preeclampsia is a significant contributor to maternal and perinatal morbidity and mortality, complicating approximately 5% to 8% of all pregnancies not terminating in first-trimester abortions (Egerman & Sibai, 1999; Martin et al., 2006; Myatt & Miodovnik, 1999). In 2004, hypertension, both chronic and pregnancy related, complicated 194,626 (4.6%) of the 4.1 million pregnancies in the United States (US; Martin et al.). For women with a history of chronic hypertension or renal disease predating pregnancy, the occurrence of preeclampsia is 25% (Jones & Hayslett, 1996).

The rate of pregnancy-related hypertension continues to rise in the United States. Pregnancy-related hypertension has increased from a rate of 35.9 per 1,000 births in 1996 to 37.4 in 2002 (Jones & Hayslett, 1996; Martin et al., 2005; Ventura et al., 2000). For the year 2004, the last year cumulative data are available, the rate of pregnancy-related hypertension was 37.9 per 1,000 births (Martin et al., 2006). Of the pregnancies complicated by hypertension, 30% of the women will have chronic hypertension and 70% will be diagnosed with gestational hypertension or preeclampsia. The rate for pregnancy-related hypertension has increased for all ages, races, and ethnic groups during the 1990s; the rates are essentially unchanged since 2000 (Martin et al., 2002, 2003, 2005). Paralleling demographics of the general population, the rate of chronic hypertension as a comorbidity during pregnancy has increased from a rate of 6.5 per 1,000 births in 1990 to a rate of 9.6 per 1,000 births in 2004 in the United States (Martin et al., 2006). The rate for eclampsia has slightly decreased since 1990 (4.0/1,000 births) to a rate of 3.0 per 1,000 births in 2003 (Martin et al., 2005).

Maternal race influences the rate of hypertension complicating pregnancy, with the highest rates seen for the American Indian, which includes births to Aleuts and Eskimos, (49.7/1,000) and African-American (40.2/1,000) women. Asian or Pacific Islander women have the lowest rate for hypertension complicating pregnancy (19.6/1,000). Non-Hispanic white and black populations approximate the African-American population for the occurrence of hypertension complicating pregnancy at 42.6 and 40.5 per 1,000 births, respectively (Martin et al., 2005; Table 6–2). Age distribution graphs as a U-shaped curve, with women younger than 20 years of age and older than 40 years of age having the highest rates of hypertension (Table 6–3).

Morbidity and Mortality

In the United States, pregnancy-associated hypertension is a leading cause of maternal death. Final mortality data for 1997 reported a total of 327 maternal deaths, producing a rate of 8.4 deaths per 100,000 live births (Hoyert, Kochanek, & Murphy, 1999). The overall rate of maternal death from preeclampsia or eclampsia is 1.6 per 100,000, which is one of the leading specific causes of death identified; the rate of obstetric pulmonary embolism-specific maternal death is also 1.6. There is a large disparity among rates of maternal death by race. African-American women are more likely to die of preeclampsia. The overall maternal death rate for African-American women was 20.8 per 100,000 in 1997, compared with 5.8 for white women and 18.3 for all other races. Of those maternal deaths from preeclampsia or eclampsia, the maternal mortality rate was 1.1 for whites, 4.5 for African Americans, and 3.8 for all other races (Hoyert, Kochanek, & Murphy, 1999).

In 2003, the Department of Health and Human Services and the Centers for Disease Control and Prevention (CDC) published data from the Pregnancy Mortality Surveillance System reporting pregnancy-related mortality from 1991 to 1999 (Chang et al., 2003). This publication examined the pregnancy-related mortality by pregnancy outcome. Hypertension remained a leading cause of maternal death, accounting for 15.7% of all maternal deaths from 1991 to 1999. For women who have hypertension as the cause of death, 19.3% gave birth to a living infant and 20% had a stillbirth; for 11.8% the pregnancy outcome was unknown (Chang et al.). The cause-specific, pregnancy-related mortality ratio was three to four times higher for African-American women diagnosed with a hypertensive disorder (Chang et al.).

Hypertension during pregnancy predisposes the woman to potentially lethal complications such as abruptio placentae, disseminated intravascular coagulation (DIC), cerebral hemorrhage, cerebral vascular accident, hepatic failure, and acute renal failure. Leading causes of maternal death from hypertension complicating pregnancy include complications from abruptio placentae, hepatic rupture, and eclampsia (Martin et al., 2006; Roberts, 2004).

Maternal hypertension contributes to intrauterine fetal death and perinatal mortality. The main causes of neonatal death are placental insufficiency and abruptio placentae (Roberts, 2004). Intrauterine growth restriction (IUGR) is common in infants of women with preeclampsia (Roberts, Taylor, Friedman, & Goldfien, 1990; Sibai, 1990a). The exact cause is

TABLE 6–2 ■ RATES OF PREGNANCY-INDUCED HYPERTENSION BY MATERNAL RACE

Maternal Race	1997	1998	1999	2000	2001	2002	2003	2004
All Races	36.8	37.6	38.2	38.8	37.7	37.8	37.4	37.9
White	37.1	37.9	38.7	39.3	38.0	38.1	38.0	43.3
African-American	39.7	40.6	40.5	41.7	40.6	41.5	40.2	42.2
America Indian (includes Aleuts and Eskimos)	48.1	46.8	48.8	48.2	47.7	46.5	49.7	Not reported
Asian or Pacific Islander								
Total	20.1	20.3	20.2	20.5	21.4	20.8	19.6	Not reported
Chinese	14.4	14.2	12.2	11.9	13.2	11.6	(only	
Japanese	18.4	17.4	21.7	16.5	22.2	16.9	reported	
Hawaiian	28.8	29.6	39.9	40.4	45.8	48.2	total)	
Filipino	28.8	30.9	30.3	30.4	32.0	30.8		
Other	18.7	18.5	18.4	19.7	19.2	19.5		
Hispanic								
Total	26.8	27.9	27.7	27.9	26.2	26.3	25.9	25.8
Mexican	25.7	26.6	26.6	27.0	24.7	24.9	24.5	
Puerto Rican	28.1	31.9	30.1	31.6	31.6	32.0	31.7	
Cuban	30.0	29.3	31.2	31.7	26.5	31.1	32.3	
Central and South America	27.1	27.5	27.7	27.2	27.7	25.1	26.5	
Other or Unknown Hispanic	36.9	36.6	36.4	35.3	35.4	38.6	34.5	
Non-Hispanic								
Total	39.1	39.9	40.8	41.7	40.8	41.0	40.8	Not reported
White	40.1	41.0	42.2	43.2	42.3	42.6	42.6	
Black	39.8	40.8	40.6	41.9	40.9	41.8	40.5	

*Rate per 1,000 live births. Rates reported as number of live births with specified medical risk factor per 1,000 live births by specified group (Martin, Hamilton et al., 2006; Martin, Hamilton et al., 2003, 2005; Martin, Hamilton, Ventura, Menacker, Park et al., 2002; Martin, Hamilton, Ventura, Menacker, & Park, 2002; Ventura, Martin, Hamilton, Curtin, & Mathews, 1999; Ventura et al., 2000).

unknown, but fetal and neonatal consequences of preeclampsia may be related to the changes in the uteroplacental unit. Histologic findings of placentas from pregnancies complicated by preeclampsia are consistent with poor uteroplacental perfusion, which can lead to chronic hypoxemia in the fetus (Roberts).

Risk Factors

Preeclampsia is a subtle and insidious disease process unique to human pregnancy. The signs and symptoms of preeclampsia become apparent relatively late in the course of the disease, usually during the third trimester of pregnancy. However, the underlying pathophysiology may be present as early as 8 weeks of gestation (Friedman, Taylor, & Roberts, 1991).

Historically, several well-defined risk factors have been identified for the development of preeclampsia (Display 6–1). Although risk factors are identified, the individual predictive values of the risk factors for screening and risk identification purposes have not been verified. Women should not be arbitrarily labeled as low- or high-risk patients based solely on historical risk factors.

Age

The incidence of preeclampsia is reported to increase in the teenage population and for the older pregnant woman. The risk of developing preeclampsia for the nulliparous adolescent younger than 19 years of age is significantly higher than that in women older than 19 years of age (Butler & Alberman, 1958; Goldberg & Craig, 1983; Guzick et al., 1987; Martin et al., 2006; Montagu, 1979; Taylor, 1988; Ventura et al., 2000). However, this association has not been identified independently of other risk factors, especially parity. Because a higher proportion of pregnancies, especially first pregnancies, are in women of younger age, more cases of preeclampsia occur in this age group. Age may be significant only in that older women are more likely to enter

TABLE 6–3 ■ RATES OF PREGNANCY-RELATED HYPERTENSION BY MATERNAL AGE

	Chronic Hypertension								Gestational Hypertension/Preeclampsia								Eclampsia						
	1997	1998	1999	2000	2001	2002	2003	2004	1997	1998	1999	2000	2001	2002	2003	2004	1997	1998	1999	2000	2001	2002	2003
All Races																							
All Ages	6.9	7.1	7.2	7.6	8.1	8.4	8.8	9.6	36.8	37.6	38.2	38.8	37.7	37.8	37.4	37.9	3.3	3.2	3.1	3.1	3.2	3.2	3.0
<20 Years	2.5	2.4	2.5	2.6	2.9	2.7	2.9	3.5	42.8	43.4	43.3	44.0	42.3	41.3	41.2	41.4	4.9	4.4	4.4	4.5	4.3	4.6	4.1
20–24 Years	4.1	4.2	4.3	4.5	4.7	4.9	5.0	5.7	37.0	37.6	38.4	38.9	37.2	37.5	36.9	37.2	3.5	3.4	3.2	3.2	3.2	3.4	3.1
25–29 Years	6.1	6.4	6.5	6.8	7.3	7.5	8.0	8.7	35.7	36.8	37.8	38.2	37.3	37.3	36.9	37.4	3.0	2.9	2.8	2.7	2.9	2.9	2.6
30–34 Years	8.6	8.9	8.7	9.4	10.0	10.3	10.9	11.8	33.6	34.5	34.9	36.1	35.4	35.6	35.5	36.1	2.7	2.6	2.6	2.6	2.7	2.8	2.6
35–39 Years	13.9	13.6	14.0	14.5	15.1	15.8	16.3	12.4	37.2	38.0	38.1	38.4	37.6	38.6	37.9	38.7	3.1	3.0	2.9	3.0	3.2	3.2	3.0
40–54 Years	23.0	24.8	24.5	23.7	25.0	25.6	26.1	26.7	46.2	48.0	47.7	47.9	47.7	47.8	47.8	48.8	4.2	4.3	4.0	3.9	4.2	4.0	3.7
White																							
All Ages	6.0	6.1	6.2	6.6	7.0	7.2	7.6	9.9	37.1	37.9	38.7	39.3	38.0	38.1	38.0	43.3	3.1	3.0	2.9	2.9	2.9	3.0	2.7
<20 Years	2.1	2.0	2.1	2.2	2.5	2.3	2.5	3.7	42.7	43.1	42.8	43.3	41.4	40.3	40.4	48.3	4.4	4.0	4.0	3.8	3.8	4.0	3.6
20–24 Years	3.5	3.7	3.8	3.9	4.1	4.3	4.3	6.1	38.0	38.5	39.5	39.9	38.0	38.0	37.4	44.8	3.3	3.2	3.0	2.9	2.9	3.1	2.9
25–29 Years	5.4	5.5	5.7	6.1	6.5	6.5	7.0	9.1	36.6	37.7	39.0	39.5	38.3	38.4	38.4	44.5	2.9	2.8	2.7	2.7	2.8	2.7	2.5
30–34 Years	7.3	7.5	7.4	8.1	8.5	8.8	9.4	11.5	33.6	34.6	35.2	36.5	35.8	36.1	36.2	40.2	2.7	2.6	2.5	2.6	2.6	2.6	2.5
35–39 Years	11.4	11.0	11.3	11.7	12.4	13.0	13.3	15.5	36.7	37.5	37.8	38.0	37.2	38.0	37.9	40.6	3.0	2.8	2.8	2.8	3.0	3.1	2.7
40–54 Years	18.7	19.8	19.2	18.9	19.6	20.4	21.0	22.2	44.8	46.8	46.8	47.3	47.2	47.0	46.9	49.4	4.1	3.8	3.6	3.7	4.0	3.8	3.6
African-American																							
All Ages	12.2	12.6	12.9	13.5	14.6	15.7	16.6	18.5	39.7	40.6	40.5	41.7	40.6	41.5	40.2	42.2	4.6	4.3	4.2	4.5	4.7	4.9	4.6
<20 Years	3.4	3.4	3.6	3.7	4.1	4.0	4.3	5.2	44.1	45.0	45.0	46.7	45.4	44.7	43.7	44.7	6.0	5.4	5.3	6.4	5.8	6.2	5.7
20–24 Years	6.5	6.2	6.4	7.1	7.4	7.9	8.2	9.5	35.2	36.2	36.5	37.3	35.6	37.2	37.0	38.4	4.5	3.9	3.7	4.1	4.3	4.5	4.2
25–29 Years	11.8	12.4	12.7	12.5	14.1	15.6	16.2	17.9	36.8	38.4	37.2	38.7	38.5	39.0	36.4	40.4	4.0	4.0	4.0	3.6	4.1	4.6	3.9
30–34 Years	20.8	21.5	21.4	23.1	25.0	25.9	27.4	30.3	41.0	41.2	41.8	42.9	42.4	42.8	42.7	43.9	3.7	3.8	3.9	4.0	4.5	4.8	4.6
35–39 Years	35.2	36.0	37.6	37.8	38.4	41.1	43.5	48.1	46.5	48.0	47.9	49.4	48.1	51.5	46.7	50.2	4.2	4.3	4.4	4.7	4.9	4.9	5.8
40–54 Years	55.8	63.1	64.1	60.3	64.5	62.0	64.6	69.1	58.4	57.7	59.4	58.2	56.5	59.3	58.2	59.1	5.4	7.1	5.9	5.6	6.6	6.1	5.1

*Rate per 1,000 live births. Table complied by author from following sources: (Martin, Hamilton et al., 2002, 2003, 2005, 2005; Ventura et al., 1999, 2000.)

DISPLAY 6-1

Risk Factors for the Development of Preeclampsia

- First pregnancy or pregnancy of a new genetic makeup (Chesley, 1986; Cunningham, 1988)
- Multiple gestations (Thompson, Lyons, & Makowski, 1987)
- Preexisting diabetes, collagen vascular disease, hypertension, or renal disease (Cunningham, Cox, Harstad, Mason, & Pritchard, 1990; Mabie, Pernoll, & Biswas, 1986; Siddiqi, Rosenn, Mimouni, Khoury, & Miodovnik, 1991)
- Hydatiform mole (Page, 1939)
- Fetal hydrops (Barron, 1991)
- Maternal age (Spellacy, Miller, & Winegar, 1986)
- African-American race (Cunningham & Leveno, 1988)
- Family history of pregnancy-induced hypertension (Chesley & Cooper, 1986)
- Antiphospholipid antibody syndrome (Branch, 1990; Branch et al., 1989)
- Angiotensin gene T235 (Ward et al., 1993)
- Socioeconomic status (Guzick et al., 1987)
- Failure to demonstrate hemodilution (Hays, Cruikshank, & Dunn, 1985)
- Failure to demonstrate a decrease in systemic vascular resistance and second-trimester mean arterial pressures (Ales, Norton, & Druzin, 1989; Gavette & Roberts, 1987).

- Use of contraceptives that prevent exposure to sperm (Klonoff-Cohen, Savitz, Cefalo, & McCann, 1989; Robillard, 2002)
- Not having oral sex (Dekker, 1999; Dekker, Robillard, & Hulsey, 1998; Dekker & Sibai, 1998)
- Pregnancy achieved through artificial donor insemination (Dekker, Robillard, & Hulsey, 1998)
- Obesity or insulin resistance (Dekker & Sibai, 1998; Khan & Daya, 1996; Schaffir, Lockwood, Lapinski, Yoon, & Alvarez, 1995)
- Thrombophilic disorders, including hyperhomocysteinemia (Branch, 1990; Branch, Silver, Blackwell, Reading, & Scott, 1989; Branch, Silver, Blackwell, Reading, & Scott, 1992; Branch, Dudley, & Mitchell, 1991; Dizon-Townson, Major, & Ward, 1998; Dizon-Townson, Nelson, Easton, & Ward, 1996; Grisaru, Zwang, Peyser, Lessing, & Eldor, 1997; Lindoff et al., 1997; Out et al., 1992; Pattinson, Kriegler, Odendaal, Muller, & Kirsten, 1989; Yamamoto, Takahaski, Geshi, Sasamori, & Mori, 1996)
- Regular physical activity (Clapp III, 2003; Jackson, Gott, Lye, Ritchie, & Clapp III, 1995; Marcoux, Berube, Brisson, & Fabia, 1992; Sorensen et al., 2003; Weissgerber, Wolfe, & Davies, 2004)
- Gestational diabetes (Barden et al., 2004; Garner, D'Alton, Dudley, Huard, & Hardie, 1990; Siddiqi, Rosenn, Mimouni, Khoury, & Miodovnik, 1991; White, 1935)
- Metabolic syndrome (Pouta et al., 2004; Ramsay et al., 2004; Solomon & Seely, 2001)
- Factor V Leiden SNP (Linn & August, 2005)

---

pregnancy with preexisting medical complications, such as undiagnosed hypertension, and the teenage population may be at risk because of coexisting lifestyle risk factors (Mittendorf, Lain, Williams, & Walker, 1996).

Race

Maternal race is often identified in conjunction with socioeconomic status; therefore, it is difficult to identify its independent significance in relation to preeclampsia. African-American women have been identified to be at a higher risk for developing preeclampsia (Cunningham & Leveno, 1988; Guzick et al., 1987; Martin et al., 2000, 2005, 2006). However, the prevalence of hypertension is generally more common among African-Americans. The association between race and preeclampsia may not be race related but more closely associated with the prevalence of unrecognized preexisting chronic hypertension (Roberts, 2004). The presence of preexisting chronic hypertension may help explain why women 35 years of age or older have a significantly (70%) greater risk of preeclampsia than their counterparts between the ages of 30 and 34 (Saftlass, Olson, Franks, Atrash, & Pokras, 1990).

Socioeconomic Status

Socioeconomic status, contrary to past belief, is not a predisposing factor to the development of preeclampsia (Baird, 1977; Chesley, 1978; Davies, 1971; Nelson, 1955). Eclampsia, however, is clearly a disease of lower socioeconomic status (Davies et al., 1970; Nelson). Lower socioeconomic status is associated with poorer diets and an increase in smoking (Redman, 1995). The association between maternal nutritional status and risk for preeclampsia is inconclusive (Belizan & Villar, 1980; Brewer, 1974, 1977; Chaudhuri, 1971; Fitzgibbon, 1922; Lu et al., 1981; Ross et al., 1954). Belizán and Villar, and Chaudhuri reported that dietary deficiencies, especially calcium and certain vitamins, are important in the pathogenesis of preeclampsia based on observations in animal models. The roles of calcium and vitamins in the pathogenesis of preeclampsia have been examined in prospective clinical trials (Levine, Esterlitz et al., 1997). Brewer reported that protein deprivation played an etiologic role in preeclampsia. However, the results reported by Brewer are in question because the incidence of preeclampsia was no different from the incidence in the general population during the study time-frame.

The role of a specific link between a nutritional deficit and the development of preeclampsia remains controversial.

Smoking has been reported to reduce the incidence of preeclampsia in several studies (Duffus & MacGillivary, 1968; Mittendorf, Lain, Williams, & Walker, 1996; Sibai et al., 1995). Although smoking increases perinatal mortality, smoking appears to diminish the maternal responses to the placental problems of preeclampsia (Redman, 1995). Like maternal age and race, the independent contribution of socioeconomic status to the risk for developing preeclampsia is unclear.

Gravidity and Parity

A woman who is pregnant for the first time is six to eight times more likely to develop preeclampsia (Chesley, 1978; Taylor, 1988) than the woman who has given birth previously. The incidence of preeclampsia ranges from 10% to 14% in the primigravid woman, compared with 5.7% to 7.3% in the multigravid woman (Long, Abell, & Beischer, 1979; Villar & Sibai, 1989). A previous pregnancy may offer a protective effect on the incidence of preeclampsia in subsequent pregnancies. Second-trimester abortion, compared with first-trimester abortion, also appears to afford some protection in subsequent pregnancies (Campbell, MacGillivray, & Carr-Hill, 1985). However, if the woman has a new partner for a subsequent pregnancy, this protective effect is not seen (Beer, 1978; Dekker, 1999; Feeney & Scott, 1980). The reported incidence for preeclampsia among nulliparous women (3.2%) and multiparous women with a change in paternity (3%) are similar but increased when compared with multiparous women with no change in paternity (1.9%; Dekker). A Norwegian study reported that men who fathered a pregnancy complicated by preeclampsia were nearly twice as likely to father a pregnancy complicated by preeclampsia in a different woman (Lie et al., 1998).

Among parous women, the risk for developing preeclampsia is increased if preeclampsia complicated a previous pregnancy (Dekker, 1999). The risk of preeclampsia in a second pregnancy is 10 to 15 times greater for women when the disease is recurrent compared with women for whom the first pregnancy was normal (Campbell, MacGillivray, & Carr-Hill, 1985; Davies et al., 1970; Dekker). One of the few factors that may help identify the woman at risk for early-onset preeclampsia is a history of previous preeclampsia (Moore & Redmon, 1983).

Gestational Age at First Prenatal Visit

Mittendorf, Lain, Williams, and Walker (1996) suggest women entering prenatal care after the first trimester are at increased risk for developing preeclampsia. The unadjusted odds ratio for beginning prenatal care after the first trimester was 1.9 (95% CI: 1.4–3.0). However, Eskenazi, Fenster, and Sidney (1991) found no association between initiation of prenatal care after the first trimester and preeclampsia.

Family History of Pregnancy-Induced Hypertension

A frequently overlooked characteristic of preeclampsia is the tendency of the condition to occur in daughters and sisters of women with a history of preeclampsia. Adams and Finlayson (1961) found a fourfold increase in the occurrence of proteinuric preeclampsia in sisters of women who had preeclampsia in their first pregnancy compared with sisters of women without the disease. Chesley and colleagues found the occurrence of preeclampsia in sisters, daughters, and granddaughters of women who had preeclampsia to be higher than the daughters-in-law (Chesley, 1984; Chesley & Cooper, 1986). The risk of eclampsia among daughters of women who were eclamptic is eight times higher than the risk among daughters of women who did not suffer from eclampsia (Chesley, Annitto, & Cosgrove, 1968). These findings may indicate a genetic predisposition for preeclampsia.

The pattern of inheritance is unclear, but researchers have suggested that a single recessive gene for which the woman is homozygous may be responsible for the susceptibility for preeclampsia (Chesley & Cooper, 1986). The single-gene theory has been challenged because identical twins do not have concordant histories (Thornton & Onwude, 1991). Several studies have also reported an association between preeclampsia and the presence of the histocompatibility leukocyte antigen DR4 (Kilpartrick, Gibson, & Liston, 1989; Redman, Bodmer, Bodmer, Beilin, & Bonnar, 1978; Simon et al., 1988). The genotype of the fetus may also be significant, suggesting the possibility that the father of the child could contribute genetically to preeclampsia (Liston & Kilpatrick, 1991).

More recently, Heiskanen, Heinonen, and Kirkinen (2003) have investigated the prognosis of obstetrical outcomes in sisters of women diagnosed with preeclampsia. Pregnancy outcomes for sister pairs in which one sister had a pregnancy complicated by preeclampsia were compared to the pregnancy outcomes for sister pairs where neither were affected by preeclampsia. For those sister pairs unaffected by preeclampsia there was a very low risk for an adverse pregnancy outcome. Among those sister pairs in which one sister had preeclampsia, the unaffected sister had pregnancy outcomes comparable to the general population. Affected sisters had pregnancy outcomes with a higher rate of prematurity, low-birth-weight infants, and small-for-gestational-age infants. Heiskanen's conclusion indicates that first-degree relatives who are unaffected by preeclampsia are at low risk for adverse outcomes and require no special antenatal care or testing; however, further investigation is required.

Chronic Disease

There is disagreement about the incidence of superimposed preeclampsia among women with chronic hypertension, but most investigators agree that preeclampsia is more common in this situation (Chesley, 1978; Chesley & Cooper, 1986). Women with chronic hypertension that predates the pregnancy are three to seven times more likely to develop superimposed preeclampsia than women who are normotensive (Chesley & Annitto, 1947; Guzick et al., 1987).

Women with a history of pregestational diabetes mellitus (Barden et al., 2004; Garner, D'Alton, Dudley, Huard, & Hardie, 1990; Siddiqi, Rosenn, Mimouni, Khoury, & Miodovnik, 1991; White, 1935) and hypertension associated with chronic renal disease are at increased risk for preeclampsia (Felding, 1969). Barden and colleagues report that with a diagnosis of gestational diabetes, significant independent predictors for the development of preeclampsia were fasting glucose, C-reactive protein (CRP), a family history of hypertension, and a history of gestational diabetes in their mothers. These same predictors have been linked to the development of metabolic syndrome, which may play a role in the development of preeclampsia (Pouta et al., 2004; Ramsay et al., 2004; Solomon & Seely, 2001).

Research has identified an association between the presence of antiphospholipid antibodies (Branch, 1990; Branch, Andres, Digre, Rote, & Scott, 1989; Branch, Dudley, LaMarche, & Mitchell, 1992; Branch, Silver, Blackwell, Reading, & Scott, 1992), angiotensinogen gene (Ward et al., 1993) and the factor V Leiden SNP (single nucleotide polymorphism; Linn & August, 2005) and preeclampsia. A history of migraine headaches may also predispose the woman to preeclampsia (Marcoux, Berube, Brisson, & Fabia, 1992) and eclampsia (Rotten, Sachtleben, & Friedman, 1959).

Pregnancy Complications

A pregnancy complicated by a multifetal gestation, fetal hydrops, or hydatidiform mole is at increased risk for the development of preeclampsia. The incidence of preeclampsia is increased five times in a pregnancy with a twin gestation (Barron, 1991; Thompson, Lyons, & Makowski, 1987). Nonimmune fetal hydrops may increase the risk for preeclampsia by as much as 50% (Barron). For the woman diagnosed with a hydatidiform mole, a well-known association exists between the molar pregnancy and the onset of preeclampsia (Page, 1939; Slattery, Khong, Dawkins, Pridmore, & Hague, 1993). Last, one report suggests that the primiparous woman who has a urinary tract infection (UTI) complicating pregnancy is five times more likely to have preeclampsia than the primiparous woman who does not have a UTI during pregnancy (Mittendorf, Lain, Williams, & Walker, 1996).

Prevention Strategies

Exercise

Regular physical activity may provide a protective effect against the development of preeclampsia (Marcoux, Berube, Brisson, & Fabia, 1992; Sorensen et al., 2003; Weissgerber, Wolfe, & Davies, 2004). Sorensen and colleagues examined the relationship of regular exercise and physical activity in the year preceding pregnancy and for the first 20 weeks of gestation to the risk of developing preeclampsia. Compared to inactive women, women who participated in physical activity and regular exercise during the first 20 weeks of gestation experienced a 35% reduced risk for developing preeclampsia (OR, 0.65; 95% CI, 0.43–0.99). As the level of physical activity or exercise increased the risk for preeclampsia decreased. Participation in light to moderate activity reduced the risk for preeclampsia by 24% (95% CI, 0.48–1.20); participation in vigorous activities by 54% (95% CI, 0.27–0.79; Sorensen et al.). Similar results were seen in women who participated in regular exercise or physical activity for the year before becoming pregnant.

Antiplatelet Therapy

Studies examining the use of antiplatelet therapy to prevent preeclampsia have failed to demonstrate a significant difference in outcomes between treatment and control groups for most women, including nulliparas (Caritis et al., 1998; Collaborative Low-Dose Aspirin Study in Pregnancy [CLASP] Collaborative Group, 1994; Duley, Henderson-Smart, Knight, & King, 2001; Estudo Collaborative para Prevencao do Pre-eclampsia com Aspirina [ECPPA] Collaborative Group, 1996; Golding, 1998; Hauth & Cunningham, 1995; Hauth et al., 1993; Institute of Medicine & Standing Committee on the Scientific Evaluation of Dietary Reference Intakes, 1997; Italian Study of Aspirin in Pregnancy, 1993; Rotchell et al., 1998; Sibai et al., 1993). Although debate exists, the use of low-dose aspirin or other antiplatelet therapy cannot be supported in women without other risk factors present.

Dietary Supplementation

To date there have been no data indicating that dietary supplementation prevents the development of preeclampsia in low-risk populations (Beazley, Ahokas, Livingston, Griggs, & Sibai, 2004; Belizan & Villar, 1980; Belizán, Villar, Gonzalez, Campodonico, & Bergel, 1991; Belizan, Villar, & Repke, 1988; Bulstra-Ramaker, Huisjes, & Visser, 1994; Chappell et al., 1999; Crowther et al., 1999; Herrera, Arevalo-Herrera, & Herrera, 1998; Institue of Medicine & Standing Committee on the Scientific Evaluation of Dietary Reference Intakes, 1997; Levine, Esterlitz et al., 1997; Levine, Hauth et al., 1997; Lopez-Jaramillo, 1996; Onwude, Lilford, Hjartardottir, Staines, & Tuffnell, 1995; Roberts & Hubel, 1999; Salvig, Olsen, & Secher, 1996; Sanchez-Ramos et al., 1997; Sibai, Villar, & Bray, 1989; Spatling & Spatling, 1988). A National Institutes of Health trial of healthy, low-risk nulliparous women failed to demonstrate a difference in the incidence or severity of preeclampsia between the treatment and placebo groups (Levine, Esterlitz et al.; Levine, Hauth et al.). Calcium supplementation in high-risk nulliparous women, however, has shown a significant reduction in the incidence of preeclampsia (Lo & Lau, 1998; Lopez-Jaramillo; Lopez-Jaramillo & de Felix, 1991; Lopez-Jaramillo et al., 1996, 1997; Lopez-Jaramillo, Narvaez, Weigel, & Yepez, 1989; Sanchez-Ramos et al., 1997).

Fish oil supplementation, like other dietary supplementation, has failed to reduce the incidence of preeclampsia in low- and high-risk populations (Bulstra-Ramaker, Huisjes, & Visser, 1994; Onwude, Lilford, Hjartardottir, Staines, & Tuffnell, 1995; Salvig, Olsen, & Secher, 1996).

Pathophysiology of Preeclampsia

Preeclampsia has been called the "disease of theories." There is not one established cause. Research is ongoing to identify the pathophysiology. Although the exact mechanism is unknown, preeclampsia is thought to occur because of changes within the maternal cardiovascular, hematologic, and renal systems.

Normal physiologic adaptations to pregnancy include an increase in plasma volume, vasodilation of the vascular bed, decreased systemic vascular resistance, elevation of cardiac output, and increased prostacyclin production. Physical assessment findings consistent with these changes are dilutional anemia, lower systemic blood pressures and mean arterial pressure, a slight increase in heart rate, and peripheral edema. In preeclampsia, these normal adaptations are altered. Instead of plasma volume expansion and hemodilution, there is a decrease in circulating plasma volume resulting in hemoconcentration. Women with preeclampsia have inadequate plasma volume expansion, with an average plasma volume 9% below expected values for mild disease and up to 40% below normal with severe disease (Duvekot, Cheriex, Pieters, Menheere, & Peters,

1993; Hays, Cruikshank, & Dunn, 1985; Sibai, Anderson, Spinnato, & Shaver, 1983). Further intravascular volume depletion may occur from endothelial injury and increased capillary permeability. The volume depletion may result in increased blood viscosity, leading to a decrease in maternal organ perfusion, including the uteroplacental unit.

Maternal intravascular volume depletion has been associated with fetal morbidity. The reduction in plasma volume may be more closely related to IUGR than hypertension (Sibai, Anderson, Spinnato, & Shaver, 1983). The vascular bed demonstrates increased sensitivity to vasoactive substances, resulting in vasoconstriction and increased vascular tone. Vasoconstriction results in increased systemic vascular resistance and hypertension. The hypertension is further aggravated by vasospasms of the arterial bed, the underlying mechanism for observed signs and symptoms of the disease process. The cumulative effect of decreased intravascular volume and vasoconstriction leads to a decreased organ perfusion. As the process worsens, hemolysis may also compromise tissue oxygen delivery.

Vasoconstriction and a further increase in cardiac output above the normal pregnancy elevation (Easterling, Benedetti, Schmucker, & Millard, 1990) result in arterial vasospasms, endothelial damage, and an imbalance in endothelial prostacyclin and thromboxane ratios (Sibai, 1991; Zeeman, Dekker, van Geijn, & Kraayenbrink, 1992). Tables 6–4 and 6–5 provide highlights of the pathophysiology of disease progression and multiple organ system involvement. Figure 6–1 demonstrates the pathophysiologic changes related to preeclampsia.

Of interest is ongoing research examining the relationship of endothelial dysfunction and alterations in the immune response with the development of preeclampsia (August, 2004; Barden et al., 2001; Belgore, Blann, Li-Saw-Hee, Beevers, & Lip, 2001; Chaiworapongsa et al., 2004; Dechend et al., 2005; Gonzalez-Quintero et al., 2004; Granger, Alexander, Llinas, Bennett, & Khalil, 2001; Harrison et al., 1997; Khalil & Granger, 2002; Kovats et al., 1990; Levesque, Moutquin, Lindsay, Roy, & Rousseau, 2004; Magnini et al., 2005; Main, Chiang, & Colbern, 1994; NHBPEP, 2000; Norris et al., 2004; Raijmakers, Dechend, & Poston, 2004; Reinhart, Bayer, Brunkhorst, & Meisner, 2002; Roberts, 2004; Taylor, 1997; Waite, Louie, & Taylor, 2005; Wang, Gu, Zhang, & Lewis, 2004; Working Group, 2000; Yamamoto, Suzuki, Kojima, & Suzumori, 2005). Vascular endothelial cells play a role in the modulation of vascular smooth muscle contractile activity and the coagulation and regulation of blood flow. Receptors within the endothelial cells respond to vasodilators and vasoconstrictors, while producing vasoactive substances such as hormones, autacoids, and mitogenic cytokines, including PGI_2, nitric oxide, and endothelin. The underlying processes are not fully

TABLE 6–4 ■ PHYSIOLOGIC AND PATHOPHYSIOLOGIC CHANGES ASSOCIATED WITH PREECLAMPSIA

Feature	Normal Pregnancy	Preeclampsia Alterations
Blood Volume	50%↑	Smaller ↑
Plasma volume	50%↑	Little or no change
Red cell mass	20%↑	Hemoconcentration
Cardiac Output	40%–50%↑	Variable
	Widening pulse pressure	↓ Vascular compliance
Blood Pressure	↓ Initially with return to prepregnant values by 3rd trimester	Hypertension
Peripheral Vascular Resistance	↓ Total peripheral resistance	↑ Resistance
		↑ Vascular reactivity
Renal Function	↑ Venous capacitance	Vasospasms
RPF	↑	↓
GFR	75%↑	↓
BUN	50%↑	↓
Creatinine clearance	↓	↑
Serum creatinine	↑	↓
Uric acid	↓	↑
Renin–Angiotensin–Aldosterone System	Markedly activated and responds appropriately to posture and salt intake	Plasma renin concentration and activity suppressed
		Loss of antagonists (vasodilators) to AII
		Increased sensitivity to vasoactive substances
Coagulation System		
Fibrinogen	↑	Normal with mild disease
Factors VII, VIII, IX, X	All ↑	Normal initially, then ↓
		Increase in ratio of von Willebrand factor to factor VII, coagulant activity increased leading to consumption of factor VI
Fibrinolytic activity	↓	↑
Platelet count	Normal	↓
Bleeding time	Normal	Prolonged

RPF, renal plasma blood flow; GFR, glomerular filtration rate; BUN, blood urea nitrogen AII, angiotensin II. Adapted from Roberts, J. (1994). Current perspectives on preeclampsia. *Journal of Nurse-Midwifery*, 39(2), 76.

understood, but women diagnosed with preeclampsia exhibit histologic evidence of increased circulating markers of endothelial activation (Roberts & Lain, 2002). Endothelial dysfunction and subsequent increased capillary permeability in turn leads to the pathway of reduced organ perfusion.

Clinical Manifestations of Preeclampsia–Eclampsia

Historically, the classic triad for preeclampsia has included hypertension, proteinuria, and edema. However, not all of these parameters must be present for the diagnosis of preeclampsia (ACOG, 2002; Australian Society for the Study of Hypertension in Pregnancy, 1993; Brown et al., 2000; Brown, Lindeheimer, Sweet, Assche, & Moutquin, 2001; Helewa et al., 1997; NHBPEP, 2000). The NHBPEP has published recommendations that clarified the differences in diagnostic criteria previously published by ACOG (1996), the Australasian Society for the Study of Hypertension in Pregnancy, and the Canadian Hypertension Society. These recommendations include elimination of the edema from the diagnostic criteria, elimination of the use blood pressure changes in defining hypertension, use of both systolic and diastolic pressures to

TABLE 6–5 ■ PREECLAMPSIA PATHOPHYSIOLOGY AS A MULTIORGAN SYSTEM DISEASE

System	Effect of Preeclampsia	Clinical Implications
Vascular Bed 1. Endothelial dysfunction 2. Altered coagulation 3. Altered response to vasoactive substances	• Increased release of cellular fibronectin, growth factors, VCAM-1, factor VIII antigen, and peptides • Endothelial cell injury initiates coagulation either by intrinsic pathway (contact adhesion) or extrinsic pathway (tissue factor) • Decreased production of prostacyclin and alteration in prostacyclin/thromboxane ratio	Endothelial dysfunction present before clinical signs of disease Increased thrombus formation, including pulmonary and cerebral emboli Vasoconstriction and vasospasm Increased sensitivity to vasoactive substance Capillary permeability, which contributes to edema formation
Cardiovascular and Pulmonary 1. ↑ Vascular resistance 2. ↑ Cardiac output and stroke volume 3. ↓ Colloid osmotic pressure	• Arteriolar narrowing • ↑ Sympathetic activity • ↑ Levels of endothelin-1, a vasoconstrictor • ↑ Sensitivity to endogenous pressors, including vasopressin, epinephrine, and norepinephrine • ↑ Capillary permeability • Further depletion of intravascular colloids through capillary permeability and renal excretion of proteins	Increased blood pressure Hyperdynamic cardiac activity Epidurals can be used safely, but must be cautious if ephedrine is used to correct hypotension Subendocardial hemorrhages are present in >50% of women who die of eclampsia At risk for pulmonary edema, myocardial ischemia, left ventricular dysfunction
Renal 1. Proteinuria 2. Altered function	• Slight decrease in glomerular size • Diameter of glomerular capillary lumen decreased • Glomerular endothelial cells are greatly enlarged and may occlude the capillary lumen • Glomerular capillary endotheliosis • Thickening of renal arterioles	Proteinuria plus hypertension is the most reliable indicator of fetal jeopardy; indicative of glomerular dysfunction ↑ Serum uric acid secondary to a ↓ urate clearance (uric acid better predictor of outcome than BP) ↓ Creatinine clearance with an elevation of serum creatinine levels ↑ BUN mirrors changes in creatine clearance and also a function of protein intake and liver function Urine sediment analysis may not be beneficial At risk for oliguria, acute tubular necrosis (ATN), renal failure
Hepatic 1. Hepatic dysfunction 2. Hepatic rupture	• Changes consistent with hemorrhage into hepatic tissue • Later changes consistent with hepatic infarction • ↑ Hepatic artery resistance • Fibrin deposition • Hepatocellular necrosis	Elevations of liver function tests; the association of microangiopathic anemia and elevations of AST/ALT carries ominous prognosis for mother and fetus HELLP syndrome Possible elevations in bilirubin Signs of liver failure: malaise, nausea, epigastric pain, hypoglycemia, hemolysis, anemia
Hematologic 1. Thrombocytopenia 2. Altered platelet function 3. Hemolysis	• ↑ Platelet destruction • ↑ Platelet aggreability • ↓ Platelet life span • Hemolytic anemia • Destruction of RBCs in microvasculature	Platelets <100,000 increased risk of coagulopathy Platelets <50,000 increased risk of hemorrhage Platelets <20,000 increased risk for spontaneous bleeding Decreased oxygen-carrying capacity and organ oxygenation

TABLE 6–5 ■ PREECLAMPSIA PATHOPHYSIOLOGY AS A MULTIORGAN SYSTEM DISEASE (Continued)

System	Effect of Preeclampsia	Clinical Implications
Central Nervous System 1. Hyperreflexia	• May indicate increasing CNS involvement, but not diagnostic of disease • Alteration of cerebral autoregulation with seizures • ↑ Intracranial pressures	Cerebral edema with severe disease Signs of CNS alterations: headache, dizziness, changes in vital signs, diplopia, scotomata, blurred vision, amaurosis, tachycardia, alteration in level of consciousness
Fetal/Neonatal 1. Fetal intolerance to labor 2. Preterm birth 3. Oligohydramnios 4. IUGR 5. IUFD 6. Abruptio placentae	• Alteration in placental function • At risk for indicated preterm birth secondary to maternal disease process	Must monitor for signs of fetal compromise Monitoring for IUGR and IUFD At risk for abruptio placentae, oligohydramnios, nonreassuring FHR patterns
Uteroplacental 1. Spiral arteries 2. Changes consistent with hypoxia	• Abnormal invasion • Retain nonpregnant characteristics • Limited vasodilatation • Vessel necrosis	Decreases in uteroplacental perfusion Increased risk for fetal compromise and IUGR

define hypertension, and to add systemic changes to the diagnostic criteria (NHBPEP; Working Group, 2000). Hypertension and proteinuria are the most significant indicators. Edema is significant only if hypertension, proteinuria, or signs of multisystem organ involvement are present.

The clinical manifestations of preeclampsia are directly related to the presence of vascular vasospasms. These vasospasms result in endothelial injury, red blood cell destruction, platelet aggregation, increased capillary permeability, increased systemic vascular resistance, renal and hepatic dysfunction, and other systemic changes.

Hypertension

Although controversy exists about the most appropriate definition of hypertension, ACOG (2002), the NHBPEP (2000), and the Working Group (2000) define hypertension as a sustained blood pressure elevation of 140 mm Hg or more systolic or 90 mm Hg or more diastolic after the 20th week of gestation that is recorded on two or more measurements. The use of elevations above baseline values, specifically a 30 mm Hg increase in the systolic blood pressure or 15 mm Hg increase in diastolic blood pressure above baseline

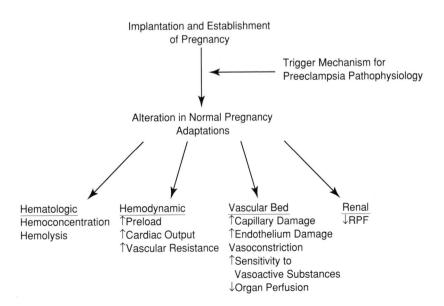

FIGURE 6–1. Pathophysiology of preeclampsia.

values, to define hypertension is of questionable value for the diagnosis of preeclampsia (MacGillivary, Rose, & Rowe, 1969; Moutquin, Fainville, & Raynauld, 1985; Villar & Sibai, 1989), and is no longer part of the diagnostic criteria for identifying hypertension (ACOG; NHBPEP; Working Group). Women who demonstrate an elevation in baseline, but fail to reach an absolute blood pressure of 140 mm Hg systolic or 90 mm Hg diastolic or higher, are not likely to suffer adverse perinatal outcomes without other risk factors. However, it is prudent to carefully observe women who have a rise of 30 mm Hg systolic or 15 mm Hg diastolic blood pressure if this change is accompanied by proteinuria or hyperuricemia (uric acid [UA] ≥6 mg/dL; NHBPEP; Working Group).

Measurement of blood pressure is important in the evaluation, diagnosis, and management of hypertension. In the past, Korotkoff 4 (K4, muffling of sound) has been used to identify the diastolic pressure. However, current recommendations are to use Korotkoff 5 (K5, disappearance of sound; NHBPEP, 2000; Working Group, 2000). It is also important to keep in mind that the diagnosis of hypertension is not made based on one blood pressure evaluation. In an ambulatory setting the diagnosis of hypertension is based on two determinations, generally within a week. The degree of suspected hypertension will determine the interval between blood pressure determinations.

In addition to the recommendation of using K5, patient position will also influence blood pressure readings. Historically blood pressure determinations were obtained in a left lateral position with the blood pressure cuff placed on the right arm. However, this position will falsely lower systolic, diastolic, and mean pressures. Current recommendations are to evaluate the blood pressure with the woman in a sitting position, with placement of the cuff on the left arm with the arm positioned at heart level. If reevaluation is required, the patient should be in the same position as the initial evaluation. If the left lateral position is being maintained by the patient, the blood pressure will still be taken in the left arm; the arm should not be under the patient or lower than heart level (Beevers, Lip, & O'Brien, 2001; Feldman, 2001).

Earlier research suggests that an increase in mean arterial pressure in the second trimester (MAP-2) of more than 85 mm Hg is useful in identifying the women at risk for developing hypertension during pregnancy (Page & Christianson, 1976). Several investigators have correlated an elevation of MAP-2 with an increased risk for maternal hypertension and for fetal and neonatal risks (Ales, Norton, & Druzin, 1989; Chesley & Sibai, 1987; Gavette & Roberts, 1987; O'Brien, 1990, 1992). However, more definitive research is needed.

Proteinuria

Proteinuria is defined as the urinary excretion of 0.3 g of protein/L (300 mg/L) in a 24-hour urine specimen (NHBPEP, 2000). Random determinations for urine protein excretion are often monitored with dipstick analysis. The stated threshold of 0.3 g/L correlates with 30 mg/dL or "1+" or greater on dipstick (NHBPEP). However, urine dipstick evaluation is a poor quantifier of protein excretion. Studies comparing traditional urine dipstick analysis to 24-hour urine protein quantitation to determine proteinuria found that in routine clinical practice a finding of "negative" or "trace" proteinuria misses significant proteinuria in up to 40% of hypertensive women. When feasible, evaluation of total protein excretion should be done by 24-hour urine protein quantitation rather than by urinalysis or dipstick analysis (Brown et al., 1995; Kuo, Loumantakis, & Gallery, 1992; Meyer, Mercer, Friedman, & Sibai, 1994; NHBPEP; Working Group, 2000). If a 24-hour urine for protein quantitation is not possible or feasible, a timed collection corrected for creatinine excretion can be performed (NHBPEP; Working Group).

Proteinuria, which should occur for the first time during the pregnancy, may indicate a worsening of the disease process and increased risk of adverse outcome for the woman and fetus. There is a positive correlation between the degree of proteinuria and the perinatal mortality and fetal growth restriction (Tervila & Vartiainen, 1975). The concentration of urine protein is extremely variable. Urinary protein concentration is influenced by factors such as contamination of the specimen with vaginal secretions, blood, or bacteria; urine specific gravity and pH; exercise; and posture.

Edema

Edema is a common finding of pregnancy and is not necessary for the diagnosis of preeclampsia (NHBPEP, 2000; Working Group, 2000). Dependent edema in the absence of hypertension or proteinuria is generally related to changes in interstitial and intravascular hydrostatic and osmotic pressures that facilitate movement of intravascular fluid into the tissues. Compression of the iliac vein increases venous hydrostatic pressure; this promotes fluid shifting into the interstitial space. Plasma volume expansion results in a decreased serum albumin levels; this lowers the colloid osmotic pressure promoting fluid leaving the intravascular space. Together, these two physiologic adaptations of pregnancy result in beguine dependent edema (Blackburn, 2003).

With preeclampsia, edema becomes pathologic when accompanied by hypertension, proteinuria, or signs of organ dysfunction. Intracellular and extracellular edema represents a generalized and excessive accumulation of fluid in tissue. As vasospasms worsen, capillary endothelial damage results in increased systemic capillary permeability (ie, leakage), which leads to hemoconcentration and increases the risk of pulmonary edema.

Hyperreflexia

Hyperreflexia is not considered diagnostic for preeclampsia or a risk factor for eclampsia (Roberts, 2004; Sibai, McCubbin, Anderson, Lipshitz, & Dilts, 1981). In healthy young women hyperreflexia can be a common finding. Deep tendon reflexes are evaluated once magnesium sulfate therapy is begun to assess for early signs of magnesium toxicity.

Mild Versus Severe Preeclampsia

The diagnosis of preeclampsia has significant implications for both maternal and fetal/neonatal well-being. Because other conditions can mimic preeclampsia it is important to look for systemic manifestations of disease progression, such as ascites, hydrothoras, increased neck vein distention, gallop rhythm, pulmonary rales, or generalized bruising or petechiae. To identify the progression of preeclampsia from mild to severe disease, or to increase the certainty of the diagnosis, nursing management requires accurate and thorough observation and assessments as well as possible preparation for birth of the infant. Display 6–2 lists criteria for confirming the diagnosis of preeclampsia and progression to severe preeclampsia. Display 6–3 lists the potential maternal and fetal complications of severe preeclampsia.

While caring for women with hypertensive disorders of pregnancy, nursing assessments focus on identification of the disease progression. Preeclampsia is a systemic disease in which one or more organ systems are involved. The wide range of symptoms and multiple organ system involvement can sometimes result in misdiagnosis and delay in treatment. Cocaine intoxication, lupus nephritis, chronic renal failure, and acute fatty liver of pregnancy are examples of conditions that may mimic preeclampsia and eclampsia (O'Brien, Mercer, Friedman, & Sibai, 1993; Simpson, Luppi, & O'Brien-Abel, 1998). Women with chronic hypertension or any preexisting medical condition that predisposes to the development of hypertension are at increased risk for superimposed preeclampsia and eclampsia. Care of the woman with severe preeclampsia or HELLP syndrome is best referred to a tertiary perinatal center.

Nursing Assessment and Interventions for Preeclampsia

Basic to the management of preeclampsia is a philosophic understanding of the disease process in that (1) birth is always the appropriate therapy for the woman, but not always so for the fetus; (2) the signs and symptoms of preeclampsia are not of pathogenetic importance; and (3) the pathogenetic changes of preeclampsia are present for an extended time before clinical signs and symptoms are present (Roberts, 2004). Once clinical signs and symptoms are observed (ie, headaches, epigastric pain, and visual disturbances), underlying pathophysiologic changes within all major organ systems are present; the degree of organ system dysfunction parallels disease progression. The only definitive therapy for preeclampsia is birth. The decision to initiate birth versus expectant management must be individualized. Decisions for management are determined by maternal and fetal status and gestational age.

Home Care Management

Mild preeclampsia may be managed at home with frequent follow-up care, including telephone contact between the woman and a high-risk perinatal nurse and periodic nurse home visits. Criteria for home management vary among primary perinatal healthcare

DISPLAY 6-2

Additional Criteria for Diagnosis of Preeclampsia and Severe Preeclampsia

- Blood pressure of 160 mm Hg or more systolic, OR 110 mm Hg or more diastolic
- Proteinuria of 2.0 g or more in 24 hours (2+ or 3+ on qualitative examination). Proteinuria should occur for the first time in pregnancy and the condition resolves postpartum.
- Increased serum creatinine (>1.2 mg/dL, unless known to be previously elevated)
- Platelet count <100,000 cells/mm^3 and/or evidence of microangiopathic hemolytic anemia (with increased lactic acid dehydrogenase [LDH])
- Elevated liver enzymes (alanine aminotransferase [ALT] or aspartate aminotransferase [AST])
- Persistent headache or other cerebral or visual disturbances
- Persistent epigastric pain
- Oliguria, 24-hour urinary output of <500 mL
- Pulmonary edema or cyanosis
- Intrauterine growth restriction (IUGR)

National High Blood Pressure Education Program [NHBPEP]. (2000). *Working group report on high blood pressure in pregnancy.* (No. NIH Publication No. 00-3029). Bethesda, MD: National Institutes of Health, National Heart, Lung, and Blood Institute, National High Blood Pressure Education Program; Walfisch, A., & Hallak, M. (2006). Hypertension. In D. James, P. Steer, C. Weiner, & B. Gonik (Eds.), *High risk pregnancy: Management options.* (3rd ed., pp. 772–789). Philadelphia: Saunders Elsevier; Working Group (2000).

DISPLAY 6-3

Potential Maternal and Fetal Complications of Severe Preeclampsia

- Cardiovascular:
  - Hypoperfusion
  - Severe hypertension
  - Hypertensive crisis
  - Pulmonary edema
  - Congestive heart failure
  - Future cardiac dysfunction
- Pulmonary:
  - Pulmonary edema
  - Hypoxemia/Acidemia
- Renal:
  - Oliguria
  - Acute renal failure
  - Impaired drug metabolism and excretion
- Hematologic:
  - Hemolysis
  - Decreased oxygen-carrying capacity
  - Thrombocytopenia

- Coagulation defects, including disseminated intravascular coagulation (DIC)
- Anemia
- Neurologic:
  - Eclampsia
  - Cerebral edema
  - Intracerebral hemorrhage
  - Stroke
  - Amaurosis (cortical blindness)
- Hepatic:
  - Hepatocellular dysfunction
  - Hepatic rupture
  - Hypoglycemia
  - Coagulation defects
  - Impaired drug metabolism and excretion
- Uteroplacental:
  - Abruptio placentae
  - Decreased uteroplacental perfusion
- Fetal:
  - Intrauterine growth restriction (IUGR)
  - Intrauterine fetal demise (IUFD)
  - Fetal intolerance to labor
  - Preterm birth
  - Low birth weight
  - Decreased oxygenation

---

providers and home care agencies. The woman must be in a stable condition with no evidence of worsening maternal or fetal status.

Inpatient Management

Women with mild preeclampsia may be evaluated in the inpatient setting and remain hospitalized. Women with severe preeclampsia or eclampsia are managed in the hospital. A woman with a fetus at an early gestational age, usually less than 34 weeks, is generally managed in a tertiary center because of the ability to provide advanced neonatal care if birth is indicated. Nursing care involves accurate and astute observations and assessments. Comprehensive knowledge regarding pharmacologic therapies, management regimens, and possible complications is also required.

The most important aspect of care for women with hypertension in pregnancy is recognition of the abilities of the facility and the obstetric and neonatal staff to handle potential emergencies. The decision to transfer a patient to a perinatal center should be based on the level of care required for the woman or should be made because the fetus is preterm and neonatal support will be required. It is best not to attempt expectant management of patients with severe preeclampsia (antepartum or postpartum) unless in a tertiary care center. However, providers of obstetric care, regardless

of level of care provided, must be able to stabilize the woman before transport.

Controversial Management Protocols: Use of Colloids and Diuretics

Some management protocols are considered to be inappropriate in the care of women with preeclampsia. Diuretics and administration of high concentrations of colloid solutions (eg, albumin, Hespan) should not be used to decrease peripheral edema or increase urine output. Preeclampsia is associated with a decrease in plasma volume expansion leading to hemoconcentration and a relative hypovolemia. The administration of diuretics further decreases intravascular volume leading to further compromise of renal perfusion and urine output. Administration of high concentrations of colloid solutions, in theory, would increase intravascular osmotic pressure causing interstitial fluid to be drawn back into the intravascular compartment; this would decrease peripheral edema. However, preeclampsia is a disease of endothelial dysfunction and capillary permeability. The increase in intravascular colloid osmotic pressure is only transient and the colloids "leak" into the interstitial space, further depleting intravascular volume. The combination of diuretics and administration of high concentrations of colloid solutions further depletes intravascular volume and increases the risk of pulmonary edema and uteroplacental insufficiency

(Clark, Cotton, Hankins, & Phelan, 1997; Dildy, Phelan, & Cotton, 1991, 1992; Repke, 1993).

Intravenous fluid therapy is not without risk in the management of a woman with preeclampsia. Administration of intravenous fluids decreases intravascular colloid osmotic pressure (Gonik & Cotton, 1984), but the administration of colloid solutions, such as Hespan or albumin, is not indicated. The administration of colloid solutions theoretically increases intravascular colloid osmotic pressure, but the proteins in these solutions leak into the tissues as a result of capillary injury and increased capillary permeability. There is a resulting alteration in the hydrostatic and osmotic forces that potentiate the development of pulmonary edema and further depletion of intravascular volume (Kirshon et al., 1988). The administration of colloids in any clinical situation in which endothelial injury and capillary permeability complicate the disease process is contraindicated.

Valium is no longer the first-line agent to stop seizure activity because of the depressant effect on the fetus and depression of the maternal gag reflex. Seizure precautions should be followed according to institution protocol. It is important to avoid insertion of a padded tongue blade to the back of the throat; a nasopharyngeal airway may be appropriate, if available. Heparin should not be administered as prophylaxis against coagulopathies, because it increases the risk for intracranial bleeding.

Antepartum Management

Antepartum management of the woman diagnosed with mild preeclampsia remains controversial. Key to the debate is whether the woman should be hospitalized or whether ambulatory management would be appropriate. In the face of severe disease, the woman should be hospitalized with the timing of birth dictated by maternal and fetal status.

Historically, women diagnosed with mild preeclampsia were admitted to the hospital for two reasons: to prevent eclampsia and to improve perinatal outcome (Gilstrap, Cunningham, & Whalley, 1978). However, researchers have questioned the practice of routine hospitalization of women diagnosed with mild preeclampsia. Mathews, Agarwal, and Shuttleworth (1980), and Crowther, Bouwmeester, and Ashurst (1992) reported no differences in maternal or perinatal outcomes for women with mild preeclampsia managed in hospitals compared with those managed expectantly on an outpatient basis. ACOG (2000) recognizes that outpatient management for women with mild preeclampsia is a viable option for those who agree to follow established protocols, can have frequent office or home visits, and can perform blood pressure monitoring.

The role of antihypertensive medication in the expectant management of women with mild preeclampsia is controversial. Antihypertensive regimens reported in prospective and retrospective studies include hydralazine, methyldopa, nifedipine, prazosin, diuretics, and beta-blockers (Cruickshank, Robertson, Campbell, & MacGillivray, 1991; Cruickshank, Robertson, Campbell, & MacGillivray, 1992; Gruppo di Studio Iperensione in Gravidanza, 1998; Plouin et al., 1988, 1990; Rubin et al., 1983; Sibai, 1996; Sibai, Barton, & Akl, 1992; Sibai, Gonzalez, Mabie, & Moretti, 1987). Although each of these studies examined the effect of different antihypertensive agents, none reported a better perinatal outcome compared with management without antihypertensives. There are insufficient data to support prophylactic use of antihypertensive therapy in the management of mild preeclampsia.

Traditionally, women diagnosed with severe preeclampsia remote from term are delivered expeditiously. Although this approach may allow recovery from the disease process for the woman, it may not improve fetal and neonatal outcomes. The use of conservative management for severe preeclampsia remote from term has suggested that pregnancy may be prolonged to gain fetal maturity without increased risk to the woman (Coppage & Sibai, 2004; Fenakel et al., 1991; Friedman, Schiff, Lubarsky, & Sibai, 1999; Haddad et al., 2004; Odendaal, Pattinson, Bam, Grove, & Kotze, 1990; Schiff, Friedman, & Sibai, 1994; Sibai, 1992, 1996; Sibai, Mercer, Schiff, & Friedman, 1994). With strict criteria for patient selection and intensive maternal and fetal surveillance, pregnancy may be prolonged. Assessments are aimed at early identification of worsening in maternal or fetal status or evidence of end-organ dysfunction. Table 6–6 provides the selection criteria for expectant management of severe preeclampsia remote from term.

Activity Restriction

Activity restriction, varying from frequent rest periods with legs elevated to complete bed rest in the full lateral position, is frequently prescribed for women with preeclampsia (ACOG, 2002). While on bed rest, blood pressure decreases, and interstitial fluid is mobilized into the intravascular space, enhancing flow to the uterus and kidneys. Controversy exists about whether the reduction of systolic blood pressure associated with bed rest improves maternal or fetal outcomes. For pregnancies complicated with nonproteinuric hypertension, bed rest does not appear to significantly improve outcome; however, for women with proteinuric preeclampsia, bed rest does seem to have some benefit. It is unclear whether bed rest in a hospital setting improves outcomes because of concurrent intensive inpatient maternal–fetal assessments and appropriate

TABLE 6–6 ■ EXPECTANT MANAGEMENT SELECTION CRITERIA FOR PATIENT WITH SEVERE PREECLAMPSIA REMOTE FROM TERM

Management Approach (if one or more of the clinical findings present)	Clinical Findings
Expeditious birth (within 72 hr)	*Maternal:* • Uncontrolled hypertension (defined as blood pressure persistently >160/110 despite maximum recommended doses of two antihypertensive medications) • Eclampsia • Platelet count <100,000 mm³ • AST or ALT >2x upper limit of normal with epigastric pain or RUQ tenderness • Pulmonary edema • Compromised renal function (rise in serum creatinine of at least 1 mg/dL over baseline values) • Abruptio placentae • Persistent severe headache or visual changes *Fetal:* • Recurrent late or variable decelerations • BPP <4 on two occasions, 4 hr apart • AFI <2 cm • Ultrasound estimated fetal weight <5th percentile • Reverse umbilical artery diastolic flow
Consider expectant management	*Maternal:* • Controlled hypertension • Urinary protein of any amount • Oliguria (<0.5 mL/kg/hr) which resolves with hydration • AST/ALT >2x upper limit of normal without epigastric pain or RUQ tenderness *Fetal:* • BPP >6 • AFI >2 cm • Ultrasound estimated fetal weight >5th percentile

AFI, amniotic fluid index; ALT, alanine aminotransferase; AST, aspartate aminotransferase; BPP, biophysical profile; RUQ, right upper quadrant.

Adapted from Coppage, K., & Sibai, B. M. (2004). Hypertensive emergencies. In M. Foley, J. T Strong & T. Garite (Eds.), *Obstetric Intensive Care Manual* (pp. 51–65). New York: McGraw-Hill; Fenakel, K., Fenakel, G., Appelman, Z., Lurie, S., Katz, Z., & Shoham, Z. (1991). Nifedipine in the treatment of severe preeclampsia. *Obstetrics and Gynecology, 77*(3), 331–337; Friedman, S., Schiff, E., Lubarsky, S., & Sibai, B. M. (1999). Expectant management of severe preeclampsia remote from term. *Clinical Obstetrics and Gynecology, 42*(3), 470–478; Haddad, B., Deis, S., Goffinet, F., Paniel, B., Cabrol, D., & Sibai, B. M. (2004). Maternal and perinatal outcomes during expectant management of 239 severe preeclamptic women between 24 and 33 weeks gestation. *American Journal of Obstetrics and Gynecology, 190*(6), 1590–1597; Odendaal, H. J., Pattinson, R. C., Bam, R., Grove, D., & Kotze, T. J. (1990). Aggressive or expectant management for patients with severe preeclampsia between 28-34 weeks gestation: A randomized controlled trial. *Obstetrics and Gynecology, 76*(6), 1070–1075; Schiff, E., Friedman, S. A., & Sibai, B. M. (1994). Conservative management of severe preeclampsia remote from term. *Obstetrics and Gynecology, 84*(4), 626–630; Sibai, B. M. (2002). High-risk pregnancy series: An expert's view. Chronic hypertension in pregnancy. *Obstetrics & Gynecology, 100*(2), 369–377; Sibai, B. M., & Hnat, M. (2002). Delayed delivery in severe preeclampsia remote from term. *OBG Management, 14*(5), 92–108; Sibai, B. M., Mercer, B. M., Schiff, E., & Friedman, S. A. (1994). Aggressive versus expectant management of severe preeclampsia at 28 to 32 weeks gestation: A randomized controlled trial. *American Journal of Obstetrics and Gynecology, 171*(3), 818–822.

medical intervention or is beneficial when considered as an independent factor (Goldenberg et al., 1994; Mathews, 1977).

Ongoing Assessment

Preeclampsia can appear to occur without warning or be recognized with the gradual development of symptoms. A key goal is early identification of women at risk for development of preeclampsia. A review of the major organ systems adds to the database for detecting changes from baseline in blood pressure, weight gain and patterns of weight gain, increasing edema, and presence of proteinuria. The nurse should note whether the woman complains of unusual, frequent, or severe headaches; visual disturbances; or epigastric pain.

Accurate and consistent blood pressure assessment is important for establishing a baseline and monitoring subtle changes throughout the pregnancy. Blood pressure readings are affected by maternal position and measurement techniques. Consistency must be ensured with the use of proper equipment and cuff size, correct maternal positioning, a rest period before recording the pressure, and recording of Korotkoff 5 (ie, disappearance of sound) Barton, Witlin, & Sibai, 1999; NHBPEP, 2000; Working Group, 2000). K4 is typically 5 to 10 mm Hg higher than K5. Ideally, blood pressure measurements should be recorded with the woman in a semi-Fowler's position with the arm at heart level. If the initial measurement indicates an elevation, the woman should be allowed to relax and have a repeat measurement performed, again in a semi-Fowler's position (ACOG, 1996, 2000; Beevers, Lip, & O'Brien, 2001). Use of electronic blood pressure devices produces different values than those obtained with a manual cuff and stethoscope. Electronic blood pressure devices systematically underestimate diastolic pressure values by approximately 10 mm Hg and overestimate systolic pressure values by approximately 4 to 6 mm Hg. These differences are related to the normal hemodynamic changes that occur during pregnancy and the subsequent changes in Korotkoff phases sounds able to be heard with the human ear compared with the electronic device. There is a widening of pulse pressure when using electronic blood pressure devices compared with manual readings; however, mean arterial pressure is unchanged (Marx, Schwalbe, Cho, & Whitty, 1993). The main points to remember are that blood pressure measurements should be taken in a consistent manner and that assessment focuses on trends, rather than on a single reading. This may support use of MAP for the diagnosis of hypertension. Since outpatient settings may use a combination of auscultation and automated technology and inpatient settings typically rely on automated technology, a common reference point allows for more consistency when comparing trends.

Presence of edema, in addition to hypertension, warrants additional investigation. Edema, assessed by distribution and degree, is described as dependent or pitting. If periorbital or facial edema is not obvious, the pregnant woman is asked if it was present when she awoke.

Deep tendon reflexes (DTRs) are evaluated if preeclampsia is suspected. The biceps and patellar reflexes and ankle clonus are assessed and the findings recorded. The evaluation of DTRs is especially important if the woman is being treated with magnesium sulfate; absence of DTR is an early indication of impending magnesium toxicity.

Proteinuria is determined from dipstick testing of a clean-catch or catheter urine specimen. A reading greater than +1 on two or more occasions at least 4 hours apart should be followed by a 24-hour urine collection (Brown et al., 1995). A 24-hour collection for protein and creatinine clearance is more reflective of true renal status, because proteinuria is a later sign in the course of preeclampsia. Urine output is assessed for volume of at least 25 to 30 mL/hour or 100 mL/4 hours. Placement of an indwelling Foley catheter with an urometer facilitates accurate assessment of urine output and may assist with the detection of early signs of renal compromise.

An important ongoing assessment is determination of fetal status. Uteroplacental perfusion decreases in women with preeclampsia, thereby placing the fetus in jeopardy. The uterine spiral arteries of the placental bed are subject to vasospasm. When this occurs, perfusion between maternal circulation and intervillous space is compromised, decreasing blood flow and oxygenation to the fetus. Oligohydramnios, IUGR, fetal compromise, and intrauterine fetal death all are associated with preeclampsia. The fetal heart rate (FHR) should be assessed for baseline rate, variability, and reassuring versus nonreassuring patterns. The presence of abnormal baseline rate, minimal or absent variability, or late decelerations may indicate fetal intolerance to the intrauterine environment. Because of the poor positive predictive value of nonreassuring fetal findings to detect fetal acidemia at birth, maternal and fetal status is evaluated to determine when birth should occur. The presence of variable decelerations, antepartum or intrapartum, may suggest decreased amniotic fluid volumes (ie, oligohydramnios), increasing the risk of umbilical cord compression, and possible fetal compromise. Biophysical or biometric monitoring for fetal well-being may be ordered. These tests include fetal movement counting, nonstress testing (NST), contraction stress test (CST), biophysical profile (BPP), and serial ultrasonography (Phelan, 1991). As long as the fetus continues to grow in an appropriate manner and biophysical findings are reassuring, it can be inferred that the placenta and uterine blood flow are appropriate.

If labor is suspected, a vaginal examination for cervical changes is indicated. Uterine tonicity is evaluated for signs of labor and abruptio placentae. Preterm contractions or a tense, tender uterus may be early indications of an abruptio placenta.

Assessments target signs of deterioration from mild preeclampsia to severe preeclampsia or eclampsia. Signs of liver involvement (eg, epigastric pain, elevated liver function test, and thrombocytopenia), renal failure, worsening hypertension, cerebral involvement, and developing coagulopathies must be assessed and documented. Lung sounds are assessed for rales (ie, crackles) or diminished breath sounds, which may indicate pulmonary edema. Noninvasive assessment parameters to assess maternal status include level of consciousness, blood pressure, hemoglobin oxygen saturation (ie, pulse oximetry), electrocardiogram (ECG) findings, and urine output. Invasive hemodynamic monitoring with a flow-directed pulmonary artery catheter (Swan-Ganz) may be indicated in selected patients (Clark, Cotton, Hankins, & Phelan, 1997).

Laboratory Tests

The nurse assists in obtaining a number of blood and urine specimens to aid in the diagnosis of preeclampsia, HELLP syndrome, or chronic hypertension. No known laboratory tests predict the development of preeclampsia (Gavette & Roberts, 1987). Laboratory abnormalities are nonspecific in preeclampsia, but changes can reflect underlying multiorgan system dysfunctions (Barton, Witlin, & Sibai, 1999; Roberts, 2004). Thrombocytopenia is the most common hematologic abnormality, but routine assessment of the other coagulation factors is not recommended until the platelet concentration is less than 100,000/mm³. Unless a preexisting coagulopathy is present, the woman is not at an increased risk for developing a coagulopathy until the platelet level falls below 100,000/mm³ (Leduc, Wheeler, Kirshon, Mitchell, & Cotton, 1992). Baseline laboratory test information is useful in the early diagnosis of preeclampsia and for comparison with results obtained to evaluate progression and severity of disease. Display 6–4 provides the common laboratory assessments for a woman with hypertension during pregnancy.

Pharmacologic Therapies

Pharmacologic therapies are instituted for two purposes: seizure prophylaxis and antihypertensive management.

Magnesium Sulfate

Magnesium sulfate is the drug of choice in the management of preeclampsia to prevent seizure activity. (Magnesium sulfate safety is presented in the section on preterm labor.) For seizure prophylaxis, magnesium sulfate is administered as a secondary infusion by an infusion-controlled device to achieve serum levels of approximately 5 to 8 mg/dL (4 to 7 mEq/dL). The loading dose is a 4- to 6-g intravenous bolus over 15 to 30 minutes, followed by a maintenance infusion of 2 to 3 g/hour.

The action of magnesium sulfate as an anticonvulsant is controversial, but it is thought to block neuromuscular transmission and decrease acetylcholine excretion at the end plate, depressing the vasomotor center and thereby depressing CNS irritability (Tatro, 2005). Magnesium circulates largely unbound to protein and is almost exclusively excreted in the urine. In

DISPLAY 6-4

Laboratory Values Assessed for Women With Hypertension During Pregnancy

Complete Blood Count
- Hemoglobin
- Hematocrit
- Platelet count

Chemistry
- Electrolytes
- Blood urea nitrogen (BUN)
- Serum creatinine
- Serum albumin
- Uric acid
- Serum calcium
- Serum sodium
- Serum magnesium
- Serum glucose
- Liver function tests: lactate dehydrogenase (LDH), asparatate aminotransferase, alanine aminotransferase
- May consider serum amylase and lipase
- May consider cardiac enzymes

Urine
- Urinalysis for protein
- 24-hour creatinine clearance may be measured in patients with chronic hypertension or renal disease
- 24-hour urine for sodium excretion
- Specific gravity

Coagulation Profile
- Platelet count and function
- Prothrombin and partial thromboplastin times
- Fibrinogen
- Fibrin split or fibrin degradation products
- Bleeding time
- D-dimer

patients with normal renal function, the half-time for excretion of magnesium is approximately 4 hours. In women with decreased glomerular filtration and renal hypoperfusion, such as seen in preeclampsia, the half-time for excretion is delayed, increasing the risk for toxicity (Chesley, 1979; Massey, 1977).

Signs and symptoms of hypermagnesemia are assessed for the duration of the infusion. Clinically significant findings of hypermagnesemia are related primarily to magnesium's cellular effects. Intravenous magnesium, more so than oral, slows or blocks neuromuscular and cardiac conducting system transmission, decreases smooth muscle contractility, and depresses central nervous system irritability. Although the desired anticonvulsant effect can be achieved easily with current dosing regimes, the nurse must be aware of the potential for untoward effects, including decreased uterine and myocardial contractility, depressed respirations, and interference with cardiac conduction which places the woman at risk for cardiac dysrhythmias or cardiac arrest (Chesley, 1979; Massey, 1977; Tatro, 2005). Contrary to popular belief, magnesium sulfate has little effect on maternal blood pressure when administered appropriately.

The effect of magnesium sulfate on fetal heart baseline variability is controversial. Fetal serum levels for magnesium will approximate maternal levels so fetal sedation is possible. However, minimal to absent baseline variability should not be seen as a side effect of maternal magnesium sulfate therapy until fetal hypoxemia has been ruled out.

Nursing responsibilities and assessments for women receiving magnesium sulfate include:

- Obtain patient history, including drug history and any known allergies; note renal function or history of heart block, myocardial damage, or concurrent use of CNS depressants, digoxin, or neuromuscular blocking agents. (Make sure anesthesia personnel are aware of infusion.)
- Assess maternal baseline vital signs, DTR, neurologic status, and urinary output before initiation of therapy and reassess per institution protocol.
- Administer magnesium sulfate according to protocol; all infusions should be prepared by the facility pharmacy, or the facility should use commercially prepared solutions.
- Establish the primary intravenous line and intravenously administer magnesium sulfate piggyback by means of a controlled-infusion device; infuse via a separate line and do not mix with other intravenous drugs unless compatibility has been established.
- Avoid administration of any solution of magnesium sulfate if particulate matter, cloudiness, or discoloration is noted.
- Document magnesium sulfate infusion in grams per hour.
- Continue fetal assessment.
- Keep calcium gluconate (1 g of a 10% solution) immediately available in a secure medication area on the unit (ie, drug dispenser system or locked emergency medication area).
- Be cautious with concurrent administration of narcotics, CNS depressants, calcium channel blockers, and beta-blockers; discontinue magnesium sulfate; and notify the physician if signs of toxicity occur.
- Monitor for signs of magnesium toxicity (e.g., hypotension, loss of DTRs, respiratory depression, respiratory arrest, oliguria, shortness of breath, chest pains, electrocardiographic changes [increased PR interval, widened QRS complex, prolonged QT interval, heart block]); if toxicity is suspected, discontinue infusion and notify provider.
- Monitor serum magnesium levels as indicated based on maternal status or if toxicity suspected; routine serum magnesium levels are not required in the absence of co-morbidities. (Depression of DTRs occurs at serum concentrations lower than those associated with adverse cardiopulmonary effects and the presence of DTRs indicates magnesium levels that are not too high.) See Table 6–7 for effects associated with various serum magnesium levels.
- Maintain strict I&O and keep patient hydrated; urine output should be at least 25 mL/hour while administering parenteral magnesium; magnesium sulfate may cause a transient osmotic diuresis.
- Maintain seizure precautions and neurologic evaluations.
- Prepare for neonatal resuscitation.

Phenytoin

Phenytoin (Dilantin) has also been proposed for eclampsia prophylaxis; however, it is not a first-line therapy in the US. Clinical studies have not demonstrated better results with phenytoin compared with magnesium sulfate (Lucas & Jordan, 1997; Lucas, Leveno, & Cunningham, 1995a, 1995b; The Eclampsia Collaborative Group, 1995). Because of a lack of experience with phenytoin and the significant maternal side effects, magnesium sulfate remains the first-line drug in the United States. However, phenytoin may be considered when the use of magnesium sulfate is associated with increased risk of maternal complications, such as with myasthenia gravis or markedly

TABLE 6–7 ■ SERUM MAGNESIUM LEVELS AND ASSOCIATED EFFECTS

Effect	Serum Level (mg/dL)
Anticonvulsant prophylaxis	5–8
Electrocardiographic changes	5–10
Loss of deep tendon reflexes	8–12
Somnolence	10–12
Slurred speech	10–12
Muscular paralysis	15–17
Respiratory difficulty	15–17
Cardiac arrest	20–35

Adapted from Coppage, K., & Sibai, B. M. (2004). Hypertensive emergencies. In M. Foley, J. T. Strong, & T. Garite (Eds.), *Obstetric intensive care manual* (pp. 51–65). New York: McGraw-Hill; and Roberts, J. M. (2004). Pregnancy-related hypertension. In R. Creasy & R. Resnik (Eds.), *Maternal-fetal Medicine* (5th ed., pp. 859–900). Philadelphia: Saunders.

reduced renal function (Lucas & Jordan, 1997; Lucas, Leveno, & Cunningham, 1995a, 1995b; The Eclampsia Collaborative Group, 1995). However, if phenytoin is used extreme care must be taken and staff must be familiar with the expected side effects and potential complications and resuscitation equipment must be immediately available.

Antihypertensive Therapy

Pharmacologic therapies directed at the control of significant hypertension include a variety of agents. Several general precautions should be considered when antihypertensive agents are ordered: antihypertensive therapy is initiated when diastolic blood pressure is sustained at greater than 110 mm Hg **or** systolic blood pressure is sustained at greater than 160 mm Hg to prevent maternal cerebral vascular accident. The effect of the antihypertensive agent may depend on intravascular volume status and hypovolemia resulting from increased capillary permeability and hemoconcentration may need correction before the initiation of therapy. Diastolic blood pressure should be maintained between 90 and 100 mm Hg to maintain uteroplacental perfusion (NHBPEP, 2000; Working Group, 2000). See Display 6–5 for indications for antihypertensive

therapy. See Table 6–8 for dosing, mechanism of action, and considerations for commonly used antihypertensive agents.

Hydralazine Hydrochloride

Hydralazine hydrochloride (Apresoline) is considered by many to be the first-line agent to decrease hypertension. Dosage regimens vary (see Table 6–8), but intermittent intravenous boluses generally work equally as well as continuous infusions; there is also less chance of rebound hypotension with intermittent boluses. Side effects of hydralazine include flushing, headache, maternal and fetal tachycardia, palpitations, and uteroplacental insufficiency with subsequent fetal tachycardia and late decelerations. Because hydralazine increases maternal cardiac output and heart rate, if hypertension is more a force issue (ie, elevated cardiac output, hypervolemia, or tachycardia) the clinical state may worsen with blood pressure either not lowering or possibly increasing.

LABETALOL HYDROCHLORIDE

Labetalol hydrochloride (Normodyne or Trandate) has been used in place of hydralazine for the management of hypertension. Dosage regimens vary, based on physician experience and preference; however, stacked dosing generally provides better results (see Table 6–8). Labetalol hydrochloride is contraindicated in women with asthma and those with greater than first-degree heart block (Chez & Sibai, 1994). Because of labetalol's alpha- and beta-adrenergic blockage, transient fetal and neonatal hypotension, bradycardia, and hypoglycemia are possible. The combined alpha- and beta-adrenergic blockade decrease the incidence of rebound maternal tachycardia, making it an attractive alternative to Apresoline, especially in women with cardiac disease who cannot tolerate tachycardia.

Postpartum Management

Immediate postpartum curettage has been associated with a more rapid recovery for women with severe preeclampsia, although more research is needed in this area (Magann et al., 1993; Magann & Martin, 1995). Most women are clinically stable within 48 hours after birth. However, because of the risk of eclampsia during the first 24 to 48 hours postpartum, careful monitoring is essential and should include frequent assessments of vital signs, level of consciousness, DTRs, urinary output, and laboratory data. Intravenous magnesium sulfate is usually continued for 24 hours postpartum. It is important to be alert for early signs and symptoms of complications of preeclampsia such as postpartum hemorrhage, DIC, pulmonary edema, HELLP syndrome, increased intracranial pressure, and intracranial hemorrhage.

DISPLAY 6 - 5

Indications for Antihypertensive Therapy

Antepartum and Intrapartum
- Persistent elevations for at least 1 hour
  - SBP ≥160 mm Hg, or
  - DBP ≥110 mm Hg, or
  - MAP ≥130 mm Hg
- Persistent elevations for at least 30 minutes
  - SBP ≥200 mm Hg, or
  - DBP ≥120 mm Hg, or
  - MAP ≥140 mm Hg
- Thrombocytopenia or congestive heart failure with persistent elevations for at least 30 minutes
  - SBP ≥160 mm Hg
  - DBP ≥105 mm Hg
  - MAP ≥125 mm Hg

Postpartum (persistent elevations for at least 1 hour)
- SBP ≥160 mm Hg
- DBP ≥105 mm Hg
- MAP ≥125 mm Hg

Coppage, K. H. & Sibai, B. M. (2004). Hypertensive emergencies. In M. R. Foley, T. H. Strong, & T. J. Garite (Eds.), *Obstetric intensive care manual* (2nd ed). New York: McGraw-Hill.

TABLE 6–8 ■ ANTIHYPERTENSIVE THERAPY FOR PREECLAMPSIA-ECLAMPSIA

Generic Name	Trade Name	Mechanism of Action	Dosage	Considerations
Hydralazine	Apresoline	• Direct-acting dilator of smooth muscle • Primary effect is arterial dilation, with minor venodilator effects • ↓ Systemic, pulmonary, and renal resistance • Systemic vasodilation results in ↓ systemic vascular resistance, ↓ arterial pressure, ↑ SV, ↑ rate of ventricular pressure rise • Reflex tachycardia may occur secondary to vasodilation • Onset of action is 15–20 min • Duration of effect is approximately 2–6 hr • Metabolized by liver	5 mg IV, Then 5–10 mg IV q20–30 min up to total dose of 30–40 mg	• Must wait 20 min for response between IV doses • Rebound hypotension • Reflex ↑ in CO and HR (Hyperdynamic circulatory changes also include ↑ LV pressure rise and SV may be dangerous in patients with certain cardiovascular disorders) • Monitor BP and HR • Maximal BP ↓ within 10 min • ↓ Dose with hepatic dysfunction, low cardiac output, and severe renal dysfunction • Use with caution in patients with coronary artery disease (reflex tachycardia can produce anginal attacks or AMI) • Contraindicated in patients with rheumatic mitral valve disease (↑ PAP) • Not recommended for blood pressure control in patients with dissecting aortic aneurysm (↑ rate of LV pressure rise stresses dissecting aortic segment and worsens aortic injury and propagates dissection) • Because of postural hypotension give with caution in patients with cerebrovascular disease • Excessive dosing may result in too rapid and too profound a reduction in BP causing ↓ uteroplacental blood flow and ↓ oxygen delivery to the fetus • May ↓ hemoglobin, neutrophil, WBC, granulocyte, platelet, and RBC counts
Labetalol	Normodyne Trandate	• Selective (α-and nonselective β-adrenergic blocking agent • Induces a controlled rapid decrease in BP • ↓ in catecholamine-induced cardiac stimulation and direct vasodilation • ↓ SVR and arterial pressure without reflex tachycardia • β-blocking effects also blunt rate of LV pressure rise usually associated with vasodilator drugs, ↓ stress on aortic wall • Hypotensive effect usually seen within 2–5 min, peaks at 10 min, and persists for 2–6 hr after IV administration	Initial dose 20 mg IV followed by stacked dosing of 40 mg–80 mg–80 mg–80 mg IV for a maximum dose of 300 mg	• Monitor HR and BP • Consider ECG monitoring for bradydysrhythmias and heart block • Monitor blood glucose levels • ↓ Amplitude and frequency of FHR accelerations; may lower FH baseline rate • Monitor newborn for hypoglycemia, hypotension, and bradycardia • Not a titratable drug; effect of increases in IV infusion rate may not be noted for approximately 10 min; diminution of the drug effect may not be noted for several hours following reduction of dose or discontinuation of drug

(continued)

TABLE 6–8 ■ ANTIHYPERTENSIVE THERAPY FOR PREECLAMPSIA-ECLAMPSIA (Continued)

Generic Name	Trade Name	Mechanism of Action	Dosage	Considerations
		• Metabolized by liver and excreted in urine and bile		• Valuable in managing hypertensive crisis as a result of dissecting aortic aneurysm or traumatic dissection of aorta • Effectively ↓ cerebral perfusion pressures without ↓ cerebral perfusion • ↓ Dose with hepatic dysfunction or hepatic hypoperfusion • ↓ Dosage necessary in patients with creatinine clearances < 10 mL/min • Adverse reactions related to α-blockade include orthostatic hypotension • Potential β-blockade reactions include bronchospasm, ↓ myocardial contractility and SV, and bradycardia (dose related) • Patient should not be quickly raised to a sitting position during therapy and for at least 2 hr after last dose • ↑ Uteroplacental perfusion and ↓ uterine vascular resistance • May exert a positive effect on early fetal lung maturation in patients remote from term • May ↑ transaminase and urea levels
Nifedipine	Procardia Adalat	• Calcium channel blocker • Thought to inhibit calcium ion influx, across cardiac and smooth-muscle cells, decreasing contractility and oxygen demand • May dilate coronary arteries and arterioles • Effect seen within 20 min, with peak action within 30–60 min with duration of 4–8 hr	10 mg PO, may be repeated × 1 after 30 min	• Oral route only; sublingual dosing can result in excessive hypotension, acute myocardial ischemia, and death • Possible exaggerated effect if used with $MgSO_4$, including severe hypotension with resulting ↓ uteroplacental perfusion and maternal neuromuscular blockade (muscle weakness, jerky movements of extremities, difficulty in swallowing, paradoxical respirations, and inability to lift head from pillow) • Principal side effects include headache and cutaneous flushing • May ↑ ALT, AST, alkaline phosphatase, and LD levels
Nitroglycerin	Nitrostat IV Tridil Nitro-Bid IV	• Relaxation of venous vascular smooth muscle, and to a lesser degree, arterial smooth muscle • Venodilatation associated with *marked* ↓ in preload; slight arterial dilator effect produces a *slight* ↓ in SVR (afterload reduction) that, in turn, is associated with an ↑ SV	Continuous IV infusion beginning at 5 micrograms /min; increase by 5–10 micrograms every 5 min until BP, wedge pressure response, or relief of pain is obtained	• Requires critical care consultation or co-management • There is no maximal dose, but most believe that if 200 micrograms/ min do not provide relief of hypertension or ischemic pain, higher doses unlikely to provide additional benefit • Monitor BP, HR, and ECG for worsening or resolution of ischemic changes

TABLE 6–8 ■ ANTIHYPERTENSIVE THERAPY FOR PREECLAMPSIA-ECLAMPSIA (Continued)

Generic Name	Trade Name	Mechanism of Action	Dosage	Considerations
		• Reflex tachycardia may occur in response to vasodilation • Also dilates the epicardial and collateral coronary arteries while preserving coronary autoregulation so that coronary blood flow is not shunted away from ischemic myocardium (coronary steal) • Onset of hypotensive effect approximately 1–5 min, duration of effect is 5–10 min • Very short hemodynamic half-life • Undergoes hepatic metabolism		• PAP and PACP should be monitored in hemodynamically unstable patients • Latent or overt hypovolemia may be associated with a marked ↓ in BP • Hypotension may worsen myocardial ischemia • Restoring circulatory volume by fluid loading generally stabilizes the patient's response to nitroglycerin • Larger doses of nitroglycerin were required following volume expansion, the ability to effect a smoother and more controlled drop in BP required prevasodilator hydration • Occasionally, bradycardia and severe hypotension occur during IV infusion (Bezold-Jarisch reflex) • May cause headache because of direct cerebral vasodilation • Methemoglobin may result from higher doses (7 micrograms/kg/min) • Patients with normal arterial oxygen saturation who appear cyanotic should be evaluated for toxicity, defined as a methemoglobin level >3% • May ↓ FH baseline variability
Sodium Nitroprusside	Nipride Nitropress	• Extremely potent direct-acting dilator of both veins and arteries of systemic, coronary, pulmonary, and renal circulations • ↓ Preload, mediated by vasodilation, associated with ↓ right and left ventricular filling volume and pressure, ↓ size and wall stress of both ventricles, and ↓ pulmonary vascular congestion and therefore pulmonary pressures • ↓ Afterload (mediated by arteriolar dilation) results in ↓ systemic and pulmonary vascular resistance and an ↑ SV • Both preload and afterload reduction ↓ myocardial oxygen consumption • Reflex tachycardia may result from ↓ BP • Titrate dosing to desired response	0.25 micrograms/kg/min infusion; increase by 0.25 micrograms/kg/min q5 min	• Critical care drug requiring critical care management • Invasive hemodynamic monitoring required • Ferrous ion in the nitroprusside molecule reacts rapidly with the sulfhydryl compounds in RBCs, resulting in release of cyanide; cyanide further metabolized in the liver to thiocyanate • Drug is photosensitive and degrades rapidly in light; IV bag should always be covered with metal foil or another opaque material; do not need to cover tubing or drip chamber • Should be observed for signs of thiocyanate and cyanide toxicity • Signs of thiocyanate toxicity include weakness, rashes, tinnitus, lactic acidosis, blurred vision, seizures, psychotic behavior, and mental confusion

(continued)

TABLE 6–8 ■ ANTIHYPERTENSIVE THERAPY FOR PREECLAMPSIA-ECLAMPSIA (Continued)

Generic Name	Trade Name	Mechanism of Action	Dosage	Considerations
		• 10 micrograms/kg/min considered usual maximal dose • Onset of effects within 30–60 sec; BP begins to rise almost immediately after discontinuation and reaches pretreatment levels within 1–10 min • Rapidly metabolized in presence of RBCs		• Metabolic acidosis one of the earliest signs of plasma accumulation of cyanide radical • Therapy should not exceed 48 hr • Does cross placenta with fetal cyanide concentrations higher than maternal levels • Transient fetal bradycardia possible • Monitor maternal serum pH, plasma cyanide, red-cell cyanide, and methemoglobin levels • Correction of hypovolemia prior to initiation of nitroprusside infusion is essential in order to avoid abrupt and often profound drops in BP

Intensity of monitoring and progression of activity are based on the patient's condition. After vital signs and mental status are stable, laboratory data indicate condition is improving, urinary output is reassuring, and intravenous magnesium sulfate is discontinued, the frequency of maternal assessments can be decreased from 1 to 2 hours to 4 to 8 hours, the Foley catheter is removed, and the patient is encouraged to ambulate. It is important to provide assistance and assess stability during initial ambulation, after bed rest, and after intravenous administration of magnesium sulfate during the intrapartum and postpartum period. Efforts should be made to initiate maternal–newborn attachment by bringing the newborn, if stable, to visit the mother. Photographs of the newborn can be taken and provided to the woman if the maternal or newborn condition prevents visitation.

HELLP Syndrome

HELLP syndrome, a multisystem disease, is a form of severe preeclampsia in which the woman presents with a variety of complaints and exhibits common laboratory markers for a syndrome of hemolysis (H), elevated liver enzymes (EL), and low platelets (LP). This subset of women progresses from preeclampsia to the development of multiple organ involvement and damage. The complaints range from malaise, epigastric pain, nausea, and vomiting to nonspecific viral–syndrome-like symptoms. On presentation, these patients are generally in the second or early third trimester and initially may show few signs of preeclampsia. Because of the presenting symptoms, these patients may receive a nonobstetric diagnosis, delaying treatment and increasing maternal and perinatal morbidity and mortality (Sibai, 1990b; Weinstein, 1982, 1985). Assessments and management of the woman diagnosed with HELLP syndrome are the same as those for the woman with severe preeclampsia.

Eclampsia

Eclampsia is the development of seizures or coma or both in a woman with signs and symptoms of preeclampsia. Other causes of seizures must be excluded. Eclampsia can occur antepartum, intrapartum, or postpartum; approximately 50% of cases occur antepartum (Fairlie & Sibai, 1993). The immediate care during a seizure is to ensure a patent airway. Once this has been attained, adequate oxygenation must be maintained by use of supplemental oxygen. Magnesium sulfate (and amobarbital sodium for recurrent convulsions) is given according to the institutional protocol (Sibai, 1990a). Aspiration is a leading cause of maternal morbidity after an eclamptic seizure. After initial stabilization and airway management, the nurse should anticipate orders for a chest radiograph and possibly arterial blood gas (ABG) determinations to exclude the possibility of aspiration. Rapid assessments of uterine activity, cervical status, and fetal status are performed. During the seizure, membranes may rupture, and the cervix may dilate because the uterus becomes hypercontractile and hypertonic. If birth is not imminent, the timing and route of delivery and the induction of labor versus cesarean birth depend on maternal and fetal status. All medications and therapy are merely temporary measures.

BLEEDING AND BLEEDING DISORDERS IN PREGNANCY

Significance and Incidence

Hemorrhagic complications during pregnancy are a significant causative factor of adverse maternal–fetal outcomes. Major blood loss predisposes the woman to an increased risk of hypovolemia, anemia, infection, and preterm labor and birth. Although bleeding can cause considerable problems for the mother, the fetus is especially at risk because significant maternal blood loss can result in negative alterations in maternal hemodynamic status and decreased oxygen carrying capacity. Maternal–fetal gas exchange decreases. When bleeding decreases blood flow to the placenta, the fetus is at risk for progressive physiologic deterioration (ie, hypoxemia, hypoxia, asphyxia, and death). This risk is directly related to the amount and duration of blood loss.

Hemorrhage during pregnancy is one of the leading causes of maternal death in the United States along with embolism and pregnancy-induced hypertension (Chang et al., 2003). The leading cause of death in women whose pregnancy ends in stillbirth is hemorrhage from placental abruption and uterine rupture (Chang et al.). Placental abruption and uterine rupture also are significant causes of fetal death (Silver, 2007). The nurse must be alert to the symptoms of hemorrhage and shock and be prepared to act quickly to minimize blood loss and hasten maternal and fetal stabilization. Up to 15% of maternal cardiac output (750 mL–1,000 mL/minute) flows through the placental bed at term; unresolved bleeding can result in maternal exsanguination in 8 to 10 minutes (Poole & White, 2003). In addition to the physiologic implications of bleeding during pregnancy, the mother experiences emotional stress as she worries about the outcome for herself and her baby. Although maternal mortality decreased approximately 99% during the 20th century, hemorrhage remains a major cause of maternal death in all parts of the world. Maternal mortality rates in the United States during the past 20 years have remained consistent at approximately 7.5 to 8.4 per 100,000 live births (Chang et al.), but hemorrhage remains a persistent risk. The risk for maternal mortality is consistently higher among African-American women, which may reflect social, economic, and cultural barriers to healthcare.

Bleeding complicates approximately one in five pregnancies; the incidence and cause of bleeding vary by trimester (MacMullen, Dulski, & Meagher, 2005). Most bleeding occurring in the first trimester of pregnancy is related to spontaneous abortion and is generally not life threatening. Ectopic pregnancy is the leading cause of life-threatening hemorrhage during the first trimester (Chang et al., 2003). Antepartum hemorrhage of unknown origin after 24 weeks gestation is associated with congenital anomalies (Chan & To, 1999). Hemorrhage during the antepartum period usually results from disruption of the placental implantation site (involving a normally implanted placenta or placenta previa) (Clark, 2004). Most serious obstetric hemorrhage occurs in the postpartum period as a result of uterine atony after placental separation (ACOG, 2006b). Other causes of postpartum hemorrhage include retained placenta, uterine rupture, uterine inversion, genital tract trauma, and coagulopathy (ACOG).

Symptomatic placenta previa is identified in approximately 0.3% to 0.5% of pregnancies (Oyelese & Smulian, 2006). Low implantation of the placenta is much more common during early pregnancy, but most of these cases resolve or are not found to be clinically significant as pregnancy progresses (Oyelese & Smulian; Frederiksen, Glassenberg, & Stika, 1999). Placentas may be classified as low-lying during the second trimester by routine ultrasonography because it is difficult to determine which placentas cross the cervical os during ultrasonographic examination in early pregnancy. Transvaginal ultrasound remains a more accurate way to diagnose placenta previa (Clark, 2004; Oyelese & Smulian).

Placenta accreta is an uncommon abnormality of placental implantation where the placenta is abnormally adherent. It is one of the most serious complications of placenta previa. In addition to placenta previa, prior uterine surgery significantly increases the risk of placenta accreta. With placenta previa, the risk of developing placenta accreta is 10% to 25% for women with a history of one prior cesarean birth and rises to more than 50% for women with two or more cesarean births or second-trimester pregnancy terminations (Clark, 2004). The incidence of placenta accreta is rising secondary to an increase in the cesarean section rate (ACOG, 2002; Oyelese & Smulian, 2006).

The incidence of abruptio placentae varies in the literature according to the population studied and diagnostic criteria. In the United States, the reported incidence is approximately 1% of all pregnancies (Anath, Oyelese, Yeo, Pradhan, & Vintzileos, 2005). Risk of recurrence in subsequent pregnancies has been reported to be as high as 5.5% to 16.6%. This rate is approximately 30 times higher than that for pregnant women without a history of prior abruptio placentae. The strongest risk factor for abruption is a history of placental abruption in a previous pregnancy (Anath, Oyelese, Yeo, Pradhan, & Vintzileos). The risk of recurrence for women with a history of two placental abruptions increases to approximately 25% (Clark, 2004).

Vasa previa is a condition in which umbilical arteries and veins abnormally implanted throughout the amnion traverse the cervical os in front of the presenting part of the fetus. It is a rare but life-threatening complication for the fetus at the time of rupture of membranes (Oyelese & Smulian, 2006). The reported incidence is approximately 1 in 3,000 births (Oyelese & Smulian; Clark, 2004). Rupture of the vessels during spontaneous or artificial rupture of membranes usually leads to fetal exsanguination or severe neurologic fetal injury secondary to fetal hemorrhage before the cause of bleeding is recognized and before an emergent cesarean birth can be accomplished (Silver, 2007). Fetal death occurs in 60% to 75% of cases of ruptured vasa previa (Oyelese & Smulian; Clark).

Uterine rupture is another significant cause of maternal hemorrhage. The risk of uterine rupture for women attempting vaginal birth after cesarean birth (VBAC) is less than 1%; however, the consequences can be catastrophic for the mother and baby (ACOG, 2004). The risk of uterine rupture depends on the number, type, and location of the previous incisions (ACOG). Although risk of uterine rupture has been reported as nearly five times greater for women with a history of two prior low transverse cesarean births when compared to women with one prior cesarean birth (ACOG), a recent large multicenter study did not find a difference in rupture rates in these two groups (Landon et al., 2006). The incidence of rupture of a vertical scar from a prior cesarean birth varies but has been reported to be as high as 7% (Shipp et al., 1999). Women with a previous low-vertical uterine incision have a similar success rate for having a VBAC as those women with a previous low transverse incision (ACOG). The risk of uterine rupture for women with a T-shaped incision from a prior cesarean birth is between 4% and 9% (ACOG).

Waiting for spontaneous labor, thus avoiding cervical ripening agents and oxytocin, appears to significantly decrease the risk of uterine rupture for women attempting VBAC (ACOG, 2004, 2006a; Aslan, Unlu, Agar, & Ceylan, 2004; Durnwald & Mercer, 2004; Landon et al., 2005; Mauldin & Newman, 2006; Zelop, Shipp, Cohen, Repke, & Leiberman, 2000). There are enough data to suggest that prostaglandins and high rates of oxytocin infusion increase the risk for rupture (ACOG, 2006c; Aslan et al., Uniu, Agar, & Ceylan, 2004; Lieberman, 2001; Durnwald & Mercer, 2004; Lydon-Rochelle, Holt, Easterling, & Martin, 2001). Uterine ruptures at the scar site and remote from the previous scar site have been reported with high doses of oxytocin (Murphy, 2006). It has been theorized that prostaglandins induce local biochemical modifications that weaken the prior uterine scar, thus predisposing it to rupture (Murphy). Due to the risk of uterine rupture with the use of misoprostol or any prostaglandin agent for cervical ripening or induction, ACOG (2004, 2006a) does not recommend

prostaglandins for women attempting VBAC. If labor needs to be induced in a patient with a previous scar for a clear and compelling clinical indication, the potential increased risk of uterine rupture with the use of prostaglandins should be discussed with the patient and documented in the medical record (ACOG 2006a).

The incidence of uterine inversion is approximately 1 case in 2,500 births, although the range varies among studies (You & Zahn, 2006). Improper management of the third stage of labor increases the likelihood of iatrogenic uterine inversion (Cunningham et al., 2005; Curran, 2003).

Postpartum hemorrhage remains one of the leading causes of maternal death worldwide (Chang et al., 2003). Early or primary postpartum hemorrhage (within 24 hours after birth) is most frequently caused by uterine atony, retained placental fragments, lower genital tract lacerations, uterine rupture, uterine inversion, placenta accreta, and coagulopathies. Late or secondary postpartum hemorrhage (>24 hours to 6 weeks after birth) is more likely to be caused by infection, placental site subinvolution, retained placental fragments, and coagulopathy (Francis, 2004). The incidence of postpartum hemorrhage after cesarean birth is approximately 6% to 8% compared with 3.9% after vaginal birth (Cunningham et al., 2005).

Definitions and Clinical Manifestations

The definitions, cause, pathophysiology, and clinical manifestations of the most frequently occurring causes of bleeding and bleeding disorders in pregnancy are described in the following sections. A diagnosis-specific summary of expected management is included. A more detailed summary of nursing interventions for bleeding during pregnancy concludes this section.

Placenta Previa

Placenta previa is the abnormal implantation of the placenta in the lower uterine segment. The reported incidence of placenta previa at birth varies widely. This variation results from differences in the time of diagnosis. Asymptomatic placenta previa is often diagnosed during routine ultrasound performed in the second trimester; most cases of placenta previa are detected before the third trimester (Oyelese & Smulian, 2006). These women are at increased risk for other obstetric complications, such as placental abruption, IUGR, and hemorrhage (Clark, 2004). It has been theorized that the placental tissue that surrounds the cervical os does not develop as well as the placental tissue that is in the myometrium (Clark; Oyelese & Smulian). By the end of 40 weeks of pregnancy, the incidence of placenta previa is approximately 0.05% (Clark). The most significant risk factors include prior uterine surgery resulting in uterine scarring and history of a prior placenta previa (Clark; Miller, Chollet, & Goodwin, 1997; Oyelese & Smulian). Late development and implantation of the ovum, more frequently occurring in older women, may also play a role in placenta previa. Display 6–6 lists the risk factors associated with placenta previa.

Placental implantation has traditionally been classified as normal, low-lying, partial placenta previa, and total placenta previa (Fig. 6–2). Clark (1999) proposed a new classification system: placenta previa: the placenta covers the internal os in the third trimester; marginal placenta previa: the placenta is within 2 to 3 cm of the internal os but does not cover the os. The rationale for this classification system is the ambiguity and lack of clinical utility of the term *low-lying placenta*. Until recently there had been no accepted definition of how close the placenta must be to mandate cesarean birth or double setup examination. It is now known that there is no increased risk of intrapartum hemorrhage if the distance from the lower margin of the placenta to the internal os is at least 2 to 3 cm. With this classification system, the term low-lying placenta would be reserved for cases in which the exact

DISPLAY 6-6

Factors Associated With Placenta Previa

- Previous placenta previa
- Previous cesarean birth
- Induced or spontaneous abortions involving suction curettage
- Multiparity
- Advanced maternal age (>35 years)
- Cigarette smoking
- Multiple gestation
- Fetal hydrops fetalis
- Large placenta
- Uterine anomalies
- Fibroid tumors
- Endometritis
- African-American or Asian ethnicity

relationship of the placenta to the cervical os has not been determined or for cases of apparent placenta previa before the third trimester. As the ability to more accurately visualize placental location increases because of advancements in ultrasound technologies,

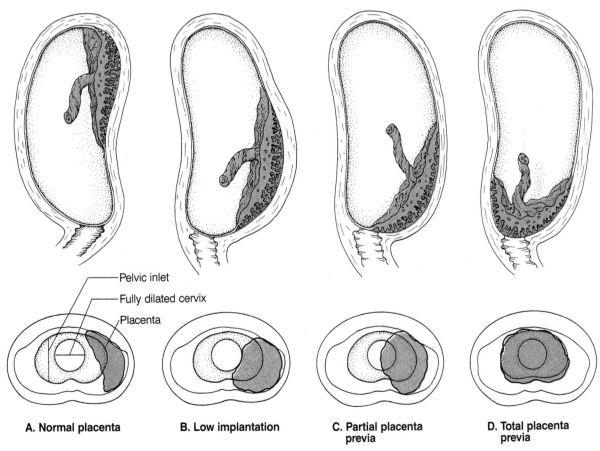

Pelvic inlet
Fully dilated cervix
Placenta

A. Normal placenta   **B. Low implantation**   **C. Partial placenta previa**   **D. Total placenta previa**

FIGURE 6–2. Placenta previa.

this classification system may be adopted in clinical practice. The term *placental migration* (a misnomer) has been used to describe the apparent movement of the placenta away from the cervical os. The placenta does not move; it remains in place as the uterus expands away from the os.

Clinical Manifestations

Painless uterine bleeding during the second or third trimester characterizes placenta previa. The first significant bleeding episode may occur before 30 weeks' gestation; some women never exhibit bleeding as a symptom until labor develops (Clark, 2004). Rarely is the first episode life threatening or a cause of hypovolemic shock. The bright red bleeding may be intermittent or continuous. After the bleeding episode, women may demonstrate "spotting" of bright red or dark brown blood on the peripad.

Diagnosis

The standard for the diagnosis of placenta previa is an ultrasound examination. It may be a transabdominal, transvaginal, or translabial ultrasound. Transvaginal ultrasound provides precise information regarding the placement of the placenta in relation to the cervical os (Clark, 2004; Oyelese & Smulian, 2006). If ultrasound reveals a normally implanted placenta, a speculum examination is performed to exclude local causes of bleeding (eg, cervicitis, polyps, carcinoma of the cervix), and a coagulation profile is obtained to exclude other causes of bleeding. Diagnosis of placenta previa increased dramatically with the advent of transabdominal ultrasound, the rate has decreased with the use of transvaginal or translabial ultrasound (Oyelese & Smulian). It is most often diagnosed before the onset of bleeding when an ultrasound examination is performed for other indications.

Management

Conservative management is usually possible when the fetus is not mature and maternal status is stable. When survival is likely and fetal lung maturity is achieved, birth can be accomplished. Most births are by cesarean section, although vaginal birth may be achieved if the placental edge does not completely cover the cervical os. This type of vaginal birth occurs in the operating room with personnel and equipment available for a cesarean birth if needed (ie, a double setup).

Patients are frequently hospitalized with the initial bleeding episode. Those with recurrent bleeding episodes, recurrent uterine activity associated with bleeding, or evidence of fetal or maternal compromise usually remain hospitalized until the birth. Some women will have a life-threatening bleeding event. For women who are unstable blood can be cross-matched

at all times and IV access maintained with an IV line. For stable patients with occasional spotting a heparin lock may be used to maintain an IV access site. In the event of sudden-onset hemorrhage a second IV line should be initiated with a large bore catheter, as it is very difficult to obtain IV access when the woman is in shock. Women who experience an initial bleeding episode that resolves, are hemodynamically stable, demonstrate fetal well-being, and have emergency services readily available to them are candidates for expectant management as outpatients (Clark, 2004; Oyelese & Smulian, 2006).

Abruptio Placentae

Abruptio placentae, or premature separation of the placenta, is the detachment of part or all of the placenta from its implantation site, typically occurring after the 20th week of pregnancy (Fig. 6–3). Premature separation of the placenta is a serious event and accounts for about 15% of all neonatal deaths (Witlin, Saade, Mattar, & Sibai, 1999). More than 50% of these deaths are the result of preterm birth. Other causes of fetal death include hypoxia and asphyxia. Risk factors associated with abruptio placentae are listed in Display 6–7. Despite these reported risk factors, the exact cause is unknown. There may be some type of disease or damage to the blood vessels; this may be of long duration. The risk of recurrence in subsequent pregnancies has been reported as high as 5% to 16% (Clark, 2004). Women with two previous placental abruptions have a risk of recurrence of 19% to 40% (Clark; Rasmussen, Irgens & Dalaker, 1997). Women with severe preeclampsia and eclampsia are at high risk for abruptio placentae. This high-risk status includes women with mild pregnancy-induced or chronic hypertension. Approximately 50% of placental abruptions severe enough to cause fetal death are associated with hypertension (Clark). A placental abruption significant enough to cause fetal death is less common (1 in 420 births), but as use of cocaine has increased, fetal death associated with abruptio placentae has risen in selected populations (Clark). Quantitative proteinuria and the degree of blood pressure elevation are not predictive of an abruption (Witlin, Saade, Mattar, & Sibai, 1999). Investigators concluded that the greatest morbidity occurred in preeclamptic women with preterm gestations not receiving prenatal care (Witlin, Saade, Mattar, & Sibai). Thrombophilias, such as factor V Leiden or the antiphospholipid antibody syndrome, are associated with an increased risk of abruption (Sibai, 2005).

Clinical Manifestations

Abruptio placenta is suspected in the woman presenting with sudden-onset, intense, often localized, uterine

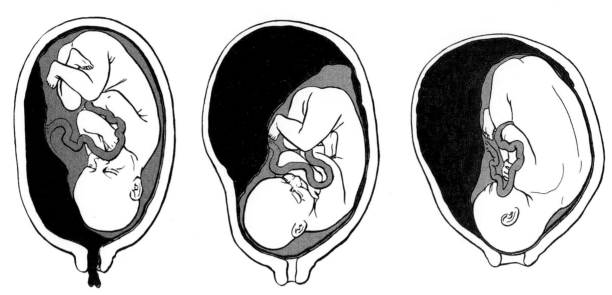

FIGURE 6–3. Abruptio placentae at various separation sites. (*Left*) External hemorrhage. (*Center*) Internal or concealed hemorrhage. (*Right*) Complete separation.

pain or tenderness with or without vaginal bleeding. Another common presentation is preterm contractions with vaginal bleeding or with an occult abruption in the absence of abdominal pain. The woman may also present with painless vaginal bleeding, although this is uncommon. In mild cases, the pain from abruption may be difficult to distinguish from the pain of labor contractions. In many cases, pain is localized to the area of the abruption. When placental implantation is

posterior, lower back pain may be more prominent than uterine tenderness. Occasionally, nausea and vomiting may occur. Vaginal bleeding from an abruptio placenta is not usually proportional to the degree of placental detachment because blood may become trapped behind the placenta. If the abruption is located centrally, no vaginal bleeding is visualized initially. Approximately 10% of women present with concealed hemorrhage (Clark, 2004). Marginal separations and large abruptions are associated with bright red bleeding and are almost always accompanied by contractions that are usually of low amplitude and high frequency (Clark). Contractions may be difficult to record if there is an increase in uterine resting tone and for women at earlier gestations. Palpation for uterine contractions or hypertonus is necessary. The contraction pattern of women with an evolving placental abruption often will show frequent contractions of short duration. Fetal assessment by electronic fetal monitoring (EFM) should be accomplished before obtaining a full uterine ultrasound because most placental abruptions cannot be accurately identified with ultrasonography. In a retrospective study of 167 patients presenting with bleeding between 13 and 26 weeks gestation, only 31% demonstrated an identifiable intrauterine clot (Signore, Sood, & Richards, 1998).

The fetal response to abruptio placentae depends on the volume of blood loss and the extent of uteroplacental insufficiency. Anticipatory nursing care includes being alert to the possibility of an abruption in the presence of any or all of the following: fetal tachycardia; bradycardia; loss of variability; presence of late decelerations; decreasing baseline (especially from tachycardia to a normal or near normal baseline with

DISPLAY 6-7

Factors Associated With Abruptio Placentae

- Partial abruption of current pregnancy
- Prior abruptio placentae
- Rapid decompression of the uterus, such as birth of the first of multiple fetuses and amniotic reduction therapy in polyhydramnios
- Hypertension
- Preterm premature rupture of membranes <34 weeks' gestation
- Prior cesarean birth
- Blunt abdominal trauma
- Thrombophilias
- Multiparity
- Cocaine use
- Cigarette smoking
- Extremely short length of the umbilical cord
- Uterine anomalies
- Uterine fibroids at the placental implantation site
- Use of intrauterine pressure catheters during labor

minimal or absent variability); a sinusoidal FHR pattern; low-amplitude, high-frequency contractions; uterine hypertonus; and abdominal pain.

The Kleihauer–Betke test may be performed on the mother's serum or vaginal blood to test for the presence of fetal red blood cells (RBCs). Fetal-to-maternal transfer of blood is documented by the presence of fetal cells in maternal serum (Silver, 2007). Depending on fetal age and size, the number of fetal RBCs present in maternal blood can be calculated to estimate the fetal blood loss. Formulas for this calculation can be found in the obstetrical literature (Cunningham et al., 2005). Cesarean birth is not always indicated. The decision to proceed with cesarean birth is usually based on fetal status. In the setting of reassuring FHR, expectant management may be appropriate for those women who are preterm and not in labor, providing the abruption is small and the mother and fetus are stable. Labor or cesarean birth, whichever mode presents the fewest risks to the woman and/or fetus, is indicated for significant bleeding or coagulopathy. The woman should be stabilized hemodynamically and hematologically before proceeding with labor initiation or cesarean birth. Some women with an abruption may demonstrate very rapid labor progress (Mahon, Chazotte, & Cohen, 1994). Chronic abruptio placentae may develop, with the woman experiencing episodic bleeding, subjecting the fetus to prolonged stress. Risk of developing disseminated intravascular coagulation (DIC) exists during placental abruption because of release of thromboplastin from the site into the maternal bloodstream.

Diagnosis

The diagnosis of abruptio placentae is based on the woman's history, physical examination, and laboratory studies. Examination of the placenta at birth or by a pathologist confirms the diagnosis. Ultrasonography is used to exclude placenta previa; however, it is not diagnostic for abruption (Clark, 2004; Lowe & Cunningham 1990). Abruptions are classified as partial, marginal (ie, only the margin of the placenta is involved), or total (ie, complete).

Management

Treatment depends on maternal and fetal status. In the presence of fetal compromise, severe hemorrhage, coagulopathy, poor labor progress, or increasing uterine resting tone, an emergent cesarean birth is performed once efforts to stabilize the woman have been initiated. In an older but reliable study, 22% of all perinatal deaths from abruption occurred after the patient was hospitalized, with 30% occurring in the first 2 hours (Knab, 1978). If the mother is hemodynamically stable, the fetus is alive with a reassuring FHR tracing, or if the fetus is dead, a vaginal birth

may be attempted. If the mother is hemodynamically unstable, attempts are first directed at maternal stabilization.

Blood replacement products and lactated Ringer's solution are infused in quantities necessary to maintain urine output of 30 to 60 mL/hour and a hematocrit of approximately 30%. Some experts suggest 1 unit of blood replacement for every 4 L of intravenous fluid or 3 ml of crystalloid solution for every milliliter of blood loss (Clark, 2004; Curran 2003). Blood loss is almost always underestimated (Oyelese & Smulian, 2006). Fluid resuscitation is aggressive in the presence of hemorrhage. With rapid volume intravenous infusions, the nurse anticipates the possibility of pulmonary edema due to lower colloid osmotic pressure in pregnancy.

Abnormal Placental Implantation

Abnormal adherence of the placenta occurs for unknown reasons but is thought to be the result of zygote implantation in an area of defective decidua basalis. The risk has greatly increased in the last 10 years with the rapidly rising rate of cesarean births (ACOG, 2002; You & Zahn, 2006). The risk of placenta accreta is increased with the number of previous cesarean births, estimated to be 0.2%, 0.3%, 0.6%, 2/1%, 2.3%, and 7.7% for women experiencing their first through their sixth cesarean births, respectively (ACOG, 2006b). When pregnancy is complicated by placenta previa, the risk of accreta is much greater, increasing to 67% for women with four or more cesarean births presenting with anterior or central placenta previa (ACOG, 2002; Clark, Koonings, & Phelan, 1985). Patients with one prior cesarean birth who present with anterior or central placenta previa in the subsequent pregnancy have a 24% risk of placenta accreta (ACOG, 2002; Clark, Koonings, & Phelan). Placenta accreta, along with uterine atony are the two most common causes of postpartum hysterectomy (ACOG, 2006b). Other risk factors include elevated maternal serum alpha-fetoprotein (MSAFP) and free ß-human chorionic gonadotropin (hCG) levels in the second trimester and advanced maternal age.

Placenta accreta occurs when there is a lack of decidua basalis, so that the placenta is implanted directly into the myometrium. Complete accreta occurs when the entire placenta is adherent; partial accreta occurs with one or more cotyledons adherent; and focal accreta occurs with one piece of a cotyledon adherent. *Placenta increta* is the abnormal invasion of the trophoblastic cells into the uterine myometrium. *Placenta percreta* occurs when the trophoblast cells penetrate the uterine musculature, and the placenta develops on organs in the vicinity of the percreta. Placenta percreta can adhere to the bladder and other

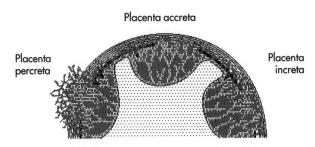

FIGURE 6–4. Abnormal adherence of the placenta.

pelvic organs and vessels. Placenta percreta accounts for only 5% of cases of abnormal adherence. Placenta increta occurs in 15% of cases, and accreta is the most common form accounting for 80% of cases (You & Zahn, 2006). Figure 6–4 demonstrates abnormal adherence of the placenta.

Elevated MSAFP in the second trimester has been associated with abnormal adherence of the placenta (Hung et al., 1999; Wheeler, Anderson, Kelly, & Boehm, 1996). Because abnormal placentation occurs in areas lacking decidua basalis, it is theorized that MSAFP can diffuse more easily over the increased surface area. Because ultrasound is routinely performed for a woman with an elevated MSAFP level, placenta accreta, increta, or percreta may be diagnosed prenatally (ACOG, 2002; Hung et al.; You & Zahn, 2006). Placenta increta has been diagnosed by ultrasound as early as 18 weeks (Wheeler, Anderson, Kelly, & Boehm), and placenta percreta has been diagnosed in the first trimester with magnetic resonance imaging (Thorp, Wells, Wiest, Jeffries, & Lyles, 1998; You & Zahn).

The diagnosis of an abnormally adherent placenta was made historically when manual separation of a retained placenta was attempted. If the placenta does not separate readily, rapid surgical intervention may be indicated. The woman with an abnormally attached placenta is at increased risk for hemorrhage; 90% of women lose more than 3,000 ml of blood intraoperatively, and the maternal mortality rate has been reported as high as 7% to 10% (Hudon, Belfort, & Broome, 1999; You & Zahn, 2006).

Women who are diagnosed before birth are treated by a multidisciplinary team to minimize complications. The goal is to prevent shock, thrombosis, infection, and adult respiratory distress syndrome (ARDS). Patients may receive erythropoietin before the surgery, and thrombosis prevention, antibiotics, and fluid resuscitation during the surgery. Invasive hemodynamic monitoring is continuous. It is recommended that 8 to 10 U of packed red blood cells be available in the operating room, with the blood bank maintaining the same amount (Hudon, Belfort, & Broome, 1999). Anesthesia, surgery, and urology services may be

involved in the cesarean hysterectomy. An interventional radiologist may be needed if selective embolization of the hypogastric arteries with an absorbable gel is performed to reduce blood loss (Dubois, Garel, Grignon, Lemay, & Leduc, 1997; Hudon, Belfort, & Broome; You & Zahn, 2006).

Planning for the potential of significant maternal blood loss and its sequelae is critical. If there is a diagnosis or strong suspicion of placenta accreta prior to birth, ACOG (2006b) recommends the following measures; the woman should be counseled about the likelihood of hysterectomy and blood transfusion; blood products and clotting factors should be available, cell savor technology should be considered if available; the appropriate location and timing of birth should be considered to allow access to adequate surgical personnel and equipment and preoperative anesthesia assessment should be obtained. These anticipatory steps improve the potential for the best possible outcome.

Women who are diagnosed at the time of birth are at higher risk for developing the previously described complications, as well as for an increased risk of death. Mobilization of nursing and medical staff, blood bank, surgery, and radiology is necessary immediately to perform the cesarean hysterectomy. In hospitals where specialized services may not be immediately available the nurse can anticipate the need for calling in extra staff, on-call physicians, obtaining uncrossed O-negative blood, and proceeding to hysterectomy.

Vasa Previa

Vasa previa is the result of a velamentous insertion of the umbilical cord. With vasa previa, the umbilical cord is implanted into the membranes rather than into the placenta. The vessels then traverse within the membrane, crossing the cervical os before reaching the placenta. The umbilical vein and arteries are not surrounded by Wharton jelly, so they have no supportive tissue which predisposes the umbilical blood vessels to laceration; this occurs most often during either spontaneous or artificial rupture of the membranes (Oyelese & Smulian, 2006). The sudden appearance of bright red blood at the time of spontaneous or artificial rupture of the membranes, coupled with the sudden onset of a nonreassuring FHR pattern, should immediately alert the nurse to the possibility of vasa previa. Bleeding that is fetal in origin is always significant because of the small volume of fetal blood. Total blood volume in the fetus is approximately 80 to 100 mL/kg, and rapid exsanguination can result in severe neurologic injury or fetal death (Silver, 2007).

Immediate cesarean birth is indicated in the presence of vasa previa. Vasa previa rupture may also occur before or after rupture of the membranes; the

DISPLAY 6-8

Factors Associated With Vasa Previa

- Succenturiate-lobed placenta
- Bilobed placenta
- Placenta previa
- In vitro fertilization
- Multiple gestation
- Fetal anomaly

diagnosis is considered for women with limited antenatal bleeding and nonreassuring FHR patterns. Risk factors associated with vasa previa are listed in Display 6–8.

Although it rarely occurs (approximately 1 in 2,500 births or 1 in 50 cases in which there is a velamentous insertion of the cord), vasa previa is associated with high incidence of fetal morbidity and mortality because fetal bleeding rapidly leads to shock and exsanguination (Oyelese et al., 2004; Sherer & Anyaegbunam, 1997). Vasa previa is occasionally diagnosed before rupture of the membranes by examiners performing an ultrasound for other indications, palpating a pulsing vessel, directly visualizing a vessel, or identifying fetal blood cells in vaginal blood. Diagnosis before birth may be made with transvaginal color Doppler ultrasound in patients with known risk factors. It has been suggested that an increased rate of diagnosis may occur if routine ultrasound examinations include an evaluation of placental cord insertion. Transvaginal ultrasound is indicated if placental cord insertion cannot be determined transabdominally (Oyelese & Smulian, 2006). If noted, planned cesarean birth is accomplished. The survival rate in one retrospective study was 56% without a prenatal diagnosis versus 97% with a prenatal diagnosis (Oyelese et al.).

In the case of an antenatal bleeding event, a number of laboratory tests are available to determine if the blood is maternal or fetal. Because the fastest test still takes 5 minutes (Odunsi, Bullough, Henzel, & Polanska, 1996; Oyelese, Turner, Lees, & Campbell, 1999), these tests have limited clinical utility during labor because of the short time required from rupture to birth to save the fetus.

Uterine Rupture

Uterine rupture may be a catastrophic event for the woman and fetus, whether related to rupture of a uterine scar from prior uterine surgery, hyperstimulation, trauma, or rarely, spontaneous rupture of the uterus. The terms *uterine rupture* and *uterine dehiscence* are sometimes used interchangeably in the literature. Uterine rupture refers to the actual separation of the uterine myometrium or previous uterine scar, with rupture of the membranes and possible extrusion of the fetus or fetal parts into the peritoneal cavity. Dehiscence refers to a separation of the old scar, usually partial, with intact membranes; the fetus usually remains inside the uterus. Excessive bleeding usually occurs with uterine rupture, whereas bleeding is generally minimal with dehiscence (Cunningham et al., 2005).

Uterine rupture occurs most frequently in women with a previous uterine incision through the myometrium and usually occurs during labor, although it can occur in the antepartum period. Hyperstimulation or hypertonus of the uterus by oxytocin or prostaglandin administration can cause uterine rupture even in the unscarred uterus (Akhan, Iyibozkurt, & Turfanda, 2001; Catanzarite, Cousins, Dowling, & Daneshmand, 2006; Cunningham et al., 2005; Khabbaz et al., 2001; Matthews, Mathal, & George, 2000; Mazzone & Woolever, 2006). Invasive or blunt trauma, seen in women after a motor vehicle accident, battery, fall, or with knife or gunshot wound, is an additional cause of uterine rupture. Uterine rupture may also occur spontaneously with no history of uterine surgery or terminations of pregnancy. The pathophysiology related to spontaneous rupture is not fully understood, although it occurs more frequently in women of high parity (Cunningham et al.). Display 6–9 describes the risk factors associated with uterine rupture.

Clinical Manifestations

The clinical presentation of the woman experiencing a uterine rupture depends on the specific type of rupture

DISPLAY 6-9

Factors Associated With Uterine Rupture

- Previous uterine surgery
- High dosages of oxytocin
- Prostaglandin preparations (eg, misoprostol, dinoprostone)
- Hyperstimulation
- Hypertonus
- Grand multiparity
- Blunt or penetrating abdominal trauma
- Midforceps rotation
- Maneuvers within the uterus
- Obstructed labor
- Abnormal fetal lie
- Previous termination(s) of pregnancy
- Vigorous pressure on the uterus at birth

and may develop over several hours, or several minutes. Impending rupture may be preceded by increasing uterine hypertonus or hyperstimulation (Sheiner et al., 2004). Contrary to earlier reports, *usually* there is no decrease in uterine tone or cessation of contractions prior to or during uterine rupture (ACOG, 2006a; Leung, Leung, & Paul, 1993), although this finding has been reported by some researchers (Sheiner et al.). Nonreassuring changes in the FHR pattern may be early signs of impending or evolving uterine rupture (Ayres, Johnson, & Hayash, 2001; Sheiner et al.). The FHR pattern prior to rupture or as the rupture is evolving may be characterized by a decrease in variability, recurrent variable, prolonged or late decelerations followed by bradycardia, or fetal bradycardia may be sudden onset (Ayres, Johnson, & Hayash; Leung, Leung, & Paul; Menihan, 1999, Ridgeway, Weyrich, & Benedetti, 2004; Sheiner et al.; Yap, Kim, & Laros, 2001). The most consistent nonreassuring FHR patterns noted with uterine rupture are recurrent late decelerations and fetal bradycardia (Ayres, Johnson, & Hayash; Ridgeway, Weyrich, & Benedetti). If the uterine rupture is preceded by late decelerations, the fetus will tolerate a shorter period of prolonged decelerations (Leung Leung, & Paul). Significant neonatal morbidity has been reported when the time between onset of prolonged decelerations and birth is equal to or greater than 18 minutes (Leung Leung, & Paul). Kirkendall, Jauregui, Kim, and Phelan (2000) reported a significant risk of brain damage, intrapartum death, and death within 1 year of life for infants who were partially or completely extruded into the maternal abdomen during uterine rupture.

The woman may complain of abdominal pain and tenderness, and/or have vomiting, syncope, vaginal bleeding, tachycardia, or pallor. Uterine contractions usually continue without a decrease in uterine tone (Menihan, 1999). If unrecognized, bleeding can quickly cause maternal hypotension and shock. A traumatic rupture may be apparent almost immediately in the woman who complains of sharp, tearing pain, "like something has given way or popped open." There may be an inability on the part of the practitioner to reach the presenting part on vaginal examination. Uterine contractions may be absent, and the fetus palpated through the abdominal wall. Bleeding may be vaginal or into the abdominal cavity or both. Intraabdominal bleeding is suspected if the woman has a tense, acute abdomen with shoulder pain. Signs of shock appear soon after a catastrophic rupture, and complete cardiovascular collapse rapidly follows without prompt intervention.

Dehiscence of a prior lower segment cesarean scar is usually asymptomatic initially. The woman may continue to have contractions without further dilation of the cervix; if an intrauterine pressure catheter is in place for labor assessments, there may be little or no change in intrauterine pressure or resting tone pressures. If the dehiscence extends past the scar tissue, the woman may begin to complain of pain in the lower abdomen that is unrelieved with analgesia or epidural anesthesia.

Common sequelae associated with uterine rupture include excessive hemorrhage requiring surgical exploration; need for hysterectomy; need for blood product transfusion; hypovolemia; hypovolemic shock; injury to the bladder or ureters bowel laceration; extrusion of any part of the fetus; cord; or placenta through the disruption; emergent cesarean birth for suspected rupture; emergent cesarean birth for nonreassuring fetal status; and general anesthesia (Guise et al., 2004; Hibbard et al., 2001; Kirkendall, Jauregui, Kim, & Phelan, 2000; Landon et al., 2004; Pare, Quinones, & Macones, 2006; Shipp, 2004). Many women with uterine rupture experience more than one of these complications (Landon et al.).

Complete or partial placental abruption usually occurs concurrently with rupture (84%), and in many cases (60%), the placenta may be at the site of the rupture (Jauregui, Kirkendall, Ahn, & Phelan, 2000). Maternal death is a rare complication (Chauhan, Martin, Henrichs, Morrison, & Magann, 2003; Guise et al., 2004; Landon et al., 2004).

Diagnosis

The key to diagnosis is suspicion that uterine rupture has occurred. The nurse immediately should inform the primary healthcare provider at the first suspicion of a uterine rupture based on characteristics of the FHR pattern and maternal condition. Diagnosis is confirmed at birth.

Management

Treatment includes maternal hemodynamic stabilization and immediate cesarean birth. If possible, the uterine defect is repaired, or hysterectomy is performed. Uterine rupture is discussed further in Chapter 7.

INVERSION OF THE UTERUS

Inversion of the uterus (ie, turning inside out) after birth is a potentially life-threatening complication. The incidence of uterine inversion is approximately 1 in 2,500 births (You & Zahn, 2006). Fundal pressure and traction applied to the cord may result in inversion. Other factors associated with inversion of the uterus are listed in Display 6–10. Partial inversion occurs when the only the fundus inverts. A complete inversion occurs when the fundus passes through the opening of the cervix (You & Zahn). Although proper management of the third stage of labor prevents most uterine inversions, some are spontaneous and otherwise

DISPLAY 6-10

Factors Associated With Uterine Inversion

- Uterine atony
- Abnormally adherent placental tissue
- Fetal macrosomia
- Fundal placentation
- Uterine anomalies
- Use of oxytocin
- Use of fundal pressure
- Traction on the umbilical cord
- Abnormally short umbilical cord

unavoidable. Regardless of the precipitating factor, once an inversion occurs, prompt recognition and correction is necessary to reduce maternal morbidity and mortality.

Clinical Manifestations

In addition to possible visualization of the inversion, the primary presenting symptoms of uterine inversion are hemorrhage and hypotension. The woman may experience sudden, acute pelvic pain. Attempts to massage the fundus are unsuccessful because the fundus has inverted into the uterus or vaginal vault, or it is visible at or through the introitus. On bimanual examination, there will be a firm mass below or near the cervix along with the absence of an identification of the uterine corpus on abdominal examination.

Management

Uterine inversion is an emergent situation associated with severe hemorrhage and requiring immediate attempts to replace the uterus. If the inversion occurs before placental separation, removal of the placenta will result in additional hemorrhage (ACOG, 2006b). The largest amounts of blood loss are those reported with delivery of the placenta prior to attempting to reposition the uterus (You & Zahn, 2006). Replacement involves the birth attendant placing the palm of the hand against the fundus (now inverted and lowermost at or through the cervix) as if holding a tennis ball, with the fingertips exerting upward pressure circumferentially (ACOG). If attempts to replace the uterus are not quickly successful, administration of tocolytics (eg, terbutaline, magnesium sulfate, nitroglycerin) or general anesthesia may be necessary (ACOG; You & Zahn). Manual replacement with or without uterine relaxants is usually successful (ACOG). Laparotomy may be required in unusual cases. Oxytocin is withheld until the uterus has been repositioned.

Monitoring of maternal vital signs is extremely important because the pharmacologic agents directed at relaxing the uterine myometrium may exacerbate maternal hypotension. Automatic blood pressure cuffs, in use in the majority of hospitals overestimate systolic values by 4 to 6 mm Hg and underestimate diastolic values by 10 mm Hg (Natarajan et al., 1999; Simpson, 2005). Fluid resuscitation should be initiated to prevent shock; there may be a vagal component from peritoneal traction (Dayan & Schwalbe, 1996). Blood replacement therapy is administered as indicated by maternal hematologic status. Broad-spectrum antibiotic therapy and placement of a nasogastric tube may be initiated as indicated. Uterine inversion may occasionally recur during a subsequent birth.

Postpartum Hemorrhage

Postpartum hemorrhage is defined as a 10% decrease in hematocrit from admission assessment to postpartum data collection or by the need to administer a transfusion of red blood cells (Cunningham et al., 2005). Estimated blood loss is traditionally underestimated (Curran, 2003; You & Zahn, 2006) and is therefore an unreliable determinant of hemorrhage or excessive blood loss. Treatment is based on clinical signs and symptoms. Postpartum hemorrhage is a leading cause of maternal morbidity and mortality (Chang et al., 2003; Cunningham et al.; You & Zahn). Complications of postpartum hemorrhage depend on the severity of the hemorrhage and range from anemia to death.

Postpartum hemorrhage can result from abnormal implantation of the placenta; lacerations of the cervix, vagina, or perineum; uterine inversion; and DIC. The most common cause of postpartum hemorrhage is uterine atony. Early postpartum hemorrhage occurs after the delivery of the placenta, up to 24 hours after birth; late postpartum hemorrhage occurs 24 hours to 6 weeks after birth. Late postpartum hemorrhage is associated with subinvolution of the uterus and with retained placental tissue that may be the result of abnormal placental implantation. Display 6–11 lists the risk factors for postpartum hemorrhage. A thorough discussion of postpartum hemorrhage is presented in Chapter 10.

UTERINE ATONY

Uterine atony is marked hypotonia of the uterus. Because of the increased blood flow to the placenta in late pregnancy (approximately 750 to 1,000 mL/minute), failure of the uterus to contract after placental separation can result in very rapid and significant blood loss. The usual methods to prevent postpartum hemorrhage are uterine massage and administration of oxytocin (10–40 units/liter [U/L] titrated to control atony).

Uterine atony is more likely to occur when the uterus is overdistended (eg, multiple gestations, macrosomia, polyhydramnios). In such conditions, the uterus is "overstretched" and contracts poorly. Other causes of atony include induction or augmentation of labor, traumatic birth, halogenated anesthesia, tocolytics, rapid or prolonged labor, intraamniotic infection, and multiparity.

LACERATIONS OF THE BIRTH CANAL

Birth canal lacerations may include injuries to the labia, perineum, vagina, and cervix. Lacerations secondary to birth trauma occur more commonly with operative vaginal birth (ie, forceps or vacuum assisted; Cunningham et al., 2005). Other risk factors include fetal macrosomia, precipitous labor and birth, and episiotomy. Prevention, recognition, and prompt, effective treatment of birth canal lacerations are vital. Lacerations may be

anticipated if the uterus is well contracted but bleeding remains brisk. Some birth canal lacerations may result in a hematoma, which may not always be immediately recognized. Severe pelvic pain may be the first reported symptom, although maternal vital signs may deteriorate as the amount of blood loss in the hematoma increases. Because hematoma formation may conceal the blood loss; the woman may develop shock in the absence of other signs of hemorrhage. Usually the pain is not covered by the usual oral analgesics.

Severe pelvic pain and continued bleeding despite efficient postpartum uterine contractions with a firm uterus warrants reexamination of the birth canal by the physician or midwife. Continuous bleeding from minor sources may be just as dangerous over time as a sudden loss of a large amount of blood.

MANAGEMENT

The first step in the treatment of postpartum bleeding is to evaluate the uterus to determine if it is firmly contracted. Intravenous access with two 16- to 18-gauge catheters may be obtained if not already established. Generally, 20 to 40 U of oxytocin in 1 L of crystalloid solution is given intravenously initially at a rate of 10 to 15 mL/min and then continued for at least 3 or 4 hours following stabilization at slower rate as determined by the provider. If the uterus initially fails to respond to oxytocin, 0.2 mg of methylergonovine may be given intramuscularly to correct uterine atony via tetanic uterine contractions. If methylergonovine fails to resolve uterine atony or is contraindicated (ie, hypertension), 15-methyl-prostaglandin $F_{2\alpha}$ may be administered intramuscularly or intrauterine as long as the woman does not have asthma or systemic lupus. Most hemorrhage is controlled with one or two injections of 0.25 mg of 15-methyl-prostaglandin $F_{2\alpha}$ by intramuscular or intramyometrial routes, depending on the type of birth (Dildy, 2002). Various dosages of misoprostol (800 to 1,000 micrograms) per rectum have been reported in the literature as a successful alternative to the traditional drugs used for postpartum hemorrhage related to uterine atony (ACOG, 2006b). Some studies show more success with misoprostal than do others due to the wide range of doses (Cunningham et al., 2005; You & Zahn, 2006). Research about misoprostol for postpartum hemorrhage is ongoing. It may be used in the woman who has asthma.

Table 6–9 lists the uterotonic agents used for postpartum hemorrhage. Blood transfusion and treatment of shock may be urgently needed. The use of autologous transfusion and cell-saver technology, in which the patient's blood is collected during surgery, washed, and transfused back to the patient, has been used since the early 1970s but has only recently been studied for use in obstetrics. Multicenter trials documented that there are no increased risks of complications in

TABLE 6–9 ■ UTEROTONIC AGENTS USED FOR POSTPARTUM HEMORRHAGE

Medical Management of Postpartum Hemorrhage

Medication	Dose/Route	Frequency	Side Effects	Comments/Contraindications
Oxytocin (Pitocin)	IV: 10–40 U in 1 L normal saline or lactated Ringer's solution IM: 10 U	Continuous	Usually none, but N&V and water intoxication have been reported	Avoid undiluted rapid IV infusion, which can cause hypotension
Methylergonovine (Methergine)	IM 0.2 mg	Every 2–4 hr	Hypertension, hypotension, N&V	Avoid if patient is hypertensive
15-methyl-prostaglandin $F_{2\alpha}$ (Carboprost, Hemobate)	IM: 0.25 mg	Every 15–90 min 8 doses maximum	N&V, diarrhea, flushing or hot flashes, chills or shivering	Avoid in asthmatic patients; relative contraindication if hepatic, renal, and cardiac disease Diarrhea, fever, and tachycardia can occur
Dinoprostone (Prostin E_2)	Suppository; vaginal or rectal 20 mg	Every 2 hr	N&V, diarrhea, fever, headache, chills or shivering	Avoid if patient is hypotensive. If available, 15-methyl-prostaglandin $F_{2\alpha}$ is preferred. Fever is common. Stored frozen, it must be thawed to room temperature.
Misoprostol (Cytotec, PGE_1)	800–1,000 micrograms rectally	1 dose	Fever, chills and shivering	Usually used when other medications have not resulted in resolution of hemorrhage

IV, intravenously; IM, intramuscularly; PG, prostaglandin; N&V, nausea and vomiting.
Adapted from American College of Obstetricians and Gynecologists. (2006b). *Postpartum hemorrhage* (Practice Bulletin No. 76). Washington, DC: Author; and from Cunningham, F. G., Leveno, K. J., Bloom, S.L., Hauth, J. C., Gilstrap, L. C., & Wenstrom, K. D. (2005). *Williams obstetrics* (22nd ed.). New York: McGraw-Hill.

patients who underwent autologous blood collection and autotransfusion during cesarean birth (Rebarber, Lonser, Jackson, Copel, & Sipes, 1998; Rebarber, Odunsi, Baumgarten, Copel, & Sipes, 1998), thus autologous transfusion is considered safe for pregnant women (ACOG, 2006b). However, it requires anticipation of a need for transfusion and the minimum hematocrit concentrations are often above those of a pregnant woman (ACOG, 2006b).

The interior of the uterus is explored so that retained products of conception can be removed and possible rupture of the uterus diagnosed. If the blood fails to clot, DIC may be developing, and prompt, appropriate treatment may be life saving. The treatment for DIC is to cure the underlying problem. Figure 6–5 provides a management plan for postpartum hemorrhage.

Nursing Assessment

A medical history is usually available in the prenatal record and can be assessed for previous bleeding or bleeding disorders in order to assist the nurse in identifying risk factors for obstetrical precursors to hemorrhage. Assessment of the woman who is bleeding begins with careful evaluation of amount and color of blood loss, character of uterine activity, presence of abdominal pain, stability of maternal vital signs, and fetal status. Bright red vaginal bleeding suggests active bleeding, and dark or brown blood may indicate past blood loss. Display 6–12 presents nursing assessments and interventions for abnormal bleeding and/or hemorrhage.

Maternal or fetal tachycardia and maternal hypotension suggest hypovolemia; however, hypotension is a late sign. Historically, the frequency of vital signs depends on patient stability. Vital signs are usually repeated every 15 minutes until the bleeding is controlled and the vital signs remain or return to normal. Vital signs are performed more frequently (every 1 to 5 minutes) when there is evidence of instability, including systolic blood pressure less than 90 mm Hg, maternal tachycardia, decreasing level of consciousness, and oligura.

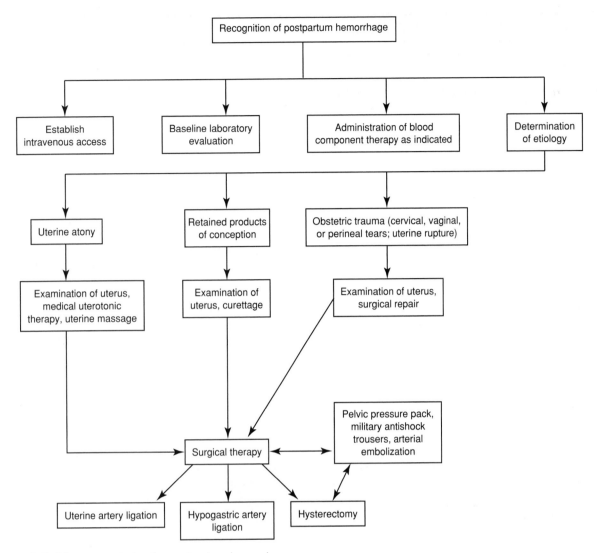

FIGURE 6–5. Management plan for postpartum hemorrhage.

When using an automatic blood pressure cuff, ensure that the Doppler is placed directly over the brachial artery for a more accurate recording. However, in severe hypotensive states, the automatic blood pressure device is less accurate. Many automatic blood pressure monitors calculate mean arterial pressure (MAP = systolic blood pressure +2 × diastolic blood pressure ÷ 3), which provides a quick number for reference and is a more stable parameter of hemodynamic function. The normal value for mean arterial pressure in the second trimester of pregnancy is approximately 80 mm Hg (Page & Christianson, 1976) and is 90 mm Hg at term (Cunningham et al., 2005).

When the blood pressure cannot be assessed with a blood pressure cuff, systolic blood pressure may be estimated by the presence of a radial, femoral, or brachial pulse. The presence of a radial pulse is associated with a systolic blood pressure of approximately 80 mm Hg, a femoral pulse with a blood pressure of 70 mm Hg, and a carotid pulse with a blood pressure of 60 mm Hg (Daddario, 1999). Placement of an arterial line in the woman who is hemorrhaging allows for continuous, accurate blood pressure monitoring and provides a means for drawing blood for arterial blood gas analysis and other laboratory values. Invasive hemodynamic monitoring with a flow-directed pulmonary artery catheter (Swan-Ganz) may be indicated in selected patients, especially in those who remain oliguric after fluid resuscitation (Clark, Greenspoon, Aldahl, & Phelan, 1986) or who have other complications such as sepsis, cardiac or pulmonary disease, or severe hypertension related to preeclampsia.

Skin and mucous membrane color is noted. Inspection also includes looking for oozing at the sites of incisions or injections and detecting petechiae or ecchymosis in areas not associated with surgery or trauma.

DISPLAY 6-12

Nursing Assessments and Interventions for Abnormal Bleeding/Hemorrhage

INITIAL NURSING INTERVENTIONS

- Notify physician and/or nurse midwife and anesthesia providers
- Secure airway, start oxygen via nonrebreather mask at 10 L/min
- Establish IV access if there is not an existing IV line: infuse lactated Ringer's solution (or normal saline) wide open, start another IV with a 16-gauge catheter (Do not infuse IV solutions containing glucose.)
- Perform uterine massage
- Obtain CBC, fibrinogen, PT, PTT, other laboratory tests.
- Draw 5 mL of the patient's blood in a clean red-top tube and observe frequently. If no clot forms within 8 to 10 minutes, suspect coagulapathy.
- Type + cross match 4 U of packed red blood cells.

- Administer oxytocin, methergine, prostaglandin $F_{2\alpha}$, cytotec as ordered.
- Administer blood products as ordered.

SECONDARY NURSING INTERVENTIONS

- Insert Foley catheter with urimeter: Assess for output of at least 30 mL/hour.
- Apply oxygen saturation monitor.
- Assess maternal vital signs per hospital policy.
- Call for additional nursing help so that one nurse can be responsible for patient care and another nurse is available for obtaining necessary medications, administering IV fluids, and monitoring intake and output if possible.
- Obtain CBC, PT, PTT, Fibrinogen, Ionized Ca, K after 5–7 U PRBC
- Anticipate surgical intervention such as exploratory laparotomy, uterine artery embolization, bilateral uterine artery ligation, B-lynch suture, hypogastric artery ligation, and hysterectomy. Notify members of the surgical team and ensure that a surgical suite is readied.

Antenatally, FHR is continuously assessed, and the uterus is palpated for contractions, especially in early gestations. In an emergent situation, use of electronic FHR and uterine monitoring provides continuous data about the fetus and uterus, allowing the nurse time to simultaneously initiate other needed treatments.

The pregnant woman is positioned in the lateral or modified Trendelenburg position, if possible. If the patient is in Trendelenburg or supine position, a wedge is placed under one hip to alleviate compression of the vena cava and aorta by the gravid uterus. Caution must be used in placing a pregnant woman in Trendelenburg because the pressure of the gravid uterus may interfere with optimal cardiopulmonary functioning. If the mother is hemodynamically unstable, oxygen is administered, preferably by nonrebreather facemask at 10 L/minute to maintain maternal–fetal oxygen saturation. Mentation is assessed frequently and provides additional indication of maternal blood volume and oxygen saturation.

Blood is drawn to assess maternal hemoglobin, hematocrit, platelet count, and coagulation profile. Display 6–13 lists the blood tests commonly ordered for the woman who is bleeding. In an emergent situation, blood may be drawn into a plain red-top (clot) tube and then visually evaluated for clot formation. Treatment for a significant coagulopathy should be initiated if no sign of clotting is evident within 8 minutes (Clark, 2004). Fresh-frozen plasma, whole blood, and cryoprecipitate may be administered; platelets are not usually given unless the

DISPLAY 6-13

Laboratory Values Assessed in Pregnant Women Who Are Bleeding

- Complete blood count
- Fibrinogen concentration
- Prothrombin time
- Activated partial thromboplastin time
- Fibrin degradation products or fibrin split products
- Platelet count
- Blood type, Rh, and antibody screen
- Clot retraction

POSSIBLY INDICATED

- Kleihauer–Betke test
- APT test
- Ivy bleeding time
- D-dimer
- Serum BUN
- Serum creatinine
- Urine creatinine clearance
- Urine sodium excretion
- Liver function test, including serum glucose
- Antithrombin III
- Arterial blood gases
- Urine or serum drug screen

TABLE 6–10 ■ BLOOD REPLACEMENT PRODUCTS

Blood Component Therapy

Product	Volume (mL)*	Contents	Effect (per unit)
Fresh whole blood	500	Red blood cells, all procoagulants	Increase hematocrit by 3 percentage points, hemoglobin by 1g/dL
Packed red blood cells	240	Red blood cells, white blood cells, plasma	Increase hematocrit by 3 percentage points, hemoglobin by 1g/dL
Platelets	50	Platelets, red blood cells, plasma; small amounts of fibrinogen, factors V and VIII	Increase platelet count 5,000–10,000/mm^3 per unit
Fresh frozen plasma	250	Fibrinogen, antithrombin III, factors V and VIII	Increase fibrinogen by 10 mg/dL to 25 mg/dL
Cryoprecipitate	40	Fibrinogen, factors VIII and XIII, von Willebrand factor	Increase fibrinogen by 10 mg/dL to 25 mg/dL

*Volume depends on individual blood bank.
Adapted from American College of Obstetricians and Gynecologists. (2006b). *Postpartum hemorrhage* (Practice Bulletin No. 76). Washington, DC: Author.

platelet count decreases to less than 30,000 cells/mm^3. Table 6–10 lists blood replacement products, factors present, and the expected effect per unit administered.

Circulating volume is usually restored with intravenous crystalloid solution administration. Two large-bore intravenous lines are needed for fluid replacement and administration of drug therapies. Blood and blood products are administered as needed or as soon as they are available. Breath sounds are auscultated before fluid volume replacement if possible to provide a baseline for future assessment. Massive fluid replacement during pregnancy or the immediate postpartum period for the woman who is hemorrhaging increases the potential for development of pulmonary edema. However, fluid replacement is necessary to restore circulatory volume, and the nurse anticipates and assesses for the development of peripheral or pulmonary edema and treatment with furosemide as ordered. Hemoglobin arterial oxygen saturation is monitored with a pulse oximeter. Pulse oximeters are an adjunct to assessment; they are not always accurate, especially in a patient in hypovolemic shock. In the hemorrhagic patient, blood flow to the extremities is decreased, and the oxygen saturation displayed may not accurately reflect tissue oxygenation status or the pulse oximeter may not be able to display a value at all. Arterial blood gas analysis may therefore be necessary to determine oxygen status. A maternal oxygen saturation level of at least 95% and a PaO$_2$ of at least 65 mm Hg as determined by blood gas analysis are necessary for the fetus to maintain adequate oxygenation.

Continuous ECG monitoring is indicated for the woman who is hypotensive or tachycardic, continuing to bleed profusely, or in shock. Maternal hypovolemia leading to hypoxia and acidosis may result in maternal heart rate dysrhythmias, including premature ventricular contractions, sinus or atrial tachycardia, and atrial or ventricular fibrillation.

A Foley catheter with an urometer is inserted to allow for hourly assessment of urine output. The most objective and least invasive assessment of adequate organ perfusion and oxygenation is urinary output of at least 30 mL/hour (Clark, 2004). Attempts should be made to maintain urine output of at least 30 mL/hour (Cunningham et al., 2005; Curran, 2003) because this is an objective and noninvasive means of evaluating adequate end-organ perfusion. In addition to volume, urine is assessed for the presence of blood and protein, and for specific gravity.

Nursing Interventions

Evaluation and management of acute episodes of bleeding during pregnancy usually occur in the inpatient setting. An exception is spotting during early gestation. After stabilization and a period of hospitalization, selected women may be managed at home.

Home Care Management

Controversy exists concerning home care management of women with placenta previa and marginal separation of the placenta; however, women in stable condition increasingly are being cared for in the home, with visits by perinatal nurses or daily provider-initiated phone contact. Criteria for home care management vary with the primary perinatal provider and home care agency. The woman must be in stable condition with no evidence of active bleeding and have resources to be able to return to the hospital immediately if active bleeding resumes. Bed rest at home remains a controversial topic; there are few data to determine how much time a women should be in bed or if bed rest affects outcome in a positive manner. Complete or partial bed rest has long-term deleterious effects on the woman physically and psychologically (Gupton, Heaman, & Ashcroft, 1997; Maloni, 1998).

Inpatient Management

When the woman is admitted to the hospital, the nurse begins assessment of the bleeding. The woman with acute bleeding requires continuous, ongoing nursing assessments and interventions. Maternal vital signs are assessed frequently according to individual clinical situations. Careful assessments are mandatory. Vital signs and noninvasive assessments of cardiac output (eg, skin color, skin temperature, pulse oximetry, mentation, urinary output) are obtained frequently to observe for signs of declining hemodynamic status.

Because a nonreassuring FHR pattern may be the first sign of maternal or fetal hemodynamic compromise, electronic FHR and uterine activity monitoring should be continuous. It is important to appreciate how rapidly maternal–fetal status can deteriorate as a result of maternal hemorrhage. Blood is shunted away from the uterus when the mother experiences hypotension or hypovolemic shock. Because of the potential for maternal–fetal mortality, it is essential to be prepared for an emergent birth at all times when caring for a pregnant woman who is bleeding. Supportive staff necessary for an emergency cesarean birth (ie, anesthesia personnel, surgical team, and neonatal resuscitation team) should be notified and on standby (if possible, in the hospital). Hemorrhage from placenta previa, abruptio placentae, or uterine rupture requires expeditious birth. Two large-bore intravenous catheters (at least 18 gauge) are placed if the woman is experiencing heavy bleeding. If consistent with institution policy, a 14- or 16-gauge intravenous catheter may be considered. The need to replace fluids and blood is determined by a number of parameters, including vital signs, amount of blood loss, mental status, laboratory values, and fetal condition.

Fluid replacement consists of administering lactated Ringer's or normal saline solution, packed red blood cells, fresh-frozen plasma, and possibly platelets. Blood product replacement therapy is anticipated, and communication with the blood bank is essential. Significant hemorrhage resulting in syncope or hypovolemic shock generally necessitates transfusion.

Blood type, Rh, and antibody screen should be obtained on admission; cross matching is ordered as necessary. The use of blood components in conjunction with crystalloid solutions, rather than with whole blood, is usually a better treatment option because it provides only the specific components needed (Cunningham et al., 2005). By using only the specific products required for the emergency, blood resources are conserved, and there is a decreased risk of blood replacement complications. Transfusion reactions may be demonstrated by chills, fever, tachycardia, hypotension, shortness of breath, muscle cramps, itching, convulsions, and ultimately cardiac arrest. The woman is assessed throughout the procedure. In the event of a reaction, the transfusion is immediately discontinued, and the intravenous line is flushed with normal saline. Treatment is then based on clinical symptoms. The development of anaphylaxis should be considered and appropriate treatment made available.

Careful fetal surveillance is critical to ensure fetal well-being during transfusion of multiple blood products. The increased incidence of uteroplacental insufficiency is related to complications of coagulation factor replacement therapy (Simpson, Luppi, & O'Brien-Abel, 1998). Administration of multiple replacement blood products leads to increased intravascular fibrin formation. Deposition of fibrin in the decidual vasculature of the chorionic villi may cause fetal compromise.

Because of the normal hemodynamic changes that occur, pregnant women may lose more than one-fourth of their fluid volume before displaying signs of shock (Clark, 2004). Women who are bleeding should be monitored carefully for the actual amount of blood loss, although this is sometimes difficult to assess in an emergent situation. Sheets or pads can be inspected and weighed. Accurate intake and output measurement and documentation are critical. Ideally, one nurse is assigned to monitor intake and output during a period of massive fluid and blood replacement. In an emergent situation in which the obstetrician and anesthesiologist may be ordering or adding replacement fluid to multiple intravenous lines, it becomes essential that one of the nurses records and maintains a running total of intake and output in addition to signing for blood products and overseeing administration.

The woman may develop a coagulopathy. Display 6–14 lists the risk factors for DIC. Pulmonary edema and renal failure, as evidenced by oliguria proceeding to anuria, must be anticipated. Systolic blood pressures of less than 60 mm Hg are associated with acute renal failure. The woman is at risk for development of acute tubular necrosis from lack of perfusion to the kidneys (ie, prerenal failure). Prolonged periods of severe hypotension may result in renal cortical necrosis. Urine output of less than 30 mL/hour should be reported to the primary care provider immediately.

In the case of severe hemorrhage, control of abdominal bleeding may be achieved by the placement of

DISPLAY 6-14

Obstetric Factors Associated With Disseminated Intravascular Coagulation

- Abruptio placentae
- Hemorrhage
- Preeclampsia or eclampsia
- Amniotic fluid embolism
- Saline termination of pregnancy
- Sepsis
- Dead fetus syndrome
- Cardiopulmonary arrest
- Massive transfusion therapy

medical antishock trousers (MAST suit), which are used in emergency and trauma units to control bleeding. Consensus does not exist about the benefits of using MAST suits; however, they are used in many institutions. Care must be taken not to put any pressure on the lower abdomen.

Hemorrhagic and Hypovolemic Shock

Hemorrhagic and hypovolemic shock is an emergent situation in which the perfusion of body organs may become severely compromised and death may ensue. Aggressive treatment is necessary to prevent adverse sequelae (eg, cellular death, fluid overload, acute respiratory distress syndrome [ARDS], oxygen toxicity). Common clinical symptoms of inadequate intravascular volume (ie, hypovolemia) that necessitates blood replacement include evidence of hemorrhage (ie, loss of a large amount of blood externally or internally in a short period of time); evidence of hypovolemic shock (ie, increasing pulse, cool clammy skin, rapid breathing, restlessness, and reduced urine output); or a decrease in hemoglobin and hematocrit below acceptable levels for trimester of pregnancy or the nonpregnant state.

Aggressive fluid and blood replacement is not without risk. The 24 hours after the shock period are critical. Observe for fluid overload, ARDS, and oxygen toxicity. Transfusion reactions may follow administration of blood or blood components. Even in an emergency, each unit should be checked per hospital protocol. Rapid transfusion with cold blood can chill the woman and cause vasoconstriction, arrhythmia, or arrest. Banked blood may be calcium deficient, increasing the risk for arrhythmias and further bleeding. Potassium levels may increase to dangerous levels. Laboratory values for other parameters are usually checked at least every 4 to 6 hours or as indicated by

the woman's condition. Display 6–15 suggests a management plan for hypovolemic shock (Clark, 1997). Infection is another complication of hemorrhage. Causes may include surgical procedures, multiple pelvic examinations, anemia, and loss of the white blood cell component of the blood. It is anticipated that the patient may receive prophylactic antibiotics or treatment for signs of infection.

Hemorrhagic disorders in pregnancy are nursing and medical emergencies requiring rapid and efficient teamwork from all members of the healthcare team. Perinatal nurses play an important role in the initial assessments, early interventions, and stabilization of the woman. Recognition that blood loss is out of proportion to the patient's clinical presentation is important because initial vital signs may remain within normal range in the presence of a significant hemorrhage.

DISPLAY 6-15

Management Plan for Obstetric Hypovolemic Shock

GOALS

- Maintain systolic blood pressure ≥90 mm Hg, urine output ≥30 mL/hr, and normal mental status.
- Eliminate source of hemorrhage.
- Avoid overzealous volume replacement that may contribute to pulmonary edema.

MANAGEMENT

- Establish two large-bore intravenous lines.
- Place woman in Trendelenburg position (wedge under hip if undelivered).
- Rapidly infuse 5% dextrose in lactated Ringer's solution while blood products are obtained.
- Infuse fresh whole blood or packed red blood cells, as available.
- Infuse platelets and fresh frozen plasma only as indicated by documented deficiencies in platelets (<30,000/mL) or clotting parameters (fibrinogen, prothrombin time [PT], partial thromboplastin time [PTT]).
- Search for and eliminate the source of hemorrhage.
- Use invasive hemodynamic monitoring if the woman fails to respond to clinically adequate volume replacement.
- Critical laboratory tests include complete blood count, platelet count, fibrinogen, PT, PTT, and arterial blood gas determinations.

Adapted from Clark, S. L. (1997). Hypovolemic shock. In S. L. Clark, D. B. Cotton, G. D. V. Hankins, & J. P. Phelan (Eds.), *Critical care obstetrics* (3rd ed., pp. 412–422). Malden MA: Blackwell Scientific.

Anticipating that a woman who is bleeding may rapidly proceed to hypovolemic shock can prevent complications and decrease maternal and fetal morbidity and mortality.

Thrombophilias in Pregnancy

Acquired and/or inherited thrombophilias in pregnancy are associated with a myriad of maternal and fetal complications including maternal thrombosis/embolism, early onset severe preeclampsia, abruption, IUGR, IUFD, nonreassuring FHR patterns, preterm birth, and recurrent miscarriage (Kutteh & Triplett, 2006; Lockwood & Silver, 2004; Silver, 2007). The most common acquired thrombophilia during pregnancy is antiphospholipid antibody syndrome (APLA syndrome; Lockwood & Silver, 2006; Sibai, 2005). Of the antiphospholipid antibodies, lupus anticoagulant (a misnomer as it causes thrombosis) and anticardiolipin antibody have the highest association with pregnancy complications. The antibodies are the result of antigenic changes in endothelial and platelet cell membranes, which promote thrombosis.

Inherited thrombophilias vary in prevalence and ability to cause thrombosis. The most common inherited thrombophilias most likely to cause thrombosis in pregnancy are mutations in Factor V Leiden, antithrombin deficiency, prothrombin gene G20210A mutation, tetrahydrofolate reductase, deficiencies in proteins C and S, and platelet collagen receptor alpha-2-beta-1 (Cohen, 2004; Lockwood & Silver, 2004; Sibai, 2005; Simpson, 2006). Other factors that contribute to thrombosis formation in pregnancy include the normal hypercoaguable state and venous stasis.

Management

Women who have been identified as having a thrombophilia need to be counseled as to current recommendations regarding anticoagulation during pregnancy. Anticoagulation is not recommended if the woman has no history of venous thromboembolism (VTE) or poor pregnancy outcome. Full- or adjusted-dose anticoagulation with unfractionated heparin (UFH), or low-molecular-weight heparin (LMWH), is recommended antenatally and 6 weeks postpartum for women who have antithrombin deficiency, homozygosity for the Factor V Leiden mutation, the prothrombin gene 20210A mutation, compound heterozygosity for both mutations, or a current VTE. The same is recommended antenatally and long term for women receiving Vitamin K antagonist therapy (Bates, Greer, Hirsh, & Ginsberg, 2004; James, Abel, & Brancazio, 2006). Women with a history of antiphospholipid antibody syndrome with a previous thrombosis (history of two or more early pregnancy losses, one or more late loss, IUGR, abruption, or preeclampsia) are offered antepartum a low dose of aspirin, a mini-moderate dose of UFH, or prophylactic LMWH. Women who have a history of a single episode of VTE and thrombophilia or a strong family history of thrombosis may receive intermediate dose LMWH, or mini-moderate dose of UFH antepartum followed with postpartum anticoagulants. For those women who have been diagnosed with APLA syndrome without a VTE or pregnancy loss surveillance, minidose UFH, prophylactic LMWH, or low-dose aspirin are recommended (Bates, Greer, Hirsh, & Ginsberg, 2004).

LMWH has fewer side effects and a longer half-life than UFH. Because of the longer half-life, women may not be able to receive regional anesthesia; many women are switched to UFH during the latter part of the third trimester. Controversy exists regarding whether to screen all women for thrombophilias or only those with poor pregnancy outcomes or preeclampsia. Until more research is done, current recommendations do not include universal screening or screening for all women with a history of preeclampsia (Robertson et al., 2006; Sibai, 2005). Individual screening is done based on the woman's history and current pregnancy.

UFH is associated with the development of osteoporosis and a 2% risk of vertebral fracture, as well as heparin-induced thrombocytopenia (HIT). LMWHs are actually fragments of UFH, which have more activity against factor Xa. There is a lower risk of developing osteoporosis and HIT (James, Abel, & Brancazio, 2006). However LMWH is very expensive, and the longer half-life increases the risk of bleeding in the intrapartum period. Neither UFH nor LMWH crosses the placenta.

Fetal surveillance may be beneficial. Serial ultrasounds for growth, and twice-weekly nonstress tests or biophysical profiles can be instituted at 24 to 25 weeks gestation. The mother can be monitored closely for the development of preeclampsia.

Maternal Trauma

The perinatal nurse may encounter pregnant women who have experienced trauma as they may be directly admitted to the labor and delivery unit or to an obstetric triage unit. In most institutions, women with major trauma are stabilized in the emergency department with the assistance of perinatal healthcare providers who are called to the department for consultation, whereas women with minor trauma may be sent directly to the labor and delivery unit. The focus of this discussion is women who present with seemingly minor or non–life-threatening trauma. A thorough knowledge of the normal physiologic changes during pregnancy, complications of bleeding and preterm labor, and maternal–fetal assessment is necessary to provide optimum care for pregnant women after trauma.

Approximately 5% to 8% of women experience trauma during pregnancy (ACOG, 1998; Mattox & Goetzl, 2005). Approximately two-thirds of all trauma events during pregnancy are the result of motor vehicle accidents. Motor vehicle accidents are the most significant cause of fetal death due to trauma (ACOG; Mattox & Goetzl). The incidence and severity of injuries can be reduced by appropriate use of automobile safety restraints, but only 46% of pregnant women use safety restraints while driving or riding as a passenger in a car (Mattox & Goetzl). Other significant causes of trauma during pregnancy are falls and direct assaults to the abdomen. Domestic violence is becoming an increasing source of trauma during pregnancy. Data about incidence of domestic violence have been difficult to accumulate because of reporting issues and the frequency of inaccurate description of the causative factors for injury given by the woman. Various sources cite rates of domestic violence ranging between 1% and 30% of pregnant women (ACOG; Mattox & Goetzl). The CDC estimates that up to 300,000 pregnant women in the United States each year are victims of domestic violence (Jones, 2000). Fetal loss resulting from blunt abdominal trauma may occur because of abruptio placentae or other placenta injury, direct fetal injury, uterine rupture, maternal shock, maternal death, or a combination of these events (ACOG).

Nursing assessment and interventions for the pregnant woman who has experienced trauma are based on the clinical situation and maternal–fetal status. A thorough history is essential and should include the nature of the trauma event, condition and symptoms at time of injury, and current clinical symptoms. The principles of management of preterm labor and complications of bleeding are applied based on the clinical situation. Ongoing maternal–fetal assessments and accurate reporting of findings to the primary healthcare provider are important.

Fortunately, most women who experience trauma suffer only minor injures that would not require inpatient evaluation for the nonpregnant population. However, approximately 5% to 25% of women who experience minor trauma have an adverse maternal or fetal outcome (Curet, Shermer, Demarest, Bieneik, & Curet, 2000; El Kady, Gilbert, Anderson, Danielsen, Towner, & Smith, 2004). Up to 50% of fetal losses and other adverse fetal outcomes related to trauma occur in women with seemingly minor or nonsignificant injuries (ACOG, 1998; El Kady, Gilbert, Anderson, Danielsen, & Smith, 2004). Careful evaluation of maternal–fetal status is warranted when pregnant women present with reports of any type of trauma. Reliability of methods to predict which women are at risk for adverse outcomes remains low. Recent retrospective data demonstrate that a positive Kleihauer–Betke (KB) test (the presence of fetal red blood cells in the maternal circulation indicating that a fetomaternal or transplacental hemorrhage has occurred) predicts preterm labor and adverse outcomes better than clinical assessment (Muench et al., 2004). The usual signs of complications, including bleeding, uterine tenderness, contractions, and loss of amniotic fluid, are valuable, but they may not be present in all cases (Curet, et al., 2000; Muench et al.). Use of ultrasound to exclude abruptio placentae has the potential to miss 50% of cases (Reis, Sander, & Pearlman, 2000). Continuous electronic fetal monitoring (EFM) is useful for ongoing evaluation of fetal status and uterine activity. Recommended duration of continuous EFM after trauma ranges from 6 hours to 24 hours based on clinical signs and symptoms and the mechanism of injury (ACOG, 1998; Curet, et al., Mattox & Goetzl, 2005). Monitoring should be continued, and further evaluation is warranted if uterine contractions, a non-reassuring FHR pattern, vaginal bleeding, significant uterine tenderness or irritability, serious maternal injury, or rupture of the membranes occurs (ACOG, 1998, Mattox & Goetzl). Women with a positive KB test may benefit greatly from continuous electronic fetal heart monitoring (EFM) and assessment of serial KB testing every 6 to 12 hours to determine if the KB value is falling. If the KB value decreases and EFM is reassuring, the woman may be evaluated for discharge. Rh immune globulin may need to be administered dependent on the results of the KB test in an Rh-negative woman. If the KB test is negative, extended EFM is not necessary (Muench et al., 2004). The decision to continue inpatient evaluation, discharge to home, or transfer to another facility is made in collaboration with the primary healthcare provider, consistent with maternal–fetal status, and as outlined in the federal Emergency Medical Treatment and Labor Act (EMTALA).

PRETERM LABOR AND BIRTH

Significance and Incidence

Preterm birth (PTB) is any birth occurring before 37 completed weeks of gestation. The rate of preterm birth in the United States has continued to rise throughout the past 2 decades, and is currently 12.7% (Hamilton, Martin, & Ventura, 2006). These data reflect an increase of 29% since 1982, and 20% since 1990. The largest contribution to the increase was births between 34 and 36 completed weeks of gestation (Raju, Higgins, Stark, & Leveno, 2006). From 1992 to 2002, two-thirds of the increase in the rate of PTBs in the United States was in this subset of preterm infants (Davidoff et al., 2006). Although the overall rate of PTB is high, the rates are different for various racial and ethnic groups (Simhan & Bodnar, 2006). The recent Institute of Medicine (IOM) report on PTB (2006) cited "troubling and persistent disparities in PTB rates among different ethnic and racial groups" (p. 1). The highest rates of PTB are in non-Hispanic blacks (18.4%). Other racial and ethnic groups have lower rates, but all are still unacceptably high. The rate of PTB for non-Hispanic whites is 11.7%; for American Indians, 13.7%; for Asians, 10.6%; and for Hispanics 12.1%. Preterm birth is cause for concern because it is the leading cause of neonatal mortality and morbidity in the US (Green et al., 2005), thus a problem that has attracted decades of research in an attempt to discover possible causes and cures.

The rising rates of PTB in the United States contrast with the drop in rates of infant mortality since the 1950s. In 2002, the rate of infant mortality for the United States was 7.0%; in 1950, by comparison, it was 29.2% (March of Dimes, 2005). This amazing change has occurred because of the emergence of the science of neonatal care, with more infants now living past their first birthday despite being born at earlier gestational ages. Sophisticated neonatal care has also allowed more preterm infants to survive, although for many of the smallest preterm infants, that survival is liable to come with significant morbidity, which could last throughout their lives.

It is important when discussing PTB that everyone is using the same definitions. Although they are different entities, often with separate etiologies, the terms *preterm birth* (PTB) and *low birth weight* (LBW) are commonly used interchangeably. In fact, most of the long-term follow-up studies of children and adults quoted in the literature are of very-low-birth weight (VLBW) or extremely-low-birth weight (ELBW) children, for assessment of gestational age was not common in perinatal care until recent decades. Birth weight has been, and continues to be, a simple and definitive assessment, thus easier to access. Preterm birth refers only to gestational age at birth, no matter the birth weight. A preterm birth is any birth <37 weeks. Although the term PTB is commonly used, other classifications in the literature of babies born preterm include moderately preterm (32–36 weeks), near term to late preterm (34–36 weeks), and very preterm birth (<32 weeks). Preterm infants may be, but do not have to be, low birth weight. A preterm infant born to a mother with gestational diabetes, for instance, might be of normal birth weight and yet be born preterm. The prematurity would then dictate the health problems of the infant, for lung, CNS, or gastrointestinal immaturity would pose health risks.

LBW refers only to weight at birth, no matter the gestational age. An infant is considered LBW if it is born <2,500 g (5½ pounds). VLBW is defined as birth <1,500 g (3½ pounds), and ELBW weight is <1,000 g (<2.2 pounds). LBW babies may be born before 37 weeks but can also be born at term (eg, a baby at 41 weeks gestational age could weigh 1,800 g because of IUGR). Risk factors, causes, and outcomes for LBW, growth restriction, and preterm birth are interrelated, but can cause some confusion when reading the literature.

The rates of LBW and PTB in the US are different. In 1990, the rate of LBW was 7.0%, but in 2005 the rate rose to 8.2% of all infants, an increase of 16% (Hamilton, Martin, & Ventura, 2006). Much research has been conducted on the sequellae of LBW, VLBW, and ELBW. The infants with the most mortality and morbidity are the VLBW and ELBW infants. An infant born at VLBW (<1,500 g) is at high risk for neonatal mortality (Morales et al., 2005), and, when compared with normal birthweight children, is at higher risk for learning disabilities and cognitive deficiencies during childhood (Litt, Taylor, Klein, & Hack, 2005). VLBW children followed through adulthood have been found to have poorer educational achievement, higher blood pressures, poorer respiratory function, and generally poorer physical abilities than their peers who were born at normal birth weight (Hack, 2006). ELBW infants demonstrate restricted growth patterns during their NICU stays and into their childhoods (Carroll, Slobodzian, & Steward, 2005). Morse, Wu, Ariet, Resnick, and Roth (2006) have also shown that there are racial and gender differences in the viability of ELBW infants, with females having a 1-year survival advantage, and black infants having a survival advantage over white infants. The outcomes for children followed to 8 years of age who had been extremely LBW infants (<1,000 g) are even worse. These children have been shown to have significantly more chronic health conditions and need for special services than normal birth weight infants; their health problems include more cerebral palsy, asthma, poor vision, low IQ (<85), poor academic skills, and poor motor skills (Hack et al., 2005; Mikkola et al., 2005).

The consequences of preterm labor and birth continue to devastate families, communities, and healthcare in general, with no cure in sight. Preterm birth is a serious and costly health problem, affecting 1 in 8 births in the US (Green et al., 2005). The healthcare community is concerned about all PTB, but the most costly births of all are those <32 weeks. Although they make up only about 2% of all births, they result in the most devastating consequences for infants and families (Green et al.). The costs to society in the United States alone for prematurity complications were estimated to be $26.2 billion in 2005 (IOM, 2006). In one state (California), Schmitt, Sneed and Phibbs (2006) found that LBW and VLBW infants were responsible for a high proportion of hospital costs: LBW infants accounted for 5.9% of the infants but 56.6% of total hospital costs; VLBW infants accounted for 0.9% of the infants, but 35.7% of the hospital costs. Clearly, this costly health problem requires further research in order to discover methods of prevention. Preterm infants are twice as likely to die by their first birthday and are more likely to suffer morbidity such as respiratory distress syndrome, intraventricular hemorrhage, and necrotizing enterocolitis than infants born at term (March of Dimes, 2005).

The Late Preterm Infant

Most PTBs are between 34 and 36 completed weeks of gestation (Davidoff et al., 2006) and do not represent infants with the most severe morbidities. However, these infants have their own set of physiologic and developmental problems, which have been poorly recognized because of the concentration on the dramatically severe difficulties encountered by the <32-week infants. Near term infants are now the focus of much research and intervention. In July 2005, the National Institute of Child Health and Human Development (NICHD) convened a panel of experts to discuss the definition and terminology, epidemiology, etiology, biology or maturation, clinical care, surveillance, and public health aspects of "near term" preterm birth and "near term" infants (Raju, Higgins, Stark, & Leveno, 2006). Along with the March of Dimes, ACOG, and the American Academy of Pediatrics (AAP), the Association of Women's Health, Obstetric and Neonatal Nurses (AWHONN) was an invited participant and has been one of the professional organizations leading the way to increase awareness among healthcare providers and the public and to promote better outcomes. Before the NICHD expert panel meeting, AWHONN established its "Near Term Initiative," a conceptual framework for optimizing the health of these babies (Medoff-Cooper, Bakewell-Sachs, Buus-Frank, & Santa-Donato, 2005; Santa-Donato, 2005). This ongoing program is focused on developing evidence-based practices for caring for this subset of preterm babies.

There is no consensus on the definition of near term. In the past, "marginally preterm," "moderately preterm," "minimally preterm," and "mildly preterm" have been used to describe this subset of preterm babies (Raju, et al., 2006). The NICHD expert panel proposed using a definition for babies born between 34 weeks and 0/7 days and 36 weeks and 6/7 days as "late preterm" and abandoning use of "near term" (Raju, et al.). Members of the NICHD expert panel felt that "near term" can be misleading,

conveying the impression that these babies are almost term, resulting in underestimation of risk and less diligent evaluation, monitoring, and follow-up (NICHD, 2005; Raju, et al.). Because there is no such thing as a normal preterm infant, "late preterm" conveys the vulnerability of these infants more than "near term."

AWHONN's examination of this issue has found that these infants are often overlooked in research, because they may not seem dramatically sick; they are, however, immature at birth, and have missed 4 to 6 weeks of the third trimester of gestation, making them at risk for many health problems. There is a growing body of evidence that compared to term babies, late preterm babies have more problems with temperature stability, feeding, hypoglycemia, respiratory distress, apnea/bradycardia, symptoms suggesting the need for sepsis evaluation, and clinical jaundice (Medoff-Cooper, et al., 2005; Raju, et al., 2006). They also are at greater risk for kernicterus, apnea, seizures, and rehospitalization (Raju, et al.). It is estimated that the brain size at 34 to 35 weeks of gestation is only 60% of that of a baby at term (Raju, et al.). Late preterm infants, once thought to be just lighter than full-term infants, are now known to be at higher risk for all of these morbidities, as well as infant mortality risk (Medoff-Cooper, et al.). See Display 6–16.

Because late preterm babies reflect such a large proportion of all preterm babies, even a modest increase in the PTB rate of this group can have a significant impact

DISPLAY 6-16

Adverse Outcomes Significantly Increased in Late Preterm Infants

- Respiratory distress syndrome (RDS)
- Transient tachypnea of the newborn
- Pulmonary infection
- Unspecified respiratory failure
- Recurrent apnea
- Temperature instability
- Jaundice as a cause for discharge delay
- Bilirubin-induced brain injury
- Clinical problems with one or more diagnoses
- Rehospitalization for all causes
- Rehospitalization for neonatal dehydration
- Feeding difficulties
- Long-term behavioral problems
- Periventricular leukomalacia
- Mortality

on healthcare costs. Possible causes for the increase in PTB of late preterm infants include increasing proportions of pregnant women over 35 years of age, multiple births, medically indicated births secondary to better surveillance of the mother and fetus, attempts to reduce stillbirths, stress from a variety of sources and early elective births for convenience (Raju, et al., 2006). Gilbert, Nesbitt, and Danielson (2003) estimated that eliminating nonmedically indicated (elective) births would have saved $49.9 million in just 1 year in California. Significant excess costs are associated with elective births before 37 completed weeks of gestation (Gilbert et al., 2003). Because estimations of the "due date" can often be miscalculated by up to 2 weeks to avoid iatrogenic preterm birth, ACOG and AAP recommend that gestational age of 39 completed weeks of gestation be confirmed by at least two methods before elective labor induction, repeat cesarean birth, or nonmedically indicated cesarean birth (AAP & ACOG, 2002; ACOG, 1999; National Institutes of Health, 2006). Late preterm infants are discussed in detail in Chapter 14.

Why Has the Rate of Preterm Birth Increased?

This is not an easy question to answer fully, although some things are known about the increase in preterm births. Some of the contributing factors, noted by Green et al. (2005), are the increasingly common use of infertility treatments producing twins and higher order multiples, more births to women at later ages (>35), more medically induced prematurity (including early labor inductions, now occurring in 20.6% of pregnancies, representing more than a doubled rate since 1990 [Martin et al., 2005], early repeat cesarean births, primary cesarean births without a medical indication), advances in maternal and fetal medicine and neonatal care (which lead providers and patients both to believe that birth at earlier gestations is not an insurmountable health hazard), more pregnancies in very-high-risk women who then require early birth, and an increase in fetal complications leading to early birth such as intrauterine growth restriction.

The issue of PTB of multiples and higher order multiples is particularly problematic. The twin birth rate in 2003 was 31.5 twins per 1,000 live births, a record high. About 55% of twins are born preterm (Kogan et al., 2000). The rate of triplet and other higher order multiple births in 2003 was 187.4 per 100,000. That number has increased by 500% since 1980 (Martin et al., 2005). Triplets are born preterm 90% of the time, and higher order multiples have a 99% rate of preterm birth (Ventura, Martin, Curtin, Mathews, & Park, 2000). In 2002, about one of every

five neonatal deaths (birth through Day 30 of life) was a multiple birth infant. It must be remembered, however, that the rising rates of preterm birth in the United States cannot be attributed solely to the rising rates of multiple births, for the preterm rate for singletons is also rising; from 10.4 to 10.6 between 2002 and 2003. This is a 9% increase since 1990 (from 9.7) (Martin et al., 2005)

What Is Preterm Labor?

Preterm labor is defined as cervical change or effacement and uterine contractions that occur between 20 and 36 weeks of pregnancy (AAP & ACOG, 2002). Display 6–17 lists the diagnostic criteria for preterm labor according to the *Guidelines for Perinatal Care* (ACOG & AAP, 2002). Nurses should know that uterine irritability without cervical dilation or effacement is not preterm labor, for patient education about this topic is essential. A woman who has an irritable uterus might not be in actual preterm labor; dilatation or effacement is necessary for that diagnosis. However, women who report these symptoms need careful assessment and follow-up to decrease the risk of progressing to active preterm labor.

Pathophysiology

Based on what has been learned from the research over the past few decades, it is doubtful that one causative factor for preterm labor will be discovered. All indications are that preterm labor has multiple causes, including social factors, physiologic factors, medical history factors, and illness factors (Green et al., 2005). The March of Dimes has characterized preterm labor as a series of complex interactions of factors and pathways (Green et al.). Figure 6–6 illustrates the determinants of preterm labor conceptualized by Green et al.

D I S P L A Y   6 - 1 7

Criteria for Diagnosis of Preterm Labor

- 20 to 36 weeks' gestation
  and
- Documented uterine contractions
  and
- Documented cervical effacement of 80%
  or
- Cervical dilation of more than 1 cm

ACOG & AAP (2002).

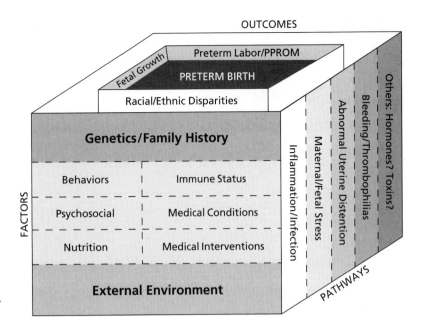

FIGURE 6–6. Determinants of preterm labor. (March of Dimes 2005.)

This conceptualization suggests that genetics, environment, stress, and psychosocial factors all play a role in the development of preterm labor leading to preterm birth. No single factor is thought to act alone, but rather to interact in as yet unknown ways to initiate the cascade of events that result in preterm labor and birth. The external environment, including personal behaviors (smoking, drug use), psychosocial factors, nutrition, immune status, medical conditions, and medical interventions interact with genetics and family history through pathways that include inflammation and infection, maternal/fetal stress, abnormal uterine distention, bleeding/thrombophilias, and other possible pathways including hormones and toxins. These factors and pathways, combined with racial and ethnic disparities, fetal growth, and preterm premature rupture of membranes finally result in preterm labor/birth. When thought of in this manner, it is clear that there is no one "cause" of preterm labor and birth, and therefore, no one single "cure." Multiple causes require research into multiple cures and preventive measures.

In fact, not all preterm births can or should be prevented. About 25% of preterm births are intentional and occur because of health problems of the mother or the fetus (eg, IUGR, preeclampsia, abruptio placentae, cardiac disease); another 25% of preterm births follow rupture of membranes (a cause not known to be preventable).

Risk Factors for Preterm Labor and Birth

Risk factors for preterm labor and birth have been published and refined since the early 1980s (IOM, 1985).

Currently, the March of Dimes (Freda & Patterson, 2004) has suggested that there are three most important known risk factors for preterm labor and birth, along with multiple categories of risk for subgroups of women. Additional risk factors include medical conditions predating the pregnancy, demographic factors, behavioral and environmental factors, illnesses occurring during the pregnancy, and genetics. These factors are listed in Displays 6–18 and 6–19.

Some of the risks have been known for decades, and some are new to the list (IOM, 1985, 2006). Knowledge of the genetics of preterm birth (see next section) is clearly a new phenomenon, as is the risk of preterm labor after the use of assisted reproductive technologies (ART), recently proposed in a study by Jackson, Gibson, & Wu, and Croughan (2004). They performed a meta-analysis of 15 studies, examining the outcomes of singletons conceived through in vitro fertilization (IVF; $n = 12,282$) compared to 1.9 million spontaneously conceived singletons. Controlling for maternal age and parity, they found significantly

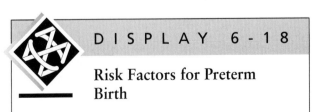

DISPLAY 6-18

Risk Factors for Preterm Birth

The three most common risk factors for preterm birth are:

- Current multifetal pregnancy
- History of a preterm birth
- Uterine/cervical abnormalities

DISPLAY   6-19

Other Possible Risk Factors for Preterm Labor

CHRONIC HEALTH PROBLEMS

- Hypertension
- Diabetes mellitus
- Clotting disorders
- Low prepregnancy weight
- Obesity

BEHAVIORAL AND ENVIRONMENTAL RISKS

- Late or no prenatal care
- Smoking
- Alcohol
- Use of illicit drugs
- DES exposure
- Domestic violence
- Lack of social support
- Stress
- Long working hours
- Long periods of standing

DEMOGRAPHIC RISKS

- Non-Hispanic black race
- <Age 17
- >Age 35
- Low socioeconomic status

GENETICS

ASSISTED REPRODUCTIVE TECHNOLOGIES

MEDICAL RISKS IN CURRENT PREGNANCY

- Infection (especially genitourinary infections)
- Short interpregnancy interval
- Fetal anomalies
- PROM
- Vaginal bleeding (especially in the second trimester or in more than one trimester)
- Periodontal disease

higher odds ratios for preterm delivery and other adverse perinatal outcomes in the singletons conceived through ART. Another risk that has received recent attention in the literature is periodontal disease (Offenbacher et al., 2006).

Clearly, the list of risk factors is lengthy. A number of these risk factors are not modifiable, but some are. Some of the current thinking in this field proposes that preconception care, or care begun before a pregnancy

has been conceived, could ameliorate some of these preexisting factors, such as smoking cessation, tight control of preexisting diabetes or hypertension, obesity, or low prepregnancy weight (ACOG, 2005b; Freda, Moos, & Curtis, 2006; Moos, 2003). The CDC held a major conference dedicated to this topic in 2005 and has published recommendations for preconception care, all aimed at reducing PTB and other poor pregnancy outcomes (Johnson et al., 2006).

Genetic Influences

In the late 1970s, when the topic of preterm labor and birth became prominent as an important entity for research and prevention, there was no thought given to the possibility that preterm labor could have a genetic component. For decades, diligent researchers in medicine, epidemiology, public health, and nursing have focused on physical symptoms, biologic pathways, and social interventions in their efforts to prevent this costly and dangerous complication of pregnancy. It was not until 2003 that the Director of the National Human Genome Research Institute at the National Institutes of Health announced that the sequencing of the human genome had been completed (Lewis, 2006). This event ushered in the genomic era of health research and has impacted the study of preterm birth in extraordinary ways. What we once thought of as strictly a social phenomenon, or a biological accident, might actually have a genetic component that could hold promise for exciting new interventions unheard of previously in history.

The possibility that preterm labor and birth has a genetic component provides us with new targets for prevention. For instance, Wang (2002) has found that infant birth weight is particularly vulnerable in women who smoke and possess a certain gene polymorphism. This could be the answer for why some women smoke during pregnancy and give birth to normal weight babies at term, and others who smoke have preterm, small babies who are at risk for more health problems. For nurses, this is truly important information, for although we would like all pregnant women to stop smoking, it could be possible to address aggressive interventions toward the smokers who possess this particular polymorphism, therefore saving those mothers and infants from the devastation of IUGR. This is just one of the many ways that genetics could transform the way we look at preterm birth.

It has been known for some time that women who were themselves born preterm have a higher chance of having preterm labors and births themselves (Porter, Fraser, Hunter, Ward, & Varner, 1997; Ward, 2003). Ward, Argyle, Meade, and Nelson (2005) have recently confirmed these data. Is it possible that these women and their sisters and mothers have a genetic predisposition toward preterm birth? If so, can it be altered? More genetic research on this topic may answer these questions.

Genetic polymorphisms have been implicated in PTB (Kalish, Vardhana, Normand, Gupta, & Witkin, 2006). Giarratano (2006) has described the effect of genetics on preterm birth, and has provided information about the genes that could possibly be implicated in preterm labor and birth. These data are reproduced here as Tables 6–11 through 6–13. These genes are the pro-inflammatory cytokines (involved in possible infection and preterm premature rupture of membranes), the labor cascade genes (being studied for their role in the initiation of labor), and the vasculopathic genes (involved in vascular problems such as preeclampsia and thrombophilas). None of these genetic studies has reached maturity, thereby making causality or interventions impossible, but they have given researchers entirely new areas in which to discover more information about how preterm labor begins, and how, possibly, to avoid it.

Risk Factors as Screening Methods to Predict Preterm Labor and Birth

Because there is as yet no known single causative factor for preterm labor, and the risk factors are numerous, and about 50% of all PTBs occurs in women with no known risk factors (Goldenberg & Rouse, 1998), it is necessary to conclude that all pregnant women are at risk for preterm labor and birth. Many studies in the 1980s and 1990s attempted to use risk-screening tools to discover the women at risk for PTB, but none of those studies produced a drop in the rate of PTB (Collaborative Group on Preterm Birth Prevention, 1993; Herron, Katz, & Creasy, 1982).

It is essential that PTB prevention efforts be directed at all pregnant women. Although specialized care for women with many risk factors may be effective in helping the small subset of women with identified risk factors to give birth closer to term, it is clear that a problem as pervasive as preterm labor and birth must be explained to all pregnant women during routine prenatal care (ie, education about signs and symptoms

TABLE 6–11 ■ PRO-INFLAMMATORY CYTOKINES

Candidate Genes	Symbol	Polymorphisms	Role of Candidate Gene in Preterm Labor and Delivery	Speculated Impact of the Polymorphism
Interleukin 6	IL-6	G-174C Other SNPs: C/C G/G G/C	Critical in the cascade of host response; activates the acute phase response, stimulates T lymphocytes, induces differentiation of B lymphocytes; increases seen in gestational tissues in PTL.	Women with C/C variation produce less IL-6 and are less likely to manifest the inflamatory cascade leading to PTL. C/C variation lacking in African-American women in PTB cases <34 weeks.
Interleukin 1 beta	IL-1β	IL-1β+3953*1 IL 1RN*2	A key pro-inflammatory cytokine correlated to prostaglandin production and increased uterine activity. Found in membranes in PTL.	Fetal carriage of these variations possibly increases the IL-1β cytokine production and risk for PTB.
Tumor Necrosis Factor-α Promotor Gene	TNF-α	G-308A (TNFA2 or Allele 2)	Pro-inflammatory cytokine. Elevated in the amniotic fluid of women experiencing preterm labor, PPROM, and positive amniotic fluid cultures.	TNFA2 allele causes elevated levels of TNF-α protein, leading to immune hyperresponsiveness to environmental factors, such as bacterial vaginosis, causing chorioamnionitis.

From Giarratano G. (2006). Genetics influences on preterm birth. MCN *The American Journal of Maternal Child Nursing*, 31(3),169–175.

TABLE 6–12 ■ LABOR CASCADE PATHWAYS

Candidate Genes	Symbol	Polymorphisms	Role of Candidate Gene in Preterm Labor and Delivery	Speculated Impact of the Polymorphism
Oxytocin Receptors	OTRs	OTR Allele1; OTR Allele 2 (Allele 2 has a 30 base pair C-A repeat)	In normal labor onset, OTRs are thought to increase myometrial sensitivity to oxytocin before labor onset. The binding of oxytocin to the myometrial receptor promotes the influx of calcium from the intracellular stores, as one pathway to activate contractions.	No published studies regarding this specific polymorphism. Continued study occurs to explore how the "normal" pathways of labor probably differ in cases of PTL and PPROM, with subsequent labor.
Corticotropin-Releasing Hormone	CRH	T255G Other SNPs: T/T T/G G/G	CRH is synthesized in the hypothalamus in response to stress, and in the placenta and membranes in pregnancy. CRH metabolic pathway promotes production of prostaglandins and PTL onset.	Research related to PTB in progress; in an obesity study, T/G variation in combination with a glucocorticoid polymorphism, increased cortisiol levels.

From Giarratano G. (2006). Genetics influences on preterm birth. MCN *The American Journal of Maternal Child Nursing, 31*(3), 169–175.

TABLE 6–13 ■ VASCULOPATHIC PATHWAYS

Candidate Genes	Symbol	Polymorphisms	Role of Candidate Gene in Preterm Labor and Delivery	Speculated Impact of the Polymorphism
Vascular Endothelial Growth Factor	VEGF	C936T Other SNP: T/T	VEGF is a major angiogenic factor and regulates endothelial cell proliferation. Threshold levels are required for fetal and placental vascular development and inhibition of cell death in the placenta.	C936T is associated with lower VEGF production; an association was found between this variation and an increased risk of spontaneous PTB.
		C677T A1298C	An abnormal vascular network is hypothesized to predispose to spontaneous abortion, or early labor and delivery.	
Methylenetra-hydrofolate reductase (enzyme)	MTHFR	Risks results from a Vitamin B-12 deficiency, plus mutation	Elevates homocysteine; a risk factor associated with many vascular disorders in adults. In pregnancy, associated with uteroplacental vasculopathy, such as thrombosis and placental infarcts, seen with PTB.	Both mutations associated with decreased MTHFR activity, which increases homocysteine concentrations, particularly with low folate. Association of this mutation with PTB is unknown.

From Giarratano G. (2006). Genetics influences on preterm birth. MCN *The American Journal of Maternal Child Nursing, 31*(3), 169–175.

of preterm labor and what to do should they occur) in order to make sure that women who have any symptoms of early labor tell their healthcare providers immediately.

Can Preterm Labor and Birth Be Prevented?

The search for prevention of preterm birth has been ongoing for decades. It would be comforting to think that simple strategies such as obtaining prenatal care could prevent preterm birth, but studies have not shown that to be true (Lu, Tache, Alexander, Kotelchuck, & Halfon, 2003). Although prenatal care is important as a healthcare strategy for all pregnant women, it is not a prevention method for PTB. At this point in time, no prevention strategy for all women has been discovered. In lieu of that, many studies have examined smaller scale prevention efforts aimed at specific subgroups of at-risk women. Other interventions, which previously had been thought to be preventive, follow.

Home Uterine Activity Monitoring

Home uterine activity monitoring (HUAM) is a system of care to detect preterm labor using a combination of recording of uterine activity with a tocodynamometer and daily telephone calls from a healthcare provider (usually a perinatal nurse) to offer the woman support and advice (ACOG, 2001, 2003a). The recording of uterine activity is transferred to the healthcare provider by telephone for rapid evaluation. The premise of HUAM is that women have an identifiable increase in uterine contractions before the onset of overt preterm labor and that pregnant women do not usually recognize these early contractions (ACOG, 1996).

For several decades it was thought that HUAM would be able to prevent preterm birth, but prospective studies were never able to confirm that premise (ACOG, 2001; Brown et al., 1999; Dyson et al., 1998). One randomized study found that women who were helped by HUAM received more benefit from the nursing telephone support they received than from the machine (Iams, Johnson, O'Shaughnessy, & West, 1987). Based on published research about efficacy, ACOG (2001, 2003a) has not recommended the use of HUAM for singleton or multiple pregnancies. According to ACOG (1996, 2001, 2003a), it has not been demonstrated that HUAM can affect the rate of preterm birth, and the use of this expensive system and subsequent treatment has the potential for substantially increasing costs.

Bed Rest

According to Maloni, Alexander, Schluchter, Shah, and Park (2004), about 700,000 women each year are placed on antepartum bed rest for risk for preterm birth. This is the most commonly ordered intervention, despite the fact that there is no evidence to support its effectiveness in actually preventing preterm birth (Maloni et al., 1993; Goldenberg & Rouse, 1998). Maloni et al. found that after only 3 days of bed rest muscle tone decreases, calcium is lost, and glucose intolerance develops. A recent study measured loss of gastrocnemius muscle tone in women on antepartum bed rest, the symptoms of which continued into the postpartum period (Maloni & Schneider, 2002). After longer periods of bed rest, women experience bone demineralization, constipation, fatigue, anxiety, and depression (Maloni et al.). Dysphoria, or negative affect, has been described in women placed on bed rest as well (Maloni, Kane, Suen, & Wang, 2002).

Bed rest may cause more harm than therapeutic benefit. Maloni et al. (2004) have described significant maternal weight loss in mothers on antepartum bed rest, as well as lower infant birth weights across all gestational ages. Goldenberg et al. (1994) showed a decade ago that bed rest had a major financial impact for families and for society in lost wages, household help expenses, and hospital costs. In addition, women who have been on bed rest suffer substantial physical and emotional symptoms during the bed rest period and after the infant's birth, including fatigue, mood changes, difficulty concentrating, back soreness, dry skin, and headaches (Maloni & Park, 2005). According to the latest review in the *Cochrane Database of Systematic Reviews*, due to the potential adverse effects of bed rest for women and their families, and the increased healthcare costs, clinicians should not routinely advise women at risk of preterm birth to rest in bed (Sosa, Althabe, Belizan, & Bergel, 2004). Despite all the literature describing the harmful effects of bed rest, it is still ordered frequently for women at risk for preterm birth. Display 6–20 describes nursing care measures for women prescribed bed rest during pregnancy.

Intravenous Hydration

One common strategy used in the inpatient setting to reduce preterm contractions is intravenous hydration. Significant amounts of intravenous fluids are usually administered to increase vascular volume and because, anecdotally, it is thought that uterine contractions are quieted by hydration. There has been no evidence found that hydration indeed can avert a preterm birth (Freda & DeVore, 1996; Lu, Tache, Alexander, Kotelchuck, & Halfon, 2003). Similar to bed rest therapy, however, intravenous fluid therapy is a traditional treatment that continues to be used. This therapy is not without side effects. Nurses should be cautious when administering intravenous fluids for this purpose, because if uterine activity continues, the next treatment could be intravenous administration of tocolytic agents, which carry a possible side effect of pulmonary edema. Careful

DISPLAY 6-20

Nursing Care for Women Prescribed Bed Rest as Therapy

- Assist the family in becoming involved in the nursing care plan.
- If the family is not available, suggest that the woman ask friends for help during this time.
- Maintaining hydration while on bed rest is important; suggest that a cooler be kept by the bed.
- Bed rest can lead to muscle wasting; teach passive limb exercises.
- Anxiety and depression are common during bed rest; teach the family to expect this and talk about their feelings.
- The woman should be in a place where she can interact with her family rather than in a bedroom alone.
- Instruct the woman not to do any nipple preparation for breastfeeding; nipple stimulation can cause uterine contractions.
- Some women find that keeping a journal helps them deal with the isolation and boredom of bed rest.
- Household jobs that can be done while in bed (eg, paying bills, mending, folding laundry) help the woman feel more a part of the family.
- This is a good time to provide short educational videotapes about all aspects of pregnancy, labor, birth, and parenting.
- A laptop computer with Internet access can help the woman keep in touch with friends and can be educational.
- Encourage the woman to develop a support system of people with whom she can talk and vent her feelings.

attention to intake and output and auscultation of the lungs are essential to monitor for the development of pulmonary edema.

According to the latest review in the *Cochrane Database of Systematic Reviews*, available data do not support any advantage of hydration as a treatment for women who present in preterm labor, although hydration may be beneficial for women with evidence of dehydration (Stan, Boulvain, Hirsbrunner-Amagbaly, & Pfister, 2002). Based on the preponderance of the evidence, therefore, according to ACOG (2003a) bed rest, hydration, and pelvic rest do not appear to improve the rate of preterm birth, and should not be routinely recommended.

Prophylactic Antibiotics and Cervical Cerclage

Both prophylactic antibiotics and placement of a cervical cerclage have been studied, and no evidence exists that they can prevent preterm birth (ACOG, 2003a; Lu, Tache, Alexander, Kotelchuck, & Halfon, 2003), although they are still used by some providers. ACOG recommends that following protocols for preventions of early onset perinatal Group B streptococcus (ACOG, 2002b) recommended by the CDC (Schrag, et al., 2002) is the best use of antibiotic therapy in women with preterm labor, for it can prevent infection in the newborn. These recommendations were reaffirmed by ACOG in 2005. Figure 6–7 presents the CDC (Schrag, et al.) recommendations for intrapartum antibiotic prophylaxis to prevent perinatal Group B streptococcal disease under a universal prenatal screening strategy based on combined vaginal and rectal cultures collected at 35 to 37 weeks of gestation from all pregnant women. Table 6–14 presents the CDC (Schrag, et al.) recommended regimens for intrapartum antimicrobial prophylaxis for perinatal Group B streptococcal disease prevention. Figure 6–8 presents a sample algorithm for Group B streptococci (GBS) prophylaxis for women with threatened preterm birth based on the CDC (Schrag, et al.) recommendations. Care of the baby exposed to GBS is presented in Chapter 14.

Progesterone

Recently, the use of progesterone for women at risk of preterm birth has been studied as a preventive measure. Meis et al. (2003) published the first randomized clinical trial of weekly injections of 250 mg of 17-alpha-hydroxyprogesterone (generally referred to in the literature as "17P"), starting at 16 to 20 weeks of gestation for prevention of PTB, and found that the group receiving 17P had significantly fewer preterm births. Although Meis et al.'s results were favorable for a selected high-risk population, according to ACOG (2003b), further research is needed because unresolved issues remain such as the optimal route of medication delivery and long-term safety of the medication. More recently, Spong et al. (2005) found that progesterone given to women who had previously given birth at <34 weeks was associated with a prolonged gestation in a subsequent pregnancy. A recent review of prenatal administration of progesterone for preventing preterm birth from the *Cochrane Database of Systematic Reviews* (Dodd, Flenady, Cincotta, & Crowther, 2006) had similar conclusions as ACOG (2003b) regarding the use of 17P for PTB prevention.

Other important maternal and fetal outcomes have been poorly reported; it is unclear if the prolongation of gestation translates into improved maternal and longer term infant health outcomes (Dodd, Crowther, Dare, & Middleton, 2006). Petrini et al. (2005) have estimated the potential reduction in PTB rate if all eligible women received progesterone. They found that progesterone could reduce PTB among eligible women, but even if it were given to all women at risk

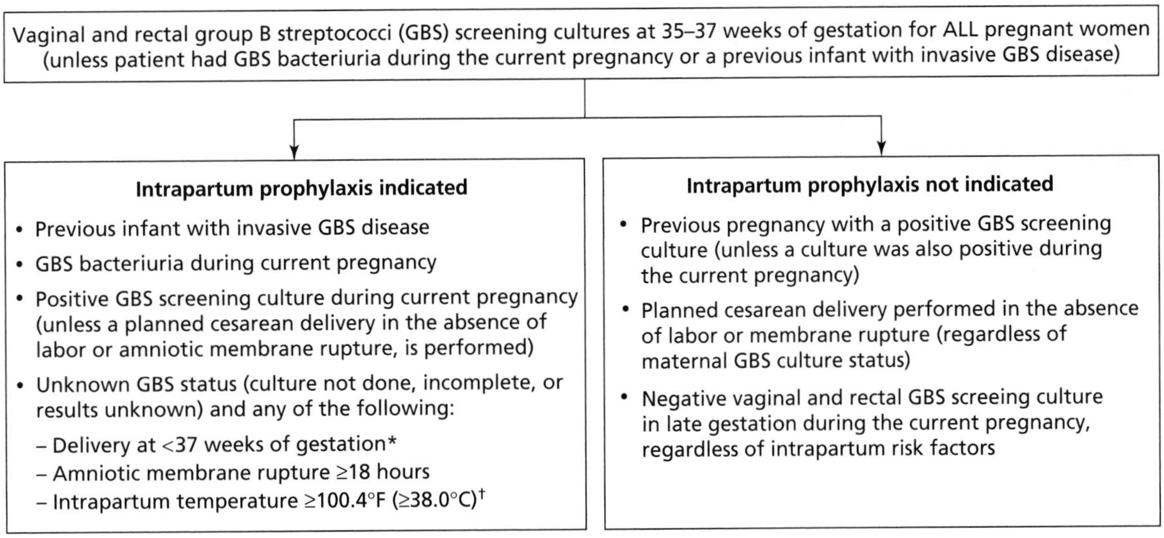

Vaginal and rectal group B streptococci (GBS) screening cultures at 35–37 weeks of gestation for ALL pregnant women (unless patient had GBS bacteriuria during the current pregnancy or a previous infant with invasive GBS disease)

Intrapartum prophylaxis indicated

- Previous infant with invasive GBS disease
- GBS bacteriuria during current pregnancy
- Positive GBS screening culture during current pregnancy (unless a planned cesarean delivery in the absence of labor or amniotic membrane rupture, is performed)
- Unknown GBS status (culture not done, incomplete, or results unknown) and any of the following:
  – Delivery at <37 weeks of gestation*
  – Amniotic membrane rupture ≥18 hours
  – Intrapartum temperature ≥100.4°F (≥38.0°C)[†]

Intrapartum prophylaxis not indicated

- Previous pregnancy with a positive GBS screening culture (unless a culture was also positive during the current pregnancy)
- Planned cesarean delivery performed in the absence of labor or membrane rupture (regardless of maternal GBS culture status)
- Negative vaginal and rectal GBS screeing culture in late gestation during the current pregnancy, regardless of intrapartum risk factors

*If onset of labor or rupture of amniotic membranes occurs at <37 weeks' gestation and there is a significant risk for preterm birth (as assessed by the clinician), follow the suggested algorithm for GBS prophylaxis as indicated by the CDC.
[†]If amnionitis is suspected, broad-spectrum antibiotic therapy that includes an agent known to be active against GBS should replace GBS prophylaxis.

FIGURE 6–7. Indications for intrapartum antibiotic prophylaxis to prevent perinatal group B streptococcal disease under a universal prenatal screening strategy based on combined vaginal and rectal cultures collected at 35–37 weeks of gestation from all pregnant women.

for preterm birth it would only have a modest effect (potentially a 2% decrease) on the national rate of PTB (Petrini et al.). Further study about the long-term effects of progesterone on both the mother and the baby and its usefulness in preventing PTB in other populations such as women with multiple gestations are needed before this therapy can be used routinely for women at risk for PTB.

TABLE 6–14 ■ RECOMMENDED REGIMENS FOR INTRAPARTUM ANTIMICROBIAL PROPHYLAXIS FOR PERINATAL GROUP B STREPTOCOCCAL DISEASE PREVENTION

Regimens	Antimicrobial
Recommended	Penicillin G, 5 million units IV initial dose, then 2.5 million units IV every 4 hr until birth
Alternative	Ampicillin, 2 g IV initial dose, then 1 g IV every 4 hr until birth
If penicillin allergic[†]	
• Patients not at high risk for anaphylaxis	Cefazolin, 2 g IV initial dose, then 1 g IV every 8 hr until birth
• Patients at high risk for anaphylaxis[‡]	
• GBS susceptible to clindamycin and erythromycin[§]	Clindamycin, 900 mg IV every 8 hr until birth OR Erythromycin, 500 mg IV every 6 hr until birth
• GBS resistant to clindamycin or erythromycin or susceptibility unknown	Vancomycin,[‖] 1 g IV every 12 hr until birth

GBS, group B streptococci; IV, intravenously.
*Broader-spectrum agents, including an agent active against GBS, may be necessary for treatment of chorioamnionitis.
[†]History of penicillin allergy should be assessed to determine whether a high risk for anaphylaxis is present. Penicillin-allergic patients at high risk for anaphylaxis are those who have experienced immediate hypersensitivity to penicillin including a history of penicillin-related anaphylaxis; other high-risk patients are those with asthma or other diseases that would make anaphylaxis more dangerous or difficult to treat, such as persons being treated with beta-adrenergic-blocking agents.
[‡]If laboratory facilities are adequate, clindamycin and erythromycin susceptibility testing should be performed on prenatal GBS isolates from penicillin-allergic women at high risk for anaphylaxis.
[§]Resistance to erythromycin often but not always is associated with clindamycin resistance. If a strain is resistant to erythromycin but appears susceptible to clindamycin, it may still have inducible resistance to clindamycin.
[‖]Cefazolin is preferred over vancomycin for women with a history of penicillin allergy other than immediate hypersensitivity reactions, and pharmacologic data suggest it achieves effective intraamniotic concentrations. Vancomycin should be reserved for penicillin-allergic women at high risk for anaphylaxis.
From Schrag, S., Gorwitz, R., Fultz-Butts, K., & Schuchat, A. (2002). Prevention of perinatal group B streptococcal disease: Revised guidelines from the CDC. *Morbidity and Mortality Weekly Report, 51*(RR11), 1–22.

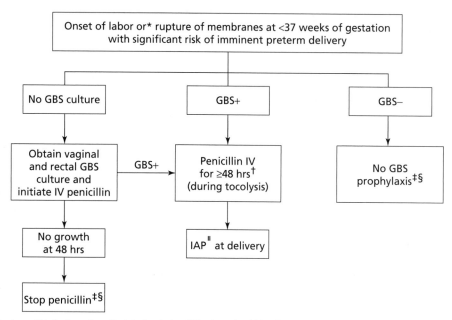

*If a hospital chooses to give antibiotics to prolong the latent period, a GBS culture should be obtained before initiating therapy and the results used to guide intrapartum management.

†Penicillin should be continued for a total of at least 48 hours, unless birth occurs sooner. At the physician's discretion, antibiotic prophylaxis may be continued beyond 48 hours in a GBS culture-positive woman if birth has not yet occurred. For women who are GBS culture positive, antibiotic prophylaxis should be reinitiated when labor likely to proceed to birth occurs or recurs.

‡If antibiotics are used to prolong the latent period, GBS cultures should be obtained prior to initiating therapy and the results used to guide intrapartum management.

§If birth has not occurred within 4 weeks, a vaginal and rectal GBS screening culture should be repeated and the patient should be managed as described, based on the result of the repeat culture.

‖Intrapartum antibiotic prophylaxis.

FIGURE 6–8. Sample algorithm for group B streptococci (GBS) prophylaxis for women with threatened preterm birth. (Adapted from Schrag, S., Gorwitz, R., Fult-Butts, K., et al. (2002). Prevention of perinatal group B streptococcal disease: revised guidelines from the CDC. *Mortality and Mortality Weekly Report, 51* (RR11), 1–22.)

Biochemical Fetal Markers

The search for early predictive factors for preterm labor and birth has included the use of biochemical markers, most notably fetal fibronectin. The US Food and Drug Administration (FDA) approved fetal fibronectin testing for preterm labor in 1995. Fetal fibronectin is an extracellular matrix glycoprotein produced in the decidual cells of the uterus (Moore, 1999). Fetal fibronectin is thought to be the trophoblastic "glue" in the formation of the uteroplacental junction. It is normally absent from vaginal secretions from 24 to 36 weeks of pregnancy. Lockwood et al. (1991) first published a study suggesting that fetal fibronectin found in vaginal secretions between 24 weeks and 34 weeks at a level greater than 50 ng/mL is a predictor of preterm labor.

It has been theorized that preterm labor breaks the bonds between the placenta and the amniotic membranes, causing a release of fetal fibronectin into the vaginal secretions. Several factors may affect the accuracy of the results of fetal fibronectin testing, however. These factors include sexual activity within 24 hours of sample collection, cervical examination within 24 hours of sample collection, vaginal bleeding, intra-amniotic and vaginal infections, and use of douches (Moore, 1999).

The discovery of this marker was initially met by much enthusiasm by the healthcare community because it fueled speculation that preterm labor could be prevented by testing women for the presence of it (ie, if present, the woman would probably give birth prematurely). Further study has shown, however, that the negative predictive value of the test is high (up to 95%), whereas the positive predictive value is low (25% to 40%). This means that the test may be most effective in predicting who will not experience preterm labor rather than who will experience it. Fetal fibronectin testing might be most useful in determining which women will not go into preterm labor within a few days, thus assisting women especially in rural areas without easy access to tertiary facilities.

Swamy, Simhan, Gammill, and Heine (2005) implemented a clinical protocol using the rapid fetal fibronectin test for women who presented with symptoms of preterm labor, and looked at pregnancy outcome. They found that a positive fetal fibronectin test was predictive of preterm birth for about 30% of women, and a negative test was predictive of no preterm labor in 98% of cases. Thus the test could be used to avoid unnecessary interventions (such as tocolysis, bed rest) in women who were not ultimately going to give birth preterm. Other researchers found that rapid fetal fibronectin testing may offer more cost savings when compared with treatment of all women with threatened preterm labor and may prevent similar numbers of cases of respiratory distress syndrome and neonatal deaths (Mozurkewich, Naglie, Krahn, & Hayashi, 2000). More data are needed about screening for preterm labor using biochemical markers before widespread use can be recommended.

Cervical Length Measurements

Measuring cervical length has been thought to be predictive of preterm birth, for in some populations it has been shown that a short cervical length can be a precursor to preterm labor. A cervical length of less than 30 mm as measured by ultrasound seems to predict some instances of preterm labor (Hartmann, Thorp, McDonald, Savita, & Granados, 1999; Tsoi, Fuchs, Rane, Geerts, Nicolaides, 2005; Yost, Bloom, Twicker, & Leveno, 1999). Schmitz et al. (2006) have found that among 359 women, the positive predictive value of cervical length measurement for preterm birth was 24%, and for positive fetal fibronectin testing was 33%. The positive predictive value of fetal fibronectin testing after a finding of shortened cervix was 36%, not significantly different from fetal fibronectin testing without measuring cervical length. Although cervical length assessment may give us some information about possible risk for preterm labor, simply knowing the cervical length does nothing to either prevent preterm labor or assist us in intervening in any meaningful way once this determination has been made.

Tocolytics

Although once thought of as the "magic bullet" for prevention of preterm birth, tocolytic drugs used to inhibit uterine contractions are now more commonly thought to be most useful in order to delay birth 24 to 48 hours, thus providing the time to allow antenatal glucocorticoids to help mature fetal lungs (ACOG, 2003a; Goldenberg & Rouse, 1998). According to ACOG (2003a) neither maintenance treatment with tocolytic drugs nor repeated acute tocolysis improves perinatal outcome; neither should be undertaken as a general practice.

Several classes of drugs have been used in an effort to stop preterm labor, although none has been shown to be effective for more than 24 to 48 hours (Goldenberg & Rouse, 1998; Sciscione et al., 1998). There are conflicting results among beta-mimetics, magnesium sulfate, calcium channel blockers, and nonsteroidal anti-inflammatory drugs (NSAIDs); all have demonstrated only limited benefit, hence there is not one first-line drug (ACOG, 2003a). If a tocolytic drug is used to stop preterm contractions, the choice of that drug can only be made based on the individual woman and her health status at the time. All of the drugs used for tocolysis have major side effects for the mother or the fetus and should only be used with extreme care. Displays 6–21, 6–22, and 6–23 describe contraindications to tocolytic therapy, complications that can arise when tocolytics are used, and nursing care for women undergoing tocolytic therapy.

Careful, expert nursing care is essential for all women who receive tocolytic therapy. In 1997 and

---

DISPLAY 6-21

Contraindications to Tocolysis for Preterm Labor

GENERAL CONTRAINDICATIONS*

- Acute fetal distress (except intrauterine resuscitation)
- Intraamniotic infection
- Eclampsia or severe preeclampsia
- Fetal demise (singleton)
- Fetal maturity
- Maternal hemodynamic instability

CONTRAINDICATIONS FOR SPECIFIC TOCOLYTIC AGENTS

Beta-mimetic Agents

- Maternal cardiac rhythm disturbance or other cardiac disease

- Poorly controlled diabetes, thyrotoxicosis, or hypertension

Magnesium Sulfate

- Hypocalcemia
- Myasthenia gravis
- Renal failure

Indomethacin

- Asthma
- Coronary artery disease
- Gastrointestinal bleeding (current or past)
- Oligohydramnios
- Renal failure
- Suspected fetal cardiac or renal anomaly
- Nifedipine
- Maternal liver disease

---

*Relative and absolute contraindications to tocolysis are based on the clinical circumstances and should take into account the risks of continuing the pregnancy versus those of birth.

From American College of Obstetricians and Gynecologists. (2003). *Management of preterm labor* (Practice Bulletin No. 43). Washington, DC: Author.

DISPLAY 6-22

Potential Complications of Tocolytic Agents

BETA-ADRENERGIC AGENTS

- Hyperglycemia
- Hypokalemia
- Hypotension
- Pulmonary edema
- Cardiac insufficiency
- Arrhythmias
- Myocardial ischemia
- Maternal death
- Fetal cardiac effects

MAGNESIUM SULFATE

- Maternal lethargy
- Drowsiness

- Double vision
- Nausea
- Vomiting
- Pulmonary edema
- Respiratory depression*
- Cardiac arrest*
- Maternal tetany*
- Profound muscular paralysis*
- Profound hypotension*

INDOMETHACIN

- Hepatitis[†]
- Renal failure[†]
- Gastrointestinal bleeding[†]
- Nifedipine
- Transient hypotension
- Premature closure of fetal ductus arteriosus

*Effect is rare and seen with toxic levels.
[†] Effect is rare and associated with chronic use.
From American College of Obstetricians and Gynecologists. (2003). *Management of preterm labor* (Practice Bulletin No. 43). Washington, DC: Author.

1998, the FDA issued warnings to healthcare providers about the potential risks of using terbutaline pumps to prevent preterm birth, citing one related maternal death and lack of evidence for clinical efficacy (Nightingale, 1998). In October 2005 and June 2006, the Institute for Safe Medication Practices (ISMP) issued Medication Safety Alerts *Preventing Magne-*

sium Toxicity in Obstetrics. Numerous cases of magnesium overdoses that resulted in maternal respiratory arrest have been reported to ISMP in the past 9 years. Maternal deaths have been reported with use of magnesium sulfate (Simpson & Knox, 2004). Available data do not support the role of tocolytic agents in reducing the incidence of preterm labor, increasing the interval from onset to birth or reducing the incidence of PTB (ACOG, 2003a), but still they are frequently used as a secondary intervention in the United States.

BETA-MIMETICS

Ritodrine hydrochloride (Yutopar) is the only agent approved by the FDA for use as a tocolytic in the United States, and continues to be used at some sites for this purpose. Terbutaline (Brethine) is used for tocolysis as well, although its use is considered "off label" (ie, used for a purpose other than that approved by the FDA). Ritodrine and terbutaline are beta agonists; they stimulate beta-receptor cells located in smooth muscle. Theoretically, these agents work by relaxing the smooth muscle, which decreases or stops uterine contractions. The beta-receptors are also located in smooth muscle in the cardiovascular, pulmonary, and gastrointestinal systems. Effects of beta-mimetic agents are related directly to dosage and route of administration. Maternal side effects are common and uncomfortable. Fetal side effects are thought to be the same as those in the mother because they rapidly cross the placenta. These

DISPLAY 6-23

Nursing Care for Women Receiving Tocolytic Therapy

- Know the contraindications and potential complications of tocolytic therapy.
- Encourage the woman to assume a sidelying position to enhance placental perfusion.
- Explain the purpose and common side effects of the medication.
- Assess maternal vital signs according to institutional protocol.
- Notify the provider if the maternal pulse exceeds 120.
- Assess for signs and symptoms of pulmonary edema.
- Assess intake and output at least every hour (unless on low-dose maintenance therapy).
- Limit intake to 2,500 mL per day (90 mL/hr).
- Provide psychosocial support.

beta-mimetic agents are contraindicated in patients with known cardiac disease. The beta-mimetic agents may be administered subcutaneously or intravenously as a secondary infusion, after baseline assessments (eg, electrolytes, blood urea nitrogen, creatinine, serum glucose, ECG status) are obtained and a meticulous intake and output record is started. The infusion is titrated according to institutional protocol until uterine activity ceases, maximum dosages are reached, or the patient experiences severe side effects. Decreases in blood pressure, a widening pulse pressure, and maternal tachycardia develop in most patients.

Terbutaline pump therapy for women is ordered in certain geographic areas of the United States. It has been studied often, but according to the most recent review of available evidence in the *Cochrane Database of Systematic Reviews*, it is not effective in prolonging pregnancy (Nanda, Cook, Gallo, & Grimes, 2002). Elliott, Istwan, Rhea, and Stanziano (2004) studied 9,359 women who received continuous terbutaline therapy and found that 15.5% had side effects, the most serious of which was pulmonary edema. Maintenance tocolytic therapy is not recommended by ACOG (2003a).

Conscientious nursing care for the woman receiving beta-mimetic therapy is essential and includes ongoing assessment and monitoring of side effects. Maternal pulse rate must be monitored for any patient who is administered a beta-mimetic agent. A heart rate of 120 beats per minute or greater may warrant continuous ECG monitoring and discontinuation of tocolytic therapy. A heart rate greater than 120 beats per minute is associated with a decreased ventricular filling time and therefore with decreased cardiac output. Over time, if the left ventricular filling time is decreased, less blood is pumped to the myocardium, resulting in decreased myocardial perfusion. This is reflected by the patient's complaints of chest heaviness, shortness of breath, or chest pain. Myocardial infarction may result if the agent is not discontinued.

There is no evidence that oral betamimetics are effective in preventing preterm birth. A recent review in the *Cochrane Database of Systematic Reviews* concerning oral beta-mimetics examined 11 randomized trials and found that available evidence does not support the use of oral beta-mimetics for maintenance therapy after threatened preterm labor (Dodd, Crowther, Dare, & Middleton, 2006).

OXYTOCIN RECEPTOR ANTAGONISTS

Atosiban, an oxytocin receptor antagonist, was tested in the United States as a tocolytic during the 1990s. It was felt that this tocolytic could be effective in stopping preterm labor, and also had few side effects for the mother or the baby. Six clinical trials were conducted, but atosiban did not reduce preterm birth significantly (Papatsonis, Flenady, Cole, & Liley, 2005) and was not approved for use in the US. This drug continues to be used in countries other than the US for tocolysis.

MAGNESIUM SULFATE

Intravenous magnesium sulfate is the most commonly used pharmacologic agent in intrapartum settings in the United States to stop preterm contractions (Grimes & Nanda, 2006). It has been estimated that approximately 80% of women in the United States each year who are administered tocolytic therapy at 34 weeks or less receive magnesium sulfate (Grimes & Nanda). Despite widespread use in the United States, magnesium sulfate therapy has not been shown to be effective as a tocolytic agent and it may be harmful to the baby (Crowther, Hiller, & Doyle, 2002; Grimes & Nanda, 2006). According to the latest review in the *Cochrane Database of Systematic Reviews*, magnesium sulfate is ineffective at delaying birth or preventing preterm birth and its use is associated with increased infant mortality (Crowther, Hiller, & Doyle).

Magnesium sulfate use for preterm labor tocolysis is considered "off-label." The exact mechanism of action is unknown. Theoretically, magnesium interferes with calcium uptake in the cells of the myometrium. Because myometrial cells are thought to need calcium to contract, decreasing the amount of calcium decreases or stops contractions. Magnesium sulfate relaxes smooth muscle throughout the body, and a decrease in blood pressure may be observed with the administration of a loading dose or at high infusion rates. Maternal side effects include flushing, headache, nausea and vomiting, shortness of breath, chest pain, and pulmonary edema. Many practitioners feel comfortable using this agent because they have experience in its administration for the prevention of eclamptic seizures. Institutional protocols differ widely for how this drug is used in women with preterm contractions.

When magnesium sulfate is being used for preterm labor prophylaxis, it is important to note any changes in uterine activity. Often, women in preterm labor receive magnesium sulfate after significant amounts of intravenous (IV) fluids have been infused in an effort to inhibit contractions. This practice increases the risk for pulmonary edema. Therefore, careful assessment of respiratory status including rate and clarity of breath sounds is required as well as accurate recording of fluid intake and output (Simpson & Knox, 2004). Signs and symptoms of pulmonary edema include shortness of breath, chest tightening or discomfort, cough, oxygen saturation below 95%, increased respiratory and heart rates, and adventitious breath sounds. Changes in behavior such as apprehension, anxiety, or restlessness may be additional signs of pulmonary edema or hypoxemia and should be closely monitored, documented, and reported (Simpson &

Knox). The physician should be notified if a woman experiences any of the following symptoms (Simpson & Knox):

- Significant changes in blood pressure (BP) from baseline values
- Double (or blurring of) vision
- Tachycardia or bradycardia
- Respiratory rate below 14 or above 24
- Oxygen saturation below 95%
- Changes in breath sounds suggestive of pulmonary edema
- Changes in level of consciousness or neurologic status
- Absent deep tendon reflexes (DTRs)
- Urinary output less than 30 mL/hr
- Nonreassuring FHR pattern

Maternal respiratory rate, oxygen saturation, DTRs, and state of consciousness should be monitored closely to detect progressive magnesium toxicity (see Table 6–7). Magnesium toxicity results in loss of DTRs and progressive muscle weakness, including the diaphragm and other respiratory muscles, leading to acute respiratory failure. In addition, an overdose of magnesium sulfate depresses the respiratory center in the brain, further inhibiting respirations. Hypotension, complete heart block, and cardiac arrest can occur. One ampule of calcium gluconate, 1 g (10 mL of a 10% solution), should be clearly labeled with directions for administration and kept in the nearest locked drug cabinet (Simpson & Knox, 2004). If respiratory depression occurs, 1 g calcium gluconate should be given IV over 3 minutes (Sibai, 2002). If respiratory arrest occurs, ventilation should be supported until the antidote takes effect (Sibai). Intravenous fluids administered at a rapid infusion rate can assist excretion of magnesium sulfate. Although significantly high values (30 to 35 mg/dL) are frequently reported as being necessary to cause cardiac arrest, it is important to remember that an untreated respiratory arrest will lead to cardiac arrest as the cardiac muscle becomes hypoxic and ischemic (Dildy et al., 2003). Thus, cardiac arrest can occur at magnesium levels consistent with respiratory failure if the respiratory failure is not identified and treated immediately. Magnesium levels causing cardiotoxicity are not required to cause cardiac arrest.

Magnesium sulfate is on the *ISMP List of High-Alert Medications* because there is serious risk of causing significant patient harm when used in error (Simpson, 2006). Although errors with these drugs may not be more common than those with other medications, consequences of errors are more devastating (ISMP, 2006). Essential components of safe nursing care for women receiving IV magnesium sulfate have been

described (ISMP, 2005, 2006; Simpson & Knox, 2004). See Display 6–24 for safe care practices when using magnesium sulfate in obstetrics. Because accidents and adverse outcomes continue to occur with magnesium sulfate in obstetrics, it is important to review important safety procedures that can minimize risk.

CALCIUM CHANNEL BLOCKERS

Calcium channel blockers are another class of drugs that have been used to suppress contractions. They cause the myometrial muscle to relax by interfering with the movement of extracellular calcium into the calcium channels of the cells. This prevents the electrical system from passing the current through the cells, preventing a contraction. These agents, especially nifedipine (Procardia) and nicardipine (Nicardipine), have been compared with ritodrine, and no differences in prolongation of pregnancy were found (Garcia-Velasco & Gonzales Gonzales, 1998). Common fetal side effects associated with its use include decreased uteroplacental blood flow, fetal hypoxia, and fetal bradycardia. Calcium channel blockers have also been associated with maternal hepatotoxicity when administered for preterm labor (Higby, Xenakis, & Pauerstein, 1993). A European comparison of nifedipine and atosiban for preterm labor cessation showed that atosiban had fewer side effects, and was warranted for use in women in whom nifedipine is contraindicated (Kashanian, Akbarian, & Soltanzadeh, 2005). vanGeijn, Lenglet, and Bolte (2005) have reviewed 40 studies on the use of nifedipine for tocolysis and shown that studies have generally been done on healthy pregnant women. Because of nifedipine's pharmacological properties, it should not be used in women with any cardiovascular compromise, intrauterine infection, multiple pregnancy, maternal hypertension, or cardiac disease (vanGeijn, Lenglet, & Bolte, 2005).

PROSTAGLANDIN INHIBITORS

Prostaglandin is a naturally produced agent that is thought to cause uterine contractions and cervical ripening in term pregnancies. Because little prostaglandin has been found in women who are not in labor, the use of drugs that inhibit the production of prostaglandin has been hypothesized as a possible treatment for preterm labor. Several types of prostaglandins affect uterine contractions and cervical ripening. The most well-known and well-studied prostaglandin inhibitor (NSAID) for use as a tocolytic agent is indomethacin (ACOG, 2003a; Besinger, Niebyl, Keyes, & Johnson, 1991). Indomethacin competes with other factors in a long-term process whereby prostacyclin is the end prod-

DISPLAY 6 - 2 4

Safe Care Practices for the Use of Magnesium Sulfate in Obstetrics

- The pharmacy should supply high-risk IV medications such as magnesium sulfate in prepackaged-premixed solutions.
- Magnesium sulfate only should be administered via controlled infusion pump.
- The infusion pump should not be preprogrammed to change the dose in the absence of direct bedside attendance of the nurse.
- A second nurse should double-check all doses and pump settings.
- Use a 100 mL(4 g)/150 mL(6 g) IVPB solution for the initial bolus instead of bolusing from the main bag with a rate change on the pump.
- Use 500-mL IV bags with 20 g of magnesium sulfate versus 1,000-mL IV bags with 40 g of magnesium sulfate for the maintenance fluids.
- Use color-coded tags on the lines as they go into the pumps and into the IV ports.
- Maternal–fetal status should be assessed and documented before the medication is administered. Assessments include maternal vital signs, oxygen saturation, level of consciousness, characteristics of the fetal heart rate, and uterine activity.
- All maternal–fetal status parameters, including how the woman is tolerating magnesium sulfate should be documented in the medical record every 15 minutes during the first hour, every 30 minutes during the second hour, and at least every hour while the maintenance dose is infusing (even for those patients who are considered to be stable).

- Signs and symptoms of magnesium toxicity should be evaluated and ruled out during each assessment. Deep tendon reflexes (DTRs) should be assessed prior to administration of the medication, at least every 2 hours thereafter and as needed based on maternal signs and symptoms. Oxygen saturation should be assessed once per hour. Continuous pulse oximetry is not recommended. Breath sounds should be auscultated before the initial administration of magnesium sulfate, then every 2 hours thereafter.
- Provide 1 to 1 nursing care at the bedside during the first hour of administration.
- Provide 1 to 2 nursing care during the maintenance dose in a clinical setting where the patient is close to the nurses' station rather than on the general antepartum or postpartum nursing unit where there is less intensive nursing care.
- Consider that a woman receiving magnesium sulfate remains high risk even when symptoms of preeclampsia or preterm labor are stable.
- When care is transferred to another nurse, have both nurses together at the bedside assess patient status, review dosage and pump settings, and review written physician medication orders.
- Once the medication therapy is completed, discontinue the medication by removing the line from the IV port to prevent accidental infusion and potential magnesium sulfate overdose.
- Conduct periodic magnesium overdose drills with airway management and calcium administration with physician and nurse team members participating together.
- Maintain calcium antidote in an easily accessible locked medication kit with the dosage and admistration (1 g of calcium gluconate should be given IV over 3 minutes) clearly printed on the kit.

Adapted from Simpson, K. R. (2006). Minimizing risk of magnesium sulfate overdose in obstetrics. *MCN The American Journal of Maternal Child Nursing, 31*(5), 340; and Simpson, K. R., & Knox, G. E. (2004). Obstetrical accidents involving intravenous magnesium sulfate: Recommendations to promote patient safety. *MCN The American Journal of Maternal Child Nursing, 29*(3), 161–171.

uct blocking the production of prostaglandin. Indomethacin is not without fetal effects, however. Although this class of drugs might have few maternal side effects (ACOG, 2003a), after 34 weeks' gestation, indomethacin may cause premature closure of the fetal ductus arteriosis, increasing the risk of fetal pulmonary hypertension (Vermillion & Robinson, 2005). Indomethacin also impairs fetal renal function that may result in oligohydramnios. The use of this drug for prevention of PTB remains controversial. Some in the research community have suggested that the risk to the fetus by using indomethacin is less than the multiple morbidities

associated with a birth at less than 32 weeks' gestation (Macones & Robinson, 1998).

Is There Any Good News?
Antenatal Glucocorticoids

Antenatal glucocorticoid use for prevention of respiratory distress syndrome in a premature infant has been endorsed by the National Institute of Child Health and Human Development (NICHD) through its consensus conferences (NIH, 1995, 2000). This class of medication does not prevent PTB; rather it prevents major complications in the neonate, which is the best outcome possible at this time. Because it is not yet possible to actively prevent PTB, ACOG (2002a) has endorsed this therapy, recommending that either of the following protocols be followed:

Betamethasone

- Given in 2 doses: 12 mg intramuscular (IM) every 24 hours

Dexamethasone

- Given in 2 doses: 6 mg IM every 12 hours

Either medication should be given to any woman at 24 to 34 weeks' gestation with signs of preterm labor, except those women with chorioamnionitis. The effects of the drug last up to 7 days. Further dosages after the 7 days are currently not advised: "Current data are insufficient to support routine use of repeat courses of antenatal corticosteroids" (NIH, 2000).

Nursing Care for the Prevention of Preterm Birth

Education About Signs and Symptoms of Preterm Labor

Educating women about signs and symptoms of preterm labor has been a hallmark of preterm birth prevention programs since the early 1980s (Herron, Katz, & Creasy, 1982). Patient education is one of nursing's core areas of practice and therefore nurses are well qualified to teach women about signs and symptoms of preterm labor. At its onset, the woman may think that preterm labor symptoms are a "normal discomfort of pregnancy," in part because physicians, nurse midwives, childbirth educators, and nurses continue to teach women about Braxton-Hicks contractions, expecting the women to decide whether the contractions experienced are normal or abnormal. Classic nursing research (Patterson, Douglas, Patterson, & Bradle, 1992) has shown that women taught in this fashion experience "diagnostic confusion" when faced with the symptoms of preterm labor and may not notify their healthcare provider because they think that the contractions they are experiencing are normal. If the goal in teaching women is to ensure prompt notification of the provider when early, subtle symptoms of preterm labor appear, use of the term *Braxton-Hicks contractions* for women before 37 weeks' gestation should be removed from prenatal teaching (Hill & Lambertz, 1990).

Because all pregnant women must be considered at risk for preterm labor, it is essential that nurses teach all pregnant women how to detect the early symptoms of preterm labor (Davies et al., 1998; Damus & Merkatz, 1991; Freda & Patterson, 2004; Moore & Freda, 1998). Nurses providing care to pregnant

women should use the literature to understand the best methods for teaching early recognition of preterm symptoms. Tiedje (2005) has described a model program for teaching women about prematurity in a clinic waiting room. Moore, Ketner, Walsh, and Wagoner (2005) have shown how listening to women can help remove barriers to effective patient education about preterm birth. Reassessment for symptoms at each subsequent prenatal visit is also essential. Patient education regarding any symptoms of contractions or cramping between 20 and 36 weeks' gestation should include telling the woman that these symptoms are not normal discomforts in pregnancy and that contractions or cramping that do not go away should prompt the woman to contact her healthcare provider.

Although many nurses teach their patients in a one-on-one manner, the use of standardized videotape for teaching women about preterm symptoms has been shown in classic nursing research to be effective in teaching women this information (Freda, Damus, Andersen, Brustman, & Merkatz, 1990). The March of Dimes videotape *Take Action* is one such example of patient education. No matter which method of patient education is used, it is imperative that nurses in prenatal settings make concerted efforts to teach all pregnant women about how to recognize early preterm labor.

Sometimes, patient education cannot be offered in person but can still be effective. A randomized clinical trial demonstrated that education offered by nurses on the telephone can result in a 26% decrease in LBW births and a 27% decrease in PTB among African-American women (Moore et al., 1998). This study demonstrates the power of nursing care, nursing support, and patient education in the care of women at highest risk for preterm birth.

Reinforcement of the signs and symptoms of preterm labor should occur at each subsequent prenatal visit along with a review of any symptoms that may have been experienced since the last visit. Research from the past 2 decades has shown that some women who experience preterm labor wait for hours or days to call a healthcare provider, significantly delaying their time of entry into the healthcare system when some proactive action could be taken (Freston et al., 1997; Iams, Johnson O'Shaughnessy, & West, 1990). Prompt notification of the healthcare provider is essential, because the use of antenatal glucocorticoids given to hasten fetal lung maturity is the most effective therapy for avoiding neonatal health problems such as respiratory distress syndrome (Leviton et al., 1999; NIH, 2000).

The message about the importance of educating pregnant women about preterm labor symptoms has not permeated the healthcare system. Davies et al. (1998) surveyed all prenatal care providers in Eastern

Ontario and found that only one-half of family physicians and obstetricians even discussed signs and symptoms of preterm labor with their prenatal patients; only 10% of family physicians and 40% of obstetricians distributed educational materials to their patients about preterm labor. In their focus groups of women who had given birth preterm, the researchers found that all of the women wished they had known more about how to recognize symptoms of preterm labor (Davies et al.).

Patient education plays an essential role in the prevention of preterm birth. Unless pregnant women know and understand the signs and early symptoms of preterm labor, they will not know to notify their provider, and could therefore lose the opportunity for obtaining antenatal corticosteroids. Nurses who work with women during the prenatal period should be prepared to educate women about the early symptoms of preterm labor. Intrapartum nurses must understand the sometimes-imperceptible nature of preterm labor to assess women who present with subtle symptoms. Waiting too long to see a healthcare provider could result in inevitable preterm birth without the added benefit of the administration of antenatal glucocorticoids and ultimately result in a baby being born at higher risk for respiratory distress syndrome and intraventricular hemorrhage. Prenatal healthcare providers need to teach women that the symptoms, when felt between 20 weeks and 37 weeks of pregnancy, should be reported to a healthcare provider promptly. In addition to teaching the symptoms in a didactic fashion, it is essential that the nurse in the antepartum or intrapartum setting establish a therapeutic relationship with the pregnant woman so she will feel comfortable reporting vague, nonspecific complaints and will come in or call her primary healthcare provider if she experiences any of the following signs or symptoms of preterm labor:

- Uterine cramping (menstrual-like cramps, intermittent or constant)
- Uterine contractions every 10 to 15 minutes or more frequently
- Low abdominal pressure (pelvic pressure)
- Dull low backache (intermittent or constant)
- Increase or change in vaginal discharge
- Feeling that the baby is "pushing down"
- Abdominal cramping with or without diarrhea

When any of these symptoms is experienced, the woman should be instructed to stop what she is doing, lie down on her side, drink two to three glasses of water or juice, and wait 1 hour. If the symptoms get worse, she should call the healthcare provider. If the symptoms go away, she should tell the healthcare provider at the next visit what happened, and if the symptoms come back, she should call the healthcare provider.

Perinatal nurses must listen carefully when pregnant women between 20 and 37 weeks' gestation complain of these symptoms, assess for cervical effacement or dilation as well as uterine contractions, and encourage them to call their provider or come back to the hospital if the symptoms reappear. Women who are between 24 and 34 weeks' gestation who present with any symptoms of preterm labor are candidates for antenatal glucocorticoid therapy.

Lifestyle Modification

Evidence exists that some women experience more preterm symptoms when engaged in certain activities. We have known for over a decade through research that when women are able to modify those lifestyle factors, they have fewer preterm births (Freda, Anderson, et al., 1990; Lynam & Miller, 1992). Activities such as stair climbing, sexual activity, riding long distances in automobiles or public transportation, carrying heavy objects, hard physical work, and inability to rest when tired have been associated with increased preterm birth (Hobel et al., 1994; Iams, Stilson, Johnson, Williams, & Rice, 1990; Papiernik, 1989). Nurses who teach women about symptoms of preterm labor should assess whether symptoms increase when these or other activities are performed and work with women to find ways to help them eliminate those activities or at least decrease their frequency.

Smoking Cessation

Smoking is a lifestyle factor strongly associated with preterm birth and LBW. It is one of the few risk factors that can be altered by pregnant women. Although the effects of smoking on risk of preterm birth and LBW have been known for more than 40 years (Simpson, 1957), between 15% and 29% of women in the United States smoke during their pregnancy (ACOG, 2005a). Ricketts, Murray, and Schwalberg (2005) have found a LBW rate of 8.5% among women who quit smoking, in comparison to a LBW rate of 13.7% in women who did not quit smoking. Magee, Hattis, and Kivel (2004) showed that LBW was 58% more likely among women who smoked than among nonsmokers. It is estimated that there would be a 10% reduction in perinatal mortality and an 11% reduction in LBW if smoking during pregnancy were eliminated (ACOG, 2005a). The risk of fetal death for pregnant women who smoke is generally 1.5-fold over that for pregnant nonsmokers (Silver, 2007). We know that even a reduction in smoking could improve perinatal outcome birth weight (England, Kendrick, Gargiullo, Zahniser, & Hannon, 2001), therefore it is incumbent on nurses to work toward helping pregnant women stop smoking completely, or at least significantly cut down on the number of cigarettes they smoke.

The physiologic effects of smoking occur as a result of transient intrauterine hypoxemia. When the pregnant woman smokes, carbon monoxide crosses the placenta and binds with maternal and fetal hemoglobin, producing carboxyhemoglobin. Carboxyhemoglobin interferes with the normal binding process of oxygen to the hemoglobin molecule, reducing the ability of the blood to carry adequate levels of oxygen to the fetus (Secker-Walker, Vacek, Flynn, & Mead, 1997). Smoking may also result in an increase in fetal vascular resistance, which can lead to impaired fetal growth and hypoxia (Silver, 2007).

An opportunity to reduce the risk of preterm birth and LBW exists if education for pregnant women about the effects of smoking on the fetus begins early in pregnancy. One of the most effective interventions to reduce smoking during pregnancy is to encourage the woman to institute a no-smoking policy at home (Mullen, Richardson, Quinn, & Ershoff, 1997).

Smoking cessation programs have been widely evaluated. Jesse, Graham, and Swanson (2006) have shown the importance of including social support and stress-relieving activities in smoking cessation programs. Ferreira-Borges (2005) has described brief counseling programs for smoking cessation with pregnant women, which had positive outcomes. The most recent review in the *Cochrane Database of Systematic Reviews* (Lumley, Oliver, Chamberlain, & Oakley, 2004) involved 64 trials of smoking cessation programs during pregnancy, and found that, no matter what type of program was initiated, smoking cessation programs can reduce the numbers of women who smoke in pregnancy, and also reduce LBW and PTB. ACOG (2005a) has promoted using the 5A's (1. Ask about tobacco use, 2. Advise to quit, 3. Assess willingness to make an attempt, 4. Assist in quit attempt, 5. Arrange follow-up) approach to smoking cessation in pregnancy for every pregnant smoker. ACOG's power point slides can be downloaded from their Web site (www.acog.org). AWHONN has also initiated a nationwide program to help women stop smoking. Their program was aimed at disseminating knowledge to nurses who work with pregnant women in order to change clinical practice by including smoking cessation strategies in nursing care. Information about this program, called "SUCCESS" (Setting Universal Cessation Counseling, Education and Screening Standards: Nursing Care for Pregnant Women Who Smoke) program can be found at www.awhonn.org

Although cessation of smoking in pregnancy is important, women should also be taught about the health hazards of postpartum smoking for their own health and the health of their children. Lawrence et al. (2005) evaluated a pregnancy smoking cessation program 18 months after the birth, and found that 86% of the women had relapsed at 18 months. Similarly, Suplee (2005) found 52% of the women who stopped smoking during pregnancy had relapsed, but her measurement was at 4 weeks after giving birth. Thyrian et al. (2006) have called for the institution of standardized interventions to help women remain smoke-free after giving birth.

Illicit Drug Use

Although not the major contributors to preterm birth, women who take illicit drugs in pregnancy are at risk for preterm birth (Kearney, 1999). It is important, therefore, for nurses to know and understand how to assess for illicit drug use, and how to intervene to best help the woman and her baby. These women are frightened and addicted and require specialized care (Hans, 1999). Nurses working in prenatal, intrapartum, or postpartum care should become aware of the treatment facilities available for drug-using women in their community so that appropriate referrals can be made, and so that the women and their infants have the best chance to improve the outcome of the pregnancy.

Domestic Violence

Parker, McFarlane, and Soeken (1994) were the first to correlate domestic violence with preterm labor and birth. Their work showed that domestic violence was a health problem, not a social problem, and that women who were battered had more LBW and PTB than women who were not. Heaman (2005) has continued this work, demonstrating again that PTB and domestic violence are related. Nursing care for women during pregnancy, therefore, should include assessment for abuse. This can be done easily and quickly with the four questions in the *Abuse Assessment Screen*, which can be found in the March of Dimes nursing module *Abuse in Pregnancy* (McFarlane, Parker, & Cross, 2001). In a recent study, Renker and Tonkin (2006) found that of 519 women screened for abuse in pregnancy, 91% were not offended, embarrassed, or angry because they were asked the questions, and that women wanted to know whether abuse, once disclosed, was reportable to legal authorities.

Intrapartum Nursing Care of the Woman in Preterm Labor

Women who seek care when they are experiencing active preterm labor will be hospitalized and probably given oral fluids or intravenous hydration in an attempt to inhibit preterm contractions. If fluid therapy is unsuccessful, one or more tocolytic drugs are likely to follow, along with bed rest and electronic fetal monitoring. Nursing care is then delivered by nurses competent to care for the high-risk pregnant woman. Simpson (2005) has described this care, especially the fetal monitoring required for a preterm fetus.

See Chapter 8 for a discussion of monitoring the preterm fetus. Although bed rest, hydration, and tocolytics have not been found to be successful in preventing preterm birth, they may contribute to prolonging the pregnancy enough to gain the benefits of antenatal steroid therapy. While the mother is in preterm labor, ongoing monitoring of maternal–fetal status is essential. If the mother is receiving IV tocolytic agents, she should not be considered "stable" or allocated to periodic assessment protocols that preclude vigilant surveillance or transferred to a less intensive level of care (Simpson & Knox, 2004). The recommended nurse to patient ratio for women with high-risk obstetrical conditions during labor is one to one (AAP & ACOG, 2002).

Women in preterm labor need emotional support and information about the potential risks to their baby if preterm labor proceeds to preterm birth. In institutions that provide special care nursery or neonatal intensive care, a visit from the neonatal nurse practitioner or neonatologist prior to the birth can be helpful in explaining what to expect and how their baby will be cared for in the nursery. This process is preferred over the neonatal resuscitation team rushing in the room at birth without prior introductions and explanations. If the baby's gestational age or condition is such that it is anticipated that an immediate admission to the nursery will be required, every effort should be made to allow the mother to see and touch the baby before the neonatal team leaves the birthing room or surgical suite. The father of the baby should be encouraged to visit the nursery as soon as possible, and the family should be provided visiting policy information. Some nurseries have cameras that can be used to provide the mother with a picture while she is in the postanesthesia recovery period before she is able to visit the nursery.

Summary

Nurses have been extremely active in the research about preterm labor and birth (Freda, 2003). They have studied everything from causes of preterm labor to effects of preterm birth on families. Because preterm labor and birth are the most pressing problems in perinatal health in the beginning of the 21st century, more research is necessary. Although research has been extensive, it has not yet found a definitive cause nor a cure for preterm labor. Green et al. (2005) have published a suggested research agenda for the future from the March of Dimes Prematurity Campaign. It consists of six specific areas for research:

1. Epidemiologic studies of ≤32-week preterm births
2. Study of genes and gene–environment interactions
3. The role of racial and ethnic disparities
4. Studies of the inflammatory responses in preterm birth
5. The role of stress in preterm birth
6. Clinical trials of the effects of biomarkers, progesterone, infection treatment, assisted reproductive technologies, multifetal pregnancies, and strategies to reduce risks.

Nurses have the ability to not only participate in this exciting research but also enhance their clinical knowledge and skills regarding this topic. One of the most important interventions that nurses can implement is their ability to effectively teach pregnant women about the symptoms of preterm labor and birth. This can result in women obtaining the essential antenatal steroids at the earliest time possible. Although we may not yet know how to prevent a preterm birth, through talking to women and sharing our knowledge nurses can make a big difference in how many babies are born with the devastating sequelae of preterm birth.

DIABETES IN PREGNANCY

Significance and Incidence

In 2005, 14.6 million people in the US were diagnosed with diabetes. It is estimated that another 6.2 million people have diabetes that has not yet been diagnosed (CDC, 2005). About 1.85 million women of reproductive age (18–44 years) have diabetes. Women of minority racial and ethnic groups, such as black, Hispanic, American Indian, and Asian/Pacific Islanders, have two to four times the rate of diabetes of white women (CDC, 2001). Approximately 7% of all pregnancies are complicated by gestational diabetes (GDM; American Diabetes Association [ADA], 2004a).

Although comprehensive obstetric care and intensive metabolic management have reduced perinatal risk in pregnancies complicated by types 1 and 2 diabetes, morbidity and mortality still remain higher than in the general population. Pregnant women with types 1 and 2 diabetes have a 2.5-fold increase in risk of fetal death (Silver, 2007). Congenital defects and unexplained fetal death account for the increased fetal and neonatal mortality in women with types 1 and type 2 diabetes (Reece & Homko, 2000) and are likely related to co-morbid conditions such as hypertension and obesity (Silver). Maternal hyperglycemia and disorders of fetal growth, metabolism, and possibly acidosis contribute to risk of fetal mortality (Silver). Preconception and early pregnancy glycemic control as evidenced by a near-normal glycosylated hemoglobin (A1C) during the period of organogenesis greatly reduces the risk of birth defects (McElvy et al., 2000; Reece & Homko, 2000; Silver). Women with poorly controlled preexisting diabetes in the early weeks of pregnancy are three to four times more likely than nondiabetic women to have a baby with a serious malformation, such as a heart defect or neural tube defect (NTD; Sheffield, Butler-Koster, Casey, McIntire, Leveno, 2002). Defects in offspring of women with preexisting diabetes have been found to be more severe, usually multiple, and more often fatal (Jovanovic, 2000b). They also are at increased risk of miscarriage and stillbirth. First-trimester control in women with pregestational diabetes also reduces the risk of macrosomia (Raychaudhuri & Maresh, 2000; Rey, Attie, & Bonin, 1999).

The rate of perinatal mortality with gestational diabetes remains similar to that for nondiabetic women, but when GDM is detected in the first trimester with an elevated A1C and fasting hyperglycemia, the risk for congenital defects has been found to approach that of women with pregestational type 2 diabetes (Schaefer-Graf et al., 1997). It is possible that these data from early diagnosed cases may actually represent type 2 diabetes that was first recognized during pregnancy rather than true gestational diabetes. According to recent data using early and appropriate screening criteria, gestational diabetes is not associated with an increased risk of fetal death when compared to outcomes of pregnancies of women without diabetes (Silver, 2007). Women with GDM are at higher risk of perinatal morbidity, such as neonatal asphyxia (15%), hypoglycemia (20%) and other metabolic abnormalities, and respiratory distress syndrome (15%; Cordero & Landon, 1993). Maintenance of euglycemia throughout pregnancy in GDM reduces the risk of these hyperglycemia-related fetal and neonatal abnormalities, but there is still an increased risk for fetal macrosomia (40%) with resultant traumatic or cesarean birth (Blank, Grave, & Metzger, 1995).

Macrosomia has been defined as a weight greater than the 90th percentile for gestational age; usually a birth weight of 4,000 g (8 pounds, 13 ounces) to 4,500 g (9 pounds, 15 ounces; ACOG, 2000). Risk of fetal injury sharply increases with birth weights above 4,500 g (ACOG). Other factors such as morbid maternal obesity and postmaturity are also associated with fetal macrosomia and, when combined with insulin-controlled diabetes, lead to an even higher occurrence. Fetal macrosomia predisposes the newborn to a variety of traumatic injuries such as shoulder dystocia with associated risk for facial palsy, cephalohematoma, subdural hemorrhage, brachial plexus injury, and clavicle fracture (ACOG; Tyrala, 1996; Uvena-Celebrezze & Catalano, 2000). Shoulder dystocia is the most common injury related to fetal macrosomia, but occurs only in approximately 1.4% of all vaginal births (ACOG). When birth weight exceeds 4,500 g, the risk of shoulder dystocia has been reported to range from 9.2% to 24% (ACOG). If the woman has

diabetes, birth weights greater than 4,500 g are associated with much higher rates of shoulder dystocia; from 19.9% to 50% (ACOG). Fetal macrosomia contributes to an excessively high rate of cesarean births (41%), with resultant increased surgical morbidity in the mother (Persson & Hanson, 1996).

The Fetal Basis of Adult Disease theory holds that events that occur during fetal development can permanently alter gene expression throughout the lifetime of the individual. A link has emerged between fetal nutrition, birth weight, and metabolic profile in adulthood. Abnormal "programming" of nutrient management increases risk for developing metabolic diseases such as obesity, hypertension, cardiovascular disease, and type 2 diabetes (Barker, 2001).

In addition to the risk of fetal macrosomia for all women with diabetes, the other extreme of weight (IUGR) with an occurrence of 20% is a significant risk for infants born to women who have vascular complications of diabetes (Tyrala, 1996). Retinopathy and nephropathy associated with hypertension and poor renal function may contribute to uteroplacental insufficiency that leads to infants that are small for their gestational age. Pregnancy-induced hypertension (PIH), to which women with diabetes (with or without vascular disease) are predisposed, also decreases uterine blood flow, compromising intrauterine fetal growth. Maintaining glucose control (average blood glucose of greater than 86 mg/dL and less than 104 mg/dL) can help to avoid IUGR (Rosenn & Miodovnik, 2000a).

Neonatal metabolic abnormalities occur with a higher frequency in offspring of women with diabetes. Hypoglycemia, defined as blood glucose of 35 mg/dL in term infants and 25 mg/dL in preterm infants, occurs during the first few hours of life in 25% to 40% of infants of mothers with uncontrolled diabetes (Reece & Homko, 1994). Preterm and large-for-gestational-age infants are at greatest risk for the development of hypoglycemia in the neonatal period. Chronic maternal hyperglycemia leads to excessive insulin production in the fetus (ie, fetal hyperinsulinemia), which lowers fetal plasma glucose and inhibits glycogen release from the fetal liver as a normal physiologic response to hypoglycemia. This combination contributes to the risk for hypoglycemia development in the first 24 hours of life when cutting the umbilical cord interrupts transplacental glucose. Early detection and prompt treatment prevent the potential severe neurologic sequelae associated with profound hypoglycemia.

Approximately 3% to 5% of infants of diabetic mothers exhibit polycythemia, which is defined as a venous hematocrit of greater than 65% (Tyrala, 1996). Polycythemia occurs as a result of chronic hyperglycemia, hyperinsulinemia, and hyperketonemia and causes increased oxygen consumption and decreased fetal arterial oxygen content. Erythropoietin production increases, increasing red blood cell production (Tyrala). Hyperbilirubinemia occurs in 20% of infants of mothers with diabetes without a definitive explanation. It is seen more frequently when maternal diabetes is severe and in the presence of neonatal polycythemia and prematurity (Uvena-Celebrezze & Catalano, 2000). Hypocalcemia and hypomagnesemia are other metabolic abnormalities frequently seen in infants of women with types 1 and 2 diabetes. The exact cause of hypocalcemia is unknown but occurs with a high frequency in cases of respiratory distress and in the presence of prematurity. Hypomagnesemia may be seen in conjunction with hypocalcemia and is believed to be the result of polyuria in association with hyperglycemia (Reece & Homko, 1994).

Strict maternal glycemic control has decreased the incidence of respiratory distress syndrome significantly, but other factors such as iatrogenic prematurity due to early delivery as a result of maternal or fetal compromise continue to contribute to the risk. Fetal surfactant production is inhibited by hyperinsulinemia, which occurs more frequently in women with poor metabolic control and is the underlying mechanism for respiratory distress syndrome in this group (Uvena-Celebrezze & Catalano, 2000; Wiznitzer & Reece, 1999).

Risks during pregnancy for the woman with type 1 or type 2 diabetes include an increased incidence of hypoglycemia (blood glucose less than 60) as a result of stricter control (Reece, Homko, & Hagay, 1995; Rosenn & Miodovnik, 2000b). Hypoglycemia does not seem to cause problems for the fetus unless blood sugar levels are chronically low, but hypoglycemia does threaten the well-being of the mother. Educational efforts focusing on prevention and appropriate management of hypoglycemia can decrease this risk.

Diabetic ketoacidosis (DKA) is a rare complication for women with diabetes. However, the occurrence of DKA carries serious morbidity and mortality for the mother and the fetus (Garner, 1995; Hagay, 1994; Kilvert, Nicholson, & Wright, 1993). Fetal loss may occur through spontaneous abortion in the first and early second trimester or as an intrauterine fetal death during an episode of DKA in late second and third trimester. Improved perinatal management has decreased the fetal loss rate to 9% (Cullen, Reece, Homko, & Sivan, 1996).

Women with microvascular complications, poor glycemic control, and a longer duration of diabetes have poorer outcomes. Retinopathy affects approximately 20% to 27% of reproductive-age women, and this microvascular complication of diabetes is frequently encountered in pregnancy (Reece, Homko, & Hagay, 1996). Retinopathy may progress during pregnancy, requiring continued surveillance and treatment with photocoagulation for proliferative retinopathy (Klein, Moss, & Klein, 1990). Nephropathy is a more serious microvascular complication that has been associated with adverse outcomes, including intrauterine growth retardation, congenital malformations, preterm delivery, and intrauterine fetal death (Rosenn & Miodovnik, 2000b).

Hypertension almost universally develops if not present at conception and may include edema, superimposed PIH, and renal failure without meticulous care (Rosenn & Miodovnik, 2000b). Macrovascular complications of diabetes such as coronary artery, peripheral vascular, and cerebral artery disease are rarely seen in reproductive-age women but are contraindications to pregnancy because of the significant maternal mortality risk (Hagay & Weissman, 1996; Wiznitzer & Reece, 1999). Gastroparesis or gastropathy is a neuropathic complication that causes delayed gastric emptying and may exacerbate nausea and vomiting. This can result in irregular absorption of nutrients, inadequate nutrition, and poor glycemic control (Rosenn & Miodovnik). Women who continue pregnancy with gastroparesis may require total parenteral nutrition. Autonomic neuropathy directed at the cardiovascular system results in a lack of compensatory response to a decrease in blood pressure, posing a serious threat to fetal and maternal well-being, and is a relative contraindication to pregnancy (Macleod et al., 1990; Rosenn & Miodovnik).

Definitions and Classification

Women with diabetes during pregnancy can be divided into two groups. The first group consists of women who have pregestational diabetes (type 1 or type 2), and the second group consists of women with gestational diabetes or diabetes diagnosed during pregnancy. The terms *insulin-dependent diabetes mellitus* (IDDM) and *non–insulin-dependent diabetes* (NIDDM) are no longer used to classifying type 1 and type 2 diabetes, respectively (ADA, 1997).

Type 1 diabetes is hyperglycemia as a result of absolute insulin deficiency. It occurs as a result of genetic autoimmunity directed at the ß cells of the pancreas after an environmental trigger turns on antibodies which attack the islet cells of the pancreas resulting in a total lack of insulin production. Exogenous insulin administration and medical nutrition therapy (MNT) are the mainstays of treatment. This disease usually occurs in people younger than 30 years of age but can develop at any age.

Insulin resistance and relative insulin deficiency characterize type 2 diabetes. Insulin resistance at the cellular level may exist because of genetic defects in insulin binding to receptor sites or in glucose transport within the cell. This demands an increase in insulin secretion from the pancreas to maintain normoglycemia. Eventually the beta cells exhaust and insulin production is diminished, resulting in hyperglycemia. Type 2 is the result of either genetic predisposition or environmental factors, such as obesity, or a combination of both. To achieve euglycemia, type 2 diabetes may require not only medical nutrition therapy and exercise but also medication. Oral medications that increase the sensitivity of cells to insulin are first-line therapy after diet and exercise for type 2 diabetes, but insulin may be and often is necessary to maintain normoglycemia. Type 2 diabetes was seen less frequently in pregnancy because the age of diagnosis is usually in women beyond the reproductive years (≥45 years of age). However, with increasing rates of obesity and type 2 diabetes in children and young adults (CDC, 2001), type 2 diabetes is becoming as common as type 1 diabetes in women of childbearing age.

Oral hypoglycemic medications are not recommended for use during pregnancy in women with type 2 diabetes. Earlier studies with first-generation sulfonylureas, which did cross the placenta, showed profound hypoglycemia in newborns because these drugs caused the fetal pancreas to secrete more insulin (Kemball et al., 1970). Earlier studies also showed an increase in malformations with oral agent use in the first trimester, but these malformations were likely due to hyperglycemia associated with ineffective control of maternal blood glucose. However, in a recent study of women with type 2 diabetes, 61% of the infants with congenital malformations were born to women taking oral antidiabetes agents at conception. Treatment with oral antidiabetes agents was independently associated with congenital anomalies (Roland, Murphy, Fall, Northcot-Wright, & Temple, 2005).

Glucose intolerance diagnosed at a gestational age of 20 weeks or less may represent undiagnosed preexisting type 2 diabetes, but this diagnosis should not be made during pregnancy. These women should be treated as if they have type 2 diabetes.

Priscilla White (1949) developed a classification system that was used to determine pregnancy prognosis for women based on the extent of microvascular disease and duration of type 1 or 2 diabetes. White's classification system is still used for descriptive purposes only, because the classification does not consider the level of glycemic control or comprehensive obstetric management, both of which greatly influence perinatal outcome.

Gestational diabetes comprises the second group and is defined as carbohydrate intolerance of any degree with onset or first recognition during pregnancy (ADA, 2004a). GDM has been subdivided further to designate those women who are diet controlled (GDM A_1) or insulin controlled (GDM A_2) (Hagay & Reece, 1992).

Pathophysiology of Diabetes in Pregnancy

Profound metabolic changes occur in normal pregnancy to allow for a continuously feeding fetus in an intermittently feeding mother. These alterations must be understood to comprehend the effects that diabetes has on a progressively changing metabolic state. In early pregnancy, ß-cell hyperplasia results in increased insulin production as a result of progesterone and estrogen increases, which also contributes to increased tissue sensitivity to insulin. This hyperinsulinemic state allows increased lipogenesis and fat deposition in early pregnancy in preparation for the dramatic rise in energy needs of the growing fetus in the latter half of pregnancy. As a result of these changes, and nausea and vomiting, the mother has an increased risk for episodes of hypoglycemia in the first trimester. In women with type 1 and insulin-controlled type 2 diabetes, exogenous insulin needs may decrease.

The second half of pregnancy is characterized by accelerated growth of the fetus and rapidly increasing levels of maternal and placental diabetogenic hormones, which include human placental lactogen, cortisol, estrogen, progesterone, and prolactin (Boden, 1996). Insulin resistance and increased insulin production result from increased circulating levels of insulin-antagonizing hormones. Increased insulin needs in women with types 1 and 2 diabetes and the appearance of glucose intolerance in women who have limited pancreatic reserve due to predisposing risk factors are the result of these normal metabolic changes of pregnancy (Buchanan & Kitzmiller, 1994). This constitutes the diabetogenic state of pregnancy—hyperglycemia in the presence of hyperinsulinemia—which allows a continuous supply of glucose to passively diffuse to the fetus transplacentally (Lesser & Carpenter, 1994).

The anabolic phase (ie, fat storage) of the first 20 weeks of pregnancy is followed by a catabolic phase (ie, fat breakdown or lipolysis) in the latter half of pregnancy (Lesser & Carpenter, 1994). This state is referred to as "accelerated starvation" because of the rapid switch from carbohydrate to lipid metabolism during fasting as a fuel source for the mother, preferentially reserving glucose and amino acids for the developing fetus (Boden, 1996). Fat breakdown increases circulating fatty acids, triglycerides, and ketones, predisposing the woman with type 1 diabetes to an increased risk for the earlier development of ketoacidosis and starvation ketosis than in women with GDM and type 2 diabetes (Buchanan & Kitzmiller, 1994). Hepatic glucose production increases by 16% to 30% during the latter half of pregnancy to meet the fetal and placental demands during maternal fasting (Butte, 2000).

In the absence of vascular disease, the pathologic manifestations of diabetes in pregnancy are usually the result of maternal hyperglycemia. Excessive hyperglycemia, as a result of insulin deficiency with a corresponding increase in counterregulatory hormones (ie, glucagon, epinephrine, growth hormone, and cortisol), contributes to the development of DKA. Factors in pregnancy that trigger the release of these hormones and development of DKA are fasting hyperglycemia, infection, stress, emesis, dehydration, steroid administration (Bouhanick, Biquard, Hadjadj, & Roques, 2000), and adrenergic agonist (ie, Terbutaline) administration for the treatment of preterm labor (Harvey, 1992). Continuous subcutaneous insulin infusion (CSII) pump failure and poor patient compliance have also led to the development of DKA during pregnancy. Nausea and vomiting of pregnancy with decreased caloric intake has been found to be a major contributor to DKA (Cullen, Reece, Homko, & Sivan, 1996). Excessive hyperglycemia results from increased hepatic glucose production and decreased peripheral glucose use (Chauhan & Perry, 1995). Urinary excretion of potassium, sodium, and water occurs as a result of osmotic diuresis due to excessive plasma glucose. Fat metabolism leads to increased circulating levels of free fatty acids and ketone bodies, which quickly overwhelm the maternal buffering system, and metabolic acidosis results (Whiteman, Homko, & Reece, 1996).

Maternal hyperglycemia during the time of organogenesis may result in spontaneous abortion or congenital malformations (Reece & Homko, 2000). Sustained or intermittent maternal hyperglycemia later in pregnancy stimulates fetal hyperinsulinemia as a normal fetal physiologic response to elevated blood glucose with pathologic consequences. Fetal hyperinsulinemia mediates accelerated fuel use and conversion of glucose to fat. Central fat deposition results in excessive growth (ie, macrosomia; Moore, 2004). Maternal hyperglycemia also contributes to fetal hypoxia. Hyperinsulinemia promotes catabolism of the extra fuel, using energy and depleting fetal oxygen stores (Moore). Fetal hyperinsulinemia also inhibits the release of surfactant that is necessary for pulmonary maturation resulting in respiratory distress syndrome. Maternal hyperglycemia is also associated with other neonatal metabolic abnormalities. Polyhydramnios, hypertension, urinary tract infections, pyelonephritis, and monilial vaginitis are other maternal complications of hyperglycemia.

Screening and Diagnosis of Gestational Diabetes Mellitus

Screening for gestational diabetes is recommended between 24 and 28 weeks' gestation, when the diabetogenic hormones are exerting a significant influence on insulin performance. Women without risk factors for GDM do not require screening (ADA, 2004a; ACOG, 2001). Display 6–25 lists characteristics of women who are at low risk for developing gestational diabetes. Women younger than 25 years of age with any other risk factor for GDM should be tested. Risk factors identifying women who should undergo early

DISPLAY 6-25

Characteristics of Women at Low Risk for Gestational Diabetes Mellitus

- Younger than 25 years of age
- Normal body weight
- No history of abnormal glucose tolerance
- No history of poor obstetric outcome
- No known diabetes in first-degree relative
- Not a member of an ethnic or racial group with higher prevalence of type 2 diabetes (eg, Hispanic, African-American, Native American, Asian, or Pacific Islander ancestry)

screening (as soon as risk is identified) are listed in Display 6–26. Women in this risk category whose early test results are negative should be retested at 24 to 28 weeks.

Evaluation for GDM may be performed in a one- or two-step approach (ADA, 2004a). The two-step approach consists of ingestion of a 50-g glucose solution (glucola) without consideration of time of day or last meal and obtaining a plasma or serum glucose level 1 hour after ingestion. If the test result is positive, a diagnostic 3-hour 100-g oral glucose tolerance test (OGTT) is administered after an 8-hour fast preceded

DISPLAY 6-26

Criteria for Early Screening for Gestational Diabetes Mellitus (Any One of the Following)

- Diabetes symptoms: polydipsia, polyuria, polyphagia, fatigue, sudden weight loss
- Persistent glycosuria
- Obesity (>150% ideal)
- Polyhydramnios
- Oral beta-mimetic therapy
- Corticosteroid therapy
- Persistent vaginal candidiasis
- Infant with congenital anomalies
- First-degree relative with type 2 diabetes
- Previous glucose intolerance
- Polycystic ovarian syndrome
- History of unexplained fetal death or stillborn
- Multiple spontaneous abortions
- History of fetal macrosomia (>4,000 g)

by 3 days of unrestricted diet and activity. Women should refrain from smoking or eating and should remain seated during testing. Plasma glucose determinations are made at fasting and at 1-, 2-, and 3-hour intervals after ingestion of the glucose solution. In the one-step approach, the screening 50-g test is omitted, and the diagnostic 3-hour OGTT is administered. The 75-g, 2-hour OGTT is another approach for diagnosis that has widespread use in Europe, but has not been endorsed by any diabetes groups in the United States (Metzger & Coustan, 1998). The Hyperglycemia and Adverse Pregnancy Outcomes (HAPO) study is a large international multicenter trial whose aim is to relate the blood glucose levels on the 75-g, 2-hour OGTT to pregnancy outcomes. The results of this trial are expected to be released in 2007.

The positive thresholds of 130 and 140 mg/dL have been used for the screening glucola. A value of 130 mg/dL identifies approximately 90% of women with gestational diabetes, whereas a cutoff of 140 mg/dL misses 10% (ACOG, 2001; ADA, 2004a). The decision for which cutoff to use should be based on cost effectiveness and risk factors in the population to be tested. A result of 200 mg/dL on the glucose challenge is considered diagnostic, alleviating the need for OGTT. However, research has challenged this diagnostic threshold (Atilano, Lee-Parritz, Lieberman, Cohen, & Barbieri, 1999; Shivvers & Lucas, 1999).

Carpenter and Coustan's (1982) criteria (Table 6–15) are recommended for diagnosis of gestational diabetes by the ADA (2004a) and ACOG (2001). Diagnosis is based on meeting or exceeding two thresholds. One abnormal value has been associated with adverse outcomes with 30% of these women exhibiting two abnormal values 1 month later (Langer, Brustman, Anyaegbunam, & Mazze, 1987; Neiger & Coustan, 1991). Women who fail the glucose challenge but pass the oral glucose tolerance test warrant closer surveillance with medical nutrition therapy and blood glucose monitoring or by repeat testing because of a much higher risk of macrosomia

without treatment (Bevier, Fischer, & Jovanovic, 1999). Women who have a fasting plasma glucose level of 120 mg/dL can be diagnosed with this cutoff after a repeat test for confirmation and should not be administered the 100-g glucola (Metztger & Coustan, 1998). Obtaining a hemoglobin A1c value is a prudent approach to determine whether hyperglycemia predates the measurement, which is very likely increasing the risk for the infant and the need for a more aggressive fetal surveillance.

Clinical Manifestations

The clinical manifestations of diabetes occur as a result of hypoglycemia and hyperglycemia. Glycemic goals for pregnancy in women with diabetes reflect the plasma blood glucose values found in pregnant women who do not have diabetes; 60 to 95 mg/dL fasting, 60 to 105 mg/dL before a meal, 140 mg/dL 1 hour after a meal, and 120 mg/dL 2 hours after a meal (ACOG, 2001, 2005). Symptoms of hyperglycemia include polyuria, polydipsia, blurred vision, and polyphagia. However, women with gestational diabetes may experience only nonspecific symptoms such as weakness, lethargy, malaise, and headache (Davidson, 2001).

Hypoglycemia is defined as a plasma glucose level of 60 mg/dL, but significant symptoms may occur at higher levels when the patient's average blood glucose level is higher. Autonomic nervous system stimulation by hypoglycemia results in adrenergic and cholinergic symptoms of pallor, diaphoresis, tachycardia, palpitations, hunger, paresthesias, and shakiness. Moderate hypoglycemia causes glucose deprivation in the central nervous system as evidenced by an inability to concentrate, confusion, slurred speech, irrational behavior, slowed reaction time, blurred vision, numbness, somnolence, or extreme fatigue (Kendrick, 1999). Disorientation, loss of consciousness, seizures, and coma may result from severe hypoglycemia and is primarily seen in type 1 diabetes and not in gestational or type 2 diabetes.

Nursing Assessments and Interventions for Diabetes Mellitus

Evaluation and management of women with diabetes, whether pregestational or gestational, generally occurs on an outpatient basis. Admission may be advisable for uncontrolled diabetes during the period of organogenesis (prior to 8 weeks) or during an episode of illness, DKA, or other obstetric complication. Nurses can have a profound role in education and monitoring of women with diabetes during pregnancy and are vital members of the multidisciplinary diabetes management team. The goal of nursing

---

TABLE 6–15 ■ DIAGNOSTIC CRITERIA FOR GESTATIONAL DIABETES MELLITUS

100-g Oral Glucose Tolerance Test	Threshold Glucose Levels (mg/dL)
Fasting	≥95
1 hr	≥180
2 hr	≥155
3 hr	≥140

Source: From Carpenter, M.W., & Coustan, D. R. (1982). Criteria for screening tests for gestational diabetes. *American Journal of Obstetrics and Gynecology, 144*(7), 768–773.

management focuses on the woman attaining and maintaining self-care behaviors, which result in near-normal blood glucose levels to improve perinatal outcome. Ideally, a team approach should be used to achieve this goal, which includes a physician with expertise in diabetes; medical nutrition therapy by a registered dietitian; exercise; education about self-monitoring of blood glucose and taking medication (as needed) by a registered nurse, preferably a certified diabetes educator (CDE); and stress reduction and management by a behavioral health specialist as needed.

Ambulatory and Home Care Management

Ideally, intensive management of diabetes should begin prior to conception in women with pregestational diabetes. Attaining an A1c <1% above normal before pregnancy will decrease the risk of congenital malformations and spontaneous abortion to that of the general population (ADA, 2004c). Unfortunately, about two thirds of pregnancies are unplanned (ADA), so care should begin immediately on discovery of the pregnancy and continue throughout the perinatal period. The assessment of women with pregestational diabetes should include a thorough history of diabetes type, duration of disease, self-care practices, acute and chronic complication assessment, and a review of current glucose values and a food history of at least 3 days. Knowledge deficits should be identified and an individualized teaching plan outlined during this initial assessment. Psychosocial issues should be explored, evaluated periodically, and appropriate referrals made. Display 6-27 lists information that should be discussed with women who have pregestational diabetes.

When women who have type 1 or type 2 diabetes become pregnant, an educational session should be scheduled as soon as possible with the diabetes educator and registered dietitian before or in conjunction with the initial prenatal visit. The session should include all aspects of medical nutrition therapy, self-monitoring of blood glucose levels, and insulin therapy, including a demonstration by the woman of the correct method for drawing up and self-injection of insulin. Injection sites should be observed for correct regional rotation, as well as for identifying evidence of lipohypertrophy or lipoatrophy, bruising, and signs and symptoms of infection.

Women with type 2 diabetes who have been using oral medications for glucose control should be converted to insulin, ideally before conception or as soon as possible thereafter. Because glycemic control is so important to prevent malformations in the first trimester, women on oral antidiabetes agents should

---

DISPLAY 6-27

Educational Guidelines for Women With Pregestational Diabetes Mellitus

- **Healthy Eating**
  - Medical Nutrition Therapy (MNT)
- **Being Active**
  - 30–60 min per day of activity such as brisk walking
- **Monitoring**
  - Self-monitoring of blood glucose levels (SMBG), 4–8 times per day,
  - Glycemic goals for pregnancy
  - Guidelines for ketone testing
- **Taking Medications**
  - Insulin/oral agent therapy
  - Prenatal vitamins with folic acid
  - Medications for other medical conditions
- **Problem Solving**
  - Sick-day management

- Appropriate treatment of hypoglycemia (correct amount & composition of snack, use of glucagon by family member)
- Signs and symptoms of diabetic ketoacidosis and contributing factors
- When and why to call the healthcare provider
- **Healthy Coping**
  - Psychosocial assessment
  - Barriers to optimal care
- **Reducing Risks**
  - Effect pregnancy has on diabetes
  - Potential for fetal or neonatal complications: intrauterine growth restriction, macrosomia, intrauterine fetal demise, birth trauma, prematurity, respiratory distress syndrome, neonatal metabolic disturbances
  - Potential for maternal complications: preterm delivery, hypertensive disorders, cesarean birth
  - Association of hemoglobin A1c to risk congenital anomalies or spontaneous abortion
  - Schedule of antenatal visits and testing

Adapted from AADE Self-Care Behaviors™. Web site: http://www.diabeteseducator.org/AADE7/index.shtml/#AADE7. Accessed December 12, 2006.

DISPLAY 6-28

Educational Guidelines for Insulin Therapy

- Glycemic goals for treatment
- Onset, peak, and duration of action of insulins to be administered
- Inspection, storage, and traveling with insulin
- Timing of injections, injection technique, site selection, and regional rotation
- Glucagon use and appropriate administration by family or significant other
- Appropriate sick-day management
- Prevention strategies and appropriate management of hypoglycemia
- Syringe disposal guidelines

not stop those agents until insulin is instituted. These women require more extensive education regarding insulin and additional support with this new aspect of their diabetes management. Display 6–28 lists issues to be reviewed in the educational session about insulin.

Treatment of Hypoglycemia

Appropriate management of hypoglycemia should be reviewed with women with pregestational diabetes. Signs and symptoms of hypoglycemia are listed in Display 6–29. They need an explanation that the occurrence will increase with intensive management during pregnancy. The level at which symptoms occur should be determined. If women have hypoglycemia unaware-

DISPLAY 6-29

Signs and Symptoms of Hypoglycemia

- Mental confusion and irritability
- Somnolence
- Slowed reaction time
- Pallor
- Diaphoresis
- Tachycardia
- Palpitations
- Hunger
- Paresthesias
- Shakiness
- Cold, clammy skin
- Blurred vision
- Extreme fatigue

ness, the risk for a potentially fatal nocturnal episode must be avoided. General guidelines for treatment of hypoglycemia during pregnancy include treatment with one carbohydrate exchange for a blood glucose of 60 mg/dL and treatment with two exchanges (liquid and solid preferably) at a level of 40 to 60 mg/dL. Blood glucose should be tested again 15 minutes after treatment of hypoglycemia. Retreatment should occur if the blood glucose level has not risen. Including protein with the carbohydrate decreases the risk for rebound hypoglycemia and provides a more consistent and stable blood glucose level after treatment. Women with evidence of gastroparesis should use liquids for initial treatment of hypoglycemia because of their slower digestion. Carbohydrates ingested for treatment of hypoglycemia should be in addition to the regularly prescribed diet so that glucagon stores may be replenished. Family members and significant others should be instructed on the use of injectable glucagon, and two kits should be readily available at all times.

Sick Day Management

Nurses should also review sick day management and provide written guidelines. Understanding appropriate self-care strategies during episodes of nausea and vomiting of early pregnancy is vital to prevent the development of ketoacidosis. Display 6–30 contains specific information that nurses should review with women about sick day management.

DISPLAY 6-30

Sick-Day Management Educational Guidelines

- Insulin should be given even with vomiting.
- Urine ketones should be checked every 4 to 6 hours and the healthcare provider notified of ≥ moderate results.
- Blood glucose levels should be checked every 1 to 2 hours.
- Healthcare provider should be notified of blood glucose levels ≥200 mg/dL.
- Liquids or soft foods should be consumed equal to the carbohydrate value of the prescribed diet (sugar free for blood glucose levels of >120 mg/dL).
- A sipping diet of 15 to 30 g CHO per hour may be consumed during periods of vomiting.
- Call the healthcare provider if liquids are not tolerated.
- Review signs and symptoms of ketoacidosis to report: abdominal pain, nausea and vomiting, polyuria, polydipsia, fruity breath, leg cramps, altered mental status, and rapid respirations.

Gestational Diabetes

Women who have been diagnosed with GDM need immediate counseling and education. Display 6–31 includes topics that nurses should discuss in the educational session. The diagnosis alone may bring excessive anxiety and fear. Appropriate education and support from the nurse educator should allay the woman's concerns and empower her with the resources she needs to adapt to the diabetic regimen, reducing the risks for perinatal complications. Including family and significant others in the education and care of women with GDM provides another source of support.

Medical Nutrition Therapy

Medical nutrition therapy (MNT) is an integral and vital component in the care of women with diabetes and is best provided by a registered dietitian whenever possible. Therapeutic goals for nutritional intervention are blunting of postprandial hyperglycemia and appropriate nourishment of mother and fetus without excessive weight gain or ketosis. Current recommendations for dietary management include 24 to 30 kcal/kg for normal-weight women, 40 kcal/kg for underweight women, and 24 kcal/kg for overweight women (Jovanovic, 2000a). These calories should be consumed in three meals and three snacks and should contain 40% to 45% carbohydrates, 20% to 25% protein, and 35% to 40% predominately monounsaturated and polyunsaturated fats (Franz et al., 2002). Pregnant women need at least 175 g of carbohydrate per day during pregnancy to support fetal growth (Institute of Medicine, 2002).

A 25- to 35-pound weight gain is encouraged for women with normal prepregnancy weight, 15- to 25-pound weight gain for overweight women, 28 to 40 pounds for underweight women, and 15 pounds or less for morbidly obese women. Nonnutritive sweeteners, including aspartame, saccharin, acesulfame-K, and sucralose appear to be safe to use during pregnancy. Saccharin can cross the placenta, although no adverse effects have been found in humans (Franz et al., 2002). Women should be taking a prenatal vitamin supplement with 400 micrograms of folic acid or 4 mg with a positive family history for neural tube defects, additional iron if anemic, and supplemental calcium for those women who do not consume enough dietary calcium.

Nutritional counseling should be individualized and culturally sensitive. Significant others and family members should be included in educational sessions to provide support. The person who prepares the meals must be a part of counseling and financial constraints determined, although a nutritional diet should not pose a financial burden. The registered dietitian should meet with the woman regularly to assess any dietary problems

---

DISPLAY 6-31

Educational Guidelines for Women With Gestational Diabetes Mellitus

- **Healthy Eating**
  - Medical Nutrition Therapy (MNT)
- **Being Active**
  - 30–60 min per day of activity such as brisk walking
- **Monitoring**
  - Technique of meter use
  - Self-monitoring of blood glucose levels (SMBG), 4 times per day
  - Glycemic goals for pregnancy
  - Guidelines for ketone testing
- **Taking Medications**
  - Insulin/oral agent therapy as needed
  - Prenatal vitamins
  - Medications for other conditions

- **Problem Solving**
  - Appropriate treatment of hypoglycemia (correct amount & composition of snack)
  - When and why to call healthcare provider
- **Healthy Coping**
  - Psychosocial assessment
  - Barriers to optimal care
- **Reducing Risks**
  - Explanation of abnormal results from prenatal glucose test
  - Role of glucose and insulin transport and effect of placental hormones
  - Potential for fetal or neonatal complications: intrauterine fetal demise, macrosomia, birth trauma, respiratory distress syndrome, neonatal metabolic disturbances
  - Potential for maternal complications: polyhydramnios, hypertensive disorders, Cesarean delivery
  - Schedule of antenatal visits and testing

Adapted from AADE Self-Care Behaviors™. Web site: http://www.diabeteseducator.org/AADE7/index.shtml/#AADE7. Accessed December 12, 2006.

and to reevaluate nutritional needs after the initial session. More frequent visits are required for women with excessive or low weight gain.

Exercise Therapy

Exercise should be used adjunctively with dietary management of diabetes (ADA, 2004b). The glucose-lowering mechanism of exercise is unknown but may be related to increased insulin sensitivity, improved first-phase insulin release, and increased caloric expenditure (Carpenter, 2000; Langer, 2000). Specific types of exercise that are most beneficial for glucose control have not been determined, although a minimum of three episodes per week for 20 minutes seems to be necessary (Langer). Sweet Success (CDAPP, 2002) recommends daily activity of 30 to 60 minutes per day. Activity can be divided into 10- to 20-minute sessions after each meal. Women with pregestational diabetes who are poorly controlled or who have vascular disease should avoid vigorous exercise during pregnancy. Walking and swimming are two forms of exercise with minimal risk and may be the exercise of choice for previously sedentary women. Safety considerations before implementing an exercise program should be thoroughly discussed, particularly for women with pregestational diabetes. Display 6–32 lists general guidelines for education of women who plan to exercise during their pregnancy. Women should be counseled to discontinue exercise if uterine activity occurs. The nurse should review the glucose log to evaluate the effect of exercise on blood sugar values and make appropriate food or insulin adjustment recommendations. The feet and lower extremities should be inspected for blisters, bruising, or other evidence of trauma. Exercise change may be required or a change in footwear needed.

Metabolic Monitoring

Metabolic monitoring during pregnancy is directed at detecting hyperglycemia and hypoglycemia and making pharmacologic, dietary, or activity adjustments to maintain euglycemia. Rather than preprandial values, postprandial blood glucose determinations appear to be the most influential in the development of fetal hyperinsulinemia (ADA, 2004a). Daily self-monitoring of blood glucose in women with gestational diabetes has been found to be superior to intermittent office monitoring (ADA). Daily self-monitoring allows the woman to know immediately the effect of food intake or activity on her blood sugar. In women with GDM, blood sugar levels should be checked at a minimum of four-times-daily fasting and 1 to 2 hours after the first bite of each meal. Table 6–16 lists the target glycemic values for pregnancy. These values are usually easily attainable in women with GDM and type 2 diabetes but may be unrealistic in women with type 1 diabetes who have hypoglycemia unawareness and are more difficult to control. Women with pregestational diabetes should check their blood sugar levels four to eight times daily, depending on their level of control. These determinations may be obtained fasting, preprandial, postprandial, bedtime, and at 2 AM to 3 AM for women with a history of nocturnal hypoglycemia. Titration of insulin is smoother when based on multiple blood glucose determinations.

Women with GDM and type 2 diabetes who are on hypocaloric diets (<1,800 kcal/day) should test their urine daily from the first void for ketones to exclude starvation ketosis (ADA, 2004a). Calories should be added at the bedtime snack if ketones are detected. Women with type 1 diabetes are asked to test their urine for ketones daily from the first void and with any blood glucose level of 200 mg/dL (Homko & Sargrad, 2003) or greater because of the increased risk for ketoacidosis. They should also be instructed to call their healthcare provider if they detect moderate levels of ketones.

DISPLAY 6-32

Exercise Guidelines

- Proper footwear with silica gel or air midsoles
- Polyester or polyester–cotton-blend socks to promote dryness and prevent blisters
- Wear a visible diabetes identification
- Carbohydrate (CHO) consumption when blood glucose <100 mg/dL and have CHO snack readily available
- Blood glucose before and after exercise (type 1)
- Adequate hydration during and after exercise
- Consult healthcare provider to assist with insulin adjustments

TABLE 6–16 ■ GLYCEMIC GOALS FOR PREGNANCY

Timing	Plasma Glucose Levels (mg/dL)
Fasting	≤95
Preprandial	≤100
Postprandial	1 hr: ≤140
	2 hr: ≤120
2 to 6 AM	60–100

Adapted from American College of Obstetricians and Gynecologists. (2005). *Pregestational diabetes mellitus* (Technical Bulletin No. 60). Washington, DC: Author.

All women with diabetes are asked to keep a log of their blood sugars, insulin doses, exercise or activity level, food intake with any abnormal values (high or low), and ketone checks when necessary. These logs allow the nurse and healthcare provider to accurately evaluate and make necessary adjustments at office visits. These visits should occur weekly for women having insulin adjustments or those with identified problems. Telephone contact may be necessary to supplement visits. Visits should occur every other week for women with well-controlled diabetes, whether pregestational or gestational, until the latter half of the third trimester.

The care and use of a blood glucose meter should be reviewed with the woman. Whole blood glucose values are approximately 14% below laboratory plasma glucose determinations. Most meters are calibrated to provide plasma values by increasing the capillary result. Nurses need to know the limits of the meters their patients are using. For women who are newly diagnosed with GDM, a more intensive instructional session should be provided. Meters that have memory capability with date and time are important so that the nurse can correlate the values in the meter to those recorded by the woman. Studies have shown that a significant number of patients supply false blood sugar values, which can be detrimental to perinatal outcome if not detected (Langer & Mazze, 1986; Mazze et al., 1984; Moses, 1986). If false blood glucose readings have been reported, fears or contributory psychosocial issues should be explored. Sometimes, an underlying fear of insulin by women with GDM contributes to this phenomenon. These women need additional support and education and possibly referral for counseling.

Pharmacologic Therapy

Insulin is the only pharmacologic agent shown to reduce fetal morbidity in conjunction with nutrition therapy in women with pregestational or gestational diabetes (ADA, 2004a, 2004c; Jovanovic, 2000b). Insulin requirements during pregnancy increase dramatically from the first to third trimester as the anti-insulin hormones rise and peripheral resistance increases.

Requirements in the first trimester may be slightly reduced because of the nausea and vomiting of pregnancy. The average insulin requirement in the first trimester is 0.7 U/kg of ideal body weight, 0.8 U/kg in the second, and 0.9 to 1.0 U/kg in the third trimester (Homko & Sargrad, 2003). These dosages are merely recommended averages requiring titration to blood glucose levels and activity for individualized management.

Glucose control during pregnancy requires intensive insulin management in women with type 1 diabetes, usually three to four injections per day. Women with type 2 or GDM may require less frequent injections.

For example, many women with GDMA$_2$ require only bedtime intermediate-acting insulin to control fasting hyperglycemia. During the day they are able to use diet and exercise to manage postmeal excursions of glucose. Morbidly obese women with GDM or type 2 diabetes may require more than 1 U/kg to achieve euglycemia.

Several rapid-acting insulin analogs (lispro, aspart, and glulisine) are now available for postmeal control. They have a quicker onset of action (10–15 minutes) and peak effect (60 minutes) than regular insulin. Lispro (Jovanovic et al., 1999) and aspart (Pettitt, Ospina, Kolaczynski, & Jovanovic, 2003) are considered safe to use during pregnancy and may help prevent hypoglycemia between meals. Intermediate-acting human NPH insulin is used for basal insulin needs. Two long-acting insulin analogs (glargine and detemir) have also been introduced. There are several case reports of glargine use during pregnancy (Devlin, Hothersall, & Wilkis, 2002; DiCianni et al., 2005; Woolderink, vanLoon, Storms, deHeide, & Hoogenber, 2005), but there are no well-controlled studies in humans. More studies are needed in this area before glargine or detemir can be recommended for use during pregnancy (Gamson, Chia, & Jovanovic, 2004).

For women with GDM who fail to achieve euglycemia (see Table 6–16) with diet and exercise, insulin therapy should be initiated. Insulin is initiated when fetal bovine serum (FBS) values are 95 mg/dL or higher, 1-hour postprandial blood glucose values are 130 to 140 mg/dL or higher and 2-hour postprandial blood glucose values are 120 mg/dL or higher (ACOG, 2001). Insulin is required for 30% to 60% of women with GDM (Langer, Conway, Berkus, Xenakis, & Gonzales, 1994). The insulin regimen should be individualized depending on what time of day blood glucose levels are elevated. Some centers may calculate doses based on body weight and gestational age, whereas others may use a standard starting dose and make adjustments based on blood glucose values (Biastre & Slocum, 2003). The educational session should follow the guidelines for insulin therapy in women with pregestational diabetes (see Display 6–28). Women who are injecting insulin for the first time are very fearful and require much support and encouragement from the nurse and family members. They need to be reassured that they have not failed to control their glucose levels.

Occasionally, a woman may not be able to correctly draw up her insulin. In those situations, a home health referral can be made, another family member can be taught, or the nurse can draw the appropriate insulin to be refrigerated before use. Prefilled syringes may be safely refrigerated for up to 30 days. Prefilled insulin pens may be an option for women who have difficulty mixing insulins in one syringe. For women with needle phobias, self-injectors may be used. Women should be educated that insulin requirements normally increase as the pregnancy progresses and reassured that rising insulin needs do not represent a failure in the woman's ability to follow such a complex medical regimen.

Continuous Subcutaneous Insulin Infusion

Another method for intensive metabolic management in pregnancy is the use of CSII, or the insulin pump. An insulin pump involves an electronic device that is programmed to deliver rapid-acting insulin subcutaneously through an implanted catheter. Lispro and aspart insulins are most commonly used in pumps. A continuous low-dose amount of basal insulin is infused, and boluses are given for meals and snacks based on carbohydrate intake. The catheter is changed every 2 to 3 days. The use of CSII in pregnancy requires careful patient selection, and only those who are very motivated and capable of using a sophisticated electronic device should be chosen. The risk for pump use during pregnancy is pump malfunction that can lead to the rapid development of DKA. This risk can be reduced by educating the woman to self-inject rapid-acting insulin and check the pump for blood glucose levels of >200 mg/dL.

Switching from conventional insulin therapy to pump therapy can be done on an inpatient or outpatient basis, individualizing the decision according to the level of family support and needs of the woman. The total daily insulin dose is reduced by 25%; 40% is given as basal insulin, and the remaining 60% is given as boluses. Boluses may be given as 20% at breakfast, 15% before lunch, and 15% before dinner (Jornsay, 1998) or calculated using an insulin-to-carbohydrate ratio (Walsh & Roberts, 2006). Another method for determining the insulin dose for CSII is based on patient weight and gestational age. Dosing is based on 0.8 U/kg in the first trimester, 1.0 U/kg in the second trimester, and 1.2 U/kg in the third trimester, and then reduced by 20% (Gabbe, 2000). Boluses for snacks may or may not be required. Single basal rates are not recommended on initiation because of the increased risk of nocturnal hypoglycemia; therefore, a lower basal rate should be infused during the early nighttime hours (Jornsay, 1998). However, because of the strong "dawn phenomenon" associated with pregnancy, an increased basal rate may be needed after 3 AM.

Self-monitoring of blood glucose (SMBG) should be done often. At a minimum, blood glucose levels should be checked while fasting, before meals, after meals, and at bedtime. Checks are required at 2 AM to 3 AM during nighttime adjustments to avoid hypoglycemia or hyperglycemia. Close contact with the diabetes management team becomes a vital component of successful insulin pump therapy during pregnancy.

Oral Antidiabetes Agents

Oral antidiabetes agents are not currently recommended by the ADA or ACOG for use during pregnancy because there is insufficient data to recommend for or against their use. Insulin is still the drug of choice to treat diabetes during pregnancy (ADA, 2004a, 2004c; ACOG 2001).

However, the use of these agents has become a focus of controversy, research, and debate. Early studies questioned whether adverse outcomes of pregnancy were due to the medication, usually first-generation sulfonylureas, or poor glycemic control at the time of conception. Many new antidiabetes medications have been introduced in recent years and research is taking place to look at the use, efficacy, and pregnancy outcomes of women using some of these agents (Slocum & Sosa, 2002).

Langer, Conway, Berkus, Xenakis, and Gonzales (2000) published the first randomized controlled trial comparing the use of glyburide and insulin in 404 women with GDM. Glyburide is a second-generation sulfonylurea, which stimulates beta cells to produce more insulin. Both groups had similar rates of macrosomia and cesarean section, and glyburide was not detected in the cord blood of any infants. They concluded that glyburide was safe to use in women with GDM. Several authors (Conway, Gonzales, & Skiver, 2004; Jacobson et al., 2005) have published their experiences with using glyburide in women with GDM. Many providers are now offering glyburide to women as an alternative to insulin therapy. This topic was discussed at the 5th International Conference/Workshop on GDM, and recommendations are expected to be published in 2007.

Metformin is a medication that works in the liver to prevent the conversion of glycogen to glucose and prevents its release into the circulation, which helps to decrease fasting glucose levels. It also reduces peripheral insulin resistance, making tissues more sensitive to insulin. Metformin may be used alone or in combination with other antidiabetes agents. If used with insulin, it can decrease the amount of insulin needed to control glucose levels. There is a great deal of research in the use of metformin in women with polycystic ovary syndrome (PCOS) (Slocum & Sosa, 2002).

PCOS is a condition characterized by hyperinsulinemia, chronic anovulation, oligomenorrhea, and hyperandrogenism. It affects approximately 5% of women of reproductive age and is a common cause of infertility (Kocak, Caliskan, Simsir, & Haberal, 2002). Some studies (Kocak, Caliskan, Simsir, & Haberal; Vandermolen et al., 2001) have shown that metformin, by improving insulin sensitivity, can restore ovulatory function and improve pregnancy rates in women with PCOS when used alone or in combination with clomiphene citrate. Other studies (Glueck, Goldenberg, Wang, Loftspring, & Sherman, 2004; Jakubowicz, Iuorno, Jakubowicz,

Roberts, & Nestler, 2002;) show that continuing met-formin can decrease the rate of first trimester miscar-riage and, if continued throughout pregnancy, can decrease the incidence of gestational diabetes in women with PCOS (Glueck, Wang, Goldenberg, & Sieve-Smith, 2002). Many women with PCOS present for prenatal care having taken metformin during organogenesis and may be reluctant to discontinue the medication. Some providers advocate discontinuing metformin on discov-ery of the pregnancy, whereas others will continue met-formin until the end of the first trimester, and still others would continue the metformin throughout pregnancy.

Metformin is also being researched for the treatment of gestational diabetes. A large trial, the Metformin in Gestational Diabetes (MiG) Study is currently under-way in Australia and New Zealand (Hague, Davoren, Oliver, & Rowan, 2003), comparing metformin with insulin therapy in the treatment of GDM. Even if these agents are found to be safe to use during pregnancy, the long-terms effects of these medications on the mother and the offspring is still unknown.

Fetal Assessment

The best method and the appropriate time to begin antepartum fetal assessment for pregnant women with diabetes have yet to be determined. Most recommend beginning some form of fetal assessment in the third trimester for women with pregestational diabetes (ACOG, 2005; Jovanovic, 2000b). Testing of women with GDM controlled by diet may be delayed until near term (Landon, 2000). Those controlled by insulin should begin earlier in the third trimester, or 32 to 36 weeks as has been suggested (Homko, 1998; Landon). Fetal movement counting is a simple, inexpensive, and appropriate test to begin in all pregnant women with diabetes in the beginning of the third trimester. Women with vascular disease need more intensive fetal and maternal surveillance, requiring a nonstress test, contraction stress testing, or biophysical profile (Lan-don). Table 6–17 provides a sample schedule to con-sider for fetal testing in women with diabetes. Display 6–33 is a summary of home care management for women with diabetes.

Inpatient Management

Women with diabetes require hospitalization during periods of poor control for intensive insulin adjustment, particularly if they are in the critical time of organogene-sis (6 to 8 weeks' gestation). Hospitalization may also be required during periods of illness for women with dehy-dration and is always required for those in diabetic ketoacidosis (DKA). Women who develop complications of pregnancy, such as preterm labor or preeclampsia may require hospitalization during the third trimester for more intensive maternal and fetal surveillance.

Diabetic Ketoacidosis

DKA is characterized by severe hyperglycemia, keto-sis, acidosis, dehydration, and electrolyte imbalance (Davidson, 2001). Kussmaul respirations develop in an effort to correct the ensuing metabolic acidosis. Acetone breath develops as ketone bodies are con-verted to acetone and excreted by the lungs. Dehydra-tion occurs as a result of hyperglycemia (Whiteman, Homko, & Reece, 1996). Altered consciousness levels, including coma, are usually present (Davidson, 2001). The diagnosis of DKA is based on the laboratory find-ings of a blood glucose level of more than 300 mg/dL, a bicarbonate level below 15 mEq/L, and an arterial pH of less than 7.2 (Davidson, 2001).

Care of women in DKA should occur in a tertiary care facility with the support services that can provide intensive care. Nurses in community hospitals should be capable of stabilizing the woman in preparation for, and during transport to, an appropriate facility.

Table 6–18 lists specific interventions nurses use in the care of women experiencing DKA. Initial treatment measures focus on rehydration, which improves tissue perfusion, insulin delivery, and a physiologic lowering of blood glucose by hemodilution. After intravenous access is established, insulin is administered as ordered to lower blood glucose. Caution should be exercised in lowering the blood glucose, because too rapid a fall results in the serious complication of cerebral edema. With improve-ment of the intravascular status, fluid shifts result in a potassium deficit that requires replacement. Nurses should continually assess the woman for signs and symptoms of hypokalemia and monitor electrolyte levels in preparation for replacement. Adequate urinary out-put must also be maintained with potassium replace-ment to avoid hyperkalemia. In addition to monitoring laboratory electrolyte status, the complete blood cell count and differential also should be monitored, as well as the clinical status for signs and symptoms of infection. Evidence of infection requires prompt and aggressive treatment for DKA treatment to be effective.

Fetal monitoring, even in previable gestations, pro-vides an indication of hydration and perfusion status and should be instituted immediately. Nonreassuring fetal status is expected but resolves as the mother is sta-bilized and should not be an indication for emergent cesarean birth, which could further compromise the mother (Chauhan & Perry, 1995). Maternal oxygena-tion status should be monitored continually and oxy-gen administered based on blood gas determinations, bedside oxygen saturation levels, and fetal status. Uter-ine activity also is associated with severe dehydration but resolves in most cases with improved perfusion. Treatment for preterm labor should not be considered in the absence of cervical change, because the use of α-adrenergic agonists or steroids worsens the clinical picture by antagonizing insulin. Magnesium sulfate is

TABLE 6–17 ■ FETAL SURVEILLANCE FOR WOMEN WITH DIABETES

Gestational Age (Weeks)	Type 1 or 2: Poorly Controlled or with Vascular Disease	Type 1 or 2: Well Controlled, No Vascular Disease	GDM A$_1$ (Diet Controlled)	GDM A$_2$ (Insulin Controlled)
6–8	Sonographic estimation of gestational age	Same		
16–19	Maternal serum alpha-fetoprotein	Same	Same	Same
20–22	High-resolution sonography, fetal echocardiography	High-resolution sonography, fetal echocardiography		
26–28	Sonographic assessment of interval growth	Same		
28	Twice-daily fetal movement counting (FMC), weekly nonstress test (NST)	Twice-daily FMC	Twice-daily FMC	Twice-daily FMC
32	Twice-weekly NST or weekly biophysical profile, sonographic assessment of interval growth	Weekly NST, then increase to twice weekly at 34–36 weeks		Weekly NST, then increase to twice weekly at 34–36 weeks
36–38	Sonographic estimation of fetal weight	Sonographic estimation of fetal weight	Sonographic estimation of fetal weight, weekly NST	Sonographic estimation of fetal weight
36–39	Consider amniocentesis and delivery with worsening disease			
39–40	Elective delivery without amniocentesis	Elective delivery without amniocentesis	Consider elective delivery if cervix favorable and for large for gestational age (LGA) fetus	Consider elective delivery if cervix favorable and for LGA fetus

the drug of choice for treatment of preterm labor because it does not interfere with the action of insulin.

After DKA has been corrected, the underlying cause—whether infection or poor self-care practices—should be discussed with the mother and family, outlining early detection and prevention strategies. For mothers whose infants did not survive, intensive grief support and follow-up should be provided.

Intrapartum Management: Pregestational and Gestational Diabetes Mellitus

Intrapartum management of women with diabetes requires skilled nursing care to prevent maternal and neonatal complications. Plasma glucose levels should be maintained at 70 to 110 mg/dL for capillary blood determinations (Homko, 1998). Hyperglycemia in labor contributes to the development of neonatal hypoglycemia. Blood glucose should be assessed on the first laboratory blood draw and then checked at the bedside every 1 to 2 hours for all women who have previously been controlled by insulin. Women with GDM who have been controlled by diet may have their blood glucose levels checked every 2 to 4 hours. Ketones should be checked with every void or every 4 hours if euglycemia is maintained.

Intravenous access should be established early so that hydration can be maintained, and insulin should be administered when necessary. Women with GDM

DISPLAY 6-33

Home Care Management of Pregnant Women With Diabetes

The following diagnostic criteria and considerations are suggested for home care management of women with diabetes:

- Patient and family willingness and ability to learn and follow diet, perform blood glucose monitoring, and insulin adjustment and administration if needed
- Family member knowledge of signs and symptoms of severe hypoglycemia and ability to administer glucagon (0.05 mg) subcutaneously if this should occur
- Family member knowledge of how and when to call for emergency assistance
- A safe and clean storage place for insulin and other supplies
- Absence of abnormal laboratory values. Glycemic control can be assessed over time (previous 4–6 weeks) using measurements of glycosylated hemoglobin (A1c). Fasting and random blood glucose levels provide information about blood glucose levels at the time of testing.

The following parameters should be assessed based on the individual clinical situation. Protocols or physician orders are used to determine threshold for each parameter:

- Diabetes care should be reviewed with the woman and family, including blood glucose monitoring, urine testing for ketones, diet, and insulin administration
- Assessment for skill in blood glucose monitoring as ordered, including trouble-shooting equipment problems
- Review of record of daily dietary intake, blood glucose levels, daily weights, urine testing for ketones, and medications
- Assessment for insulin self-injection

- Home or office visit for comprehensive maternal–fetal assessment, including fundal height, review of daily fetal movement counting log (after 24 weeks' gestation), auscultation fetal heart rate or NST one to two times weekly after 26 to 28 weeks
- Sick-day care management guidelines should be reviewed with the woman and family to ensure knowledge of how to make adjustments in insulin dosages if needed to offset altered food
- Assessment for development of complications such as preterm labor, pregnancy-induced hypertension (PIH), bleeding, or infection
- Review of warning signs to report to primary care provider: hyperglycemia (blood glucose level >200 mg/dL), decreased fetal movement, illness (especially if dietary intake is altered), skin breakdown, visual or neurologic symptoms, and signs of renal involvement

MEDICATIONS

- Insulin (as prescribed) or oral agents
- Prenatal vitamins and iron

DIET

- Invidualized meal plan as recommended by healthcare provider. Current recommendations for dietary management include 24–30 kcal/kg for normal-weight women, 40 kcal/kg for underweight women, and 24 kcal/kg for overweight women. These calories should be consumed in three meals and three snacks, comprising 40% to 50% carbohydrates, 20% to 25% protein, and 35% to 40% predominately monounsaturated and polyunsaturated fats.

ACTIVITY

- Activities of daily living
- Exercise within parameters recommended by the healthcare provider

---

and type 2 diabetes may not require insulin during labor. Those with type 1 diabetes will usually require glucose and insulin at some point. If, on admission, the blood glucose level of a woman with type 1 diabetes is 70 mg/dL or below, an infusion with 5% dextrose should be initiated at a rate of 100 to 125 mL/hour (Hagay & Reece, 1992). A main line is required, usually of normal saline, at least to keep open (TKO). All glucose-containing solutions and insulin-containing solutions should be piggybacked to the main line at ports closest to the hub of IV insertion. These are basic safety measures. Insulin administration should be initiated according to institutional protocol. Women who present in spontaneous labor who have taken their intermediate-acting insulin may not require insulin during labor but will need a glucose infusion on admission to avoid hypoglycemia.

A standardized solution of 100 U of regular human insulin (there is no advantage to using analogs when administering IV) to 100 mL of normal saline should be used—again for safety purposes. When a woman is NPO (nothing per mouth), a rate of 1 U (1 mL) per hour usually is all that is necessary. Most insulin algorithms require IV insulin adjustments according to at least hourly blood glucose levels. Polyvinyl tubing should be flushed thoroughly (at least 50 mL) to allow saturation of the insulin to the tubing, allowing the prescribed dose to be infused consistently. Glucose and insulin should be maintained on pumps to avoid overdosage of either solution. Because of the higher risk for operative birth, no oral intake should be allowed during active labor for women with diabetes.

TABLE 6–18 ■ NURSING MANAGEMENT OF DIABETIC KETOACIDOSIS

Treatment	Nursing Intervention
Fluid Resuscitation	1. Obtain large-bore peripheral access. 2. Anticipate need for hemodynamic monitoring. 3. Administer fluids as ordered, usually 1,000 to 2,000 mL of normal saline over 1 to 2 hr, then 200 to 250 mL/hr. 4. Assess for signs and symptoms of pulmonary edema—dyspnea, tachypnea, wheezing, cough. 5. Assess for hypovolemia; check vital signs every 15 min; report decrease in blood pressure, increased pulse rate, decrease in central venous and pulmonary capillary wedge pressure, and slow capillary refill. 6. Insert Foley catheter for oliguria or anuria and send specimen for urinalysis, culture, and sensitivity. 7. Hourly intake and output—report <30 mL/hr. 8. Administer 5% dextrose solution at blood glucose level of 180 mg/dL to prevent hypoglycemia.
Insulin Therapy	1. Administer intravenous insulin as ordered—10 to 20 U of regular insulin as bolus, then 5 to 10 U/hr. Follow hospital insulin/dextrose drip algorithm if established. 2. Hourly capillary blood glucose determinations (lab correlation with each draw). 3. Double dosage as ordered if 10% blood glucose decrease is not achieved in 1 hr. Follow hospital insulin/dextrose drip algorithm if established. 4. Notify physician when blood glucose level of 200 mg/dL is reached, anticipating a decrease in insulin infusion rate to 1 to 2 U/hr. 5. Monitor for hypoglycemia. 6. Monitor for cerebral edema—headache, vomiting, deteriorating mental status, bradycardia, sluggish pupillary light reflex, widened pulse pressure.
Electrolyte Replacement	1. Obtain electrocardiogram and report ST segment depression, inverted T waves, and appearance of U waves after T waves. 2. Obtain hourly laboratory electrolyte levels. 3. Anticipate potassium replacement within 2 to 4 hr.
Oxygenation	1. Establish the airway. 2. Anticipate placement of the peripheral arterial catheter. 3. Obtain initial arterial blood gases, then hourly until pH of 7.20 maintained. 4. Administer oxygen at 10 L/min by a nonrebreather facemask to maintain oxygen saturations of 95% per pulse oximeter. 5. Anticipate the need for intubation/mechanical ventilation. 6. Use continuous pulse oximetry. 7. Administer bicarbonate as ordered for pH of 7.10.
Fetal or Uterine Monitoring	1. Lateral recumbent position. 2. Apply external fetal or uterine monitoring (EFM). 3. Observe EFM for evidence of fetal compromise. 4. Observe for uterine activity. 5. Administer tocolytics as ordered (magnesium sulfate or drug of choice). 6. Avoid beta-adrenergic agonists and steroids.

Adapted from Kendrick, J. M. (2004). *Diabetes in pregnancy* (3rd ed.) (Nursing Module). White Plains, NY: March of Dimes Birth Defects Foundation.

Insulin is partially catabolized in the kidney, and in women with nephropathy, the action is unpredictable, requiring closer surveillance of blood sugar levels. Prehydration for conduction anesthesia or intravenous boluses should use non–glucose-containing solutions and be administered more slowly in the presence of vascular disease. Lactated Ringer's solution should be avoided in women with type 1 diabetes because of its gluconeogenic properties (Hirsch, McGill, Cryer, & White, 1991).

Women with diabetes may have scheduled induction or cesarean births. Early morning admissions are preferred, withholding the morning insulin dose, with IV glucose and insulin initiated.

Cervical ripening and induction procedures should follow institutional protocols and physician orders. Continuous fetal monitoring should be used and assessed for signs of fetal compromise. Labor abnormalities that would indicate potential cephalopelvic disproportion should be monitored closely. Nurses caring for women during labor with diabetes should prepare for assisted birth and the possibility of shoulder dystocia. The birth of a potentially high-risk newborn should also be anticipated and preparation made for full resuscitation. A neonatal team should be present at the birth or immediately available.

Hypoglycemia during labor is usually avoided with close monitoring but should be recognized and treated aggressively. Observation for signs and symptoms of hypoglycemia should be a continuous nursing assessment. Display 6–29 contains typical signs and symptoms of mild and moderate hypoglycemia. Concentrated dextrose solutions (10% and 50%) should be maintained at the bedside. Treatment should be initiated at a blood glucose level of 60 mg/dL by discontinuing insulin. For women with GDM A_2 or type 2 diabetes, increasing the D5 to 200 per hour for 15 minutes may be all that is required to raise the blood glucose level to 70 mg/dL. The insulin drip can then be restarted at an adjusted algorithm or when the blood glucose is 110 mg/dL. However, women with type 1 will need more aggressive treatment—administering 300 mL of 5% dextrose over 10 to 15 minutes or, if fluid restricted, 10 mL of 50% dextrose (Kendrick, 1999). The blood sugar should be rechecked after the bolus and further treatment should be administered if the blood glucose remains low. If the woman becomes unconscious, the physician should be notified immediately, and 50% dextrose should infused intravenously over 5 to 10 minutes (Kendrick). Vital signs should be assessed every 5 to 10 minutes during episodes of hypoglycemia, including blood glucose checks, until a threshold of 80 mg/dL is reached. Insulin should be resumed when the blood glucose level reaches 120 mg/dL according to a laboratory assessment or 110 mg/dL for a capillary blood glucose determination.

Postpartum Management

Pregestational Diabetes Mellitus

Insulin requirements decrease in the immediate postpartum period when the levels of circulating anti-insulin placental hormones drop (Kjos, 2000). Insulin and glucose infusions should be discontinued immediately after a vaginal birth. After cesarean births, the insulin infusion should be decreased by 50% until eating is resumed (Miller, 1994). With oral intake, subcutaneous insulin can be resumed at the prepregnancy dosage or based on postpartum weight (Neiger & Kendrick, 1994) or at one-half to one-third the pregnancy dose for women with types 1 and 2 diabetes. Strict glycemic control can be relaxed somewhat in the postpartum period.

Women with diabetes have a higher incidence of postpartum infection (mastitis, endometritis, wound infection). Therefore, nurses should observe for signs and symptoms and notify the physician if they occur. Women who have delivered a macrosomic infant or have had prolonged or induced labors should be closely monitored for hemorrhage.

Contraceptive options should be explored with the woman and her partner, and pregnancy planning should be encouraged to allow for preconception care to decrease the risks for spontaneous abortion and congenital defects in future pregnancies. Counseling and education should be provided regarding long-term consequences of diabetes and the need for glycemic control to decrease adverse sequelae.

Breastfeeding

Breastfeeding is highly recommended for at least 6 months and ideally for 12 months. Breastfeeding has been associated with reduced incidence of childhood obesity and diabetes later in life (Mayer-Davis et al., 2006). There is evidence that it may help reduce or delay the onset of type 2 diabetes in women with GDM (Kjos, Henry, Lee, Buchanan, & Mishell, 1993).

Insulin has generally been recommended for women with type 2 diabetes who choose to breastfeed their babies who cannot achieve normoglycemia by treatment with medical nutriton therapy and exercise alone (California Diabetes and Pregnancy Program [CDAPP], 2002). However, two recent studies indicate that some oral hypoglycemic agents (glyburied, glipizide, and metformin) may be safe for use while breastfeeding (Briggs, Ambrose, Nageotte, Padilla, & Wan, 2005; Feig et al., 2005). Women with type 2 diabetes who will not be breastfeeding may resume oral hypoglycemic agents.

Caloric needs mandate recalculation based on postpartum body weight and on possible lactation requirements. For obese women, a program for exercise and dietary management for weight loss should be outlined. Breastfeeding should be encouraged with adequate support from the nursing staff. Lactating mothers need assistance to prevent hypoglycemia while nursing, which may require additional snacks. Most breastfeeding mothers require less insulin due to extra calories expended with nursing (Homko & Sargrad, 2003) and the use of maternal glucose to produce the lactase in her milk (Murtaugh, Ferris, Capacchione, & Reece, 1998)

Gestational Diabetes Mellitus

Most women revert to normal glucose tolerance in the postpartum period. Reclassification of glycemic status should be obtained at the 6-week postpartum visit for all women with GDM. A fasting plasma glucose may be more convenient and less costly, but a 75-g 2-hour oral glucose tolerance test (OGTT) will more accurately identify women with impaired glucose tolerance (Conway & Langer, 1999). If the glucose level is normal, repeat testing should occur at 1 year from the birth of the baby and then at a minimum of 3-year intervals or when pregnancy is being considered (ADA, 2004a). Women with impaired fasting glucose (IFG) or impaired glucose tolerance (IGT, also known as prediabetes) should be tested yearly with a fasting blood sugar (ADA, 2004a). Sweet Success recommends repeating the 75-g 2-hour OGTT every 3 years (CDAPP, 2005) Any abnormal value requires repeat testing on another day (ADA, 2004a). Table 6–19 lists the criteria for diagnosis of diabetes mellitus from FPG, 75-g OGTT, and random testing. The risk for development of overt diabetes after GDM increases with time. Risk factors related to the development of overt diabetes include gestational age at diagnosis, degree of abnormality of the diagnostic GTT, level of glycemia at the first postpartum visit, and the presence of obesity (ACOG, 2001). Counseling should be provided to women with a history of GDM in the postpartum period for risk-reducing strategies such as weight

reduction by diet and exercise. The Diabetes Prevention Program Research Group (2002) showed that a lifestyle modification program could decrease the incidence of type 2 diabetes by 58%. Women also need to know the signs and symptoms of hyperglycemia that would warrant testing for diabetes such as polyuria, polydipsia, polyphagia, persistent vaginal candidiasis, frequent UTIs, excessive fatigue and hunger, or sudden weight loss. Women also should be informed that the risk for GDM development in subsequent pregnancies has been reported as high as 70% (Major de Veciana, Weeks, & Morgan, 1998). Testing for diabetes is encouraged before conception or in the first trimester, with early prenatal care to allow intensive management of overt diabetes, which carries a higher perinatal risk than for GDM.

CARDIAC DISEASE

Significance and Incidence

Cardiac disease is a factor in only 1% to 2% of pregnancies, yet is one of the leading causes of pregnancy-related mortality in the United States (Berg, Chang, Callaghan, & Whitehead, 2003; Chang et al., 2003; Christiansen & Collins, 2006: Horon, 2005). Approximately 15% of pregnancy-related deaths in the United States are related to cardiac disease (Berg, Chang, Callaghan, & Whitehead; Chang et al.). Although the incidence of women with cardiac disease has not changed significantly over the last 70 years in the US, the maternal mortality rate has decreased from 6% in 1930 to .05% to 2.7% in 2003 (Klein & Galan, 2004). Neonatal death secondary to underlying maternal cardiac disease ranges from 3% to 50% and also is related to an increased incidence of neonatal complications (Earing & Webb, 2005; Kafka, Johnson, & Gatzoulis, 2006; Silver, 2007; Siu et al., 2002).

Some of the more common cardiac diseases seen in pregnant women are rheumatic heart disease, congenital

---

TABLE 6–19 ■ CRITERIA FOR DIAGNOSIS OF DIABETES MELLITUS

Normoglycemia	IFG and IGT (Prediabetes)	Diabetes Mellitus

FPG <100 mg/dL
2-hr plasma glucose <140 mg/dL
	FPG ≥100 mg/dL and <126 mg/dL (IFG)
	2-hr plasma glucose ≥140 mg/dL
	    and <200 mg/dL (IGT)
		FPG ≥126 mg/dL
		2-hr plasma glucose ≥200
		    mg/dL
		Symptoms of the disease and
		    casual plasma glucose of
		    ≥200 mg/dL

FPG, fasting plasma glucose; IFG, impaired fasting glucose; IGT, impaired glucose tolerance.
Adapted from American Diabetes Association (2004a). Gestational diabetes mellitus. *Diabetes Care*, 27(Suppl. 1), S88–S90.

heart disease, cardiac arrhythmias, and cardiomyopathies (Avila et al., 2003). Despite the significantly increased risk of adverse outcomes, most pregnant women with cardiac disease do well. In a recent study of 1,000 pregnant women with various cardiac diseases, approximately 75% experienced no cardiac events during pregnancy (Avila et al.). Of those women who developed complications, the following percentages were noted: 12.3%, congestive heart failure; 6%, cardiac arrhythmias; 1.9%, thromboembolism; 1.4%, angina; 0.7%, hypoxemia; and 0.5%, infective endocarditis (Avila et al.). Careful planning and monitoring prior to, during, and after the pregnancy by an interdisciplinary healthcare team are ideal to enhance the likelihood that things will go as well as they can for the mother and the baby (Arafeh & Baird, 2006).

Two of the largest growing sectors of childbearing women are women with obesity and advanced maternal age ($\geq$35 years) (ACOG, 2005). Both complications increase risks of maternal and neonatal morbidity and mortality, as well as raise the risk of ischemic dysfunction (ACOG, 2005; Hogberg, Innala, & Sandstrome, 1994; Silver, 2007). A 35-year-old primiparous woman has a 20-fold greater risk of mortality than a multiparous woman who is younger than age 35 (Hansen, 1986). The most recent National Health and Nutrition Examination Survey (NHANES) for 1999 to 2002 found that approximately one-third of woman in the United States are obese (ACOG, 2005; Hedley et al., 2004). In childbearing years, obesity contributes to maternal complications, such as, gestational diabetes, preeclampsia, failure to progress in labor, cesarean birth, macrosomia, anesthetic complications, infection, wound dehiscence, excessive blood loss (ACOG, 2005). These complications, individually or in combination, place an additional burden on the cardiac muscle during pregnancy, labor, and birth leading to increases in potential risk.

Disease of the cardiac muscle may be acquired, congenital, structural, or functional in nature. Patients may acquire cardiac disease in the form of pulmonic and tricuspid lesions, mitral or aortic stenosis, pulmonary hypertension, or ischemic heart disease. Infection, diet, lack of exercise, hyperlipidemia, drugs (ie, fenfluramine-phentermine, known as "fen-phen"), or disease (ie, AIDS or rheumatic fever) may precipitate acquired cardiac dysfunction (Blanchard & Shaetai, 2004; Earing & Webb, 2005).

The incidence of congenital heart disease is approximately 0.8% to 1% of 100 live births (Kafka, et al., 2006). Overall, cardiac disease has decreased in the general population while survival from congenital heart disease has increased (Kafka, et al.). Advances in neonatal care and pediatric cardiac surgery have resulted in a significant improvement in survival rates for babies born with congenital heart disease. As these infants are coming of age, more women are beginning pregnancy with medical histories of significant cardiac surgical repairs from congenital heart disease (Kafka, et al.). Fifty years ago, only 25% of these infants would have survived their first year of life; however, now 85% of infants with congenital heart disease can be expected to survive to adulthood (Earing & Webb, 2005; Kafka, et al.). Based on these data, it is estimated that approximately 400,000 adult women in the US have congenital cardiac disease. When the annual birth rate of 4 million is considered, each year another 28,000 babies will be born with congenital heart disease, with 24,000 of those babies surviving to adulthood and adding to the population of women who will potentially become pregnant (Kafka, et al.).

Congenital cardiac lesions include atrial or ventricular septal defects, patent ductus arteriosus (PDA), Tetralogy of Fallot, coarctation of the aorta, pulmonmary hypertension, Eisenmenger's syndrome, or Ebstein Anomaly (Blanchard & Shabetai, 2004). Congenital syndromes may lead to defects in specific organ systems. Down syndrome, fetal alcohol syndrome, Marfan syndrome, Turner syndrome, and rubella are all examples of syndromes with congenital cardiac defects (Earing & Webb, 2005; Kafka, et al., 2006; Linker, 2001). A maternal infection of German measles (rubella) is associated with a high risk of congenital malformation of the fetal heart as well as PDA (Blanchard & Shabetai). Women with congenital heart defects are at risk for passing the defect to the baby; thus preconception counseling should include a frank discussion of these risks. Based on the most recent data, the risks of transmission of congenital cardiac defects from mother to baby are as follows: Marfan syndrome, 50%; aortic stenosis, 17%, ventricular septal defect, 17%, atrial septal defect, 6% to12%; patent ductus ateriosis, 9%; pulmonary stenosis, 7%; aortic coarctation, 6.5%; and cyanotic congenital heart disease, 6% (Klein & Galan, 2004).

Structural or functional dysfunction of the heart may appear in many forms of cardiomyopathy: dilated, peripartum, idiopathic hypertrophic, or acquired immunodeficiency syndrome (AIDS) (Blanchard & Shabetai, 2004). Dilated cardiomyopathy involves severe left ventricular dysfunction due to a possible immune response or genetics (20%), loss of cardiac output, and a 5-year survival of less than 50% without a transplant (Blanchard & Shabetai; McMinn & Ross, 1995). Peripartum cardiomyopathy is a form of dialated cardiomyopathy occurring in the last month of pregnancy until 5 months postpartum, in the absence of previous heart disease (Blanchard & Shabetai; Pearson et al., 2000). The reported incidence varies as several sources cite an incidence of 1 case per 3,000 to 4,000 live births (Blanchard & Shabetai; Clark, Cotton, Hankins, & Phelan, 2003). Other forms of cardiomyopathy, including hypertrophic obstructive cardiomyopathy, are also seen during pregnancy. Unfortunately, there is a 60% chance of recurrence in a subsequent pregnancy (Clark, et al., 2003).

Coronary artery disease (CAD) is rare in women of childbearing years because of hormonal protection against coronary atherosclerosis (Blanchard & Shabetai, 2004), yet the risk rises significantly with delayed childbirth. Risk factors for CAD include diabetes mellitus (Blanchard & Shabetai), steroid-dependent lupus erythematosus (Bruce, Urowitz, Gladman, & Hallett, 1999), cardiac transplantation (Weis & von Scheidt, 2000), and use of oral contraceptives agents (Ratnoff & Kaufman, 1982). Severe consequences from CAD leading to myocardial infarction are also rare in pregnancy. CAD predates approximately 13% of pregnant women who experience a myocardial infarction (MI) during pregnancy. Maternal mortality from an MI is approximately 20%, and death usually occurs at the time of occurrence or during labor and birth (Blanchard & Shabetai, 2004; Roth & Elkayam, 1996).

Cardiac transplant survivors rarely attempt pregnancy due to advanced age and surgical history, yet case reports exist (Key, Resnik, Dittrich, & Reisner, 1989; Kossoy, Herbert, & Wentz, 1988). Pregnancy is a state of immunologic compromise to support and promote maternal tolerance to foreign fetal tissue (Blackburn, 2003). This adaptation may also supplement tolerance of a newly transplanted organ: heart. Posttransplant treatment is complex to include immunosuppressant drugs, endomyocardial biopsies, and an uncertain prognosis (Blanchand & Shabetai, 2004).

All forms of cardiac disease are relatively infrequent but significant potential exists to limit or cause fetal demise any phase of pregnancy, labor, or birth. Perinatal morbidity and mortality attributable to underlying cardiac disease are affected by the underlying cardiac lesion, functional changes imposed by the lesion, maternal and fetal tolerance, and development of pregnancy-related complications. A summary of common cardiac diseases, risk categories, and clinical management is presented in Table 6–20.

Cardiovascular Physiology

Anatomy

The cardiovascular system functions with three components: a pump (ie, the heart), an electrical conduction system, and a vascular distribution network. The heart, or pump, has four chambers and is referenced as the right or left side. The right side of the heart pumps blood to the lungs after receiving deoxygenated blood from the periphery (ie, venous return → right atrium → right ventricle → pulmonary artery → pulmonary

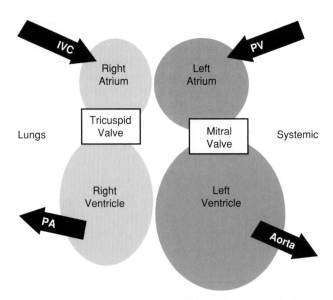

FIGURE 6–9. Linear illustration of blood flow through the heart. (Anatomic accuracy has been altered for purposes of clarity.)

capillaries → pulmonary vein) (Blackburn, 2006). The left side of the heart receives oxygenate blood expelled from the lungs and received by the periphery (ie, pulmonary vein → left atrium → left ventricle → aorta → periphery) (Blackburn, 2003; Torgersen & Curran, 2006). The left and right ventricles are separated by an interventricular septum. Valves within the heart offer assistance with forward flow while impeding backward flow. Figure 6–9 offers a conceptualization of the conduit of flow through the heart.

Once blood enters the periphery, a fine meshwork of arterioles and veins offer transportation of nutrients at the cellular level. Arteries are low-resistance vessels that function as conduits for blood flow and as a pressure reservoir that houses blood during diastole. The sympathetic nervous system innervates arterioles to vasoconstrict or vasodilate. Capillaries are thin-walled vessels with a large cross-sectional area to deliver nutrients and eliminate wastes (Blackburn, 2003). The capillaries regulate the distribution of extracellular fluid. Veins are low-resistance conduits that return blood to the heart. The sympathetic nervous system innervates venous smooth muscle and causes vasoconstriction and an increase in venous pressure.

There is a conduction system within the cardiac muscle to induce periodic contractions. The sinoartrial (SA) node is in the right atria and is established as the primary pacemaker of the heart, initiating and setting the pulse (Blackburn, 2003). An atrioventricular node offers backup if conduction through the SA node is impaired or damaged. The heart is innervated or stimulated by the autonomic nervous system (ie, sympathetic and parasympathetic nervous systems) and is affected by

TABLE 6–20 ■ CARDIAC DISEASE IN PREGNANCY

Cardiac Disease/Lesion	Risk Category	Description	Clinical Management
Atrial septal defect (ASD)	Small left to right shunt = low or minimal risk Large left to right shunt = intermediate or moderate risk	Most common congenital lesion seen during pregnancy	Physical examination systolic ejection murmur at left sternal border, wide split second heart sound Electrocardiogram (ECG): partial right bundle branch block, right axis deviation; possible right ventricular hypertrophy Common arrhythmias—atrial fibrillation or flutter Optimize preload—avoid hypovolemia or hypervolemia Oxygen during labor Avoid maternal hypotension—may increase left to right shunting Avoid maternal tachycardia—may increase left to right shunting Labor in lateral recumbent position Pain management: consider narcotic epidural
Ventral septal defect (VSD)	Small left to right shunt = low or minimal risk Large left to right shunt = intermediate or moderate risk	Size is the most important prognosticator for pregnancy: • Small → tolerated well • Larger defects → associated with CHE arrhythmia, and development of pulmonary hypertension • Left to right shunt → burdens pulmonary circulation → can lead to pulmonary hypertension	Physical examination: holosystolic thrill and murmur at left sternal border ECG: normal in most patients Echocardiogram findings: left ventricular hypertrophy may suggest large left to right shunt: right ventricular hypertrophy may suggest pulmonary hypertension Optimize preload—avoid hypovolemia or hypervolemia Oxygen during labor Labor in lateral recumbent position Avoid maternal hypotension—may increase left to right shunting Avoid maternal tachycardia—may increase left to right shunting Bacterial endocarditis prophylaxis recommended Pain management: consider narcotic epidural
Eisenmenger syndrome	High or major risk	Left to right congenital shunt, progressive pulmonary hypertension leads to reversal of shunting Most common cause is large VSD	Avoid hypotension—decrease in systemic vascular resistance causes massive right to left shunting leading to hypoxia Avoid excessive blood loss Continuous oxygen therapy: • Keep $PaO_2 \geq 70$ mm Hg • Keep $SaO_2 > 90\%$ Maintain preload—manage on "wet" side Avoid conditions that increase PVR: • Metabolic acidosis • Excess catecholamine • Hypoxemia • Hypercapnia • Vasoconstrictors • Lung hyperinflation

(continued)

TABLE 6–20 ■ CARDIAC DISEASE IN PREGNANCY (Continued)

Cardiac Disease/Lesion	Risk Category	Description	Clinical Management
Eisenmenger syndrome (continued)			High risk for thromboembolism—consider anticoagulation Pain management: consider narcotic epidural
Aortic coarctation	Uncorrected, uncomplicated = intermediate or moderate risk Complicated = high or major risk	Congenital narrowing of aorta; most common site is the origin of the left subclavian artery Associated anomalies: • VSD, PDA, aortic aneurysm. Intracranial aneurysms of the circle of Willis are relatively common	Avoid hypotension Consider assisted second stage of labor (vacuum or forceps) and/or "labor down" technique Avoid Valsalva's maneuver during pushing Oxygen therapy during labor Bacterial endocarditis prophylaxis recommended Pain management: consider epidural anesthesia
Tetralogy of Fallot	Corrected = low or minimal risk Uncorrected = intermediate or moderate risk	Congenital complex of VSD, overriding aorta, right ventricular hypertrophy, and pulmonary stenosis, surgical correction by young adulthood common	Pregnancy discouraged in uncorrected tetralogy of Fallot and/or with the following: • Hemoglobin level >20 g/L. • Hematocrit >0.65 • History of syncope or congestive heart failure • Cardiomegaly • RV pressure <120 mm Hg • Peripheral SaO$_2$ <85% Maintain preload and blood volume Avoid hypotension—decreased systemic vascular resistance may cause massive right to left shunting leading to hypoxia Bacterial endocarditis prophylaxis recommended Pain management: consider epidural anesthesia
Pulmonic stenosis	Low or minimal risk (increased transvalvular pressure gradient may increase risk)	Degree of obstruction rather than site of obstruction is determinant of clinical risk Transvalvular pressure gradient >80 mm Hg considered severe; severe stenosis can cause right-sided heart failure Peak pressure gradient, mm Hg Mild <50 Moderate 50–75 Severe >75	Optimize preload—avoid hypovolemia/hypervolemia Bacterial endocarditis prophylaxis recommended Pain management: consider epidural anesthesia
Mitral stenosis	NYHA Class I or II = Low or minimal risk NYHA Class III or IV = Intermediate or moderate risk	Most common rheumatic valvular lesion in pregnancy (25% of women first present in pregnancy) Scarring and fusion of valve apparatus	Physical examination: S1 is accentuated and snapping; low pitch diastolic rumble at the apex: presystolic accentuation Pulmonary artery catheter for class III/IV Avoid hypotension—monitor BP with arterial line

TABLE 6–20 ■ CARDIAC DISEASE IN PREGNANCY (Continued)

Cardiac Disease/Lesion	Risk Category	Description	Clinical Management

Mitral stenosis (*continued*)		Area, cm^2
		    Normal 4–6
		    Mild 1.5–2.5
		    Moderate 1–1.5
		    Severe <1
		Pressure gradient, mm Hg
		    Mild <5
		Moderate 6–12
		Severe >12
		Left arterial obstruction results in enlargement of LA and RV, and possibly pulmonary hypertension
		Atrial fibrillation possibility
		Fixed cardiac output
		Ventricular diastolic filling obstruction
			• Use phenylephrine 20–40 μg kg^{-1} min^{-1} (ephedrine will cause tachycardia)
			Optimize preload—pulmonary capillary wedge pressure (PCWP) is not an accurate reflection of LV filling pressures
			• May require elevated PCWP to maintain cardiac output: (intrapartum PCWP approximately 14 mm Hg); individualize PCWP that optimizes cardiac output
			• Maintain preload while avoiding pulmonary edema. Prepare for volume shift immediately following delivery—PCWP may rise >15 mm Hg.
			Avoid maternal tachycardia—may decrease cardiac output by decreasing left ventricular filling time
			• Consider β-blocker for pulse >90–100
			• Avoid β-adrenergic tocolytics and/or other medications that increase HR
			Atrial fibrillation—anticoagulation, digoxin, antiarrhythmics
			Bacterial endocarditis prophylaxis recommended
			Assist second-stage with vacuum or forceps; consider "labor down" technique
			Pain management: consider narcotic epidural

Aortic stenosis	NYHA Class I or II = Low or minimal risk NYHA Class III or IV = Intermediate or moderate risk	Critical stenosis with orifice has diminished to one-third or less or normal—leads to LV hypertrophy and failure: major issue is fixed cardiac output with critical stenosis; shunt gradients of >100 mm Hg are at the greatest risk Area, cm^2 • Normal 3–5 • Mild 1–2 • Moderate 0.75–1 • Severe <0.75 Maximum pressure gradient, mm Hg • Mild 16–36 • Moderate 36–50 • Moderate severe 50–75 • Severe >75 Mean pressure gradient, mm Hg • Mild <20 • Moderate 20–35 • Severe >35	Physical examination: harsh systolic ejection murmur in second right intercostals space ECG: left ventricular hypertrophy and left atrial enlargement Pulmonary artery catheter prior to labor, during labor, first 24 h postpartum Optimize preload—avoid hypovolemia • May require elevated PCWP to maintain cardiac output (intrapartum PCWP approximately 14–17 mm Hg) Avoid hypotension—decreased venous return will increase the valvular gradient and decrease cardiac output • Avoid/anticipate hemorrhage • Avoid supine position—risk of vena cava syndrome Avoid maternal tachycardia—may decrease cardiac output by decreasing left ventricular filling time • Consider β-blocker for pulse > 90–100 • Avoid β-adrenergic tocolytics and/or other medications that increase HR Oxygen during labor

(*continued*)

TABLE 6–20 ■ CARDIAC DISEASE IN PREGNANCY (Continued)

Cardiac Disease/Lesion	Risk Category	Description	Clinical Management
Aortic stenosis (*continued*)			Bacterial endocarditis prophylaxis recommended Pain management: consider narcotic epidural; avoid spinal block
Idiopathic hypertrophic subaotic stenosis (IHSS)	Intermediate or moderate	Autosomal dominant inheritance Asymmetric LV hypertrophy (especially of septum) Obstruction of LV outflow and secondary mitral regurgitation	Avoid hypotension—decreased venous return will increase the valvular gradient and decrease cardiac output • Avoid/anticipate hemorrhage • Avoid supine position—risk of vena cava syndrome Pulmonary artery catheter prior to labor, during labor, first 24 hr postpartum Optimize preload—avoid hypovolemia • May require elevated PCWP to maintain cardiac output (intrapartum PCWP approximately 14–17 mm Hg) Avoid tachycardia—may worsen obstruction • Avoid β-adrenergic tocolytics and/or other medications that increase HR Consider assisted second stage of labor (vacuum or forceps) and/or "labor down" technique • Avoid Valsalva's maneuver during pushing Bacterial endocarditis prophylaxis recommended Pain management: consider narcotic epidural: avoid spinal block
Marfan syndrome	Normal aortic root/less than 4 cm = low or minimal risk (5%) Enlarged aortic root/ ≥4 cm or valve involvement = high or major risk (up to 50%)	Autosomal dominant; generalized connective tissue weakness Can result in aneurysm formation, rupture, and dissection Sixty percent may also have mitral or aortic regurgitation	Echocardiogram needed to determine aortic root involvement Avoid maternal tachycardia—may increase shearing force on the aorta • Consider β-blocker if maternal HR >90–100 beats per minute • Avoid β-adrenergic tocolytics and/or other medications that increase HR Avoid hypertension Avoid positive inotropic medications Bacterial endocarditis prophylaxis recommended with enlarged aortic root Pain management: consider epidural anesthesia
Peripartum cardiomyopathy	High or major risk	Cardiac failure developing in pregnancy or in the first 6 mo postpartum without identifiable cause Peak incidence is 2 mo postpartum Higher incidence among older gravidas, multiparas, African-American tace, multiple gestations, and the patients with preeclampsia Manifests as biventricular failure Fifty percent go on to have dilated cardiomyopathy	Optimize cardiac output • Preload • Afterload • Contractility • HR Oxygen therapy during labor Pain management: consider narcotic epidural; keep patient comfortable to decrease oxygen utilization

TABLE 6–20 ■ CARDIAC DISEASE IN PREGNANCY (Continued)

Cardiac Disease/Lesion	Risk Category	Description	Clinical Management
Myocardial infarction (MI)	Previous MI = intermediate or moderate risk MI during pregnancy = high or major risk	Diagnosis during pregnancy is determined by ECG findings, angina, and elevated cardiac enzymes (Troponin I) Cardiac Troponin I levels are unaffected by pregnancy, labor, and delivery	MI during pregnancy—attempt to delay delivery for 2–3 wks Previous MI—advise patients to wait at least 1 yr after infarction; follow-up coronary angiography recommended Optimize cardiac output Labor in left or right lateral position Consider assisted second stage of labor (vacuum or forceps) and/or "labor down" technique Avoid Valsalva's maneuver during pushing Avoid maternal tachycardia and hypertension Bacterial endocarditis prophylaxis recommended Pain management: consider narcotic epidural; keep the patient comfortable to decrease oxygen utilization

From Arafeh, J. M., & Baird, S M. (2006). Cardiac disease in pregnancy. *Critical Care Nursing Quarterly, 29*(1), 32–52.

epinephrine secreted by the adrenal medulla (Clark, et al., 2003). Epinephrine generally stimulates ß-adrenergic receptors within the heart muscle to formulate a contraction. Dysrhythmias may accompany pregnancy and often accompany cardiac disease having an impacting on cardiac output if repetitive and prolonged (Blanchard & Shabetai, 2004)

Hemodynamics and Cardiac Output

The primary function of the human heart produces oxygenation and perfusion to the central and peripheral systems. This function, and additional parameters within the cardiovascular system, is significantly altered during pregnancy (Table 6–21). Cardiac output consists of the amount of blood ejected from the heart at a rate established by the internal conduction system (Blackburn, 2003). As a result, oxygenated blood advances into the periphery and returns deoxygenated blood to the central pump (ie, the heart; Fig. 6–9). Cardiac output is determined by four variables: preload, afterload, contractility, and heart rate. Normal hemodynamic values in pregnancy are listed in Table 6–22. Preload is the load or tension placed on the myocardium as it begins to contract at end-diastole. Preload is primarily influenced by circulating blood volume and secondarily by respiratory function (Blackburn). If the load or volume of blood returning to the heart is diminished, as in hypotension, a subsequent decrease in preload reduces cardiac output. The

intrinsic ability of the cardiac muscle to respond to variances in filling pressures is a healthy adaptation. This adaptation is challenged by the 2–3 L/minute and 40% to 50% overall rise in cardiac output during pregnancy (American College of Cardiology [ACC] et al., 2006). A commensurate increase in cardiac output usually peaks between the midportion of the second and third trimesters (ACC et al.). Preload is reported as central venous pressure in the right side of the heart and pulmonary capillary wedge pressure in the left side of the heart (Troiano, 1999).

Afterload is defined as the resistance or load that opposes ventricular ejection of blood during systole (Torgersen & Curran, 2006). Afterload is best expressed by both the pulmonary artery pressure (pulmonary vascular resistance) and the patient's blood pressure (systemic vascular resistance; Clark, et al., 2003; Troiano, 1999). Pregnancy alters afterload most directly during the second trimester (Blackburn, 2003). Under the influence of progesterone, peripheral vascular resistance decreases to accommodate this increase in vascular volume. Therefore, decreases in blood pressure during the second trimester are a common finding. Second trimester may signal the initial critical phase of maternal cardiac tolerance or intolerance during pregnancy.

Contractility is an independent intrinsic ability of the cardiac muscle to shorten aside from influences by preload and afterload (Blackburn, 2003; Troiano, 1999). This inotropic response may create a hyperdynamic,

TABLE 6–21 ■ NORMAL PHYSIOLOGIC CHANGES OF PREGNANCY

Body System	Change
Cardiovascular System	
Total blood volume	Increased 35%
Plasma volume	Increased 45%
Red cell volume	Increased 20%
Cardiac output	Increased 40% (positional)
Heart rate	Increased 15%
Systolic blood pressure	Unchanged
Systemic vascular resistance	Decreased 15%
Central venous pressure	Unchanged
Pulmonary capillary wedge pressure	Unchanged
Ejection fraction	Unchanged
Femoral venous pressure	Increased 15%
Uterine blood flow	Unchanged 20–40%
Respiratory System	
Minute ventilation	Increased 50%
Alveolar ventilation	Increased 70%
Tidal volume	Increased 40%
Respiratory rate	Increased 10–15%
Functional residual capacity	Decreased 20%
Residual volume	Decreased 20%
Oxygen consumption	Increased 20%
Arterial pH	Slightly increased (Average, 7.40–7.45)
PaO_2 (mm Hg)	Increased (104–108 mm Hg)
$PaCO_2$ (mm Hg)	Decreased (27–31 mm Hg)
Renal System	
Renal blood flow	Increased 50% (by 4th month)
Glomerular filtration rate	Increased 50% (by 4th month)
Upper limit of blood urea nitrogen	Decreased 50%
Upper limit of serum creatinine	Decreased 50%
Hepatic System	
Total plasma protein concentration	Decreased 20%
Pseudocholinesterase concentration	Decreased
Coagulation factors	Mainly increased
Gastrointestinal System	
Gastric emptying	Delayed
Gastric fluid volume/acidity	Increased
Gastroesophageal sphincter tone	Variable changes

Adapted from Luppi, C. J. (1999). Cardiopulmonary resuscitation in pregnancy. In L. K. Mandeville & N. H. Trioano (Eds.), *High risk intrapartum and critical care nursing* (2nd ed., pp. 353–379).

TABLE 6–22 ■ NORMAL HEMODYNAMIC VALUES IN PREGNANCY

Parameter	Value and Standard Deviation
Cardiac output (L/min)	6.2 ± 1.0
Systemic vascular resistance (dyne/sec/cm-5)	$1{,}210 \pm 266$
Pulmonary vascular resistance (dyne/sec/cm-5	78 ± 22
Mean pulmonary artery pressure (mm Hg)	13 ± 2
Pulmonary capillary wedge pressure (mm Hg)	7.5 ± 1.8
Central venous pressure (mm Hg)	3.6 ± 2.5
Left ventricular stroke index (g/m/m-2)	48 ± 6

normal, or failure state. Contractility is measured indirectly by the left ventricular stroke work index. Strength or contractility is inversely related to the age of a patient (ie, as age increases and contractility decreases; Troiano). Contractility may also be negatively affected by prolonged undiagnosed cardiac disease.

Heart rate is the final component of cardiac output. The speed at which the cardiac muscle pumps influences output positively or negatively. Faster rates lead to stronger contractions (Troiano, 1999). Excessively high rates lead to a decrease in filling time of the ventricles and reduction in output. Typically during trauma, dysfunction, or disease, the human heart will alter heart rate (ie, pulse) prior to detectable influences on any of the other remaining parameters (Clark, et al., 2003). In cases of severe hypovolemia, the heart rate may double before changes in the peripheral vascular resistance (ie, blood pressure) are evident. Therefore, blood pressure and pulse are two vital signs reflective of cardiac output and cardiac disease.

Cardiac Adaptations of Pregnancy

During pregnancy, normal adaptations enhance cardiac tolerance and may mimic cardiac disease. Table 6–23 outlines normal cardiac changes during pregnancy compared to abnormal signs and symptoms of cardiac disease. The outcome of hormonal-mediated alterations creates a hyperdynamic, hypervolemic, and dynamic state (Torgersen & Curran, 2006). Increases in volume, workload, and oxygen consumption during pregnancy, labor, and birth create cardiac stress (ACC et al., 2006; Curran, 2002; Torgersen & Curran). Gestational age, multiple gestations, maternal position,

TABLE 6–23 ■ NORMAL PREGNANCY SYMPTOMS VERSUS SYMPTOMS OF CARDIAC DISEASE

Pregnancy: May Be Present	Cardiac Disease From Any Cause: May Be Present
• Fatigue • Exertional dyspnea (usually limited to 3rd trimester) • Irregular or infrequent syncope • Palpations (brief, irregular, & asymptomatic) • Jugular venous distention • Mild tachycardia <15% rise • Third heart sound • Grade II/VI systolic murmur • Pedal edema	• Decreased ability to perform activities of daily living • Severe breathlessness, orthopnea, paroxysmal nocturnal dyspnea, cough, or syncope • Chest pain (not normal in pregnancy) • Systemic hypotension • Cyanosis, clubbing • Persistent jugular venous distention • Sinus tachycardia >15% normal heart rate • Fourth heart sound • Arrhythmias • Pulmonary edema • Pleural effusion

Thorne, S. (2004). Pregnancy in heart disease: Congenital heart disease. *Heart, 90*(4), 450–456; Curran, C. (2002). Multiple organ dysfunction syndrome in the obstetrical population. *Journal of Perinatal & Neonatal Nursing,* 15(4): 37–55.

stages of labor and immediate postpartum, pain, fever, and drugs increase cardiac output during pregnancy (Torgersen & Curran). An increase of as much as 50% or more may occur during routine stages of labor, critical illness, anemia, stress, or infection (Harvey, 1999). The following changes in cardiac output occur during the active phase of labor: increases 17% at ≤3 cm dilated, 23% from 4 to 7 cm dilated, and 34% at ≥8 cm dilated (Blackburn, 2003). Uterine contractions may enhance cardiac output by as much as 15% to 20% due to the increased metabolic demands (Clark et al., 2003). Uterine contractions can result in marked increases in both systolic and diastolic blood pressure (ACC et al.). The first 15 minutes following evacuation of the uterus at birth includes a return of approximately 600 to 800 cc of uterine blood to the maternal vascular compartment. Therefore, immediate postpartum is one of the most cardiovascular stressful times of all of pregnancy, labor, and birth with a 65% maximum increase in cardiac output (Blackburn, 2003).

Overall, 20% to 30% of the pregnant woman's total cardiac output is directed at blood flow to the uterus and placenta. Uterine growth to support fetal development is the primary goal of perfusion. As the pregnancy approaches term, 85% of the total uterine blood volume supplies the placental circulation. Uterine flow may be compromised by maternal positioning (ie, supine), excessive exercise, medical conditions, anesthesia, or uterine contractions.

The physiologic and hemodynamic changes of pregnancy frequently disguise, exacerbate, or mimic cardiac disease (Blanchard & Shabetai, 2004). Normal pregnancies may precipitate signs and symptoms of dizziness, dyspnea, orthopnea, fatigue, syncope, rales in the lower lung fields, jugular vein distention, systolic murmurs, dysrhythmias, and cardiomegaly (Blanchard & Shabetai; Torgersen & Curran, 2006). Symptoms indicative of heart disease include severe dyspnea, syncope with exertion, hemopotysis, paroxysmal nocturnal dyspnea, cyanosis, clubbing, diastolic murmurs, sustained cardiac arrhythmias, loud harsh systolic murmurs, and chest pain with exertion (Blanchard & Shabetai). In the later group, prompt intervention is warranted.

Obstetric Outcomes and The New York Heart Association Classifications

Favorable pregnancy outcomes are predicted and based on the preconceptional functional capacity of the women. Mortality risk is associated with the specific acquired or congenital defect and associated symptoms. Display 6–34 divides cardiac disease into three groups consisting of a mortality range between 1% and 50% (Klein & Galan, 2004; Whitty, 2002). Typically, the woman's functional ability is assessed using the New York Heart Association Criteria (Criteria Committee of the New York Heart Association [NYHA], 1979) as outlined in Table 6–24. Women are classified on the basis of their symptoms of cardiac function and failure. Up to 40% of women advance to a higher NYHA classification during pregnancy (Clark, et al., 2003). Progression to a higher NYHA classification should be addressed at any risk counseling session due to effects on maternal mortality statistics. Maternal mortality data identifies women with pulmonary hypertension, particularly associated with a right-to-left shunt in cardiac flow as in Esinmenger's syndrome, to be at greatest risk (Blanchard &

DISPLAY 6-34

Mortality Risk Associated with Pregnancy

GROUP I: MORTALITY <1%

- Atrial septal defect
- Ventricular septal defect (uncomplicated)
- Patent ductus arteriosus
- Pulmonic and tricuspid disease
- Corrected tetralogy of Fallot
- Biosynthetic valve prosthesis (porcine and human allograft)
- Mitral stenosis, New York Heart Association (NYHA) classes I & II

GROUP II: MORTALITY 5%–15%

- Mitral stenosis with atrial fibrillation
- Mechanical valve prosthesis
- Mitral stenosis, NYHA class III or NYHA IV
- Aortic stenosis
- Coarctation of the aorta (uncomplicated)
- Uncorrected tetralogy of Fallot
- Previous myocardial infarction
- Marfan syndrome with normal aorta

GROUP III: MORTALITY 25%–50%

- Eisenmenger's syndrome
- Pulmonary hypertension
- Coarctation of the aorta (complicated)
- Marfan syndrome with aortic involvement

TABLE 6–24 ■ NEW YORK HEART ASSOCIATION FUNCTIONAL CLASSIFICATION SYSTEM

Class	Description
I	Asymptomatic
	No limitation of physical activity
II	Asymptomatic at rest; symptomatic with heavy physical activity and exertion
	Slight limitation of physical activity
III	Asymptomatic at rest; symptomatic with minimal or normal physical activity
	Considerable limitation of physical activity
IV	Symptomatic at rest; symptomatic with any physical activity
	Severe limitation of physical activity

From Criteria Committee of the New York Heart Association. (1979). *Nomenclature and criteria for diagnosis of diseases of the heart and great vessels* (8th ed.). New York: New York Heart Association.

healthcare provider should counsel the women to reconsider attempting pregnancy. In conclusion, due to the incremental nature of cardiovascular adaptations, all pregnant women should be assessed for any signs

DISPLAY 6-35

Predictors of Cardiac Events

N New York Heart Association >II

O Obstruction Left Heart

Mitral valve prolapse <2 cm

Aortic valve <1.5 cm

Gradient >30 peak

P Prior Cardiac Event Before Pregnancy

Failure

Arrhythmia

Transient ischemic attack

Stroke

E Ejection Fraction <40%

Number of predictors equals risk of cardiac events during pregnancy; 0 = 5%, 1 = 27%, >1 = 75%
Adapted from Siu, S. C., Sermer, M., Colman, J. M., Alvarez, A. N., Mercier, L. A., Morton, B. C., et al. (2001). Prospective multicenter study of pregnancy outcomes in women with heart disease. *Circulation*; *104*(5), 515–521; and Thorne, S. (2004). Pregnancy in heart disease: Congenital heart disease. *Heart, 90*(4), 450–456.

Shabetai, 2004). Delay in pregnancy, termination, or close cardiac observation throughout gestation, labor, and birth are indicated (Blanchard & Shabetai). Thorne (2004) identified four cardiac conditions contraindicated to pregnancy: pulmonary hypertension of any cause, systemic ventricular dysfunction with an ejection fraction of <20%, severe left-sided, obstructive lesions, and Marfan syndrome accompanied by a dilated aortic root. Additional clinical symptomatology attributable to a 51% rise in maternal mortality may include a prepregnancy oxygen (O_2) saturation <85%, maternal hematocrit (HCT) ≥65% or hemoglobin (Hgb) >20g/dl, and/or a maternal arterial saturation level <70 mm Hg which may contribute to fetal desaturation (Clark, et al.). In Display 6–35, Siu and colleagues (2001) offer additional guidance regarding potential risk of a cardiac event during pregnancy. As the number of predictors in the NOPE acronym increase, so does the risk of a negative event. If the patient's cardiac history has all four predictors, then a of deteriorating cardiovascular function at every healthcare provider encounter.

Congenital Cardiac Disease in Pregnancy

Over the last 25 years, congenital versus acquired cardiac disease has increased due to a rise in neonatal intensive care survivors, early diagnosis, and advances in repair and treatment options (Earing & Webb, 2005; Kafka, et al., 2006). As of 1993, acquired versus congenital disease occurs at a ratio of 1:1.5 yet in 1967 the ratio difference was as high as 16:1 (deSwiet, 1993). Maternal conditions (ie, diabetes, lupus erythematosus, phenylketonuria, or drug abuse), medication ingestion (ie, Lithium, alcohol), genetics, or infections (ie, rubella, rheumatic fever, and viruses) may result in structural defects in the unborn fetus (Blanchard & Shabetai, 2004). Blood flow is critical to the development of cardiac structures during the embryonic period. If flow through cardiac structures is limited or absent, abnormal development occurs. If flow restriction occurs in early gestation during fetal cardiac development, the specific region and structures "downstream" will become small (hypoplastic) or even completely absent (atretic) (Linker, 2001). As a result, one of four structural defects may develop: hole (defect), narrowing due to stiffness causing obstruction (stenosis), underdevelopment or absence (hypoplasia or atresia), or wrong connection (transposition, inversion, anomalous connection; Linker).

Various types of cardiac defects attributed to chromosomal or congenital anomalies may appear as an atrial septal defect (ASD), ventricular septal defect (VSD), or patent ductus arteriosus (PDA; Blanchard & Shabetai, 2004). Septal defects are holes located in the designated chamber that create alterations in flow and often limits oxygenation. Holes create portals for emboli development and increase the risk of thromboembolytic injury (Linker, 2001).

Congenital heart disease may also be differentiated into acrocyanotic events (ie, coarctation of the aorta) or cyanotic events (ie, uncorrected Tetralogy of Fallot), Eisengmenger's syndrome, or transposition of the great vessels (Linker, 2001). Coarctation of the aorta comprises 9% of congenital heart disease and has a mortality rate of 3% to 6% but is usually tolerated during pregnancy (Blanchard & Shabetai, 2004; Linker). Patients with this anomaly are at risk for aortic dissection, cerebral hemorrhage, aneurysm, rupture, infective endocarditis, congenital berry aneurysm of the circle of Willis, hemorrhagic stroke, or congestive heart failure (Blanchard & Shabetai; Thorne, 2004; Linker). Typical features and diagnosis may include upper-extremity hypertension accompa-

nied by lower extremity hypotension, a late systolic murmur, visible and palpable collateral arteries in the scapular area, delayed or diminished femoral pulses as compared to the carotid, notching of the inferior rib borders via chest radiogram, and electrocardiographic (ECG) evidence of severe left ventricular hypertrophy (Blanchard & Shabetai). If indicated, corrective surgery should precede pregnancy otherwise blood pressure can be titrated with alpha-adrenergic-stimulating or blocking agents (Blanchard & Shabetai).

Tetralogy of Fallot is a right-to-left shunt without pulmonary hypertension consisting of four defects: (1) ventricular septal defect (VSD); (2) overriding aorta: dextropositon of the aorta so that the aortic orifice sits astride the VSD and overrides the right ventricle; (3) right ventricular hypertrophy; and (4) pulmonary stenosis (Blanchard & Shabetai, 2004). With an uncorrected VSD, 75% of venous return may pass directly into the aorta without being oxygenated, therefore the patient becomes cyanotic (Clark, et al., 2003). Hereditary risk of this complication is 3% to 13% if one parent has the condition (Blanchard & Shabetai). Closure of the VSD may render a maternal patient safe for pregnancy yet significant arrhythmias and conduction defects may illicit the need for cardiac pacing or implantable defibriliation years after a successful repair operation (Blanchard & Shabetai). Hence, pregnancy, labor, and birth may precipitate cardiac intolerance in the form of dysrhythmias in these patients.

Reversal of the pulmonary artery and aorta insertion leads to a second cyanotic condition known as transposition of the great vessels. Although relatively uncommon, the condition may be accompanied by additional defects such as a VSD, absent septum, or pulmonary stenosis (Clark, et al., 2003). Adult survival may require surgical correction yet some untreated women with delicately balanced lesions bear children; a collaborative approach is indicated to include cardiology and obstetric care (Blanchard & Shabetai, 2004).

Several conditions that include cardiac defects as part of a syndrome are listed in Table 6–25. The incidence of Marfan syndrome is 4 to 6 cases per 10,000 persons and is not related to sex, race, or ethnicity (Felblinger & Akers, 1998). Inherited as an autosomal dominant trait, Marfan syndrome has a wide variety of outcomes that are related to the degree of aortic root dilation (Blanchard & Shabetai, 2004; Mayet, Steer, & Somerville, 1998). Cardiovascular anomalies related to Marfan syndrome include aortic root dilation, coarctation of the aorta, aortic regurgitation, patent ductus arteriosus, hypertension, and cardiomegaly; if left untreated, life

TABLE 6–25 ■ COMMON SYNDROMES AND ASSOCIATED CARDIAC DEFECTS

Syndrome	Primary Cardiac Defects
Down	VSD, AVSD, ASD
Fetal Alcohol	VSD
Marfan	Ascending aortic aneurism, regurgitation, or coarctation; MVP, HTN, PDA
Rubella	PDA, PPS
Turner	Coarctation
Eisenmenger	Pulmonary hypertension, VSD, or PDA
Lutembacker	Mitral stenosis, ASD, heart failure

Key: VSD, ventricular septal defect; AVSD, atrioventricular septal defect; ASD, atrial septal defect; MVP, mitral valve prolapse; HTN, hypertension; PDA, patent ductus arteriosus.
Linker, D. (2001). *Practical echocardiography of congenital heart disease from fetal to adult.* New York: Churchill Livingstone; and Blanchard, D., & Shabetai, R. (2004). Cardiac diseases. In R. Creasy, R. Resnick, & J. Iams (Eds.), *Maternal-fetal medicine: Principles & practice* (5th ed., pp. 815–844). Philadelphia, PA: Saunders.

expectancy is reduced by half (Blanchard & Shabetai). The most serious maternal risk during pregnancy and birth is acute aortic dissection leading to acute hemorrhagic shock (Clark, et al., 2003).

Eisengmenger's syndrome is a collection of abnormalities that include progressive pulmonary hypertension with a congenital left to right shunt (ie, VSD or PDA) which leads to reversal of flow and decreased oxygenation to the systemic vasculature (Clark, et al., 2003). This syndrome is more common in young girls with a large VSD leading to potential pulmonary hypertension pathology symptomatic with cyanosis in the form of clubbing, hypoxemia, erythrocytosis, and high hematocrit (leads to increased viscosity of blood), and bleeding diathesis (Blanchard & Shabetai, 2004). Symptomatology of overt hypoxemia and cyanosis leads to maternal and fetal intolerance during pregnancy with a maternal mortality rate of 30% to 70% ultimately from right heart failure, pulmonary hypertension, or pulmonary hemorrhage (Blanchard & Shabetai; Linker, 2001). This state is often exacerbated by decreases in systemic vascular resistance that leads to a reduction in preload (Blanchard & Shabetai). Pregnancy, epidural anesthesia, and venal caval compression may diminish preload, therefore, caution is warranted (Torgersen & Curran, 2006). As congenital heart disease varies in pathology and symptomatology it is the responsibility of healthcare providers to continually assess for deterioration of status.

Acquired Cardiac Disease in Pregnancy

Acquired cardiac lesions include pulmonic or tricuspid lesions, mitral stenosis, mitral insufficiency or prolapse, aortic stenosis, aortic insufficiency, and myocardial infarction. Time, disease, or infection may precipitate valvular dysfunction. Although regurgitation frequently occurs during pregnancy, valvular insufficiency or stenosis contributes to alterations and limitations in flow which ultimately decreases cardiac output (Blackburn, 2003; Blanchard & Shabetai, 2004). Depending on the affected valve, right or left ventricular failure may develop. Prevalance of mitral valve prolapse is often overstated yet is considered the most frequent acquired cardiac lesion at a rate of 17% in women (Blanchard & Shabetai; Clark, et al., 2003). This anomaly may precipitate mitral regurgitation or chest pain and accompany Marfan syndrome or an ASD (Blanchard & Shabetai). Generally asymptomatic, this disease is accompanied by a systolic click noted between the first and second heart sound that varies on posture and hydration (Blanchard & Shabetai). Due to an increase in antibiotic resistance, endocarditis prophylaxis is not recommended for uncomplicated labors and births but is recommended for suspected bacteremia if regurgitation, thickened leaflets, or both exist (ACOG, 2003).

Progressive valvular calcification and gradual restriction in leaflet motion lead to stenosis of the bicuspid aortic valve, yet congenital causes may lead to severe left ventricular hypertrophy (Blanchard & Shabetai, 2004). Heart failure or sudden death may occur following an audible murmur and left ventricular hypertrophy via ECG but may be avoided by valvular replacement (Blanchard & Shabetai). Absolute contraindications to pregnancy in women with uncorrected aortic stenosis include heart failure (past or present), syncope, or a previous history of cardiac arrest (Blanchard & Shabetai).

Acute myocardial infarction (MI) is perhaps the most infrequent acquired heart disease during pregnancy at a rate of 1:10,000 with the highest risk occurring in the third trimester and in older (more than 33 years) multigravidas (Blanchard & Shabetai, 2004; Thorne, 2004). Anterior wall location is the most frequent lesion site (Roth & Elkayam, 1996). Mortality risk (20%–50%) and frequency (two-thirds) appears to be greatest if the MI occurs during the third trimester or if delivery is within 2 weeks of the infarct (Blanchard & Shabetai; Roth & Elkayam; Thorne, 2004). Cardiac troponin I is unaffected by pregnancy, labor, or birth and therefore is the investigation of choice in the diagnosis of acute coronary syndrome during pregnancy (Thorne). Treatment options may include heparin, beta-blockers (unless acute heart failure is evident), or percutaneous coronary angioplasty (often with coronary stenting; Blanchard & Shabetai). The overall treatment goal with any cardiovascular distress, congenital or acquired, is minimization of oxygen demands on the myocardium.

Cardiomyopathy

Cardiomyopathy is a subcategory of acquired heart disease with clinical examples such as hypertrophic cardiomyopathy, dilated cardiomyopathy, and peripartum cardiomyopathy. Hypertrophic disease is often of unknown cause, marked by excessive and disorganized growth of myofibrils, impaired filling of the heart (diastolic dysfunction), a reduction in the size of ventricular cavities, and often, ventricular arrhythmias and sudden death (Venes & Thomas, 2001). Hypertrophic cardiomyopathy is rarely diagnosed in early life; therefore, pregnancy may exacerbate primary symptomatology. Offspring should be screened for a genetic predisposition until they are 20 to 25 years of age (Thorne, 2004). Primary symptomatology consists of angina, dyspnea, arrhythmia, and patients with a family history (Blanchard & Shabetai, 2004). Clinical exams, ECG, and electrocardiogram data assist in the diagnosis. Treatment during pregnancy is focused on avoidance of hypovolemia; maintaining venous return; and avoiding anxiety, excitement, and strenuous activity (Blanchard & Shabetai).

Heart muscle weakness of occult or uncertain cause, possibly due to viral infections; unrecognized toxic exposures; or a genetic predisposition may lead to dilated cardiomyopathy (Venes & Thomas, 2001). Dilated cardiomyopathy is associated with acquired immunodeficiency syndrome (Bestetti, 1989; Rerkpattanapipat, Wongpraparut, Jacods, & Kotler, 2000). Progressive dyspnea, edema, fatigue, and serious ventricular arrhythmias develop as a consequence of disease (Blanchard & Shabetai, 2004). A 5-year prognosis for survival is less than 50%, yet medications may slow deterioration until transplantation is necessary (Blanchard & Shabetai).

Peripartum cardiomyopathy is defined as cardiac failure with left ventricular ejection fraction <45% occurring in the last month of pregnancy or within 5 months of delivery, in the absence of any identifiable cause of heart failure (ie, valvular, metabolic, infectious, or toxic) (Pearson et al., 2000; Clark, et al., 2003). A chest x-ray typically shows cardiomegaly with pulmonary edema. Historically, damage to cardiac chambers is caused by the rapid dilation attributed to an autoimmune response to viral myocarditis. Because pregnancy is a state of immunocompromise, infection may be enhanced. An occurrence rate of 1:3,000 to 15,000 makes this condition rare (Pearson et al.; Thorne, 2004). Adverse risk factors include age

>30 years, multiparity, twin pregnancy, and 50% of women in whom left ventricular dilation and dysfunction persist (Thorne). Approximately 60% of women who experience the disease recover, whereas up to 20% require cardiac transplants (Blanhard & Shabetai, 2004; Clark, et al.). If left ventricular dysfunction persists for 1 year following delivery, the risk of death in a subsequent pregnancy is estimated at 20% (Thorne). Due to the delay in disease within the third trimester or postpartum, fetal outcomes are usually positive.

In general, cardiac disease is poorly tolerated during pregnancy if classified as III or IV by NYHA or associated with an ejection fraction <20%, mitral regurgitation, right ventricular failure, atrial fibrillation, or systemic hypotension (Thorne, 2004). Vasodilators and anti-thromboembolics are incorporated into treatment as necessary; heparin is preferred (Blanchard & Shabetai, 2004; Venes & Thomas, 2001). Congestive heart failure is the primary morbidity leading to mortality; transplants are often necessary as outlined.

Clinical Management

The goals of clinical management for a woman whose pregnancy is complicated by cardiovascular disease mirror the goals for optimum uteroplacental perfusion. Stabilization of the mother by maintaining cardiac output stabilizes the fetal compartment. Meeting these goals requires a coordinated multidisciplinary team approach. Management strategies should include estimates of maternal and fetal risk in order for the patient and her family to make an informed decision regarding her pregnancy. The primary practitioner should discuss issues regarding maternal age at the time of pregnancy, estimations of maternal and fetal mortality, potential chronic morbidity, antepartum interventions to minimize risk, and a birth best suited to her underlying pathology (Arafeh & Baird, 2006; Blanchard & Shabetai, 2004).

The primary focus in cardiac management during pregnancy, labor, and birth maximizes cardiac output while limiting metabolic demand. Depending on underlying pathology, administration of medications and intravascular volume may be necessary to optimize or minimize preload and afterload in order to maximize cardiac output. Beta-blockers (ie, atenolol) are often used to stabilize underlying cardiomyopathy yet fetal complications exist as small for gestational age (SGA) or IUGR in the fetus (ACOG, 2001; National Institute of Health Working Group Report on High Blood Pressure in Pregnancy [NIH], 2000). If any patient experiences heart failure, traditional methods are used during pregnancy with the exception of angotensin converting enzyme (ACE) inhibitors. This class of drugs is associated with fetal and neonatal renal agenesis, failure, and death (ACOG, 2001; NIH, 2000; Thorne, 2004).

Increased intravascular volume, vasoconstricting substances or hypertension, polycythemia, and various maternal positions may all increase preload or afterload, whereas the converse decreases each factor (Elkayam, Ostrzega, Shotan, & Mehra, 1995). During the intrapartum period, ephedrine and an intravenous fluid bolus are routinely used to control hypotension following epidural analgesia to maintain cardiac output (Shnider, DeLorimier, Holl, Chapler, & Morishima, 1968). Ephedrine may promote cardiac intolerance by increasing heart rate; therefore, phenylephrine has been recommended for women with many cardiac disorders (Ralston, Shnider, & DeLorimier, 1974). Unstable ischemia may require aspirin, heparin, and intravenous nitroglycerin during pregnancy (Blanchard & Shabetai, 2004).

Additional medications may be needed when cardiac dysrhythmias are influencing heart rate and cardiac output. Commonly used antiarrhythmic medications include bretylium tosylate, digoxin, lidocaine, procainamide, propranolol, and verapamil (Clark, et al., 2003). Cardioversion, direct pacing, and defibrillation may be required to correct serious dysrhythmias (Blanchard & Shabetai, 2004) Control of anxiety, pain, temperature, and many other variables can minimize fluctuations in heart rate (Curran, 2002). Numerous medications have been shown to modify the function of the heart by increasing or decreasing contractility. Calcium, catecholamines, dopamine, dobutamine, epinephrine, digitalis, and norepinephrine have a positive inotropic effect, whereas barbiturates, propranolol, and quinidine have a negative inotropic effect (Troiano, 1999).

Often women with known heart disease are on antithrombotics or blood thinners (ie, aspirin). Heparin is the drug of choice for treatment of acute thrombotic events, prophylaxis for patients with a history of cardiac disease or thrombotic events, or for women with valvular disease (ACOG, 2000; Blanchard & Shabetai, 2004; Thorne, 2004). Heparin does not cross the placenta and is not associated with adverse fetal outcome (Ginsberg & Hirsh, 1995). Lovenox (enoxaparin sodium) therapy appears to be safe during pregnancy in candidates who need heparin prophylaxis yet it is contraindicated in pregnant women who have prosthetic heart valves (ACOG, 2002). Any anticoagulant therapy increases the risk of hemorrhage and intraspinal bleeding related to regional anesthesia (Chan & Ray, 1999) warranting preparation and a heightened awareness by the healthcare team.

The American College of Cardiology (ACC) and the American Heart Association (AHA) do not recommend routine antibiotic prophylaxis for patients with valvular heart disease having an otherwise uncompli-

cated vaginal or cesarean birth unless infection is suspected (ACC et al., 2006). Antibiotics are optional for high-risk patients with prosthetic heart valves, a previous history of endocarditis, complex, congenital heart disease, or a surgically constructed systemic-pulmonary conduit (ACC et al.). Nonetheless, many practitioners routinely prescribe antibiotics (ACC et al.; ACOG, 2003). See Table 6–26 (on page 222) for cardiovascular medications that may be administered to women with cardiac disease.

Intrapartum care and birth options need special attention to decrease maternal and fetal risk. An interdisciplinary team approach to planning intrapartum care works best. In the past, cesarean birth under general anesthesia was often chosen as the birth option with the least risks to the mother for women with congenital heart disease. However, elective cesarean birth increases the risk of hemorrhage, thrombosis, and infection and is associated with 1.2 to 1.4 times the risk of an adverse outcome when compared to vaginal birth (Kafka, et al., 2006). Current practice includes a well-planned labor and vaginal birth unless there is a specific obstetric indication for cesarean birth (Earing & Webb, 2005). See Display 6-36 for key aspects of intrapartum management and care. The stresses of labor can be managed with a low-dose slow incremental epidural anesthesia (Kafka, et al.). Initiation of epidural anesthesia early in labor inhibits or minimizes the sympathetic response to pain. Labor pain has potentially significant side effects that should be avoided for women with cardiac disease. Cardiac output can be abruptly increased with the pain and tension associated with labor (ACC et al., 2006). Minute ventilation can be increased by as much as 300%, resulting in lower $PaCO_2$ levels and rising blood lactate levels (Arafeh & Baird, 2006). Quality pain management has the additional benefits of avoiding tachycardia (important for cardiac lesions that require adequate diastolic filling or systolic ejection time), reducing myocardial workload, and the ability to shorten the second stage of labor with forceps or vacuum (Arafeh & Baird).

Spontaneous labor is preferred to induced labor; however, in selected cases labor induction may be the most feasible option to ensure that the require team members are available and present (Kafka, et al., 2006). Planned labor also may be chosen for women who live remote from the hospital and thus may not be able to get to the labor unit to benefit from early interventions in a timely manner after the initiation of spontaneous labor. Controlled labor may be necessary due to deterioration of the maternal or fetal condition; therefore, an induction of labor or scheduled cesarean birth may be indicated for selected women. Labor should progress at a reasonable pace without hyperstimulation that may lead to fetal intolerance and ultimate surgical birth. A lateral position during labor will

DISPLAY 6-36

Intrapartum Care for Women With Cardiac Disease

An interdisciplinary team should plan and participate in care (nurse and physician representatives from the following specialties, obstetrics, maternal–fetal medicine, anesthesia, cardiology, neonatology, and pediatrics). Social services and chaplain services should be consulted and available as necessary.

The unit where labor and birth occurs is based on maternal status. Most women can be managed in the labor unit with personnel from the ICU assisting with assessment of maternal hemodynamic status if invasive hemodynamic monitoring is indicated. Selected women may labor and give birth in the ICU. Personnel with expertise in fetal assessment are essential.

Labor is the most dangerous period for many pregnant women with cardiac disease since there is the period of the greatest increase in cardiac output. Therefore careful monitoring of maternal–fetal status is essential with at least a one-to-one nurse to patient ratio. Patient status and type of cardiac disease provides the basis for selection of monitoring methods.

Invasive hemodynamic monitoring should be considered for women with impaired left ventricular function, NYHA classes III and IV, severe mitral stenosis, and pulmonary hypertension.

Noninvasive monitoring includes oxygen saturation via pulse oximetry, blood pressure, heart rate, respirations, careful monitoring of fluid status, reassessment of functional status, and use of continuous ECG monitoring for women susceptible to arrhythmias.

Fetal status should be monitored continuously via EFM. Fetal status can be an indicator of maternal status. A reassuring FHR can be reflective of adequate maternal perfusion. External or internal monitoring of FHR and uterine activity is based on obstetric considerations.

Lateral positioning should be encouraged to avoid risk of venocaval compression.

Adequate and early pain management (usually via epidural anesthesia) will minimize negative effects of pain, anxiety, and tension on maternal hemodynamic parameters. Patients with severe stenotic heart defects will not tolerate sudden decreases in systemic vascular resistance; therefore, epidural anesthesia must be administered slowly and incrementally.

Supportive nursing care along with support from the patient's partner can minimize anxiety. Appropriate preparation with realistic expectations for how the labor and birth will proceed including potential complications and resultant interventions can also minimize stress and anxiety.

Labor and vaginal birth is preferred over cesarean birth for most patients because there is less risk of blood loss, fewer postpartum infections, and earlier ambulation with less risk of thrombosis and pulmonary complications.

The second stage should be managed with passive fetal descent, minimal maternal expulsive efforts, and operative (forceps or vacuum) birth as needed.

Uterine contraction after birth should be maintained to prevent postpartum hemorrhage. Women who have received anticoagulation therapy are at greater risk for hemorrhage. Oxytocic drugs have marked hemodynamic effects and should be used at the lowest effective dose. Postpartum hemorrhage should be managed aggressively to prevent hypovolemia, especially important for patients are preload dependents such as those with severe aortic stenosis or mitral stenosis. Postpartum hemorrhage should be treated with volume replacement, blood products, and plasma.

Support maternal–infant attachment by encouraging holding, touching, and breastfeeding (if the woman has chosen breastfeeding) as soon as possible.

Arafeh, J. M., & Baird, S. M. (2006). Cardiac disease in pregnancy. *Critical Care Nursing Quarterly, 29*(1), 32–52; Earing, M. G., & Webb, G. D. (2005). Congenital heart disease and pregnancy: Maternal and fetal risks. *Clinics in Perinatology, 32*(4), 913–919; Kafka, H., Johnson, M. R., & Gatzoulis, M. A. (2006). The team approach to pregnancy and congenital heart disease. *Cardiology Clinics, 24*(4), 587–605; Klein, L. L., & Galan, H. L. (2005). Cardiac disease in pregnancy. *Obstetrics and Gynecology Clinics of North America, 31*(2), 429–459; Simpson, K. R. (2006). Critical illness during pregnancy: Considerations for evaluation and treatment of the fetus as the second patient. *Critical Care Nursing Quarterly, 29*(1), 19–31.

minimize the effects of the hemodynamic fluctuations associated with uterine contractions (Earing & Webb, 2005). Approximately 500 mL of blood volume is displaced with each uterine contraction, which increases preload and cardiac output (Arafeh & Baird, 2006). See Table 6–27 for increases in cardiac output during labor and birth.

Active interventions should be limited during the second stage of labor when maternal, fetal, or combined intolerance is evident. Passive fetal descent, also known as "laboring down," in a lateral position increases oxygenation, limits maternal metabolic demands, and increases uteroplacental perfusion (Mayberry et al., 2000). Part of the plans for birth should include how long the woman will be allowed to push (if at all) without significant hemodynamic compromise, and when that limit is reached, birth is assisted by forceps or vacuum (Kafka, Johnson, & Gatzoulis, 2006). Most cardiac conditions are well tolerated by a vaginal birth under anesthesia, minimal or no pushing, and an operative vaginal birth. If appropriate, this is the safest mode of birth for the mother due to decreased blood loss and a slight decrease in hemodynamic changes when compared to a cesarean birth (Thorne, 2004).

TABLE 6–26 ■ CARDIOVASCULAR MEDICATIONS (DOSES, NURSING CARE, AND MATERNAL-FETAL IMPLICATIONS)

	Generic Name (Trade Name)	Dose	Nursing Care Specific for Pregnancy	Fetal/Neonatal Effects
Anti-arrthythmics	Adenosine (Adenocard)	6 mg IV (intravenous) bolus over 1–3 s followed by 20-mL saline bolus; may repeat with 12 mg in 1–2 min × 2		No observed fetal or newborn effects reported
	Amiodarone (Cordarone)	5 mg/kg IV over 3 min: then 10 mg/kg per day	Observe for prolonged QT	EFM: Observe for fetal bradycardia • Potential for congenital hypothyroidism • May cause IUGR • Observe for transient bradycardia and prolonged QT in the newborn
	Bretylium	5 mg/kg IV bolus; then 1–2 mg/min infusion	Observe for maternal hypotension	EFM: Potential risks for decreased uterine blood flow, fetal hypoxia, late decelerations, and bradycardia
	Lidocaine	1 mg/kg bolus; repeat one-half bolus at 10 min PRN × 4; infusion at 1–4 mg/min; total dose 3 mg/kg		EFM: Rapidly crosses placenta; potential for fetal bradycardia
	Phenytoin (Dilantin)	300 mg IV; then 100 mg every 5 min to a total of 1000 mg		Tertatogenic—fetal hydantoin syndrome: unknown fetal/newborn risk with short-term use.
	Procainamide (Pronestil)	100 mg over 30 min: then 2–6 mg/min infusion: total dose 17 mg/kg		None reported
	Quinidine	15 mg/kg IV over 60 min: then 0.02 mg kg^{-1} min^{-1} infusion	Potential oxytocic properties with high doses	Potential for eighth cranial nerve damage and thrombocytopenia.
β-Blockers	Atenolol (Tenormin)	5 mg IV over 5 min: repeat dose in 5 min: total dose 15 mg	Observe for maternal hypotension	EFM: Observe for fetal bradycardia • May cause IUGR and persistent β-blockade in the newborn
	Esmolol (Brevibloc)	500 micrograms kg^{-1} IV over 1 min with infusion rate of 50–200 micrograms kg^{-1} min^{-1}	Observe for maternal hypotension	EFM: Potential risks for decreased uterine blood flow, fetal hypoxia, late decelerations, and bradycardia
	Labetalol (Normodyne)	10–20 mg IV followed by 20–80 mg IV every 10 min: total dose of 150 mg	Observe for maternal hypotension	EFM: Observe for fetal bradycardia • May cause IUGR
	Metoprolol (Lopressor)	5 mg IV over 5 min: repeat in 10 min		Rapidly enters fetal circulation; fetal serum levels equal to maternal levels: may cause persistent β-blockade in the newborn
	Propranolol (Inderol)	1 mg IV every 2 min PRN	Observe for maternal hypotension	EFM: Observe for fetal bradycardia • May cause IUGR

TABLE 6–26 ■ CARDIOVASCULAR MEDICATIONS (DOSES, NURSING CARE, AND MATERNAL-FETAL IMPLICATIONS) (Continued)

	Generic Name (Trade Name)	Dose	Nursing Care Specific for Pregnancy	Fetal/Neonatal Effects
Calcium Channel Blockers	Diltiazem (Cardizem)	20 mg IV bolus over 2 min: repeat in 15 min		Possible teratogenic effects
	Nifedipine (Procardia)	10 mg PO; repeat every 6 h	Observe for maternal hypotension and tachycardia May cause severe hypotension and neuromuscular blockade when given with magnesium sulfate	
	Verapamil (Calan)	2.5–5 mg IV bolus over 2 min: repeat in 5 min and then q 30 min PRN to a maximum dose of 20 mg	Observe for maternal hypotension (5%–10% of patients)	Potential for reduced uterine blood flow and fetal hypoxia
Inotropic Agents	Dobutamine (Dobutrex)	Initial dose of 5.0 micrograms kg^{-1} min^{-1} titrate up to 20 micrograms kg^{-1} min^{-1}		
	Digoxin (Lanoxin)	Loading dose 0.5 mg IV over 5 min: then 0.25 IV q 6 h × 2 Maintenance dose 0.125–0.375 mg IV/PO QD	Because of increased maternal volume and elimination, increased doses are required to obtain therapeutic levels	Fetal toxicity and neonatal death have been reported
	Dopamine	Initial dose 5 micrograms kg^{-1} min^{-1}; titrate by 5–10 micrograms kg^{-1} min^{-1}; to micrograms kg^{-1} min^{-1}		
	Epinephrine	Initial bolus 0.5 mg: follow with 2–10 micrograms kg^{-1} min^{-1} infusion: endotracheal 0.5–1.0 mg q 5 min		
Vaso-constrictors	Ephedrine sulphate	10–25 mg slow IV push; repeat q 15 min PRN × 3	First-line medication in pregnancy (causes peripheral vasoconstriction w/out reducing uterine blood flow)	EFM: Observe for fetal tachycardia and decreased baseline variability following administration
	Materaminol (Aramine)	Initial dose of 0.1 mg/min: titrate to 2 mg/min	May interact with oxytocics and ergot medications to produce severe maternal hypertension	Potential for reduced uterine blood flow and fetal hypoxia

(continued)

TABLE 6–26 ■ CARDIOVASCULAR MEDICATIONS (DOSES, NURSING CARE, AND MATERNAL-FETAL IMPLICATIONS) (Continued)

	Generic Name (Trade Name)	Dose	Nursing Care Specific for Pregnancy	Fetal/Neonatal Effects
	Norephinephrine (Levophed)	Initial dose of 0.05 micrograms kg^{-1} min^{-1} titrate to maximum dose of 1.0 micrograms kg^{-1} min^{-1}	Use only with severe maternal hypotension unresponsive to other agents	May compromise uterine blood flow and cause fetal hypoxia and bradycardia
	Phenylephrine (Neosynephrine)	Initial dose of 0.1 micrograms kg^{-1} min^{-1} titrate up to 0.7 micrograms kg^{-1} min^{-1}	May interact with oxytocics and ergot medications to produce severe maternal hypertension.	Potential for reduced uterine blood flow and fetal hypoxia
Vasodilators	Hydralazine (Apressoline)	5–10 mg IV q 20 min: total dose 30 mg	Frequent, small doses preferred to avoid maternal hypotension	EFM: Potential for fetal tachycardia
	Nitroglycerine	IV infusion 10 micrograms/min: titrate up by 10–20 micrograms/min PRN: 0.4–0.8 mg sublingual; 1–2 in of dermal paste		
	Nitroprusside (Nipride)	Initial dose 0.3 micrograms kg^{-1} min^{-1}: titrate to 10 micrograms kg^{-1} min^{-1}	Monitor serum pH levels	Avoid prolonged use: potential for fetal cyanide toxicity

From Arafeh, J. M., & Baird, S M. (2006). Cardiac disease in pregnancy. *Critical Care Nursing Quarterly, 29*(1), 32–52.

It is important to consider the changes that occur immediately at birth with the relief of caval obstruction and transfusion of blood previously in the maternal placental bed. This return has the potential to overwhelm the patient's ability to cope with the extra volume load. On the other hand, failure of the uterus to contract may result in hemorrhage and blood loss. Oxytocin can have marked hemodynamic effects and should be given at the lowest effective dose with close attention to the uterine response to avoid excessive blood loss (Kafka, et al., 2006). Birth, vaginal or cesarean, may be warranted for maternal indications at any time during the antepartum or intrapartum period regardless of viability.

Risks of decompensation continue during the postpartum period, most notably during the first few hours after birth, but up to 72 hours. A period of careful monitoring should follow birth for at least 48 to 72 hours depending on the type of cardiac disease and maternal condition (Earing & Webb, 2005). Maternal death remains a risk during the postpartum period. The most common complications women with cardiac disease experience after birth include development of pulmonary edema and hemorrhage (Arafeh & Baird, 2006). Risk of pulmonary edema can persist for up to 3 to 5 days postpartum due to mobilization of interstitial fluid to the vascular space during the normal diuresis that occurs after birth (Arafeh & Baird; Blackburn, 2003). Risk of hemorrhage is increased for women who have required anticoagulation during the pregnancy (Klein & Galan, 2005). Because of the large amount of blood flow to the uterus at term (750–1,000 mL), significant blood loss can occur in a relative short period if uterine contraction is not maintained during the immediate postpartum period (Arafeh & Baird). Postpartum hemorrhage should be treated aggressively by efforts to promote hemostasis and with replacement volume, blood products, and plasma to avoid hypovolemia (Arafet & Baird; Kafka, et al., 2006; Klein & Galan, 2005).

All women with known underlying cardiac disease and dysfunction should receive care from a specialty care, Level III facility due to the risks of preterm labor and birth, SGA, IUGR, and potential for fetal or maternal compromise. Although most women with cardiac disease tolerate pregnancy and have a successful outcome, some women suffer significant hemodynamic decompensation and require comprehensive care to survive the pregnancy, labor, and birth.

TABLE 6–27 ■ INCREASES IN CARDIAC OUTPUT DURING LABOR AND BIRTH

Labor Phase or Stage	Increase Above Prelabor Values
Latent phase	15%
Active phase	30%
Second stage	45%
Immediately at birth	65%

Nursing Care

Nurses often experience the most frequent and lengthy patient encounters. Therefore, perinatal nurses should develop keen assessment techniques and skills to differentiate normal pregnancy adaptations from cardiac dysfunction and disease (Luppi, 1999). Table 6–23 compares normal adaptations of pregnancy to severe heart disease or heart failure. At any time during the antepartum, intrapartum, or postpartum periods up until 6 months following birth, the nurse should be attuned to symptoms signaling deterioration. If the pregnant woman reports progressive limitation of physical activity because of worsening dyspnea, chest pain that occurs during exercise or increased activity, or syncope that is preceded by palpitations or physical exertion, underlying cardiac disease should be suspected (Blanchard & Shabetai, 2004). As a part of the multidisciplinary team, the perinatal nurse should maintain knowledge of the current plan of care and update that knowledge with each patient encounter.

The woman's history and current physical status are analyzed in relation to cardiovascular physiology and function. The nurse should perform an initial review to include examination of her specific medical, surgical, social, and family history. A current understanding of basic pathophysiology regarding the patient's underlying cardiovascular disorder, previous therapies (ie, past hospital admissions for medical stabilization or surgery), current medications, and current NYHA classification are particularly pertinent (Blanchard & Shabetai, 2004). A woman's occupation can also provide useful information about functional status and environmental risk factors.

The nurses' knowledge of various methods and tools for cardiac assessment are prerequisites for a complete cardiovascular evaluation. Physical assessments will include a head-to-toe inspection with specific focus on cardiorespiratory interaction and subsequent systemic responses. A cardiovascular assessment minimally includes auscultation of the heart, lungs, and breath sounds; identification of pathologic edema; evaluation of respiratory rate and rhythm; evaluation of cardiac rate and rhythm; body weight assessed at the same time of day and on the same scale; assessment of skin color, temperature, and turgor; and capillary refill check. Assessment of the respiratory system reflects the function of the right heart. Auscultation of diminished breath sounds, rales, or rhonchi may reflect right cardiogenic pulmonary edema (Blackburn, 2003). Tachypnea, tachycardia, and anxiety are often early signs of edema and may be present before a cough or abnormal breath sounds appear (Clark, et al., 2003). Abnormal skin and mucous membrane color may indicate problems with oxygenation and perfusion (Curran, 2002). Assessment of the CNS may reveal signs of inadequate blood flow. Restlessness, apprehension, anxiety, or changes in level of consciousness may indicate compromised blood flow and oxygenation of the brain (Blackburn).

Observation for secondary obstetric specific complications is a primary goal in the treatment of cardiac dysfunction during pregnancy. Preeclampsia is a notable example of impaired vascular resistance and increased viscosity of the blood that alters the flow of blood. Hypertension, alone, may be a secondary complication of pregnancy or may signal worsening of the underlying cardiac disease (Blanchard & Shabetai, 2004). Proper and consistent blood pressure assessment is crucial in these patients. Changing from a supine to a sitting position may increase blood pressure by 10% to 20% enhancing cardiac output (Clark, et al., 2003). Maternal positioning, cuff size, auscultation of K4 versus K5 heart sound, device, and timing alter maternal blood pressure results during pregnancy. Electronic blood pressure may cause an enhanced widening of pulse pressure compared with manual readings; however, the mean arterial pressure remains unchanged (Marx, Schwalbe, Cho, & Whitty, 1993). It is imperative that the entire perinatal team is consistent in blood pressure technique to improve accuracy of data.

Any maternal position that causes aortocaval compression may negatively influence maternal cardiac output and blood pressure; avoidance during all phases of pregnancy, labor, and birth is indicated. Vena caval syndrome may limit maternal cardiac output by 25% to 30% and may promote maternal symptomatology in up to 15% of patients after 36 weeks gestation (Clark, et al., 2003; Torgersen & Curran, 2006). Therefore, if improved cardiac output is indicated, lateral recumbent position is optimal.

Additional noninvasive assessment techniques and equipment necessary for the treatment of cardiac disease in pregnancy may include oxygen saturation (SaO_2) via a pulse oximetry, arrhythmia assessment via 5- or 12-lead ECG, electrocardiogram, urinary output, and electronic fetal monitoring. Pulse oximetry should not be used as the ultimate diagnostic tool for hypoxemia. Blood gases offer improved accuracy when severe pulmonary compromise and systemic color changes exist (Clark, et al., 2003). Establishing a patient's baseline prior to pregnancy is optimal. All pregnant women with preexisting cardiac disease should have a baseline 12-lead ECG and may require 5-lead cardiac monitoring during labor and birth. Kidney function is also assessed for adequacy of peripheral perfusion. An indwelling Foley catheter with an urometer can assist with assessment of fluid balance and indicate signs of inadequate renal and uterine perfusion (Curran, 2002). Urinary output should be maintained at least 25 to 30 mL/hour (Clark, et al., Curran). Laboratory evaluation of renal function and perfusion includes electrolytes, blood urea nitrogen, serum creatinine, protein, and uric acid levels (Blackburn, 2003).

Fetal assessment is a sensitive indicator of adequate cardiac function (Patton et al., 1990). Electronic fetal monitoring (EFM) affords the perinatal team a means for assessing uteroplacental perfusion. Antenatal testing (ie, fetal movement counting, nonstress test, or biophysical profile) may assist in the diagnosis of uteroplacental insufficiency during the antepartum period with evidence of SGA, IUGR, or oligohydramnios (Simon, Sadovshy, Aboulafia, Ohel, & Zajicek, 1986). Prior to 23 weeks' gestation, EFM may offer guidance to deterioration in maternal status alone. Once viability is established, nonreassuring fetal heart rate patterns warrant prompt intervention in most cases. Therefore, the perinatal team must modify and maintain an ongoing plan of care which incorporates the potential immediate needs of all patients influenced by underlying cardiac disease (ie, the mother, fetus, and neonate) to include intervention by an emergent cesarean section as indicated.

Certain disorders and advanced degrees of cardiovascular illness may require invasive hemodynamic monitoring using pulmonary artery catheters, peripheral arterial catheters, or central venous pressure monitors (Troiano, 1999). Invasive hemodynamic monitoring is frequently recommended for all woman designated in the NYHA class III or IV experiencing labor. Many women require continuous cardiac rhythm monitoring during acute events and during prolonged hospitalization (Blanchard & Shabetai, 2004).

Heightened vigilance is warranted in women with cardiac disease during pregnancy, particularly the second trimester; the second stage of labor; birth; and immediate postpartum periods. Understanding and assessing for variances in normal pregnancy adaptations may signal deterioration. An interdisciplinary approach assists in overall reduction of maternal, fetal, and neonatal morbidity and mortality.

PULMONARY COMPLICATIONS

Pulmonary diseases have become more prevalent in general and during pregnancy. The increase in prevalence during pregnancy is related in part to increases among younger women, as these women comprise much of the childbearing population (Gardner & Doyle, 2004; Kwon, Triche, Belanger, & Bracken, 2006). Respiratory diseases are an important cause of maternal morbidity and mortality in pregnant women; some of the diseases are unique to pregnancy (amniotic fluid embolism, preeclampsia, and tocolytic-induced pulmonary edema), whereas others are preexisting conditions that worsen or exacerbate (pulmonary edema, peripartum cardiomyopathy, thromboembolic disease, acute respiratory syndrome, asthma, pneumonia, and HIV-related pulmonary complications (Pereira & Krieger, 2004). When pulmonary complications occur during pregnancy, an understanding of the normal physiologic changes of pregnancy and their implications for assessing maternal–fetal status is essential for developing appropriate interventions and treatment.

Anatomic and Physiologic Changes of Pregnancy That Affect the Respiratory System

Pregnant women are more susceptible to injury to the respiratory tract for several reasons, including alterations in the immune system that involve cell-mediated immunity and mechanical and anatomic changes involving the chest and abdominal cavities. The cumulative effect is decreased tolerance to hypoxia and acute changes in pulmonary mechanics. Increased circulating levels of progesterone during pregnancy result in maternal hyperventilation and an up to 50% greater tidal volume without corresponding changes in vital capacity or respiratory rate (Laibl & Sheffield, 2006; Wise, Polito, & Krishman, 2006). There are three important changes in the configuration of the thorax during pregnancy: an increase in the circumference of the lower chest wall, an elevation of the diaphragm, and a 50% widening of the costal angle (Pereira & Krieger, 2006). Oxygen consumption and minute ventilation increase as functional residual capacity and residual volume decrease with expanding abdominal girth. Total lung capacity is preserved, however, because of rib flaring and unimpaired diaphragmatic excursion. Total pulmonary resistance is reduced by 50% as a result of a reduction in airway resistance (Pereira & Krieger, 2004). The overall hemoglobin amount increases and allows for an increase in total oxygen-carrying capacity; however, the increase in blood volume is disproportionate to the increase in hemoglobin concentration thus resulting in a physiologic anemia (Laibl & Sheffield).

The increase in minute ventilation that is associated with pregnancy is often perceived as a shortness of breath. Dyspnea usually starts in the first or second trimester and is reported by up to 75% of healthy pregnant women by 30 weeks of gestation (Pereira & Krieger, 2004; Wise, et al., 2006). Dyspnea occurs secondary to the respiratory stimulation of progesterone, greater hypercapnic ventilatory response, and altered chest wall proprioceptors (Wise, Polito, & Krishman). Shortness of breath at rest or with mild exertion is so common during pregnancy that it is often referred to as "physiologic dyspnea" (Wise, et al.).

Increased estrogen levels result in mucosal edema, hyperemia, mucus hypersecretion, capillary congestion, and greater fragility of the upper respiratory tract (Pereira & Krieger, 2004). Thus, the rhinitis, with its nasal congestion and inflammation, experienced by approximately 30% of pregnant women during pregnancy is caused by hormone changes. Epistaxis, sneezing, voice changes, and mouth breathing also are common (Pereira & Krieger). Sleep disturbances also are reported frequently during pregnancy, most notably insomnia and excessive sleepiness. Sleep-disordered breathing, including obstructive and central sleep apnea, periodic breathing, and nocturnal hypoventilation is uncommon in otherwise healthy women, but occurs at rates higher than the general population in pregnant women (Wise, et al., 2006). Weight gain and upper airway resistance due to estrogen effects may cause sleep apnea to develop or worsen during pregnancy. Regular snoring is reported by approximately 9% of pregnant women. Snoring during pregnancy is not a benign condition as it has been associated with negative maternal and fetal outcomes such hypertension, preeclampsia, IUGR, and lower Apgar scores (Ellegard, 2006). Pregnancy rhinitis may cause obstructive sleep apnea in women who are predisposed to sleep apnea but who can normally breathe through their nose (Ellegard, 2006). Women with rhinitis are at greater risk for snoring and obstructive sleep apnea. The increase in nocturnal blood pressure that often accompanies snoring and obstructive sleep apnea is associated with preeclampsia (Ellegard). Pregnant women often have difficulty breathing in the supine position, but may unintendedly change to this position during sleep. Nasal congestion occurs while the patient is in the supine position because difficult breathing increases the tendency to resort to mouth breathing and snoring. Therefore, pregnancy rhinitis should be identified and treated to minimize risk of potential adverse outcomes. Women should be asked about symptoms of rhinitis routinely during prenatal care.

Pregnancy is characterized by a state of chronic compensated respiratory alkalosis (Wise, et al., 2006). Normal maternal hyperventilation during pregnancy lowers maternal PCO_2 and minimally increases blood pH. The increase in blood pH increases the oxygen affinity of maternal hemoglobin and facilitates elimination of fetal carbon dioxide, but appears to impair release of maternal oxygen to the fetus. The high levels of estrogen and progesterone during pregnancy facilitate a shift in the oxygen dissociation curve back to the right, thereby stimulating oxygen release to a fetus that has an increased affinity for oxygen. These physiologic adaptations ensure that a fetus has every advantage from increased oxygen release and adequate blood gas exchange.

The two leading causes of unexpected maternal deaths during pregnancy are thromboembolic disease and amniotic fluid embolism (Wise, Polito, & Krishman, 2006). Venous thromboembolism frequently has no symptoms, and pulmonary embolism is not suspected clinically in 70% to 80% of patients in whom it is detected postmortem (ACOG, 2000a). During pregnancy women have a fivefold increased risk of venous thromboembolism compared with nonpregnant women (ACOG, 2000b). The hypercoagulable effects of estrogen and the venous stasis that is due to increased intra-abdominal pressure during pregnancy increase the risk of venous thromboembolism. Amniotic fluid embolism may be caused by an intense response to the presence of amniotic fluid in the circulation. The pathogenesis is poorly understood; however, in many cases the clinical presentation includes abruptio placentae and fetal demise, thus disruption of the uteroplacental bed may be an associated factor (Pereira & Krieger, 2004). Amniotic fluid embolism can result in acute lung injury by causing pulmonary vascular endothelial damage, complement activation, and direct platelet aggregation effects of amniotic fluid (Wise, et al., 2006).

Asthma

Significance and Incidence

Asthma is the most common pulmonary disease noted in pregnancy, occurring in 3.5% to 8.4% of pregnant women (Kwon, et al., 2004). The incidence of asthma has risen by more than 30%, and the mortality rate from asthma has risen by 46% since the 1980s (Kwon, et al.). Appropriate management of asthma during pregnancy is important because of the significant risks for the mother and fetus. Goals when managing the woman with asthma during pregnancy include maintaining optimal respiratory status and function, preventing frequent episodes of wheezing requiring emergency therapy, and preventing repeated episodes of hospitalizations for status asthmaticus requiring intubation.

During pregnancy, approximately one-third of women with asthma will improve; one-third will experience worsening of their symptoms, most prominently between 29 and 36 weeks' gestation; and one-third remain unchanged (Beckman, 2003; Blaiss, 2004; Kwon, Belanger, & Bracken, 2003). If asthma is going to worsen, it is likely to occur between 24 and 36 weeks gestation (Gardner & Doyle, 2004). Severe asthmatics, even those under good control prior to pregnancy, are more likely to experience severe exacerbation (Gluck & Gluck, 2006). Overall, asthma is less severe in the last 4 weeks of pregnancy. After birth, 75% of asthmatic women return to their prepregnancy asthmatic status. In most women, asthma severity is the same as prepregnancy within approximately 3 months postpartum (Gluck & Gluck).

Asthma has a variable natural history, creating the variability of expression during pregnancy. History of asthma severity in previous pregnancies may predict the severity of asthma in subsequent pregnancies (Blaiss, 2004). There can be significant risks of asthma for the mother and her fetus. The relationship between asthma and pregnancy outcomes can also be influenced by demographics. Smoking, age extremes, and Hispanic and African-American races have been shown to increase perinatal risk in asthmatic women (Beckmann, 2003). Maternal complications reported among asthmatics include hyperemesis, vaginal bleeding, placenta previa, preeclampsia, hypertensive disorders, a predisposition to infections, gestational diabetes, preterm rupture of membranes, preterm labor, cesarean birth, an increased length of hospital stay, and having a LBW infant (Alexander, Dodds, & Armson, 1998; Beckmann, 2003; Cydulka, 2006; Dombrowski, 2006; Gardner & Doyle, 2006; Kallen, Rydhstroem, & Abery, 2000; Kwon, et al., 2006; Minerbi-Codish, Fraser, Avnun, Glezerman, & Heimer, 1998; National Asthma Education and Prevention Program [NAEPP], 2005; Pereira & Krieger, 2004). Potentially life-threatening complications of severe asthma include pneumothorax, pneumomediastinum, acute cor pulmonale, and respiratory arrest (Cydulka, 2006; Gardner & Doyle, 2004). Maternal mortality is reported as high as 40% when a pregnant woman with asthma requires mechanical ventilation (Gardner & Doyle).

There is little risk to the fetus with well-controlled asthma. However, exacerbations causing hypoxia, hypocapnia, alkalosis, and decreased uterine blood flow increase the incidence of IUGR, oligohydramnios, meconium-stained amniotic fluid, preterm birth, and neonatal mortality (Beckmann, 2003; Coleman & Rund, 1997). The fetus depends on its oxygen supply from maternal arterial oxygen content, venous return, and cardiac output, as well as from uterine artery and placental blood flow. Maternal hypoxia can cause fetal hypoxia directly, or the consequences of poorly controlled asthma such as hypocapnia and alkalosis can cause fetal hypoxia indirectly by reducing uteroplacental blood flow (Cydulka, 2006). The fetus is sensitive to changes in maternal respiratory status and any decrease in maternal PaO_2 may result in decreased fetal PaO_2 and fetal hypoxia (Gardner & Doyle, 2004). Asthma has been associated with a fetal death rate twice that of pregnant women without asthma (Blaiss, 2004; Silver, 2007).

Severe or uncontrolled asthma can be life-threatening for a woman and her fetus during pregnancy. The NAEPP Working Group Report on Managing Asthma during Pregnancy: Recommendations for Pharmacologic Treatment–Update 2004 (2005) defines asthma control as:

- Minimal or no chronic symptoms day or night
- Minimal or no exacerbations
- No limitations on activities
- Maintenance of (near) normal pulmonary function
- Minimal use of short-acting inhaled beta 2-agonist
- Minimal or no adverse effects from medications

Effective control can ensure a pregnancy outcome close to that of the general population (ACOG & ACAAI, 2000; Chambers, 2006; Namazy & Schatz, 2006).

Definition

Asthma is a chronic inflammatory disease of the airways in which the tracheobronchial tree is hyperresponsive to a multitude of stimuli (Gardner & Doyle, 2004). Asthma is one of the specific disease entities that is included in the general category of obstructive lung disease, which is characterized by limitation of airflow that generally is marked more during expiration than inspiration and results in a prolonged expiratory phase. Asthma has varying degrees of airway obstruction, bronchial hyperresponsiveness, and airway edema that are accompanied by eosinophilic and lymphocytic inflammation (Gardner & Doyle). This results in edema of the bronchial wall, airway diameter reduction, and secretions that are thick and tenacious. Asthma involves a complex interplay of inflammatory cells, cellular mediators, and external triggers (Gluck & Gluck, 2006). It is a chronic disease with acute exacerbations that are characterized by recurrent bouts of wheezing and dyspnea that result from airway obstruction (Gardner & Doyle). The airway of an asthmatic patient is hyperresponsive to stimuli such as allergens, viral infections, air pollutants, smoke, food additives, exercise, cold air, and emotional stress (Gardner & Doyle; Kwon, et al., 2006). Common triggers of asthma exacerbations are listed in Table 6–28.

TABLE 6–28 ■ COMMON TRIGGERS OF ASTHMA EXACERBATIONS

Allergens	Pollens, molds, animal dander, house-dust mites, cockroach antigen
Irritants	Strong odors, cigarette smoke, wood smoke, occupational dusts and chemicals, air pollution
Medical conditions	Sinusitis, viral upper respiratory infections, esophageal reflux
Drugs, additives	Sulfites, nonsteroidal antiinflammatory drugs, aspirin, beta blockers, contrast media
Other	Emotional stress, exercise, cold air, menses

Pathophysiology

The precise cause of airway inflammation and hyperresponsiveness is unknown. When triggered by external stimuli, inflammatory cells infiltrate bronchial tissue and release chemical mediators such as prostaglandins, histamine, cytokines, bradykinin, and leukotrienes. Ultimately, airway smooth muscle responsiveness is increased because of these mediators. Narrowing of the airway lumen and airway hyperresponsiveness may be a result of the development of bronchial mucosal edema, excess fluid and mucous, inflammatory cellular infiltrates, and smooth muscle hypertrophy and constriction. During asthma exacerbations, there is decreased expiratory airflow, increased functional residual capacity, increased pulmonary vascular resistance, hypoxemia, and hypercapnia. The fetus can be negatively affected during acute episodes of asthma in which there is maternal arterial hypoxemia and the potential for uterine artery vasoconstriction (Cydulka, 2006; Gardner & Doyle, 2004). Rapid and profound decreases in fetal oxygen saturation and resultant fetal hypoxia occur with clinically significant decreases in maternal PaO_2 below 60 mm Hg (Blaiss, 2004). Despite surviving in an environment of low oxygen tension, the fetus has very little oxygen reserve. Administration of oxygen to the mother may produce only small increases in fetal PaO_2, but this may increase fetal oxygen saturation significantly (Gardner & Doyle; Simpson & James, 2005). Oxygen should be administered as needed to maintain maternal oxygen saturation at 95% or higher (Cydulka).

Clinical Manifestations

The clinical manifestation of asthma is easily recognized. The woman may have only one or a combination of symptoms. Signs of respiratory distress are obvious and include shortness of breath, wheezing, nonproductive coughing, flaring nostrils, chest tightness, and use of accessory respiratory muscles. There may be scant or copious sputum, which is usually clear. Reports of nocturnal awakenings with asthma symptoms are common. Nonspecific stimuli such as an upper respiratory infection or a respiratory irritant may have provoked the exacerbation. An increase in

cough, the appearance of chest tightness, dyspnea, wheezing, decrease in fetal movement, or a 20% decrease in peak expiratory flow rate (PEFR) may signal worsening of asthma and should warrant immediate clinical attention (Cydulka, 2006). Cyanosis, lethargy, agitation, intercostal retractions, and a respiratory rate greater than 30 per minute indicate hypoxia and impending respiratory arrest. Patients with the following symptoms should be considered for intubation and mechanical ventilation using "permissive hypercapnia": (1) worsening pulmonary function tests, (2) despite vigorous bronchodilator therapy; decreasing PaO_2, increasing $PaCO_2$, or progressive respiratory acidosis, (3) declining mental status; and (4) increasing fatigue (Cydulka, 2006).

Nursing Assessment

Guidelines for assessment of the severity of asthma before therapy is initiated have been developed by the National Heart, Lung, and Blood Institute, a division of the National Institutes of Health (Scheffer, 1991). This classification system, like many others, was developed without specific consideration of pregnancy, but it may be helpful when assessing an adult patient with asthma. Patients are identified as mild, moderate, or severe asthmatics. Mild asthmatics experience exacerbations with coughing and wheezing no more than two times each week. There may be an intolerance of vigorous exercise. Women with moderate asthma experience more symptoms than women classified as having mild asthma. Severe exacerbations are infrequent with emergent care required less than three times each year. Severe asthmatics experience daily wheezing, and require emergency treatment more than three times per year. Women with severe asthma have poor exercise tolerance.

Identification of the woman with severe asthma is important so a plan of care and intensive treatment can be initiated early. Without comprehensive early treatment, there is significant risk to the mother and fetus. Characteristics of maternal history that should alert healthcare providers to an increased risk of a potentially fatal asthma exacerbation are listed in Display 6–37. Nursing evaluation of the symptoms of asthma begins with clinical assessment of signs of respiratory

DISPLAY 6-37

Markers for Potentially Fatal Asthma

- History of systemic steroid therapy >4 weeks
- Three recent emergency room visits for asthma
- History of multiple hospitalizations for asthma
- History of hypoxic seizure, hypoxic syncope, or intubation
- History of admission to an intensive care unit for asthma

DISPLAY 6-38

Clinical Findings in Asthma

SIGNS AND SYMPTOMS

- Shortness of breath, chest tightness, cough
- Recurrent episodes of symptoms
- Nocturnal awakenings from symptoms
- Waxing and waning of symptoms

AUSCULTORY FINDINGS

- Diffuse wheezes
- Diffuse rhonchi
- Longer expiratory phase than inspiratory phase

SIGNS OF RESPIRATORY DISTRESS

- Rapid respiratory rate (>30 breaths/min)
- Pulsus paradoxus >15 mm Hg
- Retractions intercostally or supraclavicularly
- Lethargy
- Confusion or agitation
- Cyanosis

distress. Significant findings include dyspnea, cough, wheezing, chest tightness, nasal flaring, presence of sputum, and tachycardia. Intercostal retractions or a respiratory rate greater than 30 per minute indicates moderate to severe asthma. Pulsus paradoxus of more than 15 mm Hg is an indication of severe asthma. If pulsus paradoxus is present, blood pressure is audible only during expiration. To make this assessment, carefully observe the woman's breathing, noting when systole first appears, and the millimeter level of mercury until pulsations are heard during inspiration and expiration. Lung auscultation usually reveals bilateral expiratory wheezing. Occasionally, on inspiration or expiration, only rhonchi are heard. Rales are rarely auscultated in asthmatics. Detailed clinical findings are listed in Display 6–38.

Clinical evaluation is an invaluable assessment parameter in asthma, but laboratory findings are also useful in determining severity of an asthma attack and distinguishing it from other respiratory conditions. The most beneficial tools are pulmonary function tests such as peak expiratory flow and measurements of oxygen saturation and arterial blood gases. Predicted values of peak expiratory flow rate are unchanged during pregnancy and range from 380 to 550 L/minute. An individual baseline should be established for each woman when her asthma is under control. Evaluation of exacerbations can be made by comparing baseline with current peak flow values. Peak expiratory flow values that are more than 50% below personal baseline require immediate attention. Maternal oxygen saturation monitoring is a simple, noninvasive measure of oxygenation. Values that remain below 95% are significant for an exacerbation of asthma that requires attention. For the fetus to maintain normal levels of oxygenation and minimize risks of fetal hypoxemia and IUGR, maternal oxygen saturation should be at least 95%.

During pregnancy, evaluations of arterial blood gases can help to establish severity of an asthma attack, with attention focused primarily on the pH and PCO_2 to define severity. A mild attack is characterized

by an elevated pH and a PCO_2 below normal for pregnancy. The combination of normal pH, low PO_2, and normal PCO_2 for pregnancy indicates a moderate asthma attack. A low PO_2, low pH, and a high PCO_2 are most significant for severe respiratory compromise. When maternal arterial PO_2 falls below 60 mm Hg, the fetus is in severe jeopardy, and risk of fetal demise is increased.

Nursing Interventions

The goals of therapeutic interventions for pregnant women with asthma are to maintain normal pulmonary function, control symptoms, prevent exacerbations, avoid adverse outcomes, avoid adverse effects of medications, and ensure the birth of a healthy baby. Four integral components are important for effective management of asthma in pregnant women: patient education, objective assessment of maternal pulmonary function and fetal well-being, control of environmental factors, and pharmacologic therapy (Blaiss, 2004; NAEPP, 2005).

Patient Education

Education should be designed to assist women to gain the motivation, confidence, and skill to keep their asthma under control. Much of the day-to-day management of asthma is the responsibility of the woman.

The pregnant woman must have an understanding of the potential adverse effects of uncontrolled asthma on herself and the fetus. Although some women may be reluctant to take prescribed medications for fear they may harm the developing fetus, the woman needs to be reassured that risks to the fetus from hypoxia related to untreated asthma are greater than risks of medications (Namazy & Schatz, 2006). It is critically important that the pregnant woman be able to recognize symptoms of worsening asthma and treat them appropriately (Namazy & Schatz). Correct inhaler technique should be reinforced, and the patient should know how to reduce her exposure to, or control, those factors that exacerbate her asthma (Namazy & Schatz). A comprehensive knowledge base and patient comfort with the management are essential. Educational topics (NAEPP, 2005) include the following:

- Signs and symptoms of asthma
- Airway changes
- Avoiding asthma triggers
- Effects of pregnancy on the disease, and the disease on pregnancy
- Peak flow meters and metered dose inhalers
- Role of medications
- Correct use of medications
- Adverse effects of medications
- Managing exacerbations
- Emergency care

Individualized education throughout pregnancy should be guided by assessment of the woman's understanding of her asthma assessment and management plan and her level of cooperation. It is essential to highlight the changes that pregnancy has on asthma and its treatment. When there is active participation by the healthcare provider, the pregnant woman, and her family, asthma control can be maximized.

Ongoing Maternal and Fetal Assessment

It is important to identify the pregnant woman with potentially fatal asthma so that maternal or fetal death can be avoided through greatly intensified treatment. Potentially fatal asthma includes a history of any one of the factors listed in Display 6–37. During pregnancy, monthly evaluations of pulmonary function and asthma history are important. These assessments should include pulmonary function testing, ideally spirometry, detailed symptom history (symptom frequency, nocturnal asthma, interference with activities, exacerbations, and medication use); and physical examination with specific attention paid to the lungs (Namazy & Schatz, 2006). In addition to the subjective and objective measurements of the severity of a woman's asthma, ongoing fetal assessment is equally important. Serial ultrasonography beginning early in pregnancy to monitor trends in fetal growth and antepartum fetal testing such as fetal movement counts (FMC), nonstress tests (NSTs), and biophysical profile (BPP) based on maternal–fetal status are essential to ensure fetal well-being for the moderate or severe asthmatic patient (NAEPP, 2005; Namazy & Schatz).

Environmental Control

Identification of triggering factors for asthma in each woman is an important aspect of nonpharmacologic management that may improve clinical status, prevent acute exacerbations, and decrease the need for pharmacologic intervention. More than 75% of asthmatics report known reactions to common inhaled allergens (Dombrowski, 1997). Historic information and prior skin testing may give important information regarding common triggers such as pollens, molds, house dust mites, animal dander, and cockroach antigens. Other common asthma irritants include air pollutants, strong odors, food additives, and tobacco smoke.

It is particularly important for the pregnant asthmatic woman to stop smoking during her pregnancy (Gluck & Gluck, 2006). Education about the risks of smoking, including an increased severity of her asthma, bronchitis, or sinusitis and the need for increased medication, can be helpful in motivating the woman to stop smoking. In addition to the association between smoking and respiratory complications, smoking increases the risk of preterm birth and LBW. Although most women indicate a desire to quit smoking during pregnancy, this goal is not often met for a number of reasons. The section about preterm labor covers risks of smoking during pregnancy and smoking cessation programs in detail.

Viral respiratory infections, vigorous exercise, and emotional stress are common stimuli of severe asthma. Drugs such as aspirin, beta-blockers, nonsteroidal antiinflammatory (NSAID) medications, radiocontrast media, and sulfites have been implicated as asthma triggers as well. Once the woman has been assisted to identify common asthma triggers, exposure to allergens or irritants can be minimized, thereby lessening exacerbations.

Pharmacologic Therapy

The goals of asthma therapy include protection of the pulmonary system from irritant stimuli, prevention of pulmonary and inflammatory response to allergen exposure, relief of bronchospasm, and resolution of airway inflammation to reduce airway hyperresponsiveness and improve pulmonary function. Undertreatment is an ongoing problem in the care of pregnant asthmatic women. Medications commonly used in asthma management are generally considered safe and effective during pregnancy and lactation, carrying FDA pregnancy risk categories of B or C (Blaiss, 2004;

Namazy & Schatz, 2006). These drugs have been widely used for many years without evidence of teratogenic effects. It is safer for pregnant women with asthma and their fetuses to take their prescribed medications than to experience an exacerbation. The effectiveness of medications for the treatment of asthma during pregnancy is assumed to be the same as in nonpregnant women (Chambers, 2006; NAEPP, 2005). Pharmacotherapy is enhanced by appropriate environmental control measures and immunotherapy for the significant number of asthmatics with an allergic component to their disease. However, environmental control of asthma is frequently inadequate, and drug therapy is the hallmark of asthma management. Inhalation therapy is usually more effective than systemic treatment, because asthma is an airway disease. Aerosolized medications are ideal because they deliver the drug directly to the airways, minimizing systemic side effects, and decreasing exposure to the fetus.

Bronchodilators

The use of short-acting beta 2-agonists for powerful bronchodilation has been the mainstay of chronic and acute asthma therapy for decades (Chambers, 2006). The onset of action is rapid, making them the preferred rescue medication for acute exacerbations of asthma. Beta 2-agonists currently available have been shown to be safe for both mother and fetus. Albuterol is commonly prescribed and an excellent safety profile has been established (NAEPP, 2005). This group of drugs causes common side effects such as maternal tachycardia, maternal tremor, widened pulse pressure, restlessness, anxiety, and increased water retention. Continuous parenteral infusions may result in more serious side effects. Adverse reactions include tachyphylaxis, cardiac arrhythmias, and paradoxical bronchoconstriction. Other than transient hypoglycemia and tachycardia, few direct adverse effects have been seen in the fetuses or neonates of women treated with beta-2-agonists (Briggs, Freeman, & Yaffe, 2005). Inhaled beta-2-agonists, taken only as needed, are usually sufficient to control women with mild, intermittent asthma. If symptoms disappear and pulmonary function normalizes, these medications can be used indefinitely. Prolonged use may result in rapid tolerance and limited usefulness. Women are candidates for antiinflammatory therapy if they require the use of a beta-2-agonist more than three times each week. In the management of moderate to severe persistent asthma, long-acting beta-agonists may be added to a regimen of inhaled corticosteroids for greater asthma control (Blaiss, 2004; NAEPP, 2005). Salmeterol and formoterol are newer long-acting beta-agonists that have not been studied enough to recommend them as safe for use during pregnancy at this time (NAEPP). Because of the success of inhalation therapy, systemic aminophylline and theophylline are rarely used today. Sustained-release theophylline may be helpful for the pregnant woman whose symptoms are primarily nocturnal, because of its long-acting properties. Although safe at recommended doses during pregnancy, theophylline treatment is associated with a higher incidence of maternal side effects than inhaled beta-agonists (NAEPP).

Antiinflammatory Therapy

One of the greatest advances in asthma treatment in the past decade has been the availability of inhaled corticosteroids (ACOG & ACAAI, 2000; Blaiss, 2004). For those with persistent mild asthma, these medications are currently the treatment of choice as they reduce the risk of asthma exacerbations associated with pregnancy, and have not been related to any increases in congenital malformations or other adverse perinatal outcomes (NAEPP, 2005). To minimize systemic effects and improve respiratory tract penetration, inhaled corticosteroids are administered with a spacer. At recommended doses, these medications act without systemic side effects to effectively reduce mucus secretion and airway edema. They may increase bronchodilator responsiveness while inhibiting many of the mediators of inflammation. Studies suggest that beclomethasone or budesonide are the inhaled steroids of choice for use during pregnancy due to reassuring safety data (ACOG & ACAAI).

Unlike the immediate-acting bronchodilators, the effects of inhaled corticosteroids are gradual. After 2 to 4 weeks of use, full effects of symptom suppression and peak expiratory flow rate improvement are seen. Patient education is vital to ensure that the woman will continue her antiinflammatory therapy until the medication achieves maximum effectiveness. The most common side effect of inhaled steroids is hoarseness; it disappears when therapy is discontinued. Other uncommon side effects include throat irritation, cough, and oral thrush. Infrequent effects such as easy bruising, skin thinning, and low serum cortisol levels have been reported. Published data have shown no evidence of teratogenicity with use of inhaled corticosteroids (Blaiss, 2004). Intranasal corticosteroids have not been studied during human pregnancy, but as their systemic effects are minimal, continued use during pregnancy appears to be safe (ACOG & ACAAI, 2000). Cromolyn and nedocromil are nonsteroidal antiinflammatory agents that work by preventing the release of inflammatory mediators through stabilization of mast cells. Neither produces any side effects. Both are FDA category B drugs (Schatz, 2001), and cromolyn data have demonstrated long-term safety (Blaiss). Neither is as effective as inhaled corticosteroids in preventing asthma symptoms.

Corticosteroids

A course of oral corticosteroids may be effective when maximum doses of bronchodilators and antiinflammatory agents fail to control asthma. If a prednisone "burst" or tapering dose fails to relieve symptoms or prevent frequent recurrence, severe asthmatics require additional therapy. Oral corticosteroids may be needed chronically or used in short tapering courses. There are documented side effects for the 5% of asthmatics who require stabilization with chronic therapy. Common unfavorable side effects include preeclampsia, gestational diabetes, or worsening of diabetes mellitus, preterm birth, and LBW (ACOG & ACAAI, 2000; Blaiss, 2004). First-trimester use of oral corticosteroids has been associated with an increased risk of cleft lip with or without cleft palate (ACOG & ACAAI, 2000; NAEPP, 2005). There is also concern for the developing fetus from long-term steroid use. When compared with chronic treatment, short-term steroid use carries a low risk of serious side effects. A 7- to 10-day course of steroids assists with rapid control of an exacerbation of asthma, while giving time for inhaled antiinflammatory agents to reach full effectiveness.

Leukotriene Modifiers

Leukotriene modifiers are a new group of medications used to treat mild to moderate asthma, although they have been shown to be less effective than inhaled corticosteroids in overall efficacy (NAEPP, 2005). These medications are currently not preferred for use during pregnancy, as minimal data are available regarding their use during gestation (ACOG & ACAAI, 2000; NAEPP).

Immunotherapy

Pregnant women with asthma who have allergens responsive to desensitization may benefit from allergen immunotherapy. Pollens, dust mites, and some fungi are aeroallergens that have been effectively suppressed with the use of allergy injections. Maintenance dose injections may continue for a pregnant woman who is not reacting regularly and continues to benefit from the immunotherapy (Blaiss, 2004). Because there is a 6- to 7-month interval before clinical benefits are seen and significant risk of a systemic reaction, pregnancy is not a time for initiation of immunotherapy.

Other Therapies

Antihistamines may be useful in the woman with a clear allergic stimulus to her asthma. The safest decongestant for use during pregnancy appears to be pseudoephedrine, although it has recently been linked to the birth defect gastroschisis (ACOG & ACAAI, 2000). Pseudoephedrine has been routinely used in the treatment of rhinitis, although intranasal corticosteroids are currently the most effective medications for this condition and carry a low risk of systemic effects. Unless absolutely necessary, avoidance of oral decongestants in the first trimester is suggested. Pregnant women with asthma should be cautioned about use of over-the-counter medications, because many of the medications contain vasoconstrictors that may cause fetal abnormalities and decreased uterine blood flow (National Heart, Lung, and Blood Institute National Asthma Education Program Working Group on Asthma and Pregnancy, 1993). The influenza vaccine is indicated for women with chronic asthma after the first trimester. Because it is an inactivated virus, the vaccine poses no risk to the fetus. Less is known about teratogenic effects on the fetus with the many newer medications, so caution must be used during pregnancy. Generally a stepwise approach to the pharmacologic management of chronic asthma is preferred (see Table 6-29).

Antepartum Care

When women have had exacerbations of asthma during pregnancy, vigilant fetal surveillance is important, especially after 20 weeks' gestation (Cousins, 1999). At each prenatal visit, confirmation that fundal height and fetal size are consistent with expected normal values based on current gestation age is crucial. Serial ultrasounds, biophysical profiles (BPPs), and electronic fetal heart monitoring are used to monitor fetal status on an ongoing basis (Namazy & Schatz, 2006). Fetal movement counting may be initiated.

Inpatient Management

Acute Exacerbations

Rapid reversal of exacerbations of asthma is critical in the pregnant woman. The following are important when caring for women with exacerbations:

- Oxygen administration initiated to maintain PaO_2 as close to normal as possible (>60 mm Hg or SaO_2 or PaO_2 >95%)
- Ongoing maternal pulse oximetry
- Baseline arterial blood gases
- Continuous EFM
- Baseline pulmonary function tests performed to gather baseline information
- Beta-agonist inhalation therapy every 20 minutes should be initiated.

If initial bronchodilator treatments fail to result in adequate response, high-dose intravenous corticosteroids are the mainstay of therapy.

Uterine contractions are not uncommon during an exacerbation of asthma. Magnesium sulfate is the tocolytic of choice if cervical change is noted. Use of magnesium sulfate therapy may enhance bronchodilation

TABLE 6–29 ■ STEPWISE APPROACH FOR THE PHARMACOLOGIC MANAGEMENT OF CHRONIC ASTHMA DURING PREGNANCY

Category	Step Therapy
Mild intermittent	Inhaled ß-agonist as needed
Mild persistent	Low-dose inhaled corticosteroid
	Alternative: cromolyn, leukotriene receptor antagonist, or theophylline
Moderate persistent	Low-dose inhaled corticosteroid and long acting ß-agonist
	Alternative: low-dose or (if needed) medium-dose inhaled corticosteroid and either theophylline or leukotriene receptor antagonist
Severe persistent	High-dose inhaled corticosteroid and long-acting ß-agonist and if needed, oral corticosteroids.
	Alternative: High-dose inhaled corticosteroid and theophylline

From National Asthma Education and Prevention Program (2005). *Working group report on managing asthma during pregnancy: Recommendations for pharmacologic treatment-update 2004.* (NIH Publication 05-3279.) Washington, DC: United States Department of Health and Human Services.

as well. Beta-agonist therapy with terbutaline may be used to control preterm labor unless the woman already uses a ß-agonist inhaler. For these women, terbutaline should be avoided to minimize the potential serious additive side effects of combined beta-agonist therapy. Nonsteroidal antiinflammatory medications such as indomethacin may exacerbate asthma and are contraindicated. Antibiotics may be used to cover atypical pneumonia or secondary bacterial infection. Strict intake and output is necessary to minimize risk of fluid overload from ß-mimetic therapy and intravenous steroids and avoid pulmonary edema. Ongoing care of the woman with an acute exacerbation is based on her response to the initial treatment plan.

Labor and Birth

Approximately 10% to 20% of women with asthma experience an exacerbation during the intrapartum period (Gluck & Gluck, 2006; Namazy & Schatz, 2006). The risk of dyspnea or wheezing can be minimized through ongoing asthma medication during labor and the postpartum period. An exacerbation during labor is treated no differently than at other times. Control of the asthma is a priority for safety of the mother and her fetus. Intravenous access should be established on admission (Gardner & Doyle, 2004). A peak flow rate should be taken on admission and then every 12 hours (Gardner & Doyle). If the woman develops symptoms of asthma, peak flows should be measured after treatments (Gardner & Doyle). If a systemic steroid has been administered in the past month, then stress-dose steroid should be given during labor to prevent maternal adrenal crisis (Namazy & Schatz). For example, intravenous hydrocortisone (100 mg every 8 hours for 24 hours) should be given to women

who have received corticosteroids during the pregnancy (Gardner & Doyle).

Continuous assessment of maternal oxygen saturation by pulse oximeter is important to attempt to maintain oxygen saturation values above 95%. Oxygen should be administered by mask if saturation values fall below this level. Additional information can be obtained from arterial blood gases. Air exchange is enhanced through patient positioning in a semi-Fowler's or high-Fowler's position. Potential for fluid overload can be avoided through strict intake and output measurements. Oxytocin is the drug of choice for the induction of labor, because prostaglandin $F_2\alpha$ is a known bronchoconstrictor (Towers, Briggs, & Rojas, 2004). The use of prostaglandin E_2 for cervical ripening intracervically or intravaginally has not been reported to result in a clinical exacerbation of asthma (Namazy & Schatz, 2006). The pain relief method of choice for women in labor with asthma is epidural analgesia (Gardner & Doyle, 2004). Epidural analgesia can reduce oxygen consumption and may enhance the effects of bronchodilators (National Heart, Lung, and Blood Institute National Asthma Education Program Working Group on Asthma and Pregnancy, 1993). Meperidine and morphine sulfate are contraindicated because of their actions on smooth muscle and the potential for respiratory depression, and they may result in bronchospasm through histamine release (Gardner & Doyle). Butorphanol or fentanyl is an appropriate substitute (Gardner & Doyle). A vaginal birth is safest for all women, but particularly for women with asthma. Maternal and fetal hypoxia that is the result of asthma can be managed medically; rarely is cesarean birth indicated. If cesarean birth is necessary for obstetric reasons, regional anesthesia is preferred;

however, if general anesthesia is required, propofol is the agent of choice (Gardner & Doyle). Use of methylergonovine (ie, Methergine) and prostaglandin $F_{2\alpha}$ for postpartum hemorrhage can cause bronchoconstriction and should be avoided.

Breastfeeding should be encouraged in women with asthma because breast milk confers some immunity to infection to the baby, especially to respiratory and gastrointestinal infections (Gardner & Doyle, 2004). Although breast milk may contain small amounts of the medications used to treat asthma, in general they are not known to be harmful to the baby (Gardner & Doyle). Corticosteroids are approximately 90% protein bound in the blood and not secreted in any significant amounts in breast milk. Inhaled beta-2-agonists (terbutaline, metapronterenol, albuterol) by metered dosage is associated with the lowest exposure to the baby. Theophylline, as with caffeine, can cause irritability and wakefulness in the baby and is no longer considered the primary treatment (Gardner & Doyle, 2004).

Pneumonia in Pregnancy

Significance and Incidence

The incidence of pneumonia during pregnancy is similar to that of the nonpregnant population, but the disease course is often more virulent, less tolerated, and the mortality rates from some pathogens is high (Laibl & Sheffield, 2006). It is the third leading cause of death in the US in pregnant women (Pereira & Krieger, 2004). The spectrum of causative pathogens is similar to that of the nonpregnant population, and the management does not differ in general from the nonpregnant state. Pneumonia is an uncommon infection in pregnant women, but the complications for mother and fetus can be serious. It is difficult to estimate the true incidence of pneumonia during pregnancy because of variability of the rates in published studies. In some studies, the incidence of viral and bacterial pneumonia during pregnancy is estimated as 0.78% to 2.7% (Munn, Groome, Atterbury, Baker, & Hoff, 1999; Yost, Bloom, Richey, Ramin, & Cunningham, 2000). Overall pneumonia is the primary diagnosis for approximately 4.2% of nonobstetric antepartum hospital admissions (Laibl & Sheffield, 2006). Pneumonia is seen more frequently in women with poor health, those who postponed childbearing, pregnant women with chronic medical conditions, and the epidemic of human immunodeficiency virus. These women are at greater risk for opportunistic lung infections. Pneumonia has also been strongly associated with asthma, HIV, cystic fibrosis, anemia, and illicit drug use (Goodnight & Soper, 2005; Lim, Macfarlan, & Colthorpe, 2001; Munn, Groome, Atterbury, Baker, & Hoff).

Antepartum pneumonia has been associated with the use of tocolytics, as well as with administration of corticosteroids for enhancement of fetal lung maturity (Goodnight & Soper, 2005). Pneumonia in pregnancy is not gestational age dependent. The average gestational age at diagnosis is 32 weeks' gestation.

Pneumonia is the leading cause of maternal mortality from nonobstetric infection in the peripartum period (Pereira & Krieger, 2004). Maternal conditions and complications that are associated with pneumonia are listed in Display 6-39. Although the introduction of antimicrobial therapy has significantly decreased maternal mortality from 23% to less than 4%, risk of maternal and fetal morbidity continues (Laibl & Sheffield, 2006). The majority of maternal deaths resulting from pneumonia are in women with preexisting cardiopulmonary disease (Goodnight & Soper, 2005). Viral pneumonias may be more virulent during pregnancy than in the nonpregnant patient.

Maternal complications of pneumonia during pregnancy include preterm labor, emphysema, bacteremia, pneumothorax, atrial fibrillation, pericardial tamponade, and respiratory failure requiring intubation (Goodnight & Soper, 2005; Madinger, Greenspoon, & Ellrodt, 1989; Munn, Groome, Atterbury, Baker, & Hoff, 1999). Pneumonia has not been related to any congenital syndrome in neonates, but antepartum respiratory infection has been associated with increased incidence

DISPLAY 6-39

Complications Associated With an Increased Risk of Pneumonia

- Coexisting chronic conditions such as asthma, diabetes, heart disease
- Altered mental status
- Vital sign abnormalities
    - Respiration ≥30 per minute
    - Temperature ≥39°C or ≤35°C
    - Hypotension
    - Pulse ≥125 beats per minute
- Laboratory data abnormalities
    - White blood cell count <4,000 mm³ or 30,000 mm³
    - Room air PaO_2 <60 mm Hg
    - Room air $PaCO_2$ >50 mm Hg
    - Serum creatinine >1.2 mg/dL
- Multiorgan dysfunction or sepsis
- Radiologic abnormalities
- Multilobe involvement
- Cavitation
- Pleural effusion

of complicated preterm birth. The loss of maternal ventilatory reserve normally seen in pregnancy coupled with maternal fever, tachycardia, respiratory alkalosis, and hypoxemia seen with respiratory infections can be adverse for fetuses. Reports of preterm labor and birth, small for gestational age infants, and fetal death have been attributed to pneumonia during pregnancy (Goodnight & Soper, 2005; Lim, Macfarlane, & Colthorpe, 2001; Nolan & Hankins, 1995; Salmon & Bruick-Sorge, 2003).

Varicella pneumonia may occur in up to 20% of adults with varicella (chickenpox) infection. The incidence of maternal varicella during pregnancy is rare (0.7 per 1,000) because more than 90% of women are immunized (Pereira & Krieger, 2004). The mortality rate for varicella pneumonia during pregnancy may exceed 35% because women with varicella pneumonia are at risk for multiple complications such as bacterial superinfection, acute respiratory distress syndrome (ARDS), endotoxin shock, and bronchiolitis obliterans organizing pneumonia (Chandra, Patel, Schiavello, & Briggs, 1998). Intrauterine infections occur in 8.7% to 26% of cases, exclusively during the first 20 weeks of gestation (Pereira & Krieger). The neonatal death rate for varicella pneumonia is between 9% and 20% (Grant, 1996). Pregnant women with varicella pneumonia should be hospitalized (Pereira & Krieger).

Fungal pneumonia from environmental organisms is rare in pregnancy, occurring most often in severely immunocompromised patients (Laibl & Sheffield, 2006). In nonimmunosuppressed patients, this disease is frequently mild, self-limiting, and usually resolves with or without treatment in women without other preexisting illnesses. Disseminated disease from *Pneumocystis carinii* develops occasionally in immunocompromised patients, and carries a high risk of preterm birth and perinatal and maternal mortality. Symptoms include fever, anorexia, dry cough, and several weeks of dyspnea. Treatment is prolonged and carries risks to the developing fetus.

Definition

Pneumonia is an inflammatory infection of the alveoli and distal bronchioles of the lower respiratory tract resulting in consolidation, exudation, and hypoxemia. It may be primary or secondary and may involve one or both lungs. The microorganisms that give rise to pneumonia are always present in the upper respiratory tract, and unless resistance is lowered, they cause no harm. Most organisms are introduced through inhalation, or aspiration of secretions from the nasopharyngeal tract. Bacterial and viral pneumonias and aspiration pneumonitis are the most commonly seen

D I S P L A Y   6 - 4 0

Causes of Pneumonia in Pregnancy

- *Streptococcus pneumococcus*
- *Haemophilus influenzae*
- *Legionella* species
- *Mycoplasma pneumoniae*
- *Chlamydia pneumoniae*
- *Pneumocystis carinii*
- Viral pathogens
  - Influenza A
  - Influenza B
  - Varicella-zoster virus (VZV)
  - Coronavirus (SARS)
- Aspiration
- Fungi

pneumonias during gestation (Salmon & Bruick-Sorge, 2003) (Display 6–40). Alteration in maternal immune status to prevent rejection of the developing fetus is the major factor predisposing women to severe pneumonic infections during pregnancy.

Pathophysiology

Pneumonia develops when host defenses are overwhelmed by an organism invading the lung parenchyma. Although a number of defense mechanisms protect lower airways from pathogens, infection leads to increased permeability of the capillaries. This causes alveolar and interstitial fluid accumulation, resulting in abnormal chest radiograph findings. Air space pneumonia, interstitial pneumonia, and bronchopneumonia are commonly seen on the chest radiograph of patients with pneumonia. Radiographic patterns differ based on the infective agent and can be helpful in diagnosing the cause of pneumonia.

Clinical Manifestations

Bacterial Pneumonia

The leading cause of pneumonia in pregnant women is bacterial (Pereira & Krieger, 2004). Risks for acquiring bacterial pneumonia include asthma, smoking, positive HIV status, poor nutrition, anemia, immunosuppressive drugs, binge drinking, and exposure to viral infections (Laibl & Sheffield, 2006). The most common causative bacterial pathogen for pneumonia in pregnancy is *Streptococcus pneumoniae*. It is responsible for approximately one-half to two-thirds of cases of bacterial pneumonia during pregnancy and approximately two-thirds of all pneumonias during pregnancy (Laibl & Sheffield). Women with bacterial pneumonia during pregnancy most often present with a history of malaise and upper respiratory infection. They frequently have abrupt onset of fever above 100°F with rigors and chills. Pleuritic chest pain, productive cough, dyspnea, and rusty sputum are other common symptoms. Blood cultures are positive in approximately 25% of cases (Neu & Sabath, 1993). *Haemophilus influenzae* is the second most common bacterium identified in patients with bacterial pneumonia, and symptoms are similar to those caused by to *S. pneumoniae*. Women with chronic obstructive pulmonary diseases and chronic bronchitis are at greatest risk. There are numerous other uncommon pneumonia pathogens that may be seen in childbearing women, including *Mycoplasma pneumoniae, Chlamydia pneumoniae, Moraxella catarrhalis, Klebsiella pneumoniae,* and *Escherichia coli*. These organisms produce an atypical pneumonia syndrome, which is characterized by gradual onset, less toxicity, lower fever, nonproductive cough, malaise, and a patchy or interstitial infiltrate (Maccato, 1991). *Legionella pneumophila* may cause pneumonia with the typical acute course or the atypical symptoms described with the less common pathogens. Underlying chronic illness, advancing age, and cigarette smoking appear to be significant predisposing factors for bacterial pneumonia. When a superimposed pulmonary infection follows a viral pneumonia, *Staphylococcus aureus* is frequently responsible. This organism may also spread by the hematogenous route related to intravenous catheters, intravenous drug abuse, or infective endocarditis. The onset of this pneumonia is usually abrupt, and the course is rapid. Pleuritic chest pain and purulent sputum production are evident.

Aspiration can cause a very serious pneumonia that carries a high mortality rate, in spite of respiratory support and aggressive management. Pneumonia from anaerobic organisms is usually caused by aspiration during induction or emergence from general anesthesia for a cesarean birth. The aspiration of particulate matter and gastric acid causes an immediate chemical pneumonitis, followed in 24 to 48 hours by a secondary bacterial infection. Fortunately, the use of nonparticulate antacids (eg, sodium citrate), regional anesthesia, and rapid sequence induction of general anesthesia with cricoid pressure have dramatically reduced the incidence of aspiration-related maternal mortality. Other causes of aspiration pneumonia include anything that may diminish consciousness, such as seizures and drug or alcohol abuse. Delayed gastric emptying, decreased esophageal sphincter tone, and elevated intragastric pressure are normal physiologic changes in the gastrointestinal tract during pregnancy that predispose a woman to aspiration (Pereira & Krieger, 2004). Acute

symptoms of aspiration include cough, significant bronchospasm, and hypoxia. Signs of chemical pneumonitis begin 6 to 24 hours after aspiration and include tachypnea, tachycardia, hypotension, and frothy pulmonary edema. Mechanical ventilation may be necessary and difficult. Resolution usually occurs over 4 to 5 days unless secondary infection develops (Pereira & Krieger). Prophylactic antibiotics and corticosteroids are not recommended. However, secondary bacterial infection must be identified and treated promptly with antibiotics to minimize significant perinatal morbidity and mortality (Pereira & Krieger).

Viral Pneumonia

Influenza and varicella are the most common pathogens causing viral pneumonia in pregnancy (Laibl & Sheffield, 2006; Ramsey & Ramin, 2001; Salmon & Bruick-Sorge, 2003). Rubeola, rubella, Hantavirus, and severe acute respiratory syndrome are also associated pathogens in viral pneumonia. Influenza-mediated viral pneumonia is most commonly caused by type A influenza, which is the most virulent strain in humans. Type A influenza attacks the lung parenchyma and causes edema, hemorrhage, and hyaline membrane formation. Chest x-ray demonstrates unilateral patchy infiltrates. Acute onset of dyspnea, tachypnea, wheezing, malaise, headache, high fever, cough, and myalgias are associated symptoms. Frequently, superimposed bacterial pneumonia develops following resolution of influenza symptoms. During pregnancy, fulminant respiratory failure may develop, requiring extended mechanical ventilation resulting in significant mortality.

Varicella pneumonia may be more common and more virulent in pregnancy than in nonpregnant patients. Smoking, late gestational age, and more than 100 skin lesions may also be risk factors for the development of this type of pneumonia, which usually occurs in the third trimester (Harger et al., 2002; Pereira & Krieger, 2004). In a patient with primary varicella symptoms, the diagnosis of varicella pneumonia is confirmed by a chest x-ray that reveals an interstitial, nodular pattern or focal infiltrates. Varicella pneumonia typically presents with fever, dyspnea, tachypnea, dry cough, pleuritic chest pain, oral mucous lesions, and hemoptysis within 2 to 7 days of the vesicular rash. Chest radiographs show a diffuse miliary or nodular pattern (Ramsey & Ramin, 2001). It is not uncommon to see rapid progression to hypoxia and respiratory failure. In addition to maternal complications, intrauterine infection occurs in up to 26% of varicella pneumonia cases (Pereira & Krieger). Congenital varicella syndrome may occur if infection occurs in the first trimester and is characterized by cutaneous scars, limb hypoplasia, chorioretinitis, cortical atrophy, cataracts, and other anomalies in the neonate (Balducci et al., 1992; Goodnight & Soper, 2005; Laibl & Sheffield, 2005). Second trimester varicella may result in congenital varicella-zoster in some infants. Premature labor and perinatal varicella infection are significant adverse effects that may result from varicella infection during pregnancy. Rubeola during pregnancy may lead to spontaneous abortion and preterm birth. Pneumonia can complicate up to 50% of cases, and bacterial superinfection is also common.

Severe acute respiratory syndrome (SARS) is a new viral illness transmitted by respiratory droplets or close personal contact (Laibl & Sheffield, 2006). It results in an atypical pneumonia that can progress to hypoxemia and respiratory failure. Chest x-ray reveals generalized, patchy, interstitial infiltrates in patients with SARS pneumonia (Laibl & Sheffield). Symptoms that are seen 2 to 7 days after exposure include headache, fever, chills, rigors, malaise, myalgia, dyspnea, and a nonproductive cough (Laibl & Sheffield). Patients are most infectious during the second week of illness (Laibl & Sheffiel). Based on limited available data, effects on pregnancy from this illness include spontaneous abortion, preterm birth, and small (for gestational-age) fetus (Wong et al., 2004). The course of SARS and clinical outcomes are worse for pregnant women when compared to nonpregnant women (Lam et al., 2004). The virus does not appear to cross the placenta and infect the fetus (Wong et al.).

Nursing Assessment

Obtaining a detailed history of the illness, including symptoms, and a physical examination are essential. All pregnant women should be questioned about immunity to varicella during the first prenatal visit. Susceptible women should be counseled to avoid contact with individuals who have chickenpox. If exposure occurs, varicella-zoster immune globulin (VZIG) in should be administered within 96 hours in an attempt to prevent maternal infection (Laibl & Sheffield, 2006). Laboratory and radiologic findings are important to help diagnose the type of pneumonia present. Chest x-ray on the majority of patients with pneumonia reflects infiltrates, atelectasis, pleural effusions, pneumonitis, or pulmonary edema. Clinical presentation and laboratory data help to determine whether the pneumonia is classic or atypical. Careful questioning about underlying chronic conditions and prior illness can identify risk factors. Physical examination usually reveals tachypnea and use of accessory muscles for respiration. Lung auscultation may identify inspiratory rales, absent breath sounds over the affected lung field, or a pleural friction rub. A sputum sample with secretions from the lower bronchial tree must be collected for Gram stain and culture. Positive blood culture results are highly specific, although they are infre-

quently performed, and rarely positive in women with pneumonia in pregnancy (Yost, Bloom, Richey, Ramin, & Cunningham, 2000). These specimens assist in identifying the pathogen responsible for the pneumonia.

Because an oxygen saturation level below 95% can adversely affect the amount of oxygen delivered to the fetus, oxygen saturation levels should be monitored continuously. Initial arterial blood gases in the pregnant woman with pneumonia usually reflect significant degrees of hypoxia without hypercapnia or acidosis (Laibl & Sheffield, 2006). The nurse must assess each woman closely for symptoms of hypoxia, including irritability and restlessness, tachycardia, hypertension, cool and pale extremities, and decreased urine output. Confusion, disorientation, and loss of consciousness can result if the hypoxia goes untreated.

Nursing Interventions

Prevention of pneumonia in pregnancy has been successful through the administration of the influenza and pneumococcus vaccines. These are safe for administration in pregnancy and should be given to high-risk women. The varicella vaccine is not safe for administration during pregnancy because it is a live vaccine (Laibl & Sheffield, 2006). In pregnant women diagnosed with pneumonia, regardless of the type of pneumonia, nursing interventions focus on close monitoring, oxygen supplementation, antipyretics, adequate hydration, control of pain, fatigue and anxiety, and ongoing fetal assessment. Positioning the woman in a semi-Fowler's or high-Fowler's position usually is most comfortable and promotes maximum oxygenation. Oxygen supplementation to maintain oxygen saturation of greater than 95% by pulse oximeter is vital to ensure adequate maternal oxygen delivery to the fetus. The most common method of oxygen administration is 2 to 4 L/minute through a nasal cannula. If the woman requires more than 4 L of oxygen to maintain adequate hemoglobin oxygen saturation, the use of a nonrebreather mask is more efficacious in delivering a higher fraction of inspired oxygen (FiO_2) (Simpson & James, 2005). Mechanical ventilation is necessary for women who are unable to maintain a PaO_2 above 60 mm Hg despite high concentrations of inspired oxygen. These women are best cared for in an intensive-care setting. Other supportive measures may have some benefit in therapy of the pregnant woman with respiratory insufficiency secondary to pneumonia. For women who are unable to cough effectively, postural drainage and tracheal suctioning can be valuable in mobilizing secretions. The use of incentive spirometry may be helpful as well.

The development of preterm labor as a complication of infection may be the result of the response of the uterus to certain mediators of inflammation and infection. Prompt attention to regular uterine contractions and cervical changes is necessary to minimize the risks of preterm birth as a result of significant maternal illness. Conversely, in patients in whom respiratory and cardiovascular statuses continue to deteriorate despite maximum supportive efforts, birth may be necessary for fetal and maternal survival.

Pharmacologic Therapy

Antimicrobial therapy must be specific to the pathogen present, along with consideration for its safety during pregnancy (Table 6–30). Until identification of the causative organism, symptoms, sputum Gram stain, and chest radiography can direct initial antibiotic use. Erythromycin has proven to be successful in treatment of pneumonia in pregnancy and is often given initially. Ampicillin may be administered if *S. pneumoniae* or *H. influenzae* is the suspected pathogen. With an increase in ampicillin-resistant pathogens, third-generation cephalosporins and trimethoprim-sulfamethoxazole are other choices for most cases of classic pneumonia (Laibl & Sheffield, 2005; Ramsey & Ramin, 2001; Yost, Bloom, Richey, Ramin, & Cunningham, 2000). These antibiotics may be the most appropriate first-line medications for sick patients when there is high probability of resistance. Varicella pneumonia must be treated promptly with acyclovir, with 8 to 10 mg/kg given intravenously every 8 hours to decrease complications and mortality. Patients who receive this medication early in the course of their illness benefit from lower temperatures and respiratory rates and from improved oxygenation without risk to their fetus. Aggressive treatment of hypoxemia and administration of corticosteroids have also shown to improve outcomes in these women (Goodnight & Soper, 2005). Varicella embryopathy may occur as a result of maternal infection, particularly in the first half of pregnancy, with an incidence of 1% to 2% (Chapman, 1998). Varicella of the newborn is a life-threatening illness that may occur when a newborn is born within 5 days of the onset of maternal illness or after postbirth exposure to varicella. Susceptible newborns should be given VZIG (Chapman, 1998).

Aspiration pneumonia is best treated with broad-spectrum antimicrobials to cover gram-negative and gram-positive bacteria that are usually present. Antiviral agents amantadine and ribavirin have been used in the treatment of influenza pneumonia and SARS pneumonia during pregnancy. Although they have shown teratogenicity in some animal studies, both have been effective in decreasing the severity of illness associated with influenza during pregnancy without adverse effects to humans. SARS pneumonia has also been effectively treated with the addition of antibiotics and corticosteroids.

Other Pulmonary Complications of Pregnancy
Tocolytic-Induced Pulmonary Edema

The use of beta-mimetic drugs for tocolysis increases the risk of pulmonary edema. Approximately 6% to 15% of women receiving tocolytics will develop pulmonary edema. Risk factors include multiple pregnancy, diabetes, preeclampsia, blood transfusions, silent cardiac disease, infections, simultaneous use of magnesium sulfate, and use of corticosteroids for more than 48 hours (Pereira & Krieger, 2004). Generally, pulmonary edema occurs during beta-agonist therapy or within 24 hours after discontinuation (Pereira & Krieger). To avoid pulmonary edema, the lowest possible dose of ß-mimetics should be used; maternal heart rate should be maintained at less than 120 beats per minute; tocolytic therapy should be limited to 48 hours or less; combination tocolytic therapy should be avoided (especially magnesium sulfate); intake and output should be carefully monitored with avoidance of a change in hematocrit less than 10%; and tocolytics should be avoided in patients with preeclampsia, pneumonia, and cardiac disease (Pereira & Krieger). Treatment involves discontinuation of the tocolytic agent, administration of oxygen, diuretics, and intravenous

---

TABLE 6–30 ■ ANTIBIOTIC THERAPY FOR PNEUMONIA PATHOGENS

Pathogen	Ampicillin	Cephalosporin	Erythromycin	Trimethoprim-Sulfamethoxazole
Streptococcus pneumoniae	+	+	+	+
Haemophilus influenzae	+	+	−	+
Mycoplasma catarrhalis	−	+	+	+
Chlamydia pneumoniae	−	−	+	−
Legionella pneumophila	−	−	+	−
Mycoplasma pneumoniae	−	−	+	−
Pneumocystis carinii	−	−	−	+

nitrates. Symptoms usually resolve within 24 hours after identification and treatment (Pereira & Krieger).

Amniotic Fluid Embolism

Amniotic fluid embolism is a rare but potentially devastating complication of pregnancy with a mortality rate of 60% to 90% (Pereira & Krieger, 2004). The incidence is 1 per 20,000 to 30,000 births in the US (Pereira & Krieger). Diagnosis should be suspected in any pregnant woman who develops profound shock and severe hypoxemic respiratory failure with bilateral pulmonary infiltrates during or immediately after labor. Treatment is mainly supportive with careful monitoring for the development of adult respiratory distress syndrome (ARDS) and coagulopathy. Mechanical ventilation using lung-protective strategies is usually initated. Cardiogenic shock requires use of inaotropic and vasoactive agents and treatment of coagulopathy requires the replacement of coagulation factors (Pereira & Krieger).

Pulmonary Embolism

Pulmonary embolism is a leading cause of maternal mortality in the US (ACOG, 2000b; Chang et al., 2003). Venous thromboembolism affects pregnant women five times more frequently than nonpregnant women of the same age (Stone & Morris, 2004). Approximately 1 in 1,000 to 2,000 pregnant women develop venous thromboembolism (Stone & Morris). The highest risk for deep-vein thrombosis is during the antepartum period with as many as one-third of cases occurring in the first trimester. The highest risk for pulmonary embolism is during the immediate postpartum period. If venous thromboembolism is suspected, objective diagnostic testing should be initiated including one or more of the following: D-dimer, compressive ultrasound, impedance plethysmography, ventilation-perfusion scanning, computed tomography (CT) scanning, and pulmonary angiography (ACOG; Stone & Morris). The diagnosis is challenging because no one diagnostic test is confirmatory and many false-positive results occur (ACOG). To prevent pulmonary embolism, anticoagulation therapy is indicated if deep vein thrombosis is diagnosed or strongly suspected, without waiting for the outcome of diagnostic tests (Pereira & Krieger). Intravenous heparin is the initial treatment of choice for pulmonary embolism during pregnancy because it does not cross the placenta and the best choice for labor because of its short half-life. Subcutaneous unfractionated heparin and low-molecular-weight heparin (LMWH) have both risks and benefits but can be used during pregnancy. Acute treatment is directed toward preserving adequate oxygenation and circulation by administration of intravenous heparin (ACOG; Stone & Morris). Pregnant patients with acute pulmonary embolism should receive intravenous heparin for 5 days. If the patient's condition is stable and labor ensues, the heparin dose can be decreased or discontinued until 4 to 8 hours after birth (ACOG).

MULTIPLE GESTATION

Over the past 25 years, multiple birth rates have increased dramatically, with the current numbers of twins, triplets, and other higher order multiples (HOM) at the highest levels in recorded history. Trends in delayed childbearing and increased use of infertility therapies and assisted reproductive technologies (ART) have contributed greatly to these increased rates (Wright, Schieve, Reynolds, & Jeng, 2005). Although multiple births represent only about 3% of the total live birth population in the United States, these births contribute disproportionately to the rates of maternal, fetal, and neonatal morbidity and mortality. Multiple birth infants are at high risk of being born too early and too small, and have strongly influenced recent increases in national rates of preterm birth (<37 weeks gestation) and low birth weight (LBW—less than 2,500 g; Martin et al., 2006). A key factor is a clear dose–response relationship: increasing plurality corresponds with higher morbidity and mortality for mothers and their infants. With these high risks, the perinatal team must be alert for potential complications during pregnancy, labor, birth, and the postpartum period.

Epidemiology

Of the more than four million United States live births in 2004, multiple births accounted for 3.3% with 132,219 twins, 7,275 triplets, 439 quadruplets, and 86 quintuplets or higher (Martin et al., 2006). Data from the National Center for Health Statistics (Martin et al.) reveal that the numbers of multiple births in 2004 were the highest ever recorded, and the multiple birth rate (live births of twins, triplets, and higher/1,000) is also at record levels (see Figures 6–10 and 6–11). From 1980 to 2004, the twin birth rate increased by 70%, whereas the rate of HOM rose more than 500%. However, the HOM birth rate seems to have stabilized after a high in 1998 of 193.5/100,000, and the number of HOM dropped 5% from 2003 to 2004 (Martin et al.). Before 1989, quadruplet and higher multiples were included in triplet data, due to low frequencies of these pregnancies. However, the number of infants born as quadruplets and quintuplets-plus doubled from 1989 to 2004, from 229 to 439, and from 40 to 86, respectively (Martin et al.).

Shifts in traditional maternal age patterns have occurred along with the rise in multiple births, mirroring the trend of delayed childbearing. Historically, twin birth rates were low for young women, rose through the age group 35 to 39 years, then declined for women

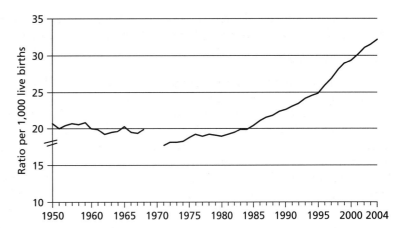

FIGURE 6–10. Twin birth rate: United States 1950 to 2004. (Based on cumulative natality data from the past 50 years from the National Center for Health Statistics.) *Note:* Break in line represents years in which data were not collected.

in their forties (Martin & Park, 1999). However, beginning in 1992, multiple birth rates rose steadily for women over age 30, and twin birth rates increased dramatically for women aged 45 to 49 years. The highest overall multiple birth rates in 2004 were for women in the 45 to 54 age group (221.2/1,000; Martin et al., 2006). Surprisingly, advanced maternal age appears to be associated with better perinatal outcomes for multiple gestationss compared with singletons (Oleszczuk, Keith, & Oleszczuk, 2005). A variety of explanations have been proposed, including greater use of donor eggs and better socioeconomic status, education, and prenatal care (Zhang, Meikle, Grainger, & Trumble, 2002). Other explanations include older women's healthier lifestyles and higher body mass index, as well as possible uterine cell proliferation or "remodeling" from prior pregnancies that may improve uterine expansion limits and fetal nourishment (Oleszczuk, Keith, & Oleszczuk).

There have also been shifts in maternal race patterns for multiple births. Historically, multiple births occurred more often in black women than in white women, but this gap has been overtaken. In 2004, twin birth rates were 36.3/1,000 for non-Hispanic white women and 35.6/1,000 for non-Hispanic black women (Martin et al.,

2006). The greatest disparities were seen in HOM. In 2004, the HOM birth rate for non-Hispanic whites (243.4.0/100,000) was more than double the rate of non-Hispanic blacks (99.7/100,000), and more than three times higher than that of Hispanic mothers (76.4/100,000; Martin et al., 2006). Overall, multiple birth rates are generally lowest in Asian and Native-American women (Martin et al., 2003). Racial rate differences are likely due to greater access and use of infertility services by white women (Abma, Chandra, Mosher, Peterson, & Piccinino, 1997).

Regardless of maternal age, a prior multiple pregnancy and higher parity increase the likelihood for spontaneous dizygotic twin conception. Twinning is about four times more likely in the fourth or fifth birth than in the first birth (Taffel, 1995).

Physiology of Twinning

Multiple gestations result from either the fertilization of a single ovum that subsequently divides into two or more zygotes (monozygotic—MZ), or the fertilization of multiple ova (dizygotic—DZ, trizygotic—TZ, etc.). The frequency of MZ twins is about 4/1,000 live births for spontaneous conceptions, or about one-third the number of DZ twins (Bomsel-Helmerich & Al Mufti, 1995; see Figure 6–12). Historically, the rate of MZ twinning has been constant; however, in recent years a frequency of 5% to 7% has been observed with reproductive technology-assisted conceptions (Blickstein, Jones, & Keith, 2003). MZ twinning occurs at a frequency of 2.3% following IVF procedures and 6.4% after ovulation induction (Blickstein, 2005).

Among MZ twin pregnancies, about 30% are dichorionic/diamniotic (DC/DA; separate placentas and amniotic sacs); about 70% are monochorionic/diamniotic (MC/DA; a single placenta with two amniotic sacs); and about 1% are monochorionic/monoamniotic (MC/MA), in which multiple fetuses

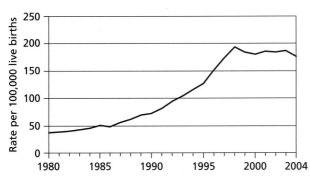

FIGURE 6–11. Higher-order multiples birth rate: United States 1980 to 2004. (Based on cumulative natality data from the past 50 years, from the National Center for Health Statistics.)

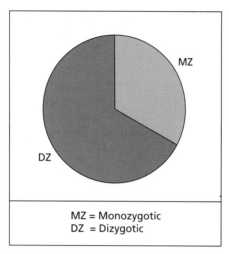

FIGURE 6–12. Zygosity distribution.

share a single placenta and one amniotic sac (Smith-Levitin, Skupski, & Chervenak, 1999; see Fig. 6–13). The degree to which structures are shared is related to the time of zygotic division after conception; early division (within 72 hours) results in DC/DA, division between Days 4 through 7 results in MC/DA, and later division results in MC/MA. Conjoined twins occur following very late; and incomplete zygotic splitting, usually after Day 13. Because they develop from a single fertilized ovum, MZ twins are always of the same gender. Dizygotic twins are always DC/DA and may be the same or different gender. Triplets and other HOM may have any combination of chorionicity/amnionicity, such as trichorionic/triamniotic (TC/TA), dichorionic/triamniotic (DC/TA), or monochorionic/triamniotic (MC/TA; see Figs. 6–14 to 6–16).

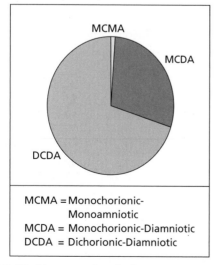

FIGURE 6–13. Monozygotic twinning.

Role of Infertility and Assisted Reproductive Technology

A significant percentage of multiple births in the United States are conceived with some type of infertility therapy, including ovulation induction and ART. Although pregnancy data submitted by ART clinics to the CDC provide a fairly accurate estimate of IVF births, exact numbers of natural and non-IVF conceptions are unknown. It is estimated that one-third of the increase in multiple births has resulted from the shift to older maternal age, with the remaining two-thirds of the increase attributable to ART procedures such as IVF (Martin & Park, 1999). In 2000, 11.8% of twin births were conceived with ART, 67.3% were estimated to have been conceived naturally, and the remaining 20.9% were unexplained and presumed to be through non-IVF infertility treatments (Reynolds, Schieve, Martin, Jeng, & Macaluso, 2003). Triplet conceptions for the same year included 42.5% from ART, 17.7% estimated from natural conceptions, and 39.7% unexplained. In 2002, 53% of the 45,751 reported infants born through ART were multiples, including 16% of twins and 44% of HOM (Wright, Schieve, Reynolds, & Jeng, 2005).

It is well known that fertility-assisted pregnancies have poorer perinatal outcomes than naturally conceived pregnancies, particularly in singletons (Lambalk & van Hooff, 2001; Zuppa, Maragliano, Scapillati, Crescimbini, & Tortorolo, 2001). However, a review of controlled trials found the effect is less on twin outcomes, and that perinatal mortality for twins was 40% lower after assisted conceptions compared with natural conceptions (Helmerhorst, Perquin, Donker, & Keirse, 2004). Although this decreased mortality may seem to be an advantage for reproductive technology-assisted twin pregnancies, this does not offset the much higher overall risks of twin pregnancy.

The high risk of multiple births with ART and other infertility therapies has generated the creation of policy recommendations and clinical guidelines. In 1998, 2004, and again in 2006, the Society for Assisted Reproductive Technology (SART) and the American Society for Reproductive Medicine (ASRM) declared that multiple gestations, especially triplets or more, is an undesirable consequence of ART and issued guidelines to assist ART programs and patients in determining the appropriate number of embryos to transfer (SART, 2006). The 2006 guidelines include the following maternal age-based embryo transfer limits for women with a favorable prognosis: a single embryo transfer for women under age 35; two embryos for women between 35 and 37 years of age; no more than three embryos for women between ages 38 and 40; and no more than five embryos for women over age 40. The guidelines may be individualized based on each woman's clinical condition, prognosis, and circumstances.

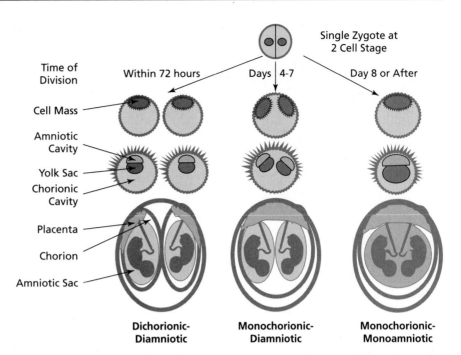

FIGURE 6–14. Monozygotic twins. (Copyright 2006 Marvelous multiples, Inc. Used by permission)

In the early 1990s, other countries instituted governmental mandates for IVF clinics to decrease the number of embryos transferred from three to two (Jain, Missmer, & Hornstein, 2004). By 2001, marked declines were seen in the rate of multiple births after IVF, especially in HOM. More importantly, the decline in multiple births had a significant impact on preterm births. Sweden had a 72% decrease in adjusted odds ratio (from 4.63 to 1.33) for preterm births (Källen, Finnstrom, Nygren, & Olausson, 2005). Sweden is further decreasing the number of embryos transferred

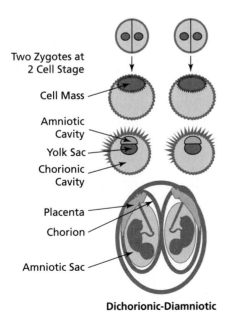

FIGURE 6–15. Dizygotic twins.

from two to one, and a further decline in multiple births from IVF is expected, without a decrease in the pregnancy rate.

Although other countries have laws restricting the number of embryos transferred, the SART/ASRM statement allows for individualized application of the guidelines depending on clinical conditions, including patient age, embryo quality, the option for cryopreservation, and the experience of the clinic (Jain, Missmer, & Hornstein, 2004). It is hoped that voluntary implementation of embryo transfer limits by US clinicians will reduce the occurrence of multiple births resulting from ART. Since the first guidelines were published by ASRM in 1998, there have been steep declines in the number of embryos transferred, with parallel decreases in the rate of HOM pregnancies (Jain, Missmer, & Hornstein). In addition, improvements in technology are increasing success rates for single embryo transfers with ART, thus decreasing the need for multiple embryo transfers. However, the estimated proportions of multiple births attributable to ART and non-IVF infertility treatments will likely continue to increase, as they have from 1997 to 2003 (from 30.1% to 45.5%, respectively; Reynolds, Schieve, Martin, Jeng, & Macaluso, 2003). Moreover, although HOM due to ART decreased during that same period (from 43.6% to 42.5%), the proportion attributable to other infertility treatments rose from 38.0% to 39.7%.

Decreasing the number of iatrogenic multiple births will not be easy. Most infertility practices are motivated by competition for patients, the desire for fertility success, and the need for rapid results (D'Alton, 2004). Infertility patients themselves often desire a multiple

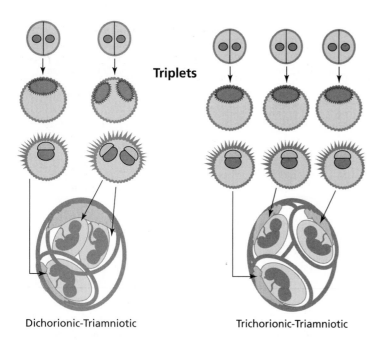

Triplets

Dichorionic-Triamniotic   Trichorionic-Triamniotic

FIGURE 6–16. Triplets. (Copyright 2006 Marvelous Multiples, Inc. Used by permission.)

pregnancy. In a Canadian study, 41% of infertility clinic questionnaire respondents considered multiple pregnancy an ideal treatment outcome, and their desire increased with longer duration of treatment (Child, Henderson, & Tan, 2004). In a similar study of 464 infertile women in a United States university-based clinic, 20.3% listed a multiple pregnancy as their most desired treatment outcome, and 94% of these wanted twins (Ryan, Zhang, Dokras, Syrop, & Van Voorhis, 2004). In this study, fewer than half of the women knew of the increased risk of cerebral palsy and infant mortality associated with twins. In one study, women could accurately recall infertility counseling and precise statistics about various treatment options as long as 4 years later (Collopy, 2004). However, these women were insistent that the information had no meaning for them because they were so focused on overcoming infertility, not on avoiding multiple births. It has been concluded that significant change in the US will not occur without political and social changes among consumers and providers to view treatment success in terms of singleton pregnancies and births (Wright, Schieve, Reynolds, & Jeng, 2005).

Multifetal Pregnancy Reduction

Multifetal pregnancy reduction (MFPR) is a pregnancy termination procedure that reduces the number of fetuses in a HOM pregnancy to a lower and potentially more viable number, thus increasing the chances for a positive pregnancy outcome. The rise in use of MFPR has paralleled the rising number of HOM pregnancies. Currently, an estimated 70% of patients seeking reduction have conceived HOM with ovulation induction medications and 30% with ART (Evans, Ciorica, Britt, & Fletcher, 2005). MFPR is typically

performed in the late first trimester and terminates one or more fetuses by potassium chloride injection into the fetal thoracic cavity. Nearly all procedures performed today use transabdominal needle insertion under ultrasound guidance (Evans et al., 2005). Although MFPR is sometimes called selective reduction, this terminology should be used when a specific fetus is targeted for reduction because of a known anomaly, aneuploidy, or a risk identified with nuchal translucency screening.

There have been many studies comparing pregnancy outcomes from MFPR with twins conceived spontaneously or following ART, as well as studies comparing MFPR with expectantly managed triplet pregnancies. Generally, outcomes following reduction to twins appear comparable with outcomes for twins conceived spontaneously or by ART, but study findings about the risks and benefits associated with reduction procedures are not as clear (Dodd & Crowther, 2005a). Complications include procedural (eg, infection or incomplete procedure), total pregnancy loss, and a continued risk for preterm birth. Collaborative data from several centers have shown that higher starting numbers of fetuses (≥6) correspond with poorer outcomes after reduction; total pregnancy loss rates prior to 24 weeks' gestation are 4.5% for triplets, 8% for quadruplets, 11% for quintuplets, and 15% for sextuplets or more (Evans et al., 2005). All reduced pregnancies have been shown to have an ongoing increased risk for preterm birth, except for pregnancies reduced to singletons (Evans et al.). Some studies have shown an increased risk for IUGR in the remaining fetuses post-MFPR (ACOG, 2004a). Without prenatal diagnostic testing prior to MFPR, there is the possibility of terminating a healthy fetus, while leaving an abnormal one.

MFPR presents a difficult dilemma for most couples. They often face conflicting values as they consider reduction after years of desiring fertility and must weigh the medical/obstetric/neonatal risks and the psychosocial/moral/economic impact on their family (Elliott, 2005a). The seemingly (and often actual) arbitrary choice as to which fetus should live and which should die is distressing (Bryan, 2005). Further, the decision for reduction must be made in a short time between diagnosis and the optimal timing for the procedure. The decision has been described as highly stressful, psychologically traumatic, frightening, painful, overwhelming, confusing, and a surreal experience (Bergh, Möller, Nilsson, & Wikland, 1999; Bryan, 2005; Collopy, 2004). The following responses from women indicate their inner conflicts about the decision: "I believe reduction saved one of my children. It's the not knowing that kills me." "If I tried to carry all of the babies, I would most definitely lose them all. I also look at my survivor knowing she probably would have been chosen for reduction. This also wracks me with guilt" (from a mother who spontaneously lost some of her fetuses and did not have to reduce) (Pector, 2004, p. 716). There is also evidence from interviews with patients that viewing fetuses on ultrasound just prior to or during reduction made the reduction more difficult (Maifeld, Hahn, Titler, & Mullen, 2003; Schreiner-Engel, Walther, Mindes, Lynch, & Berkowitz, 1995). Studies have shown that persistent feelings of sadness and guilt may continue after the MFPR procedure; however, most women believe their choice was correct and that reduction was necessary for them to achieve their goal of motherhood (Collopy, 2004). The grief response with MFPR may not fit the classic process, and may be more complicated or delayed. More research is needed to determine long-term psychological outcomes, including effects on parent–child bonding and responses of child survivors.

The reduction debate also can be problematic for clinicians. Some studies have found no difference in outcomes of women with triplet gestations who are managed expectantly when compared to those who have MFPR (Leondires, Ernst, Miller, & Scott, 2000). With these data, and the improvements in neonatal care and long-term outcomes for preterm infants, some clinicians may be unwilling to accept that medical risks are sufficient grounds for reducing a triplet pregnancy (Bryan, 2005). Another consideration is the first trimester spontaneous loss rate for multiple gestationss, which might make MFPR unnecessary. One study found that spontaneous loss of one or more gestational sacs or embryos occurred before the 12th week of gestation in 65% of quadruplet pregnancies, 53% of triplets, and 36% of twins (Dickey et al., 2002).

The controversy is likely to continue. Based on reports that pregnancy outcomes for cases starting at triplets or quadruplets reduced to twins do nearly as well as those for cases of nonreduced twins, cautious aggressiveness in infertility treatments has been suggested (Evans, Ciorica, Britt, & Fletcher, 2005). Some have also proposed that future debates will no longer be over reduction of HOM and triplets, but over a routine offer of reduction of all twins (Evans et al., 2004).

Nurses have much to contribute in the care of women considering and undergoing MFPR, Establishing a rapport, exploring treatment options, and assisting with decision making with a consistently available primary nurse has been recommended (Collopy, 2004).

Diagnosis of Multiple Gestations

First trimester ultrasound is highly accurate in diagnosing multiple gestations; the earliest gestation for determining chorionicity is 5 weeks; for fetal number, 6 weeks; and for amnionicity, 8 weeks (Shetty & Smith, 2005). Diagnosis is confirmed when multiple embryos or embryonic parts are seen in the gestational sac(s). Women at high risk of conceiving multiples, such as those using infertility therapies, should have an ultrasound early in the first trimester. Ultrasound is highly accurate in determining chorionicity and amnionicity when performed between 10 and 14 weeks (Newman & Luke, 2000). Thickness and numbers of membrane layers can be counted, and ultrasound markers can be visualized. The triangular lambda sign predicts DZ chorionicity, a T-shaped junction is present in MC placentas, and a Y-shaped ipsilon zone is characteristic of the three interfetal membranes of TZ triplet gestations (Shetty & Smith, 2005; Smith-Levitin, Skupski, & Chervenak, 1999). First trimester ultrasonography has 100% sensitivity, 97.9% specificity, and a positive predictive value of 88.2% in determining chorionicity, but accuracy decreases as the pregnancy progresses and varies with sonographer skill and experience (Menon, 2005). Early identification of MC and MA pregnancies is important in planning appropriate management of these high-risk pregnancies.

Clinical examination may also assist in diagnosis. With an accurate menstrual history, a fundal height 2 cm to 4 cm larger than the expected gestational age suggests multiple gestation. Other signs include palpation during the Leopold maneuver that reveals multiple fetal parts or fetal poles, or when there is more than one fetal heart sound, particularly with a difference of 10 beats per minute (Bowers & Gromada, 2006).

Maternal perceptions may also provide clues to the presence of more than one fetus. These include excessive fatigue, hyperemesis or increased appetite and weight gain (especially in early pregnancy), exaggerated pregnancy discomforts, increased fetal activity, the feeling that the pregnancy is different from previous singleton pregnancies, and peculiar insights about the pregnancy (Bowers & Gromada, 2006).

Not all women are psychologically prepared for the diagnosis of twins, and even fewer for the discovery of HOM. Ambivalence is normal, even when a pregnancy has been greatly desired or after years of infertility treatments (Klock, 2001). Revealing the diagnosis of multiple pregnancy should be done with sensitivity to each woman's situation, with a factual nonemotional approach and guarded enthusiasm (Bowers & Gromada, 2006). Many couples are at first overwhelmed with joy by the announcement of multiples, then simply overwhelmed by the physical, emotional, and financial demands ahead.

Maternal Adaptation

Nearly every maternal structure and body system is affected by the physiologic changes that occur in multiple gestations, with symptoms often more exaggerated than with a singleton pregnancy. General complaints of pregnancy such as urinary frequency, constipation, difficulty sleeping, fatigue, and varicose veins tend to be magnified and occur earlier with multiples.

Gastrointestinal

Paralleling high hormonal levels in early pregnancy, as many as half of women pregnant with multiples experience nausea and vomiting in the first trimester, with symptoms persisting throughout pregnancy in up to 20% of women. Of these, 1% to 3% suffer with hyperemesis gravidarum (Rohde, Dembenski, & Dom, 2003); this is approximately double the risk in singletons (Fell, Dodds, Joseph, Allen, & Butler, 2006). If prolonged, these conditions can affect weight gain and nutritional status of the mother, as well as increase the risk for LBW infants (ACOG, 2004b). Interestingly, one study found that women carrying a combination of male and female fetuses have the highest risk for hyperemesis, with risks decreasing for all males followed by all females (Fell, Dodds, Joseph, Allen, & Butler). Women may also complain of gastroesophageal reflux early in pregnancy, which is consistent with decreased lower esophageal sphincter tone of pregnancy, and increasing mechanical pressure due to the rapidly growing uterus and slowed gastrointestinal transit time (Richter, 2003).

Hematologic

Plasma volume increases by 50% to 100% with multiple gestations, and results in a dilutional anemia (Malone & D'Alton, 2004). Evaluations of iron status in multiple gestations have found lower hemoglobin levels in the first and second trimesters and increased rates of iron-deficiency anemia (Luke, 2005).

Cardiovascular

Women experience significant cardiovascular changes with a multiple pregnancy. Heart rate and stroke volume are increased over that of singleton gestations, resulting in higher cardiac output and cardiac index in the second and third trimesters (Norwitz, Edusa, & Park, 2005). Combined with increased plasma volume, these cardiovascular changes increase the risk of pulmonary edema in multiple gestations (Rao, Sairam, & Shehata, 2004). The large uterus may increase a woman's susceptibility to supine hypotension syndrome; and aortocaval compression should be avoided.

Respiratory

Respiratory changes in a multiple gestations are similar to singletons, but with greater tidal volumes and oxygen consumption, and a more alkalotic arterial pH (Malone & D'Alton, 2004). Increased abdominal distention and loss of abdominal muscle tone may require women to use their accessory muscles during respiration, resulting in greater dyspnea and shortness of breath (Norwitz, Edusa, & Park, 2005).

Musculoskeletal

The rapidly growing uterus of a multiple gestations magnifies typical pregnancy complaints of back and ligament pain, and women often experience symptoms much earlier in their pregnancy. Women may benefit from a pregnancy support garment and many find that increased rest helps relieve back pain. Women also need instructions in good body mechanics, posture, and placement of supportive pillows while sleeping.

Dermatologic

Approximately 2.9% of twin and 14% of triplet pregnancies develop pruritic urticarial papules and plaques of pregnancy (PUPPP; Elling, McKenna, & Powell, 2000). This dermatosis is thought to be related to abdominal distention and presents with redness and itching in the abdominal striae and urticarial papules on the lower abdomen. In severe cases, the papules merge into pruritic plaques, extend to the buttocks and thighs, and may be generalized. PUPPP usually responds to treatment with topical antipruritics, topical steroids, or oral antihistamines or steroids, and then quickly disappears postpartum. Other causes of abdominal itching should be considered, including normal striae/stretching skin or pruritis secondary to intrahepatic cholestasis, which are both more likely in multiple gestations.

Perinatal Complications

Despite their overall small numbers and incidence, multiple gestations represent a substantial proportion of poor perinatal outcomes. Compared to their counterparts with singleton gestations, women pregnant with multiples are more likely to experience more frequent and severe pregnancy complications and have infants that are smaller, born earlier, less likely to survive the first year of life, and more likely to suffer lifelong disability. It has been observed that multiple births account for 21% of all LBW infants, 19% to 24% of VLBW infants, 20% of preterm births before 32 weeks, 20% of all NICU admissions, 26% of all perinatal deaths, and 16% of neonatal deaths (Newman & Luke, 2000).

Maternal Morbidity and Mortality

Studies have shown significant increases in adverse maternal outcomes in multiple compared with singleton gestations. The combination of physiologic changes and perinatal pathologies that are unique or more likely in twin gestations contribute to this increased risk. Increased adverse outcomes include anemia, cardiac morbidity, amniotic fluid embolus, preeclampsia, eclampsia, gestational diabetes, preterm labor, abruptio placentae, urinary tract infection, cesarean birth, postpartum hemorrhage, puerperal endometritis, prolonged hospital stay, need for obstetric intervention, hysterectomy, and blood transfusion (Conde-Agudelo, Belizan, & Lindmark, 2000; Wen, Demissie, Yang, & Walker, 2004; Walker, Murphy, Pan, Yang, & Wen, 2004).

As compared to women with twins, women carrying HOM are at even greater risk for pregnancy-related morbidities, including anemia, diabetes mellitus, gestational hypertension, eclampsia, abruptio placentae, preterm premature rupture of membranes (PPROM), and increased rate of cesarean birth (Wen, Demissie, Yang, & Walker, 2004). Dose–response relationships of several complications have also been shown with increasing plurality.

There are few studies on maternal deaths in multiple gestations, and national data are likely to be underreported. However, one review found a substantially higher risk of maternal death in multiple gestations compared to singleton pregnancies (MacKay, Berg, & King, 2004). In this report, the maternal mortality ratio for singletons was 4.0/100,000 pregnancies in 1980 and nearly doubled to 7.9/100,000 in 1997. In contrast, for the same years, the maternal mortality ratio for multiples more than tripled, from 11.4/100,000 pregnancies to 36.6/100,000; the relative risk increased from 2.9 to 4.6. These increased mortality ratios are consistent with the rising rates of multiple births and the disproportionate share of adverse pregnancy outcomes associated with these pregnancies (see Fig. 6–17).

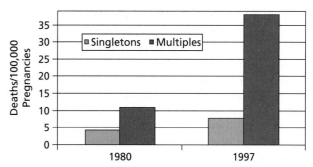

FIGURE 6–17. Maternal mortality for multiple-gestation-related deaths, United States 1980 and 1997. (Based on data from Martin, J. A., Hamilton, B. E., & Sutton, P. D., et al. [2006]. Births: Final data for 2004. *National Vital Statistical Reports, 55*[1], 1–102.)

Preterm Labor

Preterm labor (PTL) is a significant and frequent complication for multiple gestations, occurring in 50% of twins, 76% of triplets, and 90% of quadruplets (Elliott, 2005b). Because unchecked PTL can lead to preterm birth, prevention, early detection, and effective treatment of PTL are essential to the care of women with multiple gestations. Prevention and early detection of PTL in multiples include educating women in signs and symptoms of PTL, cervical assessment, reduction of risk factors for PTL, and possible use of hormonal therapies. Women should receive formal preterm labor education by 18 weeks gestation (Lam & Gill, 2005a) with continual reinforcement at prenatal visits. Although routine hospital admission for bed rest has been advocated to prevent preterm birth in twins, this practice was actually found to increase the likelihood of preterm birth (Dodd & Crowther, 2005a). A recent meta-analysis of bed rest and hospitalization for triplets also found there is no benefit of routine hospitalization and bed rest for women with a triplet pregnancy to reduce the risk of preterm birth, contradicting prior findings (Dodd & Crowther, 2005b). However, women with a history of, or risk for preterm labor or IUGR should reduce their activity in the second and third trimesters (AAP & ACOG, 2002).

Multiple studies have confirmed that prophylactic betamimetic agents do not reduce the incidence of preterm labor and birth in twins (Dodd & Crowther, 2005a). Although use of home uterine activity monitoring (HUAM), along with frequent nurse contact, has been shown to reduce preterm birth in twins, it is not known whether the monitor or the nurse contributes most to preterm birth reduction (Morrison & Chauhan, 2003), and HUAM is not routinely used for twins. Suggested criteria for use of HUAM include higher-order multiple gestations, women with a cervical score of ≤0 or cervical length <25 mm before 30 weeks' gestation, a prior premature singleton birth, or preterm labor in the current pregnancy (Newman and Luke, 2000).

Prophylactic cervical cerclage has not been found to prevent preterm birth of twins (Rao, Sairam, & Shehata, 2004; Dodd & Crowther, 2005a), nor has it been shown to improve pregnancy or neonatal outcomes in women with triplet pregnancies (Rebarber, Roman, Istwan, Rhea, & Stanziano, 2005). However, cerclage is indicated for women with a history of cervical incompetence, and rescue or emergency cerclage is sometimes used in HOM gestations with premature cervical dilatation or as part of the management of a delayed-interval birth (Bowers & Gromada, 2006).

For HOM, an aggressive proactive management approach to preventing PTL has been advocated, including patient education in PTL signs and symptoms, HUAM, decreased activity (bed rest), psychologic reassurance, and prophylactic tocolytic therapy (Elliott, 2005a).

One preterm birth prevention therapy that holds promise is 17-alpha-hydroxyprogesterone caproate (17P) given in weekly injections or daily suppositories beginning early in the second trimester. This therapy has been shown to be safe and effective in women with singletons at high risk for preterm labor (Meis, 2005). Although there is no current evidence for the use of 17P to prevent preterm birth in women with a multiple gestations, clinical trials are under way.

Predicting PTL is difficult as most known risk factors for spontaneous preterm birth in singletons are not significantly associated with spontaneous preterm birth of twins (Goldenberg et al., 1996). However, assessment of cervical length is effective in identifying at-risk women with twins. At 24 weeks, cervical length ≤25 mm was the best predictor of spontaneous preterm birth at <32 weeks, <35 weeks, and <37 weeks (Goldenberg et al.). Other studies have shown that a cervical length ≤25 mm at 18 weeks and ≤22 mm at 24 weeks were the best predictors of birth before 35 weeks gestation (Gibson et al., 2004). Fetal fibronectin testing may also be an effective tool in preterm birth prediction for multiple pregnancies, especially in its negative predictive value, but studies are inconsistent (Goldenberg et al.; Gibson et al.).

Cervical length also appears to be predictive of preterm birth risk in triplets. Studies have shown that a cervical length <25 mm between 14 and 20 weeks' gestation is associated with preterm birth of twins before 32 weeks' gestation (Maslovitz et al., 2004; Poggi et al., 2002). In one study, cervical length of <2.5 mm for triplets between 15 and 20 weeks' gestation had both a specificity and a positive predictive value of 100% for birth at <28 weeks' gestation (Guzman et al., 2000). Because of the value of cervical measurement in predicting preterm birth in multiples, routine assessments appear prudent, beginning with a

baseline exam in the early second trimester for comparison purposes. Although the frequency of performing cervical assessments is not clear (Crowther, 1999), regular exams to detect changes have been suggested for high-risk pregnancies including multiples (Hoesli, Tercanli, & Holzgreve, 2003). Ultrasound has the advantages of objective measurement, as well as visualization of the internal os and proximity of the presenting fetal part and membranes. Digital assessment is most successful when performed by the same clinician who would notice subtle changes in the woman's cervix over time (Bowers & Gromada, 2006).

There are several challenges in managing preterm labor with multiples. These include increased incidence of preterm labor at earlier gestations, greater tocolytic latency than in singletons, less maternal perceptions of uterine activity, higher risk of tocolytic-related complications, and failure of therapy resulting in multiple infants affected by potential morbidities and mortality of preterm birth (Lam & Gill, 2005b).

Treatment of PTL in multiples includes use of tocolytics and corticosteroid therapies. However, the application for multiples may be different from singletons. Multiple gestations have been observed to have different uterine activity patterns compared with singleton pregnancies, including increased contraction frequencies, a significant crescendo in uterine activity 24 hours before the development of clinical preterm labor, and a higher prevalence of low-amplitude, high-frequency (LAHF) contractions (Morrison & Chauhan, 2003). Lam and Gill (2005a) described a characteristic pattern of recurring preterm labor in twins in Display 6–41.

Dosing and titration of tocolytics for multiple gestations is also challenging due to the higher plasma volumes and increased renal clearance; thus, higher dosages

DISPLAY 6-41

Characteristics of Recurring Preterm Labor in Twins

- Return of excessive levels of (LAHF) precursor uterine activity patterns
- Return of a circadian, nocturnal pattern of organized, high-amplitude uterine contractions
- Rapidly increasing need for increased frequency and dosage of terbutaline
- Acceleration of frequency of uterine contractions 48 to 72 hours before the episode of active recurrent preterm labor

Lam, F., & Gill, P. (2005a). *β*-Agonist tocolytic therapy. *Obstetrics and Gynecology Clinics, 32*(3), 457–484.

may be required. Women receiving beta-mimetic agents such as terbutaline should be carefully monitored for adverse effects including maternal and fetal tachycardia and systolic blood pressure below 90 torr (Lam & Gill, 2005b). Women receiving magnesium sulfate should also be assessed for signs of neurologic depression by evaluating deep tendon reflexes hourly, monitoring of bowel sounds and function, and frequently reviewing the status of each fetal. Emergency resuscitation equipment should be easily accessible and calcium gluconate (10 mL in 10% solution) for magnesium toxicity reversal should be in an easily accessible locked medication cabinet (Lam & Gill, 2005b). Magnesium sulfate safety is discussed in detail in the section on preterm labor. Other tocolytic agents may be used sequentially or in conjunction with β-mimetic therapy. These include prostaglandin synthetase inhibitors, such as indomethacin, and calcium channel blockers, such as nifedipine. Side effects of indomethacin include increased fetal pulmonary vasculature and ductal constriction and should not be used after 32 weeks' gestation or for treatment >72 hours (Lam & Gill). Another side effect of indomethacin is decreased fetal renal function, which can lead to oligohydramnios; thus twin-to-twin transfusion syndrome is a contraindication for this therapy.

The greatest complication of tocolytic therapy for women with multiple gestations is the high risk for pulmonary edema, particularly if complicated by fluid overload or underlying infection. Maximum fluid administration should not exceed 2000 mL per 24 hours, and a strict intake and output must be maintained (Lam & Gill, 2005a). Nursing assessments should include signs and symptoms of pulmonary edema by observation (shortness of breath, coughing or wheezing) and auscultation; daily weights; and metabolic evaluations including blood glucose, CBC, and electrolyte status (Lam & Gill, 2005b).

Antenatal steroids should be administered to women with multiple gestations who experience preterm labor or rupture of membranes before 34 weeks' gestation (AAP & ACOG, 2002). However, corticosteroids may be less effective in prevention of RDS in twins. Betamethasone appears to have a shorter half-life and greater maternal clearance in mothers of twins compared with singletons, which may lead to suboptimal therapeutic levels (Ballabh et al., 2003). No safety or efficacy data are available to support the use of repeated or rescue corticosteroid dosing in multiple gestations (National Institutes of Health, 2000). Increases in uterine contractions following corticosteroid administration have been observed in HOM pregnancies (Elliott & Radin, 1995).

Hypertension

Pregnancy-related hypertensive disease has a dose–response relationship with plurality. Data from a cohort of 34,374 pregnancies showed that hypertensive conditions occur in 6.5% of singletons, 12.7% of twins, 20.0% of triplets, and 19.6% of quadruplet pregnancies (Day, Barton, O'Brien, Istwan, & Sibai 2005). Hypertensive disease included gestational hypertension, preeclampsia, eclampsia, and HELLP syndrome. Other studies have reported similar findings, whereas some have found rates as high as 40% in quadruplets (Newman & Luke, 2000).

Preeclampsia tends to develop earlier in a multiple pregnancy and become more severe than in singleton gestations. It is thought that fetal number and placental mass are somehow involved in the pathogenesis of preeclampsia (Gyamfi, Stone, & Eddleman, 2005). Symptoms of severe preeclampsia with laboratory changes may indicate HELLP syndrome. In HOM, the signs and symptoms of hypertensive disorders are often atypical, without the classic elevations of blood pressure or proteinuria (Newman & Luke, 2000). In a review of triplet and quadruplet pregnancies, of 16 women delivered for preeclampsia, only 8 had elevated blood pressure; whereas 10 had epigastric pain, visual disturbances, and/or headache; 9 had elevated liver enzymes; and 7 had low platelet counts (Hardardottir et al., 1996). Careful assessment of maternal signs and symptoms, in addition to laboratory evaluations, are important in the diagnosis and early treatment of hypertensive disease. Nurses should also be alert to the often-subtle signs of HELLP syndrome (Bowers & Gromada, 2006). When magnesium sulfate is used, fluid balance should be carefully monitored because of the increased risk of pulmonary edema.

Preterm Premature Rupture of Membranes

The incidence of preterm premature rupture of membranes (PPROM) is increased in multiple gestations, with rates reported from 6% to 15% in twins and 11% to 20% in triplets, compared with 2% to 4% in singletons (Gyamfi, Stone, & Eddleman, 2005; Newman & Luke, 2000; Smith-Levitin, Skupski, & Chervenak, 1999; Wen, Demissie, Yang, & Walker, 2004). PPROM in multiples also has a shorter latency to birth than singletons (Norwitz, Edusa, & Park, 2005). Although membrane rupture usually occurs in the presenting sac, rupture of a nonpresenting sac may occur, especially after invasive procedures such as amniocentesis (Norwitz, Edusa, & Park). It is difficult to assess for PPROM in a nonpresenting sac, and intermittent leakage of fluid is the typical clinical presentation. Rupture of the separating membrane in a twin gestation is a unique complication in MC/DA twins, creating a monoamniotic twin risk scenario. Clinical management of PPROM in multiples is similar to that in singletons, with expectant management including antibiotics, and birth for signs and symptoms of chorioamnionitis at 32 to 36 weeks (Gyamfi, Stone, & Eddleman).

Gestational Diabetes

The increased placental mass with multiple fetuses and subsequent increase in diabetogenic hormones are thought to influence the incidence of gestational diabetes mellitus (GDM) in multiple gestations (Ben-Haroush, Yogev, & Hod, 2003). However, studies are inconsistent in demonstrating an increased risk for GDM in multiple gestations (Gyamfi, Stone, & Eddleman, 2005). Some studies have found no increase in GDM; others have shown a clear dose–response relationship with increasing plurality. A population-based study by Walker and colleagues (2004) found a statistically significant relative risk of 1.12 for twins compared with singletons. Wen, Murphy, Pan, Yang, and Wen (2004) reported an adjusted odds ratio of 1.56 for GDM in triplets compared to twins, and 1.81 in quadruplets compared to twins. Newman and Luke (2000) reported GDM rates of 4% for singletons, 7% for twins, 9% for triplets, and 11% for quadruplets. Diagnosis and management of GDM are similar to that in singleton pregnancies (Norwitz, Edusa, & Park, 2005).

Intrahepatic Cholestasis

The incidence of intrahepatic cholestasis in women with a multiple pregnancy is two to five times that of singletons (Rao, Sairam, & Shehata, 2004; Glantz, Marshall, & Mattsson, 2004). The increased risks of preterm birth and fetal death with this condition warrant careful investigation into pruritis without a rash that occurs in the late second and early third trimesters (Nichols, 2005).

Acute Fatty Liver

In a recent multicenter review of 16 cases of acute fatty liver of pregnancy (AFPL), 18% were multiple gestations including one triplet pregnancy (Fesenmeier, Coppage, Lambers, Barton, & Sibai, 2005). Nausea and vomiting in the third trimester were the most common symptoms (75%). Although AFPL is very rare, the high associated morbidity and mortality indicate a need for careful surveillance. Women with nausea, vomiting, or epigastric pain in the third trimester should be carefully assessed.

Peripartum Cardiomyopathy

Approximately 13% of cases of peripartum cardiomyopathy (PPCM) are twins, and several risk factors for this condition are more likely in multiple gestations, including maternal age >30 years and gestational hypertension (Elkayam et al., 2005). Women with multiple pregnancy who have dyspnea, orthopnea, persistent weight retention or weight gain, peripheral edema, nocturnal cough, and profound fatigue, especially postpartum, should be carefully assessed for this life-threatening condition (Murali & Baldisseri, 2005). Maternal mortality with PPCM was 9% in one study,

and 4% required heart transplantation (Elkayam et al., 2005).

Antepartum Hemorrhage

Placenta previa does not appear to occur more frequently in multiple gestations; however, placental abruption is significantly more common. Salihu et al. (2005a) found a rate of abruption of 6.2/1,000 in singletons, 12.2/1,000 in twins, and 15.6/1,000 in triplets, indicating a dose–response relationship. However, there was an inverse relationship with perinatal mortality and plurality; as the number of fetuses increased from one to three, the risk of placental abruption rose, whereas the risk of abruption-related perinatal mortality declined. Odds ratios for perinatal mortality among singletons were 14.3, 4.4 for twins, and 3.0 for triplets. The authors suggested this is partly explained by the different circumstances in which abruption is diagnosed in singleton as opposed to multiple gestations, such as more frequent cesarean birth of multiples.

Pulmonary Embolism

A multiple pregnancy is a risk factor for pulmonary embolism. The mechanical obstruction of the enlarged uterus contributes to venous stasis, particularly for women on bed rest. Thromboembolism is associated with cesarean birth, birth before 36 weeks of gestation, a body mass index (BMI) of 25 or higher, and maternal age of 35 years or older (ACOG, 2004a), all of which are more common in multiple gestations. Therapeutic levels of anticoagulation may be more difficult to achieve with multiple gestations because of the larger volume of distribution.

Fetal Morbidity and Mortality

Zygosity, chorionicity, and fetal growth are important predictors of fetal health and survival in multiples. The inherent physiology associated with the twinning process, along with sharing of uterine space and placental resources, increases the risks for fetal morbidity. Perinatal morbidity and mortality rates for MZ twins are estimated to be 3 to 10 times higher than those for DZ twins (Trevett & Johnson, 2005). Fetal mortality also increases with plurality and late gestational age. Analysis of linked birth and death US population data found the prospective risk (a proportion of all fetuses still at risk at a given gestational age) of fetal death for singletons, twins, and triplets at 24 weeks was 0.28/1000, 0.92/1,000, and 1.30/1,000, respectively (Kahn et al., 2003). In comparison, the corresponding risk was 0.57/1,000 for singletons and 3.09/1,000 for twins at 40 weeks, and 13.18/1,000 for triplets at 38 or more weeks (see Fig. 6–18). These data are consistent with the accelerated placental aging and earlier lung maturation in multiples (Newman & Luke,

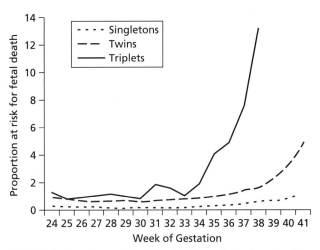

FIGURE 6–18. Prospective risk of fetal mortality by plurality and gestational age. (Based on data from Kahn, B., Lumey, L. H., Zybert, P. A., Lorenz J. M., Cleary-Goldman, J., D'Alton, M. E., & Robinson. J. N. [2003]. Prospective risk of fetal death in singleton, twin, and triplet gestations: implications for practice. *Obstetrics and Gynecolog, 102*[4] 685–692.)

2000). Because of the increased risks for fetal death at late gestational ages, some clinicians are electing to deliver multiples at earlier gestations.

Intrauterine Growth Restriction

Overall, the incidence of IUGR is greater in multiple birth infants than in singletons. This is likely due to placental insufficiency and competition for nutrients. IUGR is associated with increased mortality rates at all gestational ages (Garite, Clark, Elliott, & Thorp, 2004). Recent studies indicate that slowed or compromised fetal growth in both twins at 20 to 28 weeks and from 28 weeks to birth is highly associated with very preterm birth (30–32 weeks; Hediger et al., 2006). Twins and singletons have similar fetal growth rates until about 30 to 32 weeks, when twin fetal weights decrease to the 10th to 50th percentiles (Newman & Luke, 2000). Significant differences in growth begin in triplets at about 29 weeks and in quadruplets, at approximately 27 weeks (Garite, Clark, Elliott, & Thorp, 2004). Fetal growth and subsequent birth weight are also influenced by zygosity and chorionicity. Birth weights are highest in DZ twins with DC placentas, slightly less in MZ twins with DC placentas, and lowest in MZ twins with a MC placenta (Derom, Derom, & Vlietinck, 1995).

A sizable proportion of multiples have discordant growth, in which the weight of one multiple differs significantly from that of the other(s), usually ≥25%. Discordancy is more common in MC twins and is characteristic of Twin to Twin Transfusion Syndrome (TTTS). Maternal age, parity, sex discordance, and gestational age also affect the amount of birth weight discordance (Wen, Demissie, Yang, & Walker, 2004).

A review of 59,034 Canadian twin births found 53% had 0% to 9% birth weight difference; 30% had 10% to 19% discordance; 11% had 20% to 29% discordance; and 6% had ≥30% discordance (Wen et al., 2005). In HOM, two or more fetuses may be concordant but have discordant co-multiple(s). Among triplets, 30% have weight differences ≥25% (Newman & Luke, 2000).

Congenital Anomalies

Multiples are more likely to have structural congenital defects as well as chromosomal and genetic anomalies. Structural abnormalities may be related to the process of embryonic splitting, aberrant vascular or placental physiology, maternal and obstetric factors, or genetic or chromosomal defects. Major structural deformities occur in an estimated 2% of twins, with a higher prevalence in same-sex twins and MZ twins (Newman & Luke, 2000). The most common defects are cardiac malformations, neural tube defects, facial clefts, and gastrointestinal anomalies, with the rate of cardiac defects and gastrointestinal abnormalities in multiples twice that in singletons (Newman & Luke). The excess incidence of congenital anomalies in all twins is due almost exclusively to the higher rate of anomalies in MZ twins (Newman & Luke).

Certain abnormalities are unique to multiple gestations. Conjoined twins occur at a rate of 1/50,000 to 1/100,000 births (Newman & Luke, 2000) and are three times more common in female fetuses than in male fetuses (Graham & Gaddipati, 2005). Survival of conjoined twins is usually dependent on the extent of shared organs. Acardiac malformations (defects in which one multiple has no defined cardiac structure and survives using the co-multiple's cardiac pump mechanism) occur exclusively in MZ multiples at a rate of 1/100 MZ births or 1/35,000 births (Meyers, Elias, & Arrabal, 1995). This condition is also referred to as "twin reversed arterial perfusion (TRAP) sequence" because of the reversal of circulation in the acardiac fetus. Although the acardiac twin of a MZ pair has 100% mortality, the co-twin's survival depends on the discordance in weights between the two, with higher mortality associated with increasing discordance (Newman & Luke, 2000).

Abnormal Vascular/Placental Changes

TTTS is a condition unique to twins and develops in about 15% of MC pregnancies (Galea, Jain, & Fisk, 2005). It occurs when there is unequal shunting of blood from donor fetus to the co-twin recipient through vascular connections in a shared (MC) placenta. Dichorionic TTTS has also been reported (Malone & D'Alton, 2004). Fetofetal transfusion can also occur in HOM with shared placental beds. Vascular anastomoses occur in more than three-fourths of all MC placentas and may be arteriovenous, venovenous, or arterial–arterial (Crowther, 1999). However, many connections appear to be protectively bidirectional as only about one third show clinical evidence (Newman & Luke, 2000).

Fetal compromise occurs when there is significant single direction vascular flow. The recipient twin becomes hypervolemic and polycythemic, progressing to polyhydramnios, congestive heart failure, and death. The donor twin becomes hypovolemic, anemic, and growth restricted. The pathophysiology of TTTS appears to be more complex than just volume shifts between twins. There is evidence that hypertensive mediators renin and angiotensin also play an important role in TTTS (Harkness & Crombleholme, 2005). The most severe form of TTTS is the stuck twin, when the donor twin is depleted of amniotic fluid. The stuck twin complicates 8% of all twin pregnancies, up to 35% of MC/DA gestations, and carries a mortality rate of over 80% (Crowther, 1999). If left untreated, the mortality rate for TTTS is 80% to 100%, especially when it presents earlier than 20 weeks' gestation (Harkness & Crombleholme). More than 30% of survivors have associated neurodevelopmental anomalies (Fox, Kilby, & Khan, 2005). TTTS accounts for 15% to 17% of all twin perinatal mortality (Newman & Luke, 2000).

Diagnosis of TTTS may include the following sonographic findings: (1) monochorionicity, (2) discrepancy in amniotic fluid between the amniotic sacs with polyhydramnios in one sac (largest vertical pocket >8 cm) and the oligohydramnios in the other sac (largest vertical pocket <2 cm), (3) discrepancy in umbilical cord size, (4) presence of cardiac dysfunction in the polyhydramniotic twin, (5) abnormal umbilical artery or ductus venosus Doppler velocimetry, and (6) significant growth discordance (often >20%; Harkness & Crombleholme, 2005). Cases are often described using Quintero's staging criteria, but this classification does not necessarily correlate with prognosis (Quintero et al., 1999). See Display 6-42.

Treatment for TTTS includes serial amnioreduction, selective fetoscopic laser photocoagulation, intertwin amniotic membrane septostomy, and umbilical cord coagulation. Of these treatments, serial amnioreduction has been the most common, as it is a simple outpatient procedure, easily performed by a trained obstetrician. The procedure involves removal of large amounts of amniotic fluid, often more than 1 to 2 L on a recurring basis. In addition to the paradoxical effect of fluid increasing in the oligohydramniotic sac, side benefits of this therapy include prevention of preterm labor related to polyhydramnios, improved fetal hemodynamics, and uteroplacental blood flow (Harkness & Crombleholme, 2005). Yet the procedure is not without problems. Despite reported success rates as high as 83% with amnioreduction, 5% to 58% of survivors suffer neurodevelopmental handicaps (Fox, Kilby, & Khan, 2005).

DISPLAY 6-42

Quintero Staging for Twin to Twin Transfusion Syndrome

Stage 1—Donor twin bladder is visible, normal Doppler studies.

Stage 2—Bladder of the donor twin is no longer visible, Doppler studies not critically abnormal.

Stage 3—Critically abnormal cardiovascular function in either twin with absent or reverse end-diastolic velocity in the umbilical artery, pulsatile umbilical venous flow, or reverse flow in ductus venosus.

Stage 4—Evidence of overt heart failure/hydrops (ascites, pericardial or pleural effusion, scalp edema) in either fetus.

Stage 5—Intrauterine death of either fetus.

Quintero, R. A., Morales, W. J., Allen, M. H., Bornick, P. W., Johnson, P. K., & Kruger, M. (1999). Staging of twin-twin transfusion syndrome. *Journal of Perinatology, 19*(8 Pt. 1), 550–555.

Once considered experimental, selective fetoscopic laser photocoagulation or fetoscopic laser therapy has gained acceptance as a treatment for moderate and severe TTTS. This procedure uses fetoscopy to visualize, and laser to coagulate vascular anastomoses at the intertwin membrane. It is used as a primary intervention or for cases with deteriorating cardiac and hemodynamic changes unresponsive to amnioreduction (Harkness & Crombleholme, 2005). Risks of the procedure include neurologic morbidity or death of one or both twins. In a prospective study of 200 severe midtrimester (median gestation 20.7 weeks) TTTS cases treated with fetoscopic laser therapy, the overall survival rate was 71.5%, with 59.5% survival of both fetuses and 83.5% survival of at least one twin; however, survival rates decreased with increasing stage severity (Huber, Diehl, Bregenzer, Hackelöer, & Hecher, 2006). Lopriore et al. (2006) reported that 10% of survivors of laser-treated TTTS had severe cerebral ultrasound findings, which the researchers believed occurred antenatally; however, fetal cranial imaging was not performed prior to the laser treatment. A meta-analysis of existing studies compared serial amnioreduction with selective fetoscopic laser therapy and concluded that laser ablation in early-onset TTTS significantly increases survival in at least one fetus, while reducing long-term neurodevelopmental morbidity (Fox, Kilby, & Khan, 2005).

Abnormal umbilical cord insertion is a common finding in multiple gestations, especially in those with

MC placentas. Velamentous cord insertion (directly into the membranes) occurs in 13% to 21% of twin gestations, compared with 1% to 2% of singleton pregnancies (Hanley et al., 2002). Higher numbers of fetuses may create a crowding effect on cord implantation sites (Machin, 2002). One study found that only 23.8% of MC/DA twins had a normal disc insertion for both twins, compared with 56.1% of DC/DA twins (Hanley et al.). Velamentous insertion is estimated to occur in 25% of triplet pregnancies, and represents a 25- to 50-fold increase compared with singleton gestations (Feldman et al., 2002). Velamentous cord insertions may contribute to poor uteroplacental perfusion and birth weight discordancy.

Fetal Loss

Spontaneous loss early in a multiple pregnancy is often termed the "vanishing twin" and is associated with bleeding in approximately 25% of cases (Newman & Luke, 2000). This type of early loss has no adverse effects on the remainder of the pregnancy, and there is usually no visual evidence of the vanished fetus at birth. However, grief responses are possible because of first trimester ultrasound diagnosis and mothers' early prenatal attachment.

Later intrauterine death of one fetus in a set of multiples is a unique situation and carries both physiologic and psychologic risks. Fetal death at 20 weeks or later occurs in 2.6% of twin and 4.3% of triplet gestations (Johnson & Zhang, 2002). The surviving twin is at increased risk of fetal death, neonatal death, and severe long-term morbidity. The overall risk of severe neurological defect (including cerebral palsy) for the survivor has been estimated at 20% (Pharoah & Adi, 2000). The risks are greater for MZ twins; however, a review of 41 sets of multiples complicated by single fetal death found that 21% of the survivors with known neurologic damage were from dichorionic placentations (Liu, Benirschke, Scioscia, & Mannino, 1992). Although MA twins are rare (1% of MZ twins), these fetuses have an extremely high risk of death during pregnancy and at birth, primarily due to cord entanglement. Perinatal mortality rates for MA twins have historically ranged from 40% to 70%, but more recent reports have found fetal mortality rates of 10% to 12% with intensive surveillance (Motew & Ginsberg, 1995; Allen, Windrim, Barrett, & Ohlsson, 2001).

Management of fetal death depends on multiple factors, including chorionicity, gestational age, and condition of the surviving fetus(es). Generally, after a fetal death at 20 weeks' gestation or later, the survival of the remaining fetuses is inversely related to the time the death occurred and survivors of opposite-sex twin pairs are more likely to survive than remaining twins of same-sex twin pairs (Johnson & Zhang, 2002).

Antepartum Management

Antepartum management of multiple pregnancy should be a collaborative effort of the members of the perinatal healthcare team, including perinatologists, obstetricians, nurse midwives, registered nurses, advanced practice nurses, perinatal educators, ultrasonographers, social workers, and dietitians.

Prenatal Diagnosis and Genetic Testing

Because of the increased risk of congenital abnormalities in multiples, and the higher maternal age for many women, prenatal diagnostic testing is frequently offered. The maternal-age-related risk for aneuploidy is approximately the same for MZ twins as for singletons (Rustico, Baietti, Coviello, Orlandi, & Nicolini, 2005). However, for DZ twins, the risk of aneuploidy in one of the twins is double that of singletons, because the independent risk for each twin is additive. The risk of aneuploidy occurring in both DZ twins is the singleton risk squared (Bush & Malone, 2005). In practical terms, a 33-year-old woman with twins has the same risk of Down syndrome as a 35-year-old woman with a singleton (ACOG, 2004a). In a 28-year-old woman with triplets, the risk of at least one fetus having Down syndrome is similar to the risk of a 35-year-old with a singleton (Malone & D'Alton, 2004). It has been recommended that invasive prenatal diagnosis should be offered to all women with a twin pregnancy at 31 years of age (Rodis et al., 1990). However, using maternal age alone to calculate risk has been questioned due to low sensitivity and high false-positive rate in singletons, as well as overestimation of risk in twins (Odibo, Lawrence-Cleary, & Macones, 2003). Further, it is difficult to estimate risk for HOM.

First trimester nuchal translucency (NT) screening appears to be as accurate in twins and HOM as in singletons (Cleary-Goldman, D'Alton, & Berkowitz, 2005). Detection rates for NT screening in twins are approximately 75% to 85%, with a 5% false-positive rate (Bush & Malone, 2005). Each fetus is individually assessed and the pregnancy risk is calculated.

Second trimester maternal serum screening in twin gestations is associated with a high false-positive rate, particularly in ART pregnancies (Maymon, Neeman, Shulman, Rosen, & Herman, 2005), as an unaffected co-twin may mask the abnormal maternal serum levels associated with an aneuploid fetus. Even if screening suggests the presence of an affected fetus, biochemical markers cannot specify which twin is abnormal (Bush & Malone, 2005). Because ultrasound is needed to confirm which fetus is affected following a positive result, many centers are not routinely offering serum screening for multiples (Cleary-Goldman, D'Alton, & Berkowitz, 2005). Regardless of other screening tests, a targeted ultrasound examination for fetal anomaly detection is suggested for all multiples between 18 and 20 weeks gestation (Dodd & Crowther, 2005a).

Invasive prenatal diagnostic techniques may be indicated when prenatal screening tests identify increased risks for genetic or chromosomal abnormalities. Genetic amniocentesis between 15 and 20 weeks has been found to be accurate in twin gestations. Some authors report an increased risk of fetal loss associated with genetic amniocentesis of approximately 6%, whereas others suggest a procedure-related loss rate similar to or slightly higher than that in singletons (Dodd & Crowther, 2005a; Cleary-Goldman, D'Alton, & Berkowitz, 2005). Use of a marker dye such as indigo carmine helps prevent cross-contamination of fluids when tapping multiple sacs.

Chorionic villus sampling (CVS) may be offered when genetic results are needed earlier in pregnancy than second trimester amniocentesis can provide. CVS appears to be safe in multiple gestations, although there are technical difficulties in accessing multiple fetuses, a higher risk of uncertain results compared with singletons, and risks for sample cross contamination. The associated loss rates are comparable to amniocentesis when performed by experienced clinicians; however, loss rates as high as 4.5% have been reported (Cleary-Goldman, D'Alton, & Berkowitz, 2005).

Prenatal diagnosis presents unique challenges for parents, especially if one fetus is abnormal, as they may face the dilemma of selective reduction. Parents may also worry about the status of the unaffected twin throughout pregnancy, highlighting a potential need for regular pre- and postnatal examination and ongoing reassurance, or invasive prenatal testing in the surviving fetuses after reduction (Bryan, 2005).

Prenatal Care

The *Guidelines for Perinatal Care* (AAP & ACOG, 2002) recommends referral of twin gestations to a board-certified obstetrician. In practice, many clinicians also refer women with complicated multiple pregnancies, especially those with HOM, to a consulting perinatologist (maternal–fetal medicine specialist) (Bowers & Gromada, 2006). These specialists typically coordinate care with the primary obstetrician or may provide primary obstetrical care. Although most clinicians increase the number of antenatal care visits for women with multiple pregnancy, there is no consensus as to the frequency of visits that constitutes optimal care (Dodd & Crowther, 2005a). However, in light of the higher risks for perinatal complications in these pregnancies, regular and frequent antenatal visits increase the likelihood for early detection and treatment. Newman's (2005) recommendations for antepartum management of twins are listed in Table 6-31.

TABLE 6–31 ■ COMPONENTS OF ROUTINE ANTEPARTUM CARE OF TWINS

Conception to 12 weeks	Early diagnosis Confirm viability Determine placentation Patient education
12 to 20 weeks	Identify anomalies Prenatal diagnostic testing Cervical length and integrity Nutritional counseling
20 to 26 weeks	Cervical length and score Fetal fibronectin Activity modification as needed BMI-specific weight gain Serial ultrasound assessment
26 to 32 weeks	Preterm birth prevention efforts Serial ultrasound assessment Screening for GDM BMI-specific weight gain
32 to 38 weeks	Preeclampsia surveillance Weekly fetal testing Serial ultrasound assessment Determine fetal positions Determine optimal birth time

Newman, R. B. (2005). Routine antepartum care of twins. In I. Blickstein & L. G. Keith (Eds.), *Multiple pregnancy: Epidemiology, gestation and perinatal outcome* (2nd ed., pp. 405–419). New York: Taylor and Francis.

Specialized multiple-birth clinics (twin clinics) have reported improved perinatal morbidity and neonatal outcomes (Luke et al., 2003; Ruiz, Brown, Peters, & Johnston, 2001; Newman & Luke, 2000; Papiernik, Keith, Oleszczuk, & Cervantes, 1998; Newman & Ellings, 1995). Interventions in such clinics include consistent care providers, intensive education about prevention of preterm birth, individualized modification of maternal activity, increased attention to nutrition, ultrasonography, tracking of clinic nonattendees, and a supportive clinical environment. Cited benefits include improved maternal education, increased maternal weight gain and birth weights, longer gestations, lowered rates of VLBW, NICU admissions, and perinatal mortality, shortened hospital stays, and lower hospital charges.

In an assessment of the impact of aggressive antepartum management on twin birth outcomes, United States vital statistics data from 1981 to 1997 were reviewed (Kogan et al., 2000). Ironically, the steepest increases in twin preterm birth rates were among women who received the most intensive prenatal care, compared with those given adequate care. (Care levels were calculated using the time prenatal care began, the number of visits, and adjusted for length of gestation). A surprising finding was that the mortality rate for the infants of mothers who received the most intensive care declined significantly, from 27.6/1,000 to 17.8/1,000. This increase in preterm births yet decreased infant mortality, despite greater utilization of prenatal care, appears to be a paradox. However, it may be explained by more aggressive management and medically indicated earlier births for complicated cases, along with better access to and improvements in neonatal care (Kogan et al., 2000).

Management of HOM gestations involves more intensive surveillance, attention, and interventions. Although there is no consensus as to content or frequency of prenatal care for these high-risk pregnancies, some suggested strategies for prenatal management of HOM are listed in Table 6-32.

Prenatal Education

Parents expecting multiples have unique perinatal educational needs. The high-risk nature and extraordinary aspects of their pregnancy, along with the unknowns of parenting multiple infants, present a need for specialized education (Bryan, 2002). As the goal of patient education for women with high-risk pregnancies is to assist them in the improvement of their own health (Freda, 2000), providing education about their condition and healthcare options allows women expecting multiples to make informed decisions concerning treatment. The increasing number of multiple gestations makes providing specialized multiple birth classes both feasible and practical. Such classes offer detailed information about the differences in multiple pregnancy and birth, educate about potential complications, enhance coping skills, teach parenting skills, and provide an immediate support system for expectant families with other parents of multiples (Bowers & Gromada, 2006). Multiple birth class topics include physical and emotional changes, variations in labor and birth and postpartum care, and detailed education about nutrition. Common pregnancy complications, especially preterm labor, should also be included. Parents will need advice in practical skills for coping with more than one newborn, breastfeeding multiples, and choosing appropriate layette and infant equipment (Bowers & Gromada). A hospital tour should include the NICU, optimally allowing couples to meet neonatologists and nurses, and seeing premature infants in intensive care (Bryan, 2002). Because so many women with multiples are at risk for complications and potential bed rest, they should attend classes in their early second trimester. Options include a mini-class to supplement standard childbirth classes offering tips and practical advice on handling multiple newborns, or a complete multiples-specific prenatal education curriculum, such as that offered through Marvelous Multiples, Inc.

Nutrition and Weight Gain

Luke (2005, p. 348) described a multiple pregnancy as "a state of magnified nutritional requirements, resulting in a greater nutrient drain on maternal resources and an accelerated depletion of nutritional reserves." Evidence is growing that optimal maternal nutrition and weight gain are linked with positive perinatal outcomes for multiples, including reduced incidence of LBW and VLBW infants (Roem, 2003). The shortened length of gestation for most multiples limits the time for intrauterine growth, and the more rapid aging of multiple birth placentas shortens the period for effective transfer of nutrients to the developing fetuses. Thus, higher weight gains during early

---

TABLE 6–32 ■ SUGGESTED COMPONENTS OF ANTEPARTUM CARE OF HIGHER ORDER MULTIPLES

- Discontinue working between 20 and 24 weeks' gestation
- Modified bed rest at home beginning in the second trimester; strict bed rest for quadruplets and higher
- Frequent prenatal visits with cervical evaluation using digital or ultrasound examination
- Contraction monitoring for evidence of increased uterine activity or signs of preterm labor beginning at 20 weeks' gestation
- Serial ultrasound studies for fetal growth evaluation, beginning at 20 weeks, then every 2 to 3 weeks from 28 weeks to delivery
- Selected use of home uterine activity monitoring
- Weekly monitoring beginning at 24 to 32 weeks' gestation, using nonstress tests (NSTs) or biophysical profile (BPP) testing
- Weekly Doppler flow studies for discordant fetal growth
- Hospitalization for evidence of preterm labor or other complications
- Tocolysis for confirmed preterm labor
- Elective cesarean birth at onset of labor near term or at 36 completed weeks' gestation with documentation of lung maturity

Chitkara, U., & Berkowitz, R. L. (2002). Multiple gestations. In S. G. Gabbe, J. R. Niebyl, & J. L. Simpson (Eds.), *Obstetrics: Normal and problem pregnancies* (4th ed., pp. 827–867). Philadelphia: Churchill Livingstone; Newman, R. B., & Luke, B. (2000). *Multifetal pregnancy*. Philadelphia: Lippincott Williams & Wilkins; Bowers, N. A., & Gromada, K. K. (2006). *Care of the multiple-birth family: Pregnancy and birth* (Nursing Module). White Plains, NY: March of Dimes Birth Defects Foundation.

gestation may influence the structural and functional development of the placenta and subsequently augment fetal growth through more effective placental function as well as the transfer of a higher level of nutrients (Luke, 2005).

Women with multiple gestation require additional calories, micronutrient supplementation, and a higher gestational weight gain than women with singletons (Brown & Carlson, 2000; Luke, 2005; Roem, 2003; Rosello-Soberon, Fuentes-Chaparro, & Casanueva, 2005). Energy expenditures are increased in women carrying multiples as evidenced by significantly higher resting basal metabolic rates in twin pregnancies compared with singletons (1,636 ± 174 kcal/day and 1,456 ± 158 kcal/day, respectively; Shinagawa, 2005). Because of these increased energy demands, an additional 300 calories are recommended over and above the 2,400 calories for a singleton pregnancy (AAP & ACOG, 2002). However, official dietary standards for nutrient and energy intake for multiple gestations have not been established, other than the long-standing recommendations for increases in micronutrients by the Institute of Medicine (1992) that include zinc, copper, calcium, vitamin B6, folate, and iron after 12 weeks' gestation. Many clinicians recommend a supplement containing iron and folate in addition to a regular prenatal vitamin. One nutritional intervention program for twin and triplet pregnancies recommends a diet with 20% of calories from protein, 40% of calories from carbohydrates, and 40% of calories from fat to provide additional calories with less bulk (Luke, 2004). This diet emphasizes low glycemic index carbohydrates to prevent wide fluctuations in blood glucose concentrations. Compared with singleton pregnancies, multiple gestations have a faster depletion of glycogen stores and increased metabolism of fat between meals and overnight (Luke, 2005). Women should be counseled to eat frequent, small meals, similar to a diabetic diet; this may also aid digestion as the rapidly growing uterus crowds the stomach.

Studies have shown that pregravid maternal weight, weight gain patterns, and total amounts of gain in multiple pregnancy are linked to fetal weight gain, length of gestation, and eventual infant birth weights (Luke et al., 2003; Brown & Carlson, 2000; Luke, 2005; Rosello-Soberon, Fuentes-Chaparro, & Casanueva, 2005). Maternal nutrient stores deposited in early pregnancy are utilized in late pregnancy for placental growth. This is demonstrated in studies showing that poor early maternal weight gain is associated with inadequate intrauterine growth and increased perinatal morbidity in twins (Rosello-Soberon, Fuentes-Chaparro, & Casanueva). Early maternal weight gain in multiple gestations appears to have a stronger effect on infant birth weights than do mid- and late-pregnancy gains (Luke, 2004).

Using maternal pregravid body mass index (BMI) status, Luke and colleagues (2003) formulated maternal weight gain guidelines associated with optimal fetal growth and birth weights in twins. These guidelines promote higher overall weight gain for underweight women and lower overall gain for overweight and obese women (see Table 6–33).

Few studies have examined weight gain and nutritional recommendations for HOM pregnancies. A 50-pound total weight gain for triplet pregnancy, approximately 1.5 pounds/week, has been suggested (Brown & Carlson, 2000). Available data indicate that the associations of maternal weight gain with fetal growth and infant birth weights are even more important for these pregnancies, as early pregnancy weight gain and higher total gain in underweight women with HOM appear to have an even greater effect on outcomes (Luke, 2005). See Display 6-43.

TABLE 6–33 ■ MATERNAL WEIGHT GAIN PATTERN AND TOTAL RECOMMENDED GAIN FOR TWIN GESTATIONS

Prepregnant BMI	Rate of Gain (Lbs/Week)				
	0–20 Weeks	Gain by 28 Weeks	20–28 Weeks	28 Weeks to Delivery	Total Weight Gain (lbs)
Underweight (BMI <19.8)	1.25–1.75	37–49 lbs	1.50–1.75	1.25	50–62 lbs
Normal Weight (BMI 19.8–26.0)	1.0–1.50	30–44 lbs	1.25–1.75	1.0	40–54 lbs
Overweight (BMI 26.1–29.0)	1.0–1.25	28–37 lbs	1.0–1.50	1.0	38–47 lbs
Obese (BMI >29.0)	0.75–1.0	21–30 lbs	0.75–1.25	0.75	29–38 lbs

Luke, B., Brown, M. B., Misiunas, R., Anderson, E., Nugent, C., van de Ven, C., et al. (2003). Specialized prenatal care and maternal and infant outcomes in twin pregnancy. *American Journal of Obstetrics and Gynecology* 189(4), 934–938.

DISPLAY 6-43

Nutrition and Weight Gain in Multiple Gestation

Optimal maternal nutrition and weight gain are linked with positive perinatal outcomes for multiples.

Women pregnant with multiples need:
- Increased caloric intake
- Micronutrient supplementation (IOM, 1989 recommendations):
  - 15 mg zinc
  - 2 mg copper
  - 250 mg calcium
  - 2 mg vitamin B_6
  - 300 mcg folate (current recommendations are for 400 μg)
  - 50 mg vitamin C
  - 5 mcg (200 IU) vitamin D
  - 30 mg iron after the 12th week

- Nutrition education, counseling, referral to services for basic food supplements

Weight gain counseling in multiple gestation includes:
- Higher weight gains than for singleton pregnancies
- Early (first trimester) weight gain to build maternal stores for later placental growth.
- Assessment of pregravid weight status and adjustment of weight gain goals

Weight gain recommendations for twin pregnancy:
- Overall gain of 40–45 lb
- Gain approximately 1.5 lb per week in the second and third trimesters.
- Underweight women should gain at higher end of range.
- Overweight and obese women should gain at lower end of range.
- First trimester weight gain (4 to 6 lb)

Weight gain recommendations for triplet pregnancy:
- Overall gain of at least 50 lb
- Steady rate of gain of approximately 1.5 lb per week throughout pregnancy

---

Bed rest appears to have a negative effect on maternal weight gain. A study of 31 women hospitalized with a twin or triplet pregnancy found the weekly rate of maternal weight gain during hospitalization was significantly less than recommended weight gain amounts, although infant birth weights were appropriate for gestational age (Maloni, Margevicius, & Damato, 2006). The study found 65% of women with twins and 86% with triplets either lost or gained no weight in the first week, and 43% of women with twins and 57% of those with triplets either lost or did not gain weight over the entire hospitalization. It is unknown whether nutritional interventions are effective in countering weight loss for women on bed rest, either at home or in the hospital, and additional studies are needed.

Nutrition counseling and weight gain advice is a simple, low-cost, and effective intervention for improving perinatal outcome in multiple gestations (Brown & Carlson, 2000). However, surveys showed that more than one-fourth of pregnant women, including those with twins received no advice regarding weight gain, and among women who did receive guidance, more than one-third received inappropriate advice (Luke, 2004). A consult with a registered dietitian specializing in perinatal nutrition is helpful for all expectant mothers of multiples, especially for those who are underweight for height, vegetarian (particularly vegans who consume no animal proteins), and pregnant with HOM (Bowers & Gromada, 2006).

Fetal Surveillance

Due to the increased incidence of fetal morbidity and mortality in multiples, assessment of fetal well-being is often incorporated into routine antenatal care. Additional testing is advised for multiple gestations at increased risk including those with maternal complications, as well as for fetuses with MC or MA chorionicity, IUGR, and growth discordance. Fetal movement counting may be a useful adjunct with other antepartum fetal surveillance (AAP & ACOG, 2002). Emphasis should be placed on a woman's perception of a decrease in fetal activity relative to previous levels, rather than on a precise number of movements. However, some women may have difficulty differentiating movement among fetuses. For multiples with IUGR, fetal surveillance often includes twice-weekly nonstress testing (NST) and follow-up biophysical profile (BPP) for nonreactive patterns (Bowers & Gromada, 2006). Both tests are considered reliable in twin and triplet gestations (ACOG, 2004a). Doppler velocimetry frequently is used in the diagnosis and assessment of growth discordancy and has been associated with improved perinatal outcomes (Dodd & Crowther, 2005a). A suggested plan for antenatal surveillance is listed in Display 6–44.

For all surveillance techniques, fetal positions should be consistently documented using a uterine mapping system. This allows comparisons with prior assessments and accurate clinical reporting. The presenting

DISPLAY 6-44

Suggested Plan for Fetal Surveillance of Multiples

- Ultrasound at 10 to 14 weeks' gestation for fetal number and chorionicity
- Targeted ultrasound at 18 to 20 weeks' gestation for gestational age, amniotic fluid assessment, and anatomic survey for anomalies
- DC/DA twins with normal prior scans, subsequent ultrasound at 24 to 26 weeks, and every 3 to 4 weeks if no problems
- MC placentation: subsequent ultrasounds a minimum of every 2 weeks
- MC/MA: add frequent NST after viability is reached
- IUGR, growth or fluid discordance, intensified fetal surveillance, BPP and Doppler velocimetry studies
- Further testing for any nonreassuring result

Chitkara, U., & Berkowitz, R. L. (2002). Multiple gestations. In S. G. Gabbe, J. R. Niebyl, & J. L. Simpson (Eds.), *Obstetrics: Normal and problem pregnancies* (4th ed., pp. 827–867). Philadelphia: Churchill Livingstone.

fetus is always "A," and remaining fetuses ("B," "C," etc.) are identified by relative ascending positions (Bowers & Gromada, 2006). Notations should also be made of fetal position changes, such as when female fetus B moves to C position, and when male fetus C moves to B position.

Intrapartum Management

The high risks of twin and HOM pregnancies require a hospital-based birth in a facility that is capable of emergent cesarean birth and neonatal resuscitation. Antepartum transfer to a specialty or subspecialty level care facility ensures access to appropriate neonatal care (AAP & ACOG, 2002). This also assures that mother and babies stay together. Ideally, births prior to 34 to 35 weeks' gestation occur in a facility with a level III NICU. Despite some proponents of home birth for multiples, this alternative lacks the obstetric, anesthetic, and surgical care needed for emergency interventions (Bowers & Gromada, 2006).

On admission, ultrasound should be used to confirm viability, placental location, and fetal presentation (Healy & Gaddipati, 2005). Although there is excellent correlation between fetal presentations at 32 to 36 weeks and those at birth, some twins undergo spontaneous version in the third trimester. Cephalic-presenting twins at 28 weeks are fairly stable, but non–vertex-presenting twins are more likely to spontaneously

convert to a vertex presentation before birth (Chasen, Spiro, Kalish, & Chervenak, 2005).

Expectant parents' birth plans and desires should be respected as much as possible, acknowledging the unique aspects of the birth for many of these families. They should be given anticipatory guidance for all labor and birth procedures. Many are surprised at the large perinatal team that typically attends the birth of multiples. For a preterm cesarean birth of twins, it is not uncommon for as many as 15 people to be present: 2 obstetricians, 2 to 3 labor and delivery nurses, 1 or 2 neonatologists, a NICU team for each infant, 1 or 2 anesthesia staff, and the parents (Bowers & Gromada, 2006). Essential personnel for intrapartum management of multiple births include experienced obstetricians, nurses, anesthesiologists, operating room technicians, and neonatal staff. Women may labor in labor rooms/labor–delivery–recovery rooms (LDRs), but vaginal births should be performed in a surgical suite with a double setup in case of emergent cesarean birth (Healy & Gaddipati, 2005; Simpson, 2004). The increased risk for cesarean birth of multiples warrants interventions such as a large-bore IV, withholding oral liquids and solid food, evaluating the woman's airway, and providing an antacid to prevent gastric aspiration (Bowers & Gromada, 2006). Recommendations for labor and birth procedures and management are listed in Display 6–45.

Timing of Birth

There is current debate over the optimal timing for birth of multiples. In view of the increasing risk of fetal death beginning at 37 weeks for twins and 35 weeks for HOM (Kahn et al., 2003), as well as studies indicating optimal birth weights at near-term gestations (Luke, 1996), some clinicians electively deliver multiples before the spontaneous onset of term labor. Luke determined optimal timing for birth by examining rates of fetal deaths in twins and triplets by birth weight and gestational age. The lowest fetal mortality rates were at 36 to 37 weeks for twins weighing 2,500 to 2,800 g, and at 34 to 35 weeks for triplets weighing 1,900 to 2,200 g. However, a Cochrane review of existing studies found that there are insufficient data available to support a practice of elective birth at 37 weeks' gestation for women with an otherwise uncomplicated twin pregnancy (Dodd & Crowther, 2003). Others warn that effecting an early birth exclusively for maternal and/or physician convenience risks iatrogenic complications related to induction and prematurity (Ramsey & Repke, 2003).

Thus, consideration must be given to each clinical situation. Evidence of appropriate fetal size for gestational age and sustained intrauterine growth, with normal amniotic fluid volume and reassuring tests of fetal

Labor and Birth Recommendations for Multiple Births

- Hospital birth with a Level II or III NICU
- Antenatal maternal transport if appropriate maternal or neonatal services are not available
- Two experienced obstetricians or an obstetrician and a certified nurse–midwife
- Obstetric nurses to circulate and assist and provide support to the woman
- Anesthesiologist and assistant to provide epidural and general anesthesia
- Neonatal team with nurses and respiratory care personnel sufficient for all infants—pediatricians/ neonatologists available if fetal problems occur or birth is preterm or operative
- Delivery in room large enough to accommodate personnel and equipment
- Cesarean birth access immediately available
- Neonatal resuscitation beds available with individual oxygen and suction supplies
- Neonatal transport protocol in place
- Forceps or vacuum extraction immediately available
- Qualified ultrasonographer present with real-time ultrasound
- Continuous electronic fetal monitoring of all fetuses; scalp electrode on each presenting fetus, when possible
- Large-bore (16- to 18-gauge) IV access
- Oxytocin infusion, premixed
- Typed and cross-matched blood immediately available
- Agents for hemorrhage management available
- Cord blood samples for blood gas analysis obtained routinely
- All placentas sent for pathological examination

Bowers, N. A., & Gromada, K. K. (2006). *Care of the multiple-birth family: Pregnancy and birth* (Nursing Module). White Plains, NY: March of Dimes Birth Defects Foundation. With permission.

well-being, in the absence of maternal complications, warrant allowing the pregnancy to continue (ACOG, 2004a). Another approach is to weigh the risks of continuing the pregnancy for mother and fetuses with the risks to the infants once they are born. One clinical strategy based on this premise is to deliver DC twins at 37 to 38 weeks, MC/DA twins at 36 to 37 weeks, MC/MA twins at 32 to 34 weeks, triplets at 35 to 36 weeks, and quadruplets at 34 weeks (Elliott, 2005b).

Fetal pulmonary maturity should be documented if prenatal care is uncertain, for both scheduled births and cases with preterm labor or PPROM (ACOG, 2004a). Tapping of both sacs is recommended due to inconsistent lecithin/sphingomyelin levels between twins, and especially if lung maturity testing will affect clinical management (Malone & D'Alton, 2004).

Labor with Multiples

Labor in multiple gestations appears to differ in length from that of singletons. Most data are from twin labors, with limited information from triplets. Early studies evaluated cervical dilatation on admission and found significant differences between twins and singletons (Friedman & Sachtleben, 1964). However, a multiple pregnancy is frequently complicated by preterm labor and will have advanced cervical dilatation long before entering active labor. More recent reports have evaluated the length of labor from the onset of the active phase at 4 or 5 cm. One study of 1,821 twin births in a single institution found cervical effacements and vertex stations on admission were similar for twins and matched singleton controls (Schiff et al., 1998). Interestingly, women with twins had less cervical dilatation on admission. In this study, the time for cervical progression from 4 cm to 10 cm was less in nulliparous women with twins (3.2 ± 1.3 hours) than those with singletons (4.7 ± 2.6 hours; $P < .001$), but there were no differences for multiparous women. No significant differences in the mean length of the second stage of labor were observed for twins (0.8 hours) and singletons (0.7 hours). Silver et al. (2000) reported similar findings, and included triplets in their analysis (32 triplets, 64 twins, and 64 singletons; all at approximately 34 weeks' gestation). The mean rate of cervical dilatation in hours from 5 cm to complete was 1.8 ± 1.2 for triplets, 1.7 ± 1.3 for twins, and 2.3 ± 1.5 for singletons ($P < .05$). Factors affecting labor progress may include fetal weights, presentations, and use of epidural anesthesia.

Fetal Monitoring

All multiples should have continuous FHR monitoring during labor (AAP & ACOG, 2002; ACOG, 2005). Dual-channel electronic fetal monitors allow simultaneous heart rate recordings, eliminating the need to synchronize several monitors for tracing comparisons. Monitors may display each FHR in a different color and/or by printing one in a bold line and the other in a faint line. Each FHR should be clearly labeled to indicate the corresponding ultrasound transducer and fetus that is being monitored. For example, the nurse should monitor one fetus long enough to get a tracing and then identify on the tracing (either electronically or directly on the paper version) and nurses' notes, "Bold line = fetus in LLQ or A" (Bowers & Gromada, 2006). Ultrasound may be helpful in locating fetal hearts for transducer placement. A fetal scalp electrode should be applied to the presenting fetus in early labor if membranes are already ruptured (Chitkara & Berkowitz, 2002; Rao, Sairam, & Shehata, 2005).

Eganhouse and Peterson (1998) explained the phenomenon of fetal synchrony in multiples. This is a similarity in frequency and timing of FHR accelerations, baseline oscillations, and periodic changes with contractions that occur in healthy twins more than 50% of the time. Some electronic monitors address synchrony with discrimination technology that uses printing of signal marks on the tracing, separate monitoring scales, or artificial separation of single-scale tracings into two separate tracings (Bowers & Gromada, 2006). However, these system cues do not replace careful nursing assessment of each FHR pattern (Simpson, 2004). Bakker, Colenbrander, Verstraeten, and Van Geijn (2004) reported a higher incidence of signal loss in twins compared with singletons and cited abnormal twin positions, polyhydramnios, and twin–twin interactions as factors contributing to signal loss.

Clinicians must be familiar with principles of monitoring preterm fetuses because many multiples present in labor before 37 weeks' gestation. Preterm fetuses typically have baseline FHR in the upper range of normal (150 to 160 beats per minute), and accelerations are shorter in duration and of lower amplitude than in more mature fetuses (Eganhouse & Peterson, 1998). Nonreassuring FHR patterns, including deceleration, bradycardia, tachycardia, and minimal to absent variability may occur in up to 60% of preterm fetuses, and variable decelerations are more common among preterm than term births (ACOG, 2005). However, published data are limited to monitoring preterm twins during antepartum testing, so these conditions and FHR patterns may or may not be applicable to intrapartum monitoring (Simpson, 2004). A full discussion of fetal assessment during labor is presented in Chapter 8.

After birth of the first infant, ultrasound should be used to assess presentation of the second twin and to exclude a funic presentation (cord between the fetal vertex and the internal cervical os; Malone & D'Alton, 2004). Membrane rupture of the second twin should be delayed until contractions are reestablished and the presenting part is engaged in the pelvis to minimize the risk of cord prolapse (Rao, Sairam, & Shehata, 2004). Once the presenting part of the next fetus is accessible and membranes are ruptured, a scalp electrode should be applied. An intrauterine pressure catheter may be used for accurate monitoring of uterine contraction activity (Bowers & Gromada, 2006).

Labor Induction and Augmentation

There are limited data pertaining to the safety and efficacy of labor induction methods, including prostaglandins, mechanical dilators, and medications to stimulate uterine contractions in twin pregnancies (Healy & Gaddipati, 2005). However, standard protocols for cervical ripening and labor induction appear to be appropriate for twin pregnancies (Ramsey & Repke, 2003; Malone & D'Alton, 2004). Oxytocin is often used for uterine inertia following the birth of the first twin (Rao, Sairam, & Shehata, 2004).

Mode of Birth

There are three routes of birth of twins: vaginal delivery for both, cesarean delivery for both, or a combined vaginal/cesarean birth. The choice of birth mode varies with fetal presentations, estimated fetal weights, and maternal and fetal health, as well as clinician experience and preferences of mother and clinician. Perinatal outcomes for vaginal and cesarean births also vary depending on gestational age and birth weight, as well as fetal presentation. Some studies have shown higher rates of adverse perinatal outcome for the second twin in a vaginal birth, and for twins at or near term with vaginal birth, especially for those weighing >3,000 g, when compared with twins born via cesarean (Barrett, 2004). Twins born via cesarean between 36 and 38 weeks' gestation have a greater incidence of neonatal respiratory disease compared with twins born vaginally between 38 and 40 weeks' gestation, and have a greater risk of death due to respiratoy distress syndrome (RDS) following cesarean birth (Dodd & Crowther, 2005a).   An algorithm for birth management of twins is shown in Figure 6–19.

Twin A Vertex/Twin B Vertex

Approximately 43% to 45% of twins present vertex–vertex, and the general recommendation is for vaginal birth, including those with estimated fetal weights less than 1,500 g (Chitkara & Berkowitz, 2002; Dodd & Crowther, 2005; Robinson & Chauhan, 2004). In one large population-based study, the vaginal/vaginal route carried the lowest neonatal and postneonatal mortality rates for vertex–vertex twins ≥34 weeks (Kontopoulos, Ananth, Smulian, & Vintzileos, 2004). In this study, combined vaginal/cesarean birth for vertex–vertex twin pairs had the highest neonatal, postneonatal, and infant mortality rates. This is consistent with the potential for prolonged fetal heart rate deceleration, cord prolapse, vaginal bleeding, or placental abruption in the second twin that may require cesarean birth. These complications may also explain the increased infant mortality rates in this subset of twins (Kontopoulos, Ananth, Smulian, & Vintzileos, 2004). Fetal weight may influence outcomes for vertex–vertex presentations. A review of a US 1995 to 1997 matched twin registry found significantly higher risks of mortality and morbidity in vertex second twins with birth weights ≥2,500 g whose co-twins were born vaginally compared with

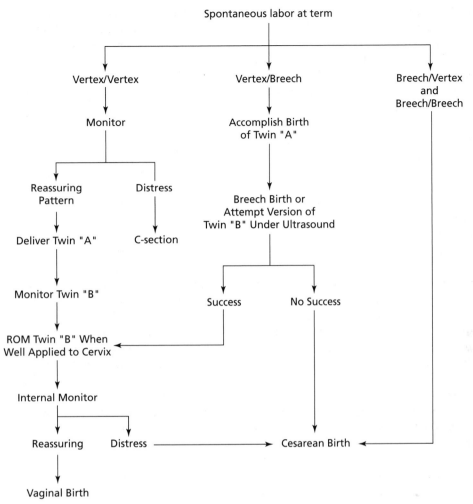

FIGURE 6–19. Management of the birth of twins.

risks for second twins after primary cesarean section of both twins (Yang et al., 2006). In a study of 41 vertex–vertex twin pairs weighing less than 1,500 g, cesarean birth was significantly associated with the incidence of RDS (Ziadeh, Sunna, & Badria, 2000).

A trend is emerging for elective/non-medically indicated cesarean birth of vertex–vertex presenting twins, despite the estimate that 70% to 86% of vertex–vertex twins may be safely born vaginally (ACOG, 2000; Healy & Gaddipati, 2005). Kontopoulos, Ananth, Smulian, and Vintzileos (2004) found that 87.4% of cesarean twin births had vertex–vertex presentations. Just as with the trend toward elective cesarean birth for singleton births (Meikle, Steiner, Zhang, & Lawrence, 2005), consumer choice may play a role in the increase in cesarean births of twins. Clinicians may be turning to non–medically indicated cesarean births of vertex–vertex twins due to concerns over possible intrapartum changes in fetal presentation and subsequent fetal compromise (ACOG, 2000; Barrett, 2004), as well as fears over potential malpractice litigation.

However, spontaneous version of the second twin has been reported to occur following birth of the first twin in only 2% of vertex–vertex twins (Robinson & Chauhan, 2004). It has been suggested that obstetric practitioners not comfortable with vaginal birth of the second twin should consider referral to, or co-management with an experienced obstetrician (ACOG, 2000).

Twin A Vertex/Twin B Nonvertex

Approximately 34% to 38% of twins present vertex–nonvertex (Chitkara & Berkowitz, 2002; Robinson & Chauhan, 2004). There is no consensus for the mode of birth for vertex–nonvertex (breech or transverse) twins (ACOG, 2000; Dodd & Crowther, 2005). Options for delivery include cesarean for both, vaginal birth of Twin A and external cephalic version of Twin B, vaginal birth of Twin A and breech extraction of Twin B, or vaginal birth of Twin A with emergent cesarean birth of Twin B. Numerous retrospective studies have examined outcomes for management of vertex–nonvertex twins. In the population-based report by Kontopoulos,

Ananth, Smulian, and Vintzileos (2004), the cesarean/cesarean route carried the lowest neonatal and post-neonatal mortality rates for vertex–breech pairs. External cephalic version (ECV) of Twin B was associated with increased incidence of cord prolapse, fetal distress, and cesarean birth when compared with breech extraction (Healy & Gaddipati, 2005; Rao, Sairam, & Shehata, 2004). A review of 15,185 vertex–nonvertex twin births found the combined vaginal/cesarean birth rate was 24.8%, much higher than the 9.5% rate when vertex second twins were included in the analysis (Yang et al., 2005).

Twin A Nonvertex

The first twin presents as nonvertex in approximately 19% to 21% of cases (Chitkara & Berkowitz, 2002; Robinson & Chauhan, 2004). Although rare, the primary risk is interlocking of the heads of breech–vertex twins during a vaginal birth. Cesarean birth is generally recommended for this presentation (ACOG, 2000; Healy & Gaddipati, 2005). Planned cesarean section may decrease the risk of a low 5-minute Apgar score when Twin A is breech (Hogle, Hutton, McBrien, Barrett, & Hannah, 2003).

Triplet Birth

A review of US triplet births for 1995 to 1998 found that 95% of triplets were born by cesarean section (Vintzileos, Ananth, Kontopoulos, & Smulian, 2005). In the report, vaginal birth was associated with the highest gestational age-adjusted relative risks for stillbirth (6.04), neonatal death (2.92), and infant death (2.38), compared with cesarean birth of all three triplets (1.0). There was no association between birth order and mortality rates, except that the stillbirth rate was increased for the third fetus, regardless of the mode of birth. However, vaginal birth may be an option for select triplet pregnancies. Recent prospective studies using a standardized protocol have reported improved or similar Apgar scores, cord pH, and length of maternal and neonatal stays compared with cesarean births (Ramsey & Repke, 2003). In addition to standard considerations for a safe birth of multiple gestations, criteria for vaginal birth of triplets include gestational age ≥28 weeks, presenting triplet is vertex, fetal monitoring for all three fetuses, no obstetric contraindications, and informed consent (Ramsey & Repke).

Interdelivery Interval

No clear guidelines are established for the interdelivery interval between births of twins. However, with increasing time, risks increase in the second twin for complications such as umbilical cord prolapse, abruption, and malpresentation (Healy & Gaddipati, 2005). The risk for asphyxia-related mortality increases if the birth interval between twins is greater than 30 minutes (Dodd & Crowther, 2005a). Umbilical cord arterial and venous pH of the second twin has been found to decline in a continuous linear fashion with increasing intertwin birth interval time (McGrail & Bryant, 2005). Lengthy interdelivery intervals also increase the chances of a fully dilated cervix to contract down, limiting birth options for the second fetus (Malone & D'Alton, 2004). It has been suggested that with reassuring fetal status, progressive descent, and stable maternal condition, an interval beyond 30 minutes may be reasonable with judicious oxytocin use (Healy & Gaddipati). Continuous fetal monitoring of the remaining fetus(es) is essential in the interdelivery interval.

Delayed-Interval Birth

Delayed-interval birth, or asynchronous birth, occurs when one or more very preterm multiples are vaginally born, and births of the remaining fetus(es) are delayed in hopes of improving neonatal survival and decreasing neonatal morbidity. Lengthy interdelivery time intervals (up to 153 days) have been reported in the literature, with a median ranging from 6 to 31 days (Cristinelli, Fresson, André, & Monnier-Barbarino, 2005; Zhang, Hamilton, Martin, & Trumble, 2004). Population-based reviews of multiple births from 1995 to 1998 found 56% had delays from 2 to 7 days (Zhang, Hamilton, Martin, & Trumble, 2004), whereas 6.0% of twins had delayed birth ≥1 week (Oyelese, Ananth, Smulian, & Vintzileos, 2005). Decreases in perinatal and infant mortality were seen only when the first twin was born at 22 to 23 weeks and when the birth interval was ≤3 weeks. However, there was no benefit in perinatal or infant mortality for intervals ≥4 weeks or when the first twin was born at 24 to 28 weeks (regardless of birth interval). Further, delayed birth of ≥4 weeks was associated with increased risk of SGA in the second twin, regardless of gestational age at birth of the first (Oyelese, Ananth, Smulian, & Vintzileos, 2005).

The optimal clinical management of delayed-interval births is unknown. Fetal pathology, monochorionicity, placenta previa, placental abruption, and preeclampsia have been cited as contraindications (Cristinelli, Fresson, André, & Monnier-Barbarino, 2005). Clinical reports include use of aggressive tocolysis, cervical cerclage, corticosteroids, and prophylactic and therapeutic antibiotics (Oyelese, Ananth, Smulian, & Vintzileos, 2005; Zhang, Hamilton, Martin, & Trumble, 2004). Although there appear to be benefits for delaying birth of the remaining fetuses after a very preterm birth, this practice bears significant risk. Delayed-interval birth is associated with a high risk of intrauterine infection (approximately 36%) and maternal sepsis (about 5%), and data on long-term outcomes of surviving infants are lacking (Zhang, Hamilton, Martin, & Trumble).

Vaginal Birth After Cesarean

A multicenter retrospective review of 535 twin pregnancies with a prior cesarean birth found that women with twin pregnancies were just as likely to be successful in a vaginal birth after cesarean (VBAC) attempt as women with singleton pregnancies (Cahill et al., 2005). However, women with twins were less likely to undergo a VBAC trial, and those who did had slightly increased maternal morbidity compared with twin gestations that deliver by repeat cesarean. Major maternal morbidities were no more likely than in women with singletons; uterine rupture occurred in 1.1% of twin pregnancies versus 0.9% in singletons. Women desiring VBAC should be evaluated with criteria and counseling similar to that used for women with singleton gestations.

Anesthesia

The choice of anesthesia should be made with anticipation of the potential need for uterine manipulation, operative birth, version of the second twin, emergent cesarean birth, and the increased risks for uterine atony and postpartum hemorrhage (Dodd & Crowther, 2004; Ramsey & Repke, 2003). Epidural anesthesia is commonly used for vaginal and cesarean births of twins. Both epidural and spinal anesthesia are safely used for triplet cesarean births, but spinal anesthesia has been associated with a larger initial decrease in systolic blood pressure (Marino, Goudas, Steinbok, Craigo, & Yarnell, 2001). Sublingual or intravenous nitroglycerin may be used for acute uterine relaxation for situations such as head entrapment of the second breech twin or retained placenta (Ramsey & Repke, 2003).

Although nonmedicated vaginal births of twins are uncommon, the woman's preferences must be balanced with potential risks and need for interventions. For example, an option for a woman desiring a nonmedicated birth is to have an epidural catheter placed, but not have medication infused through the catheter (Bowers & Gromada, 2006).

Postpartum Management

Hemorrhage

Blood loss with twin vaginal births is approximately 1,000 mL, similar to that of singleton cesarean section; blood loss with triplet cesarean section is typically much more than 1,000 mL due to increased risk of uterine atony (Klein, 2002). The incidence of postpartum hemorrhage is 6% for twins, 12% for triplets, and 21% for quadruplets, compared with 1.2% for singletons (Newman & Luke, 2000). A Canadian population-based study of maternal complications reported mothers of multiples were 1.66 times more likely to need blood transfusion than mothers of singletons (1.0; Walker, Murphy, Pan, Yang, & Wen, 2004).

Uncontrollable hemorrhage may lead to hysterectomy. A historical review of 100 peripartum hysterectomies performed in one clinical center found a significant increase in risk for twins (0.44%) and HOM (3.48%) compared with singletons (0.15%; Francois, Ortiz, Harris, Foley, & Elliott, 2005). Others have found similar rates (Walker, Murphy, Pan, Yang, & Wen, 2004). In the review by Francois, Ortiz, Harris, Foley, and Elliott, all the hysterectomies in multiple gestations were performed emergently, and all but one were for uterine atony.

Hemorrhage prevention includes anticipation of risk, recognition of uterine atony, and use of uterotonic agents in the third stage of labor. Type and cross-matched blood and blood products should be on hand. Nurses should make careful postpartum assessments of bleeding, uterine tone, and vital signs to detect later hemorrhage. A comprehensive discussion of postpartum hemorrhage is presented in Chapter 10.

Maternal Recovery

Multiple pregnancy and birth increase stresses on a woman's body, and these are intensified by antepartum, intrapartum, and postpartum complications (Gromada & Bowers, 2005). Having an infant in the NICU or caretaking responsibilities for multiple infants at home can also increase physical and emotional stress. In particular, women who have had extended antepartum bed rest may have difficulty recuperating after birth. A study of 31 women with twins and triplets who had been hospitalized during pregnancy reported a higher mean number and longer duration of postpartum symptoms than women with singleton pregnancies (Maloni, Margevicius, & Damato, 2006). Although many symptoms decreased over the days and weeks after birth, a high percentage persisted at 6 weeks postpartum, including back muscle soreness, dry skin, fatigue, tenseness, mood changes, and difficulty concentrating. Muscle atrophy also occurs, particularly in the weight-bearing muscles of the legs and back (Maloni & Schneider, 2002). These continuing symptoms increase the difficulty for these mothers as they remobilize after birth to care for themselves and their infants. Women need anticipatory guidance that their recovery will be slower than expected. They may also benefit from a physical therapy assessment and rehabilitation plan for their physical limitations due to bed-rest-induced muscle atrophy and cardiovascular deconditioning.

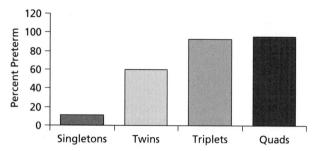

FIGURE 6–20. Percentage of preterm births by plurality: United States 2004.

Multiple Birth Infants

Infant Morbidity and Mortality

Preterm birth and LBW are the greatest predictors of infant morbidity and mortality in all infants including multiples (Mathews, Menacker, & MacDorman, 2004). In 2004, preterm birth occurred in 10.8% of singletons, 59.7% of twins, 93.0% of triplets, and 95.9% of quadruplets (Martin et al., 2006; see Fig. 6–20). The gestational age distribution by plurality is shown in Figure 6–21. Compared with 6.3% of singletons, 56.6% of twins, 94.1% of triplets, and 98.4% of quadruplets were born LBW in 2004 (Martin et al., 2006). In 2002, 24% of all LBW infants in the United States were born in a twin, triplet, or other higher order birth (Martin et al., 2003). Twins are 9 times, and triplets 30 times more likely than singletons to be born to VLBW (less than 1,500 g; see Fig. 6–22).

Increased use of labor induction and/or cesarean birth in recent years has increased the rate of preterm birth among twins, especially at 34 to 36 weeks of gestation (Ananth, Joseph, & Kinzler, 2004). In one study, investigators found a 235% increase in the rate of preterm labor induction (from 1.7% to 5.7%) and a 40% increase in the rate of preterm cesarean birth of twins (from 23.5% to 33.0%; Ananth, Joseph, & Kinzler, 2004).

Multiples appear to have higher overall risks for neonatal complications when compared with singletons. A review of numerous studies found odds ratios for selected complications in multiples were 2 to nearly 80 times higher than those in singletons (Newman & Luke, 2000). See Figure 6–23. However, several studies have found no differences in neonatal outcomes among singletons, twins, and triplets. Ballabh and colleagues (2003) analyzed outcomes of 116 sets of triplets matched with the same number of twins and singletons over 7 years in a tertiary center. Of 9 respiratory and 22 nonrespiratory outcome variables, there were no statistically significant differences among triplets, twins, and singletons. This study had several limitations, including use of a single tertiary center, and inclusion of only those infants admitted to the NICU. Infants were matched only for gestational age, and not for race, use of ART, or mode of birth. Another analysis of 36,931 singletons, 12,302 twins, and 2,155 triplets in a prospectively recorded database from 24 NICUs from 1997 to 2002 also found no significant differences in neonatal outcomes (Garite, Clark, Elliott, & Thorp, 2004). Although this study drew from a large and diverse database, the infants studied were all in NICUs and did not include multiple birth infants who died, were stillborn, or were not admitted to the NICU because of stable health.

According to national data for 2002, the infant mortality rate (IMR) for all multiple births was 32.3/1,000, more than five times the rate for singleton births (6.1/1,000; Mathews, Menacker, & MacDorman, 2004). The rate increased with plurality; the IMR for quadruplets was 160.4/1,000 and 60.1/1,000 for triplets, more than five times and about twice, respectively, the rate for twin births (30.2/1,000). Compared with singletons, IMRs for triplets and quadruplets were nearly 10 times and more than 26 times higher, respectively. Infant mortality rates also differ by race. Black infants have the highest IMR for all pluralities compared with whites and Hispanics (Salihu et al., 2005b). Interestingly, Hispanic singletons and twins have

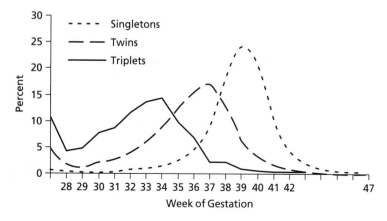

FIGURE 6–21. Gestational age distribution by plurality: United States 2002. (Based on data from Martin, J. A., Hamilton, B. E., Sutton, P. D., Ventura, S. J., Menacker, F., & Munson, M. L. [2003]. Births: final data for 2002. *National Vital Statistics Reports, 55*[1], 1–102.)

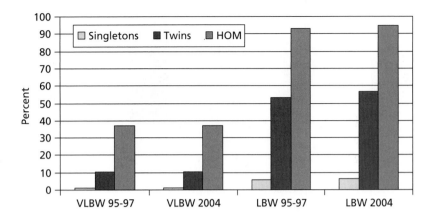

FIGURE 6–22. Low birth weight and very low birth weight by plurality: United States 1995 to 1997 and 2004. (Based on data from Martin, J. A., Hamilton, B. E., Sutton, P. D., Ventura, S. J., Menacker, F., Kirmeyer, S. [2006]. Births: final data for 2004. *National Vital Statistics Reports, 55*[1], 1–102.)

slightly improved survival over whites, but infant mortality for Hispanic triplets is 20% higher (see Fig. 6–24). The association of maternal age with infant mortality in multiple births is a paradox. In singletons, infant mortality is higher at the extremes of maternal age, producing a U-shaped curve, but in multiples, IMRs are highest at young maternal ages, but continue to decrease with rising maternal age (Misra & Ananth, 2002). See Figure 6–25.

Long-Term Morbidities

Multiple birth infants are more likely than singletons to suffer long-term serious morbidities, including cerebral palsy (CP), severe learning disabilities (LD), behavioral difficulties, and chronic respiratory disease (Pharoah, 2002; Rand, Eddleman, & Stone, 2005). Overall, twins have a five times higher prevalence of CP than singletons (Pharoah). In the United States, it is estimated that 8% of the increase in the prevalence of CP is due solely to the rise in multiple births, with rates for CP in singletons, twins, and triplets of 1.6 to 2.3, 7.3 to 12.6, and 28 to 44.8 per 1,000, respectively (Blickstein, 2001).

The increased prevalence of CP is due in part to a combination of a higher proportion of LBW infants among twins and the significantly higher prevalence of CP in normal birth weight twins (Pharoah, 2002). However, multiple birth appears to be an independent risk factor for CP, as the excess risk for death, and severe morbidity in twins cannot be explained by their greater rates of prematurity and LBW alone (Rand, Eddleman, & Stone, 2005). It has been suggested that cerebral impairment occurring during intrauterine development and attributable to the twinning process may lead to preterm birth. Or, preterm birth of a vulnerable infant might lead to an impairment that occurred in the perinatal period (Pharoah, 2002). The fetal death of one multiple increases the risk for CP in the survivor(s), especially in MC gestations. Long-term serious neurologic impairment or cerebral palsy has also been observed when both MC twins are born alive, but one dies in infancy (Rand, Eddleman, & Stone). Assisted reproductive technology also poses a risk for CP. The estimated incidence of CP is significantly higher after the transfer of three embryos than after the transfer of two, or after multifetal reduction from three to two embryos (Blickstein, 2005).

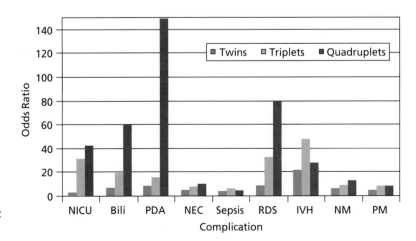

FIGURE 6–23. Risk of neonatal complications by plurality as odds ratio compared to singletons. (Based on data from Newman, R. B., & Luke, B. [2000]. *Multifetal pregnancy.* Philadelphia: Lippincott Williams & Wilkins.)

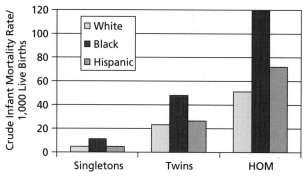

FIGURE 6–24. Race-specific infant mortality by plurality: United States 1995 to 1999. (Based on data from Salihu, H. M., Garces, I. C., Sharma, P. P., Kristensen, S., Ananth, C. V., & Kirby, R. S. [2005b]. Stillbirth and infant mortality among Hispanic singletons, twins, and triplets in the United States. *Obstetrics and Gynecology, 106*[4], 789–796.)

Multiple birth infants appear to have higher risks for chronic lung disease. A study of VLBW infants including 4,754 singletons, 2,460 twins, and 906 triplets examined the incidence of RDS and the use of antenatal corticosteroid treatment (Blickstein, Shinwell, Lusky, & Reichman, 2005). After adjustment for confounders, the investigators found that the risk for RDS increased with plurality whether corticosteroid therapy was complete, partial, or not given at all. The authors suggested that standard antenatal corticosteroid treatment in multiples might be inadequate to prevent RDS to the same degree as in singleton infants.

Others have examined morbidities associated with poor long-term outcomes in premature infants, including necrotizing enterocolitis (NEC), severe retinopathy of prematurity (ROP), severe intraventricular hemorrhage (IVH); and the need for ventilator use and respiratory support at 28 days of age, but found no differ-

ences in these morbidities at any gestational age among singletons, twins, and triplets (Blickstein, Shinwell, Lusky, & Reichman; Israel Neonatal Network, 2005).

Deformational plagiocephaly (asymmetrically shaped head) has been found to occur more frequently in newborn twins than in singletons (56% versus 13%; Peitsch, Keefer, LaBrie, & Mulliken, 2002). It has been suggested that positioning in utero may be the initial cause of plagiocephaly, with sleep positions worsening the condition (positional plagiocephaly) (Langkamp & Girardet, 2006). Vertex-presenting first twins, identical twins, and the smaller of a twin pair appear to have more severe involvement.

Studies conflict on the risk of SIDS in twins. Analysis of linked birth and infant death files for 1995 to 1998 found twins are at higher risk for SIDS than are singletons, and that the epidemiology of SIDS in twins was similar to that seen in singletons (Getahun, Demissie, Lu, & Rhoads, 2004). A similar analysis of an earlier data set (1987–1991) found that although the incidence of SIDS in twins is higher than in singletons, independent of birth weight, twins do not appear to be at greater risk for SIDS compared with singletons (Malloy & Freeman, 1999). The authors concluded that the increased risk is a function of the higher prevalence of LBW infants among twins. A review of 2,349 British SIDS cases observed that heavier twins (birth weight >3,000 g) were at significantly greater risk of SIDS than singletons of the same weight group (Platt & Pharoah, 2003).

Newborn Hospital Care

Newborn in-hospital care of healthy full-term multiples is similar to the care of singletons. However, meticulous care should be taken to maintain the exact identities of each baby, especially when the babies are MZ, such as double-checking of identification bracelets and crib cards (Gromada & Bowers, 2005).

A sizable proportion of multiple birth infants can be classified as late preterm infants with 36.3% of twins and 29.9% of HOM born between 34 and 37 weeks' gestation according to national data from 2000 to 2002 (NCHS, personal communication, February 10, 2006). See Table 6–34. Such infants are at increased risk for neonatal mortality and morbidity in the newborn period, and nurses should be alert to the subtle signs of difficulty, including temperature instability, hypoglycemia, need for intravenous infusions, respiratory distress, apnea and bradycardia, symptoms prompting a sepsis evaluation, and clinical jaundice (Medoff-Cooper, Bakewell-Sachs, Buus-Frank, & Santa-Donato, 2005). Additional nursing time, attention, and special skills may be needed to help mothers with breastfeeding, as late preterm infants may have a weak and ineffective suck, resulting in delays in latching on at the breast, establishing successful nutritive breastfeeding, or achieving adequate oral intake from either the bottle or the

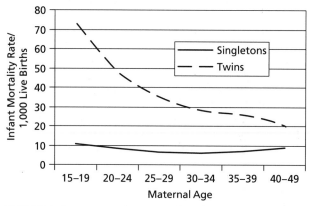

FIGURE 6–25. Maternal age-specific infant mortality by plurality, United States 1985 to 1986, 1990 to 1991, 1995 to 1996. (Based on data from Misra, D. P., & Ananth, C. V. [2002]. Infant mortality among singletons and twins in the United States during 2 decades: Effects of maternal age. *Pediatrics, 110*[6], 1163–1168.)

TABLE 6-34 ■ PERCENTAGE OF LATE-TERM TWINS AND TRIPLETS/+ BY GESTATIONAL AGE: UNITED STATES, COMBINED YEARS 2000–2002

	Twins	Triplets/+
Gestational Age		
34 weeks	8.48%	13.55%
35 weeks	12.12%	10.08%
36 weeks	15.67%	6.25%
Total percentage 34–36 weeks	36.27%	29.87%
Total twins or triplets w/stated GA	365,296	22,197

Personal communication; National Center for Health Statistics (February 10, 2006).

breast (Medoff-Cooper, Buus-Frank, & Santa-Donato; Near-Term Infant Advisory Panel, 2005).

Rooming-in with newborn multiples is optimal, as long as a support person is with the new mother in her hospital room. As some mothers may not be physically ready or will be overwhelmed with all the infants at once, having only one infant in the room at a time may be helpful at first. However, a mother should be encouraged to assume care for all healthy infants together as soon as she is able before discharge (Gromada & Bowers, 2005).

Cobedding Multiple Neonates

Cobedding is the practice of placing multiple birth infants together in the same bed, based on the concept of continuing the womb-sharing experience. Cobedding allows prenatal interaction to continue, thus providing comfort and decreasing stress to the co-multiples. It is a form of developmentally supportive care and one way to foster the continuity between the intrauterine and extrauterine life of multiple birth infants (Leonard, 2002). Cobedding literature and research are limited, and most studies are of preterm multiples. Generally, the in-hospital practice is safe, with no increases in infection or major complications (Gromada & Bowers, 2005). Tables 6–35 and 6–36 provide information on the advantages and disadvantages of cobedding and a list of interventions for providing cobedding in the NICU.

Limited data are available on home cobedding practices. A British study of 60 twin pairs found that the majority of infants were cobedded at one month of age, and 40% were still cobedding at 4 months (Ball, 2002). The study observed that in-hospital infant sleeping practices strongly influenced at-home practices; cobedded infants did not wake more frequently than separated infants; and closely cobedded infants did not have increased core body temperatures. The infants were also found to have more synchronous sleep patterns. The researcher concluded that parents should receive advice regarding use of coverings and blankets, as well as potentially dangerous practices such as separating barriers and swaddling.

Currently, there is no evidence to establish cobedding of multiples outside the NICU as a safe or unsafe sleep practice. The recommendations from the AAP Task Force on Sudden Infant Death Syndrome (2005) state that infants should not bed share with other children,

TABLE 6-35 ■ IN-HOSPITAL COBEDDING ADVANTAGES AND DISADVANTAGES

Advantages may include:	Disadvantages may include:
• Improved heart rate	• Potential for injury or dislodging of medical equipment
• Improved temperature control	• One or both infants may become physiologically unstable (heart rate, breathing, temperature control)
• Fewer apneic periods	• Infants may disturb one another, resulting in more crying, restlessness, less sleep, and added stress
• Lower oxygen requirements	• Nursing difficulty caring for multiple infants
• Greater weight gain	• Potential for medication/treatment errors
• Improved motor development	• No studies about cobedding healthy multiples
• Coregulation (balancing and supporting of one another)	• No studies about cobedding at home
• Facilitation of state control such as sleep and alertness	• May result in difficulty separating infants
• Improved infant growth and development	
• Faster movement from isolettes to open cribs	
• Shorter hospital stay	
• Decreased hospital costs	
• Improved parent-nurse communication	
• More consistent care	
• Decrease in the number of rehospitalizations	
• Enhanced parent-infant attachment	
• Easier transition to home	

Leonard, L. G. (2002). Prenatal behavior of multiples: implications for families and nurses. *Journal of Obstetric, Gynecologic and Neonatal Nursing, 31*(3), 248–255.

TABLE 6–36 ■ NEONATAL INTENSIVE CARE UNIT COBEDDING INTERVENTIONS

- Educate parents about benefits of cobedding preterm multiples in the NICU
- Initiate co-bedding immediately or when multiples are stable
- Allow IVs, gavage feeding, cardiopulmonary monitoring, oximetry, and phototherapy
- Color-code each infant, equipment, and charts. Infants should wear ID bands at all times.
- Simulate intrauterine positions when possible (data from prenatal ultrasound reports). Positions may include side by side; facing; tandem; head-to-toe in the same incubator, warmer, or crib
- Lightly swaddle one blanket around multiples, leaving their hands free; place boundaries around all infants
- Provide clustered/simultaneous care
- Allow babies to cobed until discharge
- Exclusion criteria may include:
  - Mechanical ventilation. However, oxygen via nasal cannula is permitted.
  - Umbilical catheter, arterial line, or pleural drainage
  - Risk of infection transmission between infants
  - Insufficient space for infants and equipment
  - Surgery in one infant that precludes contact with the other(s) for safe healing

Gromada, K. K., & Bowers, N. A. (2005). *Care of the multiple-birth family: Postpartum through infancy* (Nursing Module). New York: March of Dimes Birth Defects Foundation. With permission.

but do not specifically address multiples. Parents of multiples may desire cobedding at home for various reasons, including convenience, cost savings, or because the infants were cobedded in the NICU. When discussing at-home sleeping arrangements, the high incidence of prematurity and LBW in multiple birth infants and the corresponding risks for SIDS should be considered. As with all families, parents of multiples should be taught SIDS risk-reduction practices including supine positioning, babies sleeping in parents' room, firm bedding surface, no loose coverings/items in bed, and no smoke exposure (AAP, 2005). Use of barriers between infants in the same bed is an unsafe practice due to the potential for entrapment or entanglement. More research is needed to define safe at-home sleeping practices for both preterm and term multiples.

Discharge Planning

Frequently, multiple babies cannot be discharged at the same time due to illness or differences in growth and feeding abilities. This can place a physical and emotional burden on parents, especially on postpartum mothers recuperating from multiple pregnancy and birth who must travel back and forth to the hospital (Gromada & Bowers, 2005). Parents will need a place for daytime visits and privacy for breastfeeding, and ideally, rooms are available for overnight stays. Policies should be in place to clarify issues such as bringing the well multiple(s) back to the hospital. Discharging infants separately may be easier for families with HOM. When infants go home one or two at a time, the parents can become acquainted with each infant individually before facing the overwhelming tasks of caring for all of the infants together (Gromada & Bowers, 2005).

Feeding Multiples

Just as for singleton infants, breast milk is the ideal food for multiple birth infants, especially those who are born preterm. However, it is common for mothers of multiples to be unaware that breastfeeding is an option, and many question whether they can produce enough milk to meet the needs of two or more infants. Mothers also report that care providers are unaware or are discouraging of breastfeeding multiples. Fortunately, the challenges of managing multiple newborns do not dissuade most mothers of multiples from breastfeeding. Results from a convenience sample of mothers in a twin support group showed 89.4% initiated breastfeeding or initiated a milk supply by pumping (Damato, Dowling, Madigan, & Thanattherakul, 2005). The investigators reported that mothers who were breastfeeding exclusively or almost exclusively at an average of age of about 9 weeks were significantly more likely to still be breastfeeding at about 28 weeks. The same sample also provided information about cessation of breastfeeding in mothers of twins (Damato, Dowling, Standing, & Schuster, 2005). Reasons cited included unique issues related to infants' behaviors, challenges presented by growth and development, and time commitments that interfered with breastfeeding continuation. In particular, inadequate milk supply was reported as a leading reason for breastfeeding cessation; however, the survey responses did not clarify whether concerns about milk production were real or perceived. The study authors noted that long-term use of a breast pump, whether to initiate a milk supply or to obtain milk to store for future use was beneficial in prolonging the provision of breast milk. However, this practice had the potential to become an extreme burden for a mother who was also breastfeeding or bottle-feeding two infants. These reports emphasize the need for ongoing lactation support after birth to manage challenges of new breastfeeding issues with twin growth and development.

Several breastfeeding principles must be recognized and communicated to mothers of multiples. First, mothers need to be informed early in pregnancy that breastfeeding is not only an option for feeding multiple infants but also the recommended feeding method. Second, establishing an adequate milk supply for multiple babies begins with babies at the breast as soon as possible after birth. Third, a continuing and adequate milk supply is dependent on frequent feedings or pumpings that effectively remove milk from the breasts; ineffective milk removal is associated with inadequate milk production. Fourth, meeting a mother's goal of successful breastfeeding requires support from everyone around her, including her care providers. The British Columbia Reproductive Care Program (2006) has developed guidelines for breastfeeding multiples for use by health care providers. The guidelines describe best practices based on current research as well as empirical and anecdotal evidence from professionals and multiple birth families and are listed in Display 6–46.

Breastfeeding management of healthy newborn multiples born at term is similar to singleton care. Usually, mothers begin with one infant at a time in order to monitor each infant as both learn to breastfeed. Breasts can be alternated on a per-feeding or daily basis. Once one infant is able to achieve a deep, comfortable latch and is feeding effectively, the second infant can be positioned for simultaneous feedings. Mothers and/or infants may not be ready for simultaneous feedings in the first few days, or even weeks. However, nurses or lactation consultants should help mothers with positioning options before they leave the hospital. These positions include the double football, parallel/cradle-clutch combo, and double cradle/criss-cross holds (see Fig. 6–26). At home, infants can be fed on cue, feeding each when he or she demonstrates feeding cues, or feeding together, with the mother actively waking the second twin

DISPLAY 6-46

Guidelines for Breastfeeding Multiples

1. Families need opportunities to become informed about and prepared for breastfeeding term and preterm multiple birth infants.
2. Families require access to multiple-specific and general breastfeeding resources.
3. Families should be supported to initiate lactation and provide breast milk to their infants and the earliest opportunity.
4. Families should be assisted in the ongoing development of a breastfeeding plan that considers the needs of the mother, each infant, and the family as a whole.
5. Families should receive evidence-based and skilled breastfeeding assistance throughout the postpartum and early childhood periods.
6. Families should receive coordinated, comprehensive, consistent, and seamless breastfeeding care throughout pregnancy and early childhood.

British Columbia Reproductive Care Program. (2006). *Breastfeeding multiples, nutrition, Part III.* Retrieved December 11, 2006, from http://www.rcp.gov.bc.ca/guidelines/General/Gen3CBreastfeedingMultiplesNovember2006.pdf

when the first one shows feeding cues. This method of feeding takes less time than feeding the infants separately or based solely on individual infant feeding cues. Many mothers use a combination of individual and simultaneous feedings. For HOM, a mother may rotate infants and breasts so that each has the optimal time at the breast, or she may have a helper bottle-feed one or two infants while she breastfeeds the other two (Gromada & Bowers, 2005).

Breastfeeding premature or sick multiples is more complex, yet there are clear benefits of providing breast milk for these infants. Mothers whose infants are

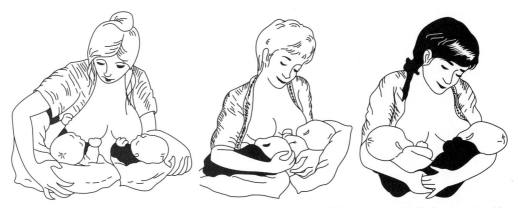

FIGURE 6–26. Breast-feeding positions for mothers of multiples. (Copyright 2006 Marvelous Multiples, Inc. Used by permission.)

unable to breastfeed should begin pumping as soon as possible, within hours after birth (Biancuzzo, 2003). This provides sick infants with antibody-rich colostrum, may have a long-term impact on milk production and volumes obtained, and facilitates the establishment of a pumping routine. Pumped colostrum or milk should be distributed among the infants; however, priority is often given to the sickest of the infants (Gromada & Bowers, 2005). Mothers will need instructions about pumping and storage of breast milk, as well as resources for obtaining a hospital-grade breast pump after discharge. A plan for breastfeeding well and sick or premature multiples is provided in Table 6–37.

Parenting Newborn Multiples

In addition to the physical demands of their own recovery, mothers of multiple newborns face challenges in parenting several babies at once. In the first weeks at home, it is essential that tasks of housekeeping, laundry, cooking, grocery shopping, and sibling care are delegated to friends and family, so that the mother is permitted time for recovery and interaction with her infants. The first month is hardest, as parents learn skills and routines for infant care, feedings, and sleep. Usually, parents of healthy twins can successfully care for their infants along with occasional help from family and friends. Parents with HOM, or infants with a health problem will need formal help for a much longer time. In simplest terms, one person cannot hold three infants at once. Helpers should assume non–baby care responsibilities, such as household chores and assisting the mother with feedings or diaper changes. Whether helpers are friends, family, or employed, their roles and responsibilities should be clearly outlined.

With the help of their pediatrician, parents can establish routines for feeding, sleep, and activities. This is particularly important for preterm infants who may need frequent feedings. Simultaneous feeding can be helpful, but requires waking a sleeping infant when another is ready to eat. Feeding routines also help develop similar sleep/waking patterns. Nurses should stress flexible routines, allowing for differences in each baby's temperament and needs. Some infants are high-need, requiring constant cuddling or touch, whereas others are content with a feeding and a few visual toys. A daily log of

TABLE 6–37 ■ PLAN FOR BREASTFEEDING MULTIPLES (INFORMATION FOR MOTHERS)

For Well Newborns	For Preterm or Sick Newborns
• After birth (vaginal or cesarean), put each baby to breast within the first 30–90 min or as soon as any baby cues to feed.	• Begin breast pumping using an electric breast pump with double-collection kit setup as soon as possible after delivery (vaginal or cesarean). Ideally, begin within 6 hr.
• Avoid using bottles, pacifiers, and other intraoral objects if possible.	• Apply the pump to both breasts at least 8 times each 24 hr. Night-time pumping can be limited if babies' discharge is unlikely, but do not allow more than 5–6 hr between pumpings. Pump more often during the day to achieve at least 8 pumping sessions per 24 hr.
• Room-in with your babies at least 8 hr each day. (You may need a support person to stay with you).	
• Ask your nurse or lactation consultant to help you the first few times you breastfeed.	• Pump on a regular schedule. As your babies' discharge nears, pump more often and add night pumping, to achieve up to 10–12 times in 24 hr.
• Initially feed each baby separately. Make sure each baby can latch-on to the breast and has correct tongue placement and suck.	• Learn how to safely collect, store, and transport your beast milk.
• Nurse each baby when any demonstrates feeding cues, which should be 8–12 times over 24 hr by their second 24 hr after birth.	• Let your babies' nurses and doctors know that you want to start Kangaroo Care (KC) skin-to-skin as soon as possible. Let each baby have mouth/nose to nipple contact as soon as possible. Allow the babies to progress to breastfeeding as soon as medically possible.
• Alternate breasts at each feeding or daily for each baby or offer your fullest breast to the hungriest baby.	
• If babies are nursing well, you can feed them together. Your nurse or lactation consultant can show you different positions. Practice with all babies before discharge.	• Preterm babies must physically mature before they can sustain effective breastfeeding. Gradually, they will improve so you can nurse your babies as with well babies.
• If you are concerned about your milk supply, call a lactation consultant or breastfeeding support leader, feed your babies more frequently, and use an electric breast pump after feedings, between feedings or as needed to help increase milk supply.	• Use your breast pump at home after feedings if needed to help with milk supply.
• Know the number of your lactation consultant breast-feeding support leader if you need help at home.	• Know the number of your lactation consultant or breastfeeding support leader if you need help at home.

Marvelous Multiples, Inc., used by permission.

feedings and diaper counts for each infant is important until growth and weight gain are well established (Gromada & Bowers, 2005).

Referral of expectant families to both local and national multiple birth support groups provides an instant network among other expectant parents of multiples, as well support from experienced parents who have "been there." A list of support groups is provided at the end of this chapter.

Psychologic Issues with Multiple Gestations

During pregnancy, birth, and the months following the birth of multiples, each family experiences "a constellation of stresses which jeopardize physical and mental health and family functioning" (Malmstrom & Biale, 1990). These stresses cut across all socioeconomic and educational levels and include increases in child abuse, marital troubles, and family dysfunction.

Prenatal Attachment

The prenatal attachment process for multiples is complex, with maternal/fetal interactions woven together with interfetal interactions. Just as an expectant mother relates to her fetuses through fetal movement, intrauterine tactile stimulation between multiples plays a role in attachment among infants. Each multiple develops an individual temperament and each set of multiples establishes their own patterns of tactile communication. The same behaviors, traits, and intermultiple interactions seen in pregnancy also have been observed in infancy and beyond (Leonard, 2002).

Maternal attachment with multiples is similar to attachment processes in singleton pregnancies. Interestingly, women who were younger, with lower income, a history of infertility, greater self-esteem, who had experienced quickening, and were further along in their pregnancy reported greater prenatal attachment to their twins (Damato, 2004a). Postpartum depression, cesarean birth, and the experience of a NICU admission for one or both twins negatively influenced mothers' postnatal attachment compared with their prenatal attachment (Damato, 2004b).

Fetal movements enable a woman expecting multiples to relate to her unborn children, affirm that each one is alive and healthy, and attach to them individually and as a unit (Leonard, 2002). Nurses can promote prenatal attachment by encouraging expectant mothers to observe fetal movements and patterns, to differentiate between individual multiples, identify behavioral similarities and differences, recognize intermultiple contacts (during ultrasound examinations and fetal monitoring), and ask questions during fetal testing (Leonard). Nurses should provide support and follow-up, especially for older, higher-income women with low self-esteem and provide prenatal education and counseling to help build confidence and develop effective parenting strategies (Damato, 2004a). Postnatal attachment can be supported by implementing measures to increase a mother's opportunities for proximity with her twins such as promotion of breastfeeding, skin-to-skin contact, and encouraging complete access to and participation in her infants' NICU care (Damato, 2004b).

Prenatal Family Adjustments

Preparation for multiple infants requires significant adjustments for families even before the babies are born. Depending on the pregnancy, women may need to reduce or stop working, be limited in activities, or be placed on bed rest at home or in the hospital. There is evidence that women on bed rest with multiples may have even greater emotional and physical needs than those with singletons. A recent study revealed that women with multiple gestations had many more antepartum symptoms during hospitalization and treatment with bed rest than women with singleton gestations (Maloni, Margevicius, & Damato, 2006). The number of symptoms reported by women with multiples appears to be higher than those reported by women with singleton gestations. Over half of the women in the study had very high depressive symptom scores on admission, and they identified concerns for their family and being separated as major stressors. The average number and persistence of postpartum symptoms reported during the first weeks also appear to be higher than those for women with singleton pregnancies. The authors concluded that women have many physical and psychological discomforts during a multiple gestation, and experience continuing symptoms indicative of underlying postpartum morbidity that are not completely recovered by 6 weeks.

Families with a mother on bed rest often experience difficulty assuming maternal responsibilities, anxiety about outcomes for mother and infants, and adverse emotional effects on the children (Maloni, Brezinski-Tomasi, & Johnson, 2001). Expectant fathers often receive the brunt of family and household responsibilities during a multiple pregnancy and are often required to "be all things to all family members, including father and mother, financial provider, cook, maid and the emotional support system" (Bowers & Gromada, 2006 p. 36). In addition to their concerns about the health of the mother and fetuses, fathers must cope with the effects of increased family responsibilities and emotional pressures in their own lives. If a mother's income is eliminated due to pregnancy complications, finances may become a concern, even in economically advantaged families. Fathers may be at increased risk for depression, especially those who have a history of depression, are unemployed, and have an unsupportive partner or one with perinatal depression (Leonard, 1998).

Children may be affected by the strains of a high-risk pregnancy as well. Young children whose mothers are on bed rest may be unable to fully comprehend maternal restrictions, the need to reallocate childcare, or maternal absence during hospitalization (Maloni, Brezinski-Tomasi, & Johnson, 2001).

Nurses play an integral role in providing psychosocial support for families expecting multiples. Anticipatory guidance includes the expected physical and emotional changes of a multiple pregnancy; the need for contingency planning at home for children and household management; nutritional assessment and counseling; plans for testing, interventions, and treatment options; referrals to support organizations such as local parents of twins groups; and information about multiple birth prenatal education classes. It is also important to ensure that hospitalized women and those on bed rest at home have access to education; this may include provision of in-home classes, videos, reading materials, and resources. Measures to decrease the stressors of hospitalization may include liberal visitation with husband and other children; home-cooked food from family and friends; provision of technology for in-room videos, music, and Internet access; and opportunities for networking with other expectant mothers of multiples (Bleyl, 2002).

Postnatal Attachment

Parent–infant attachment with multiple infants is complex and evolves through various processes. Ultimately, parents need to view each infant as an individual with a unique personality and characteristics. Initially, a unit-attachment is formed, with parents focusing on the concept of the set of twins or triplets prenatally and after birth. Individual attachments follow, often with brief periods of attachment to one infant before shifting to another (Gromada & Bowers, 2005). Some parents develop preferential feelings for a particular infant. If this is consistently demonstrated, there can be long-term cognitive and behavioral effects for all the infants. Unequal attachments are more likely when one infant is healthier than the other, or one is more responsive (Gromada & Bowers, 2005). Nurses should observe parent–infant interactions noting behaviors indicative of progression toward individualization. Signs of positive attachment/individualization behaviors include acknowledgment and response to each infant's cues; initiating verbalization, touching, soothing, cuddling, and so forth, with each infant; alternating eye contact among infants; and referring to each infant by name (Gromada & Bowers, 2005).

The demands of multiple infants can limit parent–infant interactions. Frequent, slow feedings, repeated diaper changes, and constant cries of multiple infants are exhausting. To compensate, parents may focus more on physical care than on their infants' emotional needs. This exposes multiple birth infants to a unique risk—the deprivation of the parents' exclusive focus and involvement (Feldman & Eidelman, 2004). A study of preterm twins and singletons found that mothers of twins exhibited fewer initiatives toward their infants and were less responsive to both positive signals and to crying (Ostfeld, Smith, Hiatt, & Hegyi, 2000). The twin mothers lifted or held, touched, patted, and talked to their infants less, and their infants had lower cognitive scores at 18 months than singletons. The child who is less effective in eliciting parental care or who may be less rewarding during interactions appears to be at an especially high risk. A study of social–emotional development of triplets found the infant with birth weight discordance >15% received the lowest levels of parent response and displayed the poorest behavior outcomes among the set. Parenting difficulties appeared to be related to the lack of emotional resources for adapting to each infant's individual patterns (Feldman & Eidelman). Multiple birth children also appear to be at increased risk for child abuse. One long-standing study found a ninefold higher risk of reported abuse/neglect among twins compared with singletons (Groothuis et al., 1982).

Anxiety and Depression

The very nature of a high-risk pregnancy increases stress and anxiety for expectant mothers and may be intensified by the unknowns of a multiple pregnancy. Around-the-clock needs of multiple infants, sleep deprivation, inconsistent support, and a sense of isolation may contribute to maternal stress (Gromada & Bowers, 2005). It has been estimated that as many as 25% of multiple birth parents (including fathers) are affected by perinatal depression and anxiety disorders (Leonard, 1998). Evidence indicates that stress and depression in pregnant and postpartum women are of considerable concern due to the association with adverse obstetrical outcomes, postpartum depression, and emotional and behavioral problems in the children (Mian, 2005). The additive effects of infertility history, multiple birth, and first-time parenting may increase the risk for psychological resource depletion (Klock, 2004). Nurses have a key role in identifying parents at risk; early recognition and support of women and families affected by these disorders; and providing prevention-focused health, education, and social support programs at the family and community levels (Leonard).

Beck (2002) found that "life on hold" was the basic social psychological problem during the first year for mothers of twins in a multiple birth support group.

Mothers in the study experienced four phases: (1) draining power, a demanding, sleep-deprived period, when mothers had no time and were torn between infants' needs; (2) pausing own life, which involved a blurring of days and nights with confinement and self-surrender; (3) striving to reset, when mothers began to develop coping strategies such as routines, schedules, prioritizing tasks, recruiting family help, and problem solving; (4) resuming own life, which was achieved when mothers felt their lives were more manageable, and when milestones such as sleeping through the night or twins beginning to self-feed were reached. It was in this last phase that mothers were able to relate the blessings of having twins. Beck (2002) concluded that the most vulnerable period for these mothers was 3 months' postpartum.

A study of mothers of multiples who conceived with ART identified children's health, unmet family needs, maternal depression, and parental stress as key areas of concern (Ellison & Hall, 2003). The study revealed that the inordinate stresses of raising multiple birth infants strengthened some marriages when there was greater paternal participation in childcare and household tasks. Marriages weakened when couples were unable to equitably divide family and household labor, or were unable to work together as a team. The psychosocial risks associated with iatrogenic multiple births appear to increase with plurality. In another study, parents of ART multiples reported significant difficulty in providing basic material needs for their families, decreased quality of life, social stigma, and maternal depression (Ellison et al., 2005). Such distress may decrease their willingness to seek help or admit their distress to their care providers.

Grief and Loss

Parents who experience the death of a complete set of multiples have been found to grieve more intensely than parents who lose a singleton; they are at significant risk for depression, and may experience grief 6 months longer (Pector & Smith-Levitin, 2002). However, the grieving process becomes more complex with the death of a part of a set of multiples. These parents experience the difficult paradox of grieving for the infants that died while feeling joy for their living infants. Studies have shown that grief is often delayed for 1 to 3 years while parents focus on survivors, bonding is sometimes impaired, and some parents may even resent the survivors (Pector & Smith-Levitin). The intensity of grief after a multiple's death equals that with a singleton, yet parents rarely receive as much sympathy (Pector & Smith-Levitin). It is important to validate parents' loss with healing actions and responses. A fundamental concept with loss in multiple births is that no matter how many infants survive, the parents remain parents of multiples (Gromada & Bowers, 2005). Recommendations for clinicians to help

grieving parents of multiples are listed in Display 6–47. Peer support can be especially helpful at the time of the loss. Multiple birth organizations such as Center for Loss in Multiple Birth (CLIMB) and the Triplet Connection have information and support to help parents cope with the death of one or more multiples.

DISPLAY 6-47

Recommendations to Help Grieving Parents of Multiples

- Provide opportunities for parents to see and/or hold all babies of a set, together, and separately
- Mementos such as photographs, videos, monitor strips, locks of hair, and footprints should be collected for all babies.
- Do not place beds of surviving multiples beside intact sets in the nursery or NICU.
- After a prenatal loss or multifetal reduction, ask how parents want to refer to the pregnancy: by the number conceived or by the number remaining.
- After neonatal loss, most parents consider living children to be survivors and are comfortable with saying they had triplets or twins.
- Parents should have input into labeling for two or more remaining multiples; generally, triplets B and C should retain their designation of B & C after triplet A's death.
- Allow mothers to wear all their infants' bracelets throughout the hospital stay.

- **Suggested helpful and healing responses include:**
  - This must be very hard for you.
  - I'm so sorry your twins died.
  - I have no idea how you must feel.
  - How are you feeling? What would help your family through this?
  - How are you coping with everything?

- **Hurtful responses to be avoided include:**
  - You're young, you could have other multiples.
  - You couldn't handle them all.
  - At least it happened before you were too attached.
  - It's for the best. They would have been severely disabled.
  - Set your grief aside. You must be strong for your survivors.
  - At least you have two living babies. Some parents can't have any!
  - Multiples are so expensive. Think of the money you'll save.

Pector, E. A., & Smith-Levitin, M. (2002). Mourning and psychological issues in multiple birth loss. *Seminars in Neonatology, 7*(3), 247–256. Gromada & Bowers, 2005). Gromada, K. K., & Bowers, N. A. (2005). *Care of the multiple-birth family: Postpartum through infancy* (Nursing Module). New York: March of Dimes Birth Defects Foundation.

Multiple Birth Resources and Support Organizations

Organizations for multiple birth families provide a supportive environment for parents to network and learn from others (see Display 6–48). National organizations often offer free brochures and handouts that can be included in packets created especially for the expectant parents of multiples. See Figure 6–27 for pictures of twins in utero, at birth, and at 3 years old.

Multiples can truly be marvelous.

DISPLAY 6-48

Multiple Birth Resources and Support Organizations

Center for Loss in Multiple Birth, Inc. (CLIMB)
P.O. Box 91377
Anchorage, AK 99509
907-222-5321
E-mail climb@pobox.alaska.net
www.climb-support.org

The Center for Study of Multiple Birth
333 East Superior Street, Suite 464
Chicago, IL 60611
312-926-7498
Fax 312-926-7780
E-mail lgk@northwestern.edu
www.multiplebirth.com

International Society for Twin Studies (ISTS)
www.ists.qimr.edu.au

Marvelous Multiples, Inc.
P.O. Box 381164
Birmingham, AL 35238-1164
205-437-3575
Fax 205-437-3574
E-mail marvmult@aol.com
www.marvelousmultiples.com

Monoamniotic Monochorionic Support Site
www.monoamniotic.org

MOST (Mothers of Supertwins)
PO Box 306
East Islip, NY 11730
631-859-1110
E-mail info@MOSTonline.org
www.mostonline.org

**Multiple Births Canada (MBC)/
Naissances Multiples Canada**
(formerly Parents of Multiple Births Association
   [POMBA] Canada)
PO Box 432
Wasaga Beach, Ontario, Canada L9Z 1A4
705-429-0901, 866-228-8824 (toll-free in Canada)
Fax 705-429-9809
E-mail office@multiplebirthscanada.org
www.multiplebirthscanada.org

National Organization of Mothers of Twins Clubs, Inc. (NOMTC)
NOMOTC Executive Office
PO Box 700860
Plymouth, MI 48170-0955
248-231-4480
877-540-2200
E-mail info@nomotc.org
www.nomotc.org

The Triplet Connection
P.O. Box 429
Spring City, UT 84662
435-851-1105
Fax 435-462-7466
E-mail TC@tripletconnection.org
www.tripletconnection.org

***TWINS* Magazine**
11211 E. Arapahoe Road, Suite 101
Centennial, CO 80112-3851
303-290-8500
888-55-TWINS
www.twinsmagazine.com

The Twin to Twin Transfusion Syndrome (TTTS) Foundation, Inc.
411 Longbeach Parkway
Bay Village, OH 44140
440-899-TTTS (8887)
800-815-9211
Fax 440-899-1184
E-mail info@tttsfoundation.org
www.tttsfoundation.org

Twinless Twins Support Group
P.O. Box 980481
Ypsilanti, MI 48198
888-205-8962
E-mail contact@twinlesstwins.org
twinlesstwins.org

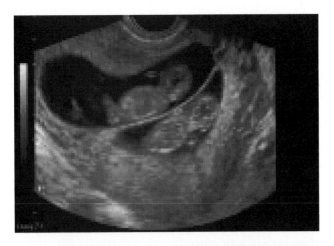

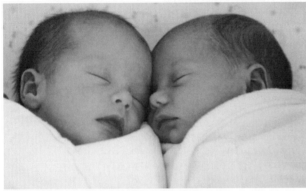

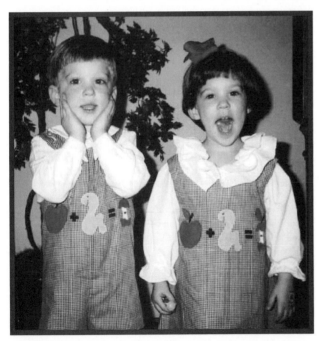

FIGURE 6–27. Twins from pregnancy, birth, and as toddlers. (Courtesy of photographer [and proud new father] Robert Hammer. Used with permission.)

MATERNAL TRANSFER

Maternal transfer from a level I or level II institution to a level III institution is an option in the care of pregnant women. Each case is considered individually. Suggested guidelines for transfer of care of the mother are provided in Display 6–49. Before transfer, the severity of the clinical situation and the time and distance to the receiving hospital are considered.

DISPLAY 6-49

Guidelines for Maternal Transfer

FROM A LEVEL I INSTITUTION*

- Labor with cervical change less than 34–36 weeks' gestation
- Preterm premature rupture of membranes (PPROM) less than 34–36 weeks' gestation
- Labor and/or PPROM when dating data are uncertain
- Preterm labor with maternal or fetal complications
- Bleeding less than 34–36 weeks' gestation
- Twin or triplet gestation with contractions or labor less than 34–36 weeks
- Severe preeclampsia
- Eclampsia if maternal condition stabilized
- Intrauterine growth restriction
- Oligohydramnios
- Polyhydramnios (severe or uncertain origin)
- Fetal hydrops
- Fetal anomalies, especially at gestational ages less than 34–36 weeks, that require specialized neonatal intervention (eg, diaphragmatic hernia, oomphalocele, severe neural tube defects)
- Fetal conditions requiring cordocentesis and/or transfusion
- Maternal medical conditions outside of the scope of medical and nursing care available (eg, liver transplant, renal dialysis, severe mitral stenosis, cancer, active lupus, pulmonary embolism)
- Maternal (and possibly fetal) trauma
- Unusual fetal heart dysrhythmia (eg, complete fetal heart block)

FROM A LEVEL II INSTITUTION

- Any fetus requiring long-term ventilatory support as a newborn
- Any fetus requiring neonatal care less than 30–34 weeks' gestation depending on the institution resources
- Maternal complications listed above

*All guidelines assume maternal and fetal stability.

Maternal transport can be accomplished by a one-way or two-way transfer of care. One-way transfer of care occurs when a referring hospital calls a receiving hospital to ask to transfer a pregnant patient. After the patient is accepted verbally and the initial physician report is given, the originating or referring hospital provides care throughout the transport process until the patient arrives at the receiving facility. Two-way transport occurs when the receiving facility accepts the patient verbally and then sends a team, including a registered nurse and possibly a physician, to transport the woman to the receiving facility. In this case, the transferring facility turns over the care and responsibility of the patient once the patient is under transport. Transport is accomplished by a variety of methods, including private ambulance, public rescue vehicles, helicopters, and airplanes.

An accurate, thorough nursing report is a critical element of transfer of care. A photocopy of the original record accompanies the patient. Any nursing or medical action performed en route (eg, vital signs, palpating for contractions) is documented, and a copy is left with the receiving hospital. Many institutions have specific forms for the transfer of obstetric patients. The decision about the necessity of a nurse, physician, or both accompanying the patient in transfer is made in each case. Transfers require a physician's order and a physician who is willing to accept care at the receiving hospital. Should the physician not agree to transport the patient or if the nurse feels it inappropriate to transfer a specific patient without a physician present and one has not been provided, the institutional chain of command can provide a method for conflict resolution (see Chapter 1).

Based on an assessment of maternal–fetal status, appropriate equipment is required to ensure patient safety during the transfer process. For the woman with preeclampsia, a nasal airway, Ambu bag, and anticonvulsant and antihypertensive agents should be included. Transport vehicles routinely are stocked with intravenous solutions and emergency equipment. Maternal transfer is less often initiated for women who are bleeding unless the patient is hemodynamically stable (ie, the blood pressure and pulse are within normal limits, and the FHR tracing is reassuring). When transferring women at risk for preterm labor, a birth kit from the originating hospital should be included; the rescue kits on the ambulance are usually minimally stocked. A full birth kit with suction catheters, suction bulb, blankets, and hat for the newborn is necessary. One-quart zip-lock plastic bags are useful to place the newborn in immediately after birth, with the zip-lock closed on either side around the newborn's neck to prevent body heat loss. It is recommended that all patients have at least two infusion lines because attempting to start an intravenous line en route is extremely difficult.

SUMMARY

Perinatal nurses may be challenged by the complications of pregnancy, especially when they occur unexpectedly in the low-risk setting. A thorough knowledge of the nursing care for common perinatal complications, including timely identification and appropriate interventions, is required to ensure optimal outcomes for mothers and babies.

REFERENCES

Hypertensive Disorders

Adams, E. M., & Finlayson, A. (1961). Familial aspects of preeclampsia and hypertension in pregnancy. *Lancet, 2,* 1375–1378.

Ales, K. L., Norton, M. E., & Druzin, M. L. (1989). Early prediction of antepartum hypertension. *Obstetrics and Gynecology, 73*(6), 928–933.

American College of Obstetricians and Gynecologists. (1996). *Management of preeclampsia (ACOG Technical Bulletin No. 219).* Washington, DC: Author.

American College of Obstetricians and Gynecologists. (2002). *Diagnosis and management of preeclampsia and eclampsia (ACOG Practice Bulletin No. 33).* Washington, DC: Author.

August, P. (2004). Hypertensive disorders in pregnancy. In G. Burrow, T. Duffy & J. Copel (Eds.), *Medical complications during pregnancy* (6th ed., pp. 43–68). Philadelphia: Elsevier.

Australasian Society for the Study of Hypertension in Pregnancy. (1993). Consensus statement. Management of hypertension in pregnancy: Executive summary. *Medical Journal of Australia, 158*(May 17), 700–702.

Baird, D. (1977). Epidemiological aspects of hypertensive pregnancy. *Clinical Obstetrics and Gynaecology, 4*(3), 531–548.

Barden, A., Ritchie, J., Walters, B., Michael, C., Rivers, J., Mori, T., et al. (2001). Study of plasma factors associated with neutrophil activation and lipid peroxidation in preeclampsia. *Hypertension, 38*(4), 803–808.

Barden, A., Singh, R., Walters, B., Ritchie, J., Roberman, B., & Beilin, L. (2004). Factors predisposing to preeclampsia in women with gestational diabetes. *Journal of Hypertension, 22*(12), 2371–2378.

Barron, W. M. (1991). Hypertension. In W. M. Barron & M. D. Lindheimer (Eds.), *Medical Disorders in Pregnancy* (pp. 1–42). Chicago: Mosby–Year Book.

Barton, J. R., Witlin, A. G., & Sibai, B. M. (1999). Management of mild preeclampsia. *Clinical Obstetrics and Gynecology, 42*(3), 455–469.

Beazley, D., Ahokas, R., Livingston, J., Griggs, M., & Sibai, B. M. (2004). Vitamin C and E supplementation in women at high risk for preeclampsia: A double-blind, placebo-controlled trial. *American Journal of Obstetrics and Gynecology, 192*(2), 520–521.

Beer, A. E. (1978). Possible immunologic bases of preeclampsia/eclampsia. *Seminars in Perinatology, 2*(1), 39–59.

Beevers, G., Lip, G. Y. H., & O'Brien, E. (2001). ABC of hypertension. Blood pressure measurement. Part I—Sphygmomanometry: Factors common to all techniques. *British Medical Journal, 322,* 981–985.

Belgore, F., Blann, A., Li-Saw-Hee, F., Beevers, D., & Lip, G. (2001). Plasma levels of vascular endothelial growth factor and its soluble receptor (SFlt-1) in essential hypertension. *American Journal of Cardiology, 87*(6), 805–807.

Belizan, J. M., & Villar, J. (1980). The relationship between calcium intake and edema-proteinuria and hypertension-getosis: An hypothesis. *American Journal of Clinical Nutrition, 33*(10), 2202–2210.

Belizán, J. M., Villar, J., Gonzalez, L., Campodonico, L., & Bergel, E. (1991). Calcium supplementation to prevent hypertensive disorders of pregnancy. *New England Journal of Medicine, 325*(20), 1399–1405.

Belizan, J. M., Villar, J., & Repke, J. (1988). The relationship between calcium intake and pregnancy-induced hypertension: Up-to-date evidence [see comments]. *American Journal of Obstetrics and Gynecology, 158*(4), 898–902.

Blackburn, S. (2003). *Maternal, fetal, and neonatal physiology: A clinical perspective* (2nd ed.). St. Louis: Saunders.

Branch, D. W. (1990). Antiphospholipid antibodies and pregnancy: Maternal implications. *Seminars in Perinatology, 14*(2), 139–146.

Branch, D. W., Andres, R., Digre, K. B., Rote, N. S., & Scott, J. R. (1989). The association of antiphospholipid antibodies with severe preeclampsia. *Obstetrics and Gynecology, 73*(4), 541–545.

Branch, D. W., Dudley, D. J., LaMarche, S., & Mitchell, M. D. (1992). Sera from preeclamptic patients contain factor(s) that stimulate prostacyclin production by human endothelial cells. *Prostaglandins, Leukotrienes, and Essential Fatty Acids, 45*(3), 191–195.

Branch, D. W., Dudley, D. J., & Mitchell, M. D. (1991). Preliminary evidence for homeostatic mechanism regulating endothelin production in preeclampsia. *Lancet, 337*(8747).

Branch, D. W., Silver, R. M., Blackwell, J. L., Reading, J. C., & Scott, J. R. (1992). Outcome of treated pregnancies in women with antiphospholipid syndrome: An update of the Utah experience. *Obstetrics and Gynecology, 80*(4), 614–620.

Brewer, T. (1974). Metabolic toxemia of late pregnancy in a county prenatal nutrition education project. *Journal of Reproductive Medicine, 13*(5), 175–176.

Brewer, T. (1977). Role of malnutrition in preeclampsia and eclampsia. *American Journal of Obstetrics and Gynecology, 125*(2), 281.

Brown, M., Hague, W., Higgins, J., Lowe, S., Mcowan, L., Oates, J., et al. (2000). The detection, investigation and management of hypertension in pregnancy. Full consensus statement of recommendations from the Council of the Australasian society for the Study of Hypertension in Pregnancy (ASSHP). *Australian and New Zealand Journal of Obstetrics and Gynaecology.*

Brown, M., Lindeheimer, M., Sweet, M. d., Assche, A. v., & Moutquin, J. M. (2001). The classification and diagnosis of the hypertensive disorders of pregnancy: Statement from the International Society for the Study of Hypertension in Pregnancy (ISSHP). *Hypertension in Pregnancy, 20*(1), ix–xiv.

Brown, M. A., Buddle, M. L., Bennett, M., Smith, B., Morris, R., & Whitworth, J. A. (1995). Ambulatory blood pressure in pregnancy: Comparison of the Spacelabs 90207 and Accutracker II monitors with intraarterial recordings. *American Journal of Obstetrics and Gynecology, 173*(1), 218–223.

Bulstra-Ramaker, M., Huisjes, J., & Visser, G. (1994). The effects of 3G eicosapentaenoic acid daily on recurrence of intrauterine growth retardation and pregnancy-induced hypertension. *British Journal of Obstetrics and Gynaecology, 92*(2), 131–140.

Butler, N. R., & Alberman, E. D. (1958). *Perinatal problems. Second report of the British Perinatal Mortality Survey.* Edinburgh: E S Livingstone.

Campbell, D. M., MacGillivray, I., & Carr-Hill, R. (1985). Preeclampsia in second pregnancy. *British Journal of Obstetrics and Gynaecology, 92*(2), 131–140.

Caritis, S., Sibai, B., Hauth, J., Lindheimer, M. D., Klebanoff, M., Thom, E., et al. (1998). Low-dose aspirin to prevent preeclampsia in women at high risk. National Institute of Child Health and Human Development Network of Maternal-Fetal Medicine Units. *New England Journal of Medicine, 338*(11), 701–705.

Chaiworapongsa, T., Romero, R., Espinoza, J., Bujpold, E., Kim, Y., Concalves, L., et al. (2004). Evidence supporting a role for blockade of the vascular endothelial growth factor system in the pathophysiology of preeclampsia. *American Journal of Obstetrics and Gynecology, 190*(6), 1541–1550.

Chang, J., Elam-Evans, L., Berg, C., Hendon, J., Flowers, L., Seed, K., et al. (2003). Pregnancy-related mortality surveillance—United States, 1991-1999. *Surveillance Summaries, Morbidity and Mortality Weekly Report (MMWR), 52*(SS-2), 1–8.

Chappell, L., Seed, P., Briley, A., Kelly, F., Lee, R., Hunt, B., et al. (1999). Effect of antioxidants on the occurrence of preeclampsia in women at increased risk: A randomised trial. *Lancet, 354*(9181), 810–816.

Chaudhuri, S. (1971). Role of nutrition in the eiology of toxemias of pregnancy. *American Journal of Obstetrics and Gynecology, 110*(1), 46–48.

Chesley, L., & Annitto, J. (1947). Pregnancy in the patient with hypertensive disease. *American Journal of Obstetrics and Gynecology, 53*, 372–381.

Chesley, L., Annitto, J., & Cosgrove, R. (1968). The familial factor in toxemia of pregnancy. *Obstetrics and Gynecology, 32*(3), 303–311.

Chesley, L. C. (1978). *Hypertensive disorders in pregnancy.* New York: Appleton–Century–Crofts.

Chesley, L. C. (1979). Parenteral magnesium sulfate and the distribution, plasma levels, and excretion of magnesium. *American Journal of Obstetrics and Gynecology, 133*(1), 1–7.

Chesley, L. C. (1984). History and epidemiology of preeclampsia-eclampsia. *Clinical Obstetrics and Gynecology, 27*(4), 801–820.

Chesley, L. C., & Cooper, D. W. (1986). Genetics of hypertension in pregnancy: Possible single gene control of pre-eclampsia and eclampsia in the descendants of eclamptic women. *British Journal of Obstetrics and Gynaecology, 93*(9), 898–908.

Chesley, L. C., & Sibai, B. M. (1987). Blood pressure in the midtrimester and future eclampsia. *American Journal of Obstetrics and Gynecology, 157*(5), 1258–1261.

Chez, R., & Sibai, B. M. (1994). Labetalol for intrapartum hypertension. *Contemporary OB/GYN, 39*, 37–38.

Clapp III, J. (2003). The effects of maternal exercise on fetal oxygenation and feto-placental growth. *European Journal of Obstetrics, Gynecologic, and Reproductive Biology, 110*(Suppl. 1), S80–S85.

Clark, S., Cotton, D., Hankins, G., & Phelan, J. (Eds.). (1997). *Critical Care Obstetrics* (3rd ed.). Malden, MS: Blackwell Science.

CLASP (Collaborative Low-Dose Aspirin Study in Pregnancy) Collaborative Group. (1994). CLASP: A randomised trial of low-dose aspirin for the prevention and treatment of pre-eclampsia among 9364 pregnant women. *Lancet, 343*, 619–629.

Coppage, K., & Sibai, B. M. (2004). Hypertensive emergencies. In M. Foley, J. T Strong & T. Garite (Eds.), *Obstetric intensive care manual* (pp. 51–65). New York: McGraw-Hill.

Crowther, C., Hiller, J., Pridmore, B., Bryce, R., Duggan, P., Hague, W. M., et al. (1999). Calcium supplementation in nulliparous women for the prevention of pregnancy-induced hypertension, preeclampsia, and preterm birth: An Australian randomized trial. FRACOG and the ACT Study Group. *Australian and New Zealand Journal of Obstetrics and Gynaecology, 39*(1), 12–18.

Cruickshank, D. J., Robertson, A. A., Campbell, D. M., & MacGillivray, I. (1991). Maternal obstetric outcome measures in a randomised controlled study of labetalol in the treatment of hypertension in pregnancy. *Clinical and Experimental Hypertension —Part B Hypertension in Pregnancy, B10*(3), 333–344.

Cruickshank, D. J., Robertson, A. A., Campbell, D. M., & MacGillivray, I. (1992). Does labetalol influence the development of proteinuria in pregnancy hypertension? A randomised controlled study. *European Journal of Obstetrics Gynecologic Reproductive Biology, 45*(1), 47–51.

Cunningham, F. G., Cox, S. M., Harstad, T. W., Mason, R. A., & Pritchard, J. A. (1990). Chronic renal disease and pregnancy outcome. *American Journal of Obstetrics and Gynecology, 163*(2), 453–459.

Cunningham, F. G., & Leveno, K. J. (1988). Management of pregnancy-induced hypertension. In P. C. Rubin (Ed.), *Handbook of hypertension* (Vol. X). Amsterdam: Elsevier Science.

Davies, A. G. (1971). *Geographical epidemiology of the toxemias of pregnancy.* Springfield IL: Charles C Thomas.

Davies, A. M., Czaczkes, J. W., Sadovsky, E., Prywes, R., Weiskopt, P., & Stesk, W. (1970). Toxemia of pregnancy in Jerusalem. I. Epidemiological studies of a total community. *Israeli Journal of Medical Science, 6*(2), 253–266.

Dechend, R., Gratze, P., Wallukat, G., Shagdarsuren, E., Plehm, R., Brasen, J., et al. (2005). Agnoistic autoantibodies to the AT1 receptor in a transgenic rat model of preeclampsia. *Hypertension, 45*(Part 2), 742–746.

Dekker, G. (1999). Risk factors for preeclampsia. *Clinical Obstetrics and Gynecology, 42*(3), 422–435.

Dekker, G. A., Robillard, P. Y., & Hulsey, T. C. (1998). Immune maladaptation in the etiology of preeclampsia: a review of corroborative epidemiologic studies. *Obstetric and Gynecologic Survey, 53*(6), 377–382.

Dekker, G. A., & Sibai, B. M. (1998). Etiology and pathogenesis of preeclampsia: Current concepts. *American Journal of Obstetrics and Gynecology, 179*(5), 1359–1375.

Dildy, G. A., Phelan, J. P., & Cotton, D. B. (1991). Complications of pregnancy-induced hypertension. In S. L. Clark, D. B. Cotton, G. D. V. Hankins, & J. P. Phelan (Eds.), *Critical care obstetrics* (2nd ed., pp. 251–288). Boston: Blackwell Scientific Publications.

Dildy, G. A., Phelan, J. P., & Cotton, D. B. (1992). Complications of pregnancy-induced hypertension. In S. L. Clark, D. B. Cotton, G. D. V. Hankins & J. P. Phelan (Eds.), *Critical Care Obstetrics* (2nd ed., pp. 251–288). Boston: Blackwell Scientific Publications.

Dizon-Townson, D. S., Major, H., & Ward, K. (1998). A promoter mutation in the tumor necrosis factor alpha gene is not associated with preeclampsia. *Journal of Reproductive Immunology, 38*(1), 55–61.

Dizon-Townson, D. S., Nelson, L. M., Easton, K., & Ward, K. (1996). The factor V Leiden mutation may predispose women to severe preeclampsia. *American Journal of Obstetrics and Gynecology, 175*(4, Pt. 1), 902–905.

Duffus, G., & MacGillivary, I. (1968). The incidence of pre-eclamptic toxaemia in smokers and non-smokers. *Lancet, 1*(7550), 994–995.

Duley, L., Henderson-Smart, D., Knight, M., & King, J. (2001). Antiplatelet drugs for prevention of preeclampsia and its consequences: Systematic review. *British Journal of Medicine, 322*(7282), 329–333.

Duvekot, J., Cheriex, E., Pieters, F., Menheere, P., & Peters, L. (1993). Early pregnancy changes in hemodynamics and volume homeostasis are consecutive adjustments triggered by a primary fall in systemic vascular tone. *American Journal of Obstetrics and Gynecology, 169*(6), 11382–11392.

Easterling, T. R., Benedetti, T. J., Schmucker, B. C., & Millard, S. P. (1990). Maternal hemodynamics in normal and preeclampsia pregnancies: A longitudinal study. *Obstetrics and Gynecology, 76*(6), 1061–1069.

ECPPA (Estudo Colaborativo para Prevencao do Pre-eclampsia com Aspirina) Collaborative Group. (1996). ECPPA: Randomized trial of low dose aspirin for the prevention of maternal and fetal complications in high risk pregnant women. *British Journal of Obstetrics and Gynaecology, 103*(7), 39–47.

Egerman, R. S., & Sibai, B. M. (1999). HELLP syndrome. *Clinical Obstetrics and Gynecology, 42*(2), 381–389.

Eskenazi, B., Fenster, L., & sidney, S. (1991). A multivariate analysis of risk factors for preeclampsia. *Journal of the American Medical Association, 266*(2), 237–241.

Fairlie, F. M., & Sibai, B. M. (1993). Hypertensive diseases in pregnancy. In E. A. Reece, J. C. Hobbins, M. J. Mahoney, & R. H. Petrie (Eds.), *Medicine of the fetus and mother.* Philadelphia: Lippincott.

Feeney, J., & Scott, J. (1980). Pre-eclampsia and changed paternity. *European Journal of Obstetrics, Gynecology and Reproductive Biology, 11*(1), 35–38.

Felding, C. (1969). Obstetric aspects in women with histories of renal disease. *Acta Obstetricia et Gynecologica Scandinavica, 48*(Suppl 2), 1–43.

Feldman, D. M. (2001). Blood pressure monitoring during pregnancy. *Blood Pressure Monitoring, 6*(1), 1–7.

Fenakel, K., Fenakel, G., Appelman, Z., Lurie, S., Katz, Z., & Shoham, Z. (1991). Nifedipine in the treatment of severe preeclampsia. *Obstetrics and Gynecology, 77*(3), 331–337.

Fitzgibbon, G. (1922). The relationship of eclampsia to other toxemias of pregnancy. *British Journal of Obstetrics and Gynaecology, 29*, 402.

Friedman, S., Schiff, E., Lubarsky, S., & Sibai, B. M. (1999). Expectant management of severe preeclampsia remote from term. *Clinical Obstetrics and Gynecology, 42*(3), 470–478.

Friedman, S. A., Taylor, R. N., & Roberts, J. M. (1991). Pathophysiology of preeclampsia. *Clinics in Perinatology, 18*(4), 661–682.

Garner, P. R., D'Alton, M. E., Dudley, D. K., Huard, P., & Hardie, M. (1990). Preeclampsia in diabetic pregnancies. *American Journal of Obstetrics and Gynecology, 163*(2), 505–508.

Gavette, L., & Roberts, J. (1987). Use of mean arterial pressure (MAP-2) to predict pregnancy-induced hypertension in adolescents. *Journal of Nurse-Midwifery, 32*(6), 357–364.

Gifford, R., August, P., Cunningham, G., Green, L., Lindeheimer, M., McNellis, D., et al. [Working Group]. (2000). *National High Blood Pressure Education Program Working Group National High Blood Pressure in Pregnancy.* NIH Publication No. 00-3029. Bethesda, MD: National Institutes of Health, National Heart, Lung, Blood Institute.

Gilstrap, L. C., Cunningham, G. F., & Whalley, P. J. (1978). Management of pregnancy induced hypertension in the nulliparous patient remote from term. *Seminars of Perinatology, 2*(1), 73–81.

Goldberg, G. L., & Craig, C. J. T. (1983). Obstetric complications in adolescent pregnancies. *South African Medical Journal, 64*(22), 863–864.

Goldenberg, R. L., Cliver, S. P., Bronstein, J., Cutter, G. R., Andrews, W. W., & Mennenmeyer, S. T. (1994). Bed rest in pregnancy. *Obstetrics and Gynecology, 84*(1), 131–136.

Golding, J. (1998). A randomised trial of low dose aspirin for primiparae in pregnancy. The Jamaica Low Dose Aspirin Study Group. *British Journal of Obstetrics and Gynaecology, 105*(3), 293–299.

Gonik, B., & Cotton, D. B. (1984). Peripartum colloid osmotic pressure changes: Influence of intravenous hydration. *American Journal of Obstetrics and Gynecology, 150*(1), 90–100.

Gonzalez-Quintero, V., Smarkusky, L., Jimenez, J., Mauro, L., Jy, W., Hortsman, L., et al. (2004). Elevated plasma endothelial microparticles: Preeclampsia versus gestational hypertension. *American Journal of Obstetrics and Gynecology, 191*(4), 1418–1424.

Granger, J., Alexander, B., Llinas, M., Bennett, W., & Khalil, R. (2001). Pathophysiology of hypertension during preeclampsia linking placental ischemia with endothelial dysfunction. *Hypertension, 38*(Pt. 2), 718–722.

Grisaru, D., Zwang, E., Peyser, M. R., Lessing, J. B., & Eldor, A. (1997). The procoagulant activity of red blood cells from patients with severe preeclamspia. *American Journal of Obstetrics and Gynecology, 177*(6), 1513–1516.

Gruppo di Studio Iperensione in Gravidanza. (1998). Nifedipine versus expectant management in mild to moderate hypertension in pregnancy. *British Journal of Obstetrics and Gynaecology, 105*(7), 718–722.

Guzick, D. S., Klein, V. R., Tyson, J. E., Lasky, R. E., Gant, N. F., & Rosenfeld, C. R. (1987). Risk factors for the occurrence of pregnancy-induced hypertension. *Clinical and experimental hypertension—Part B Hypertension of pregnancy, B6*(2), 281–297.

Haddad, B., Deis, S., Goffinet, F., Paniel, B., Cabrol, D., & Sibai, B. M. (2004). Maternal and perinatal outcomes during expectant management of 239 severe preeclamptic women between 24 and 33 weeks gestation. *American Journal of Obstetrics and Gynecology, 190*(6), 1590–1597.

Harrison, G. A., Humphrey, K. E., Jones, N., Badenhop, R., Guo, G., Elakis, G., et al. (1997). A genomewide linkage study of preeclampsia/eclampsia reveals evidence for a candidate region on 4q. *American Journal of Human Genetics, 60*(5), 1158–1167.

Hauth, J., & Cunningham, F. (1995). *Williams obstetrics supplement no. 14: Low-dose aspirin during pregnancy.* Norwalk, CT: Appleton & Lange.

Hauth, J., Goldenberg, R., Parker, R., Philips, J., Copper, R., DuBard, M., et al. (1993). Low-dose aspirin therapy to prevent preeclampsia. *American Journal of Obstetrics and Gynecology, 168*(4), 1083–1093.

Hays, P. H., Cruikshank, D. P., & Dunn, L. J. (1985). Plasma volume determination in normal and preeclamptic outcomes. *American Journal of Obstetrics and Gynecology, 151*(7), 958–966.

Heiskanen, N., Heinonen, S., & Kirkinen, P. (2003). Obstetric prognosis in sisters of preeclamptic women—Implications for genetic linkage studies. *BMC Women's Health, 3*, 1–5.

Helewa, M., Burrows, R., Smith, J., Williams, K., Brian, P., & Rabkin, S. (1997). Report of the Canadian Hypertension Society Consensus Conference: 1. Definitions, evaluation, and classification of hypertensive disorders in pregnancy. *Canadian Medical Association Journal, 157*(6), 715–725.

Herrera, J. A., Arevalo-Herrera, M., & Herrera, S. (1998). Prevention of preeclampsia by linoleic acid and calcium supplementation: a randomized controlled trial. *Obstet Gynecol, 91*(4), 585–590.

Hoyert, D., Kochanek, K., & Murphy, S. (1999). Deaths: Final data for 1997. *National Vital Statistics Report, 47*(19), 1–104.

Institute of Medicine, & Standing Committee on the Scientific Evaluation of Dietary Reference Intakes. (1997). *Dietary reference intakes: For calcium, phosphorus, magnesium, vitamin D, and fluoride.* Washington, DC: Author.

Italian Study of Aspirin in Pregnancy. (1993). Low-dose aspirin in prevention and treatment of intrauterine growth retardation and pregnancy-induced hypertension. *Lancet, 341*(8842), 396–400.

Jackson, M., Gott, P., Lye, S., Ritchie, J., & Clapp III, J. (1995). The effects of maternal aerobic exercise on human placental development: Placental volumetric compostion and surface areas. *Placenta, 16*(2), 179–191.

Jones, D. C., & Hayslett, J. P. (1996). Outcome of pregnancy in women with moderate or severe renal insufficiency. *New England Journal of Medicine, 335*(4), 226–232.

Khalil, R., & Granger, J. (2002). Vascular mechanisms of increased arterial pressure in preeclampsia: Lessons from animal models. *American Journal of Physiology Regulatory Integrative Comparative Physiology, 283*(1), R29–R45.

Khan, K. S., & Daya, S. (1996). Plasma glucose and pre-eclampsia. *International Journal of Gynaecology and Obstetrics, 53*(2), 111–116.

Kilpartrick, D. C., Gibson, F., & Liston, W. A. (1989). Association between susceptibility to pre-eclampsia within families and HLA DR4. *Lancet, 2*(8671), 1063–1065.

Kirshon, B., Moise, K. J., Jr., Cotton, D. B., Longmire, S., Jones, M., Tessem, J., et al. (1988). Role of volume expansion in severe preeclampsia. *Surgery, Gynecology, and Obstetrics, 167*(5), 367–371.

Klonoff-Cohen, H. S., Savitz, D. A., Cefalo, R. C., & McCann, M. F. (1989). An epidemiologic study of contraception and preeclampsia. *Journal of the American Medical Association, 262*(22), 3143–3147.

Kovats, S., Main, E., Librach, C., Stubblebine, M., Fisher, S., & DeMars, R. (1990). A class I antigen, HLA-G, expressed in human trophoblasts. *Science, 248*(4952), 220–223.

Kuo, V. S., Loumantakis, G., & Gallery, E. D. (1992). Proteinuria and its assessment in normal and hypertensive pregnancy. *American Journal of Obstetrics and Gynecology, 167*(3), 723–728.

Leduc, L., Wheeler, J. M., Kirshon, B., Mitchell, P., & Cotton, D. B. (1992). Coagulation profile in severe preeclampsia. *Obstetrics and Gynecology, 79*(1), 14–18.

Levesque, S., Moutquin, J., Lindsay, C., Roy, M., & Rousseau, F. (2004). Implication of an AGT haplotype in a multigene association study with pregnancy hypertension. *Hypertension, 43*(1), 71–78.

Levine, R. J., Esterlitz, J. R., Raymond, E. G., DerSimonian, R., Hauth, J. C., Ben Curet, L., et al. (1997, January 20–25, 1997). *Calcium for preeclampsia prevention (CPEP): A double-blind, placebo-controlled trial in healthy nulliparas.* Paper presented at the Society of Perinatal Obstetricians, 1997 17th Annual Meeting, Anaheim, CA.

Levine, R. J., Hauth, J. C., Curet, L. B., Sibai, B. M., Catalano, P. M., Morris, C. D., et al. (1997). Trial of calcium to prevent preeclampsia. *New England Journal of Medicine, 337*(2), 69–76.

Lie, R. T., Rasmussen, S., Brunborg, H., Gjessing, H. K., Lie-Nielsen, E., & Irgens, L. M. (1998). Fetal and maternal contributions to risk of pre-eclampsia: A population based study. *British Medical Journal, 316*(7141), 1343–1347.

Lindoff, C., Ingemarsson, I., Martin, Hamiltonsson, G., Segelmark, M., Thysell, H., & Astedt, B. (1997). Preeclampsia is associated with a reduced response to activated protein C. *American Journal of Obstetrics and Gynaecology, 176*(2), 457–460.

Linn, J., & August, P. (2005). Genetic thrombophilias and preeclampsia: A meta-analysis. *Obstetrics and Gynecology, 105*(1), 182–192.

Liston, W. A., & Kilpatrick, D. C. (1991). Is genetic susceptibility to pre-eclampsia conferred by homozygosity for the same single recessive gene in mother and fetus? *British Journal of Obstetrics and Gynaecology, 98*(11), 1079–1086.

Lo, K. W., & Lau, T. K. (1998). Cushing's syndrome in pregnancy secondary to adrenal adenoma. A case report and literature review. *Gynecologic Obstetrics Investigation, 45*(3), 209–212.

Long, P. A., Abell, D. A., & Beischer, N. A. (1979). Parity and preeclampsia. *Australian and New Zealand Journal of Obstetrics and Gynaecology, 19*(4), 203–206.

Lopez-Jaramillo, P. (1996). Prevention of preeclampsia with calcium supplementation and its relation with the L-arginine:nitric oxide pathway. *Brazilian Journal of Medical Biologic Research, 29*(6), 731–741.

Lopez-Jaramillo, P., & de Felix, M. (1991). Prevention of toxemia of pregnancy in Ecuadorian Andean women: experience with dietary calcium supplementation. *Bulletin of the Pan American Health Organization, 25*(2), 109–117.

Lopez-Jaramillo, P., Delgado, F., Jacome, P., Teran, E., Ruano, C., & Rivera, J. (1997). Calcium supplementation and the risk of preeclampsia in Ecuadorian pregnant teenagers. *Obstetrics and Gynecology, 90*(2), 162–167.

Lopez-Jaramillo, P., Narvaez, M., Calle, A., Rivera, J., Jacome, P., Ruano, C., et al. (1996). Cyclic guanosine 3',5' monophosphate concentrations in pre-eclampsia: Effects of hydralazine. *British Journal of Obstetrics and Gynaecology, 103*(1), 33–38.

Lopez-Jaramillo, P., Narvaez, M., Weigel, R. M., & Yepez, R. (1989). Calcium supplementation reduces the risk of pregnancy-induced hypertension in an Andes population. *British Journal of Obstetrics and Gynaecology, 96*(6), 648–655.

Lu, J. Y., Cook, D. L., Javia, J. B., Kirmani, Z. A., Liu, C. C., Makadia, D. N., et al. (1981). Intake of vitamins and minerals by pregnant women with selected symptoms. *Journal of the American Dietary Association, 78*(5), 477–482.

Lucas, L. S., & Jordan, E. T. (1997). Phenytoin as an alternative treatment for preeclampsia. *Journal of Obstetric, Gynecologic, and Neonatal Nursing, 26*(3), 263–269.

Lucas, M., Leveno, K., & Cunningham, F. (1995a). A comparison of magnesium sulfate with phenytoin for the prevention of eclampsia. *New England Journal of Medicine, 333*(4), 201–205.

Lucas, M., Leveno, K., & Cunningham, F. (1995b). Magnesium sulfate versus phenytoin for the prevention of eclampsia—Reply. *New England Journal of Medicine, 333*, 1639.

Mabie, W. C., Pernoll, M. L., & Biswas, M. K. (1986). Chronic hypertension in pregnancy. *Obstetrics and Gynecology, 67*(2), 197–205.

MacGillivary, I., Rose, G. A., & Rowe, B. (1969). Blood pressure survey in pregnancy. *Clinical Science, 37*(2), 395–407.

Magann, E., & Martin, J. J. (1995). Complicated postpartum preeclampsia-eclampsia. *Obstetrics and Gynecology Clinics of North America, 22*(2), 337–356.

Magann, E. F., Hamilton, J. M., Isaacs, J. D., Perry, K. G., Martin, Hamilton, R. W., & Meydrech, E. F. (1993). Immediate postpartum curettage: Accelerated recovery from severe preeclampsia. *Obstetrics and Gynecology, 81*(4), 502–506.

Magnini, L., Latthe, P., Villar, J., Kilby, M., Carroli, G., & Khan, K. (2005). Mapping the theories of preeclampsia: The role of homocysteine. *Obstetrics and Gynecology, 105*(2), 411–425.

Main, E., Chiang, M., & Colbern, G. (1994). Nulliparous preeclampsia (PE) is associated with placental histocompatibility gene: HLA-G (abstract). *American Journal of Obstetrics and Gynecology, 170*(5), 289.

Marcoux, S., Berube, S., Brisson, J., & Fabia, J. (1992). History of migraine and risk of pregnancy-induced hypertension. *Epidemiology, 3*(1), 53–56.

Martin, J. A., Hamilton, B. E., Sutton, P. D., Ventura, S. J., Menacker, F., & Kormeyer, S. (2006). Births: Final data for 2004. *National Vital Statistics Reports, 55*(1), 1–102.

Martin, J. A., Hamilton, B. E., Sutton, P. D., Ventura, S. J., Menacker, F., & Munson, M. (2003). Births: Final data for 2002. *National Vital Statistics Reports, 52*(10), 1–116.

Martin, J. A., Hamilton, B. E., Sutton, P. D., Ventura, S. J., Menacker, F., & Munson, M. (2005). Births: Final data for 2003. *National Vital Statistics Reports, 54*(2), 1–116.

Martin, J. A., Hamilton, B. E., Ventura, S. J., Menacker, F., & Park, M. M. (2002). Births: Final data for 2000. *National Vital Statistics Reports, 50*(5), 1–102.

Martin, J. A., Hamilton, B. E., Ventura, S. J., Menacker, F., Park, M., & Sutton, P. D. (2002). Births: Final data for 2001. *National Vital Statistics Reports, 51*(2), 1–104.

Marx, G. F., Schwalbe, S. S., Cho, E., & Whitty, J. E. (1993). Automated blood pressure measurements in laboring women: Are they reliable? *American Journal of Obstetrics and Gynecology, 158*(3, Pt. 1), 796–798.

Massey, S. (1977). Pharmacology of magnesium. *Annual Review of Pharmacology, 17*, 67.

Mathews, D. (1977). A randomized controlled trial of bed rest and sedation or normal activity and non-sedation in the management of nonalbuminuric hypertension in late pregnancy. *British Journal of Obstetrics and Gynaecology, 84*(2), 108–114.

Mathews, D. D., Agarwal, V., & Shuttleworth, T. P. (1980). The effect of rest and ambulation on plasma urea and urate levels in pregnant women with proteinuric hypertension. *British Journal of Obstetrics and Gynaecology, 87*(12), 1095–1098.

Meyer, N. L., Mercer, B. M., Friedman, S. A., & Sibai, B. M. (1994). Urinary dipstick protein: A poor predictor of absent or severe proteinuria. *American Journal of Obstetrics and Gynecology, 170*(1, Pt. 1), 137–141.

Mittendorf, R., Lain, K. Y., Williams, M. A., & Walker, C. K. (1996). Preeclampsia: A nested, case-control study of risk factors and their interactions. *Journal of Reproductive Medicine, 41*(7), 491–496.

Montagu, M. F. A. (1979). *Reproductive development of the female* (3rd ed.). Littleton, MA: John Wright-PSG Publishing.

Moore, M. P., & Redmon, C. W. G. (1983). Case-control study of severe pre-eclampsia of early onset. *British Medical Journal, 287*(6392), 580–583.

Moutquin, J. M., Fainville, R. N., & Raynauld, P. (1985). A prospective study of blood pressure in pregancy: Prediction of preeclampsia. *American Journal of Obstetrics and Gynecology, 151*(2), 191–196.

Myatt, L., & Miodovnik, M. (1999). Predicition of preeclampsia. *Seminars in Perinatology, 23*(1), 45–57.

National High Blood Pressure Education Program Working Group on High Blood Pressure in Pregnancy [Working Group]. (2000). Report of the National High Blood Pressure Education Program Working Group on high blood pressure in pregnancy. *American Journal of Obstetrics and Gynecology, 183*(1), S1–S22.

National High Blood Pressure Education Program [NHBPEP]. (2000). *Working group report on high blood pressure in pregnancy.* (NIH Publication No. 00-3029). Bethesda, MD: National Institutes of Health, National Heart, Lung, and Blood Institute, National High Blood Pressure Education Program.

Nelson, T. R. (1955). A clinical study of preeclampsia, Parts I and II. *Journal of Obstetrics and Gynaecology in the British Empire, 64,* 48–66.

Norris, M., Todeschini, M., Cassis, P., Pasta, F., Cappellini, A., Bonazzola, S., et al. (2004). L-Arginine depletion in preeclampsia orients nitric oxic synthase toward oxidant species. *Hypertension, 43*(3), 247–250.

O'Brien, J. M., Mercer, B. M., Friedman, S. A., & Sibai, B. M. (1993). Amniotic fluid index in hospitalized hypertensive patients managed expectantly. *Obstetrics and Gynecology, 82*(2), 247–250.

O'Brien, W. F. (1990). Predicting preeclampsia. *Obstetrics and Gynecology, 75*(3, Pt. 1), 445–452.

O'Brien, W. F. (1992). The prediction of preeclampsia. *Clinical Obstetrics and Gynecology, 35*(2), 351–364.

Odendaal, H. J., Pattinson, R. C., Bam, R., Grove, D., & Kotze, T. J. (1990). Aggressive or expectant management for patients with severe preeclampsia between 28-34 weeks' gestation: A randomized controlled trial. *Obstetrics and Gynecology, 76*(6), 1070–1075.

Onwude, J., Lilford, R., Hjartardottir, H., Staines, A., & Tuffnell, D. (1995). A randomised double blind placebo controlled trial of fish oil in high risk pregnancy. *British Journal of Obstetrics and Gynaecology, 102*(2), 95–100.

Out, H. J., Bruinse, H. W., Christaens, G. C., Vliet, M. V., George, P. G. D., Nieuwenhuis, H. K., et al. (1992). A prospective, controlled multicenter study on the obstetric risks of pregnant women with antiphospholipid antibodies. *American Journal of Obstetrics and Gynecology, 167*(1), 26–32.

Page, E. W. (1939). The relation between hydatid moles, relative ischemia of the gravid uterus, and the placental origin of eclampsia. *American Journal of Obstetrics and Gynecology, 37,* 291–293.

Page, E. W., & Christianson, R. (1976). The impact of mean arterial pressure in the middle trimester upon the outcomes of pregnancy. *American Journal of Obstetrics and Gynecology, 125*(6), 740–745.

Pattinson, R. C., Kriegler, E., Odendaal, H., Muller, L. M., & Kirsten, G. (1989). Increased placental resistance and late decelerations associated with severe proteinuric hypertension predicts poor fetal outcome. *South African Medical Journal, 75*(5), 211–214.

Phelan, J. (1991). Fetal considerations in the criticaly ill obstetric patient. In S. L. Clark, D. B. Cotton, G. D. V. Hankins & J. P. Phelan (Eds.), *Critical care obstetrics* (2nd ed., pp. 634–658). Boston: Blackwell Scientific Publications.

Plouin, P. F., Breart, G., Llado, J., Dalle, M., Keller, M. E., Goujon, H., et al. (1990). A randomized comparison of early with conservative use of antihypertensive drugs in the management of pregnancy-induced hypertension. *British Journal of Obstetrics and Gynaecology, 97*(2), 134–141.

Plouin, P. F., Breart, G., Maillard, F., Papiernik, E., Relier, J. P., & The Labetalol Methyldopa Study Group. (1988). Comparison of antihypertensive efficacy and perinatal safety of labetalol and methyldopa in the treatment of hypertension in pregnancy: A randomized controlled trial. *British Journal of Obstetrics and Gynaecology, 95*(9), 868–876.

Pouta, A., Hartikainen, A., Sovio, U., Gissler, M., Laitinen, J., McCarthy, M., et al. (2004). Manifestations of metabolic syndrome after hypertensive pregnancy. *Hypertension, 43*(4), 825–831.

Raijmakers, M., Dechend, R., & Poston, L. (2004). Oxidative stress and preeclampsia: Rationale for antioxidant clinical trials. *Hypertension, 44*(4), 374–380.

Ramsay, J., Ferrell, W., Crawford, L., Wallace, A., Greer, I., & Sattar, N. (2004). Divergent metabolic and vascular phenotypes in preeclampsia and intrauterine growth restriction: Relevance of adiposity. *Journal of Hypertension, 22*(11), 2177–2183.

Redman, C. (1995). Hypertension in pregnancy. In G. Chamberlain (Ed.), *Turnbull's obstetrics* (2nd ed., pp. 441–479). Edinburgh: Churchill Livingstone.

Redman, C. W., Bodmer, J. G., Bodmer, W. F., Beilin, L. J., & Bonnar, J. (1978). HLA antigens in severe pre-eclampsia. *Lancet, 2*(8086), 397–399.

Reinhart, K., Bayer, O., Brunkhorst, F., & Meisner, M. (2002). Markers of endothelial damage in organ dysfunction and sepsis. *Critical Care Medicine, 30*(5), S302–S312.

Repke, J. T. (1993). Hypertension and preeclampsia. In T. R. Moore, R. C. Reiter, R. W. Rebar & V. V. Baker (Eds.), *Gynecology & obstetrics: A longitudinal approach* (pp. 463–477). New York: Churchill Livingstone.

Roberts, J., & Hubel, C. (1999). Is oxidative stress the link in the two-stage model of preeclampsia? *Lancet, 354*(9186), 788–789.

Roberts, J., & Lain, K. (2002). Recent insights into the pathogenesis of preeclampsia. *Placenta, 23*(5), 359–372.

Roberts, J. M. (2004). Pregnancy-related hypertension. In R. Creasy & R. Resnik (Eds.), *Maternal-fetal medicine* (5th ed., pp. 859–900). Philadelphia: Saunders.

Roberts, J. M., Taylor, R. N., Friedman, S. A., & Goldfien, A. (1990). New developments in preeclampsia. *Fetal Medicine Review, 2*, 125.

Robillard, P. (2002). Interest in preeclampsia for researchers in reproduction. *Journal of Reproductive Immunology, 53*(1–2), 279–287.

Ross, R., Perizweig, W., Taylor, H., McBryde, A., Yates, A., & Kondutyer, A. (1954). A study of certain dietary factors of possible etiologic significance in toxemias of pregnancy. *American Journal of Obstetrics and Gynecology, 351*, 426.

Rotchell, Y. E., Cruickshank, J. K., Gay, M. P., Griffiths, J., Stewart, A., Farrell, B., et al. (1998). Barbados Low Dose Aspirin Study in Pregnancy (BLASP): A randomised trial for the prevention of preeclampsia and its complications. *British Journal of Obstetrics Gynaecology, 105*(3), 286–292.

Rotten, W., Sachtleben, M., & Friedman, E. (1959). Migraine and eclampsia. *Obstetrics and Gynecology, 14*, 322–330.

Rubin, P. C., Butters, L., Clark, D. M., Reynolds, B., Sumner, D. J., Steedman, D., et al. (1983). Placebo-controlled trial of atenolol in treatment of pregnancy-associated hypertension. *Lancet, 1*(8322), 431–434.

Saftlass, A. F., Olson, D. R., Franks, A. L., Atrash, H. K., & Pokras, R. (1990). Epidemiology of preeclampsia and eclampsia in the United States, 1979-1986. *American Journal of Obstetrics and Gynecology, 163*(2), 460–465.

Salvig, J., Olsen, S., & Secher, N. (1996). Effects of fish oil supplementation in late pregnancy on blood pressure: A randomised controlled trial. *British Journal of Obstetrics and Gynaecology, 103*, 529–533.

Sanchez-Ramos, L., Briones, D., Kaunitz, A., Delvalle, G., Gaudier, F., & Walker, C. (1997). Calcium supplementation and the risk of preeclampsia in Ecuadorian pregnant teenagers. *Obstetrics and Gynecology, 90*, 162–167.

Schaffir, J. A., Lockwood, C. J., Lapinski, R., Yoon, L., & Alvarez, M. (1995). Incidence of pregnancy-induced hypertension among gestational diabetes. *American Journal of Perinatology, 12*(4), 252–254.

Schiff, E., Friedman, S. A., & Sibai, B. M. (1994). Conservative management of severe preeclampsia remote from term. *Obstetrics and Gynecology, 84*(4), 626–630.

Sibai, B. (1996). Treatment of hypertension in pregnant women. *New England Journal of Medicine, 335*(4), 257–265.

Sibai, B., Barton, J., & Akl, S. (1992). A randomized prospective comparison of nifedipine and bed rest versus bed rest alone in the management of preeclampsia remorte from term. *American Journal of Obstetrics and Gynecology, 167*, 879.

Sibai, B. M. (1990a). Eclampsia VI. Maternal-periantal outcome in 254 consecutive cases. *American Journal of Obstetrics and Gynecology, 163*(3), 1049–1054.

Sibai, B. M. (1990b). The HELLP syndrome (hemolysis, elevated liver enzymes, and low platelets): Much ado about nothing? *American Journal of Obstetrics and Gynecology, 162*(2), 311–316.

Sibai, B. M. (1991). Immunologic aspects of preeclampsia. *Clinical Obstetrics and Gynecology, 34*(1), 27–34.

Sibai, B. M. (1992). Management and counseling of patients with preeclampsia remote from term. *Clinical Obstetrics and Gynecology, 35*(2), 426–436.

Sibai, B. M. (2002). High-risk pregnancy series: An expert's view. Chronic hypertension in pregnancy. *Obstetrics & Gynecology, 100*(2), 369–377.

Sibai, B. M., Anderson, G. D., Spinnato, J. A., & Shaver, D. C. (1983). Plasma volume findings in patients with mild pregnancy-induced hypertension. *American Journal of Obstetrics and Gynecology, 147*(1), 16–19.

Sibai, B. M., Caritis, S. N., Thom, E., Klebanoff, M., McNellis, D., Rocco, L., et al. (1993). Prevention of preeclampsia with low-dose aspirin in healthy, nulliparous pregnant women. *New England Journal of Medicine, 329*(17), 1213–1218.

Sibai, B. M., Gonzalez, A. R., Mabie, W. C., & Moretti, M. (1987). A comparison of labetalol plus hospitalization versus hospitalization alone in the management of preeclampsia remote from term. *Obstetrics and Gynecology, 70*(3, Pt 1), 323–327.

Sibai, B. M., Gordon, T., Thom, E., Caritis, S. N., Klebanoff, M., McNellis, D., et al. (1995). Risk factors for preeclampsia in healthy nulliparous women: A prospective multicenter study. *American Journal of Obstetrics and Gynecology, 172*(2, Pt. 1), 642–648.

Sibai, B. M., & Hnat, M. (2002). Delayed delivery in severe preeclampsia remote from term. *OBG Management, 14*(5), 92–108.

Sibai, B. M., McCubbin, J., Anderson, G., Lipshitz, J., & Dilts, P. (1981). Eclampsia I: Observation from 67 recent cases. *Obstetrics and Gynecology, 58*(5), 601–613.

Sibai, B. M., Mercer, B. M., Schiff, E., & Friedman, S. A. (1994). Aggressive versus expectant management of severe preeclampsia at 28 to 32 weeks' gestation: A randomized controlled trial. *American Journal of Obstetrics and Gynecology, 171*(3), 818–822.

Sibai, B. M., Villar, M. A., & Bray, E. (1989). Magnesium supplementation during pregnancy: a double-blind randomized controlled clinical trial. *American Journal of Obstetrics and Gynecology, 161*(1), 115–119.

Siddiqi, T., Rosenn, B., Mimouni, F., Khoury, J., & Miodovnik, M. (1991). Hypertension during pregnancy in insulin-dependent diabetic women. *Obstetrics and Gynecology, 77*(4), 514–519.

Simon, P., Fauchet, R., Pilorge, M., Calvez, C., Le Fiblec, B., Cam, G., et al. (1988). Association of HLA DR4 with the risk of recurrence of pregnancy hypertension. *Kidney International Supplement, 25*, S125–S128.

Simpson, K. R., Luppi, C. J., & O'Brien-Abel, N. (1998). Acute fatty liver of pregnancy. *Journal of Perinatal and Neonatal Nursing, 11*(4), 35–44.

Slattery, M. A., Khong, T. Y., Dawkins, R. R., Pridmore, B. R., & Hague, W. M. (1993). Eclampsia in association with partial molar pregnancy and congenital abnormalities. *American Journal of Obstetrics and Gynecology, 169*(6), 1625–1627.

Solomon, C., & Seely, E. (2001). Hypertension in pregnancy: A manifestation of the Insulin resistance syndrome? *Hypertension, 37*(2), 232–239.

Sorensen, T., Williams, M., Lee, I., Dashow, E., Thompson, M., & Luthy, D. (2003). Recreational physical activity during pregnancy and risk of preeclampsia. *Hypertension, 41*(6), 1273–1280.

Spatling, L., & Spatling, G. (1988). Magnesium supplementation in pregnancy. A double-blind study. *British Journal of Obstetrics and Gynaecology, 95*(2), 120–125.

Spellacy, W. N., Miller, S. J., & Winegar, A. (1986). Pregnancy after 40 years of age. *Obstetrics and Gynecology, 68*(4), 452–454.

Tatro, D. (2005). *A to Z drug facts.* St. Louis: Wolters Kluwer Health.

Taylor, D. J. (1988). Epidemiology of hypertension during pregnancy. In P. C. Rubin (Ed.), *Handbook of hypertension: Hypertension in Pregnancy* (pp. 223–240). New York: Elsevier.

Taylor, R. N. (1997). Review: Immunobiology of preeclampsia. *American Journal of Reproductive Immunology, 37*(1), 79–86.

Tervila, L., & Vartiainen, E. (1975). Acid-base relationship between mother and fetus in gestosis (pre-eclampsia) and in pregnant women with a labile blood pressure. *Acta Obstetricia et Gynecologica Scandinavia, 54*(3), 251–253.

The Eclampsia Collaborative Group. (1995). Which anticonvulsant for women with eclampsia? Evidence from the collaborative eclampsia trial. *Lancet, 345*(89623), 1455–1463.

Thompson, S. A., Lyons, T. L., & Makowski, E. L. (1987). Outcomes of twin gestations at the University of Colorado Health Sciences Center, 1973-1983. *Journal of Reproductive Medicine, 32*(5), 328–339.

Thornton, J., & Onwude, J. (1991). Pre-eclampsia: Discordance among identical twins. *British Medical Journal, 303*(6812), 1241–1242.

Ventura, S., Martin, J., Curtin, S., & Mathews, T. (1999). Births: Final data for 1997. *National Vital Statistics Reports, 47*(18), 1–96.

Ventura, S. J., Hamilton, J. A., Curtin, S. C., Mathews, T. J., & Park, M. M. (2000). Births: Final data for 1998. *National Vital Statistics Reports, 48*(3), 1–100.

Villar, M. A., & Sibai, B. M. (1989). Clinical significance of elevated mean arterial blood pressure in second trimester and threshold increase in systolic and diastolic blood pressure during third trimester. *American Journal of Obstetrics and Gynecology, 160*(2), 419–423.

Waite, L., Louie, R., & Taylor, R. (2005). Circulating activators of peroxisome proliferator-activated receptors are reduced in preeclamptic pregnancy. *Journal of Clincial Endocrinology and Metabolism, 90*(2), 620–626.

Walfisch, A., & Hallak, M. (2006). Hypertension. In D. James, P. Steer, C. Weiner, & B. Gonik (Eds.), *High risk pregnancy: management options.* (3rd ed., pp. 772–789). Philadelphia: Saunders Elsevier.

Wang, Y., Gu, Y., Zhang, Y., & Lewis, D. (2004). Evidence of endothelial dysfunction in preeclampsia: Decreased endothelial nitric oxide synthases expression is associated with increased cell permeability in endothelial cells from preeclampsia. *American Journal of Obstetrics and Gynecology, 190*(3), 817–824.

Ward, K., Hata, A., Jeunemaitre, X., Helin, C., Nelson, L., Namikawa, C., et al. (1993). A molecular variant of angiotensinogen associated with preeclampsia. *Nature Genetics, 4*(1), 59–61.

Weinstein, L. (1982). Syndrome of hemolysis, elevated liver enzymes, and low platelet count: A severe consequence of hypertension in pregnancy. *American Journal of Obstetrics and Gynecology, 142*(2), 159–167.

Weinstein, L. (1985). Preeclampsia/eclampsia with hemolysis, elevated liver enzymes, and thrombocytopenia. *Obstetrics and Gynecology, 66*(5), 657–660.

Weissgerber, T., Wolfe, L., & Davies, G. (2004). The role of regular physical activity in preeclampsia prevention. *Medicine & Science in Sports & Exercise, 36*(12), 2024–2031.

White, P. (1935). Pregnancy complicating diabetes. *Surgical Gynecology and Obstetrics, 61*, 324–332.

Yamamoto, T., Suzuki, Y., Kojima, K., & Suzumori, K. (2005). Reduced flow-mediated vasodilation is not due to a decrease in production of nitric oxide in preeclampsia. *American Journal of Obstetrics and Gynecology, 192*(2), 558–563.

Yamamoto, T., Takahaski, Y., Geshi, Y., Sasamori, Y., & Mori, H. (1996). Anti-phospholipid antibodies in preeclampsia and their binding ability for placental villous lipid fractions. *Journal of Obstetrics and Gynaecologic Research, 22*(3), 275–283.

Zeeman, G. G., Dekker, G. A., van Geijn, H. P., & Kraayenbrink, A. A. (1992). Endothelial function in normal and pre-eclamptic pregnancy: A hypothesis. *European Journal of Obstetric and Gynecologic Reproductive Biology, 43*(2), 113–122.

Bleeding

Akhan, S. E., Iyibozkurt, A. C., Turfanda, A. (2001). Unscarred uterine rupture after induction of labor with misoprostol: A case report. *Clinical and Experimental Obstetrics and Gynecology, 28*(2), 118–120.

American College of Obstetricians and Gynecologists. (1998). *Obstetric aspects of trauma management* (Educational Bulletin No. 251). Washington, DC: Author.

American College of Obstetricians and Gynecologista. (2002). *Placenta accreta* (Committee Opinion No. 266). Washington, DC: Author.

American College of Obstetricians and Gynecologists. (2004). *Vaginal birth after previous cesarean delivery* (Practice Bulletin No. 54). Washington, DC: Author.

American College of Obstetricians and Gynecologists. (2006a). *Induction of labor for vaginal birth after cesarean delivery* (Committee Opinion No. 342). Washington, DC: Author.

American College of Obstetricians and Gynecologists. (2006b). *Postpartum hemorrhage* (Practice Bulletin No. 76).Washington, DC: Author.

Ananth, C. V., Oyelese, Y., Yeo, L., Pradhan, A., & Vintzileos, A. M. (2005). Placental abruption in the United States, 1979 through 2001: Temporal trends and potential determinants. *American Journal of Obstetrics and Gynecology, 192*(1), 191–198.

Aslan, H., Unlu, E., Agar, M., & Ceylan, Y. (2004). Uterine rupture associated with misoprostol labor induction in women with a previous cesarean delivery. *European Journal of Obstetrics, Gynecology, and Reproductive Biology, 113*(1), 45–48.

Ayres, A. W., Johnson, T. R., & Hayashi, R. (2001). Characteristics of fetal heart rate tracings prior to uterine rupture. *International Journal of Gynaecology and Obstetrics, 74*(3), 235–240.

Bates, S. M., Greer, I. A., Hirsh, J., & Ginsberg, J. S. (2004). Use of antithrombotic agents during pregnancy: The seventh ACCP conference on antithrombotic and thrombolytic therapy. *Chest, 126*(3S), 627S–644S.

Catanzarite, V., Cousins, L., Dowling, D., & Daneshmand, S. (2006). Oxytocin-associated rupture of an unscarred uterus in a primagravida. *Obstetrics and Gynecology, 108*(3, Pt. 1), 723–725.

Chan, C. C., & To, W. W. (1999). Antepartum hemorrhage of unknown origin—What is its clinical significance? *Acta Obstetricia et Gynecologica Scandinavica, 78*(3), 186–190.

Chang, J., Elam-Evans, L., Berg, C., Herndon, J., Flowers, L., Seed, K., et al. (2003). Pregnancy-related mortality Surveillance, United

States, 1991-1999. *Morbidity and Mortality Weekly Report, 52*(2), 1–8.

Chauhan, S. P., Martin, J. N. Jr., Hendricks, C. E., & Morrison, J. C. (2003). Maternal and perinatal complications with uterine rupture in 142,075 patients who attempted vaginal birth after cesarean delivery: A review of the literature. *American Journal of Obstetrics and Gynecology, 189*(2), 408–417.

Clark, S. L. (1997). Hypovolemic shock. In S. L. Clark, D. B. Cotton, G. D. V. Hankins, & J. P. Phelan (Eds.), *Critical care obstetrics* (3rd ed. pp. 412–422). Malden MA: Blackwell Scientific.

Clark, S. L. (1999). Placenta previa and abruptio placentae. In R. K. Creasy, R. Resnick, & J. Iams (Eds.), *Maternal-fetal medicine* (4th ed., pp. 616–631). Philadelphia: Saunders.

Clark, S. L. (2004). Placenta previa and abruptio placentae. In R. K. Creasy, R. Resnick, & J. Iams (Eds.), *Maternal-fetal medicine* (5th ed., pp. 707–722). Philadelphia: Saunders.

Clark, S. L., Koonings, P. P., & Phelan, J. P. (1985). Placenta previa/accreta and prior cesarean section. *Obstetrics and Gynecology, 66*(1), 89–92.

Clark, S. L., Greenspoon, J. S., Aldahl, D., & Phelan, J. P. (1986). Severe preeclampsia with persistent oliguria: Management of hemodynamic subsets. *American Journal of Obstetrics and Gynecology, 154*(3), 490–494.

Cohen, S. M. (2004). Factor V Leiden Mutation in Pregnancy. *Journal of Obstetric, Gynecological & Neonatal Nursing, 33*(3), 348–353.

Cunningham, F. G., Leveno, K. J., Bloom, S. L., Hauth, J. C., Gilstrap, L. C., & Wenstrom, K. D. (2005). *Williams obstetrics* (22nd ed.). New York: McGraw-Hill.

Curet, M. J., Schermer, C. R., Demarest, G. B., Bieneik, E. J., III, & Curet, L. B. (2000). Predictors of outcome in trauma during pregnancy: Identification of patients who can be monitored for less than 6 hours. *Journal of Trauma, 49*(1), 18–25.

Curran, C. A. (2003). Intrapartum emergencies. *Journal of Obstetric, Gynecological & Neonatal Nursing, 32*(6), 802–813.

Daddario, J. (1999). Trauma in pregnancy. In L. Mandeville & N. Troiano (Eds.), *High-risk and critical care intrapartum nursing* (2nd ed., pp. 322–352). Philadelphia: Lippincott.

Dayan, S. S., & Schwalbe, S. S. (1996). The use of small-dose intravenous nitroglycerin in a case of uterine inversion. *Anesthesia and Analgesia 82*(5), 1091–1093.

Dildy, G. (2002). Postpartum hemorrhage: New management options. *Clinical Obstetrics and Gynecology, 45*(2), 330–344.

Dubois, J., Garel, L., Grignon, A., Lemay, M., & Leduc, L. (1997). Placenta percreta: Balloon occlusion and embolization of the internal iliac arteries to reduce intraoperative blood losses. *American Journal of Obstetrics and Gynecology, 176*(3), 723–726.

Durnwald, C., & Mercer, B. (2004). Vaginal birth after cesarean delivery: Predicting success, risks of failure. *Journal of Maternal-Fetal and Neonatal Medicine, 15*(6), 388–393.

El Kady, D., Gilbert, W.M., Anderson, J., Danielsen, B., & Smith, L.H. (2004). Trauma during pregnancy: An analysis of maternal and fetal outcomes in a large population. *American Journal of Obstetrics & Gynecology, 190*(6), 1661–1668.

Francis, K. (2004). Postpartum hemorrhage. In M. R. Foley, T. H. Strong, & T. J. Garite (Eds.), *Obstetric intensive care manual* (2nd ed. pp. 24–37).

Frederiksen, M. C., Glassenberg, R., & Stika, C. S. (1999). Placenta previa: A 22 year analysis. *Obstetrics and Gynecology, 180*(6, Pt. 1), 1432–1437.

Guise, J. M., Berlin, M., McDonagh, M., Osterwell, P., Chan, B., & Helfand, M. (2004). Safety of vaginal birth after cesarean: A systematic review. *Obstetrics and gynecology, 103*(3), 420–429.

Gupton, A., Heaman, M., & Ashcroft, T. (1997). Bed rest from the perspective of the high-risk pregnant woman. *Journal of Obstetric, Gynecologic and Neonatal Nursing, 26*(4), 423–430.

Hibbard, J. U., Ismail, M. A., Wang, Y, Te, C., Karrison, T., Ismail, M. A. (2001). Failed vaginal birth after cesarean section: How risky is it? I. Maternal morbidity. *American Journal of Obstetrics and Gynecology, 184*(7), 1365–1371.

Hudon, L., Belfort, M. A., & Broome, D. R. (1999). Diagnosis and management of placenta percreta: A review. *Obstetrical and Gynecological Survey, 54*(11), 156–164.

Hung, T. H., Shau, W. Y., Hsieh, C. C., Chiu, T. H., Hsu, J. J., & Hsieh, T. T. (1999). Risk factors for placenta accreta. *Obstetrics and Gynecology, 93*(4) 545–550.

James, A. H., Abel, D. E., & Brancazio, L. R. (2006). Anticoagulants in pregnancy. *Obstetrical & Gynecological Survey, 61*(1), 59–69.

Jauregui, I., Kirkendall, C., Ahn, M. O., & Phelan, J. (2000). Uterine rupture: A placentally mediated event? *Obstetrics and Gynecology, 95*(4 Suppl 1), S75.

Jones, W. K. (2000). *Safe motherhood: Preventing pregnancy-related illness and death.* Washington, DC: National Center for Chronic Disease Prevention and Health Promotion.

Khabbaz, A.Y., Usta, I. M., El-Hajj, M. I., Abu-Musa, A., Seoud, M., & Nassar, A. H. (2001). Rupture of an unscarred uterus with misoprostol induction: Case report and review of the literature. *Journal of Maternal-Fetal and Neonatal Medicine, 10*(2), 141–145.

Kirkendall, C., Jauregui, I., Kim, J. O., & Phelan, J. (2000). Catastrophic uterine rupture: Maternal and fetal characteristics. *Obstetrics and Gynecology, 95*(4 Suppl), S74.

Knab, D. R. (1978). Abruptio placenta: An assessment of the time and method of delivery. *Obstetrics and Gynecology, 52*(5), 625–629.

Kutteh, W. H., & Triplett, D. A. (2006). Thrombophilias and recurrent pregnancy loss. *Seminars in Reproductive Medicine, 24*(1), 54–65.

Landon, M. B., Hauth, J. C., Leveno, K. J., Spong, C. Y., Leindecker, S., Varner, M. W., et al. (2004). Maternal and perinatal outcomes associated with a trial of labor after prior cesarean delivery. *New England Journal of Medicine, 351*(25), 2581–2589.

Landon, M. B., Leindecker, S., Spong, C. Y., Hauth, J. C., Bloom, S., Varner, M. W., et al. (2005). The MFMU cesarean delivery registry: Factors affecting the success of a trial of labor after previous cesarean delivery. *American Journal of Obstetrics and Gynecology, 193*(3, Pt. 2), 1016–1023.

Landon, M. B., Spong, C. Y., Thom, E., Hauth, J. C., Bloom, S. L., et al. for the National Institute of Child Health and Human Development Maternal-Fetal Medicine Units Network. (2006). Risk of uterine rupture with a trial of labor in women with multiple and single prior cesarean delivery. *Obstetrics and Gynecology, 108*(1), 12–20.

Leung, A., Leung, E., & Paul, R. (1993). Uterine rupture after previous cesarean delivery: Maternal and fetal consequences. *American Journal of Obstetrics and Gynecology, 169*(4), 945–950.

Lieberman, E. (2001). Risk factors for uterine rupture during a trial of labor after cesarean. *Clinical Obstetrics and Gynecology, 44*(3), 609–621.

Lockwood, C. J., & Silver, R. (2004). Thrombophilias in pregnancy. In R. K. Creasy, R. Resnick, & J. Iams (Eds.), *Maternal-fetal medicine* (5th ed., pp. 1005–1021). Philadelphia: Saunders.

Lowe, T. W., & Cunningham, F. G. (1990). Placental abruption. *Clinical Obstetrics and Gynecology, 33*(3), 406–413.

Lydon-Rochelle, M., Holt, V. L., Easterling, T. R., & Martin, D. P. (2001). Risk of uterine rupture during labor among women with a prior cesarean delivery. *New England Journal of Medicine, 345*(1), 3–8.

MacMullen, N. J., Dulski, L. A., & Meagher, B. (2005). Red alert: Perinatal hemorrhage. *MCN The American Journal of Maternal Child Nursing, 30*(1), 46–51.

Mahon, T. R., Chazotte, C., & Cohen, W. R. (1994). Short labor: Characteristics and outcome. *Obstetrics and Gynecology, 84*(1), 47–51.

Maloni, J. H. (1998). *Antepartum bedrest: Case studies, research and nursing care* (Symposium). Washington, DC: Association of Women's Health, Obstetric and Neonatal Nurses.

Mathews, J. E., Mathai, M., & George, A. (2000). Uterine rupture in a multiparous woman during labor induction with oral misoprostol. *International Journal of Gynaecology and Obstetrics, 68*(1), 43–44.

Mattox, K. L., & Goetzl, L. (2005). Trauma in pregnancy. *Critical Care Medicine 33*(10), S385–S389.

Mauldin, J. G., & Newman, R. B. (2006). Prior cesarean: A contraindication to labor induction? *Clinical Obstetrics and Gynecology, 49*(3), 684–697.

Mazzone, M. E., & Woolever, J. (2006). Uterine rupture in a patient with an unscarred uterus: A case study. *Wisconsin Medical Journal, 105*(2), 64–66.

Menihan, C. A. (1999). The effect of uterine rupture on fetal heart rate patterns. *Journal of Nurse-Midwifery, 44*(1), 40–46.

Miller, D. A., Chollet, J. A., & Goodwin, T. M. (1997). Clinical risk factors for placenta previa-placenta accreta. *American Journal of Obstetrics and Gynecology, 177*(1), 210–214.

Muench, M. V., Baschat, A. A., Reddy, U. M., Mighty, H. E., Weiner, C. P., Scalea, T. M., & Harman, C. R. (2004). Kleihauer-Betke testing is important in all cases of maternal trauma. *Journal of Trauma: Injury, Infection & Critical Care, 57*(5), 1094–1098.

Murphy, D. J. (2006). Uterine rupture. *Current Opinion in Obstetrics and Gynecology, 18*(2), 135–140.

Natarajan, P., Shennan, A. H., Penny, J., Halligan, A. W., de Swiet, M., & Anthony, J. (1999). Comparison of auscultatory and oscillometric automatic blood pressure monitors in the setting of preeclampsia. *American Journal of Obstetrics & Gynecology 181*(5, Pt.1) 1203–1210.

Odunsi, K., Bullough, C., Henzel, J., & Polanska, A. (1996). Evaluation of chemical tests for fetal bleeding from vasa previa. *International Journal of Obstetrics and Gynecology, 55*(3), 207–212.

Oyelese, Y., Catanzarite, V., Prefumo, F., Lashley, S., Schachter, M., Tovbin, Y. et al., (2004). Vasa previa: The impact of prenatal diagnosis on outcome. *Obstetrics & Gynecology, 103*(5, Pt. 1), 937–942.

Oyelese, Y., & Smulian, J. (2006). Placenta previa, placenta accreta and vasa previa. *Obstetrics & Gynecology, 107*(4), 927–941.

Oyelese, K. O., Turner, M., Lees, C., & Campbell, S. (1999). Vasa previa: An avoidable obstetric tragedy. *Obstetrical and Gynecological Survey, 54*(2), 138–145.

Page, E. W., & Christianson, R. (1976). The impact of mean arterial pressure in the middle trimester upon the outcome of pregnancy. *American Journal of Obstetrics and Gynecology, 125*(6), 740–746.

Pare, E., Quinones, J. N., & Macones, G. A. (2006). Vaginal birth after cesarean section versus elective repeat cesarean section: Assessment of maternal downstream health outcomes. *British Journal of Obstetrics and Gynaecology, 113*(1), 75–85

Plaut, M. M., Schwartz, M. L., & Lubarsky, S. L. (1999). Uterine rupture associated with use of misoprostol in the gravid patient with a previous cesarean section. *American Journal of Obstetrics and Gynecology, 180*(6, Pt. 1), 1535–1542.

Poole, J. H., & White, D. (2003). *Obstetrical emergencies for the perinatal nurse* (Nursing Module). White Plains, NY: March of Dimes Birth Defects Foundation.

Rasmussen, S., Irgens, L. M., & Dalaker, K. (1997). The effect on the likelihood of further pregnancy of placental abruption and the rate of its recurrence. *British Journal of Obstetrics and Gynecology, 104*(11), 1292–1295.

Rebarber, A., Odunsi, K., Baumgarten, A., Copel, J., & Sipes, S. (1998). In vitro assessment of fetal contamination of human blood processed through the Cell-Saver 5 (CS5) at cesarean section (C/S). *American Journal of Obstetrics and Gynecology, 178* (Suppl. 1), 80S.

Rebarber, A., Lonser, R., Jackson, S., Copel, J., & Sipes, S. (1998). The safety of intraoperative autologous blood collection and autotransfusion during cesarean section. *American Journal of Obstetrics and Gynecology, 179*(3, Pt. 1), 715–720.

Reis, P. M., Sander, C. M., & Pearlman, M. D. (2000). Abruptio placentae after auto accidents: A case control study. *Journal of Reproductive Medicine, 45*(1), 6–10.

Ridgeway, J. J., Weyrich, D. L., & Benedetti, T. J. (2004). Fetal heart rate changes associated with uterine rupture. *Obstetrics and Gynecology, 103*(3), 506–512.

Robertson, L., Wu, O., Langhorne, P., Twaddle, S., Clark, P., Lowe, G. D., et al. (2006). Thrombophilia in pregnancy: A systematic review. *British Journal of Haematology, 132*(2), 171–196.

Sheiner, E., Levy, A., Ofir, K., Hadar, A., Shoham-Verdi, I., Hallak, M., et al. (2004). Changes in fetal heart rate and uterine patterns associated with uterine rupture. *Journal of Reproductive Medicine, 49*(5), 373–378.

Sherer, D. M., & Anyaegbunam, A. (1997). Perinatal ultrasonographic morphologic assessment of the umbilical cord: A review, Part I. *Obstetrical and Gynecological Survey, 52*(8), 506–514.

Shipp, T. D. (2004). Trial of labor after cesarean: So, what are the risks? *Clinical Obstetrics and Gynecology, 47*(2), 365–377.

Shipp, T., Zelop, C., Repke, J., Cohen, A., Caughey, A., & Lieberman, E. (1999). Uterine rupture during a trial of labor comparing a lower segment vertical incision to a lower segment transverse incision. *American Journal of Obstetrics and Gynecology, 180* (Suppl. 1), S112.

Sibai, B. (2005). Thrombophilia and severe preeclampsia: Time to screen and treat in future pregnancies? *Hypertension, 46*(6), 1252–1253.

Signore, C. C., Sood, A. K., & Richards, D. S. (1998). Second-trimester vaginal bleeding: Correlation of ultrasonographic findings with perinatal outcome. *American Journal of Obstetrics and Gynecology, 178*(2), 336–340.

Silver, R. M. (2007). Fetal death. *Obstetrics and Gynecology, 109*(1), 153–167.

Simpson, K. R. (2005). The context and clinical evidence for common nursing practices during labor. *MCN The Journal of Maternal Child Nursing, 30*(6), 356–363.

Simpson, K. R. (2006). Venous thromboembolism during pregnancy and postpartum: An inherited risk. *MCN The Journal of Maternal Child Nursing, 31*(3), 208.

Simpson, K. R., Luppi, C. J., & O'Brien-Abel, N. (1998). Acute fatty liver of pregnancy. *Journal of Perinatal and Neonatal Nursing, 11*(4), 35–44.

Thorp, J. M., Jr., Wells, S. R., Wiest, H. H., Jeffries, L., & Lyles, E. (1998). First-trimester diagnosis of placenta previa percreta by magnetic resonance imaging. *American Journal of Obstetrics and Gynecology, 178*(3), 616–618.

Wheeler, T. C., Anderson, T. L., Kelly, J., & Boehm, F. H. (1996). Placenta previa increta diagnosed at 18 weeks gestation: Report of a case with sonographic and pathologic correlation. *Journal of Reproductive Medicine, 41*(3), 198–200.

Witlin, A. G., Saade, G. R., Mattar, F., & Sibai, B. M. (1999). Risk factors for abruptio placentae and eclampsia: Analysis of 445 consecutively managed women with severe preeclampsia and eclampsia. *American Journal of Obstetrics and Gynecology,* 180(6, Pt. 1), 1322–1329.

Yap, O. W., Kim, E. S., & Laros, R. K., Jr. (2001). Maternal and neonatal outcomes after uterine rupture in labor. *American Journal of Obstetrics and Gynecology,* 184(7), 1576–1581.

You, W. B., & Zahn, C. M. (2006). Postpartum hemorrhage: Abnormally adherent placenta, uterine inversion, and puerperal hematomas. *Clincal Obstetrics & Gynecology,* 49(1), 184–197.

Zelop, C., Shipp, T., Cohen, A., Repke, J. T., & Lieberman, E. (2000). Outcomes of trial of labor following previous cesarean beyond the estimated date of delivery. *Obstetrics and Gynecology,* 94(4, Suppl. 1), S79.

Preterm Labor and Birth

American Academy of Pediatrics & American College of Obstetricians and Gynecologists. (2002). *Guidelines for perinatal care* (5th ed.). Elk Grove Village, IL: Author.

American College of Obstetricians and Gynecologists. (1996). *Home uterine activity monitoring* (Committee Opinion No. 172). Washington, DC: Author.

American College of Obstetricians and Gynecologists. (1998). *Special problems of multiple gestations* (Educational Bulletin No. 253). Washington, DC: Author.

American College of Obstetricians and Gynecologists. (1999). *Induction of labor* (Practice Bulletin No. 10). Washington, DC: Author.

American College of Obstetricians and Gynecologists. (2001). *Assessment of risk factors for preterm birth* (Practice Bulletin No. 31). Washington DC: Author.

American College of Obstetricians and Gynecologists. (2002a). *Antenatal corticosteroid therapy for fetal maturation* (Committee Opinion No. 273). Washington, DC: Author.

American College of Obstetricians and Gynecologists. (2002b). *Prevention of early-onset group B streptococcal disease in newborns* (Committee Opinion No. 279; Reaffirmed in 2005). Washington, DC: Author.

American College of Obstetricians and Gynecologists. (2003a). *Management of preterm labor* (Practice Bulletin No. 43). Washington DC: Author.

American College of Obstetricians and Gynecologists. (2003b). *Use of progesterone to reduce preterm birth* (Committee Opinion No. 291). Washington DC: Author.

American College of Obstetricians and Gynecologists. (2005a). *Smoking cessation during pregnancy* (Committee Opinion No. 316). Washington, DC: Author.

American College of Obstetricians and Gynecologists. (2005b). *The importance of preconception care in the continuum of women's health care* (Committee Opinion No. 313). Washington DC: Author.

Besinger, R. E., Niebyl, J. R., Keyes, W. G., & Johnson, T. R. (1991). Randomized comparative trial of indomethacin and ritodrine for the long term treatment of preterm labor. *American Journal of Obstetrics and Gynecology,* 164(4), 981–988.

Brown, H. L., Britton, K. A., Brizendine, E. J., Hiett, A. K., Ingram, D., Turnquest, M. A., et al. (1999). A randomized comparison of home uterine activity monitoring in the outpatient management of women treated for preterm labor. *American Journal of Obstetrics and Gynecology,* 180(4), 798–805.

Carroll, J., Slobodzian, R., & Steward, D. K. (2005). Extremely low birth weight infants: Issues related to growth. *MCN The American Journal of Maternal Child Nursing,* 30(5), 312–318, quiz 319–320.

Collaborative Group on Preterm Birth Prevention. (1993). Multicenter randomized controlled trial of a preterm birth prevention program. *American Journal of Obstetrics and Gynecology,* 169(2, Pt. 1), 352–366.

Crowther, C. A., Hiller, J. E., & Doyle, L. W. (2002). Magnesium sulphate for preventing preterm birth in threatened preterm labour. *Cochrane Database of Systematic Reviews* (4), CD001060.

Davidoff, M. J., Dias, T., Damus, K., Russell, R. Bettegowda, V. R. Dolan, S., Schwartz, R. H., Green, N. S., & Petrini, J. (2006). Changes in the gestational age distribution among U.S. singlton births: Impact on rates of late preterm births, 1992 to 2002. *Seminars in Perinatology,* 30(1), 8–15.

Davies, B. L., Stewart, P. J., Sprague, A. E., Niday, P. A., Nimrod, C. A., & Dulberg, C. S. (1998). Education of women about the prevention of preterm birth. *Canadian Journal of Public Health,* 89(4), 260–263.

Dildy, G. A., Belfort, M. A., Saade, G. R., Phelan, J. P., Hankins, G. D. V., & Clark, S. L. (2003). *Critical care obstetrics* (4th ed.). Malden, MA: Blackwell Science.

Dodd, J., Crowther, C., Dare, M., & Middleton, P. (2006). Oral betamimetics for maintenance therapy after threatened preterm labour. *Cochrane Database of Systematic Reviews* (1), CD003927.

Dodd, J., Flenady, V., Cincotta, R., & Crowther, C. (2006). Prenatal administration of progesterone for preventing preterm birth. *Cochrane Database of Systematic Reviews,* (1), CD004947.

Dyson, D. C., Danbe, K. H., Bamber, J. A., Crites, Y. M., Field, D. R., Maier, J. A., et al. (1998). Monitoring women at risk for preterm labor. *New England Journal of Medicine,* 338(1), 15–19.

Elliott, J. P., Istwan, N. B., Rhea, D., & Stanziano, G. (2004). The occurrence of adverse events in women receiving continuous subcutaneous terbutaline therapy. *American Journal of Obstetrics and Gynecology,* 191(4), 1277–1282.

England, L. J., Kendrick, J. S., Wilson, H. G., Merritt, R. K., Gargiullo, P. M., & Zahniser, S.C. (2001). Effects of smoking reduction during pregnancy on the birth weight of term infants. *American Journal of Epidemiology,* 154(8), 694–701

Ferreira-Borges, C. (2005). Effectiveness of a brief counseling and behavioral intervention for smoking cessation in pregnant women. *Preventive Medicine,* 41(1) 295–302.

Freda, M. C., Moos, M. K., & Curtis, M. (2006). The history of preconception care: Evolving standards and guidelines. *Maternal Child Health Journal,* 10(7), 43–52.

Freda, M. C., Anderson, H. F, Damus, K., Poust, D., Brustman, L., & Merkatz, I. R. (1990). Lifestyle modification as an intervention for inner city women at risk for preterm birth. *Journal of Advanced Nursing,* 15(3), 364–372.

Freda, M. C., Damus, K., Andersen, H. F., Brustman, L. E., & Merkatz, I. R. (1990). A "PROPP" for the Bronx: Preterm birth prevention education in the inner city. *Obstetrics and Gynecology,* 76(1, Suppl.), S93–S96.

Freda, M. C., Damus, K., & Merkatz, I. R. (1991). What do pregnant women know about the prevention of preterm birth? *Journal of Obstetric, Gynecologic, and Neonatal Nursing,* 20(2), 140–145.

Freda, M. C., & DeVore, N. (1996). Should intravenous hydration be the first line of defense with threatened preterm labor? A critical review of the literature. *Journal of Perinatology,* 16(5), 385–389.

Freda, M. C. (2003). Nursing's contributions to the literature on preterm labor and birth. *Journal of Obstetric, Gynecologic and Neonatal Nursing,* 32(5), 659–667.

Freda M. C., & Patterson E. T. (2004). *Preterm labor and birth: Prevention and management* (Nursing Module). White Plains, NY: March of Dimes Birth Defects Foundation.

Freston, M. S., Young, S., Calhoun, S., Fredericksen, T., Salinger, L., Malchodi, C., et al. (1997). Responses of pregnant women to potential preterm labor symptoms. *Journal of Obstetric, Gynecologic, and Neonatal Nursing,* 26(1), 35–41.

Garcia-Velasco, J. A., & Gonzalez Gonzalez, A. (1998). A prospective, randomized trial of nifedipine vs. ritodrine in threatened preterm labor. *International Journal of Gynecology and Obstetrics, 61*(3), 239–244.

Giarratano, G. (2006). Genetics influences on preterm birth. *MCN The American Journal of Maternal Child Nursing, 31*(3), 169–75.

Gilbert, W. M., Nesbitt, T. S., & Danielsen, B. (2003). The cost of prematurity: Quantification by gestational age and birth weight. *Obstetrics and Gynecology, 102*(3), 488–492.

Goldenberg, R. L., Cliver, S. P., Bronstein, J., Cutter, G. R., Andrews, W. W., & Mennemeyer, S. T. (1994). Bed rest in pregnancy. *Obstetrics and Gynecology, 84*(1), 131–136.

Goldenberg, R. L., & Rouse, D. J. (1998). Prevention of premature birth. *New England Journal of Medicine, 339*(5), 313–320.

Green, N. S., Damus, K., Simpson, J. L., Iams, J., Reece, E. A., Hobel, C. J., et al., and the March of Dimes Scientific Advisory Committee on Prematurity. (2005). Research agenda for preterm birth: Recommendations from the March of Dimes. *American Journal of Obstetrics and Gynecology, 193*(3, Pt. 1), 626–635.

Grimes, D. A., & Nanda, K. (2006). Magnesium sulfate tocolysis: Time to quit. *Obstetrics and Gynecology, 108*(4), 986–989.

Hack, M. (2006). Young adult outcomes of very-low-birth-weight children. *Seminars in Fetal and Neonatal Medicine, 11*(2), 127–137.

Hack, M., Taylor, H. G., Drotar, D., Schluchter, M., Cartar, L., Andreias, L., et al. (2005). Chronic conditions, functional limitations, and special health care needs of school-aged children born with extremely low-birth-weight in the 1990s. *Journal of the American Medical Association, 294*(3), 318–325.

Hamilton, B. E., Martin, J. A., & Ventura, S. J. (2006). Births: Preliminary data for 2005. Retrieved January 2, 2007, from www.cdc.gov/nchs

Hans, S. L. (1999). Demographic and psychosocial characteristics of substance-abusing pregnant women. *Clinical Perinatology, 26*(1), 55–74.

Heaman, M. I. (2005). Relationships between physical abuse during pregnancy and risk factors for preterm birth among women in Manitoba. *Journal of Obstetric, Gynecologic, and Neonatal Nursing, 34*(6), 721–731.

Hartmann, K., Thorp, J. M., Jr., McDonald, T. L., Savitz, D. A., & Granados, J. L. (1999). Cervical dimensions and risk of preterm birth: A prospective cohort study. *Obstetrics and Gynecology, 93*(4), 504–509.

Herron, M. A., Katz, M., & Creasy, R. K. (1982). Evaluation of a preterm birth prevention program: A preliminary report. *Obstetrics and Gynecology, 59*(4), 442–446.

Higby, K., Xenakis, E. M., & Pauerstein, C. J. (1993). Do tocolytic agents stop preterm labor? A critical and comprehensive review of efficacy and safety. *American Journal of Obstetrics and Gynecology, 168*(4), 1247–1256.

Hill, W. C., & Lambertz, E. L. (1990). Let's get rid of the term "Braxton-Hicks contractions." *Obstetrics and Gynecology, 75*(4), 709–710.

Hobel, C. J., Ross, M. G., Bemis, R. L., Bragonier, J., Jr., Nessim, S., Sandhu, M., et al. (1994). The West Los Angeles Preterm Birth Preventions Project I: Program impact on high-risk women. *American Journal of Obstetrics and Gynecology, 170*(1, Pt. 1), 54–62.

Iams, J. D., Johnson, F. F., O'Shaughnessy, R. W., & West, L. C. (1987). A prospective random trial of home uterine activity monitoring in pregnancies at increased risk of preterm labor. *American Journal of Obstetrics and Gynecology, 157*(3), 638–643.

Iams, J. D., Stilson, R., Johnson, F. F., Williams, R. H., & Rice, R. (1990). Symptoms that precede preterm labor and preterm premature rupture of the membranes. *American Journal of Obstetrics and Gynecology, 162*(2), 486–490.

Institute of Medicine. (1985). *Preventing low birth weight.* Washington, DC: National Academy Press.

Institute of Medicine. (2006). *Preterm birth: Causes, consequences and prevention.* New York: National Academies Press.

Institute for Safe Medication Practices. (2005). Preventing magnesium toxicity in obstetrics. *ISMP Medication Safety Alert, 10*(21), 1–2.

Institute for Safe Medication Practices. (2005). Preventing magnesium toxicity in obstetrics. *Nurse Advise-ERR: ISMP Medication Safety Alert, 4*(3), 1–2.

Jackson, R. A., Gibson, K. A., & Wu Y. W., & Croughan, M. S. (2004). Perinatal outcome in singletons following IVF: A meta-analysis. *Obstetrics & Gynecology, 103*(3), 551–563.

Jesse, E. D., Graham, M., & Swanson, M. (2006). Psychosocial and spiritual factors associated with smoking and substance use during pregnancy in African American and white low-income women. *Journal of Obstetric, Gynecologic, and Neonatal Nursing, 35*(1), 68–77.

Johnson, K., Posner, S., Bierman, J., Cordero, J. F., Atrash, H. K., Parker, C. S., et al. (2006). Recommendations to improve preconception health and health care—United States, A report of the CDC/ATSDR Preconception Care Work Group and the Select Panel on Preconception Care. *Morbidity and Mortality Weekly Report, 55*(RR06), 1–23.

Kalish, R. B., Vardhana, S., Normand, N. J., Gupta, M., & Witkin, S. S. (2006). Association of a maternal CD14-159 gene polymorphism with preterm premature rupture of membranes and spontaneous preterm birth in multi-fetal pregnancies. *Journal of Reproductive Immunology, 70*(1–2), 109–117.

Kashanian, M., Akbarian, A. R., & Soltanzadeh, M. (2005). Atosiban and Nifedipin for the treatment of preterm labor. *International Journal of Gynaecology and Obstetrics, 91*(1), 10-4.

Kearney, M. (1999). *Perinatal impact of alcohol, tobacco and other drugs* (Nursing Module). White Plains, NY: March of Dimes Birth Defects Foundation.

Kogan, M. D., Alexander, G. R., Kotelchuck, M., MacDorman, M. F., Buekens, P., Martin, J. A., et al. (2000). Trends in twin birth outcomes and prenatal care utilization in the United States, 1981–1997. *Journal of the American Medical Association, 284*(3), 335–341.

Lawrence, T., Aveyard, P., Cheng, K. K., Griffin, C., Johnson, C., & Croghan, E. (2005). Does stage-based smoking cessation advice in pregnancy result in long-term quitters? 18-month postpartum follow-up of a randomized controlled trial. *Addiction, 100*(1) 107–116.

Leviton, L. C., Goldenberg, R. L., Baker, C. S., Schwartz, R. M., Freda, M. C., Fish, L. J., et al. (1999). Methods to encourage the use of antenatal corticosteroid therapy for fetal maturation: A randomized controlled trial. *Journal of the American Medical Association, 281*(1), 46–52.

Lewis J. A. (2006). Genetics: Another nursing specialty. *MCN The American Journal of Maternal Child Nursing, 31*(3), 142.

Litt, J., Taylor, H. G., Klein, N., & Hack, M. (2005). Learning disabilities in children with very low birth weight: Prevalence, neuropsychological correlates, and educational interventions. *Journal of Learning Disabilities 38*(2), 130–141.

Lockwood, C. J., Senyei, A. E., Desche, M. R., Casal, D., Shah, K. D., Thung, S. N., et al. (1991). Fetal fibronectin in cervical and vaginal secretions as a predictor of preterm delivery. *New England Journal of Medicine, 325*(10), 669–674.

Lumley J., Oliver S. S., Chamberlain C., & Oakley L. (2004). Interventions for promoting smoking cessation during pregnancy. *Cochrane Database of Systematic Reviews, 18*(4), CD001055.

Lynam, L. E., & Miller, M. A. (1992). Mothers' and nurses' perceptions of the needs of women experiencing preterm labor. *Journal of Obstetric, Gynecologic, and Neonatal Nursing, 21*(2), 126–136.

Lu, M. C., Tache V., Alexander, G. R., Kotelchuck, M., & Halfon, N. (2003). Preventing low birth weight: Is prenatal care the answer? *The Journal of Maternal-Fetal Neonatal Medicine, 13*(6), 362–380.

Macones, G. A., & Robinson, C. A. (1998). Is there justification for using indomethacin in preterm labor? An analysis of neonatal risks and benefits. *American Journal of Obstetrics and Gynecology, 177*(4), 819–824.

Magee, B. D., Hattis, D., & Kivel, N. M. (2004). Role of smoking in low birth weight. *The Journal of Reproductive Medicine, 49*(1), 23–27.

Maloni, J. A., & Park, S. (2005). Postpartum symptoms after antepartum bed rest. *Journal of Obstetric, Gynecologic and Neonatal Nursing, 34*(2), 163–171.

Maloni, J. A., Alexander, G. R., Schluchter, M. D., Shah, D. M., & Park, S. (2004). Antepartum bed rest: Maternal weight change and infant birth weight. *Biological Research for Nursing, 5*(3), 177–186.

Maloni, J. A., Kane, J. H., Suen, L. J., & Wang, K. K. (2002). Dysphoria among high-risk pregnant hospitalized women on bed rest: A longitudinal study. *Nursing Research, 51*(2), 92–99.

Maloni, J. A., & Schneider, B. S. (2002). Inactivity: Symptoms associated with gastrocnemius muscle disuse during pregnancy. *AACN Clinical Issues, 13*(2), 248–262.

Maloni, J. A., Chance, B., Zhang, C., Cohen, A. W., Betts, D., & Gange, S. J. (1993). Physical and psychosocial side effects of antepartum hospital bed rest. *Nursing Research, 42*(4), 197–203.

March of Dimes. (2005). Perinatal Data Center. Retrieved February 14, 2006, from www.marchofdimes.com

Martin, J. A., Hamilton, B. E., Sutton, P. D., Ventura, S. J., Menacker, F., & Munson, M. L. (2005). Births: Final data for 2003. *National Vital Statistics Report, 54*(2), 1–116.

McFarlane, J., Parker, B., & Cross, B. (2001). *Abuse during pregnancy: A protocol for prevention and intervention* (Nursing Module, 2nd edition). White Plains, NY: March of Dimes Birth Defects Foundation.

McFarlane, J., & Gondolf, E. (1998). Preventing abuse during pregnancy: A clinical protocol. *MCN The American Journal of Maternal Child Nursing, 23*(1), 22–27.

Medoff-Cooper B., Bakewell-Sachs S., Buus-Frank M., & Santa-Donato A. (2005). The AWHONN near term initiative: A conceptual framework for optimizing the health of near term infants. *Journal of Obstetric, Gynecologic and Neonatal Nursing, 34*(6), 666–671.

Meis, P. J., Klebanoff, M., Thom, E., Dombrowski, M. P., Sibai, B., Moawad, A. H., et al. for the National Institute of Child Health and Human Development Maternal-Fetal Medicine Units Network. (2003). Prevention of recurrent preterm delivery by 17 alpha-hydroxyprogesterone caproate. *New England Journal of Medicine, 348*(24), 2379–2385.

Mikkola, K., Ritari, N., Tommiska, V., Salokorpi, T., Lehtonen, L., Tammela, O., et al. (2005). Neurodevelopmental outcome at 5 years of age of a national cohort of extremely low birth weight infants who were born in 1996-1997. *Pediatrics, 116*(6), 1391–4000.

Moore, M. L., Meis, P. J., Ernest, J. M., Wells, H. B., Zaccaro, D. J., & Terrell, T. (1998). A randomized trial of nurse intervention to reduce preterm and low birth weight births. *Obstetrics and Gynecology, 91*(5, Pt. 1), 656–661.

Moore, M. L., & Freda, M. C. (1998). Reducing preterm and low birth weight births: Still a nursing challenge. *MCN The American Journal of Maternal Child Nursing, 23*(4), 200–209.

Moore, M. L. (1999). Biochemical markers for preterm birth: What is their role in caring for pregnant women? *MCN The American Journal of Maternal Child Nursing, 24*(2), 80–86.

Moore, M. L., Ketner, M. Walsh, K., & Wagoner, S. (2005). Listening to women at risk for preterm birth: Their perceptions of barriers to effective care and nurse telephone interventions.

MCN The American Journal of Maternal-Child Nursing, 29(6), 391–297.

Moos, M. K. (2003). *Preconception health promotion: a focus for women's wellness* (Nursing Module). White Plains, NY: March of Dimes Birth Defects Foundation.

Morales, L. S., Staiger, D., Horbar, J. D., Carpenter, J., Kenny, M., Geppert, J., et al. (2005). Mortality among very low-birth weight infants in hospitals serving minority populations. *American Journal of Public Health, 95*(12), 2206–2212.

Morse, S. B., Wu, S. S., Ma, C., Ariet, M., Resnick, M., & Roth, J. (2006). Racial and gender differences in the viability of extremely low birth weight infants: A population-based study. *Pediatrics, 117*(1), e106–e312.

Mozurkewich, E. L., Naglie, G., Krahn, M. D., & Hayashi, R. H. (2000). Predicting preterm birth: A cost effective analysis. *American Journal of Obstetrics and Gynecology, 182*(6), 1589–1598.

Mullen, P. D., Richardson, M. A., Quinn, V. P., & Ershoff, D. H. (1997). Postpartum return to smoking: Who is at risk and when. *American Journal of Health Promotion, 11*(5), 323–330.

Nanda, K., Cook, L. A., Gallo, M. F., & Grimes, D. A. (2002). Terbutaline pump maintenance therapy after threatened preterm labor for preventing preterm birth. *Cochrane Database of Systematic Reviews, (4),* CD003933.

National Institutes of Health Consensus Development Panel on the Effect of Corticosteroids for Fetal Lung Maturation and Perinatal Outcomes. (1995). Effect of corticosteroids for fetal maturation on perinatal outcomes. *Journal of the American Medical Association, 273*(5), 413–418.

National Institutes of Health. (2000). Antenatal Corticosteroids Revisited: Repeat courses. Retrieved February 16, 2006, from http://consensus.nih.gov/cons/112/112_statement.htm

National Institute of Child Health and Human Development. (2005). *Optimizing care and long term outcomes of near-term pregnancy and near-term newborn infants*. Bethesda, MD: Author.

National Institutes of Health. (2006). *State of the science conference statement: Cesarean delivery on maternal request*. Bethesda, MD: Author.

Nightingale, S. L. (1998). Warning on use of terbutaline sulfate for preterm labor: From the food and drug administration. *Journal of the American Medical Association, 279*(1), 9.

Offenbacher, S., Boggess, K. A., Murtha, A. P., Jared, H. L., Lieff, S., McKaig, R. G., et al. (2006). Progressive periodontal disease and risk of very preterm delivery. *Obstetrics and Gynecology, 107*(1) 29–36.

Papatsonis, D., Flenady, V., Cole S., & Liley, H. (2005). Oxytocin receptor antagonists for inhibiting preterm labour. *Cochrane Database of Systematic Reviews, 20*(3), CD004452.

Papiernik, E. (1989). *Effective prevention of preterm birth: The French experience at Hagenau*. New York: March of Dimes Birth Defects Foundation.

Parker, B., McFarlane, J., & Soeken, K. (1994). Abuse during pregnancy: Effects on maternal complications and birth weight in adult and teenage women. *Obstetrics and Gynecology, 84*(3), 323–328.

Patterson, E. T., Douglas, A. B., Patterson, P. M., & Bradle, J. B. (1992). Symptoms of preterm labor and self-diagnostic confusion. *Nursing Research, 41*(6), 367–372.

Petrini, J. R., Callaghan, W. M., Klebanoff, M., Green, N. S., Lackritz, E. M., Howse, J. L., et al. (2005). Estimated effect of 17 alpha-hydroxyprogesterone caproate on preterm birth in the United States. *Obstetrics and Gynecology, 105*(2), 267–272.

Porter, T. F., Fraser, A. M., Hunter C. Y., Ward, R. H., & Varner, M. W. (1997). The risk of preterm births across generations. *Obstetrics and Gynecology, 90*(1), 63–67.

Raju, T. N. K., Higgins, R. D., Stark, A. R., & Leveno, K. J. (2006). Optimizing care and outcomes for late preterm (near-term) infants: A summary of the workshop sponsored by the National

Institute of Child Health and Human Development. *Pediatrics, 118*(3), 1207–1214.

Renker, P. R., & Tonkin P. (2006). Women's views of prenatal violence screening: Acceptability and confidentiality issues. *Obstetrics and Gynecology, 107*(2), 348–354.

Ricketts, S. A., Murray, E. K., & Schwalberg, R. (2005). Reducing low birth weight by resolving risks: Results from Colorado's prenatal plus program. *American Journal of Public Health, 95*(11), 1952–1957.

Santa-Donato, A. (2005). Near-term infants: What experts say health care providers and parents need to know. *AWHONN Lifelines, 9*(6), 456–461.

Schmitz, T., Maillard, F., Bessard-Bacquaert, S., Kayem, G., Fulla, Y., Cabrol, D., et al. (2006). Selective use of fetal fibronectin detection after cervical length measurement to predict spontaneous preterm delivery in women with preterm labor. *American Journal of Obstetrics and Gynecology, 194*(1), 138–143.

Schrag, S., Gorwitz, R., Fultz-Butts, K., & Schuchat, A. (2002). Prevention of perinatal group B streptococcal disease: Revised guidelines from the CDC. *Morbidity and Mortality Weekly Report, 51*(RR11), 1–22.

Sciscione, A. C., Stamilio, D. M., Manley, J. S., Shlossman, P. A., Gorman, R. T., & Colmorgen, G. H. (1998). Tocolysis of preterm contractions does not improve preterm delivery rates or perinatal outcomes. *American Journal of Perinatology, 15*(3), 177–181.

Secker-Walker, R. H., Vacek, P., Flynn, B., & Mead, P. (1997). Smoking in pregnancy, exhaled carbon monoxide and birth weight. *Obstetrics and Gynecology, 89*(5, Pt. 1), 648–653.

Schmitt, S. K., Sneed, L., & Phibbs, C. S. (2006). Costs of newborn care in California: A population-based study. *Pediatrics, 117*(1), 154–160.

Sibai, B. M. (2002). Hypertension. In S. G. Gabbe, J. R. Niebyl, & J. L. Simpson (Eds.). *Obstetrics: Normal and problem pregnancies* (4th ed., pp. 945–1004). New York: Churchill Livingstone.

Silver, R. M. (2007). Fetal death. *Obstetrics and Gynecology, 109*(1), 153–167.

Simhan, H. N., & Bodnar, L. M. (2006). Prepregnancy body mass index, vaginal inflammation, and the racial disparity in preterm birth. *American Journal of Epidemiology, 163*(3), 459–466.

Simhan, H. N. & Bodnar, L. M. (2006). Prepregnancy body mass index, vaginal inflammation, and the racial disparity in preterm birth. *American Journal of Epidemiology, 163*(5), 459–466.

Simpson, W. J. (1957). A preliminary report on cigarette smoking and the incidence of prematurity. *American Journal of Obstetrics and Gynecology, 73*, 808–815.

Simpson R. (2005). Monitoring the preterm fetus during labor. *MCN, The American Journal of Maternal Child Nursing, 29*(6), 380–390.

Simpson, K. R. (2006). Minimizing risk of magnesium sulfate overdose in obstetrics. *MCN The American Journal of Maternal Child Nursing, 31*(5), 340.

Simpson, K. R., & Knox, G. E. (2004). Obstetrical accidents involving intravenous magnesium sulfate: Recommendations to promote patient safety. *MCN, The American Journal of Maternal Child Nursing, 29*(3), 161–171.

Sosa, C., Althabe, F., Belizan, J., & Bergel, E. (2004). Bed rest in singleton pregnancies for preventing preterm birth. *Cochrane Database of Systematic Reviews*, (1), CD003581

Spong, C. Y., Meis, P. J., Thom, E. A., Sibai, B., Dombrowski, M. P., Moawad, A.H., et al., and the National Institute of Child Health and Human Development Maternal Fetal Medicine Units Network. (2005). Progesterone for prevention of recurrent preterm birth: Impact of gestational age at previous delivery. *American Journal of Obstetrics and Gynecology, 193*(3, Pt. 2), 1127–1131.

Stan, C., Boulvain, M., Hirshbrunner-Amagbaly, P., & Pfister, R. (2002). Hydration for treatment of preterm labour. *Cochrane Database of Systematic Reviews*, (2), CD003096.

Suplee, P. D. (2005). The importance of providing smoking relapse counseling during the postpartum hospitalization. *Journal of Obstetric, Gynecologic and Neonatal Nursing, 34*(6), 703–712.

Swamy, G. K., Simhan, H. N., Gammill, H. S., & Heine, R. P. (2005). Clinical utility of fetal fibronectin for predicting preterm birth. *Journal of Reproductive Medicine, 50*(11), 851–856.

Thyrian, J. R., Hannover, W., Grempler, J., Roske, K., John, U., & Hapke, U. (2006). An intervention to support postpartum women to quit smoking or remain smoke free. *Journal of Midwifery, 51*(1), 45–50.

Tiedje, L. B. (2005). Teaching is more than telling: education about prematurity in a prenatal clinic waiting room. *MCN, The American Journal of Maternal Child Nursing. 29*(6), 373–379.

Tsoi, E., Fuchs, I . B., Rane, S., Geerts, L., & Nicolaides, K. H. (2005). Sonographic measurement of cervical length in threatened preterm labor in singleton pregnancies with intact membranes. *Ultrasound in Obstetrics & Gynecology, 25*(4), 353–356.

VanGeijn, J. P., Lenglet, J . E., & Bolte, A. C. (2005). Nifedipine trials: Effectiveness and safety aspects. *British Journal of Obstetrics and Gynaecology, 112*(Suppl 1), 79–83.

Ventura, S. J., Martin, J. A., Curtin, S. C., Mathews, T. J., & Park, M. M. (2000). Births: Final data for 1998. *National Vital Statistics Report, 48*(3), 1–100.

Vermillion, S. T., & Robinson, C. J. (2005). Antiprostaglandin drugs. *Obstetrics and Gynecology Clinics of North America, 32*(3), 501–517.

Wang, X., Zuckerman, B., Pearson, C., Kaufman, C., Chen, C., & Wang, G. (2002). Maternal cigarette smoking, metabolic gene polymorphism, and infant birth weight. *Journal of the American Medical Association, 287*(2), 195–202.

Ward, K., Argyle, V.A., Meade, M., & Nelson, L. (2005). The heritability of preterm delivery. *Obstetrics and Gynecology, 106*(6), 1235–1239.

Ward, K. (2003). Genetic factors in preterm birth. *British Journal of Obstetrics and Gynecology, 110*(Suppl 20), 117.

Yost, N. P., Bloom, S. L., Twickler, M. D., & Leveno, K. L. (1999). Pitfalls in ultrasonic cervical length measurement for predicting preterm birth. *Obstetrics and Gynecology, 93*(4), 510–516.

Diabetes

American College of Obstetricians and Gynecologists. (2000). *Fetal macrosomia* (Practice Bulletin No. 22). Washington, DC: Author.

American College of Obstetricians and Gynecologists. (2001). *Gestational diabetes* (Practice Bulletin No. 30). Washington, DC: Author.

American College of Obstetricians and Gynecologists. (2005). *Pregestational diabetes mellitus* (Practice Bulletin No. 60). Washington, DC: Author.

American Diabetes Association. (1997). Report of the expert committee on the diagnosis and classification of diabetes mellitus. *Diabetes Care, 20*(7), 1183–1197.

American Diabetes Association. (2004a). Gestational diabetes mellitus. *Diabetes Care, 27*(Suppl. 1), S88–S90.

American Diabetes Association. (2004b). Physical activity/exercise and diabetes mellitus. *Diabetes Care, 27*(Suppl. 1), S58–S62.

American Diabetes Association. (2004c). Preconception care of women with diabetes. *Diabetes Care, 27*(Suppl. 1), S76–S78.

Atilano, L. C., Lee-Parritz, A., Lieberman, E., Cohen, A. P., & Barbieri, R. L. (1999). Alternative methods of diagnosing gestational diabetes mellitus. *American Journal of Obstetrics and Gynecology, 181*(5, Pt. 1), 1158–1161.

Barker, D. J. (2001). A new model for the origins of chronic disease. *Medicine, Health Care & Philosophy, 4*(1), 31–35.

Bevier, W. C., Fischer, R., & Jovanovic, L. (1999). Treatment of women with an abnormal glucose challenge test (but a normal oral glucose tolerance test) decreases the prevalence of macrosomia. *American Journal of Perinatology, 16*(6), 269–275.

Biastre, S. A., & Slocum, J. M. (2003). Gestational diabetes. In M. J. Franz (Ed.), *A core curriculum for diabetes education: Diabetes in the life cycle and research* (5th ed., pp. 143–176). Chicago: American Association of Diabetes Educators.

Blank, A., Grave, G. D., & Metzger, B. E. (1995). Effects of gestational diabetes on perinatal morbidity reassessed. *Diabetes Care, 18*(1), 127–129.

Boden, G. (1996). Fuel metabolism in pregnancy and gestational diabetes mellitus. *Obstetrics and Gynecology Clinics of North America, 23*(1), 1–10.

Bouhanick, B., Biquard, F., Hadjadj, S., & Roques, M. (2000). Does treatment with antenatal glucocorticoids for the risk of premature delivery contribute to ketoacidosis in pregnant women with diabetes who receive continuous subcutaneous insulin infusion (CSII)? *Archives in Internal Medicine, 160*(2), 242–243.

Briggs, G. G., Ambrose, P. J., Nageotte, M. P., Padilla, G., & Wan, S. (2005). Excretion of metformin into breast milk and the effect of nursing infants. *Obstetrics and Gynecology, 105*(5), 1437–1441.

Buchanan, T. A., & Kitzmiller, J. L. (1994). Metabolic interactions of diabetes and pregnancy. *Annual Review of Medicine, 45,* 245–260.

Butte, N. F. (2000). Carbohydrate and lipid metabolism in pregnancy: Normal compared with gestational diabetes mellitus. *American Journal of Clinical Nutrition, 71*(Suppl. 5), S1256–S1261.

California Diabetes and Pregnancy Program. (2002*). Sweet success guidelines for care.* Sacramento: State of California, Maternal & Child Health Branch.

California Diabetes and Pregnancy Program. (2005*). Sweet success guidelines for care: Updates.* Retrieved December 11, 2006, from www.llu.edu/llumc/sweetsuccess/updates.html

Carpenter, M. W. (2000). The role of exercise in pregnant women with diabetes mellitus. *Clinical Obstetrics and Gynecology, 43*(1), 56–64.

Carpenter, M. W., & Coustan, D. R. (1982). Criteria for screening tests for gestational diabetes. *American Journal of Obstetrics and Gynecology, 144*(7), 768–773.

Centers for Disease Control and Prevention. (2001). *Diabetes & women's health across the life stages: A public health perspective.* Atlanta, GA: Author.

Centers for Disease Control and Prevention. (2005). *National diabetes fact sheet: General information and national estimates on diabetes in the United States, 2005.* Atlanta, GA: Author.

Chauhan, S. P., & Perry, K. G. (1995). Management of diabetic ketoacidosis in the obstetric patient. *Obstetrics and Gynecology Clinics of North America, 22*(1), 143–155.

Conway, D. L., Gonzales, O., & Skiver, D. (2004). Use of glyburide for the treatment of gestational diabetes: The San Antonio experience. *Journal of Maternal-Fetal and Neonatal Medicine, 15*(1), 51–55.

Conway, D. L., & Langer, O. (1999). Effects of new criteria for type 2 diabetes on the rate of postpartum glucose intolerance in women with gestational diabetes. *American Journal of Obstetrics and Gynecology, 81*(3), 610–614.

Cordero, L., & Landon, M. B. (1993). Infant of the diabetic mother. *Clinics in Perinatology, 20*(3), 635–648.

Cullen, M. T., Reece, E. A., Homko, C. J., & Sivan, E. (1996). The changing presentations of diabetic ketoacidosis during pregnancy. *American Journal of Perinatology, 13*(7), 449–451.

Davidson, M. B. (2001). Hyperglycemia. In M. J. Franz (Ed.), *A core curriculum for diabetes education: Diabetes and complications* (4th ed., pp. 21–44). Chicago: American Association of Diabetes Educators.

Devlin, J. T., Hothersall, L, & Wilkis, J. L. (2002). Use of insulin glargine during pregnancy in a type 1 diabetic woman. *Diabetes Care, 25*(6), 1095–1096.

Diabetes Prevention Program Research Group. (2002). Reduction in the incidence of type 2 diabetes with lifestyle intervention or metformin. *New England Journal of Medicine, 346*(6), 393–403.

DiCianni, G., Volpe, L., Lencioni, C., Chatzianagnostou, K., Cuccuru, I., Chio, A. et al. (2005) Use of insulin glargine during the first weeks of pregnancy in five type 1 diabetic women. *Diabetes Care, 28*(4), 982–983.

Feig, D. S., Briggs, G. G., Kraemer, J. M., Ambrose, P. J., Moskovitz, D. N., Nageotte, M., et al. (2005). Transfer of glyburide and glipizide into breast milk. *Diabetes Care, 28*(8), 1851–1855.

Franz, M. J., Bantle, J. P., Beebe, C. A., Brunzell, J. D., Chiasson, J., Garg, A., et al. (2002). Evidence-based nutrition principles and recommendations for the treatment and prevention of diabetes and related complications. *Diabetes Care, 25*(1), 148–198.

Gabbe, S. G. (2000). New concepts and applications in the use of the insulin pump during pregnancy. *Journal of Maternal Fetal Medicine, 9*(1), 42–45.

Gamson, K., Chia, S., & Jovanovic, L. (2004). The safety and efficacy of insulin analogues in pregnancy. *Journal of Maternal-Fetal & Neonatal Medicine, 15*(1), 26–34.

Garner, P. (1995). Type 1 diabetes mellitus and pregnancy. *Lancet, 346*(8968), 157–159.

Glueck, C. J., Goldenberg, N., Wang, P., Loftspring, M., & Sherman, A. (2004). Metformin during pregnancy reduces insulin, insulin resistance, insulin secretion, weight, testosterone and development of gestational diabetes: prospective longitudinal assessment of women with polycystic ovary syndrome from preconception through pregnancy. *Human Reproduction, 19*(3), 210–521.

Glueck, C. J., Wang, P., Goldenberg, N., & Sieve-Smith, L. (2002). Pregnancy outcomes among women with polycystic ovary syndrome treated with metformin. *Human Reproduction, 17*(11), 2858–2864.

Hagay, Z. J. (1994). Diabetic ketoacidosis in pregnancy: Etiology, pathophysiology, and management. *Clinical Obstetrics and Gynecology, 37*(1), 39–49.

Hagay, Z. J., & Reece, E. A. (1992). Diabetes mellitus in pregnancy. In E.A. Reece, J.C. Hobbins, M.J. Mahoney, & R. H. Petrie (Eds.), *Medicine of the fetus and mother* (pp. 982–1020). Philadelphia: Lippincott.

Hagay, Z., & Weissman, A. (1996). Management of diabetic pregnancy complicated by coronary artery disease and neuropathy. *Obstetrics and Gynecology Clinics of North America, 23*(1), 205–220.

Hague, W. M., Davoren, P. M., Oliver, J., & Rowan, J. (2003). Metformin may be useful in gestational diabetes. *British Medical Journal, 326*(7392), 762–763.

Harvey, M. G. (1992). Diabetic ketoacidosis during pregnancy. *Journal of Perinatal and Neonatal Nursing, 6*(1), 1–13.

Hirsch, I. B., McGill, J. B., Cryer, P. E., & White, P. F. (1991). Perioperative management of surgical patients with diabetes mellitus. *Anesthesiology, 74*(2), 346–359.

Homko, C. J. (1998). Gestational diabetes: A screening and management update. *Advance for Nurse Practitioners, 6*(12), 59–61, 63.

Homko, C. J., & Sargrad, K. R. (2003). Pregnancy with preexisting diabetes. In M. J. Franz (Ed.), *A core curriculum for diabetes education: Diabetes in the life cycle and research* (5th ed., pp. 97–142). Chicago: American Association of Diabetes Educators.

Institute of Medicine of the National Academies. (2002). *Dietary reference intakes: Energy, carbohydrate, fiber, fat, fatty acids, cholesterol, protein, and amino acids.* Washington, DC: The National Academies Press.

Jacobson, G. F., Ramos, G. A., Ching, J. Y., Kirby, R. S., Ferrara, A., & Field, D. R. (2005). Comparison of glyburide and insulin for the management of gestational diabetes in a large managed care organization. *American Journal of Obstetrics and Gynecology, 193*(1), 118–124.

Jakubowicz, D. J., Iuorno, M. J., Jakubowicz, S., Roberts, K. A., & Nestler, J. E. (2002). Effects of metformin on early pregnancy loss in the polycystic ovary syndrome. *Journal of Clinical Endocrinology & Metabolism, 87*(2), 524–529.

Jornsay, D. L. (1998). Continuous subcutaneous insulin infusion (CSII) therapy during pregnancy. *Diabetes Spectrum, 11*(1), 26–32, 51.

Jovanovic, L. (2000a). Role of diet and insulin treatment of diabetes in pregnancy. *Clinical Obstetrics and Gynecology, 43*(1), 46–55.

Jovanovic, L. (Ed.). (2000b). *Medical management of pregnancy complicated by diabetes* (3rd ed.). Alexandria VA: American Diabetes Association.

Jovanovic, L., Ilic, S., Pettitt, D. J., Hugo, K., Gutierrez, M., Bowsher, R. R., & Bastyr, E. J. (1999). Metabolic and immunologic effects of insulin Lispro in gestation diabetes. *Diabetes Care, 22*(9), 1422–1427.

Kemball, M., McIver, C., Milner, R., Nourse, C., Schiff, D., & Tiernan, J. (1970). Neonatal hypoglycemia in infants of diabetic mothers given sulphonylurea drugs in pregnancy. *Archives of Disease in Childhood, 45*, 696–670.

Kendrick, J. M. (2004). *Diabetes in pregnancy* (3rd ed.) (Nursing Module). White Plains, NY: March of Dimes Birth Defects Foundation.

Kendrick, J. M. (1999). Diabetes mellitus in pregnancy. In L. K. Mandeville & N. H. Troiano (Eds.), *High risk and critical care intrapartum nursing* (pp. 224–254). Philadelphia: Lippincott Williams & Wilkins.

Kilvert, J. A., Nicholson, H. O., & Wright, A. D. (1993). Ketoacidosis in diabetic pregnancy. *Diabetic Medicine, 10*(3), 278–281.

Kjos, S. L. (2000). Postpartum care of women with diabetes. *Clinical Obstetrics and Gynecology, 43*(1), 75–86.

Kjos S. L., Henry, O., Lee, R. M., Buchanan, T. A., & Mishell, D. R. (1993). The effect of lactation on glucose and lipid metabolism in women with recent gestational diabetes. *Obstetrics and Gynecology, 82*(3), 451–455.

Klein, B. E., Moss, S. E., & Klein, R. (1990). Effect of pregnancy on progression of diabetic retinopathy. *Diabetes Care, 13*(1), 34–40.

Kocak, M., Caliskan, E., Simsir, C., & Haberal A. (2002). Metformin therapy improves ovulatory rates, cervical scores, and pregnancy rates in clomiphene citrate-resistant women with polycystic ovary syndrome. *Fertility and Sterility, 77*(1), 101–106.

Landon, M. B. (2000). Obstetric management of pregnancies complicated by diabetes mellitus. *Clinical Obstetrics and Gynecology, 43*(1), 65–74.

Langer, O. (2000). Management of gestational diabetes. *Clinical Obstetrics and Gynecology, 43*(1), 106–115.

Langer, O., Conway, D. L., Berkus, M. D., Xenakis, E. M. J., & Gonzales, O. (2000). A comparison of glyburide and insulin in women with gestational diabetes. *New England Journal of Medicine, 343*(16), 1134–1138.

Langer, O., & Mazze, R. S. (1986). Diabetes in pregnancy: Evaluating self-monitoring performance and glycemic control with memory-based reflectance meters. *American Journal of Obstetrics and Gynecology, 155*(3), 635–637.

Langer, O., Brustman, L., Anyaegbunam, A., & Mazze, R. (1987). The significance of one abnormal glucose tolerance test value on adverse outcome in pregnancy. *American Journal of Obstetrics and Gynecology, 157*(3), 758–763.

Langer, O., Rodriguez, D. A., Xenakis, E. M., McFarland, M. B., Berkus, M. D., & Arrendondo, F. (1994). Intensified versus conventional management of gestational diabetes. *American Journal of Obstetrics and Gynecology, 170*(4), 1036–1046, discussion 1046–1047.

Lesser, K. B., & Carpenter, M. W. (1994). Metabolic changes associated with normal pregnancy and pregnancy complicated by diabetes mellitus. *Seminars in Perinatology, 18*(5), 399–406.

Macleod, A. F., Smith, S. A., Sonksen, P. H., & Lowy, C. (1990). The problem of autonomic neuropathy in diabetic pregnancy. *Diabetic Medicine, 7*(1), 80–82.

Major, C. A., de Veciana, M., Weeks, J., & Morgan, M. A. (1998). Recurrence of gestational diabetes: Who is at risk? *American Journal of Obstetrics and Gynecology, 179*(4), 1038–1042.

Mayer-Davis, E. J., Hu, F. B., Rifas-Shiman, S. L., Colditz, G. A., Zhou, L., & Gillman, M. W. (2006). Breast-feeding and risk for childhood obesity. *Diabetes Care, 29*(10), 2231–2237.

Mazze, R. S., Shamoon, H., Pasmantier, R., Lucido, D., Murphy, J., Hartmann, K., et al. (1984). Reliability of blood-glucose monitoring by patients with diabetes mellitus. *American Journal of Medicine, 77*(2), 211–217.

McElvy, S. S., Miodovnik, M., Rosenn, B., Khoury, J. C., Siddiqi, T., Dignan, P. S., & Tsang, R. C. (2000). A focused preconceptional and early pregnancy program in women with type 1 diabetes reduces perinatal mortality and malformation rates to general population levels. *Journal of Maternal-Fetal Medicine, 9*(1), 14–20.

Metzger, B. E., & Coustan, D. R. (1998). Summary and recommendations of the Fourth International Workshop-Conference on Gestational Diabetes Mellitus: The Organizing Committee. *Diabetes Care, 21*(Suppl. 2), B161–B169.

Miller, E. H. (1994). Metabolic management of diabetes in pregnancy. *Seminars in Perinatology, 18*(5), 414–431.

Moore, T. R. (2004). Diabetes in pregnancy. In R. K. Creasy & R. Resnik (Eds.), *Maternal-fetal medicine: Principles and practice* (5th ed., pp. 1023–1063). Philadelphia: Saunders.

Moses, R. G. (1986). Assessment of reliability of patients performing SMBG with a portable reflectance meter with memory capacity (M-Glucometer). *Diabetes Care, 9*(6), 670–671.

Murtaugh, M. A., Ferris A., Capacchione C. M., & Reece, E. A. (1998). Energy intake and glycemia in lactating women with type 1 diabetes. *Journal of the American Dietetic Association, 98*(6), 642–648.

Neiger, R., & Coustan, D. R. (1991). The role of repeat glucose tolerance tests in the diagnosis of gestational diabetes. *American Journal of Obstetrics and Gynecology, 165*(4, Pt. 1), 787–790.

Neiger, R., & Kendrick, J. (1994). Obstetric management of diabetes in pregnancy. *Seminars in Perinatology, 18*(5), 432–450.

Persson, B., & Hanson, U. (1996). Fetal size at birth in relation to quality of blood glucose control in pregnancies complicated by pregestational diabetes mellitus. *British Journal of Obstetrics and Gynaecology, 103*(5), 427–433.

Pettitt, J., Ospina, P., Kolaczynski, J. W., Jovanovic, L. (2003). Comparison of an insulin analog, insulin aspart, and regular human insulin with no insulin in gestational diabetes mellitus. *Diabetes Care, 26*(1), 183–186.

Raychaudhuri, K., & Maresh, M. J. (2000). Glycemic control throughout pregnancy and fetal growth in insulin-dependent diabetes. *Obstetrics and Gynecology, 95*(2), 190–194.

Reece, E. A., & Homko, C. J. (1994). Infant of the diabetic mother. *Seminars in Perinatology, 18*(5), 459–469.

Reece, E. A., & Homko, C. J. (2000). Why do diabetic women deliver malformed infants? *Clinical Obstetrics and Gynecology, 43*(1), 32–45.

Reece, E. A., Homko, C. J., & Hagay, Z. (1995). When the pregnancy is complicated by diabetes. *Contemporary OB/GYN, 40*(7), 43–61.

Reece, E. A., Homko, C. J., & Hagay, Z. (1996). Diabetic retinopathy in pregnancy. *Obstetrics and Gynecology Clinics of North America, 23*(1), 161–171.

Rey, E., Attie, C., & Bonin, A. (1999). The effects of first-trimester diabetes control on the incidence of macrosomia. *American Journal of Obstetrics and Gynecology, 181*(1), 202–206.

Roland, J. M., Murphy, H. R., Fall, V., Northcot-Wright, J., & Temple, R. C. (2005). The pregnancies of women with type 2 diabetes: Poor outcomes but opportunities for improvement. *Diabetic Medicine, 22*(2), 1774–1777.

Rosenn, B. M., & Miodovnik, M. (2000a). Glycemic control in diabetic pregnancy: Is tighter always better? *Journal of Maternal Fetal Medicine, 9*(1), 29–34.

Rosenn, B. M., & Miodovnik, M. (2000b). Medical complications of diabetes mellitus in pregnancy. *Clinical Obstetrics and Gynecology, 43*(1), 17–31.

Schaefer-Graf, U. M., Songster, G., Xiang, A., Berkowitz, K., Buchanan, T. A., & Kjos, S.L. (1997). Congenital malformations in offspring of women with hyperglycemia first detected during pregnancy. *American Journal of Obstetrics and Gynecology, 177*(5), 1165–1171.

Sheffield, J. S., Butler-Koster, E. L., Casey, B. M., McIntire, D. D., & Leveno, K. J. (2002). Maternal diabetes mellitus and infant malformations. *Obstetrics and Gynecology, 100*(5), 925–930.

Shivvers, S. A., & Lucas, M. J. (1999). Gestational diabetes: Is the 50-g screening result > or = 200 mg/dL diagnostic? *Journal of Reproductive Medicine, 44*(8), 685–688.

Silver, R. M. (2007). Fetal death. *Obstetrics and Gynecology, 109*(1), 153–167.

Slocum, J. M., & Sosa, M. E. B. (2002). Use of antidiabetes agents in pregnancy: Current practice and controversy. *Journal of Perinatal and Neonatal Nursing, 16*(2), 40–53.

Tyrala, E. E. (1996). The infant of the diabetic mother. *Obstetric and Gynecology Clinics of North America, 23*(1), 221–241.

Uvena-Celebrezze, J., & Catalano, P. M. (2000). The infant of the woman with gestational diabetes mellitus. *Clinical Obstetrics and Gynecology, 43*(1), 127–139.

Vandermolen, D. T., Ratts, V. S., Evans, W. S., Stovall, D. W., Kauma, S. W., & Nestler, J.E. (2001). Metformin increases the ovulatory rate and pregnancy rate from clomiphene citrate in patients with polycystic ovary syndrome who are resistant to clomiphene citrate alone. *Fertility and Sterility, 75*(2), 310–315.

Walsh, J., & Roberts, R. (2006). *Pumping insulin* (4th ed) San Diego: Torrey Pines Press.

White, P. (1949). Pregnancy complicating diabetes. *American Journal of Medicine, 7,* 609.

Whiteman, V. E., Homko, C. J., & Reece, E. A. (1996). Management of hypoglycemia and diabetic ketoacidosis in pregnancy. *Obstetrics and Gynecology Clinics of North America, 23*(1), 87–107.

Wiznitzer, A., & Reece, E.A. (1999). Assessment and management of pregnancy complicated by pregestational diabetes mellitus. *Pediatric Annals, 28*(9), 605–613.

Woolderink, J. M., vanLoon, A. J., Storms, F., deHeide, L, & Hoogenber, K. (2005). Use of insulin glargine during pregnancy in seven type 1 diabetic women. *Diabetes Care, 28* (10), 2594–2595.

Cardiac Disease

American College of Cardiology/American Heart Association Task Force on Practice Guidelines, Society of Cardiovascular Anesthesiologists, Society for Cardiovascular Angiography and Interventions, Society of Thoracic Surgeons, Bonow, R. O., Carabello, B. A., et al. (2006). ACC/AHA 2006 guidelines for the management of patients with valvular heart disease: A report of the American College of Cardiology/American Heart Association task force on practice guidelines (writing committee to revise the 1998 guidelines for the management of patients with valvular heart disease): Developed in collaboration with the Society of Cardiovascular Anesthesiologists: endorsed by the Society for Cardiovascular Angiography and Interventions and the Society of Thoracic Surgeons. *Circulation, 114*(5), e84–e231.

American College of Obstetricians and Gynecologists. (2000). *Thromboembolism in pregnancy* (Practice Bulletin No. 29). Washington, DC: Author.

American College of Obstetricians and Gynecologists. (2001). *Chronic hypertension in pregnancy* (Practice Bulletin No. 29). Washington, DC: Author.

American College of Obstetricians and Gynecologists. (2002). *Safety of lovenox in pregnancy* (Committee Opinion No. 276). Washington, DC: Author.

American College of Obstetricians and Gynecologists. (2003). *Prophylactic antibiotics in labor and delivery* (Practice Bulletin No. 47). Washington, DC: Author.

American College of Obstetricians and Gynecologists. (2005). *Obesity in pregnancy* (Committee Opinion No. 315). Washington, DC: Author.

Arafeh, J. M., & Baird, S. M. (2006). Cardiac disease in pregnancy. *Critical Care Nursing Quarterly, 29*(1), 32–52.

Avila, W. S., Rossi, E. G., Ramires, J. A., Grinberg, M., Bortolotto, M. R., Zugaib, M., et al. (2004). Pregnancy in patients with cardiac disease: Experience with 1,000 cases. *Clinical Cardiology, 26*(3), 135–142.

Berg, C. J., Chang, J., Callaghan, W. M., & Whitehead, S. J. (2003). Pregnancy-related mortality in the United States, 1991-1997. *Obstetrics and Gynecology, 101*(2), 289–296.

Bestetti, R. B. (1989). Cardiac involvement in the acquired immune deficiency syndrome. *International Journal of Cardiology, 22*(2), 143–146.

Blackburn, S. (2003). *Maternal, fetal, & neonatal physiology: A clinical perspective.* St. Louis, MO: Saunders.

Blanchard, D., & Shabetai, R. (2004). Cardiac diseases. In R. Creasy, R. Resnick, & J. Iams (Eds.), *Maternal-fetal medicine: Principles & practice* (5th ed., pp. 815–844). Philadelphia, PA: Saunders.

Bruce, I. N., Urowitz, M. B., Gladman, D. D., & Hallet, D. C. (1999). Natural history of hypercholesterolemia in systemic lupus erythematosus. *Journal of Rheumatology, 26*(10), 2137–2143.

Chan, W. S., & Ray, J. G. (1999). Low molecular weight heparin use during pregnancy: Issues of safety and practicality. *Obstetrical and Gynecological Survey, 54*(10), 649–654.

Chang, J., Elam-Evans, L., Berg, C., Herndon, J., Flowers, L., Seed, K., & Syverson, C. (2003). Pregnancy-related mortality Surveillance, United States, 1991–1999. *Morbidity and Mortality Weekly Report, 52*(2), 1–8.

Christiansen, L. R., & Collins, K. A. (2006). Pregnancy-related deaths: A 15 year retrospective study and overall review of maternal pathophysiology. *American Journal of Forensic Medicine and Pathology, 27*(1), 11–19.

Clark, S., Cotton, D., Hankins, G., & Phelan, J. (2003). *Critical care obstetrics* (4th ed.). Malden, MA: Blackwell Science.

Criteria Committee of the New York Heart Association. (1979). *Nomenclature and criteria for diagnosis of diseases of the heart and great vessels* (8th ed.). New York: New York Heart Association.

Curran, C. (2002) Multiple organ dysfunction syndrome in the obstetrical population. *Journal of Perinatal & Neonatal Nursing, 15*(4): 37–55.

deSwiet, M. (1993). Maternal mortality from heart disease in pregnancy. *British Heart Journal, 69*(6), 524.

Earing, M. G., & Webb, G. D. (2005). Congenital heart disease and pregnancy: Maternal and fetal risks. *Clinics in Perinatology, 32*(4), 913–919.

Elkayam, U., Ostrzega, E., Shotan, A., & Mehra, A. (1995). Cardiovascular problems in pregnant women with the Marfan syndrome. *Annals of Internal Medicine 123*(2), 117–122.

Felblinger, D. M., & Akers, M. C. (1998). Marfan's syndrome in pregnancy: Implications for advanced practice nurses. *AACN Clinical Issues, 9*(4), 563–568.

Ginsberg, J. S., & Hirsh, J. (1995). Use of antithrombotic agents during pregnancy. *Chest, 108*(4, Suppl.), 305S–311S.

Hansen, J. P. (1986). Older maternal age in pregnancy outcome: A review of the literature. *Obstetrical and Gynecological Survey, 41*(11), 726–742.

Harvey, M. (1999). Physiologic changes during pregnancy. In L. K. Mandeville & N. H. Troiano (Eds.), *AWHONN's High-risk intrapartum nursing* (2nd ed, pp 2–31). Philadelphia, PA: Lippincott.

Hedley, A., Ogden, C., Johnson, C., Carroll, M., Curtin, L., & Flegal, K. (2004). Prevalence of overweight and obesity among US children, adolescents, and adults, 1999-2002. *Journal of the American Medical Association, 291*(23), 2847–2850.

Hoffman, J. I. (1995). Incidence of congenital heart disease: II. Perinatal incidence. *Pediatric Cardiology, 16*(4), 155–165.

Hogberg, U., Innala, E., & Sandstrom, A. (1994). Maternal mortality in Sweden, 1980–1988. *Obstetrics and Gynecology, 84*(2), 240–244.

Homans, D. C. (1985). Peripartum cardiomyopathy. *New England Journal of Medicine, 312*(23), 1432–1437.

Horon, I. L. (2005). Underreporting of maternal deaths on death certificates and the magnitude of the problem of maternal mortality. *American Journal of Public Health, 95*(3), 478–482.

Kafka, H., Johnson, M. R., & Gatzoulis, M. A. (2006). The team approach to pregnancy and congenital heart disease. *Cardiology Clinics, 24*(4), 587–605.

Key, T. C., Resnik, R., Dittrich, H. C., & Reisner, L., (1989). Successful pregnancy following cardiac transplantation. *American Journal of Obstetrics and Gynecology, 160*(2), 356–361.

Klein, L. L., & Galan, H. L. (2005). Cardiac disease in pregnancy. *Obstetrics and Gynecology Clinics of North America, 31*(2), 429–459.

Kossoy, L., Herbert, C., & Wentz, A. (1988). Management of heart transplant recipients: Guidelines for obstetrician-gynecologist. *American Journal of Obstetrics and Gynecology, 159*(2), 490–499.

Linker, D. (2001). *Practical echocardiography of congenital heart disease from fetal to adult.* New York: Churchill Livingstone.

Luppi, C. J. (1999). Cardiopulmonary resuscitation in pregnancy. In L. K. Mandeville & N. H. Troiano (Eds.), *High risk intrapartum and critical care nursing* (2nd ed., pp. 353–379). Philadelphia: Lippincott Williams & Wilkins.

Marx, G. F., Schwalbe, S. S., Cho, E., & Whitty, J. E. (1993). Automated blood pressure measurements in laboring women: Are they reliable? *American Journal of Obstetrics and Gynecology, 168*(3, Pt. 1), 796–798.

Mayberry, L., Gennaro, S., Strange, L., Lee, L., Heisler, D., & Nielsen-Smith, K. (2000). *Second stage labor management: Promotion of evidence-based practice and a collaborative approach to patient care* (Practice Monograph). Washington, DC: Association of Women's Health, Obstetric, & Neonatal Nursing.

Mayet, J., Steer, P., & Somerville, J. (1998). Marfan syndrome, aortic dilatation, and pregnancy. *Obstetrics and Gynecology, 92* (4, Pt. 2), 713.

McMinn, T. R., Jr., & Ross, J., Jr. (1995). Hereditary dilated cardiomyopathy. *Clinical Cardiology, 18*(1), 7–15.

NIH Working Group Report on High Blood Pressure in Pregnancy. (2000). *National high blood pressure education program.* National Institute of Health National Heart, Lung, and Blood Institute: No. 00–3029.

Patton, D. E., Lee, W., Cotton, D. B., Miller, J., Carpenter, R. J., Jr., Huhta, J., & Hankins, G. (1990). Cyanotic maternal heart disease in pregnancy. *Obstetrical and Gynecological Survey, 45*(9), 594–600.

Pearson, G. D., Veille, J. C., Rahimtoola, S., Hsia, J., Oakley, C. M., Hosenpud, J. D., et al. (2000). Peripartum cardiomyopathy: National Heart, Lung, and Blood Institute and Office of Rare Diseases (National Institutes of Health) workshop recommendations and review. *Journal of the American Medical Association, 283*(9), 1183–1188.

Ralston, D. H., Shnider, S. M., & DeLorimier, A. A. (1974). Effects of equipotent ephedrine, metaraminol, mephentermine and methoxamine on uterine blood flow in the pregnant ewe. *Anesthesiology, 40*(4), 354–370.

Ratnoff, O. D., & Kaufman, R. (1982). Arterial thrombosis in oral contraceptive users. *Archives of Internal Medicine, 142*(3), 447–448.

Rerkpattanapipat, P., Wongpraparut, N., Jacods, L. E., & Kotler, M. N. (2000). Cardiac manifestations of acquired immunodeficiency syndrome. *Archives of Internal Medicine, 160*(5), 602–608.

Roth, A., & Elkayam, U. (1996). Acute myocardial infarction associated with pregnancy. *Annals of Internal Medicine; 125*(9), 751–762.

Shnider, S. M., DeLorimier, A. A., Holl, J. W., Chapler, F. K., & Morishima, H. O. (1968). Vasopressors in obstetrics: Correction of fetal acidosis with ephedrine during spinal hypotension. *American Journal of Obstetrics and Gynecology, 102*(7), 911–919.

Silver, R. M. (2007). Fetal death. *Obstetrics and Gynecology, 109*(1), 153–167.

Simon, A., Sadovshy, E., Aboulafia, Y., Ohel, G., & Zajicek, G. (1986). Fetal activity in pregnancies complicated by rheumatic heart disease. *Journal of Perinatal Medicine, 14*(5), 331–334.

Simpson, K. R. (2006). Critical illness during pregnancy: Considerations for evaluation and treatment of the fetus as the second patient. *Critical Care Nursing Quarterly, 29*(1), 19–31.

Siu, S. C., Sermer, M., Colman, J. M., Alvarez, A. N., Mercier, L. A., Morton, B. C., et al. (2001). Prospective multicenter study of pregnancy outcomes in women with heart disease. *Circulation, 104*(5), 515–521.

Sui, S. C., Colman, J. M., Sorensen, S., Smallhorn, J. F., Farine, D., Amankwah, K. S., et al. (2002). Adverse neonatal and cardiac outcomes are more common in pregnant women with cardiac disease. *Circulation, 105*(18), 2179–2184.

Thorne, S. (2004). Pregnancy in heart disease: Congenital heart disease. *Heart, 90*(4), 450–456.

Torgersen, K., & Curran, C. (2006). A systematic approach to the physiologic adaptations of pregnancy. *Critical Care Nursing Quarterly, 29*(1), 2–18.

Troiano, N. (1999). Invasive hemodynamic monitoring in obstetrics. In L. K. Mandeville & N. H. Troiano (Eds.), *AWHONN's high-risk intrapartum nursing* (2nd ed, pp. 66–83), Philadelphia, PA: Lippincott Company.

Venes, D., & Thomas, C. (Eds.). (2001). *Taber's Cyclopedic Medical Dictionary* (19th ed.). Philadelphia, PA: F. A. Davis Company.

Weis, M., & von Scheidt, W. (2000). Coronary artery disease in the transplanted heart. *Annual Review of Medicine, 51*, 81–100.

Weitz, J. I. (1997). Low molecular weight heparins. *New England Journal of Medicine, 337*(10), 688–698.

Whitty, J. (2002). Maternal cardiac arrest in pregnancy. *Clinical Obstetrics and Gynecology, 45*(2), 377–392.

Pulmonary Complications

Alexander, S., Dodds, L., & Armson, B. A. (1998). Perinatal outcomes in women with asthma during pregnancy. *Obstetrics and Gynecology, 92*(3), 435–440.

American College of Obstetricians and Gynecology. (2000a). *Prevention of deep vein thrombosis and pulmonary embolism* (Practice Bulletin No. 21). Washington, DC: Author.

American College of Obstetricians and Gynecology. (2000b). *Thromboembolism in pregnancy* (Practice Bulletin No. 19). Washington, DC: Author.

American College of Obstetricians and Gynecologists & American College of Allergy, Asthma and Immunology. (2000). The use of newer asthma and allergy medications during pregnancy (Position Statement). *Annals of Allergy, Asthma, and Immunology, 84*(5), 475–480.

Balducci, J., Rodis, J. F., Rosengren, S., Vintezileos, A. M., Spivey, G., & Vosselles, C. (1992). Pregnancy outcome following first-trimester varicella infection. *Obstetrics and Gynecology, 79*(1), 5–6.

Beckman, C. A. (2003). The effects of asthma on pregnancy and perinatal outcomes. *Journal of Asthma, 40*(2), 171–180.

Blaiss, M. S. (2004). Management of asthma during pregnancy. *Allergy and Asthma Proceedings, 25*(6), 375–379.

Briggs, G. G., Freeman, R. K., & Yaffe, S. J. (2005). *Drugs in Pregnancy and lactation* (7th ed.). Philadelphia: Lippincott Williams & Wilkins.

Chambers, C. (2006). Safety of asthma and allergy medications in pregnancy. *Immunology and Allergy Clinics of North America, 26*(1), 13–28.

Chandra, P. C., Patel, H., Schiavello, H. J., & Briggs, S. L. (1998). Successful pregnancy outcome after complicated varicella pneumonia. *Obstetrics and Gynecology, 92*(4, Pt. 2), 680–682.

Chang, J., Elam-Evans, L., Berg, C., Herndon, J., Flowers, L., Seed, K., & Syverson, C. (2003). Pregnancy-related mortality surveillance, United States, 1991-1999. *Morbidity and Mortality Weekly Report, 52*(2), 1–8.

Chapman, S. J. (1998). Varicella in pregnancy. *Seminars in Perinatology, 22*(4), 339–346.

Coleman, M. T., & Rund, D. A. (1997). Nonobstetric conditions causing hypoxia during pregnancy: Asthma and epilepsy. *American Journal of Obstetrics and Gynecology, 177*(1), 1–7.

Cousins, L. (1999). Fetal oxygenation, assessment of fetal well-being, and obstetric management of the pregnant patient with asthma. *Journal of Allergy and Clinical Immunology, 103*(2, Pt. 2), S343–S349.

Cydulka, R. K. (2006). Acute asthma during pregnancy. *Immunology and Allergy Clinics of North America, 26*(1), 103–117.

Dombrowski, M. P. (1997). Pharmacologic therapy of asthma during pregnancy. *Obstetrics and Gynecology Clinics of North America, 24*(3), 559–574.

Dombrowski, M. P. (2006). Outcomes of pregnancy in asthmatic women. *Immunology and Allergy Clinics of North America, 26*(1), 81–92.

Ellegard, E. K. (2006). Pregnancy rhinitis. *Immunology and Allergy Clinics of North America, 26*(1), 119–135.

Gardner, M. O., & Doyle, N. M. (2004). Asthma in pregnancy. *Obstetrics and Gynecology Clinics of North America, 31*(2), 385–413.

Gluck, J. C., & Gluck, P. A. (2006). The effect of pregnancy on the course of asthma. *Immunology and Allergy Clinics of North America, 26*(1), 63–80.

Goodnight, W. H., & Soper, D. E. (2005). Pneumonia in pregnancy. *Critical Care Medicine, 33*(10), S390–S397.

Grant, A. (1996). Varicella infection and toxoplasmosis in pregnancy. *Journal of Perinatal and Neonatal Nursing, 10*(2), 17–29.

Harger, J. H., Ernest, J. M., Thurnau, G. R., Moawald, A., Momirova, V., Landon, M. B., et al. (2002). Risk factor and outcome of varicella-zoster pneumonia in pregnant women. *Journal of Infectious Disease, 185*(4), 422–427.

Kallen, B., Rydhstroem, H., & Aberg, A. (2000). Asthma during pregnancy: A population based study. *European Journal of Epidemiology, 16*(2), 167–171.

Kwon, H. L., Belanger, K., & Bracken, M. B. (2003). Effect of pregnancy and stage of pregnancy on asthma severity: A systematic review. *American Journal of Obstetrics and Gynecology, 190*(5), 1201–1210.

Kwon, H. L., Triche, E. W., Belanger, K., & Bracken, M. B. (2006). The epidemiology of asthma during pregnancy: Prevalence, diagnosis and symptoms. *Immunology and Allergy Clinics of North America, 26*(1), 29–62.

Lam, C. M., Wong, S. F., Leung, T. N., Chow, K. M., Yu, W. C., Wong, T. Y., et al. (2004). A case-controlled study comparing clinical course and outcomes of pregnant and non-pregnant women with severe acute respiratory syndrome. *British Journal of Obstetrics and Gynaecology, 111*(8), 771–774.

Laibl, V. R., & Sheffield, J. S. (2005). Influenza and pneumonia in pregnancy. *Clinics in Perinatology, 32* (2), 727–738.

Laibl, V. R., & Sheffield, J. S. (2006). The management of respiratory infections during pregnancy. *Immunology and Allergy Clinics of North America, 26*(1), 155–172.

Lim, W. S., Macfarlane, J. T., & Colthorpe C. L. (2001). Pneumonia and pregnancy. *Thorax, 56*(5), 398–405.

Maccato, M. L. (1991). Respiratory insufficiency due to pneumonia in pregnancy. *Obstetrics and Gynecology Clinics of North America, 18*(2), 289–299.

Madinger, N. E. Greenspoon, J. S., & Ellrodt, A. G. (1989). Pneumonia during pregnancy: Has modern technology improved maternal and fetal outcome? *American Journal of Obstetrics and Gynecology, 161*(3), 657–662.

Minerbi-Codish, I., Fraser, D., Avnun, L., Glezerman, M., & Heimer, D. (1998). Influence of asthma in pregnancy on labor and the newborn. *Respiration, 65*(20), 130–135.

Munn, M. B., Groome, L. J., Atterbury, J. L., Baker, S. L., & Hoff, C. (1999). Pneumonia as a complication of pregnancy. *Journal of Maternal-Fetal Medicine, 8*(4), 151–154.

Namazy, J. A., & Schatz, M. (2006). Current guidelines for the management of asthma during pregnancy. *Immunology and Allergy Clinics of North America, 26*(1), 93–102.

National Asthma Education and Prevention Program. (2005). *Working group report on managing asthma during pregnancy: Recommendations for pharmacologic treatment-update 2004.* (NIH Publication 05-3279). Washington, DC: United States Department of Health and Human Services.

National Heart, Lung, and Blood Institute National Asthma Education Program Working Group on Asthma and Pregnancy. (1993). *Management of asthma during pregnancy* (NIH Pub. No. 93-3279). Washington, DC: Department of Health and Human Services.

Neu, H. C., & Sabath, L. D. (1993). Criteria for selecting oral antibiotic therapy for common acquired pneumonia. *Infectious Medicine, 10*(Suppl. 2), 33S.

Nolan, T. E., & Hankins, G. D. V. (1995). Acute pulmonary dysfunction and distress. *Obstetrics and Gynecology Clinics of North America, 22*(1), 39–54.

Pereira, A., & Krieger, B. (2004). Pulmonary complications of pregnancy. *Clinics in Chest Medicine, 25*(2), 299–310.

Ramsey, P. S., & Ramin, K. D. (2001). Pneumonia in pregnancy. *Obstetrics and Gynecology Clinics, 28*(3), 1–11.

Salmon, B., & Bruick-Sorge, C. (2003). Pneumonia in pregnant women. *AWHONN Lifelines, 7*(1), 48–52.

Schatz, M. (2001). The efficacy and safety of asthma medications during pregnancy. *Seminars in Perinatology, 25*(3), 145–152.

Scheffer, A. L. (1991). Guidelines for the diagnosis and management of asthma (National Heart, Lung, and Blood Institute, National Asthma Education Program, Expert Panel Report). *Journal of Allergy and Clinical Immunology, 88*(3, Pt. 2), 425–534.

Silver, R. M. (2007). Fetal death. *Obstetrics and Gynecology, 109*(1), 153–167.

Simpson, K. R., & James, D. C. (2005). Efficacy of intrauterine resuscitation techniques in improving fetal oxygen status during labor. *Obstetrics and Gynecology, 105*(6), 1362–1368.

Stone, S. E., & Morris, T. A. (2004). Pulmonary embolism and pregnancy. *Critical Care Clinics, 20*(4), 661–677.

Towers, C. V., Briggs, G. G., & Rojas, J. A. (2004). The use of prostaglandin E2 in pregnant patients with asthma. *American Journal of Obstetrics and Gynecology, 190*(6), 1777–1780.

Wise, R. A., Polito, A. J., & Krishman, V. (2006). Respiratory physiologic changes in pregnancy. *Immunology and Allergy Clinics of North America, 26*(1), 1–12.

Wong, S. F., Chow, K. M., Leung, T. N., Ng, W. F., Ng, W. F., Shek, C. C., et al. (2004). Pregnancy and perinatal outcomes of women with severe acute respiratory syndrome. *American Journal of Obstetrics and Gynecology, 191*(1), 292–297.

Yost, N. P., Bloom, S. L., Richey, S. D., Ramin, S. M., & Cunningham, F. G. (2000). An appraisal of treatment guidelines for Antepartum community-acquired pneumonia. *American Journal of Obstetrics and Gynecology, 183*(1), 131, 135.

Multiple Gestation

Abma, J., Chandra, A., Mosher, W., Peterson, L., & Piccinino, L. (1997). Fertility, family planning, and women's health: New data from the 1995 National Survey of Family Growth. *Vital and Health Statistics, 23*(19), 1–125.

Allen, V. M., Windrim, R., Barrett, J., & Ohlsson. A. (2001). Management of monoamniotic twin pregnancies: A case series and systematic review of the literature. *BJOG: An International Journal of Obstetrics and Gynaecology, 108*(9) 931–936.

American Academy of Pediatrics (AAP) Task Force on Sudden Infant Death Syndrome. (2005). The changing concept of sudden infant death syndrome: diagnostic coding shifts, controversies regarding the sleeping environment, and new variables to consider in reducing risk. *Pediatrics, 116*(5), 1245–1255.

American Academy of Pediatrics & American College of Obstetricians and Gynecologists. (2002). *Guidelines for perinatal care* (5th ed.). Elk Grove Village, IL: Author.

American College of Obstetricians and Gynecologists. Task Force on Cesarean Delivery Rates. (2000). *Evaluation of cesarean delivery*. Washington, DC: Author.

American College of Obstetricians and Gynecologists. (2004a). *Multiple gestations: Complicated twin, triplet, and high-order multifetal pregnancy* (Practice Bulletin No. 56). Washington, DC: Author.

American College of Obstetrics and Gynecology. (2004b). *Nausea and vomiting of pregnancy.* (Practice Bulletin No. 52). Washington, DC: Author.

American College of Obstetrics and Gynecology. (2005) *Intrapartum fetal heart rate monitoring.* (Practice Bulletin No. 70). Washington, DC: Author.

Ananth, C. V., Joseph, K. S., & Kinzler, W. L. (2004). The influence of obstetric intervention on trends in twin stillbirths: United States, 1989-99. *The Journal of Maternal-Fetal & Neonatal Medicine, 15*(6), 380–387.

Bakker, P. C., Colenbrander, G. J., Verstraeten, A. A., & Van Geijn, H. P. (2004). Quality of intrapartum cardiotocography in twin deliveries. *American Journal of Obstetrics and Gynecology 191*(6), 2114–2119.

Ball, H. L. (2002). Sleeping arrangements in twin infants. *Final project report prepared for the foundation for the study of infant deaths* (Project 237). Retrieved February 12, 2006, from http://www.dur.ac.uk/sleep.lab/Sleeping%20arrangements%20in%20twin%20infants%20%20formatted[1].pdf

Ballabh, P., Kumari, J., AlKouatly, H. B., Yih, M., Arevalo, R., Rosenwaks, Z., et al. (2003). Neonatal outcome of triplet versus twin and singleton pregnancies: a matched case control study.

European Journal of Obstetrics, Gynecology, and Reproductive Biology, 107(1), 28–36.

Barrett, J. F. R. (2004). Delivery of the term twin. *Best Practice & Research Clinical Obstetrics & Gynaecology, 18*(4), 625–630.

Beck, C. T. (2002). Releasing the pause button: mothering twins during the first year of life. *Qualitative Health Research, 12*(5), 593–608.

Ben-Haroush, A., Yogev, Y., & Hod, M. (2003). Epidemiology of gestational diabetes mellitus and its association with Type 2 diabetes. *Diabetic Medicine, 21*(2), 103–113.

Bergh, C., Möller, A., Nilsson, L., & Wikland, M. (1999). Obstetrical outcome and psychological follow-up of pregnancies after embryo reduction. *Human Reproduction, 14*(8), 2170–2175.

Biancuzzo, M. (2003). *Breastfeeding the newborn: Strategies for nurses* (2nd ed.). St. Louis: Mosby.

Bleyl, J. (2002). Familial and psychological reaction in triplet families. In L. G. Keith & I. Blickstein (Eds.), *Triplet pregnancies and their consequences* (pp. 361–369). New York: The Parthenon Publishing Group.

Blickstein, I. (2001). The risk of cerebral palsy after assisted reproductive technologies. In I. Blickstein & L. G. Keith (Eds.). *Iatrogenic multiple pregnancy: Clinical implications* (p. 26). New York: The Parthenon Publishing Group.

Blickstein, I. (2005). Estimation of iatrogenic monozygotic twinning rate following assisted reproduction: Pitfalls and caveats. *American Journal of Obstetrics and Gynecology, 192*(2), 365–368.

Blickstein, I., Jones, C., & Keith, L. G. (2003). Zygotic-splitting rates after single-embryo transfers in in vitro fertilization. *New England Journal of Medicine, 348*(23), 2366–2367.

Blickstein, I., Shinwell, E. S., Lusky, A., & Reichman, B., & Israel Neonatal Network. (2005). Plurality-dependent risk of respiratory distress syndrome among very-low-birth-weight infants and antepartum corticosteroid treatment. *American Journal of Obstetrics and Gynecology, 192,* 360–364.

Bomsel-Helmerich, O., & Al Mufti, W. (1995). The mechanism of monozygosity and double ovulation. In L. G. Keith, E. Papiernik, D. M. Keith, & B. Luke (Eds.), *Multiple pregnancy: epidemiology, gestation and perinatal outcome* (pp. 25–40). New York: The Parthenon Publishing Group.

Bowers, N. A., & Gromada, K. K. (2006). *Care of the multiple-birth family: Pregnancy and birth* (Nursing Module). White Plains, NY: March of Dimes Birth Defects Foundation.

British Columbia Reproductive Care Program. (2006). *Breastfeeding multiples, nutrition, Part III.* Retrieved December 11, 2006, from http://www.rcp.gov.bc.ca/guidelines/General/Gen3CBreastfeedingMultiplesNovember2006.pdf

Brown, J. E., & Carlson, M. (2000). Nutrition and multifetal pregnancy. *Journal of the American Dietetic Association, 100*(3), 343–348.

Bryan, E. (2002). Educating families, before, during and after a multiple birth. *Seminars in Neonatology, 7*(3), 241–246.

Bryan, E. (2005). Psychological aspects of prenatal diagnosis and its implications in multiple pregnancies. *Prenatal Diagnosis, 25*(9), 827–834.

Bush, M. C., & Malone, F. D. (2005). Down syndrome screening in twins. *Clinics in Perinatology, 32*(2), 373–386.

Cahill, A., Stamilio, D. M., Pare, E., Peipert, J. P., Stevens, E. J., Nelson, D. B., et al. (2005). Vaginal birth after cesarean (VBAC) attempt in twin pregnancies: Is it safe? *American Journal of Obstetrics and Gynecology, 193*(3 Pt 2), 1050–1055.

Chasen, S. T., Spiro, S. J., Kalish, R. B., & Chervenak, F. A. (2005). Changes in fetal presentation in twin pregnancies. *The Journal of Maternal-Fetal and Neonatal Medicine, 17*(1), 45–48.

Child, T. J., Henderson, A. M., & Tan, S. L. (2004). The desire for multiple pregnancy in male and female infertility patients. *Human Reproduction, 19*(3), 558–561.

Chitkara, U., & Berkowitz, R. L. (2002). Multiple gestations. In S. G. Gabbe, J. R. Niebyl, & J. L. Simpson (Eds.), *Obstetrics: Nor-*

mal and problem pregnancies (4th ed., pp. 827–867). Philadelphia: Churchill Livingstone.

Cleary-Goldman, J., D'Alton, M. E., & Berkowitz, R. L. (2005). Prenatal diagnosis and multiple pregnancy. *Seminars in Perinatology, 29*(5), 312–320.

Collopy, K. S. (2004). "I couldn't think that far": Infertile women's decision making about multifetal reduction. *Research in Nursing & Health, 27*(2), 75–86.

Conde-Agudelo, A., Belizan, J. M., & Lindmark, G. (2000). Maternal morbidity and mortality associated with multiple gestations. *Obstetrics and Gynecology, 95*(6 Pt 1), 899–904.

Cristinelli, S., Fresson, J., André, M., & Monnier-Barbarino, P. (2005). Management of delayed-interval delivery in multiple gestations. *Fetal Diagnosis and Therapy, 20*(4), 285–290.

Crowther, C.A. (1999). Multiple pregnancy. In D. K. James, P. J. Steer, C. P. Weiner, & B. Gonik (Eds.), *High risk pregnancy: Management options* (pp. 129–151). London: Harcourt Brace and Company Limited.

D'Alton, M. (2004). Infertility and the desire for multiple births. *Fertility and Sterility, 81*(3), 523–525.

Damato, E. G. (2004a). Prenatal attachment and other correlates of postnatal maternal attachment to twins. *Advances in Neonatal Care, 4*(5), 274–291.

Damato, E. G. (2004b). Predictors of prenatal attachment in mothers of twins. *Journal of Obstetric, Gynecologic and Neonatal Nursing, 33*(4), 436–445.

Damato, E. G., Dowling, D. A., Madigan, E. A., & Thanattherakul, C. (2005). Duration of breastfeeding for mothers of twins. *Journal of Obstetric, Gynecologic and Neonatal Nursing, 34*(2), 201–209.

Damato, E. G., Dowling, D. A., Standing, T. S., & Schuster, S. D. (2005). Explanation for cessation of breastfeeding in mothers of twins. *Journal of Human Lactation, 21*(3), 296–304.

Day, M. C., Barton, J. R., O'Brien, J. M., Istwan, N. B., & Sibai, B. M. (2005). The effect of fetal number on the development of hypertensive conditions of pregnancy. *Obstetrics and Gynecology, 106*(5 Pt 1), 927–931.

Derom, R., Derom, C., & Vlietinck, R. (1995). Placentation. In L. G. Keith, E. Papiernik, D. M. Keith, & B. Luke (Eds.), *Multiple pregnancy: Epidemiology, gestation and perinatal outcome.* (pp. 113–128). New York: The Parthenon Publishing Group.

Dickey, R. P., Taylor, S. N., Lu, P. Y., Sartor, B. M., Storment, J. M., Rye, P. H. et al. (2002). Spontaneous reduction of multiple pregnancy: Incidence and effect on outcome. *American Journal of Obstetrics and Gynecology, 186*(1), 77–83.

Dodd, J. M., & Crowther, C. A. (2003). Elective delivery of women with a twin pregnancy from 37 weeks gestation. *Cochrane Database of Systemic Reviews, (1),* CD003582.

Dodd, J. M., & Crowther, C. A. (2005a). Evidence-based care of women with a multiple pregnancy. *Best Practice & Research Clinical Obstetrics and Gynaecology, 19*(1), 131–153.

Dodd, J. M., & Crowther, C. A. (2005b). Hospitalisation for bed rest for women with a triplet pregnancy: An abandoned randomised controlled trial and meta-analysis. *BMC Pregnancy and Childbirth, 5*:8. Retrieved on January 23, 2005, from http://www.biomedcentral.com/1471-2393/5/8

Eganhouse, D. J., & Peterson, L. A. (1998). Fetal surveillance in multifetal pregnancy. *Journal of Obstetric, Gynecologic and Neonatal Nursing, 27*(3), 312–321.

Elkayam, U., Akhter, M. W., Singh, H., Khan, S., Bitar, F., Hameed, A., et al. (2005). Pregnancy-associated cardiomyopathy: Clinical characteristics and a comparison between early and late presentation. *Circulation. 111*(16), 2050–2055.

Elling, S. V., McKenna, P., & Powell, F. C. (2000). Pruritic urticarial papules and plaques of pregnancy in twin and triplet pregnancies. *Journal of the European Academy of Dermatology & Venereology, 14*(5), 378–381.

Ellison, M. A., & Hall, J. E. (2003). Social stigma and compounded losses: Quality-of-life issues for multiple-birth families. *Fertility and Sterility, 80*(2), 405–414.

Ellison, M. A., Hotamisligil, S., Lee, H., Rich-Edwards, J. W., Pang, S. C., & Hall, J. E. (2005). Psychosocial risks associated with multiple births resulting from assisted reproduction. *Fertility and Sterility, 83*(5), 1422–1428.

Elliott, J. P. (2005a). Management of high-order multiple gestations. *Clinics in Perinatology, 32*(2), 387–402.

Elliott, J. P. (2005b). Preterm labor in twins and high-order multiples. *Obstetrics and Gynecology Clinics, 32*(3), 429–439.

Elliott, J. P., & Radin, T. G. (1995). The effect of corticosteroid administration on uterine activity and preterm labor in high-order multiple gestations. *Obstetrics and Gynecology, 85*(2), 250–254.

Evans, M. I., Ciorica, D., Britt, D. W., & Fletcher, J. C. (2005). Update on selective reduction. *Prenatal Diagnosis, 25*(9), 807–813.

Evans, M. I., Kaufman, M. I., Urban, A. J., Krivchenia, E. L., Britt, D. W., & Wapner. R. J. (2004). Fetal reduction from twins to a singleton: a reasonable consideration. *Obstetrics and Gynecology, 104*(1), 102–109.

Feldman, D. M., Borgida, A. F., Trymbulak, W. P., Barsoom, M. J., Sanders, M. M., & Rodis, J. F. (2002). Clinical implications of velamentous cord insertion in triplet gestations. *American Journal of Obstetrics and Gynecology, 186*(4), 809–811.

Feldman, R., & Eidelman, A. I. (2004). Parent–infant synchrony and the social–emotional development of triplets. *Developmental Psychology, 40*(6), 1133–1147.

Fell, D. B., Dodds, L., Joseph, K. S., Allen, V. M., & Butler, B. (2006). Risk factors for hyperemesis gravidarum requiring hospital admission during pregnancy. *Obstetrics and Gynecology, 107*(2 Pt. 1), 277–284.

Fesenmeier, M. F., Coppage, K. H., Lambers, D. S., Barton, J. R., & Sibai, B. M. (2005). Acute fatty liver of pregnancy in 3 tertiary care centers. *American Journal of Obstetrics and Gynecology, 192*(5), 1416–1419.

Fox, C., Kilby, M. D., & Khan, K. S. (2005). Contemporary treatments for twin-twin transfusion syndrome. *Obstetrics and Gynecology, 105*(6), 1469–1477.

Francois, K., Ortiz, J., Harris, C., Foley, M. R., & Elliott, J. P. (2005). Is peripartum hysterectomy more common in multiple gestations? *Obstetrics and Gynecology, 105*(6), 1369–1372.

Freda, M. C. (2000). Educational interventions in high-risk pregnancy. In W. R. Cohen (Ed.), *Cherry and Merkatz's complications of pregnancy* (pp. 177–184). Philadelphia: Lippincott Williams & Wilkins.

Friedman, E. A., & Sachtleben, M. R. (1964). The effect of uterine overdistention on labor: Multiple pregnancy. *Obstetrics and Gynecology, 23,* 164–172.

Galea, P., Jain, V., & Fisk, N. M. (2005). Insights into the pathophysiology of twin-twin transfusion syndrome. *Prenatal Diagnosis, 25*(9), 777–785.

Garite, T. J., Clark, R. H., Elliott, J. P., & Thorp, J. A. (2004). Twins and triplets: the effect of plurality and growth on neonatal outcome compared with singleton infants. *American Journal of Obstetrics and Gynecology, 191*(3), 700–707.

Getahun, D., Demissie, K., Lu, S. E., & Rhoads, G. G. (2004). Sudden infant death syndrome among twin births: United States, 1995–1998. *Journal of Perinatology, 24*(9), 544–551.

Gibson, J. L., Macara, L. M., Owen, P., Young, D., Macauley, J., & Mackenzie. F. (2004). Prediction of preterm delivery in twin pregnancy: A prospective, observational study of cervical length and fetal fibronectin testing. *Ultrasound in Obstetrics and Gynecology, 23*(6), 561–566.

Glantz, A., Marschall, H. U., & Mattsson, L. A. (2004). Intrahepatic cholestasis of pregnancy: Relationships between bile acid levels and fetal complication rates. *Hepatology, 40*(2), 467–474.

Goldenberg, R. L., Iams, J. D., Miodovnik, M., Van Dorsten, J. P., Thurnau, G., Bottoms, S., et al. (1996). The preterm prediction study: Risk factors in twin gestations. National Institute of Child Health and Human Development Maternal-Fetal Medicine Units Network. *American Journal of Obstetrics and Gynecology, 175*(4 Pt. 1), 1047–1053.

Graham, 3rd, G. M., & Gaddipati, S. (2005). Diagnosis and management of obstetrical complications unique to multiple gestations. *Seminars in Perinatology, 29*(5), 282–295.

Gromada, K. K., & Bowers, N. A. (2005). *Care of the multiple-birth family: Postpartum through infancy* (Nursing Module). New York: March of Dimes Birth Defects Foundation.

Groothuis, J. R., Altemeier, W. A., Robarge, J. P., O'Connor, S., Sandler, H., Vietze, P., et al. (1982). Increased child abuse in families with twins. *Pediatrics, 70*(5), 769–773.

Guzman, E. R., Walters, C., O'Reilly-Green, C., Meirowitz, N. B., Gipson, K., Nigam, J., et al. (2000). Use of cervical ultrasonography in prediction of spontaneous preterm birth in triplet gestations. *American Journal of Obstetrics and Gynecology, 183*(5), 1108–1113.

Gyamfi, C., Stone, J., & Eddleman, K.A. (2005). Maternal complications of multifetal pregnancy. *Clinics in Perinatology, 32*(2), 431–442.

Hanley, M. L., Ananth, C. V., Shen-Schwarz, S., Smulian, J. C., Lai, Y. L., & Vintzileos, A. M. (2002). Placental cord insertion and birth weight discordancy in twin gestations. *Obstetrics and Gynecology, 99*(3), 477-482.

Hardardottir, H., Kelly, K., Bork, M. D., Cusick, W., Campbell, W. A., & Rodis, J. F. (1996). Atypical presentation of preeclampsia in high-order multifetal gestations. *Obstetrics and Gynecology, 87*(3), 370–374.

Harkness, U. F., & Crombleholme, T. M. (2005). Twin–twin transfusion syndrome: Where do we go from here? *Seminars in Perinatology, 29*(5), 296–304.

Healy, A. J., & Gaddipati, S. (2005). Intrapartum management of twins: truths and controversies. *Clinics in Perinatology, 32*(2), 455–473.

Hediger, M. L., Luke, B., Gonzalez-Quintero, V. H., Martin, D., Nugent, C., Witter, F. R., et al. (2006). Fetal growth rates and the very preterm delivery of twins. *American Journal of Obstetrics and Gynecology, 193*(4), 1498–1507.

Helmerhorst, F. M., Perquin, D. A., Donker, D., & Keirse, M. J. (2004). Perinatal outcome of singletons and twins after assisted conception: A systematic review of controlled studies. *British Medical Journal, 328*(7434), 261–266.

Hogle, K. L., Hutton, E. K., McBrien, K. A., Barrett, J. F., & Hannah, M. E. (2003). Cesarean delivery for twins: A systematic review and meta-analysis. *American Journal of Obstetrics and Gynecology, 188*(1), 220–227.

Hoesli, I., Tercanli, S., & Holzgreve W. (2003). Cervical length assessment by ultrasound as a predictor of preterm labour—is there a role for routine screening? *BJOG: An International Journal of Obstetrics and Gynaecology, 110*(Suppl 20), 61–65.

Huber, A., Diehl, W., Bregenzer, T., Hackelöer, B. J., & Hecher, K. (2006). Stage-related outcome in twin-twin transfusion syndrome treated by fetoscopic laser coagulation. *Obstetrics and Gynecology, 108*(2), 333–337.

Institute of Medicine (U.S.). Subcommittee for a Clinical Application Guide. (1992). *Nutrition during pregnancy and lactation: An implementation guide / Subcommittee for a Clinical Application Guide.* Washington, DC: National Academy Press.

Jain, T., Missmer, S. A., & Hornstein, M. D. (2004). Trends in embryo-transfer practice and in outcomes of the use of assisted reproductive technology in the United States. *New England Journal of Medicine, 350*(16), 1639–1645.

Johnson, C. D., & Zhang, J. (2002). Survival of other fetuses after a fetal death in twin or triplet pregnancies. *Obstetrics and Gynecology, 99*(5 Pt 1), 698–703.

Kahn, B., Lumey, L. H., Zybert, P. A., Lorenz, J. M., Cleary-Goldman, J., D'Alton, M. E., et al. (2003). Prospective risk of fetal death in singleton, twin, and triplet gestations: Implications for practice. *Obstetrics and Gynecology, 102*(4), 685–692.

Källen, B., Finnstrom, O., Nygren, K. G., & Olausson, P.O. (2005). Temporal trends in multiple births after in vitro fertilisation in Sweden, 1982-2001: A register study. *British Medical Journal, 331*(7513), 382–383.

Klein, V. R. (2002). Maternal complications. In L. G. Keith & I. Blickstein (Eds.), *Triplet pregnancies and their consequences* (pp. 215–224). New York: The Parthenon Publishing Group.

Klock, S. C. (2001). The transition to parenthood. In I. Blickstein & L. G. Keith (Eds.), *Iatrogenic multiple pregnancy: Clinical implications* (pp. 225–234). New York: The Parthenon Publishing Group.

Klock, S. C. (2004). Psychological adjustment to twins after infertility. *Best Practice & Research Clinical Obstetrics & Gynaecology, 18*(4), 645–656.

Kogan, M. D., Alexander, G. R., Kotelchuck, M., MacDorman, M. F., Buekens, P., Martin, J. A., et al. (2000). Trends in twin birth outcomes and prenatal care utilization in the United States, 1981-1997. *Journal of the American Medical Association, 284*(3), 335–341.

Kontopoulos, E. V., Ananth, C. V., Smulian, J. C., & Vintzileos, A. M. (2004). The impact of route of delivery and presentation on twin neonatal and infant mortality: A population-based study in the USA, 1995-97. *Journal of Maternal-Fetal & Neonatal Medicine, 15*(4), 219–224.

Lam, F., & Gill, P. (2005a). β-Agonist tocolytic therapy. *Obstetrics and Gynecology Clinics, 32*(3), 457–484.

Lam, F., & Gill, P. (2005b). Inhibition of preterm labor and subcutaneous terbutaline therapy. In I. Blickstein & L. G. Keith (Eds.), *Multiple pregnancy: Epidemiology, gestation and perinatal outcome* (2nd ed., pp. 601–620). New York: Taylor and Francis.

Lambalk, C. B., & van Hooff, M. (2001). Natural versus induced twinning and pregnancy outcome: A Dutch nationwide survey of primiparous dizygotic twin deliveries. *Fertility and Sterility, 75*(4), 731–736.

Langkamp, D. L., & Girardet, R. G. (2006). Primary care for twins and higher order multiples. *Current Problems in Pediatric and Adolescent Health Care, 36*(2), 47–67.

Leonard, L. G. (1998). Depression and anxiety disorders during multiple pregnancy and parenthood. *Journal of Obstetric, Gynecologic and Neonatal Nursing, 27*(3), 329–337.

Leonard, L. G. (2002). Prenatal behavior of multiples: implications for families and nurses. *Journal of Obstetric, Gynecologic and Neonatal Nursing, 31*(3), 248–255.

Leondires, M. P., Ernst, S. D., Miller, B. T., & Scott, R. T., Jr. (2000). Triplets: Outcomes of expectant management versus multifetal reduction for 127 pregnancies. *American Journal of Obstetrics and Gynecology, 183*(2), 454–459.

Liu, S., Benirschke, K., Scioscia, A. L., & Mannino, F. L. (1992). Intrauterine death in multiple gestations. *Acta Geneticae Medicae et Gemellologiae, 41*(1), 5–26.

Lopriore, E., van Wezel-Meijler, G., Middeldorp, J. M., Sueters, M., Vandenbussche, F. P., & Walther, F. J. (2006). Incidence, origin, and character of cerebral injury in twin-to-twin transfusion syndrome treated with fetoscopic laser surgery. *American Journal of Obstetrics and Gynecology, 194*(5), 1215–1220.

Luke, B. (1996). Reducing fetal deaths in multiple births: Optimal birth weights and gestational ages for infants of twin and triplet births. *Acta Geneticae Medicae et Gemellologiae, 45*(3), 333–348.

Luke B. (2004). Improving multiple pregnancy outcomes with nutritional interventions. *Clinical Obstetrics and Gynecology, 47,* 146–162.

Luke, B. (2005). Nutrition and multiple gestations. *Seminars in Perinatology, 29*(5), 349–354.

Luke, B., Brown, M. B., Misiunas, R., Anderson, E., Nugent, C., van de Ven, C., et al. (2003). Specialized prenatal care and maternal and infant outcomes in twin pregnancy. *American Journal of Obstetrics and Gynecology 189*(4), 934–938.

Luke, B., Hediger, M. L., Nugent, C., Newman, R. B., Mauldin, J. G., Witter, F. R., et al. (2003). Body mass index—Specific weight gains associated with optimal birth weights in twin pregnancies. *The Journal of Reproductive Medicine, 48,* 217–224.

Machin, G. A. (2002). Triplet zygosity and chorionicity. In L. G. Keith & I. Blickstein (Eds.), *Triplet pregnancies and their consequences* (pp. 17–32). New York: The Parthenon Publishing Group.

MacKay, A. P., Berg, C., & King. J. C. (2004). *Pregnancy-related mortality among women with multiple gestations: Trends and risk factors, United States, 1980-97.* Reproductive Health Poster Session: Issues in Maternal and Perinatal Health, The 132nd Annual Meeting (November 6–10, 2004) of APHA, Washington, DC. Retrieved September 21, 2005, from http://apha.confex.com/apha/132am/techprogram/paper_91037.htm

Maifeld, M., Hahn, S., Titler, M. G., & Mullen, M. (2003). Decision making regarding multifetal reduction. *Journal of Obstetric, Gynecologic, and Neonatal Nursing, 32*(3), 357–369.

Malone, F. D., & D'Alton, M. E. (2004). Multiple gestations: Clinical characteristics and management. In R. K. Creasy & R. Resnik (Eds.), *Maternal fetal medicine* (5th ed. pp 513–538). Philadelphia: WB Saunders Co.

Malloy, M. H., & Freeman, D. H., Jr. (1999) Sudden infant death syndrome among twins. *Archives of Pediatrics & Adolescent Medicine, 153*(7), 736–740.

Maloni, J. A., & Schneider, B. S. (2002). Inactivity: Symptoms associated with gastrocnemius muscle disuse during pregnancy. *AACN Clinical Issues, 13*(2), 248–262.

Maloni, J. A., Brezinski-Tomasi, J. E., & Johnson, L. A. (2001). Antepartum bedrest: Effect upon the family. *Journal of Obstetrics, Gynecologic and Neonatal Nursing, 30*(2), 165–173.

Maloni, J. A., Margevicius, S. P., & Damato, E. G. (2006). Multiple gestations: Side effects of antepartum bed rest. *Biological Research for Nursing, 8*(2), 115–128.

Malmstrom, P. M., & Biale, R. (1990). An agenda for meeting the special needs of multiple birth families. *Acta Geneticae Medicae et Gemellolgiae, 39*(4), 507–514.

Marino, T., Goudas, L. C., Steinbok, V., Craigo, S. D., & Yarnell, R. W. (2001). The anesthetic management of triplet cesarean delivery: A retrospective case series of maternal outcomes. *Anesthesia and Analgesia, 93*(4), 991–995.

Martin, J. A., Hamilton, B. E., Sutton, P. D., Ventura, S. J., Menacker, F., & Munson, M. L. (2003). Births: Final data for 2002. *National Vital Statistics Reports, 52(10),* 1–113.

Martin, J. A., & Park, M. M. (1999). Trends in twin and triplet births: 1980–97. *National Vital Statistics Reports, 47*(24), 1–16.

Martin, J. A., Hamilton, B. E., Sutton, P. D., Ventura, S. J., Menacker, F., & Kirmeyer, S. (2006). Births: Final data for 2004. *National Vital Statistics Reports, 55*(1), 1–102.

Maslovitz, S., Hartoov, J., Wolman, I., Jaffa, A., Lessing, J. B., & Fait, G. (2004). Cervical length in the early second trimester for detection of triplet pregnancies at risk for preterm birth. *Journal of Ultrasound in Medicine, 23*(9), 1187–1191.

Mathews, T. J., Menacker, F., & MacDorman, M. F. (2004). Infant mortality statistics from the 2002 period linked birth/infant death data set. *National Vital Statistics Reports, 53*(10): 1–30.

Maymon, R., Neeman, O., Shulman, A., Rosen, H., & Herman, A. (2005). Current concepts of Down syndrome screening tests in assisted reproduction twin pregnancies: Another double trouble. *Prenatal Diagnosis, 25*(9), 746–750.

Maslovitz, S., Hartoov, J., Wolman, I., Jaffa, A., Lessing, J. B., & Fait, G. (2004). Cervical length in the early second trimester for detection of triplet pregnancies at risk for preterm birth. *Journal of Ultrasound in Medicine, 23*(9), 1187–1191.

McGrail, C., & Bryant, D. (2005). Intertwin time interval: How it affects the immediate neonatal outcome of the second twin. *American Journal of Obstetrics and Gynecology, 192*(5), 1420–1422.

Medoff-Cooper, B., Bakewell-Sachs, S., Buus-Frank, M. E., & Santa-Donato, A., Near-Term Infant Advisory Panel. (2005). The AWHONN Near-Term Infant Initiative: a conceptual framework for optimizing health for near-term infants. *Journal of Obstetric, Gynecologic and Neonatal Nursing, 34*(6), 666–671.

Meikle, S. F., Steiner, C.A., Zhang, J., & Lawrence, W. L. (2005). A national estimate of the elective primary cesarean delivery rate. *Obstetrics and Gynecology, 105*(4), 751–756.

Meis, P. J. (2005). 17 hydroxyprogesterone for the prevention of preterm delivery. *Obstetrics and Gynecology, 105*(5 Pt 1), 1128–1135.

Menon, D. K. (2005). A retrospective study of the accuracy of sonographic chorionicity determination in twin pregnancies. *Twin Research and Human Genetics, 8*(3), 259–261.

Meyers, C., Elias, S., & Arrabal, P. (1995). Congenital anomalies and pregnancy. In L. G. Keith, E. Papiernik, D. M. Keith, & B. Luke (Eds.), *Multiple pregnancy: Epidemiology, gestation and perinatal outcome* (pp. 73–92). New York: The Parthenon Publishing Group.

Mian, A. I. (2005). Depression in pregnancy and the postpartum period: Balancing adverse effects of untreated illness with treatment risks. *Journal of Psychiatric Practice, 11*(6), 389–396.

Misra, D. P. & Ananth, C. V. (2002). Infant mortality among singletons and twins in the United States during 2 decades: Effects of maternal age. *Pediatrics, 110*(6), 1163–1168.

Morrison, J. C., & Chauhan S. P. (2003). Current status of home uterine activity monitoring. *Clinics in Perinatology, 30*(4), 757–801.

Motew, M., & Ginsberg, N. A. (1995). Clinical management of monoamniotic twins. In L. G. Keith, E. Papiernik, D. M. Keith, & B. Luke (Eds.), *Multiple pregnancy: Epidemiology, gestation and perinatal outcome* (pp. 527–534). New York: The Parthenon Publishing Group.

Murali, S., & Baldisseri, M. R. (2005). Peripartum cardiomyopathy. *Critical Care Medicine, 33*(Suppl. 10), 340–346.

National Institutes of Health (NIH). (2000). Antenatal corticosteroids revisited: Repeat courses. *NIH Consensus Statement, 17*(2), 1–18.

Newman, R. B. (2005). Routine antepartum care of twins. In I. Blickstein & L. G. Keith (Eds.), *Multiple pregnancy: Epidemiology, gestation and perinatal outcome* (2nd ed., pp. 405–419). New York: Taylor and Francis.

Newman, R. B., & Ellings, J. M. (1995). Antepartum management of the multiple gestations: The case for specialized care. *Seminars in Perinatology, 19*(5), 387–403.

Newman, R. B., & Luke, B. (2000). *Multifetal pregnancy.* Philadelphia: Lippincott Williams & Wilkins.

Nichols, A. A. (2005). Cholestasis of pregnancy: A review of the evidence. *Journal of Perinatal & Neonatal Nursing, 19*(3), 217–226.

Norwitz, E. R., Edusa, V., & Park, J. S. (2005). Maternal physiology and complications of multiple pregnancy. *Seminars in Perinatology 29*(5), 338–348.

Odibo, A. O., Lawrence-Cleary, K., & Macones, G. A. (2003). Screening for aneuploidy in twins and higher-order multiples: Is first-trimester nuchal translucency the solution? *Obstetrical and Gynecological Survey, 58*(9), 609–614.

Oleszczuk, J. J., Keith, L. G., & Oleszczuk, A. K. (2005). The paradox of old maternal age in multiple pregnancies. *Obstetric and Gynecologic Clinics of North America, 32*(1), 69–80.

Ostfeld, B. M., Smith, R. H., Hiatt, M., & Hegyi, T. (2000). Maternal behavior toward premature twins: Implications for development. *Twin Research, 3*(4), 234–241.

Oyelese, Y., Ananth, C. V., Smulian, J. C., & Vintzileos, A. M. (2005). Delayed interval delivery in twin pregnancies in the United States: Impact on perinatal mortality and morbidity. *American Journal of Obstetrics and Gynecology, 192*(2), 439–444.

Papiernik, E., Keith, L., Oleszczuk, J. J., & Cervantes, A. (1998). What interventions are useful in reducing the rate of preterm delivery in twins? *Clinical Obstetrics and Gynecology, 41*(1), 12–23.

Pector, E. A. (2004). How bereaved multiple-birth parents cope with hospitalization, homecoming, disposition for deceased, and attachment to survivors. *Journal of Perinatology, 24*(11), 714–722.

Pector, E. A., & Smith-Levitin, M. (2002). Mourning and psychological issues in multiple birth loss. *Seminars in Neonatology, 7*(3), 247–256.

Peitsch, W. K., Keefer, C. H., LaBrie, R. A., & Mulliken, J. B. (2002). Incidence of cranial asymmetry in healthy newborns. *Pediatrics, 110*(6), e72.

Pharoah, P. O., & Adi, Y. (2000). Consequences of in-utero death in a twin pregnancy. *Lancet, 355*(9215), 1597–1602.

Pharoah, P. O. (2002). Neurological outcome in twins. *Seminars in Neonatology, 7*(3), 223–230.

Platt, M. J., & Pharoah, P. O. (2003). The epidemiology of sudden infant death syndrome. *Archives of Disease in Childhood, 88*(1), 27–29.

Poggi, S. H., Ghidini, A., Landy, H. J., Alvarez, M., Pezzullo, J. C., & Collea, J. V. (2002). *Journal of Maternal-Fetal and Neonatal Medicine, 12*(1), 46–49.

Quintero, R. A., Morales, W. J., Allen, M. H., Bornick, P. W., Johnson, P. K., & Kruger, M. (1999). Staging of twin-twin transfusion syndrome. *Journal of Perinatology, 19*(8 Pt 1), 550–555.

Ramsey, P. S., & Repke, J. T. (2003). Intrapartum management of multifetal pregnancies. *Seminars in Perinatology, 27*(1), 54–72.

Rand, L., Eddleman, K. A., & Stone, J. (2005). Long-term outcomes in multiple gestations. *Clinics in Perinatology, 32*(2), 495–513.

Rebarber, A., Roman, A. S., Istwan, N., Rhea, D., & Stanziano, G. (2005). Prophylactic cerclage in the management of triplet pregnancies. *American Journal of Obstetrics and Gynecology, 193*(3 Pt. 2), 1193–1196.

Rao, A., Sairam, S., & Shehata, H. (2004). Obstetric complications of twin pregnancies. *Best Practice & Research Clinical Obstetrics & Gynaecology, 18*(4), 557–576.

Reynolds, M. A., Schieve, L. A., Martin, J. A., Jeng, G., & Macaluso, M. (2003). Trends in multiple births conceived using assisted reproductive technology, United States, 1997-2000. *Pediatrics, 111*(5 Pt 2), 1159–1162.

Rebarber, A., Roman, A. S., Istwan, N., Rhea, D., & Stanziano, G. (2005). Prophylactic cerclage in the management of triplet pregnancies. *American Journal of Obstetrics and Gynecology, 193*(3 Pt. 2), 1193–1196.

Richter, J. E. (2003) Gastroesophageal reflux disease during pregnancy. *Gastroenterology Clinics of North America, 32*(1), 235–261.

Robinson, C., & Chauhan, S. P. (2004). Intrapartum management of twins. *Clinical Obstetrics and Gynecology, 47*(1), 248–462.

Rodis, J. F., Egan, J. F., Craffey, A., Ciarleglio, L. Greenstein, R. M., & Scorza, W. E. (1990). Calculated risk of chromosomal abnormalities in twin gestations. *Obstetrics and Gynecology, 76*(6), 1037–1041.

Roem, K. (2003). Nutritional management of multiple pregnancies. *Twin Research, 6*(6), 514–519.

Rohde, A., Dembinski, J., & Dorn, C. (2003). Mirtazapine (Remergil) for treatment resistant hyperemesis gravidarum: Rescue of a twin pregnancy. *Archives of Gynecology and Obstetrics, 268*(3), 219–221.

Rosello-Soberon, M. E., Fuentes-Chaparro, L., & Casanueva, E. (2005). Twin pregnancies: eating for three? Maternal nutrition update. *Nutrition Reviews, 63*(9), 295–302.

Ruiz, R. J., Brown, C. E., Peters, M. T., & Johnston, A. B. (2001). Specialized care for twin gestations: Improving newborn outcomes and reducing costs. *Journal of Obstetric, Gynecologic and Neonatal Nursing, 30*(1), 52–60.

Rustico, M. A., Baietti, M. G., Coviello, D., Orlandi, E., & Nicolini, U. (2005). Managing twins discordant for fetal anomaly. *Prenatal Diagnosis, 25*(9), 766–771.

Ryan, G. L., Zhang, S. H., Dokras, A., Syrop, C. H., & Van Voorhis, B. J. (2004). The desire of infertile patients for multiple births. *Fertility and Sterility, 81*(3), 500–504.

Salihu, H. M., Bekan, B., Aliyu, M. H., Rouse, D. J., Kirby, R. S., & Alexander, G. R. (2005a). Perinatal mortality associated with abruptio placenta in singletons and multiples. *American Journal of Obstetrics and Gynecology, 193*(1), 198–203.

Salihu, H. M., Garces, I. C., Sharma, P. P., Kristensen, S., Ananth, C. V., & Kirby, R. S. (2005b). Stillbirth and infant mortality among Hispanic singletons, twins, and triplets in the United States. *Obstetrics and Gynecology, 106*(4), 789–796.

Schreiner-Engel, P., Walther, V. N., Mindes, J., Lynch, L., & Berkowitz, R. L. (1995). First-trimester multifetal pregnancy reduction: Acute and persistent psychologic reactions. *American Journal of Obstetrics and Gynecology, 172*(2 Pt. 1), 541–547.

Schiff, E., Cohen, S. B., Dulitzky, M., Novikov, I., Friedman, S. A., Mashiach, S., et al. (1998). Progression of labor in twin versus singleton gestations. *American Journal of Obstetrics and Gynecology, 179*(5), 1181–1185.

Shetty, A., & Smith, A.P. (2005). The sonographic diagnosis of chorionicity. *Prenatal Diagnosis, 25*(9), 735–739.

Shinagawa, S., Suzuki, S., Chihara, H., Otsubo, Y., Takeshita, T., & Araki, T. (2005). Maternal basal metabolic rate in twin pregnancy. *Gynecologic and Obstetric Investigation, 60*(3), 145–148.

Silver, R. K., Haney, E. I., Grobman, W. A., MacGregor, S. N., Casele, H. L., & Neerhof, M. G. (2000). Comparison of active phase labor between triplet, twin and singleton gestations. *Journal of the Society for Gynecologic Investigation, 7*(5), 297–300.

Simpson, K. R. (2004). Monitoring the preterm fetus during labor. *MCN The American Journal of Maternal Child Nursing, 29*(6), 380–388.

Smith-Levitin, M., Skupski, D. W., & Chervenak, F. A. (1999). Multifetal pregnancies: Epidemiology, clinical characteristics and management. In E. A. Reece & J. C. Hobbins (Eds.), *Medicine of the fetus and mother* (2nd ed., pp. 243–264). Philadelphia: Lippincott-Raven Publishers.

Society for Assisted Reproductive Technology and the Practice Committee of the American Society for Reproductive Medicine. (2006). Guidelines on number of embryos transferred. *Fertility and Sterility, 86*(5), S51–S52.

Taffel, S. M. (1995). Demographic trends: USA. In L. G. Keith, E. Papiernik, D. M. Keith, & B. Luke (Eds.), *Multiple pregnancy: Epidemiology, gestation and perinatal outcome* (pp. 133–144). New York: The Parthenon Publishing Group.

Trevett, T., & Johnson, A. (2005). Monochorionic twin pregnancies. *Clinics in Perinatology, 32*(2), 475–494.

Vintzileos, A. M., Ananth, C. V., Kontopoulos, E., & Smulian, J. C. (2005). Mode of delivery and risk of stillbirth and infant mortality in triplet gestations: United States, 1995 through 1998. *American Journal of Obstetrics and Gynecology, 192*(2), 464–469.

Walker, M. C., Murphy, K. E., Pan, S., Yang, Q., & Wen, S. W. (2004). Adverse maternal outcomes in multifetal pregnancies.

BJOG: An International Journal of Obstetrics and Gynaecology, 111(11), 1294–1296.

Wen, S. W., Demissie, K., Yang, Q., & Walker, M. C. (2004). Maternal morbidity and obstetric complications in triplet pregnancies and quadruplet and higher-order multiple pregnancies. *American Journal of Obstetrics and Gynecology,* 191(1), 254–258.

Wen, S.W., Fung, K.F., Huang, L., Demissie, K., Joseph, K.S., Allen, A.C., et al., Fetal and Infant Health Group of the Canadian Perinatal Surveillance System. (2005). Fetal and neonatal mortality among twin gestations in a Canadian population: The effect of intrapair birth weight discordance. *American Journal of Perinatology,* 22(5), 279–286.

Wright, V. C., Schieve, L. A., Reynolds, M. A., & Jeng, G. (2005). Assisted reproductive technology surveillance–United States, 2002. *Morbidity and Mortality Weekly Report. Surveillance Summaries,* 54(2), 1–24.

Yang, Q., Wen, S. W., Chen, Y., Krewski, D., Fung, K. F., & Walker, M. (2005). Neonatal death and morbidity in vertex-nonvertex second twins according to mode of delivery and birth weight. *American Journal of Obstetrics and Gynecology,* 192(3), 840–847.

Yang, Q., Wen, S. W., Chen, Y., Krewski, D., Fung, K. F., & Walker, M. (2006). Neonatal mortality and morbidity in vertex–vertex second twins according to mode of delivery and birth weight. *Journal of Perinatology,* 26(1), 3–10.

Zhang, J., Hamilton, B., Martin, J., & Trumble, A. (2004). Delayed interval delivery and infant survival: A population-based study. *American Journal of Obstetrics and Gynecology,* 191(2), 470–476.

Zhang, J., Meikle, S., Grainger, D. A., & Trumble, A. (2002). Multifetal pregnancy in older women and perinatal outcomes. *Fertility and Sterility,* 78(3), 562–568.

Ziadeh, S. M., Sunna, E., & Badria, L. F. (2000). The effect of mode of delivery on neonatal outcome of twins with birth weight under 1500 grams. *Journal of Obstetrics and Gynaecology,* 20(4), 389–391.

Zuppa, A. A., Maragliano, G., Scapillati, M. E., Crescimbini, B., & Tortorolo, G. (2001). Neonatal outcome of spontaneous and assisted twin pregnancies. *European Journal of Obstetrics, Gynecology and Reproductive Biology,* 95(1), 68–72.

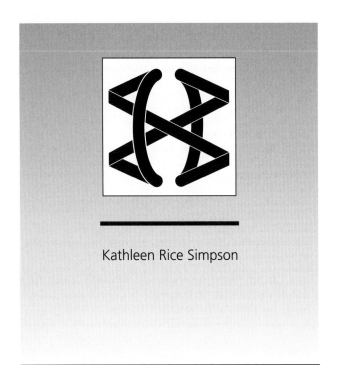

Kathleen Rice Simpson

CHAPTER 7

Labor and Birth

INTRODUCTION

Labor and birth are natural processes. Most women do well with support and minimal selected intervention. The minimal intervention philosophy acknowledges that most pregnancies, labors, and births are normal and that intervention creates the potential for iatrogenic maternal–fetal injuries. Interventions should move forward on a continuum from noninvasive to least invasive and from nonpharmacologic to pharmacologic according to the wishes of the woman and the discretion of healthcare providers based on individual clinical situations. A philosophy of minimal intervention works best in the context of a well-designed safety net, allowing for intervention when necessary in a clinically timely manner.

During the intrapartum period, nurses use knowledge of physiologic and psychosocial aspects of birth and selected pharmacologic therapies to provide comprehensive care for women and families. The focus of this chapter is on nursing interventions that facilitate the labor and birth process. A brief overview of the physiology of labor and birth is discussed. Maternal–fetal assessments, influence of maternal positioning on labor progression, second-stage care practices and opportunities for providing supportive care, and promoting family attachment throughout the birth process are described. Clinical interventions, including cervical ripening, labor induction and augmentation, and amnioinfusion, are also presented. Strategies to ensure consistency with perioperative standards of care for cesarean births are included, as well as controversial issues such as fundal pressure, perineal mas-

sage, and cesarean birth without a medical indication. The evidence (or lack thereof) for each of these topics are discussed with recommendations for practices that contribute to the best possible outcomes for mothers and babies.

OVERVIEW OF LABOR AND BIRTH

Onset of Labor

Multiple theories have been proposed to explain the biophysiological factors that initiate labor; however, this process is not yet fully understood. A combination of maternal–fetal factors influence labor onset (see Display 7-1). It is likely that a parturition cascade occurs in humans that results in the removal of the mechanisms that maintain uterine quiescence and the initiation of factors that promote uterine activity (Liao, Buhimschi, & Norwitz, 2005). Labor and birth are multifactorial processes that involve interconnected positive feedforward and negative feedback loops that are linked in a carefully time-regulated fashion (Nathanielsz, 1998). These pathways in the fetus, placenta, and mother require sequential initiation and include redundancy that can prevent a single factor from prematurely initiating labor or preventing the initiation of labor (Liao et al., 2005). Animal studies suggest that the fetus determines the duration of gestation while the mother determines the time of day at which labor begins (Nathanielsz, 1998).

A complex series of events must occur during labor and birth that represent a reversal of role for the uterus and cervix during pregnancy. The myometrium,

DISPLAY 7-1

Possible Causes of the Onset of Labor

Maternal Factor Theories

Uterine muscles are stretched, causing release of prostaglandin.

Pressure on cervix stimulates nerve plexus, causing release of oxytocin by maternal posterior pituitary gland (the Ferguson reflex).

Oxytocin stimulation in circulating blood increases slowly during pregnancy, rises dramatically during labor, and peaks during second stage. Oxytocin and prostaglandin work together to inhibit calcium binding in muscle cells, raising intracellular calcium and activating contractions.

Estrogen/progesterone ratio change: estrogen excites uterine response, and progesterone quiets uterine response. Decrease of progesterone allows estrogen to stimulate the contractile response of the uterus.

Fetal Factor Theories

Placental aging and deterioration triggers initiation of contractions.

Fetal cortisol concentration, produced by the fetal adrenal glands, rises and acts on the placenta to reduce progesterone formation and increase prostaglandin. Anencephalic fetuses (no adrenal glands) tend to have prolonged gestation.

Prostaglandin, produced by fetal membranes (amnion and chorion) and the decidua, stimulates contractions. When arachidonic acid stored in fetal membranes is released at term, it is converted to prostaglandin.

---

which has remained relatively quiet for many months, has to become active, and the cervix, which has functioned to prevent birth, must lose its resistance. This involves an integrated set of changes within the maternal tissues (myometrium, deciduas, and cervix) that occur gradually over a period of days to weeks (Liao et al., 2005). Despite extensive research, knowledge of the exact mechanism for spontaneous labor remains incomplete. Most of what is known is from animal studies and in vitro investigations of biopsies obtained from the myometrium and cervix at cesarean birth (Bernal, 2003; Liao et al., 2005).

The forces of labor are uterine contractions acting on the resistance of the cervix. The uterine walls are flexible, expanding over time until the onset of labor, when the myometrium converts from a quiet state to a highly active contractile organ. The cervix, composed of connective tissue, remains firmly closed until it is

time for labor to begin; then it undergoes rapid, dramatic changes, including ripening, effacement, and dilation (Liao et al., 2005). The conditions and processes that result in term labor are regulated by several compounds and biochemical systems, including progesterone withdrawal and prostaglandin synthesis (Bernal, 2003). Activation of the myometrium requires receptor sites, increased production of prostaglandin, and formation of gap junctions. Gap junctions are specialized protein units located within the cell membrane that connect neighboring cells and provide communication channels (Ulmsten, 1997). The number of gap junctions and their permeability and performance have a direct influence on myometrial function during labor (Bernal, 2003).

It is theorized that after the preparation and activation period, the myometrium is ready to be stimulated for contractions (Liao et al., 2005). Prostaglandin and oxytocin are the most important biochemical factors in stimulating term myometrial activity (Olah & Gee, 1996; Slater, Zervou, & Thornton, 2002). Prostaglandin synthesis during the cervical ripening period also prepares the myometrium to respond to oxytocin (Sheehan, 2006). It is known that oxytocin alone cannot induce formation of gap junctions. The oxytocin hormone is synthesized by the hypothalamus, then transported to the posterior lobe of the pituitary gland, where it is released into maternal circulation.

The release of oxytocin is caused by stimuli such as breast stimulation, sensory stimulation of the lower genital tract, and cervical stretching. The milk-ejection reflex results from oxytocin released due to breast stimulation. Oxytocin released in response to vaginal and cervical stretching results in uterine contractions through Ferguson's reflex. There are differences in reported plasma concentrations of oxytocin during pregnancy and spontaneous labor, which can be attributed in part to individual variations among pregnant women and methodologies used to measure levels of oxytocin; however, it is generally accepted that in addition to a tonic baseline release of oxytocin, there is a pulsatile release action that may increase in amplitude and frequency during labor (Brindley & Sokol, 1988; Fuchs et al., 1991).

Two types of oxytocin receptors have been identified and quantified in the human uterus: myometrial and decidual (Liao et al., 2005). Both play an important part in the initiation of spontaneous labor and birth. Oxytocin receptors are present in low concentrations until the later part of the third trimester, during which their numbers increase dramatically. This lack of receptors until late pregnancy probably is the cause for the lack of uterine response to oxytocin other than during the third trimester (Sultatos, 1997). Oxytocin receptors in the myometrium and decidua reach their peak levels at slightly different times during pregnancy and labor. During pregnancy, as weeks of gestation increase, there is a steady increase in the number of oxytocin receptors in the myometrium (Calderyo-Barcia & Poseiro, 1960). As pregnancy progresses, the number of oxytocin receptor site in the myometrium increases by 100-fold at 32 weeks and by 300-fold at the onset of labor (Arias, 2000). Myometrial receptors are thought to peak in early spontaneous labor and significantly contribute to the initiation of uterine activity (Fuchs, Fuchs, Husslein, & Soloff, 1984). It is likely that the concentration of myometrial receptors play a dominant role in uterine response to endogenous and exogenous oxytocin.

Over an approximate two-week period before the onset of labor, contraction frequency and intensity increase in a pre-labor synchronization of uterine activity. However, these contractions are usually not perceived by the pregnant woman because they are less than 20 mm Hg in intensity (Newman, 2005). As intensity increases beyond 20 to 30 mm Hg, the woman gradually becomes aware of uterine activity, especially via palpation, although these contractions are not noted as painful by most women (Newman, 2005). When contraction intensity is above 30 mm Hg, some women may perceive discomfort. This type of contraction pattern is usually characterized by infrequent contractions and periodic episodes until active labor begins (Newman, 2005). Early labor contractions are concentrated in the lower and middle uterine segments, while active labor contractions originate in the fundal area of the uterus (Newman, 2005).

Oxytocin receptors in the decidua are thought to increase as labor progresses and reach peak levels during birth (Fuchs, Husslein, & Fuchs, 1981). During labor, oxytocin stimulates the production and release of arachidonic acid and prostaglandin F_2 by the decidua that has been sensitized to oxytocin, thus potentiating oxytocin-induced uterine activity (Husslein, Fuchs, & Fuchs, 1981). All oxytocin-receptor site interactions do not result in uterine muscle contraction. Although oxytocin does occupy myometrial and decidual receptor sites during labor, the uterus is not in a constant state of contraction. Labor contractions are rhythmic and coordinated, providing evidence that some smooth muscle cells have their oxytocin receptor site occupied without stimulating contraction (Bernal, 2003; Sultatos, 1997).

The exact mechanism of muscle cell coordination during labor remains unknown. One theory is that a signal from pacemaker cells, possibly located in the uterine fundus, is transmitted to other myometrial cells by cell-to-cell communication through gap junctions (Sultatos, 1997). Another theory is that although there is a tonic baseline release of oxytocin from the posterior lobe of the pituitary gland, it is the pulsatile release action that may increase in amplitude and frequency during labor, which could be responsible for the rhythmic nature of uterine contractions (Brindley & Sokol, 1988; Fuchs et al., 1991). More data are needed to confirm or dispute these theories.

During the first stage of spontaneous labor, maternal circulating concentrations of endogenous oxytocin are approximately that which would be achieved with a continuous infusion of exogenous oxytocin at 2 to 4 mU/min (Dawood, Ylikorkala, Trivedi, & Fuchs, 1979). The fetus is thought to secrete oxytocin during labor at a level similar to an infusion of oxytocin at approximately 3 mu/min (Dawood, Wang, Gupta & Fuchs, 1978). Thus, the combined effects of maternal–fetal contributions to maternal plasma oxytocin concentration is equivalent to a range of about 5 to 7 mU/min (Shyken & Petrie, 1995a). Plasma clearance of oxytocin is through the maternal kidneys and liver by the enzyme oxytocinase, with only a small amount excreted unchanged in the urine. Maternal metabolic clearance rate of oxytocin at term is 19 to 21 mL/kg/min and is unaffected by pregnancy (Zeeman, Kahn-Dawood, & Dawood, 1997).

Due to lack of knowledge about the exact physiology of labor, it is difficult to determine the most optimum dosages to be used to correct abnormal labor with artificial pharmacologic compounds. Hyperstimulation with oxytocin and other prostaglandin compounds is often evident during cervical ripening and stimulation of labor as a result of knowledge gaps in this area. While hyperstimulation can be the result of endogenous oxytocin or prostaglandins, it is more often seen with exogenous pharmacologic agents (Crane, Young, Butt, Bennett, & Hutchens, 2001). Each woman has an individual myometrial sensitivity to oxytocin and prostaglandin (Ulstem, 1997).

Premonitory signs, such as lightening, urinary frequency, pelvic pressure, changes in vaginal discharge, bloody show, loss of mucous plug, and irregular contractions, are frequently reported several weeks before actual labor begins. Some women also describe changes in sleep patterns and increased energy levels in the final weeks of pregnancy. True labor is characterized by contractions that produce progressive effacement and dilation of the cervix with fetal descent into the maternal pelvis (see Display 7–2).

Duration of Labor

Wide variations in labor progress and duration exist among childbearing women. There is no consensus among perinatal experts on appropriate length of labor and its potential relationship to risks of adverse maternal–fetal outcomes (Ness, Goldberg, & Berghella, 2005). Classic research by Friedman in 1955 described characteristics of labor of nulliparous women. This research was later expanded to include a series of

D I S P L A Y   7 - 2

Comparison of False and True Labor

FALSE LABOR

- Regular contractions
- Decrease in frequency and intensity; longer intervals
- Discomfort in lower abdomen and groin
- Activity has no effect or decreases contractions; disappear with sleep
- No appreciable change in cervix
- Sedation decreases or stops contractions
- Show usually not present

TRUE LABOR

- Regular contractions
- Progressive frequency and intensity; closer intervals
- Discomfort begins in back, radiating to the abdomen
- Activity such as walking increases contractions; continue even when sleeping
- Progressive effacement and dilation of cervix
- Sedation does not stop contractions
- Show usually present

definitions of labor protraction and arrest (Friedman, 1978). The Friedman labor curve is still commonly used in the clinical setting to assess normal progression of labor. Generally, characteristics of most unmedicated labors will be similar in length, progression, cervical changes, and fetal descent as outlined by Friedman (1955, 1978) and Friedman, Niswander, Bayonet-Rivera, and Sachtleben (1966); however, this early research was done before the nearly universal application of electronic fetal monitoring (EFM) during labor and the significant increase in use of pharmacologic agents to ripen the cervix and stimulate uterine contractions, as well as the popularity of regional analgesia/anesthesia in the United States and Canada. Other clinical conditions with potential to influence labor progress also have changed. Body mass of laboring women is significantly higher than it was 50 years ago and with the reduction in smoking as well as other factors, babies are bigger (Silbar, 1986; Young & Woodmansee, 2002; Zhang, Troendle, & Yancey, 2002). These factors combined have contributed to a lengthening of what can be expected for the course of "normal" labor.

There are significant differences in length of spontaneous labor and induced labor (Hoffman, Vahratian, Sciscione, Troendle, & Zhang, 2006; Rouse, Owen, Savage, & Hauth, 2001; Simon & Grobman, 2005; Vahartian, Zhang, Troendle, Sciscione, & Hoffman,

2005). Spontaneous labor is generally shorter with less risk of cesarean birth; however, pre-induction cervical ripening can minimize risk of cesarean birth associated with electively induced labor for nulliparous women (Vahratian et al., 2005). When the admission Bishop score is less than 6, elective induction for nulliparous women significantly increases risk of cesarean birth (Vrounenraets et al., 2005). A latent phase as long as 18 hours during labor induction for nulliparous women is not unusual, and most of these women will give birth vaginally if time is allowed to achieve active labor (Simon & Grobman, 2005). Regional analgesia/anesthesia lengthens the active phase of labor by approximately 60 to 90 minutes (ACOG, 2002a; Alexander, Sharma, McIntire, & Leveno, 2002).

Based on available data (Albers, 1999; Albers, Schiff, & Gorwoda, 1996; Cohen, 1977; Menticoglou, Manning, Harman, & Morrison, 1995; Moon, Smith, & Rayburn, 1990; Rouse et al., 2001; Schiessl et al., 2005; Zhang et al., 2002), it is likely that previously held arbitrary time frames for duration of labor (Friedman, 1955; Friedman, 1978; Friedman et al., 1966; Hellman & Prystowsky, 1952) are no longer valid for all women. Multiple factors, including parity, timing and dosage of epidural analgesia/anesthesia; use of oxytocin or misoprostol; amniotomy; fetal size and position; and maternal psyche, age, body mass, labor positions, and pelvic structure influence progress of labor (Hoffman et al., 2006; Malone et al., 1996; Rojansky, Tanos, Reubinoff, Shapira, & Weinstein, 1997; Rouse et al., 2001; Zhang et al., 2002). Generally, active labor of a nulliparous woman progresses slower (0.5 to 1 cm/hr) than labor of a multiparous woman (>1 cm/hr).

Although multiparous women usually experience faster labor than nulliparous women, additional childbearing generally has no further effect on labor progression (Vahratian, Hoffman, Troendle, & Zhang, 2006). There also is a relationship between parity and type of labor progression variances. It is known that women in labor with their first child are more likely to experience hypertonic uterine dysfunction, primary inertia, or a prolonged latent phase in early labor (Freidman, 1978). During second and subsequent labors, deviations from the Friedman criteria during active labor, such as hypotonic uterine dysfunction, secondary inertia, and protraction or arrest of the active phase, are more common (Ness et al., 2005).

The Friedman (1955, 1978) curve likely represented the ideal labor progression of women of during the time these data were collected and analyzed rather than the average labor progression (Zhang et al., 2002). Figure 7–1 provides graphic representations of an expected labor pattern and commonly seen deviations based on Friedman's 1955 and 1978 data. Figure 7–2A represents data comparing Friedman's original work with

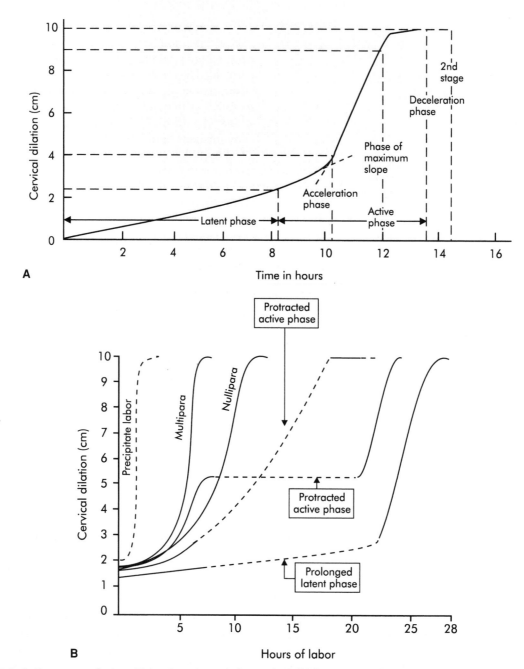

FIGURE 7–1. A, Partogram of normal labor based on Friedman's (1955) labor curve. **B**, Major types of deviation from normal progress of labor based on Friedman's (1978) curve. (From Bobak, I. M., & Jensen, M. D. [1991]. *Essentials of maternity nursing* [p. 765]. St. Louis, MO: Mosby–Year Book. Copyright 1991 by Mosby–Year Book. Reprinted with permission.)

more contemporary data (Zhang et al., 2002). Figure 7–2B represents data regarding patterns of cervical dilation and fetal descent for nulliparous women based on clinical conditions occurring in the present obstetrical environment (Zhang et al., 2002). These data are averages; each woman progresses in labor based on individual factors and clinical conditions.

Although previously it was thought that limiting the second stage of labor to 2 hours was essential to decrease risks of fetal morbidity and mortality (Hellman & Prystowsky, 1952; Wood, Ng, Hounslow, &

Benning, 1973), it is now known that waiting beyond two hours for the fetus to descend spontaneously is safe for the fetus. The 2-hour recommendation was made before the widespread use of continuous EFM and epidural anesthesia. Based on a substantial body of literature, the arbitrary 2-hour time frame is no longer clinically valid. As long as the fetal heart rate (FHR) is reassuring and there is evidence of fetal descent, there is no risk to the fetus in waiting a reasonable time for spontaneous birth (Cheng, Hopkins, & Caughey, 2004; Hagelin & Leyon, 1998; Janni et al.,

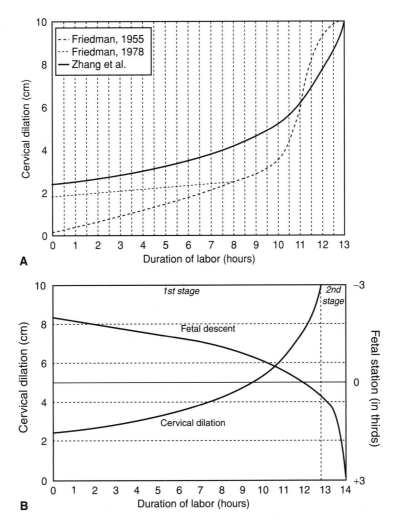

FIGURE 7–2. A: Comparison between the Friedman curve and the pattern of cervical dilation based on current data. **B**: Patterns of cervical dilation (left) and fetal descent (right) in nulliparous women based on contemporary clinical conditions. (From Zhang, J., Troendle J. F., & Yancey, M. K. [2002]. Reassessing the labor curve in multiparous women. *American Journal of Obstetrics and Gynecology, 187*(4), 824–828.)

2002; Myles & Santolaya, 2003). Although earlier studies have suggested that the length of the second stage does not influence maternal outcomes (Albers, 1999; Albers et al., 1996; Cohen, 1977; Derham, Crowhurst, & Crowther, 1991; Maresh, Choong, & Beard, 1983; Menticoglou et al., 1995; Moon et al., 1990; Paterson, Saunders, & Wadsworth, 1992; Thomson, 1993), later data suggest a prolonged second stage beyond 4 hours may increase maternal risk of operative vaginal birth and perineal trauma (Cheng et al., 2004; Myles & Santolaya, 2003; Sheiner et al., 2006).

The American College of Obstetricians and Gynecologists (ACOG) (2000b) recommends that operative vaginal birth be considered for nulliparous women when there is lack of continuing progress for 2 hours with regional anesthesia or for 2 hours without regional anesthesia. For multiparous women, operative vaginal birth should be considered after lack of continuous progress for 2 hours with regional anesthesia or

for 1 hour without regional anesthesia (ACOG, 2000b). These recommendations are for consideration, and are not an absolute necessity for operative vaginal birth. In other words, after these time periods, a complete evaluation of patient progress, maternal–fetal status, and the likelihood that more pushing will safely accomplish vaginal birth should be undertaken.

The ACOG (2000b) recommendations are based on timing of determination of complete cervical dilation and fetal head engagement. Supportive evidence is based on when patients were noted to be completely dilated via vaginal examination rather than when they were actually 10 cm, so these data are inexact. Frequency of vaginal examinations during labor has a significant effect on accuracy of determination of the beginning of second-stage labor. Other maternal factors, such as length of active pushing and efficacy of maternal pushing efforts, should be considered as well when determining the safest method of birth. Some women may need to individualize pushing efforts based on the fetal response (eg, pushing with every other or every third contraction or discontinuing pushing temporarily to maintain a reassuring FHR pattern). Other women may become fatigued after repetitive sustained pushing efforts and request a period of rest. Therefore, maternal–fetal status and individual clinical situations provide the best data for labor assessment and management.

Stages of Labor and Birth

Labor and birth have traditionally been divided into four stages. The first stage is subdivided into the latent, active, and transition phases of labor. Cervical changes are used in assessing progression through each phase: latent phase, 0–3 cm; active phase, 4–7 cm; and transition, 8–10 cm. Women laboring for the first time usually experience complete cervical effacement prior to dilation. Increasing effacement usually occurs simultaneously with dilation in multiparous women. The second stage of labor begins at complete cervical dilation and ends with the birth of the baby. This stage of labor is subdivided into the initial latent phase (passive fetal descent, laboring down) and the active pushing phase (Roberts, 2002, 2003). The third stage of labor begins with the birth of the baby and ends with the delivery of the placenta. The fourth stage of labor begins with the delivery of the placenta and lasts until the woman is stable in the immediate postpartum period, usually within the first hour after birth. Table 7–1 summarizes stages of labor, including average duration, cervical changes, uterine activity, maternal activity, and physical sensations.

Nursing Assessments

Admission Assessment of Maternal–Fetal Status

Major roles of the perinatal nurse caring for laboring women include a thorough admission assessment and ongoing maternal–fetal assessments. This chapter's Appendix 7–A contains a sample intrapartum admission assessment as outlined in a traditional paper format. In many hospitals, these data are entered electronically into the medical record. Either method is appropriate; however, the content should generally be the same. The focus of this assessment is on prior obstetric history, current pregnancy, and labor symptoms. Usually a complete history and physical examination has been conducted by the primary care provider during the prenatal period and included in the prenatal records that become part of the hospital's medical record. By 36 weeks of gestation, a copy of the prenatal record should be on file in the perinatal unit so pertinent data can easily be accessed when the woman presents in labor. If the woman has received

prenatal care and data regarding a recent history and physical examination confirming normal progress of pregnancy are available for review, the admission evaluation may be limited to an interval history and physical examination directed at the presenting condition. If the woman has not had prenatal care, or no prenatal care records are available, a more comprehensive assessment including appropriate laboratory data is advised. *Guidelines for Perinatal Care* (American Academy of Pediatrics [AAP] & ACOG, 2002) provides recommendations for the components of a comprehensive admission assessment for pregnant women.

Pregnant women may come to the hospital's labor and birth unit not only for perinatal care, but also for treatment of any sign or symptom of illness. Any pregnant woman presenting to a hospital for care should, at a minimum, be assessed for the following: FHR (as appropriate for gestational age), maternal vital signs, and uterine contractions (AAP & ACOG, 2002). The responsible perinatal healthcare provider should be informed promptly if any of the following findings are present: vaginal bleeding, acute abdominal pain, temperature of 100.4°F or higher, preterm labor, preterm premature rupture of membranes, hypertension, and nonreassuring FHR (AAP & ACOG, 2002). When a pregnant woman is evaluated for labor, the following factors should be assessed and recorded: blood pressure (BP), pulse, temperature, frequency and duration of uterine contractions, fetal well-being, urinary protein and glucose, cervical dilatation and effacement (unless contraindicated [eg, placenta previa]), fetal presentation and station of the presenting part, status of the membranes, date and time of the woman's arrival and notification of the provider (AAP & ACOG, 2002). The provider should assess and document the maternal pelvis and estimated fetal weight (AAP & ACOG, 2002). Previously identified risk factors should be recorded in the prenatal record. If no new risk factors are found, attention may be focused on the following historical factors: time of onset and frequency of contractions; status of the membranes; presence or absence of bleeding; fetal movement; history of allergies; the time, content, and amount of most the recent food or fluid ingestion; and use of any medication (AAP & ACOG, 2002).

At times, pregnant women may come to the hospital before labor is established. They may be experiencing uterine contractions that have not yet resulted in cervical changes or they may be in very early labor. Onset of labor is established by observing progressive cervical change; thus, differentiation between true and false labor status may require two or more cervical examinations that are separated by an adequate period to observe change (AAP & ACOG, 2002). A policy that

TABLE 7–1 ■ STAGES OF LABOR

Stage	Duration	Contraction Frequency	Contraction Duration	Contraction Intensity	Physical Sensations	Maternal Behavior
First Stage Latent, 0–3 cm	Primigravida, 8.6 hr; multigravida, 5.3 hr	3–30 min; may be irregular	30–40 sec	Mild by palpation; 25–40 mm Hg by intrauterine pressure catheter (IUPC)	Menstrual-like cramps; low, dull backache; light bloody show; diarrhea; possible rupture of membranes	Pain controlled fairly well; able to ambulate and talk through most contractions; range of emotions—excited, talkative, and confident versus anxious, withdrawn, and apprehensive
Active, 4–7 cm	Primigravida, 4.6 hr; multigravida, 2.4 hr	2–5 min	40–60 sec	Moderate to strong by palpation; 50–70 mm Hg by IUPC	Increasing discomfort; trembling of thighs and legs; pressure on bladder and rectum; persistent backache with occipitoposterior fetal position	Begins to work at maintaining control during contractions; accepts "coaching" efforts of perinatal staff and support persons; quieter
Transition, 8–10 cm	Primigravida, 3.6 hr; multigravida, variable	1.5–2 min	60–90 sec	Strong by palpation; 70–90 mm Hg by IUPC	Increased bloody show; urge to push; increased rectal pressure; membranes may rupture if they have not already	Ambulation difficult with uterine contractions; may be irritable and agitated; self-absorbed and may appear to sleep between contractions; need for support increases; verbalizes feelings of discouragement and doubts her ability to cope
Second Stage 10 cm to birth	Primigravida, up to 3 hr; multigravida, 0–30 min	2–3 min	40–60 sec	Strong by palpation; 70–100 mm Hg by IUPC	As presenting part descends, urge to push increases; increased rectal and perineal pressure; sensation of burning, tearing, and stretching of vagina and perineum	Excited and eager to push; reluctant, ineffective at pushing
Third Stage Birth of the infant to birth of the placenta	5–30 min				Mild uterine contractions; feeling of fullness in vagina as placenta is expelled	Attention is focused on the newborn; feelings of relief

allows for adequate evaluation for patients in labor and prevents unnecessary admissions to the perinatal unit is advisable (AAP & ACOG, 2002). When false or early labor is diagnosed, the woman should be given instructions regarding when to return to the hospital. Reassuring fetal status should be determined prior to discharge, ideally using a reactive nonstress test (NST). If a thorough maternal–fetal assessment results in the decision to discharge the woman, it is important to insure that assessment and discharge processes are consistent with federal regulations as per the Emergency Medical Treatment and Labor Act.

The initial interaction during the admission process is used to develop rapport with the woman and her family and to get a sense of their expectations for their birth experience. Ideally, the amount of childbirth preparation and type of pain management anticipated during labor is covered during the admission assessment. A review of preferences for childbirth, including a discussion of options that are available at the institution, works best to facilitate a positive experience (Perez, 2005). Although some labor nurses, physicians, and other members of the perinatal team may have negative feelings toward written birth plans, a birth plan can be valuable in helping the nurse meet the couple's expectations and indicates that the woman has given considerable thought to how she would like the labor and birth to proceed (Lothian, 2006). Birth plans that have been discussed previously with the woman's primary healthcare provider can promote her participation in and satisfaction with her care (AAP & ACOG, 2002).

Ongoing Assessment of Maternal–Fetal Status

Limited data are available to support prescribed frequencies of maternal–fetal assessments during labor and birth. No prospective studies have been published concerning how often to assess the mother and fetus during labor. Therefore, a reasonable approach to determining frequency of assessment is based on individual clinical situations, guidelines, and standards from professional organizations and unit policies. ACOG recommends that maternal temperature, pulse, respirations, and BP be assessed and recorded at regular intervals during labor or least every 4 hours (AAP & ACOG, 2002). This frequency may be increased, particularly as active labor progresses, according to clinical signs and symptoms.

When using EFM during the active phase of the first stage of labor, the FHR should be assessed at 30-minute intervals, and during the active pushing phase of the second stage of labor, at 15-minute intervals, unless fetal risk status or response to labor indicates

the need for more frequent assessment (AAP & ACOG, 2002; ACOG, 2005). If risk factors are present on admission or develop during the course of labor, the FHR should be assessed every 15 minutes during the active phase of the first stage of labor and every 5 minutes during the active pushing phase of the second stage of labor (AAP & ACOG, 2002). Continuous EFM is recommended for patients with high-risk conditions (eg, suspected intrauterine growth restriction, preeclampsia, and type 1 diabetes). When EFM is used to record FHR data permanently, periodic documentation can be used to summarize fetal status, as outlined by institutional protocols. A reasonable approach is to include a summary of assessment data every 30 minutes.

If intermittent auscultation of the FHR is selected as the method of fetal assessment during labor, ACOG (2005) recommends assessment and documentation of the FHR every 15 minutes during the active phase of the first stage of labor and every 5 minutes during the second stage of labor. Regional analgesia/anesthesia, oxytocin dosage rate, and intervals between increases in oxytocin dosage rate are additional considerations when determining how often to assess maternal–fetal well-being during labor.

Guidelines for ongoing labor assessments are described in AWHONN's Symposiums *Cervical Ripening and Induction and Augmentation of Labor* (Simpson, 2002) and *Fetal Heart Rate Auscultation* (Feinstein, Sprague, & Trepanier, 2000) and AWHONN's Evidence-Based Clinical Practice Guidelines *Nursing Management of the Second Stage of Labor* (2000) and *Nursing Care of the Woman Receiving Regional Analgesia/Anesthesia in Labor* (2001). *Guidelines for Perinatal Care* (AAP & ACOG, 2002), *Intrapartum Fetal Heart Rate Monitoring* Practice Bulletin (ACOG, 2005), *Guidelines for Regional Anesthesia in Obstetrics* (American Society of Anesthesiologists [ASA], 2000), *Practice Guidelines for Obstetric Anesthesia* (ASA, 2006), perinatal nursing textbooks, and some state board of health publications are other resources that provide guidelines for initial and ongoing nursing assessments of women in labor. Based on these standards and guidelines, each perinatal center should have expectations for maternal–fetal assessment during labor in the form of clinical policies, protocols, or algorithms. See Display 7–3 and Table 7–2 for suggested guidelines for maternal and fetal assessment during labor, birth, and immediately postpartum and Chapter Appendix 7–B for a sample medical record form for documentation during labor.

While most providers in the United States currently choose continuous or intermittent EFM, the institution's policy should include guidelines for intermittent auscultation based on the ACOG (2005)

TABLE 7–2 ■ MATERNAL–FETAL ASSESSMENT AND DOCUMENTATION GUIDELINES

	Active Labor	Oxytocin	Cervidil/Cytotec	Second-Stage Labor (Active Pushing)	First hour of Magnesium Sulfate and Any Change in Dose	Magnesium Sulfate Maintenance Dose	All Other Patients
	Every 30 min*	Assessment each time rate is increased or at least every 15 min if rate is unchanged*; summary notes every 30 min	Every 30 min first two hr; then every hr*	Assessment every 15 min*; summary notes every 30 min	Every 15 min*	At least every hr*	At least every hr*
Maternal Vital Signs	P, R, BP every hr; temp every 2 hr unless ROM, then every hr	P, R, BP every hr; temp every 2 hr unless ROM, then every hr	P, R, BP every hr; temp every 2 hr unless ROM, then every hr	P, R, BP every hr; temp every 2 hr unless ROM, then every hr	P, R, BP every 15 min; temp every 2 hr unless ROM, then every hr	P, R, BP every hr; temp every 2 hr unless ROM, then every hr	T, P, R, BP every 4 hr
FHR	*	*	*	*	*	*	*
Uterine Activity	*	*	*	*	*	*	*
Pain Status	*	*	*	*	*	*	*
Response to Labor	*	*	*	*	*	* if applicable	*
Comfort Measures	*	*	*	*	*	*	*
Position	*	*	*	*	*	*	*
Oxytocin Rate (mU/min)		*					
Vaginal Exam/Fetal Station/Progress in Descent	As needed	As needed	As needed	As needed, at least every 30 minutes			
Magnesium Sulfate Rate (g/hr)					*	*	
Any Signs and Symptoms of Side Effects of Magnesium Sulfate					*	*	
Intake and Output	Every 8 hours	Every 8 hours	Every 8 hours	Every 8 hours	Every hour	Every hour	Every 8 hours

T, temperature; P, pulse; R, respirations; BP, blood pressure; FHR, fetal heart rate.

FHR characteristics include baseline rate, variability, and presence or absence of accelerations and decelerations.

Uterine activity includes contraction frequency, duration, intensity, and uterine resting tone.

DISPLAY 7-3

Maternal–Fetal–Newborn Assessments During Labor, Birth, and the Immediate Postpartum Period

MATERNAL VITAL SIGNS

Maternal vital signs should be assessed and recorded at regular intervals, at least every 4 hours. This frequency may be increased, particularly as active labor progresses according to clinical signs and symptoms (AAP & ACOG, 2002).

FETAL HEART RATE

In the absence of risk factors:
• The standard practice is to evaluate and record the FHR at least every 30 minutes during the active phase of the first stage of labor and at least every 15 minutes during the active pushing phase of the second stage of labor.

When risk factors are present, continuous EFM is recommended:
• During the active phase of the first stage of labor the FHR should be evaluated every 15 minutes.
• During the active pushing phase of the second stage of labor the FHR should be evaluated at least every 5 minutes. (AAP & ACOG, 2002).

During oxytocin induction or augmentation, the FHR should be evaluated every 15 minutes during the active phase of the first stage of labor and every 5 minutes during the active pushing phase of the second stage of labor (AAP & ACOG, 2002).

When EFM is used to record FHR data permanently, periodic documentation can be used to summarize fetal status as outlined by institutional protocols. During oxytocin induction or augmentation, at a minimum, the FHR should be documented before each dose increase. If the dosage is maintained at the same rate, a reasonable approach is for nurses to document the FHR at least every 30 minutes during the first stage of labor and during the active pushing phase of the second stage of labor while oxytocin is being administered (Simpson, 2002).

Misoprostol should be administered at or near the labor and birth suite, where the FHR can be monitored continuously (ACOG, 1999b).

Cervidil (prostaglandin E$_2$ [PGE$_2$] vaginal insert [Forest Pharmaceuticals, St. Louis, MO]) should be administered at or near the labor and birth suite, where the FHR can be monitored continuously while in place and for at least 15 minutes after removal (ACOG, 1999b).

Prepidil (PGE$_2$ gel [Pharmacia and Upjohn Co., Peapack, NJ] should be administered at or near the labor and birth suite, where the FHR can be monitored continuously for 30 minutes to 2 hours after administration (ACOG, 1999b).

UTERINE ACTIVITY/LABOR PROGRESS

For women who are at no increased risk for complications, evaluation of the quality of uterine contractions should be sufficient to detect abnormalities in the progress of labor (AAP & ACOG, 2002).

Generally, uterine activity should be assessed each time the FHR is assessed, because uterine activity has implications for fetal status.

When EFM is used to record uterine activity data permanently, periodic documentation can be used to summarize uterine activity as outlined by institutional protocols.

During oxytocin induction or augmentation, at a minimum, uterine contractions should be assessed before every dosage increase. If the dosage is maintained at the same rate, a reasonable approach is for nurses to document uterine activity at least every 30 minutes during the first stage of labor and during the active pushing phase of the second stage of labor while oxytocin is being administered (Simpson, 2002).

Misoprostol should be administered at or near the labor and birth suite, where uterine activity can be monitored continuously (ACOG, 1999b).

Cervidil should be administered at or near the labor and birth suite, where uterine activity can be monitored continuously while in place and for at least 15 minutes after removal (ACOG, 1999b).

Prepidil should be administered at or near the labor and birth suite, where uterine activity can be monitored continuously for at least 30 minutes to 2 hours after placement (ACOG, 1999b).

Vaginal examinations and evaluation of the quality of uterine contractions should be sufficient to detect abnormalities in the progress of labor (AAP & ACOG, 2002). Vaginal examinations include assessment of dilation and effacement of the cervix and station of the fetal presenting part.

MONITORING AND ASSESSMENT DURING REGIONAL ANALGESIA/ANESTHESIA

Women who receive epidural analgesia should be monitored in a manner similar to that used for any patient in labor.

For women in labor receiving regional anesthesia, vital signs and FHR should be monitored and documented by a qualified individual (ASA, 2000).

When regional anesthesia is administered during labor, maternal vital signs should be monitored at regular intervals by a qualified member of the healthcare team (AAP & ACOG, 2002).

Before epidural anesthesia/analgesia is initiated, the nurse should assess and document maternal vital signs. The FHR should be assessed before and after the procedure, either intermittently or continuously, and as possible during the procedure. Additional monitoring of the patient should be provided during epidural anesthesia/analgesia when the patient's condition warrants (AWHONN, 2001). A suggested protocol includes assessing "the FHR after the initiation or re-bolus of a regional block, including PCEA. FHR may be assessed every 5 minutes for the first 15 minutes. More or less frequent monitoring may be indicated based on consideration of factors such as the type of analgesia/anesthesia, route and dose of medication used, the maternal-fetal response to medication, maternal-fetal consideration, the stage of labor or facility protocol" (AWHONN, 2001, p. 13).

ADDITIONAL PARAMETERS

Assess character and amount of amniotic fluid (eg, clear, bloody, meconium stained, odorous).

Assess character and amount of bloody show/vaginal bleeding.

Assess maternal and fetal response to labor.

Assess level of maternal discomfort and effectiveness of pain management/pain relief measures.

Assess labor support person(s)' abilities.

ASSESSMENTS DURING THE IMMEDIATE POSTPARTUM PERIOD

Maternal Assessments

During the period of observation immediately after birth, maternal vital signs and additional signs or events should be monitored and recorded as they occur. Maternal blood pressure and pulse should be assessed and recorded immediately after birth and repeated every

15 minutes for the first hour. These evaluations may be undertaken more frequently if warranted by the woman's condition or findings. The amount of vaginal bleeding should be evaluated often, and the uterine fundus should be identified and massaged and its size and degree of contraction noted (AAP & ACOG, 2002).

Newborn Assessments

Apgar scores should be obtained at 1 minute and 5 minutes after birth. If the 5-minute Apgar score is less than 7, additional scores should be assigned every 5 minutes up to 20 minutes. Temperature, heart and respiratory rates, skin color, adequacy of peripheral circulation, type of respiration, level of consciousness, tone, and activity should be monitored and recorded at least once every 30 minutes until the newborn's condition has remained stable for at least 2 hours (AAP & ACOG, 2002).

Summary

When determining frequency of maternal–fetal assessments during labor, factors such as stage of labor; maternal–fetal risk status; and institutional policies, procedures, and protocols should be taken into consideration. As new standards and guidelines are published, these assessment parameters will need to be reviewed and updated.

---

recommendations if electronic monitoring is not the preference of the woman, physician, or certified nurse midwife (CNM). Women with high-risk conditions (eg, suspected fetal growth restriction, preeclampsia, type 1 diabetes, abnormal antepartum test [NST, biophysical profile, modified biophysical profile, contraction stress test, blood flow studies] results, receiving prostaglandin agents for cervical ripening or labor induction) should be monitored continuously via EFM (ACOG, 1999b, 2005) The AWHONN symposium *Fetal Heart Rate Auscultation* (Feinstein et al., 2000) provides a comprehensive discussion about technique, rationale, interpretation, and clinical decision making when using intermittent auscultation during labor.

Maternal–fetal assessment should occur at the bedside by laying hands on the pregnant woman rather than using data obtained from the central monitoring station. Characteristics of FHR patterns may be different when obtained by direct observation of the EFM tracing at the bedside. Direct observation allows assessment of maternal anxiety or pain, contractions, and positioning, all of which have potential to affect vital signs. For example, maternal anxiety or pain can result in increases in BP, pulse, and respirations, while maternal supine positioning can result in hypotension. Repositioning from semi-Fowler's position to a lateral position may result in a decrease in diastolic BP of up to 10 mm Hg. Changes (increase or

decrease) in maternal heart rate may occur during contractions (Murray, 2004). Maternal pushing efforts that involve the Valsava maneuver result in an initial increase, then a decrease in BP (Caldeyro-Barcia et al., 1981).

Use of automatic BP devices should be avoided, as they may record inaccurate data during pregnancy and specifically during labor. Use of a manual BP cuff and stethoscope is the more accurate method of assessing BP in pregnant and laboring women (Green & Froman, 1996; Hasan, Thomas, & Prys-Roberts, 1993; Marx, Schwalbe, Cho, & Whitty, 1993; Natarajan et al., 1999; Pomini et al., 2001). Automatic BP devices tend to overestimate systolic BP by 4–6 mm Hg and underestimate diastolic BP by 10 mm Hg when used for pregnant women (Brown et al., 1994; Franx et al., 1994). Inaccuracies in BP data can lead to inappropriate treatment. For example, a diastolic BP of 95 mm Hg obtained by a nurse using a manual BP cuff and stethoscope would be recorded as 85 mm Hg by an automatic BP device, so an elevated BP would potentially be missed and not treated appropriately or in a timely manner. In contrast, an underestimated diastolic BP could result in treatment for hypotension following epidural dosage potentially leading to fetal compromise if a vasopressor is given for hypotension that does not actually exist. Many women report discomfort when automatic BP cuffs are used frequently during labor.

Standards of care, inaccuracy issues, costs, and patient discomfort should be important considerations in discontinuing routine use of automatic BP devices, cardiac monitors, and pulse oximeters for healthy women during labor. If the woman's clinical condition requires more intensive and frequent monitoring, use of these devices may be appropriate and can provide valuable data about maternal well-being. Data from automatic BP devices may be used for evaluating trends in maternal BP for women who need more intensive and frequent assessment, but should be used in the context of what is known about the differences in readings obtained from mercury BP cuffs and a stethoscope as compared to these devices.

Evaluation of routine practices for healthy women who desire regional analgesia during labor and/or are receiving pharmacologic agents to stimulate uterine contractions should be based on available literature and publications from ACOG (2002a), AWHONN (2001), and ASA (2000, 2006). A standards-based protocol contributes to appropriate levels of care according to individual clinical situations, while avoiding unnecessary interventions and technology.

There are no standards or guidelines from AWHONN or ACOG about how often BP should be assessed when women are receiving oxytocin, yet in many institutions, protocols are in place that require every 15-minute BP assessment. These protocols are not based on any sound scientific data; however, they contribute to the routine use of automatic BP devices during labor because intrapartum nurses find it difficult to manually assess maternal BP every 15 minutes if they are responsible for more than one patient. These protocols have not been shown to contribute to better outcomes during labor. If the nurse has responsibility for more than one patient in labor, many times the automatic BP device is activated according to programmed intervals while the nurse is not at the bedside. The automatic BP device can be initiated and data recorded during a uterine contraction. Maternal pain and anxiety during the height of a contraction can alter BP. The woman in labor may have repositioned herself while the nurse was out of the room. It is well known that maternal positions affect BP. These data are either automatically recorded on the EFM strip or manually recorded in the medical record by the nurse when she has time to return to the bedside. Thus, BP data obtained by automatic devices are not used in a clinically timely manner and may have been obtained during a uterine contraction or following a maternal position change unknown to the nurse. Retrospective evaluation and documentation of a series of BPs recorded by an automatic BP device while the nurse was out of the room is not consistent with timely assessment during labor. If an automatic BP device is chosen to evaluate trends in maternal status, the nurse should activate it at the bedside so

a complete assessment can be made, rather than setting the device at preprogrammed intervals with the risk of activation when the nurse is away from the bedside.

In many institutions, routine care for healthy women during epidural analgesia includes cardiac monitoring, pulse oximetry, and frequent BP assessment using an automatic BP device. Use of these monitoring devices are not required (AAP & ACOG, 2002; ACOG, 2002a; ASA, 2000, 2006; AWHONN, 2001) and may lead to increased cost and unnecessary technologic interventions for women without identified risk factors. Discourage continuous maternal oxygen saturation (SpO2) monitoring because it often produces inaccurate data due to maternal movement and dislocation of the device. Often, long periods of erroneous recordings of low SpO2 are automatically entered into the electronic medical record and printed on the paper version of the FHR tracing without nursing confirmation that these data accurately reflect maternal condition. Pulse oximeters are designed to measure SpO2 rather than heart rate. Continuous tracing of maternal heart rate on the FHR tracing often obscures the FHR, particularly during second-stage pushing. Spot checks of maternal SpO2 are more appropriate if there is a concern regarding maternal oxygen status. Manual assessment of maternal pulse is more appropriate for differentiating between maternal heart rate and FHR is there is a concern regarding the origin of heart rate tracing as maternal versus fetal. Unless risk factors have been identified, care for a woman with epidural analgesia may be similar to that of any other woman in labor. Regular assessment of maternal–fetal status should be performed by a qualified healthcare provider during epidural analgesia for labor and birth (ASA, 2000, 2006).

Vaginal Examinations

Nurses should develop proficiency in performing vaginal examinations to assess labor progress, and determine the need for nursing interventions such as position change and timing of medication. They must first be able to identify situations in which a vaginal examination is required and also recognize when a vaginal examination is contraindicated, such as with unexplained vaginal bleeding or with premature rupture of the membranes. Developing clinical proficiency in performing vaginal examinations requires practice and assistance from a knowledgeable preceptor. Because full assessment may require more time than usual during the period when vaginal examination skills are being acquired, an ideal patient for nurses to learn the technique has adequate regional anesthesia and intact membranes so she can tolerate the potentially longer vaginal examination and there is less risk of infection with the confirmation examination by the preceptor. Usually, patients who are fully informed that the examiner is learning will consent to this type of examination.

Women undergoing a vaginal examination should be minimally exposed and should be advised of the necessity of the examination and the findings. The woman should also be positioned on her back with her head slightly elevated. The vaginal examination should be as quick as possible, but systematic, beginning with assessment of dilation and effacement, then fetal presentation, station, and position. The normal length of the pregravid cervix is 3.5–4 cm. The length of the cervix may vary in women who have had any cervical surgery, such as conization or laser excision procedures.

Assessment of station and position of the fetal head requires more skill. The ischial spines must be identified to assess station in relation to the biparietal diameter of the fetal head. The ischial spines may be identified by pressing in the sidewall of the vagina approximately 1 inch, with the examining fingers at approximately 3 and 9 o'clock, respectively. It is not necessary to identify both spines to assess station. The occiput of the fetal head should be at the level of the ischial spines, to be engaged or zero station. The examiner should not be confused by caput formation but instead identify the fetal skull for this assessment.

The most difficult determination to make is that of fetal head position: occiput anterior or posterior. The examining nurse must be familiar with the location of the suture lines in the fetal skull more so than the shape of the anterior or posterior fontanelle because distortion or overlapping bones will alter fontanelle shape. The nurse should first identify the sagittal suture and then slide fingers to a fontanelle and count the number of suture lines extending from it exclusive of the sagittal suture. This can be accomplished by sweeping the examining finger 180° at a right angle to the sagittal suture. The anterior fontanelle has three suture lines extending from it, and the posterior fontanelle has two suture lines. It is not necessary to palpate the posterior fontanelle to determine position of the fetal head. Determination of the position of the fetal head becomes necessary primarily during the second stage when descent is slow. Repositioning the woman to a squatting, side-lying, or hands and knees position to push or using the towel pull technique during pushing may facilitate rotation of the fetal head.

Perineal hygiene is important during periodic vaginal examinations. Attention to clean technique is critical, particularly if membranes are ruptured. Sterile water-soluble lubricants may be used to decrease discomfort during vaginal examinations; however, antiseptics such as povidone-iodine and hexachlorophene should be avoided. These antiseptics have not been shown to decrease infections acquired during the intrapartum period, but they may cause local irritation and are absorbed through maternal mucous membranes and fetal skin (AAP & ACOG, 2002). Thus, lubricants containing these agents, and sprays or liquids delivering them directly to the introitus, are not recommended for use during labor (AAP & ACOG, 2002).

Leopold Maneuvers

Leopold maneuvers provide a systematic assessment of fetal position and presentation and should be performed prior to application of EFM, as part of the admission assessment by appropriately educated licensed personnel. Information obtained while performing these maneuvers supports assessments made during vaginal examinations and assists in determining the best position to locate the FHR (see Figure 7–3). Leopold maneuvers may be difficult with women who are obese, have tense or guarded abdominal muscles, or have polyhydramnios. In these situations, an ultrasound may be necessary to determine fetal position and presentation.

Fetal Heart Rate Assessment

Systematic assessment of the FHR via EFM includes determination of the baseline rate, variability, and presence or absence of accelerations and decelerations. Intermittent auscultation of the FHR via stethoscope or handheld ultrasound device includes determination of the rate and presence or absence of accelerations and decelerations. If decelerations are noted, further assessment is required to determine the type and duration. Clinical interventions are based on comprehensive assessment of all of the characteristics of the FHR pattern depicted via EFM or noted during auscultation and the individual clinical situation of the mother and fetus including, but not limited to, gestational age and medications administered to the mother. The FHR can be determined by use of the external ultrasound device of the EFM in most situations. If the clinical situation is such that more accurate data are needed about fetal status, an internal fetal scalp electrode (FSE) may be applied. See Chapter 8 for a comprehensive discussion about FHR assessment.

Uterine Activity Assessment

A thorough and accurate assessment of the frequency, duration, and intensity of contractions and the uterine resting tone between contractions is an important component of nursing assessments during labor. An assessment of uterine activity begins with direct palpation. Contraction frequency is measured from the beginning of one contraction to the beginning of the next and is described in minutes. Duration is assessed

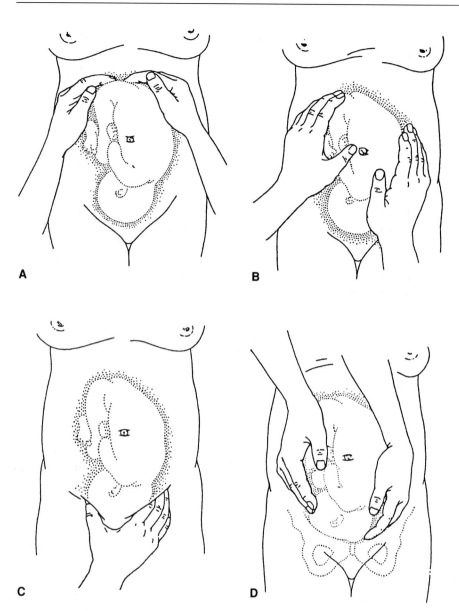

FIGURE 7–3. Leopold maneuvers. **A,** First maneuver. **B,** Second maneuver. **C,** Third maneuver. **D,** Fourth maneuver.

by the length of the contraction and is described in seconds. Intensity refers to the strength of the contraction and is described as mild, moderate, or strong by palpation, or millimeters of mercury (mm Hg) of intraamniotic pressure with an intrauterine pressure catheter. Uterine resting tone is assessed in the absence of contractions or between contractions. By direct palpation, resting tone is described as soft or hard, and by intrauterine pressure catheter (IUPC) in terms of mm Hg of intraamniotic pressure.

The external tocodynamometer detects abdominal wall changes during contractions and uterine relaxation. This method provides information about frequency and duration; however, resting tone and intensity must be determined by palpation. Contraction frequency, duration, intensity, and uterine resting tone can be evaluated by both palpation and an IUPC. The

IUPC is more accurate because direct measurement of intraamniotic pressure is recorded but requires ruptured membranes for insertion. The cervix should be at least 2–3 cm dilated before insertion of an IUPC or FSE. As with any procedure, the least invasive approach is preferred unless maternal–fetal status indicates need for more objective data.

Intravenous Fluids and Oral Intake During Labor and Birth

Before the 1940s, women in the United States were encouraged to eat and drink during labor to maintain their stamina for the work of childbirth (American College of Nurse Midwives [ACNM], 2000). In 1946, Mendelson suggested that maternal aspiration of gastric contents during general anesthesia for cesarean birth was a significant cause of maternal morbidity. This was based on his theory that the delay in gastric emptying during labor contributed to aspiration pneumonitis and that the acidity of the gastric contents determined the severity of maternal complications and risk of death (Mendelson, 1946). For the next 50 years, to prevent aspiration should a cesarean birth be necessary, fasting became the norm for laboring women in most hospitals in the United States. It is now known that regardless of the time of the woman's last meal, the stomach is never completely empty and that fasting does not eliminate stomach contents but rather increases the concentration of hydrochloric acid (ACNM, 2000).

Risks of general anesthesia–related maternal morbidity have decreased significantly since the 1940s but have remained constant over the past 20 years (Hawkins, 2003). Decreased use of general anesthesia for cesarean birth, use of cricoid pressure, and routine tracheal intubation with improved technique have contributed to decline in maternal mortality (Sommer, Norr, & Roberts, 2000). In the cases of anesthesia-related maternal deaths that have been reported in the literature, complications such as poor physical status, obesity, emergent procedures, hypertension, embolism, and hemorrhage appear to be co-existing factors (ACNM, 2000; Hawkins, 2003; Ross, 2003). Most women in the United States who have a cesarean birth are given regional anesthesia. The case fatality rate for regional anesthesia between 1991 and 1996 was recently reported to be 2.5 per million regional anesthetics during cesarean birth (Hawkins, 2003). The case fatality rate for general anesthesia during the same period was 16.8 per million general anesthetics for cesarean birth (Hawkins, 2003). Although rare, the number-one cause of maternal death in obstetric anesthesia is aspiration of gastric contents frequently associated with a difficult or failed intubation (Hawkins, 2003). Failed intubation is much more common in obstetrics than in the general population (1 in 280 obstetrics versus 1 in 2,230 in all other patients); therefore, all members of the perinatal team should be familiar with the ASA (2003) *Difficult Airway Algorithm*.

The physiologic requirements for glucose increase during active labor (Wasserstrum, 1992). Fasting depletes the carbohydrates available; thus, women in labor who not allowed oral intake may have to metabolize fat for energy (Keppler, 1988). Although there has been limited research about specific nutritional needs during labor, it has been suggested that 50 to 100 calories per hour are needed during active labor (ACNM, 2000). The energy needs of the laboring woman have been compared to those of athletes in competition. Pregnancy and labor are characterized by an exaggerated response to starvation, reflected in part by more rapid development of hypoglycemia and hyperketonemia

(Wasserstrum, 1992). Thus, modest amounts of oral intake during labor may be beneficial for women without complications or risks of complications. When women are allowed oral intake during labor, the amount of food and fluids they chose generally decrease as labor progresses (Ludka & Roberts, 1994). Few women choose to eat solid food beyond the latent phase of labor (Parsons, Bidewell, & Nagy, 2006).

In light of the data about the rarity of anesthesia-related maternal mortality and other evidence about nutritional needs of laboring women, in 1999 ASA revised its recommendations for oral intake during labor. These recommendations are supported by ACOG (2002a) and were reaffirmed by ASA in 2006. Examples of clear liquids recommended by ASA (2006) during labor include water, fruit juices without pulp, carbonated beverages, clear tea, black coffee, and sports drinks. Flavored gelatin, fruit ice, popsicles, and broth also are many times offered. The volume of liquid is less important than the type of liquid. ASA (2006) recommends restricting oral fluids on a case-by-case basis for women who are at risk for aspiration (eg, morbidly obese, diabetic, difficult airway) and for women at risk for operative birth (eg, nonreassuring fetal heart rate patterns and nonprogression of labor). A fasting time for solid food that is predictive of maternal anesthesia complications has not been determined, so there is insufficient evidence to support safe recommendations for solid intake during labor (ASA, 2006). A fasting time for solid food of at least 6 to 8 hours prior to elective cesarean birth is recommended (ASA, 2006). A risk assessment of women in labor should determine whether oral fluid and/or solid intake is appropriate (ACNM, 2000).

Each institution should have a policy for oral nutrition during labor that has been developed in collaboration with anesthesia providers. This policy should not arbitrarily restrict oral and solid intake during labor but rather be based on what is known about complications that increase the risk of general anesthesia. Inform women of the small, but potentially serious, risks of aspiration related to oral intake during labor (ACNM, 2000). Make it clear that it is the anesthesia that is the risk, not the oral intake, and if labor deviates from the normal she may be asked to refrain from oral intake (ACNM, 2000).

Normal healthy women at term have at least 2 liters of water stored in their extravascular spaces and have accumulated fat and fluids over the course of the pregnancy (Sleutel & Golden, 1999). A long labor with the woman fasting may deplete those energy resources. Maternal fluid loss occurs with perspiration, use of various breathing techniques, and vomiting. When fasting during labor became the norm after the 1940s, administration of intravenous (IV) fluids became routine practice. Prophylactic IV access was advocated in anticipation of administration of rapid volume expanders and blood products in the case of emergencies that can result in maternal hypovolemia and hemorrhage, such as uterine rupture, abruptio placentae, regional anesthesia complications, and immediate postpartum hemorrhage.

IV fluids are thought to increase maternal blood volume, leading to increased blood flow (oxygen) to the placenta and resulting in more oxygen available at the placenta site for maternal–fetal exchange. Therefore, non-glucose-containing IV fluid boluses are often given during a nonreassuring FHR pattern (Simpson, 2007). In a recent study, fetuses of mothers who were given an IV fluid bolus of either 500 mL or 1,000 mL of lactated Ringer's solution over 20 minutes had significant increases in fetal SpO2 that persisted at least 30 minutes after the IV fluid bolus was completed (Simpson & James, 2005b). The greatest increase occurred in the fetuses of mothers who received 1,000 mL. The women in this study were normotensive and adequately hydrated, and their fetuses had reassuring FHR patterns. Therefore, an IV fluid bolus can result in a transfer of maternal oxygen to the fetus even if the woman is not experiencing hypotension or dehydration (Simpson & James, 2005b). It is likely that the benefits of an IV fluid bolus would be greater if the FHR pattern were nonreassuring because of the transfer of oxygen through the placenta by passive diffusion from high concentration to low concentration, but more data are needed regarding this common intervention.

Administration of IV solutions containing glucose during labor is controversial and probably causes more harm than good (Sleutel & Golden, 1999). In theory, administration of glucose averts maternal hypoglycemia and starvation ketosis; however, there is evidence to suggest that maternal IV administration of glucose can have potentially detrimental effects on fetal status including increased fetal lactate and decreased fetal pH (Philpson, Kalhan, Riha, & Pimentel, 1987). If the fetus is hypoxic, relatively small elevations in glucose can lead to lactate acidosis (Philpson et al., 1987; Wasserstrum, 1992). IV solutions with glucose can cause fetal hyperglycemia and subsequent reactive hypoglycemia, hyperinsulinism, hyponatremia, acidosis, jaundice, and transient tachypnea in the newborn after birth (Carmen, 1986; Grylack, Chu, & Scanlon, 1984; Mendiola, Grylack, & Scanlon, 1982; Singhi, 1988; Sleutel & Golden, 1999; Sommer et al., 2000). A bolus of IV solution containing glucose can cause marked maternal hyperglycemia (Mendiola et al., 1982; Wasserstrum, 1992). Thus, when the clinical situation is such that a bolus of IV fluids may be necessary to expand plasma volume (eg, initial treatment for preterm labor, before administration of epidural anesthesia, or during hypovolemic maternal emergencies), the IV fluids should not contain glucose (Cerri et al., 2000; Hawkins, 2003). Glucose requirements vary depending on weight, use of anesthesia, phase of labor, fetal status, and other factors, so it is difficult to determine the optimal rate of glucose infusion during labor.

Despite the controversy about glucose administration during labor, occasionally lactated Ringer's solution with 5% dextrose (D5L/R) may be administered during labor. One liter of D5L/R IV solution provides 225 calories (ACNM, 2000). The most common IV solution used during labor is lactated Ringer's (L/R). An isotonic IV solution should be used to dilute oxytocin during induction and augmentation of labor (ACOG, 1999b). Two randomized controlled trials suggest that the usual amount of IV fluids during labor (125 mL/hr) may be insufficient to meet the needs of women and that inadequate hydration during labor may cause complications of labor (Eslamian, Marsoosi, & Pakneeyat, 2006; Garite, Weeks, & Peters-Phair, 2000). These researchers found that women who received 125 mL/hr of L/R solution had longer labors, more oxytocin, and higher rates of cesarean birth when compared with women who received 250 mL/hr of L/R IV fluids. A study of pregnant women comparing different amounts of oral intake considering the same outcome variables would add to what is known about how much and what method of hydration during labor is appropriate.

Individual clinical situations should guide the selection of IV fluids during labor. More data are needed about the appropriate amount and type of IV fluids during labor. This area of intrapartum care has not been well researched, so practice is based on tradition rather than solid evidence. Current resources for guidelines about IV fluids and oral intake during labor include *Practice Guidelines for Obstetrical Anesthesia* (ASA, 2006) and the *Intrapartum Nutrition Clinical Bulletin* (ACNM, 2000).

Maternal Positioning During Labor and Birth

Unit culture, clinician preferences, and patient cultural background often determine the position women assume during labor and childbirth, such as lying down, squatting, sitting, standing, kneeling, or on all fours (Engleman, 1884; Liu, 1989). Recumbency, a Western cultural tradition for the convenience of obstetricians, began when more women were hospitalized for childbirth. Early medical research challenging the recumbent position was ignored (Mengert & Murphy, 1933; Vaughn, 1937). Many women today are confined to bed during the majority of labor as a result of the widespread use of EFM, IVs, oxytocin, and regional analgesia/anesthesia. However, even while in bed, women may be assisted to various positions for labor and birth that may improve maternal and fetal outcomes.

Ambulation during labor has been shown to decrease the rate of operative birth by 50% (Albers et al., 1997). Women who are encouraged to be mobile during labor report greater comfort and ability to tolerate labor, as well as decreased use of analgesia and anesthesia (Bloom et al, 1998; Lupe & Gross, 1986). Although recent tradition in the United States is confining women in active labor to bed, there is no greater risk of adverse maternal–fetal outcomes when women are encouraged to ambulate during labor (Bloom et al, 1998). If continuous EFM has been selected as the method of fetal assessment during labor, use of EFM via telemetry can allow the woman to ambulate while being monitored, even while Cervidil is in place or oxytocin is being administered.

An upright position shortens labor. Duration of both first- and second-stage labor are shorter in women who labor 30° upright as compared to those in a flat recumbent position (Liu, 1989; Terry, Wescott, O'Shea, & Kelly, 2006). An upright position can also decrease the use of pain medication and the need for oxytocin (Bodner-Adler et al., 2003). In one study, the second stage of labor was decreased when women were in a squatting position (primiparous women, 23 minutes; multiparous women, 13 minutes), and there was less use of oxytocin, fewer mechanically assisted births, and fewer and less-severe lacerations and episiotomies compared to semirecumbent births (Golay, Vedam, & Sorger, 1993). More recent data support these early findings. Evidence suggests that any upright or lateral position during second-stage labor results in less pain, less perineal trauma, fewer episiotomies, fewer operative-assisted births, and fewer FHR abnormalities (Bodner-Adler et al., 2003; de Jong et al., 1997; Downe, Garrett, & Renfrew, 2004; Ragnar, Altman, Tyden, & Olsson, 2006; Roberts, Algert, Cameron, & Torvaldsen, 2004; Schiessl et al., 2005). Sitting on the toilet may be an acceptable and comfortable alternative to squatting for women who are fatigued (Shermer & Raines, 1997). Perineal edema and pelvic congestion can be prevented when using the toilet for first- or second-stage labor by position changes every 10 to 15 minutes (Shermer & Raines, 1997).

It is important to avoid the supine position during labor because of the relationship between lying flat and maternal hypotension and impedance of utero–placental blood flow. When the woman in labor is supine, the pressure of the uterus against the spine causes compression of the inferior vena cava, aorta, and iliac arteries. If the woman prefers to lie down, a left or right lateral position promotes maternal–fetal exchange at the placental level and enhances fetal well-being (Simpson & James, 2005b). Research has been done to enhance fetal rotation from occiput posterior (OP) to occiput anterior (OA) because there is an association between adverse neonatal outcomes and a persistent OP position (Cheng, Shaffer, & Caughey, 2006). Preliminary data suggest a hands-and-knees position for at least 30 minutes during labor may be beneficial in promoting rotation from OP to OA (Stremler et al., 2005). Other methods that may be beneficial are lateral positioning during labor and using the towel-pull technique during second-stage pushing efforts. The hands-and-knees position can help to reduce back pain for women in labor and may be useful during both first- and second-stage labor (Stremler et al., 2005). Women are often assisted to hands-and-knees position for certain nonreassuring FHR patterns but returned to a more standard position for birth. Last-minute change of maternal position for birth may be unwarranted, because birth may be just as easily accomplished in hands-and-knees position (Brunner, Drummond, Meenan, & Gaskin, 1998; Gannon, 1992). Some women may benefit from use of a birth ball for relieving pressure and facilitating a more comfortable position during labor. Figures 7–4 A–V depict positions for labor and birth.

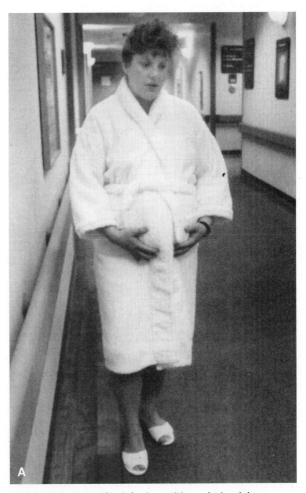

FIGURE 7–4, A–V. Physiologic positions during labor. **A,** Walking.

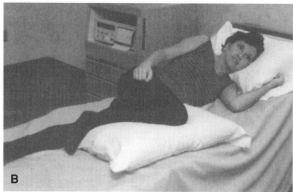

FIGURE 7–4B. Sidelying with pillow support.

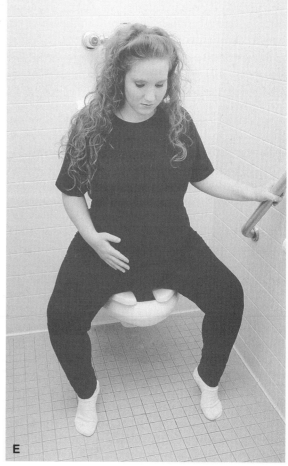

FIGURE 7–4D. Using birthing ball while standing.

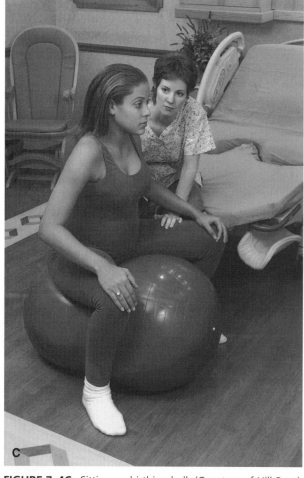

FIGURE 7–4C. Sitting on birthing ball. (Courtesy of Hill-Rom)

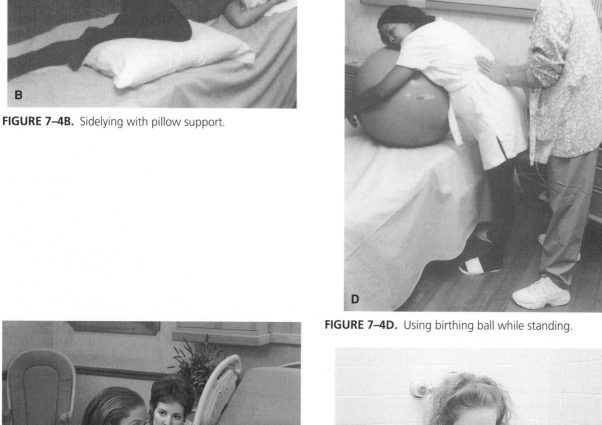

FIGURE 7–4E. Sitting on toilet; also can be used for pushing.

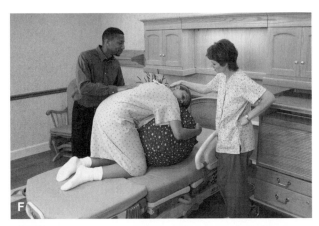

FIGURE 7–4F. Kneeling in bed using birthing ball. (Courtesy of Hill-Rom)

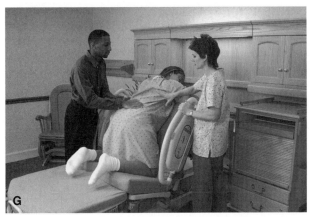

FIGURE 7–4G. Kneeling in bed with head of bed elevated and chest supported; partner applying counter-pressure. (Courtesy of Hill-Rom)

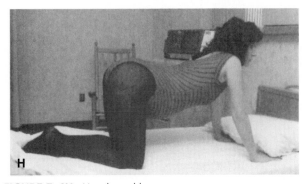

FIGURE 7–4H. Hands and knees.

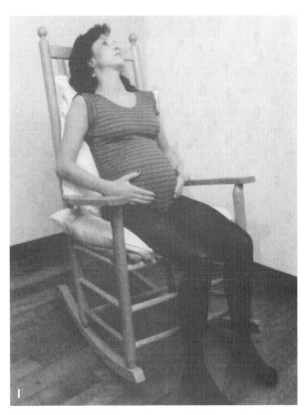

FIGURE 7–4I. Rocking.

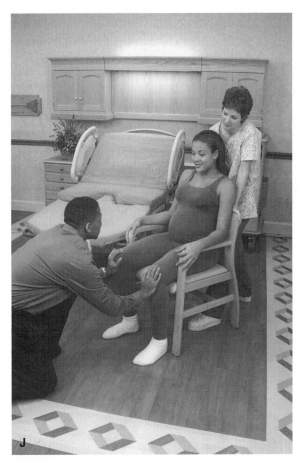

FIGURE 7–4J. Sitting with partner massaging legs. (Courtesy of Hill-Rom)

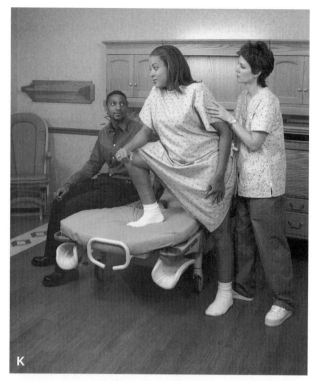

FIGURE 7–4K. Lunging using foot of bed. (Courtesy of Hill-Rom)

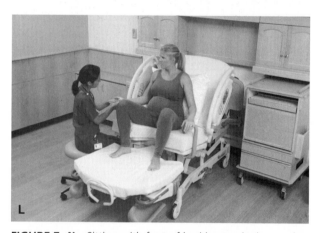

FIGURE 7–4L. Sitting with foot of bed lowered; also can be used for pushing. (Courtesy of Hill-Rom)

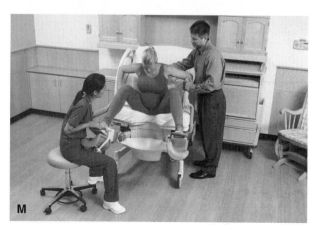

FIGURE 7–4M. Pushing using foot rests as support. (Courtesy of Hill-Rom)

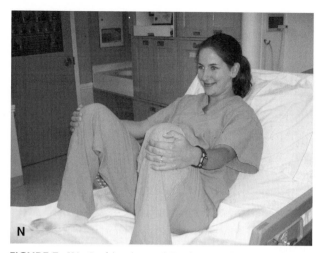

FIGURE 7–4N. Pushing in semi-Fowler's position with feet flat on bed.

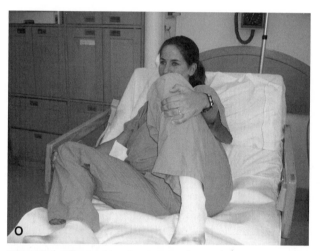

FIGURE 7–4O. Pushing in semi-Fowler's position with right tilt.

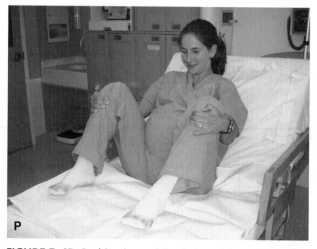

FIGURE 7–4P. Pushing in semi-Fowler's position with mother holding knees back slightly.

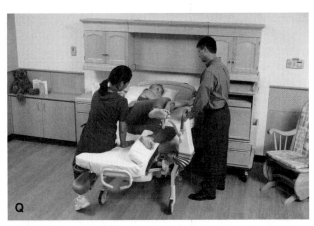

FIGURE 7–4Q. Pushing in sidelying position. (Courtesy of Hill-Rom)

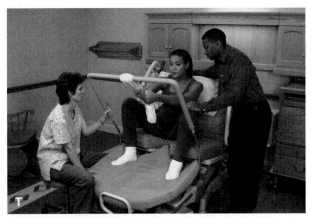

FIGURE 7–4T. Pushing using towel-pull technique with squatting bar and feet flat on bed. (Courtesy of Hill-Rom)

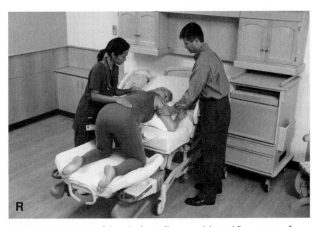

FIGURE 7–4R. Pushing in kneeling position. (Courtesy of Hill-Rom)

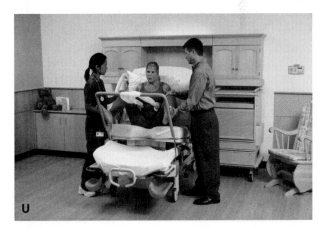

FIGURE 7–4U. Pushing using towel-pull technique with squatting bar and feet supported against bar. (Courtesy of Hill-Rom)

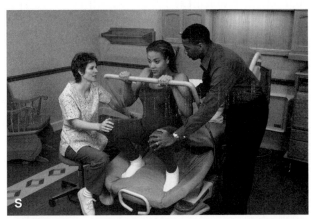

FIGURE 7–4S. Pushing using squatting bar. (Courtesy of Hill-Rom)

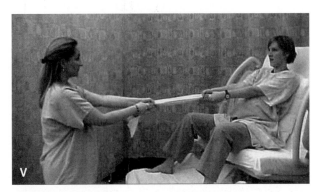

FIGURE 7–4V. Pushing using towel-pull technique with counter pull of nurse.

Regional anesthesia/analgesia may limit the use of some positions for labor and birth, particularly if there is significant enough motor blockade to prevent easy repositioning or ambulation. Epidurals that produce less motor block and intrathecal narcotics are becoming more prevalent and are more efficient because they can provide excellent pain management without as much of a limit to mobility (Cohen, Yeh, Riley, & Vogel, 2000; Collis, Harding, & Morgan, 1999; Manning, 1996). Using medication dosages that provide an analgesic rather than an anesthetic level of epidural allows the woman to move about more freely and feel pressure as the fetal head descends (Cohen et al, 2000; Collis et al., 1999; Driver, Popham, Glazebrook, & Palmer, 1996; Olofsson, Ekblom, Ekman-Ordeberg, & Irestedt, 1998; Roberts, 2002). Feeling pressure will facilitate spontaneous maternal bearing down efforts during the second stage of labor (Roberts, 2002). Nurses should be innovative with use of positioning techniques for women with epidurals to facilitate birth while maintaining maternal safety (Gilder, Mayberry, Gennaro, & Clemmens, 2002). If the mother is confined to bed, sitting may still be accomplished by adjusting the birthing bed to a more upright position, dropping the lower section or by helping the mother sit on the side of the bed with a stool for support (Mayberry, Strange, Suplee, & Gennaro, 2003). The use of a bean bag in the bed may also assist with an upright position in women whose epidurals have resulted in decreased motor sensation in the extremities.

Supportive care techniques during labor and interventions to manage the pain most women experience related to labor and birth are covered in detail in Chapter 9.

Care During Second-Stage Labor

The second stage of labor begins when the cervix is completely dilated. However, women often begin to have an involuntary urge to push prior to complete cervical dilation (Roberts, 2002). This urge to push is triggered by the Ferguson reflex as the presenting fetal part stretches pelvic floor muscles (Ferguson, 1941). Stretch receptors are then activated, releasing endogenous oxytocin, supporting the hypotheses that the urge to push is dependent more on station than dilation (Cosner & deJong, 1993; Noble, 1981). Women report well-defined urges to push that occur before, during, and after complete dilation (McKay, Barrows, & Roberts, 1990). These findings suggest that "when to push" should be individualized to the maternal response rather than labor routines that dictate pushing at complete dilation (AWHONN, 2000, 2006; Roberts, 2002). The goals

during the second stage of labor should be to support, rather than direct, the woman's involuntary pushing efforts leading to movement of the fetus down and out of the pelvis and to minimize the use of the Valsalva maneuver with its associated negative maternal hemodynamic effects and resultant adverse implications for the fetus (AWHONN, 2000, 2006; Simpson & James, 2005a). Preparing women who attend childbirth classes to anticipate and actively participate in a physiologic-based second stage of labor may be beneficial in promoting optimal care (Simpson, 2006).

There are generally two approaches to coaching women to push during the second stage of labor: open- and closed-glottis pushing. The traditional approach is to begin pushing and bearing down instructions at complete dilation whether or not the woman feels the urge to push. This technique has been used more frequently since the widespread incidence of epidural anesthesia, yet it has no scientific basis and is known to be harmful to maternal–fetal well-being (Aldrich et al., 1995; Caldeyro-Barcia, 1979; Langer et al, 1997; Simpson & James, 2005a; Thomson, 1993). Typically, women are coached to take a deep breath and hold it for at least 10 seconds while bearing down three to four times during each contraction. Women are instructed not to make a sound and to bring their knees up toward their abdomen with their elbows outstretched while pushing. Many clinicians will assist by holding the woman's legs back against her abdomen and counting to 10 with each pushing effort. These approaches are outdated and physiologically inappropriate (AWHONN, 2000, 2006).

When the woman takes a deep breath and holds it (closed glottis), the Valsalva maneuver is instituted. This technique increases intrathoracic pressure, impairs blood return from lower extremities, and initially increases and then decreases blood pressure, resulting in a decrease in uteroplacental blood flow (Barnett & Humenick, 1982; Bassell, Humayun, & Marx, 1980; Caldeyro-Barcia et al., 1981). In the newborn, iatrogenic hypoxemia, acidemia, and lower Apgar scores may result. Sustained pushing of 9–15 seconds can result in significant decelerations in the FHR (Caldeyro-Barcia et al., 1981) and decreases in fetal SpO2 (Aldrich et al., 1995; Langer et al., 1997; Simpson & James, 2005a) (see Fig. 7–5).

Transient and permanent peroneal nerve damage have been reported following prolonged periods of coached pushing with the woman in the supine lithotomy position. When the woman and/or care provider applies pressure to the peroneal nerve during pushing over a prolonged period, nerve damage resulting in numbness and tingling of the legs, inability to bear

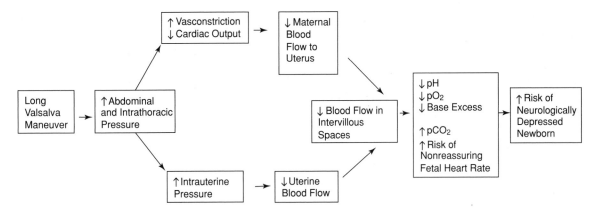

FIGURE 7–5. Coached closed-glottis (Valsalva) pushing during second stage: effect on maternal hemodynamics and fetal status.

weight, and transient loss of feeling may result (Colachis, Pease, & Johnson, 1994; Turbridy & Redmond, 1996). This type of iatrogenic injury can be prevented by encouraging the woman to keep her feet flat on the bed during second-stage pushing. Healthcare providers should avoid forcibly pushing the woman's legs against her abdomen and placing the woman's legs in stirrups while pushing, as these techniques increase the risk of peroneal nerve damage (Colachis et al. 1994; Turbridy & Redmond, 1996).

The length and type of pushing, as well as maternal position during pushing, has a direct impact on the fetal response to the second stage of labor and newborn transition to extrauterine life. Avoid sustained closed-glottis pushing if at all possible. The practice of the caregiver counting to 10 with each pushing effort to encourage prolonged breath-holding should be abandoned. There are strategies that can be used to decrease the impact of pushing on fetal well-being. If the fetus is not responding well to maternal pushing efforts, the most appropriate intervention is to stop pushing temporarily, assist the woman to a lateral position, and let the fetus recover (AWHONN, 2006; Simpson, 2004b). If the fetus continues to respond poorly, as evidenced by recurrent late and/or variable FHR decelerations, and there is a compelling reason to continue pushing, try pushing with alternate contractions while the woman is on her side (Freeman, Garite, & Nageotte, 2003). It may be necessary to encourage the woman to push with every other contraction or every third contraction to maintain a reassuring FHR pattern. A baseline should be able to be identified between contractions. If the fetus does not tolerate pushing and the woman has an epidural, the passive fetal descent approach works best. Discuss concerns with the physician/CNM if there is pressure or a sense of urgency (unrelated to maternal or fetal status) to get the baby delivered. There is evidence to suggest that for women with epidurals, coached push-

ing does not result in a clinically significant decrease in the length of the second stage (Fraser, Marcoux, et al, 2000; Hansen et al., 2002; Mayberry, Hammer, Kelly, True-Driver, & De, 1999). Passive fetal descent will result in a similar length of the second stage for women with epidural analgesia/anesthesia as compared with the coached closed-glottis pushing approach.

At present, there is no reliable method to know which fetuses can tolerate continued physiologic stress of sustained coached closed-glottis pushing. Therefore, the FHR pattern must be used as the indicator as to how well the fetus is responding (Simpson, 2004b). It is known that recurrent late and/or variable decelerations during the second stage are associated with respiratory acidemia at birth (Kazandi, Sendag, Akercan, Terek, & Gundem, 2003). Some fetuses may develop metabolic acidemia if this type of pattern continues over a long period (Parer, King, Flanders, Fox, & Kilpatrick, 2006; Shifrin & Ater, 2006). These babies are difficult to resuscitate and may not transition well to extrauterine life. Repetitive, sustained pushing efforts in the presence of a nonreassuring FHR pattern during second-stage labor characterized by recurrent late and/or variable decelerations, a rising baseline rate, and decreasing variability increase risk of fetal harm, such as fetal hypoxic and ischemic injuries (Shifrin & Ater, 2006).

In contrast, physiologic second-stage management is based on the principles that the second stage of labor is a normal physiological event and that women should push spontaneously and give birth with minimal intervention (AWHONN, 2000, 2006). Second-stage labor has been divided into two phases with the first described as the period from complete dilatation to spontaneous bearing down (Roberts, 2002). The second phase is characterized by vigorous expulsive efforts based on the woman feeling pressure and the urge to push (Roberts & Woolley, 1996). More effective expulsive efforts are associated with delaying pushing until the mother feels the urge to do so (Roberts, 2002).

Women who give birth in an upright position without bearing-down instructions experience a shorter labor, compared with women who receive routine bearing-down instructions in upright (26.4 minutes shorter) and recumbent (48.2 minutes shorter) positions (Liu, 1989). Women prefer encouragement and assistance with breathing, relaxation, pushing techniques, and imagery (McKay & Smith, 1993). However, confusion can occur if several caregivers' pushing directions are different or at odds with body sensations (McKay & Smith, 1983; Roberts, 2002). Individualized, consistent coaching (in coordination with the woman's expulsive efforts) that provides necessary instructions, support, and encouragement is important (Sampselle, Miller, Luecha, Fischer, & Rosten, 2005). Figure 7–6 provides an algorithm for physiologic second-stage management. Display 7–4 lists suggestions for optimal second-stage labor care.

With involuntary pushing, women are observed to hold their breath for 6 seconds while bearing down, and take several breaths in between bearing-down efforts (Roberts, Goldstein, Gruener, Maggio, & Mendez-Bauer, 1987). When pushing spontaneously without instructions, women do not instinctively take a deep breath; they do not start expulsive efforts at the beginning of the contraction, and they use both open- and closed-glottis pushing (Thomson, 1995). This is in contrast to the traditional second-stage coaching instructions that encourage holding breath for 10 seconds

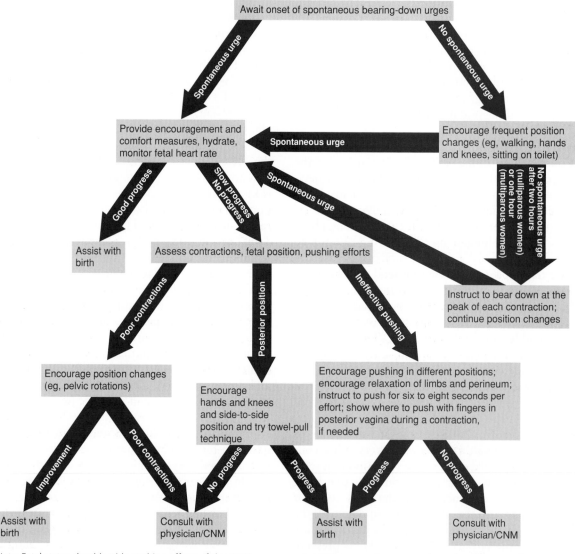

Note: Fetal status should guide pushing efforts. If the FHR is nonreassuring, encourage the woman to push with every other or every third contraction to promote fetal wellbeing. It may be necessary to stop pushing temporarily to allow the fetus to recover.

FIGURE 7–6. Flow sheet for second stage management. (Adapted from Cosner, K. R., & deJong, E. [1993]. Physiologic second-state labor. *Maternal Child Nursing, 18*[1], 41.)

DISPLAY 7-4

Second Stage of Labor Nursing Care

- Use upright positioning with the woman's feet flat on the bed. Change to lateral or other positions of comfort as necessary. Encourage pushing in various other positions such as semi-Fowler's, squatting, or hands and knees.
- Avoid forcing the woman's legs back against her abdomen.
- Use the towel-pull technique to minimize maternal fatigue and promote fetal descent.
- Avoid pushing in the supine lithotomy position.
- Avoid pushing in stirrups; use foot rests instead.
- For women who do not feel the urge to push when they are completely dilated (often occurs with regional analgesia/anesthesia), delay pushing until the urge to push is felt (up to 2 hours for nulliparous women and up to 1 hour for multiparous women).
- Discourage prolonged breath-holding. Instead, instruct the woman to bear down and hold it as long as she can and/or to do what ever comes naturally. Allow her to choose whether to hold her breath while pushing.
- Discourage more than three to four pushing efforts with each contraction and more than 6–8 seconds of each pushing effort (avoid counting to ten with each pushing effort).
- Take steps to maintain a reassuring FHR pattern while pushing. Push with every other or every third contraction if necessary to avoid recurrent FHR decelerations and maintain a stable baseline FHR. Reposition as necessary to treat FHR decelerations. If the FHR remains nonreassuring, stop pushing temporarily until the fetus recovers. Use the fetal response to pushing as a guide for second-stage care.
- Decrease or discontinue oxytocin to simulate a naturally occurring second-stage contraction pattern.
- Make sure that contractions are no closer than every 2 to 3 minutes while pushing. Titrate oxytocin accordingly. Use an IV fluid bolus of lactated Ringer's solution and reposition to decrease contraction frequency. Discontinue oxytocin if the FHR is nonreassuring.
- Avoid uterine hyperstimulation during the second stage of labor and treat appropriately if it occurs without waiting until the FHR becomes nonreassuring.
- Allow the woman's perineum to stretch naturally rather than using manual massage or stretching.
- Avoid use of an arbitrary 2-hour time limit for the second stage if there is evidence of progress and maternal–fetal status is reassuring.
- Operative vaginal births outside of the guidelines recommended by ACOG (2000b), FDA (1998), SOGC (2004), or the vacuum manufacturer should be avoided.

---

while bearing down and allowing only one quick breath between pushes. Open-glottis or gentle pushing avoids fetal stress, has less impact on uteroplacental blood flow, allows for perineal relaxation, and is more physiologically appropriate (AWHONN, 2000, 2006; Caldeyro-Barcia et al., 1981; McKay & Roberts, 1985; Simpson & James, 2005a). The woman is more in control and responding to her body's own pushing cues, enhancing maternal confidence and satisfaction with the birth experience. Open-glottis pushing as compared to closed-glottis pushing can shorten the length of the second stage of labor (Parnell, Langhoff-Roos, Iversen, & Damgaard, 1993). Avoid counting to 10 with each pushing effort and telling the woman to hold her breath while she pushes. Encourage her to bear down as long as she can or to do what ever comes naturally (Bloom, Casey, Schaffer, McIntire, & Leveno, 2006).

Delayed Pushing (Laboring Down/Passive Fetal Descent) for Women with Regional Analgesia/Anesthesia

When women have regional analgesia/anesthesia, they may not feel the urge to push when they are completely dilated. In this situation, an alternative approach to the second stage is to delay pushing while the fetus descends passively. Various researchers have described success with a protocol allowing nulliparous women to wait 2 hours or until the urge to push and allowing multiparous women 1 hour or until the urge to push (Hansen et al., 2002; Mayberry et al, 1999). A lateral position will facilitate passive fetal descent until the presenting part is low enough to stimulate the Ferguson reflex. There are significantly fewer FHR decelerations when the fetus is allowed to descent spontaneously when compared to coached closed-glottis pushing (Hansen et al., 2002; Simpson & James, 2005a). Maternal fatigue is less when women are allowed a period of passive descent when compared to immediate pushing when there is no urge to push (Hansen et al., 2002).

Risk of operative vaginal birth is less with delayed pushing until urge to push when compared to pushing immediately at 10 cm (Fraser Marcoux et al., 2000; Roberts, Torvaldsen, Cameron, & Olive, 2004). Injuries to the structure and function of the pelvic floor are less likely when a passive second stage results in a decreased period of maternal expulsive efforts (Devine, Ostergard, & Noblett, 1999). Delaying pushing and avoiding closed-glottis pushing has been shown to decrease risk of perineal injuries (Albers, Sedler,

Bedrick, Teaf, & Peralta, 2006; Sampselle & Hines, 1999; Simpson & James, 2005a). When compared to spontaneous bearing down efforts, coached pushing results in greater risk of urodynamic stress incontinence, decreased bladder capacity, decreased first urge to void, and detrusor over-activity (Shaffer et al., 2005).

There are no benefits for the mother and fetus to a policy involving immediate and continued pushing when compared to allowing a variable period of rest with spontaneous fetal descent (Bloom et al. 2006; Handa, Harris, & Ostergard, 1996; Hansen et al., 2002; Maresh et al., 1983; Mayberry et al, 1999; Simpson & James, 2005a; Vause, Congdon, & Thorton, 1998). The active pushing phase is the most physiologically stressful part of labor for the fetus, so shorting pushing time can promote fetal well-being (Robert, 2002; Simpson & James, 2005a). Laboring down avoids maternal fatigue and the nonreassuring FHR patterns associated with sustained coached closed-glottis pushing. Allowing maternal rest and passive fetal descent will not result in a clinically significant increase in the duration of the second stage of labor.

Maintaining Adequate Pain Relief While Pushing for Women with Labor Epidurals

In the past, some care providers have discontinued the labor epidural infusion when women are unable to push effectively and/or do not feel an adequate urge to push. The efficacy and ethics or this practice should be questioned (Roberts, 2002). There has been an erroneous assumption by some care providers that discontinuation of epidural analgesia/anesthesia could speed the second-stage process and avoid an operative vaginal birth or cesarean birth. However, often the opposite occurs. Women who have been receiving adequate regional pain relief and then have discontinuation of the epidural infusion experience significant pain and are at risk for fetal malrotations, dysfunctional uterine activity, a longer second stage, and forceps- or vacuum-assisted birth (Phillips & Thomas, 1983; Roberts, 2002). The increased catecholamine levels related to severe pain can adversely affect uterine activity and fetal status as well as a prolong second stage (Roberts, 2002). There is no evidence to support the hypothesis that discontinuing epidural analgesia/anesthesia late in labor benefits the mother or baby (Torvaldsen, Roberts, Bell, & Bell-Greenow, 2004). If women often have difficulty feeling urge to push and effectively working with the pressure as the baby descends, review the level of motor block and type and amount of medications routinely used for regional labor analgesia/anesthesia in the perinatal unit. Consult with anesthesia providers to develop a more appropriate combination of medications that will result in adequate pain relief without an overly dense motor block.

Fundal Pressure

Because there are limited published data about maternal–fetal injuries related to the use of fundal pressure to shorten the second stage of labor, it is difficult to accurately quantify the risks to the mother and baby (Merhi & Awonuga, 2005). The limited data about many known or reported adverse outcomes associated with fundal pressure application during the second stage of labor should not be used to suggest that this practice is acceptable or risk-free (Simpson & Knox, 2001). The consequences of not choosing clinical management with least-associated risk become understood only when the rare serious injury occurs.

Fundal pressure refers to the application of steady pressure with one hand on the fundus of the uterus at a 30° to 45° angle to the maternal spine in the direction of the pelvis (Rommal, 1999) (see Fig. 7–7). The pressure is applied in a longitudinal direction with careful avoidance of downward pressure on the maternal spine because of the risk of direct vena cava compression and maternal hypotension (Rommal, 1999).

Perinatal nurses may feel pressured by physicians to use fundal pressure to shorten an otherwise normal second-stage labor even when they feel it is not in the best interest of the woman and fetus. There is no evidence that this procedure is beneficial to shorten an otherwise normal second-stage labor for maternal or provider convenience, while there is evidence of potential harm to the mother and baby. The perinatal nurse has the right to refuse to participate in fundal pressure application in this clinical context.

Fundal pressure may be appropriate in limited clinical situations. For example, fundal pressure is sometimes used to guide the fetal head into the pelvis against the cervix if fetal station is high when artificial rupture of the membranes is indicated. Fundal pressure in this situation may decrease the risk of a prolapsed

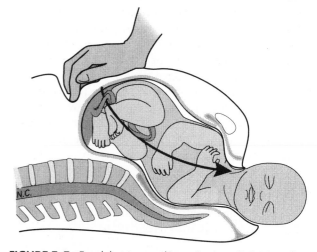

FIGURE 7–7. Fundal pressure. (From Penney, D. S., & Perlis, D. W. [1992]. When to use suprapubic or fundal pressure. *American Journal of Maternal Child Nursing, 17,* 34–36)

umbilical cord. If the FHR is nonreassuring or difficult to trace electronically, or when there is indication for more accurate fetal assessment, some healthcare providers will opt to place an internal FSE. When fetal station is such that application is difficult, gentle fundal pressure may make it easier to apply the FSE. Finally, there are situations when the fetal head is crowning, maternal pushing efforts are insufficient to effect birth, and the FHR is nonreassuring, suggesting an expeditious birth is indicated. In this case, fundal pressure may be the quickest option for birth. However, a careful analysis of risks and benefits is required based on the individual clinical situation (Simpson & Knox, 2001). An alternative option is to stop pushing, allow fetal recovery, and proceed with cesarean birth.

The potential use of fundal pressure in selected clinical situations requires well-researched guidelines for practice. These guidelines may contain descriptions of the techniques, indications, contraindications, and criteria for medical record documentation, along with suggestions on how to handle clinical disagreements related to fundal pressure that may arise in the clinical setting (Rommal, 1999).

Fundal pressure should not be applied during shoulder dystocia, as it can result in further impaction of the shoulder and increase risk of fetal injuries (ACOG, 2002b). There are data to suggest that fundal pressure may actually cause shoulder dystocia if applied concurrently with vacuum extraction because the head of the fetus does not descend on its own (Bahar, 1996; Bofill et al., 1997b). Nesbitt, Gilbert, and Herrchen (1998) found that shoulder dystocia increased 35% to 45% in vacuum- or forceps-assisted births to nondiabetic mothers of infants weighing more than 3,500 grams. When fundal pressure is used during shoulder dystocia, the risk of permanent brachial plexus injury is significantly increased (Phelan, Ouzounian, Gherman, Korst, & Goodwin, 1997). Hankins (1998) reported a severe lower thoracic spinal cord injury to a fetus with permanent neurologic sequelea when fundal pressure was applied in an attempt to relieve shoulder dystocia. Subgaleal hemorrhage has been reported in at least four cases where fundal pressure application was combined with use of vaccuum (Simpson & Knox, 2001). This type of fetal injury can result in acute blood loss and shock. Excessive fundal pressure can increase fetal intracranial pressure to such a degree as to result in significant decreases in cerebral blood flow and nonreassuring FHR patterns (Amiel-Tison, Sureau, & Shnider, 1988). Cord compression and functional alterations in intervillous space blood flow caused by the mechanical forces of fundal pressure compromise fetal status and can lead to fetal hypoxemia and asphyxia (Amiel-Tison et al., 1988). The perinatal nurse has the right to refuse to participate in fundal pressure application during shoulder dystocia.

In addition to an increased risk of fetal injuries, application of fundal pressure increases the risk of injuries to the mother (Simpson & Knox, 2001). Maternal perineal injuries such third- and fourth-degree lacerations and anal sphincter tears have been found to be associated with use of fundal presure (Cosner, 1996; Zetterstrom et al., 1999). Cases of uterine rupture and uterine inversion have also been reported as a result of the use of fundal pressure (Drummond, 1998; Lee, Baggish, & Lashgari, 1978; Rommal, 1996). Other maternal injuries and complications reported include pain, hypotension, respiratory distress, abdominal bruising, fractured ribs, and liver rupture (Simpson & Knox, 2001).

Based on evidence in the literature, case reports and reviews of malpractice cases that resulted in adverse outcomes, it must be concluded that fundal pressure, used either in cases of shoulder dystocia or to shorten the second stage of an otherwise normal labor, presents an increased—but not at this time quantifiable—risk to mothers and babies and to perinatal providers using it (Merhi & Awonuga, 2005; Simpson & Knox, 2001). Each institution should review clinical risk management guidelines provided by its professional liability insurance carrier as part of the process of developing unit guidelines for fundal pressure application (Simpson & Knox, 2001).

Shoulder Dystocia

Shoulder dystocia is an unpredictable obstetric emergency. However, reasonable steps can be undertaken once shoulder dystocia is identified. A thorough knowledge of what to do should this crisis occur is essential for perinatal nurses to ensure the best possible outcomes for the woman and fetus. Key nursing interventions include calling for additional help, calm supportive actions, and working in sync with the physician or CNM who is directing the maneuvers to deliver the impacted shoulder (Simpson, 1999). In July 2004, JCAHO's Sentinel Event Alert *Preventing Infant Death and Injury During Delivery* recommended conducting periodic drills for obstetrical emergencies such as shoulder dystocia (JCAHO, 2004b). The ACOG (1995) video *Shoulder Dystocia* provides details concerning how to plan and implement shoulder dystocia drills.

Interventions that have been described in the literature to relieve the impacted shoulder include suprapubic pressure; the McRoberts, Woods, Rubin (reverse Woods), Schwartz-Dixon, Gaskin, and Zavanelli maneuvers; and symphisiotomy (see Fig. 7–8 and Fig. 7–9). There is no clear evidence-based order of these maneuvers; however, most clinicians use McRoberts as the initial intervention, followed by suprapubic pressure (ACOG, 2002b). Although suprapubic pressure and

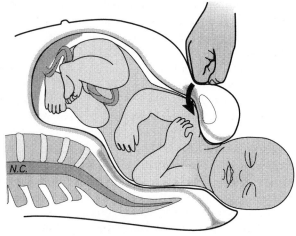

FIGURE 7–8. Suprapubic pressure. (From Penney, D. S., & Perlis, D. W. [1992]. When to use suprapubic or fundal pressure. *American Journal of Maternal Child Nursing, 17,* 34–36)

McRoberts are often used prophylactically for women considered to be at high risk for shoulder dystocia, there is no evidence that these interventions reduce the incidence of shoulder dystocia or neonatal adverse outcomes (Beall, Spong, & Ross, 2003). The essential issue during shoulder dystocia is to continue to intervene using an organized expeditious series of steps until the infant has been delivered. If an injury occurs as a result of shoulder dystocia despite the best efforts of the obstetric providers, it is likely that litigation will follow (Gherman, 2002).

Shoulder dystocia is diagnosed when attempts at gentle downward traction on the fetal head are unsuccessful in delivering the shoulders. The classic "turtle sign," in which the head appears to retract into the perineum, may or may not occur simultaneously. It has been difficult to evaluate studies describing shoulder dystocia in a systematic process because of the various definitions used by researchers. Most authors define shoulder dystocia as birth-requiring maneuvers in addition to gentle downward traction on the fetal head. An objective method of defining shoulder dysto-

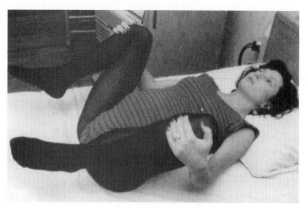

FIGURE 7–9. McRoberts maneuver.

cia is a prolonged head-to-body birth interval of ≥60 seconds and/or the use of ancillary obstetric maneuvers (Spong, Beall, Rodrigues, & Ross, 1995). Because the average head-to-body birth interval is approximately 24 seconds for normal vaginal birth, this definition seems reasonable (Gherman et al., 2006). A universally used definition of shoulder dystocia would enhance the ability of researchers to advance science and knowledge about risk factors and appropriate interventions.

Numerous antepartum and pregnancy risk factors associated with shoulder dystocia have been discussed in the literature, including previous birth of a macrosomic baby, pre-existing or gestational diabetes mellitus, a previous pregnancy complicated by gestational diabetes, obesity, muliparity, history of a prior shoulder dystocia, excessive weight gain and post-dates gestation, macrosomic fetus, and disproportionate fetal growth with increased abdominal and chest circumference (ACOG, 2000a; Gherman, 2002). Intrapartum risk factors that have been reported include labor induction; abnormal labor progress, including prolonged second-stage labor; and operative vaginal birth (ACOG, 2000a; Gherman, 2002).

Widely quoted, but not scientifically based, risk factors include male fetus, advanced maternal age, short maternal stature, maternal birth-weight, abnormal pelvic size or shape, and molding of the fetal head (Gherman et al., 2006). It is important to note that none of these risk factors individually or in combination is predictive of shoulder dystocia (ACOG, 2002b). The two risk factors most strongly associated with shoulder dystocia are fetal macrosomia and maternal diabetes (ACOG, 2002b). However, the vast majority of women with one or more of these risk factors go on to have an uncomplicated labor and birth. Most cases of shoulder dystocia occur in the context of lack of a significant risk factor (Gherman, 2002).

One of the most significant factors in shoulder dystocia is a macrosomic fetus (ACOG, 2000a). Macrosomia is usually defined as an infant weight more than 4,000 g (8 lbs, 13 oz) or 4,500 g (9 lbs, 15 oz) (ACOG, 2000a). According to ACOG (2000a), 4,500 g is the most appropriate estimated fetal weight beyond which the fetus should be considered macrosomic. In the United States, approximately 10% of all infants weigh more than 4,000 g, and about 1.5% weigh more than 4,500 g (ACOG, 2000a). The risk of shoulder dystocia significantly increases when birth weight exceeds 4,500 g, with reported rates for this weight category ranging from 9.2% to 24% (ACOG, 2002b). In the presence of diabetes, birth weights above 4,500 g have been associated with rates of shoulder dystocia from 19.9% to 50% (ACOG, 2002b). However, not all macrosomic fetuses will experience shoulder dystocia and not all cases of shoulder dystocia involve macrosomic fetuses. Shoulder dystocia is a rare event (0.06% to 1.4% of vaginal births) even among macrosomic infants. Approximately 70% to 90% of macrosomic infants (even those >5,000 grams) will be born without experiencing shoulder dystocia (Gherman et al., 2006). Approximately 40% to 60% of cases of shoulder dystocia occur in infants weighing less than 4,000 g (Gherman et al., 2006). No birth-weight category is completely free of risk for shoulder dystocia. Brachial plexus injuries can occur without shoulder dystocia (ACOG, 2002b).

There have been numerous attempts to develop criteria that would accurately diagnose macrosomia prior to birth, including clinical estimation of fetal weight by abdominal palpation and ultrasonographic parameters. These clinical factors have been statistically associated with shoulder dystocia using retrospective analyses; however, none of these factors or criteria has been shown to have a high positive predictive value for the individual patient when attempting to predict macrosomia or shoulder dystocia prospectively (ACOG, 2002b). The likelihood of an inaccurate prediction of fetal weight increases with the size of the fetus. Birth weight is underestimated by approximately 0.5 kg (1 lb) or more in 50% of cases where the fetus is larger than 4,000 g and in as many as 80% of cases where the fetus is larger than 4,500 g.

Maternal diabetes is consistently related to risk of shoulder dystocia (ACOG, 2002b). While it is known that women with diabetes tend to have larger infants, there are also anthropometric differences in infants of diabetic mothers that may explain the propensity for shoulder dystocia in this population (Gherman et al., 2006). Macrosomic infants of diabetic mothers tend to have larger shoulder and extremity circumferences, a decreased head-to-shoulder ratio, significantly higher body fat, and thicker upper extremity skinfolds when compared to nondiabetic infants of similar birth weight and birth length (Gherman et al., 2006). The risk of shoulder dystocia for women with diabetes is at least double that of women who do not have diabetes, with a further increase in risk with use of vacuum or forceps (Gherman et al., 2006).

Although the diagnosis of fetal macrosomia is imprecise, prophylactic cesarean birth may be considered for suspected fetal macrosomia with estimated fetal weights >5,000 g in women without diabetes and >4,500 g in women with diabetes (ACOG, 2002b). This is a decision made by the CNM or physician in collaboration with the pregnant woman and her family. Individual clinical situations vary, however, and not all women may agree to this course. Macrosomia is relative to maternal pelvic structures and size and fetal presentation and position. For all practical purposes, shoulder dystocia cannot be predicted with any degree of accuracy (ACOG, 2002b; Beall, Spong, &

Ross, 2003). The important issue is for perinatal nurses to be aware of maternal–fetal risk factors for individual patients and be prepared if shoulder dystocia should occur.

Once the diagnosis of shoulder dystocia is made, the nurse assists with maneuvers to disimpact the shoulder under the direction of the physician or CNM. Calmly assisting the woman to the appropriate positions during the maneuvers will help her feel confident that necessary interventions are being done as quickly as possible by competent healthcare providers.

Fundal pressure should be avoided during shoulder dystocia because it can further impact the fetal shoulder, resulting in an inability to deliver the fetal body as well as contributing to fetal brachial plexus injuries and fractures of the humerus and clavicle (ACOG, 2002b; Gherman et al., 2006). Gross and colleagues (1987) reported a 77% fetal injury rate when fundal pressure was the only maneuver used to relieve shoulder dystocia. Fundal pressure during shoulder dystocia has been associated with a high rate of permanent brachial plexus injuries (Phelan et al., 1997).

The McRoberts maneuver (a knee-chest position while supine) is usually the first maneuver initiated, and it involves hyperflexion of the woman's thighs against her abdomen. This position can ease delivery of the shoulder by changing the relationship of the maternal pelvis to the lumbar spine. This maneuver may not actually increase birth canal dimensions, but it does result in flattening of the sacrum relative to the maternal lumbar spine (Gherman, Tramont, Muffley, & Goodwin, 2000). In many cases, the McRoberts maneuver alone or along with suprapubic pressure will result in birth. If the McRoberts maneuver is not immediately successful, the next approach is usually suprapubic pressure.

Firm suprapubic pressure using the palm of the hand will usually dislodge the impacted shoulder while gentle downward pressure is applied by the physician or CNM. Suprapubic pressure is directed away from the pubic bone to either the left or the right side following directions from the physician or CNM based on which way they are attempting to rotate the shoulders.

If birth does not occur immediately with McRoberts and suprapubic pressure, a call for the help of other available nurses and physicians should be considered. If the woman has epidural anesthesia or she is uncomfortable, another provider may be needed to help support her legs and maintain proper positioning. Preparations for newborn resuscitation are warranted if additional maneuvers are required after application of suprapubic pressure and the McRoberts maneuver or if several minutes have elapsed since delivery of the fetal head.

During shoulder dystocia, the umbilical cord may be partially or completed occluded between the fetal body and maternal pelvis. Compression of the fetal neck, resulting in cerebral venous obstruction, excessive vagal stimulation, and bradycardia, may be combined with reduced arterial oxygen supply to cause clinical deterioration out of proportion to the duration of hypoxia (Kwek & Yeo, 2006). The normally oxygenated fetus can tolerate several minutes of cord compression without significant adverse effects. However, most experts note that a >5-minute head-to-body interval may result in acid-base deterioration in a fetus whose condition was normal prior to the onset of shoulder dystocia (Benedetti, 1995). If fetal status was nonreassuring prior to the shoulder dystocia, the fetus may have less physiologic reserve (Kwek & Yeo, 2006; Shifrin & Ater, 2006). Persistent coached pushing efforts for a prolonged period with recurrent late and variable decelerations can result in fetal oxygen desaturation, fetal metabolic acidemia, and risk of fetal hypoxic and ischemic injuries (Parer et al, 2006; Shifrin & Ater, 2006; Simpson & James, 2005a). In this case, the fetus may have less ability to tolerate additional insult such as shoulder dystocia. In one study using neonatal brain injury as the outcome, brain injury cases were associated with a significantly prolonged head-to-body interval of >10 minutes and ≥7 minutes had a sensitivity of 67% and specificity of 74% in predicting brain injury (Ouzounian, Korst, Ahn, & Phelan, 1998).

If possible, an assessment of fetal status via EFM or handheld ultrasound devices will provide information about how the fetus is tolerating the interventions. However, time should not be lost attempting to locate the FHR if it is not readily identified. It is better to direct attention to dislodging the fetal shoulder by assisting the woman to the appropriate positions and following the direction of the physician or CNM.

During the Woods maneuver, the physician or CNM exerts downward pressure on the uterine fundus with one hand while inserting two fingers of the other hand on the anterior aspect of the posterior shoulder and gently rotating clockwise. Ideally this will deliver the posterior shoulder. With continued synchronized downward pressure on the fundus by the physician or CNM, two fingers make gentle counter-clockwise pressure upward around the circumference of the pelvic arc to and beyond 12 o'clock, which will unscrew and deliver the remaining shoulder. This is the only time fundal pressure is appropriate during a shoulder disimpaction maneuver.

The Schwartz-Dixon maneuver may be used to deliver the posterior arm, thus easing delivery of the body. Physicians or CNMs gently insert their hand along the curvature of the fetal sacrum and their fingers follow along the humerus to the antecubital fossa. The fetal forearm is flexed and swept across the chest and face and out the vagina. Ideally the anterior shoulder

will slide under the symphysis after the posterior arm is delivered. There is a risk of fracture of the humerus with this technique. The physician or CNM may need to rotate the baby to achieve delivery using a technique similar to the Woods maneuver.

The all-fours maneuver described by Ina May Gaskin (Brunner et al, 1998) appears to be a rapid, safe, and effective method for reducing shoulder dystocia. For the Gaskin maneuver, the woman is assisted to her hands and knees. The exact mechanism by which this maneuver relieves shoulder dystocia is unknown. However, in a recent report of 82 consecutive cases of shoulder dystocia, the Gaskin maneuver contributed to a successful vaginal birth in all cases (Brunner et al., 1998). It is possible that the simple act of repositioning may be enough to dislodge the shoulder. An advantage to this position is the ability to continue other maneuvers if the position change does not reduce the shoulder dystocia. The women in the Brunner et al. (1998) study received no anesthesia for labor or birth. For women with epidural analgesia/ anesthesia, it may be difficult, but not impossible, to assist the woman to this position.

Episiotomy as an intervention for shoulder dystocia is controversial. Because shoulder dystocia is considered a "bony dystocia" and therefore not caused by obstructing soft tissue, its use may not be helpful (ACOG, 2002b). Episiotomy or proctoepisiotomy has been associated with nearly a seven-fold increase in the rate of severe perineal trauma without benefit of reducing the occurrence of neonatal depression or brachial plexus injury (Gherman et al., 2006).

While performance of a symphysiotomy is described in the literature, most practitioners have not had experience with this procedure (Gherman et al., 2006). Risks to the mother include major bladder and urethra damage, long-term pain, and difficulty walking. This procedure is rarely used in the United States (ACOG, 2002b). Deliberate fracture of the clavicles is also described as a method to reduce shoulder width; however, many practitioners find this procedure technically difficult (Gherman et al., 2006).

In the event that these or other maneuvers do not result in birth, the physician or CNM may attempt to replace the fetal head into the vagina and proceed with cesarean birth. This is known as the Zavanelli maneuver or cephalic replacement. It is important that the head be returned to the occipitoanterior or occipitoposterior position, then flexed and slowly pushed back into the birth canal. A review of 103 published cases of the Zavanelli maneuver from 1985 to 1997 revealed a 92% success rate, with no reports of fetal injuries in those eventually born via cesarean section (Sandberg, 1999). Others have reported fetal injuries such as Erb's palsy, paresis of the lower extremities, seizures, brain damage, delayed motor development, quadriplegia, cerebral palsy, and death as a result of the Zavanelli maneuver (Gherman et al., 2006). If the Zavanelli maneuver is successful, when possible, an assessment of fetal status via EFM or a handheld ultrasound device is desired while preparing for emergent cesarean birth. Personnel skilled in neonatal resuscitation should be in attendance at the cesarean birth.

Once the shoulder has been disimpacted and birth has occurred, the nurse can direct attention to newborn care and assessment. After the newborn and mother are stabilized, documentation about the events surrounding the birth involving shoulder dystocia is possible. See Display 7–5 for suggestions for medical record documentation following birth complicated by shoulder dystocia.

Support and communication with the family is important after birth. The woman and her family will likely be concerned about the condition of the baby and have questions about what occurred. As part of the discussion, the woman should be informed that she is at risk of shoulder dystocia recurrence in subsequent birth.

The Perineum

Episiotomy is a median or mediolateral incision into the perineum. According to the latest data based on 2004 hospital procedures, episiotomy is performed during approximately 23% of births in the United States (DeFrances & Podgornik, 2006). The episiotomy rate has steadily decreased over the past years from 54% in 1992 to 33% in 2000 to 23% in 2004, the latest year for which these data are available (ACOG, 2006b; DeFrances & Podgornik, 2006). Although this surgical technique has long been thought to permit easier passage of the baby and to decrease risk of perineal trauma, there is little supportive evidence for these beliefs (ACOG, 2006b; Scott, 2005).

Those who consider routine episiotomy to be beneficial cite the following advantages: prevention of perineal tearing; ease of repair when compared to lacerations; reduction in the time and stress of the second stage of labor; decreased compression of fetal head, especially for preterm infants; and allowance of easier

---

DISPLAY 7-5

Suggestions for Medical Record Documentation After a Birth Complicated by Shoulder Dystocia

- Provide emergent nursing care to the woman and newborn as a first priority.
- A narrative note, summarizing the series of interventions and clinical events with a focus on a logical step-by-step approach to relieving the impacted shoulder and resuscitating the newborn, works best in most situations.
- Avoid documenting a minute-by-minute account of the emergency unless it is absolutely certain that the times included are accurate.
- Attempt to closely approximate the time interval between delivery of fetal head and body.
- Review the electronic fetal monitoring strip, and talk with other providers in attendance to insure most accurate details of clinical circumstances.
- Include fetal assessment data or attempts to obtain data about fetal status during the maneuvers.
- List the order of each maneuver used in clear and precise terms.
- Note that nursing assistance with these maneuvers were under the direction of the physician or certified nurse midwife (CNM).

- If suprapubic pressure was used, make sure it is noted as such to avoid later allegations of fundal pressure.
- If fundal pressure is used during the Woods maneuver or after the shoulder is disimpacted, clearly note when and how it was used.
- Include times for calls for assistance and when other providers arrived.
- Carefully note the condition of the newborn at birth and during the immediate newborn period.
- Describe any resuscitation efforts and those who attended the newborn.
- Make sure that neonatal personnel in attendance understand the difference between suprapubic pressure and fundal pressure to avoid a neonatal note indicating fundal pressure was applied if this is inaccurate.
- If umbilical blood gases were obtained, make sure they become part of the record.
- If a discussion between the physician or CNM and the woman and her family about the shoulder dystocia and subsequent newborn condition occurred after birth, include a note about the content of this conversation and those who were present.
- It may be helpful to compose the note on a separate paper and review it for accuracy before entering these data into the medical record.
- Attempt to document in the medical record within a reasonable time after the mother and newborn are stabilized.
- If possible, avoid late entries many hours or days after birth.

From Simpson, K.R. (1999). Shoulder dystocia: Nursing interventions and risk management strategies. *MCN The American Journal of Maternal Child Nursing*, 24(6), 305–311. Used with permission.

manipulation during breech or operative vaginal birth. However, the benefits of routine episiotomy have not been demonstrated by rigorous research (ACOG, 2006b; Carroli & Belizan, 2000; Eason & Feldman, 2000; Eason, Labrecque, Wells, & Feldman, 2000; Hartmann et al., 2005). It appears that personal beliefs, education, and experience of the practitioner, rather than evidence, influence clinical judgment about whether to perform an episiotomy (ACOG, 2006b; Low, Seng, Murtland, & Oakley, 2000).

Based on available data, giving birth over an intact perineum results in less blood loss, less risk of infection, and less perineal pain postpartum (ACOG, 2006b; Eason & Feldman, 2000). Methods to prevent perineal trauma during birth include upright positioning, avoidance of episiotomy, avoidance of forceps or vacuum extractors, passive fetal descent, avoidance of Valsalva pushing, slowing birth of the fetal head to allow the perineum time to stretch, and birth between contractions (Albers et al., 2006; Andrews, Sultan, Thakar, & Jones, 2006; Eason & Feldman, 2000; FitzGerald, Weber, Howden, Cundiff, & Brown, 2007; Kudish et al., 2006; Mayerhofer et al., 2002; Sampselle, & Hines, 1999; Schaffer et al., 2005; Simpson & James, 2005a).

Episiotomy is often performed when the physician or CNM feels that there is a risk of lacerations of the perineum or vagina during birth. The goal is to protect the perineum and maintain future perineal function and integrity; however, supportive evidence is lacking that these goals can be achieved with routine episiotomy (ACOG, 2006b; Scott, 2005). The use of episiotomy is associated with significant risks such as increased risk of third- and fourth-degree lacerations (Aukee, Sundstrom, & Kairaluoma, 2006; Hudelist et al., 2005; Ogunyemi, Manigat, Marquis, & Bazargan, 2006), anal sphincter injuries (Andrews et al., 2006; Clemons, Trowers, McClure, & O'Boyle, 2005; Dandolu et al., 2005; FitzGerald et al., 2007; Hudelist et al., 2005; Kurdish et al., 2006), severe lacerations and injuries in subsequent births (Edwards, Grotegut, Harmanli, Rapkin, & Dandolu, 2006; Peleg, Kennedy, Merrill, & Zlatnik, 1999; Spydslaug, Trogstad, Skrondal, & Eskild, 2005), infection, delayed healing (McGuinness, Norr, & Nacion, 1991), breakdown in repair (Williams & Chames, 2006), increased blood loss (Eason & Feldman, 2000), scarring (Koger, Shatney, Hodge, & McClenathan, 1993), increased pain, (Macarthur & Macarthur, 2004), sexual dysfunction (Stamp, Kruzins, & Crowther, 2001), and higher costs secondary to time and suture. Episiotomy does not protect against problems with perineal muscle function postpartum (Fleming, Newton, & Roberts, 2003). Lacerations of the vagina and perineum are classified according to degree as listed in Display 7–6.

DISPLAY 7-6

Perineal Lacerations

TYPE OF LACERATION	INVOLVEMENT
First degree	Perineal skin and vaginal mucous membrane
Second degree	Skin and mucous membrane plus fascia and muscle of perineum
Third degree	Skin, mucous membrane, muscle of perineum; extends into rectal sphincter
Fourth degree	Extends into rectal mucosa to expose lumen of rectum

Nursing interventions during labor can have a direct impact on the use and perceived need for episiotomy. Upright position and open-glottis, gentle pushing that coincide with the woman's natural urges and sensations, aids gradual perineal stretching with less pain, thus avoiding the need episiotomy and resultant perineal trauma (Devine et al, 1999; Eason et al., 2000; Flynn, Franick, Janssen, Hannah, & Klein, 1997; Sampselle & Hines, 1999; Simpson & James, 2005a). Women who give birth in lithotomy position are more likely to have an episiotomy than women who give birth in squatting, hands-and-knees, standing, or sitting positions (Bodner-Adler et al., 2003; de Jong et al., 1997; Gupta & Hofmeyr, 2004; Terry et al., 2006). Passive fetal descent and spontaneous bearing down efforts versus directed Valsalva pushing result in fewer episiotomies and perineal lacerations (Albers et al., 2006; Devine et al., 1999; Sampselle & Hines, 1999; Simpson & James, 2005a).

Other measures that have been proposed to enhance perineal stretching and decrease perineal trauma are the application of warm compresses, gentle perineal massage and stretching, and warm oil perineal massage during the second stage of labor. There is no evidence from any randomized clinical trial that use of warm compresses and second-stage perineal massage with or without oil decrease the need for episiotomy or decrease the risk of perineal trauma (Albers, Sedler, Bedrick, Teaf, & Peralta, 2005; Eason et al., 2000). One study found that perineal massage during the second stage was associated with a greater risk of perineal trauma (Aikins-Murphy & Feinlan, 1998), and another study suggested that some women in labor are uncomfortable with this technique (Albers et al., 2005). There is significant disagreement among providers as to whether second-stage perineal massage should be used (Mayerhofer et al., 2002; Stamp, 1997;

Stamp et al. 2001). Perineal massage has not shown to increase the likelihood of an intact perineum or reduce the risk of pain, dyspareunia, or urinary or fecal problems (Albers et al., 2005; Stamp et al. 2001). Absent data to suggest benefit along with limited data to suggest harm, perineal massage during the second stage should be used with caution, if at all, until more evidence is available about risks and benefits.

Antepartum perineal massage has also been studied as a method to decrease risk of perineal trauma at birth. Usually, women who choose perineal massage are taught to use the technique daily during the third trimester (Labrecque et al., 1999; Shipman, Boniface, Tefft, & McCloghery, 1997). Very limited data exist to support the role of antepartum perineal massage in reducing the rate of episiotomies and perineal trauma (Eason et al., 2000; Renfrew, Hannah, Albers, & Floyd, 1998). In one study, women who were taught perineal massage reported pain, discomfort, irritation, fatigue, uneasiness with the concept, and negative physician comments (Mynaugh, 1991). The women who practiced perineal massage also experienced more perineal lacerations than those in the control group (Mynaugh, 1991). In another study, perineal massage was effective in reducing the rate of episiotomy for first-time mothers only (Labrecque et al, 1999). In a recent study, antenatal perineal massage did not reduce the incidence of episiotomy or abnormal continence scores (Eogan, Daly, & O'Herlihy, 2006). Perineal massage during pregnancy has been shown to neither impair nor substantially protect perineal function at three months postpartum (Labrecque, Eason, & Macrcoux, 2000). Based on the latest systematic review from the Cochrane Database of Systematic Reviews, antenatal perineal massage may decrease the incidence of episiotomy in women giving birth vaginally for the first time (Beckmann & Garrett, 2006). Perhaps women who practice perineal massage antenatally are more likely to request that episiotomy be avoided unless necessary. More research is needed to determine whether perineal massage performed by the woman in the weeks before labor and birth is effective in avoiding the medical need for episiotomy or reducing the extent of lacerations. If women choose to practice perineal massage during pregnancy, there appears to be no harm in doing so.

EMOTIONAL AND PHYSICAL SUPPORT DURING LABOR AND BIRTH

Impact of the Psyche on Childbirth

The psyche plays a major role in the process of labor and birth. A high level of anxiety has been associated with increased catecholamine secretion that can result in ineffective uterine activity and longer and dysfunctional labor (Lederman, Lederman, Work, & McCann, 1985). Anxiety, uncertainty, loss of control, loss of self-confidence, patterns of coping, support systems, fatigue, optimism, fatalism, and aloneness are some of the psychosocial factors to consider when caring for women in labor. Previous birth experiences, present support systems, concerns/questions, anxiety or fear, and cultural considerations further contribute to attitudes and expectations for the current pregnancy experience.

Facilitating Labor and Birth

Nursing care during childbirth includes providing information so the woman knows what to expect, interpreting physical sensations, encouraging maternal position changes, reinforcing breathing and other relaxation efforts, support during the second stage, and continued pain management. Women expect that their nurse will provide physical comfort and informational and emotional support, as well as technical nursing care and ongoing monitoring of maternal–fetal status during labor (Tumlin & Simkin, 2001). They appreciate the nurse's being there for them (Mackinnon, McIntyre, & Quance, 2005). In a recent systematic review of women's satisfaction with their childbirth experience, women whose experiences were better than expected and women with high expectations were more likely to be satisfied, whereas women with low expectations that were subsequently met had lower levels of satisfaction (Hodnett, 2002). One-to-one nursing care during labor is a significant patient satisfier, although that type of care is not always feasible in a busy labor unit (Hodnett et al., 2002). Nursing behaviors that demonstrate valuing and respecting childbearing women are essential in enhancing the quality of the birth experience (Matthews & Callister, 2003).

Supportive Care by Partners, Family, and Friends

Attention also should be given to the woman's partner/support person, family members, and friends in attendance. Every effort should be made to support and encourage those in attendance to assist the woman during labor and to allow as many support persons as the woman desires. Arbitrary rules prohibiting more than one support person during labor are contrary to the philosophy that the birth experience belongs to the woman and her family rather to those providing clinical care. Although healthcare providers are sometimes inclined to attempt to control this aspect of the birth process using various arguments for safety and convenience, when examined critically, these arguments have little scientific merit. Women should be able to choose who will be with them during this special and unique life experience. Family-centered care supports the concept that the "family" is defined by the childbearing woman.

Women who have continuous intrapartum support are less likely to have intrapartum analgesia, have operative birth, or report dissatisfaction with their childbirth experiences (Hodnett, Gates, Hoymeyr, & Sakala, 2003). Continuous labor support is associated with greater benefits when the provider of that support is not a member of the hospital staff (Campbell, Lake, Falk, & Backstrand, 2006; Hodnett et al., 2002; Hodnett et al., 2003). Fewer perinatal complications, fewer newborns with 5-minute Apgar scores less than 7, fewer newborns admitted to the neonatal intensive care unit (NICU), lower rates of analgesia and anesthesia, lower operative birth rates, and shorter labors result when women have a support person as compared to women without support (Campbell et al., 2006; Klaus, Kennel, Robertson, & Sosa, 1986; Norbeck & Anderson, 1989; Pascoe, 1993; Sauls, 2002). Presence of a lay support person has also been found to reduce the rate of cesarean births (Klaus, Kennel, McGrath, Robertson, & Hinkley 1988, 1991). There is adequate research to validate the significance of promoting support from family members/coaches during the labor and birth experience; thus, all women should have support throughout labor and birth (Hodnett et al., 2003). See Chapter 9 for a more detailed discussion of labor support.

Families should be free to take still pictures and record video and/or audio tapes during labor and birth. Policies restricting cameras are in conflict with the philosophy that the birth experience should be what the woman and her family desire within reason. There is no evidence that videotapes of labor and birth later produced as part of a legal claim increase liability. Video or still pictures showing that the perinatal team provided excellent care in a challenging situation could prove to be beneficial to a situation known to suffer from hindsight bias. Concerns about safety, liability, privacy, and space limitations can be adequately addressed without restrictive policies about visitors and use of cameras during labor and birth if care providers are committed to meeting the needs of childbearing women and their support persons (AAP & ACOG, 2002).

Caring for Women Who Have Been Sexually Abused

It has been estimated that approximately 27% of women have a history of childhood sexual abuse (Heritage, 1998; Roussillon, 1998). The abuse has a lifelong impact on survivors and has been shown to have a negative effect on birth outcomes and the childbearing experience

(Heimstad, Dahloe, Laache, Skogvoll, & Schel, 2006; Hobbins, 2004). Women with a history of sexual abuse have unique needs during the intrapartum period. Routine screening can assist in identifying victims; however, not all women report or remember sexual abuse (Hobbins, 2004). Sensations of labor and birth can mimic physical experiences of the abuse and sometimes cause flashbacks and extreme anxiety (Rhodes & Hutchison, 1994). Common experiences and procedures during childbirth can trigger child sexual abuse memories. These include bodily fluid odors, nausea, gagging, vomiting, ambivalence, embarrassment, lack of control of body sensations, pain, fear, vaginal bleeding or bloody show, rupture of membranes or fluid leaking from the vagina, perineal injury or trauma, breast exposure or suckling, feeling overpowered or helpless, and begging for release or help (Hobbins, 2004). When the woman feels of lack of choice, it can feel similar to the experience of sexual trauma (Chalfen, 1993). Pelvic examinations may evoke feelings of depersonalization and powerlessness (Kitzinger, 1990).

Nurses caring for women with a history of sexual abuse should have a heightened awareness of potential behavior during labor (Hobbins, 2004). The woman may choose to discuss her history of sexual abuse with the nurse. This type of acknowledgment may be a sign of healing and indicate that the woman believes her feelings will be taken seriously (Chalfen, 1993). There is evidence that survivors want to be asked how the abuse is affecting them (Hobbins, 2004). It is important to respond therapeutically in a calm, nonjudgmental, empathetic manner if the woman does choose to share the abuse with the nurse (Hobbins, 2004). Appropriate, affirming, comforting responses suggested by Hobbins (2004) include "You are not to blame for what has happened," "You have done nothing wrong," "I'm glad you shared your experiences with me," "I believe you," "I'm sorry that happened to you," "I imagine it is very difficult to for you to tell me these things. I admire your courage and respect you for it," "I will do my best to help you," and "Do you feel unsafe or fearful of anything?" Inappropriate, traumatizing responses reported by Hobbins (2004) include "Are you kidding me?", "How did you ever live through that?", "Are you sure that happened?", "You were awfully young," "Why did you have sex with him?", "Why didn't you tell your mother?", "What else did he do to you?", "Well, that was a long time ago. It sounds like you've resolved the issue, so let's focus on concerns you have today for yourself and your baby." Not all women will be able to share the history of abuse with the nurse but may exhibit difficulty and anxiety during pelvic examination. This behavior is a sign of possible previous sexual trauma requiring further exploration.

Nurses should help the woman feel empowered to make choices about labor and birth by assuring the woman that she is in control and her wishes will be respected. Provide thorough explanations of all procedures and treatment and obtain permission before touching the woman. Minimal exposure and talking to the patient during a pelvic examination is vital. Examinations should not be forced. Allow the woman to have a choice in procedures, even if that means "breaking the rules" a bit (Hobbins, 2004). Some common procedures during labor and birth can engender helplessness and fear. These include IVs, blood drawing, vaginal and other examinations, draping, surgical straps, restraints, and anesthesia mask application during cesarean birth (Hobbins, 2004). Be sensitive to the potential impact of these interventions and procedures as labor progresses and birth occurs. Trust that each woman knows her needs and what she is able to tolerate. Do not disregard or discount the woman's perceptions (Hobbins, 2004). If the woman has not had counseling or is not presently in counseling, with her consent, a referral would be appropriate.

Supporting Maternal and Family Attachment

At birth, skin-to-skin contact between mother and baby has positive benefits. Although babies were traditionally separated from their mothers immediately after birth for assessment and temperature stabilization and regulation by placing babies in warmers in the delivery room, this practice is not necessary for newborn well-being. Immediate skin-to-skin contact with the baby on the mother's chest after birth and continued contact during the first few days of life can promote normal temperature stabilization and regulation in the newborn and decrease risk of neonatal hypothermia and hypoglycemia (Britton, 1980; Bystova et al., 2003; Fransson, Karlsson, & Nilsson, 2005; Mzurek et al., 1999). Duration of breastfeeding and the baby's recognition of the mother's milk odor are enhanced with early skin-to-skin contact immediately after birth (Anderson, Moore, Hepworth, & Bergman, 2003; de Chateau & Wiberg, 1984; Mikiel-Kostryra, Boltruszko, Mazur, & Zielenska, 2001; Mikiel-Kostryra, Mazur, & Boltruszko, 2002; Mizuno, Mizuno, Shinohara, & Noda, 2004). Early breastfeeding has similar benefits, so mothers should be encouraged to breastfeed as soon as possible after birth (de Chateau & Wiberg, 1984; Mikiel-Kostyra, et al., 2001; Mikiel-Kostyra et al., 2002). Positive long-term effects of early contact include greater communication between mother and baby and encouraging behavior by the mother to the baby (Renfrew, Lang, & Woolbridge, 2000). Most mothers enjoy the experience and would choose skin-to-skin contact for future births (Carfoot, Williamson, & Dickson, 2005).

Women's expectations and desires regarding who will be present at their birth vary widely. Some women prefer that their partner be the sole participant, while others choose to have more family members and friends share this important event. The desires of the woman should guide this process rather than arbitrarily determined visitor policies. As long as space permits and the safety of the mother and baby are not a consideration, the woman should be able to have as many family members and support persons as she requests (AAP & ACOG, 2002). Every effort should be made to have the woman's partner next to her as she is giving birth and to be able to see and touch the baby immediately after birth. If newborn resuscitation is required or unexpected, encourage the partner to be close to the baby as soon as possible. As the baby's condition is stabilized, encourage the woman and her partner to hold and examine their baby.

Sibling presence during labor and birth also presents a unique opportunity for nurses to promote family attachment. Parents report that children present during labor and birth show a greater number of mothering and caretaking behaviors than did children not present (DelGiudice, 1986). Sibling classes to prepare children for the birth experience are imperative. These classes should be age-related and include films on childbirth, discussion of maternal behavior and sounds in labor, and reassurance that pain experienced by the mother is temporary. Additionally, each child needs a support person to accompany the child and be familiar with the child's developmental level, so that both the child's curiosity and concerns for his/her mother and new brother/sister are answered.

As the family is introduced to their newborn immediately at birth, explanation of umbilical cord clamping/cutting and inspection of the placenta help the family understand the final physiological separation of the newborn from the mother's life-support system. During skin-to-skin contact, allow the family, support persons, and siblings to be close to the mother to see and touch the baby. After stabilization, if the baby has been wrapped, the nurse can unwrap the newborn and describe normal physical characteristics. Siblings can count fingers and toes. Encouraging interaction with the newborn sets the stage for successful attachment and integration into the family unit. All family members can hold the newborn after birth as desired, and opportunities for photographs and videos should be provided.

CLINICAL INTERVENTIONS FOR WOMEN IN LABOR

The majority of pregnancies, labors, and birth are normal, requiring little or no intervention. However, some women require clinical interventions to optimize outcomes in pregnancies with identified maternal or fetal risk factors. The risk status for the woman and fetus may increase at any time during the pregnancy, labor and birth, or postpartum period (AAP & ACOG, 2002). Nurses in perinatal settings must be able to quickly assess and identify changes in maternal–fetal status and adjust nursing care accordingly. For example, nursing management during labor may require intrauterine resuscitation techniques when a nonreassuring FHR is noted, or plans for vaginal birth may be quickly changed when an emergent cesarean birth becomes the safest option for the mother and baby. Knowledge of appropriate nursing interventions for common maternal–fetal complications during labor is essential. The nurse must also be aware of changes in maternal–fetal status requiring physician or CNM notification. The next section focuses on the clinical interventions of cervical ripening, induction and augmentation, operative vaginal birth, and amnioinfusion. Implications for nursing care are presented with key points for assessment.

Cervical Ripening and Induction and Augmentation of Labor

Definition of Terms

Cervical ripening is the process of effecting physical softening and distensibility of the cervix in preparation for labor and birth. *Induction of labor* is the stimulation of uterine contractions before the spontaneous onset of labor for the purpose of accomplishing vaginal birth. *Augmentation of labor* is the stimulation of uterine contractions when spontaneous contractions have failed to result in progressive cervical dilation or descent of the fetus.

Various terminology and definitions have been used in the literature to describe excessive uterine activity that results from pharmacologic agents used for cervical ripening and induction or augmentation of labor. The imprecise and inconsistent use of these terms and definitions has contributed to inaccurate data about risks and benefits of each agent and makes it difficult to compare adverse effects among agents. For the purposes of this chapter, the term *hyperstimulation* will be used to describe excessive uterine activity. A clear definition of hyperstimulation is essential in each institution, because clinical management strategies, policies, and protocols should include what actions are expected when hyperstimulation is identified. All members of the perinatal team in each institution should be aware of the clinical criteria their institution has established for hyperstimulation and the expected actions. Hyperstimulation is a series of single contractions lasting 2 minutes or more, contractions of normal duration occurring within 1 minute of each other or a contraction frequency of more than five in 10 minutes (ACOG, 1999b, 2003a, 2005; Simpson, 2002). In Canada, excessive uterine activity is defined as five or more contractions in 10 minutes or contractions lasting 2 minutes or more (Society of Obstetricians and Gynecologists of Canada [SOGC], 2001). In the United Kingdom, excessive uterine activity is considered to be more than three to four contractions in 10 minutes (Royal College of Obstetricians and Gynaecologists [RCOG], 2001).

Other terms that have been used to describe excessive uterine activity are *tachysystole* and *hypertonus*. There is more variation in the definition and use of these terms than for hyperstimulation, and they are not used in all areas of the United States and Canada. Some authors reserve the term *hyperstimulation* for a contraction frequency of more than five in 10 minutes with evidence that the fetus is not tolerating this contraction pattern, as demonstrated by late decelerations or fetal bradycardia. Definitions of hyperstimulation that include evidence of nonreassuring fetal status are not clinically appropriate because such definitions may delay interventions to reduce uterine activity while fetal status deteriorates.

Incidence

According to the National Center for Health Statistics (NCHS) (Martin et al., 2006), in 2004 (the most recent year for which natality data are available) the rate of induction of labor in the United States was approximately 21.1%. This is more than twice the rate in 1990 (9.5%) and represents an all-time high since these data have been recorded from birth certificates (Martin et al., 2006). The latest natality data can be accessed at http://www.cdc.gov/nchs/births.htm. Most perinatal care providers would note that these data seem low when compared to actual clinical practice. The induction rate is calculated based on all women who give birth (Martin et al., 2006). If women who had a planned or repeat cesarean birth are excluded from the denominator and the figures are calculated based on all others who potentially could have had labor induction, the reported rate of induction would be significantly higher (Zhang, Yancey, & Henderson, 2002). Induction rates based on NCHS data consistently do not match data from hospital discharge data (Kirby, 2004). It is likely these data are significantly underreported by those completing birth certificate information. It has been estimated that between one-half and two-thirds of labor inductions are for nonmedical indications (Moore & Rayburn, 2006; Ramsey, Ramin, & Ramin, 2000); however, the comparison range for elective versus medically indicated varies widely based on type of institution (community or academic), area of the country (region, state, rural, or urban), and individual care providers (Glantz, 2005).

Indications

Because spontaneous labor is associated with fewer complications than induced labor, induction without a medical indication should be discouraged. Common medical indications for induction in the United States noted on birth certificates include premature rupture of membranes, intraamniotic infection, severe preeclampsia, pregnancy-associated hypertension, and diabetes. Induction of labor has merit as a therapeutic option when the benefits of expeditious birth outweigh the risks of continuing the pregnancy (ACOG, 1999b; SOCG, 2001). Controversy exists in the literature and in clinical practice about the exact nature and intensity of some risks and benefits. Multiple factors influence the decision to induce labor. Not all of the indications are clinical. Display 7–7 lists criteria, indications, and contraindications for cervical ripening and induction and augmentation of labor. Macrosomia is not a recommended indication for labor induction because this factor alone as an indication increases risk of cesarean birth (ACOG, 2000a, 2002b; Chauhan et al., 2005).

According to ACOG (1999a), labor may be induced for logistic reasons, such as a history of rapid labor, distance from the hospital or "psychosocial indications." The interpretation of psychosocial indications varies widely among providers and is most commonly noted for an elective (ie, nonmedical indication) induction of labor. When labor is induced for logistic reasons or psychosocial indications, the pregnant woman should be at 39 completed weeks of gestation to avoid the risk of iatrogenic prematurity (ACOG, 1999b; National Institute of Child Health and Human Development [NICHD], 2005). There is a common obstetrical misperception that babies born a few weeks before their time are not at any more risk of adverse outcomes than babies born at term. However, compared to term babies, late preterm (near-term) babies have higher incidence of prematurity-related medical and surgical conditions, such as respiratory distress syndrome, transient tachypnea, patent ductus arteriosus, hypothermia, apnea, infection, feeding difficulty, necrotizing enterocolitis, hyperbilirubinemia and kernicterus, seizures, and intracranial hemorrhage (NICHD, 2005; Raju, Higgins, Stark, & Leveno, 2006). There is an approximate doubling of the rates of respiratory symptoms and other problems related to newborn adaptation as well as NICU admissions for babies born via cesarean section for each week under 39 to 40 weeks of gestation (National Institutes of Health [NIH], 2006). Late preterm babies need closer monitoring than term babies, often requiring special care or intensive care nursery admissions, or readmissions after initial hospital discharge, and result in significantly more hospital costs (NICHD, 2005). Therefore, elective birth before 39 completed weeks of gestation is not recommended (ACOG, 1999b).

According to SOGC (2001), because elective induction of labor is associated with potential complications, it should be discouraged and undertaken only after fully informing the woman of the risks and establishing accurate gestational age. Culture may influence the incidence and request for elective induction. In the United States, there is controversy about elective induction prior to 39 weeks, how to dissuade patients from requesting elective birth, and how to prevent some providers from scheduling elective births for their convenience before this time, while in the UK, these same issues are related to births before 41 completed weeks of gestation (RCOG, 2001).

Risk-Benefit Analysis and Informed Consent

There is compelling evidence that elective induction of labor significantly increases the risk of cesarean birth, especially for nulliparous women (Kaul et al., 2004; Moore & Rayburn, 2006; Shin, Brubaker, & Ackerson, 2004; Vahratian et al., 2005; Vrouenraets et al., 2005). When the vertex is unengaged prior to initiation of induction, the risk of cesarean birth is even higher (Shin et al., 2004). Nulliparous women who have elective labor induction are a higher risk of requiring a blood transfusion, a longer length of stay, and their babies being admitted to the NICU when compared to nulliparous women who have spontaneous labor (Vrouenraets et al., 2005). Elective labor induction increases risk of significant pain requiring pain relief as well as operative vaginal birth (van Gemund, Hardeman, Scherjo, & Kanhai, 2003). Use of pharmacologic agents required for induction of labor increases the risk of complications related to hyperstimulation, nonreassuring FHR patterns, and cesarean birth for nonreassuring fetal status and failure to progress in labor. Failure to progress, also known as dystocia, is the number-one reason for primary cesarean birth in the United States (ACOG, 2003a). Women often have a cesarean birth during the latent phase of labor before they achieve active labor (Gifford et al., 2000; Lin & Rouse, 2006; Simon & Grobman, 2005). Cesarean birth after labor is associated with increased maternal and neonatal morbidity and mortality as well as an increase in inpatient length of stay and healthcare costs (Allen, O'Connell, & Baskett, 2006a, 2006b; Deneux-Tharaux, Carmona, Bouvier-Colle, & Breart, 2006; Getahun, Oyelese, Salihu, & Ananth, 2006).

Labor induction is not an isolated intervention. The decision for labor induction often results in a cascade of other interventions and activities that have the potential to negatively affect the childbirth process. Labor induction in the United States leads to an IV line, bedrest, and

DISPLAY 7-7

Criteria, Indications, and Contraindications for Cervical Ripening and Induction and Augmentation of Labor

CRITERIA FOR CERVICAL RIPENING AND INDUCTION OF LABOR

- Gestational age, cervical status, pelvic adequacy, fetal size, and fetal presentation should be assessed.
- Any potential risks to the mother and fetus should be considered.
- The medical record should document that a discussion was held between the pregnant woman and her healthcare provider about the indications, agents, and methods of labor induction, including the risks, benefits, and alternative approaches, and the possible need for repeat induction or cesarean birth.
- Personnel familiar with the effects of uterine stimulants on the mother and fetus should be available because uterine hyperstimulation may occur with induction of labor.
- Cervical ripening agents should be administered at or near the labor and birth suite where uterine activity and FHR can be monitored continuously.
- FHR and uterine contractions should be monitored during induction and augmentation as for any high-risk patient in active labor.
- A physician capable of performing a cesarean birth should be readily available.

INDICATIONS FOR CERVICAL RIPENING AND INDUCTION OF LABOR

Indications for induction of labor are not absolute, but should take into account maternal and fetal conditions, gestational age, cervical status, and other factors. Following are examples of maternal or fetal conditions that may be indications for induction of labor:

- Abruptio placentae
- Chorioamnionitis (intraamniotic infection)
- Fetal demise
- Pregnancy-induced hypertension
- Premature rupture of membranes
- Postterm pregnancy
- Maternal medical conditions (such as diabetes mellitus, renal disease, chronic pulmonary disease, or chronic hypertension)
- Fetal compromise (such as severe fetal growth restriction or isoimmunization)
- Preeclampsia, eclampsia

Labor may also be induced for logistic reasons, such as risk of rapid labor, distance from the hospital, or psychosocial indications. In such circumstances, at least one of the following criteria should be met or fetal lung maturity should be established:

- Fetal heart tones have been documented for 20 weeks by nonelectronic fetoscope or for 30 weeks by Doppler.
- It has been 36 weeks since a positive serum or urine human chorionic gonadotropin pregnancy test was performed by a reliable laboratory.
- An ultrasound measurement of the crown–rump length, obtained at 6–12 weeks, supports a gestational age of at least 39 weeks.
- An ultrasound examination performed between 13 and 20 weeks of gestation confirms the gestational age of at least 39 weeks determined by clinical history and physical examination.

CONTRAINDICATIONS TO INDUCTION OF LABOR

Generally, the contraindications for labor induction are the same as those for spontaneous labor and vaginal birth. They include, but are not limited to, the following:

- Vasa previa or complete placenta previa
- Transverse fetal lie
- Umbilical cord prolapse
- Previous transfundal uterine incision

OBSTETRIC CONDITIONS THAT ARE NOT CONTRAINDICATIONS TO INDUCTION BUT MAY REQUIRE SPECIAL ATTENTION

- One or more previous low-transverse cesarean births
- Breech presentation
- Maternal heart disease
- Multifetal pregnancy
- Polyhydramnios
- Presenting part above the pelvic inlet
- Severe hypertension
- Abnormal FHR patterns not requiring emergent birth
- A trial of labor after a previous cesarean birth or history of a prior uterine scar

INDICATIONS FOR AUGMENTATION OF LABOR

Uterine hypocontractility should be augmented only after both the maternal pelvis and fetal presentation have been assessed.

- Dystocia
- Uterine hypocontractility

CONTRAINDICATIONS TO AUGMENTATION OF LABOR

Contraindications to augmentation of labor are similar to those for induction of labor and may include, but are not limited to, the following:

- Placenta or vasa previa
- Umbilical cord presentation
- Prior classical uterine incision
- Active genital herpes infection
- Pelvic structural deformities
- Invasive cervical cancer

Adapted from American College of Obstetricians and Gynecologists (2003). *Dystocia and augmentation of labor.* (Practice Bulletin No. 49.) Washington, DC: Author; American College of Obstetricians and Gynecologists (1999a). *Induction of labor* (Practice Bulletin No. 10). Washington, DC: Author; and American College of Obstetricians and Gynecologists (2006). *Induction of labor for vaginal birth after cesarean birth* (Committee Opinion No. 342). Washington, DC: Author.

continuous EFM, as well as amniotomy, significant discomfort, epidural analgesia/anesthesia and a prolonged stay on the labor unit. Although it was once believed that amniotomy decreased the risk of cesarean birth and significantly shortened labor, it is now known that early amniotomy actually increases the risk of cesarean birth and is associated with at most, a modest nonclinically significant decrease in the length of labor (ACOG, 1999b; Fraser, Turcot, Krauss, & Brisson-Carrol, 2000; Segal, Sheiner, Yohai, Shodam-Vardi, & Katz, 1999; Sheiner et al., 2000). Risks of amniotomy include the possibility of umbilical cord prolapse, intraamniotic infection, fetal injury, bleeding from an undiagnosed vasa previa, and commitment to labor with an uncertain outcome (Hadi, 2000; Usta, Mercer, & Sibai, 1999). Intraamniotic infection, umbilical cord prolapse, and bleeding from an undiagnosed vasa previa are significant causes of fetal death (Silver, 2007). Elective amniotomy has been shown to result in "severe" variable decelerations of the FHR and an increased rate of cesarean birth for nonreassuring fetal status (Dilbaz et al., 2006; Garite, Porto, Carlson, Rumney, & Reimbold, 1993; Goffinet et al., 1997; Sheiner et al., 2000). Obstetric interventions such as amniotomy, fetal scalp electrode placement, and intrauterine pressure catheter insertion are responsible for nearly half of the cases of umbilical cord prolapse (Usta et al., 1999).

The use of oxytocin and prostaglandin agents increases the risk of fetal compromise during labor and birth. Hyperstimulation alone and hyperstimulation accompanied by a nonreassuring FHR pattern are significantly more common during cervical ripening and labor induction than in spontaneous labor (Crane et al., 2001). Each woman has individual myometrial sensitivity to oxytocin and prostaglandin (Ulstem, 1997). Because of the lack of knowledge about the exact physiology of labor, it is difficult to determine the optimal dosages necessary to correct abnormal labor with artificial pharmacologic compounds. From the perspective of maternal–fetal safety, prolonged periods of hyperstimulation of hyperstimulation should be avoided to minimize risk of progressive deterioration in fetal status and subsequent nonreassuring FHR patterns. Thus interventions for hyperstimulation should not be delayed until there is evidence of nonreassuring fetal status.

The discomfort and frequency of oxytocin-induced contractions sets the stage for epidural analgesia/anesthesia, which in turn increases the risk of complications such as hypotension, fever, and FHR decelerations (ACOG, 2002b). Epidural analgesia/anesthesia prolongs labor by 40–90 minutes, and approximately 50% of women who are not receiving oxytocin before epidural placement will receive oxytocin to maintain labor progress after epidural dosage (Alexander et al., 2002; Halpern, Leighton, Ohlsson, Barrett, & Rice, 1998; Howell, 2000). Epidural analgesia/anesthesia

also increases risk of an operative vaginal birth with vacuum or forceps application (ACOG, 2002b). The operative vaginal birth associated with the epidural increases the risk of third- and fourth-degree perineal lacerations (ACOG, 2006b; Eason & Feldman, 2000). The perceived need to cut an episiotomy due to the increased length of the second stage associated with epidurals and the perineal lacerations from the operative vaginal birth can result in other complications, such as anal sphincter injuries, severe lacerations in subsequent births, infection, delayed healing, increased blood loss, scarring, increased pain, and sexual dysfunction (ACOG, 2006b). A cesarean birth that results from any of these induction-related complications is likely to be followed by another cesarean birth in a subsequent pregnancy (Martin et al., 2006). The additional risk of iatrogenic prematurity and potential admission to the NICU if estimations of gestational age are inaccurate must be considered as well (ACOG, 1999b).

Because of these risks, a risk–benefit analysis is recommended before the procedure as well as a discussion by the provider with the patient of the agents, methods, advantages, disadvantages, and alternative approaches, including the risk of cesarean birth and a repeat induction (ACOG, 1999b; Joint Commission on Accreditation of Healthcare Organizations [JCAHO], 2007a; SOGC, 2001). Following this discussion, when the woman has enough information to participate in the decision-making process, the provider should obtain informed consent (ACOG, 1999b). The medical record should contain documentation that this discussion occurred and that the woman consented to proceed (ACOG, 1999b; JCAHO, 2007a).

The perinatal nurse may face a dilemma when women are admitted for cervical ripening or induction of labor but do not seem to know the indication for the procedure. It is not the nurse's responsibility to provide the required information; however, advocating for the woman and fetus includes ensuring that the woman has been fully informed by her primary healthcare provider before beginning the procedure. One way to enhance compliance with ACOG (1999a), SOGC (2001), and JCAHO (2007a) recommendations is to establish a unit policy requiring evidence of informed consent before elective cervical ripening and labor induction is initiated. See Appendix 7–C for a sample form that can be included in the medical record as documentation of informed consent and indications.

The Nurse's Role

The nurse providing care for the woman during cervical ripening and induction of labor must be aware of appropriate indications for the use of each mechanical method and pharmacologic agent, as well as their actions, expected results, and potential risks. Before any cervical ripening or labor induction agent is used, maternal status and fetal well-being should be established, and cervical status should be assessed and documented in the medical record (ACOG, 1999b; SOGC, 2001). Estimation of fetal weight and assessment of maternal pelvis should be determined and documented by the provider (AAP & ACOG, 2002). The indications for preinduction cervical ripening and induction of labor also should be documented. Ongoing maternal–fetal assessments during labor induction are presented in Display 7–3. Avoidance of potential complications such as uterine hyperstimulation and fetal compromise is an important aspect of the nurse's role during cervical ripening, labor induction, and labor augmentation. Absence of fetal well-being necessitates direct evaluation by a physician or CNM, and interdisciplinary discussion and written documentation of further clinical management plans.

Clinical Protocol and Unit Policy Development

Most institutions have policies and/or protocols in place for cervical ripening and induction and augmentation of labor. Suggestions for key concepts to be included are presented in Display 7–8. A sample protocol for labor induction and augmentation is presented in Appendix 7–D. Both ACOG (1999a) and SOGC (2001) recommend that healthcare providers at each institution develop a policy or protocol for cervical ripening and induction and augmentation of labor. Ideally physicians, nurse midwives, and nurses jointly develop these policies or protocols on the basis of current evidence and published guidelines from professional organizations such as ACOG, AWHONN, SOGC, and JCAHO. The best approach is to develop a single unit policy or protocol rather than allowing each provider to have his or her own policy or protocol with individual variations. For example, the group should come to consensus

---

DISPLAY 7-8

Suggestions for Key Concepts to Include in Clinical Protocols and Unit Policies

PRIORITIZATION AND DOCUMENTATION

- Criteria for designating patient priority for cervical ripening and induction based on the nature and intensity of the indication that can be used as a framework for decision-making during periods of limited staffing.
- Documentation of indication by primary care provider
- Documentation of risk–benefit analysis discussion with pregnant woman by primary healthcare provider and informed decision-making process, as recommended by ACOG (1999a), SOGC (2001), and JCAHO (2007a)
- Specific recommendations for care of women with a prior history of cesarean birth or uterine scar

STAFFING CONSIDERATIONS

- Experience of registered nurse
- Availability of registered nurses to meet recommended nurse-to-patient ratios
- Acuity of patient
- Ongoing evaluation of labor status
- Availability and skill level of support personnel
- Contingency plans such as on-call list

PATIENT ASSESSMENT

- Establishment of maternal and fetal well-being
- Documentation of cervical status

- Method of fetal assessment
- Frequency of maternal–fetal assessments

METHODS AND DOSAGES

- Cervical ripening agents to be used
- Initial oxytocin or misoprostol dosage
- Intervals and amounts for oxytocin dosage increases
- Intervals and amounts for misoprostol dosages
- Orders for oxytocin and documentation in milliunits per minute (mU/min)
- Titration of oxytocin dosage based on progress of labor and maternal–fetal response
- Dosage of misoprostol based on progress of labor and maternal–fetal status
- Maintenance or decrease in oxytocin dosage if labor is progressing

COMPLICATIONS

- Definition of hyperstimulation
- Interventions for hyperstimulation
- Interventions for nonreassuring fetal status
- Criteria for provider notification

UNIT POLICY

- Algorithm/chain of command for addressing clinical disagreements
- Methods for documenting all of the key concepts and interventions outlined in the policy/protocol
- An expectation that the policy will be followed by all members of the healthcare team

Adapted from Simpson, K. R. (2002). *Cervical ripening and induction and augmentation of labor.* (Practice Monograph). Washington, DC: Association of Women's Health, Obstetric and Neonatal Nurses.

on the IV concentrations, rate of dosage increases, and interval between increases in dosage rate on the basis of available evidence and published guidelines. Once the interdisciplinary team agrees on a policy or protocol, it should be expected that all providers will practice within the established unit parameters.

Staffing Considerations

The number of women who are scheduled for cervical ripening and induction of labor influences nursing staff requirements for labor and birth units. Because induction of labor is likely to occur during the day, more nurses may be needed during this time than during the late evening or early morning. A record maintained on the unit of women who are scheduled for labor induction is essential to plan staffing and personnel needs based on expected volume. Many units place a limit on the number of scheduled labor inductions that can be performed on any given day to ensure that adequate staff and rooms are available to provide the appropriate level of care. Development of criteria for designating patient priority for induction of labor based on the nature and intensity of the indication can provide a useful decision-making framework when conflicts arise. Ideally, these criteria are developed jointly by physician and nurse members of a unit practice committee. Requiring documentation of indications and having these data available on the unit before admission using a method such as the *Cervical Ripening and Induction of Labor Analysis* form in Appendix 7–C may be helpful in designating patient priority when resources are limited. Elective induction of labor may need to be postponed or rescheduled at times, especially if there are not enough resources available. Establishment of a perinatal nurse on-call system may facilitate securing staffing resources as needed in a timely manner.

The appropriate number of qualified professional registered nurses should be in attendance during cervical ripening and induction or augmentation of labor (Simpson, 2002). The current recommendations for the nurse-to-patient ratio during induction or augmentation of labor in the United States is 1:2 (AAP & ACOG, 2002); in Canada, it is 1:1 (SOGC, 2001). These recommendations are for women in labor who are healthy and have no significant maternal or fetal complications. It is important to consider that some clinical situations may warrant more intense nursing care during induction or augmentation of labor. Staffing requirements for labor and birth are dynamic; thus, assessment of the appropriate balance between available resources and patient care needs is an ongoing process. If a nurse cannot clinically evaluate the effects of medication at least every 15 minutes or a physician who has privileges to perform a cesarean birth is not readily available, oxytocin infusion should be discontinued or the initial or subsequent doses of misoprostol delayed until this level of maternal–fetal care can be provided (AAP & ACOG, 2002; ACOG, 1999b).

Cervical Status

Cervical assessment includes documentation of the Bishop score (Bishop, 1964) and the presence or absence of uterine activity. Cervical status is the most important factor predicting the success of induction of labor. It is assessed most commonly by using the Bishop pelvic scoring system (Bishop, 1964) (see Table 7–3). Perinatal nurses are qualified to assess and document cervical status based on the Bishop scoring system. If the total score is more than 8, the probability of vaginal birth following induction of labor is similar to that of spontaneous labor (ACOG, 1999b). For women at term, a Bishop score of 6 or more may be useful in predicting onset of spontaneous labor within 7 days (Rozenberg, Goffinet, & Hessabi, 2000). Despite efforts by many researchers to modify the Bishop score, it remains the most reliable and cost-effective method of predicting likelihood of successful induction. The factor with the strongest association with successful induction seems to be cervical dilation; however, all components collectively can be quite useful in selecting appropriate candidates for labor induction (Baacke & Edwards, 2006). Other factors that have been shown to influence successful labor induction are

---

TABLE 7–3 ■ BISHOP SCORE FOR ASSESSING READINESS FOR INDUCTION

Factor	Assigned Value			
	0	*1*	*2*	*3*
Cervical dilation	0	1–2 cm	3–4 cm	5 cm or more
Cervical effacement	0–30%	40–50%	60–70%	80% or more
Fetal station	−3	−2	−1,0	+1,+2
Cervical consistency	Firm	Moderate	Soft	
Cervical position	Posterior	Midposition	Anterior	

From Bishop, E. H. (1964). Pelvic scoring for elective induction. *Obstetrics and Gynecology, 24,* 266.

maternal age, parity, weight, and height. Younger women, women who are normal weight, women who are tall, and women who are multiparous are more likely to have success with labor induction (Crane, 2006).

Outdated Methods of Stimulating Labor

There is no evidence that enemas or castor oil are effective methods of labor induction; however, women report pain and discomfort with both methods and embarrassment if they result in diarrhea during labor and birth (Cuervo, Bernal Mdel, & Mendoza, 2006; Kelly, Kavanagh, & Thomas, 2001; Summers, 1997; Tenore, 2003). These methods are not part of contemporary evidence-based practice and have been virtually eliminated in the United States and Canada (Tenore, 2003).

Cervical Ripening

Many mechanical and pharmacologic methods have been used to induce cervical ripening. The ideal ripening agent or procedure should be simple to use, noninvasive,

and effective within a reasonable time period; it should not stimulate or induce labor during the ripening process nor increase maternal, fetal, or neonatal morbidity. Unfortunately, the ideal agent or procedure for cervical ripening has not yet been identified.

Mechanical Methods

Mechanical methods of cervical ripening have been used for hundreds of years. Current mechanical methods include insertion of dilators such as *Laminaria* (*Laminaria japonica*), synthetic hygroscopic dilators (eg, Lamicel and Dilapan), and balloon catheters that soften the cervix, change the Bishop score, and facilitate amniotomy when compared with no pretreatment (see Display 7-9). There is no evidence that mechanical methods of cervical ripening are associated with a reduced cesarean birth rate or a decrease in the induction-to-birth interval; however, the risk of hyperstimulation is much less when compared with the use of pharmacologic agents (Boulvain, Kelly, Lohse, Stan, & Irion, 2001, Gelber & Sciscione, 2006). Thus, mechanical dilation may be an ideal method in women for whom pharmacologic agents are contraindicated and for those who have an increased risk of uterine rupture,

---

DISPLAY 7-9

Mechanical Methods of Cervical Ripening

ALL DEVICES

- Perineum and vagina are prepped with antiseptic
- Placed in endocervical canal under direct visualization using aseptic technique
- Inserted by physician or CNM
- May be appropriate for women for whom pharmacologic agents for cervical ripening are contraindicated

LAMINARIA TENTS

- Desiccated stems of cold water seaweed (*Laminaria japonica*)
- Available in various sizes from 2–6 mm in diameter and approximately 60 mm in length
- Progressively placed until the cervix is "full"
- The "tails" are allowed to fall into the vagina for ease of identification and removal
- Sterile gauze pad is placed in the vagina to hold the dilators in place
- Absorb fluid from the cervical tissues
- Swell two to three times diameter in 6–12 hours
- Cause mechanical dilation and local prostaglandin release

SYNTHETIC OSMOTIC DILATORS (LAMICEL AND DILAPAN)

- Polyvinyl alcohol polymer sponge soaked in 450 mg of magnesium sulfate
- Progressively placed until the cervix is "full"
- The "tails" are allowed to fall into the vagina for ease of identification and removal
- Sterile gauze pad is placed in the vagina to hold the dilators in place
- Absorb fluid from cervical tissues
- Swell three to four times diameter in 2–4 hours
- Multiple serial applications possible
- Cause mechanical dilation and local prostaglandin release

BALLOON CATHETERS

- Balloon catheters: 14–26 g Foley catheter balloon inflated above internal os with 30–50 mL of sterile water
- Extraamniotic saline infusion: Balloon catheter with normal saline infusion at 1 mL/min into extraamniotic space (the addition of extraamniotic saline infusion has not been found to enhance the process when compared to use of the balloon catheter alone)
- Cause direct pressure and overstretching of the lower uterine segment and cervix as well as local prostaglandin release
- Results are usually seen within 8–12 hours after insertion
- Balloon catheter usually falls out when cervical dilation occurs

Adapted from Simpson, K. R. (2002). *Cervical ripening and induction and augmentation of labor.* (Practice Monograph). Washington, DC: Association of Women's Health, Obstetric and Neonatal Nurses.

such as women with a history of prior uterine scar who are attempting a trial of labor. Balloon catheters have been found to be as efficacious as pharmacologic agents in cervical ripening (Gelber & Sciscione, 2006). Mechanical dilators do not appear to result in an increase in neonatal complications, but they have been associated with a slight increase in peripartum infections (ACOG, 1999b).

Mechanical dilators are usually used for women with an indication for induction but have little or no cervical effacement (Gelber & Sciscione, 2006). Physicians and CNMs insert *Laminaria* tents, hygroscopic dilators, and balloon catheters using direct visualization of the cervix and antiseptic technique. Following placement, documentation should include the number of dilators placed in the cervix and the number of sponges placed in the vagina. Note the type and size of the balloon catheter along with the amount of fluid instilled in the balloon. Because the woman is positioned to facilitate placement of the dilators, take care to minimize the effects of supine hypotension. Encourage the woman to assume a lateral position as soon as possible following insertion.

After the appropriate time (usually 6–12 hours), the physician or CNM can remove the sponges and examine the cervix. If cervical dilation is determined to be adequate, the dilators are removed and an oxytocin infusion is initiated to induce labor. If cervical dilation is determined not to be adequate, either the dilators can be removed and fresh ones inserted or additional dilators can be placed around those already in position. Regardless of whether the dilators are removed and replaced or additional dilators are inserted, all dilators and sponges must be accounted for after their use. The balloon catheter usually falls out when the cervix begins to dilate, and this event should be noted in the medical record. Additional nursing assessment and documentation includes notation of the onset of regular painful contractions, nonreassuring fetal status, maternal fever, rupture of membranes, bleeding, or continuous uterine pain, should any of these occur. There are no data or published guidelines regarding the frequency of maternal–fetal assessments during mechanical dilation for cervical ripening; thus, maternal–fetal status and institutional policies and procedures determine frequency of assessment.

Pharmacologic Methods

Various hormonal preparations are available to induce cervical ripening. These agents include prostaglandin E_1 (PGE_1): misoprostol (Cytotec) and PGE_2 preparations: dinoprostone (Prepidil gel or Cervidil insert). Nurses caring for women receiving any of these agents should be aware that they may lead to the onset of labor, particularly if the cervix is favorable. When the cervix is unfavorable, cervical softening and thinning are more likely to occur. Table 7–4 summarizes key points about the use of prostaglandins for cervical ripening.

PROSTAGLANDIN E_2

Dinoprostone (PGE_2) is one of the most frequently prescribed medications for cervical ripening. The mechanism of action is similar to the natural ripening process, and women often go into spontaneous labor following administration. The prostaglandin preparations used successfully for cervical ripening today produce the desired cervical changes, but all tend to increase myometrial contractility. For this reason, prostaglandins for cervical ripening must be viewed as the first step in labor induction. Dinoprostone induces cervical ripening by directly softening the cervix, relaxing the cervical smooth muscle, and producing uterine contractions. An added benefit is the facilitation of postcervical ripening induction by preparing the uterus to produce coordinated contractions with lower doses of oxytocin (Kierse, 2006). Dinoprostone preparations appear to be as efficacious as other methods of cervical ripening (Kierse, 2006).

In December 1992, the U.S. Food and Drug Administration (FDA) approved the first commercially prepared dinoprostone gel preparation (Prepidil) for cervical ripening for intracervical administration in women at or near term who have a medical indication for labor induction. In 1995, the FDA approved a dinoprostone vaginal insert (Cervidil) for cervical ripening.

The use of dinoprostone in women with a history of asthma; reactive airway disease; glaucoma; or pulmonary, hepatic, cardiac or renal disease has been debated. Concern exists about the vascular and pulmonary effects of prostaglandins in inducing maternal compromise. Unlike $PGF_2\alpha$, which is a potent bronchoconstrictor, PGE_2 is a bronchodilator and thus does not cause bronchial constriction, risk of asthma exacerbation, or significant blood pressure changes (ACOG, 1999b).

PREPIDIL

Prepidil is packaged as a single-dose syringe containing 0.5 mg of dinoprostone gel in 2.5 mL of a viscous gel composed of colloidal silicon dioxide in triacetin. The syringe is packaged with two soft plastic catheters for intracervical administration. The catheter is shielded to prevent application above the internal cervical os. Cervical effacement determines the appropriate catheter tip to use for placement of the gel. The cervix is visualized using a speculum, and a physician or CNM then introduces the gel into the cervical canal just below the level of the internal os. Positioning of the woman should minimize the risk of hypotension during placement of the gel and for the initial period of bedrest following application. The cervix is reexamined after six hours. If there is no response to the initial dose, a repeat dose is administered, up to three doses over a 24-hour period

TABLE 7–4 ■ PHARMACOLOGIC AGENTS USED FOR CERVICAL RIPENING/LABOR INDUCTION AND AUGMENTATION

Factor	Pitocin (Oxytocin)	Prepidil (Dinoprostone)	Cervidil (Dinoprostone)	Cytotec (Misoprostol)
Storage and Preparation	Room temperature storage. Available in 20-unit ampules. There are many variations in the dilution rate. Some protocols suggest adding 10 units of oxytocin to 1,000 mL of an isotonic electrolyte IV solution, resulting in an infusion dosage rate of 1 mU/min = 6 mL/hr. Other commonly reported dilutions are 20 units of oxytocin to 1,000 mL IV fluid (1 mU/min = 3 mL/hr) and 30 units of oxytocin to 500 mL of IV fluid or 60 units of oxytocin to 1,000 mL IV fluid (1 mU/min = 1 mL/hr). One advantage to using 30 units in 500 mL IV fluid or 60 units in 1,000 mL IV fluid is that a 1 to 1 concentration results that requires no mathematical conversion from mL per hour to mU per min when documenting the amount of oxytocin infused. The key issues are documentation in mU per min of oxytocin infused and consistency in practice within each institution.	Store in refrigerator (stable up to 2 y when stored at 2–8°C). Bring to room temperature just before administration. Do not use warm water bath, microwave or other methods to speed the process of bringing gel to room temperature, as heat may cause inactivation.	Keep frozen (–20°C) until immediately before use. No warming required.	Available in 100 micrograms & 200 microgram tablets. 100-μg tablet is not scored; dose should be prepared by hospital pharmacy.
Initial Administration	Administered IV in an isotonic electrolyte solution, piggybacked into the main IV line at the port most proximal to the venous site. Start at 0.5 to 1 mU/min.	0.5 mg of dinoprostone in 2.5 mL of viscous gel. If cervix is not effaced, use 20-mm shielded endocervical catheter. If cervix is ≥50% effaced, use 10-mm catheter. Perform speculum exam, insert gel just below cervical os.	10 mg dinoprostone in a controlled-release vaginal insert with removable cord is easy to administer and does not require speculum exam.	Various dosing regimens have been reported: safest approach is 25 micrograms (1/4 tablet) as the initial dose inserted into the posterior vaginal fornix and repeated every 3–6 hr, up to six doses in 24 hr as needed. Not enough data are available to recommend oral administration.

Patient Considerations	Patient need not remain in bed during infusion. Intermittent auscultation of the FHR at prescribed intervals or EFM telemetry can be used during ambulation or sitting on a chair or birthing ball. Careful close monitoring for women with a history of a prior cesarean birth or uterine scar, using the lowest dose possible to achieve labor progress.	Patient should remain recumbent for at least 30 min after administration. Not recommended for use in women with a history of a prior cesarean birth or uterine scar.	Patient should remain supine for 2 hr following insertion and then may ambulate if EFM telemetry is used. Not recommended for use in women with history of prior cesarean birth or uterine scar.	Not recommended for use in women with history of prior cesarean birth or uterine scar.
Effects	There are wide variations in time from initial dose to uterine activity. The biologic half-life is approximately 10–12 min. 3–4 half-lives are need to reach physiologic steady state (30 to 60 min) at which the full effect of the dosage on the uterine response can be assessed.	Uterine contractions usually occur within 1 hr of administration. Peak activity occurs within 4 hr.	Uterine contractions usually occur within 5–7 hr.	Wide variations exist in time of onset of uterine contractions. Peak action is approximately 1 to 2 hr when administered intravaginally, but can be up to 4 to 6 hours for some women.
Adjusting Dosage	Advance by 1 to 2 mU/min at intervals no less than every 30 to 60 min until adequate labor progress is achieved. Titrate dose to the maternal–fetal response to labor. Use the lowest dose possible to achieve adequate progress of labor (progressive cervical effacement and approximately 0.5 cm to 1 cm per hr cervical dilation). Reevaluate the clinical situation if the oxytocin dosage rate reaches 20 mU/min. Contractions should not be closer than every 2 min. Avoid hyperstimulation. Discontinue if nonreassuring FHR pattern develops.	If no response, increase dose by 0.5 mg every 6 hr. Maximum *cumulative* dose is 1.5 mg (three doses) over 24 hr.	Remove after 12 hr or at onset of labor. Remove if hyperstimulation and/or nonreassuring FHR pattern occurs.	Redosing is permissible if (1) cervical condition remains unfavorable, (2) uterine activity is minimal, (3) FHR is reassuring, and (4) it has been at least 3 h since the last dose. Observe for up to 2 h after spontaneous rupture of membranes before redosing. Redosing is *withheld* if there are two or more contractions in 10 min, adequate cervical ripening is achieved (Bishop score $\geq$8 or cervix is 80% effaced and 3 cm dilated), patient enters active labor, or FHR is nonreassuring.

(continued)

TABLE 7–4 ■ PHARMACOLOGIC AGENTS USED FOR CERVICAL RIPENING/LABOR INDUCTION AND AUGMENTATION (Continued)

Factor	Pitocin (Oxytocin)	Prepidil (Dinoprostone)	Cervidil (Dinoprostone)	Cytotec (Misoprostol)
Monitoring	Administer in the labor and birth suite, where uterine activity and FHR can be recorded continuously via EFM and evaluated at a minimum every 15 min during the 1st stage of labor and every 5 min during the 2nd stage of labor. If using intermittent auscultation, determine and record the FHR and palpate uterine contractions at least every 15 min during the 1st stage of labor and every 5 min during the second stage of labor.	Administer at or near labor and birth suite, where uterine activity and FHR can be monitored continuously for 30 min to 2 hr after dosage.	Administer at or near the labor and birth suite, where uterine activity and FHR can be monitored continuously while in place and for at least 15 min after removal.	Administer at or near labor and birth suite, where uterine activity and FHR can be monitored continuously.
Use With Oxytocin, if Needed	NA	Oxytocin should be delayed for 6–12 hr after last dose.	Oxytocin should be delayed for at least 30–60 min after removal of insert.	Oxytocin should be delayed until at least 4 hr after last dose.
Complications	Risk of hyperstimulation is dose-related. 50% of cases of hyperstimulation will result in a nonreassuring FHR pattern.	Rate of hyperstimulation is 1%–5%; usually occurs within 1 hr of administration.	Rate of hyperstimulation is about 5%; usually occurs within 1 hr of administration but may occur up to 9.5 hr after administration.	Hyperstimulation is more common with misoprostol as compared to Prepidil, Cervidil, and Oxytocin. Rates of hyperstimulation are lower with lower dosages (25 micrograms) and when dosed less frequently (i.e., every 6 hr instead of every 3 hr).

Adapted from: Simpson, K. R. (2002). *Cervical ripening and induction and augmentation of labor:* (AWHONN Practice Monograph). Washington, DC: Association of Women's Health, Obstetric, and Neonatal Nurses. Used with permission.

(for a cumulative dose of 1.5 mg in 24 hours). Previous exposure to PGE_2 attenuates the contractile response to oxytocin (Maul, Mackay, & Garfield, 2006). After the final dose of dinoprostone or once cervical ripening is accomplished, it is recommended that use of IV oxytocin be delayed for at least 6–12 hours, because the effects of PGE_2 may be heightened with oxytocin (ACOG, 1999b).

Prior to placement of the gel, the woman should be afebrile, with no vaginal bleeding and without regular contractions. Dinoprostone is rapidly absorbed, with maximum concentrations reported within 15–45 minutes; half-life ranges from approximately 2.5–5 minutes (Albrecht, 1997; Rayburn, Records, & Swanson, 1996). After gel application, plasma concentration increases rapidly within 20–30 minutes and remains high for more than 4 hours (Winkler & Rath, 1999). ACOG (1999b) recommends continuous monitoring of the FHR and uterine activity for 30 minutes to 2 hours after placement of the gel. Monitoring of the FHR and uterine activity should continue if regular contractions persist (ACOG, 1999b). Research is limited on maternal–fetal assessment techniques other than EFM.

If no increase in uterine activity is noted and the FHR is reassuring after the recommended period of observation, continuous monitoring may be discontinued, and the patient may be transferred elsewhere (ACOG, 1999b). In an uncomplicated pregnancy, the woman may be encouraged to ambulate after the initial period of observation. Assessments should focus on uterine activity, monitoring for hyperstimulation, and fetal response to therapy. If hyperstimulation occurs, the woman may be placed in a lateral position and given tocolytic therapy (0.25 mg of terbutaline subcutaneously), based on the clinical condition and fetal response (Albrecht, 1997; Witter, 2000). Irrigation of the cervix and vagina is not beneficial (ACOG, 1999b). There is a risk of uterine rupture when prostaglandins are used for women attempting a vaginal birth following a previous cesarean birth (VBAC), thus Prepidil is not recommended for these patients (ACOG, 2006c).

CERVIDIL

The Cervidil vaginal insert is a thin, flat, rectangular-shaped, cross-linked polymer hydrogel that releases dinoprostone from a 10-mg reservoir at a controlled rate of approximately 0.3 mg/hr in vivo (Forest Pharmaceuticals, 1995). The reservoir chip is encased within a pouch of knitted Dacron® polyester with a removal cord. The entire system comes preassembled and prepackaged in sterile foil packets.

Cervidil may be inserted by the perinatal nurse when the nurse has demonstrated competence in insertion and the activity is within the scope of practice as defined by state and provincial regulations. Institutional guidelines should be established for the nurse's

role related to the use of Cervidil. Unlike the transcervical preparations, Cervidil does not require visualization of the cervix for insertion. The insert is placed into the posterior fornix of the vagina, with its long axis transverse to the long axis of the vagina. The ribbon end of the retrieval system may be allowed to extrude distally from the vagina or tucked into the vagina. Once placed, Cervidil absorbs moisture, swells, and releases dinoprostone at a controlled rate. The system makes Cervidil relatively simple to insert and requires only a single digital examination.

Cervidil is removed after 12 hours, or when active labor begins (ACOG, 1999b). Regular contractions (three in 10 minutes lasting 60 seconds or more with moderate patient discomfort) will occur in approximately 25% of women after Cervidil placement (Rayburn, Tassone, & Pearman, 2000). One major advantage of Cervidil is that the system can be easily and quickly removed in the event of uterine hyperstimulation or other complications. If uterine hyperstimulation occurs, complete reversal of the prostaglandin-induced uterine pattern usually occurs within 15 minutes of removal. If necessary, the woman may be given tocolytic therapy (0.25 mg of terbutaline subcutaneously). Previous exposure to PGE_2 attenuates the contractile response to oxytocin (Maul et al., 2006), so careful maternal–fetal monitoring is warranted when oxytocin is administered after Cervidil has been used for cervical ripening. Oxytocin administration should be delayed until at least 30 to 60 minutes after removal of the Cervidil insert (ACOG, 1999b). Continuous monitoring of the FHR and uterine activity is indicated while Cervidil is in place and for 15 minutes after removal (1999b). Ambulation while Cervidil is in place is an option if continuous EFM via telemetry is available. There have been no studies using methods other than continuous EFM for maternal–fetal assessment.

Because of the high rate of initiation of regular contractions and the 5% rate of hyperstimulation, Cervidil is not appropriate for outpatient cervical ripening (ACOG, 1999b; Rayburn et al., 2000). There is a risk of uterine rupture when prostaglandins are used for women attempting VBAC, thus Cervidil is not recommended for these patients (ACOG, 2006c).

PROSTAGLANDIN E₁

Misoprostol (PGE_1) is a synthetic prostaglandin E_1 analogue that has been used for cervical ripening and induction of labor. Misoprostol was originally approved by the FDA for prevention of peptic ulcers, not for cervical ripening or induction of labor. In August 2000, Searle sent a letter to healthcare providers titled, *Important Drug Warning Concerning Unapproved Use of Intravaginal or Oral Misoprostol in Pregnant Women for Induction of Labor or Abortion.* Searle was concerned that its medication was being used off-label for indications and patients not approved by the FDA and wanted to issue a written warning about the potential adverse effects for pregnant women and their fetuses. This letter caused considerable controversy, and some healthcare providers and institutions temporarily or permanently stopped using the drug for pregnant women. Several months later, ACOG (2000c) responded with a Committee Opinion reaffirming their earlier statements about the safety and efficacy of misoprostol as described in its 1999 Practice Bulletin *Induction of Labor*. Off-label use of drugs is not uncommon during pregnancy and labor when there is a substantial body of supportive literature and experience. For example, terbutaline is not approved by the FDA for preterm labor prophylaxis but is used as such in many perinatal centers in the United States.

In April 2002, the FDA removed the contraindication for the use of misoprostol for women during pregnancy because it was widely used for cervical ripening and labor induction and was part of an FDA-approved regime for use with mifepristone to induce abortion in pregnancies of 49 days or less. The FDA (2002) included warnings about potential adverse effects of misoprostol when used for cervical ripening, labor induction, and treatment of serious postpartum hemorrhage in the presence of uterine atony. According to the FDA (2002), a major adverse effect of the obstetrical use of misoprostol is hyperstimulation of the uterus, which may progress to uterine tetany with marked impairment of uteroplacental blood flow, uterine rupture, or amniotic fluid embolism. The FDA (2002) further noted that pelvic pain, retained placenta, severe genital bleeding, shock, fetal bradycardia, and fetal and maternal death have been reported. As more data are published from ongoing clinical research studies, a clearer understanding of safety and appropriate dosages will emerge.

The controversy about misoprostol for cervical ripening and labor induction centers in part on whether there is enough evidence to support its safe use for women and their fetuses. This controversy and the lack of consensus among experts are not limited to the United States. RCOG (2001) and SOGC (2001) have recommended that use of misoprostol be confined to clinical trials because of the risks of hyperstimulation and the lack of evidence about the best dose and route for labor induction.

When used for cervical ripening or induction of labor, 25 micrograms placed in the posterior vaginal fornix should be considered for the initial dose (ACOG, 1999b, 1999c). Higher dosages have been associated with an increased rate of hyperstimulation (ACOG, 1999b, 1999c; Kierse, 2006; Wing & Lyons, 2006). However, it is important to consider that hyperstimulation and nonreassuring FHR changes are associated with both the 25- and 50-microgram doses (Crane et al., 2001; Kierse, 2006). Recent systematic reviews found that uterine hyperstimulation with and without nonreassuring FHR changes is significantly higher with use of misoprostol when compared with Cervidil, Prepidil and oxytocin (Hofmeyr & Gulmezoglu, 2003; Wing & Lyons, 2006). A 4- to 6-hour interval between doses has been associated with less uterine hyperstimulation than the 3-hour interval (ACOG, 1999b, 1999c; Hofemeyr & Gulmezoglu, 2003; Wing & Lyons, 2006).

Uterine rupture is a complication of the use of misoprostol for cervical ripening and labor induction, especially those who have a uterine scar (Hofmeyr & Gulmezoglu, 2003; Lydon-Rochelle, Holt, Easterling, & Martin, 2001b; Wing & Lyons, 2006). However, it is important to consider that uterine rupture after misoprostol (or oxytocin) can occur in the unscarred uterus, although the risk is lower than for women with a previous uterine scar (Akhan, Iyibozkurt, & Turfanda, 2001; Bennett, 1997; Catanzarite, Cousins, Dowling, & Danshmand, 2006; Khabbaz et al., 2001; Mazzone & Woolever, 2006). Misoprostol is contraindicated in women with a history or prior uterine surgery or cesarean birth because of the risk of uterine rupture (ACOG, 1999b, 1999c, 2006c; Lydon-Rochelle et al., 2001b; Wing & Lyons, 2006).

Because the 100 microgram tablet is unscored, there is no assurance that the PGE_1 is uniformly dispersed throughout the tablet. It is possible that one-quarter of a tablet may contain more or less than 25 micrograms of PGE_1. The hospital pharmacist should prepare the tablet in four equal parts before administration of a quarter of a tablet intravaginally (Simpson, 2002). Individual providers attempting to break the small tablet into four equal parts increases the risk of inaccurate dose administration.

Advocates of misoprostol for cervical ripening and induction of labor cite the low cost, ease of insertion, and quick action as its main advantages (Sanchez-Ramos, 2005; Wing & Lyons, 2006). The most commonly reported adverse effects are hyperstimulation, meconium passage, neonatal cord pH below 7.16, low 5-minute Apgar scores, admission to the NICU, nonreassuring FHR patterns, and a higher rate of cesarean birth related to nonreassuring FHR patterns from hyperstimulation (ACOG, 1999b, 1999c; Bennett, Butt, Crane, Hutchens, & Young, 1998; Buser, Mora, & Arias, 1997; Farah et al., 1997; Hofmeyr & Gulmezoglu, 2003; Sanchez-Ramos & Kaunitz, 2000; Wing & Lyons, 2006). These adverse effects can be minimized by using the lowest dose (25 micrograms) no more than every 3–6 hours (ACOG, 1999b, 1999c; Wing & Lyons, 2006). If uterine hyperstimulation and a nonreassuring FHR pattern occur with misoprostol and there is no response to routine corrective measures (maternal repositioning and supplemental oxygen administration), consider cesarean birth (ACOG, 1999b). Terbutaline, 0.25 mg subcutaneously, also can be used in an attempt to correct the nonreassuring FHR pattern or the uterine hyperstimulation (ACOG, 1999b).

If induction or augmentation of labor is required after cervical ripening with misoprostol, some providers opt to use oxytocin. Plasma concentration of misoprostol after vaginal administration of misoprostol rises gradually, reaching peak levels between 1 and 2 hours and declining slowly to an average of 61% of peak level at 4 hours (Arias, 2000; Goldberg, Greenberg, & Darney, 2001; Song, 2000; Zeiman, Fong, Benowitz, Banskter, & Darney, 1997). Some women will have increased plasma concentrations 4 to 6 hours after vaginal administration (Zeiman et al., 1997). Based on these pharmacologic data, administration of oxytocin should be delayed for at least 4 hours after the last dose of misoprostol (ACOG, 2000c).

Misoprostol can be administered by perinatal nurses; however, in many institutions, this practice is deferred to physicians or CNMs. If misoprostol administration is delegated to perinatal nurses, they must have demonstrated competence in insertion and the activity must be within the scope of practice as defined by state and provincial regulations.

There is insufficient evidence regarding oral misoprostol to support this route of administration (ACOG, 199b). Due to a relatively high rate of uterine hyperstimulation and lack of data concerning dosing regimens, oral misoprostol is not recommended for cervical ripening and labor induction (ACOG, 1999a; Alfirevic & Weeks, 2006).

Induction and Augmentation of Labor

Mechanical Methods of Induction of Labor

Stripping the Membranes

Digital separation of the chorioamnionic membrane from the wall of the cervix and lower uterine segment during a vaginal examination, commonly referred to as *stripping* or *sweeping* the membranes, is sometimes used to induce labor. This procedure is performed by inserting a finger into the internal cervical os and rotating through 360°. Although the exact mechanism of action is not fully understood, the procedure is thought to release prostaglandins produced locally from the amnion and chorion and the adjacent decidua (Hadi, 2000; Sellers et al., 1980). The amount of prostaglandins released correlates to the area of the membranes stripped (Mitchell et al., 1977) and may also cause release of maternal oxytocin from the posterior pituitary gland (Norwitz, Robinson & Repke, 2002). The best results are seen if the vertex is well

applied to the cervix in a term pregnancy. The procedure appears to be most beneficial for women who are pregnant for the first time and who have an unripe cervix at term (Boulvain, Stan, & Irion, 2005).

There has been little research comparing stripping the membranes with awaiting spontaneous labor; thus, the efficacy of the technique remains unknown. Available data are inconsistent, and most studies suffer from small sample size. Studies of nearly identical design in terms of randomization, weeks of gestation when the procedure was performed, and outcome measures produced different results (Kashanian, Akbarian, Baradaran, & Samiee, 2006; Tan, Jacob, & Omar, 2006). On the basis of current evidence, a decrease in the interval from membrane stripping to onset of labor is probably limited to pregnant women of at least 41 weeks of gestation or greater with no increase in adverse maternal–fetal outcomes. There is evidence that membrane sweeping is more efficacious than other types of mechanical dilation such as balloon catheters (Ifnan & Jameel, 2006). More data are needed, including studies with larger sample sizes, to further evaluate efficacy and potential for maternal–fetal complications related to membrane stripping (Boulvain et al., 2005).

Risks of membrane stripping include the potential for intraamniotic infection, unplanned rupture of membranes, disruption of an undiagnosed placenta previa, and precipitous labor and birth (ACOG, 1999b; Hadi, 2000; Sanchez-Ramos, 2005). The unpredictable nature of membrane stripping and lack of supportive data have prompted some experts to suggest this procedure should not be used routinely as a method of induction (Norwitz et al., 2002). However, there is no consensus in the literature or in clinical practice about routine membrane stripping. A recent review of the evidence to date suggests that membrane stripping was associated with shorter duration of pregnancy and less likelihood that pregnancy would continue beyond 41 or 42 weeks (Boulvain et al., 2005). It should be noted that most women find the procedure uncomfortable (Wong, Hui, Choi, & Ho, 2002). Potential benefits include relative ease of the procedure during routine vaginal examination at term and the fact that it incurs no additional cost if performed during a scheduled prenatal visit. Probably the greatest potential benefit of membrane stripping is the possible avoidance of other methods of induction if the procedure is successful (Boulvain et al., 2005).

Generally, membrane stripping is a procedure reserved for qualified physicians and perinatal nurses in advanced practice roles, such as CNMs, nurse practitioners, and clinical nurse specialists. Patient preparation should include a discussion of the expected results of the procedure as well as the possible complications. The patient should be aware that the procedure will likely be uncomfortable. She needs to know that she should call her physician or CNM or come to the hospital if the membranes rupture, bleeding occurs, fetal activity decreases, fever develops, regular contractions begin, or discomfort persists between uterine contractions.

AMNIOTOMY

Amniotomy is more frequently used for augmentation in women in active labor, but can also be successful as a method of induction when the woman has a favorable cervix and the cervix is adequately dilated (Pates & Satin, 2005; Sheiner et al., 2000). Amniotomy is particularly successful in multiparous women with cervical dilation greater than 2 cm. For some women, amniotomy may preclude the need for oxytocin. In contrast, early amniotomy before active labor is established increases risk of nonreassuring FHR patterns and cesarean birth (Segel, Sheiner, Yohai, Shoham-Vardi, & Katz, 1999). Early amniotomy is contraindicated when maternal infection, such as HIV, an active perineal herpes simplex viral infection, and possibly viral hepatitis, is present (Norwitz et al., 2002). There have been several reports over the past three decades about the efficacy and safety of amniotomy for labor induction. Most of the research has included oxytocin and other methods of induction in addition to amniotomy. Few data compare amniotomy alone with no intervention (Bricker & Luckas, 2000). More data are needed about the efficacy of amniotomy alone as a method of induction.

The potential benefit of amniotomy is the possible avoidance of oxytocin if rupture of membranes results in uterine contractions adequate to effect normal labor progress (Bricker & Luckas, 2000). Risks include the possibility of umbilical cord prolapse, intraamniotic infection, fetal injury, bleeding from an undiagnosed vasa previa and commitment to labor with an uncertain outcome (Hadi, 2000). Amniotomy results in more variable FHR decelerations and an increased risk of cesarean birth for nonreassuring fetal status (Garite et al., 1993; Fraser, Turcot et al., 2000; Goffinet et al., 1997). Obstetric interventions such as amniotomy, fetal scalp electrode placement, and intrauterine pressure catheter insertion are responsible for nearly half of the cases of umbilical cord prolapse (Usta et al., 1999). Unless there is an urgent reason for labor induction, the most reasonable approach is to await sufficient cervical dilation before rupturing membranes because of the potential risks of umbilical cord prolapse and the lack of a solid body of evidence to support efficacy and maternal–fetal outcomes (Fraser, Turcot et al, 2000).

Performance of amniotomy is reserved for qualified physicians and CNMs. Application of an internal fetal electrode in the presence of intact amniotic membranes is amniotomy. Amniotomy should not be performed by staff nurses for the convenience of other healthcare providers. Some institutions allow nurses to rupture membranes in rare cases in which the benefits of more data about fetal well-being clearly outweigh the risks associated with the nurse's inability to perform an emergency cesarean birth if prolapse of the umbilical cord should occur. If perinatal nurses are allowed to perform amniotomy, the individual nurse should demonstrate competence in the procedure and an institutional policy, procedure, or protocol should be in place that meets the criteria of the scope of nursing practice defined by the state board of nursing (AWHONN, 2004).

Medical record documentation should include the indication for amniotomy; amount, color, and odor of amniotic fluid; characteristics of the FHR before amniotomy; fetal response following the procedure; cervical status; and fetal station. If the amniotomy was difficult or uncomfortable for the woman, additional support and reassurance are appropriate.

Pharmacologic Methods of Induction of Labor

Oxytocin

Oxytocin is the most commonly used induction agent in the United States and worldwide (Smith & Merrill, 2006). Oxytocin is a peptide consisting of nine amino acids. Endogenous oxytocin is synthesized by the hypothalamus, then transported to the posterior lobe of the pituitary gland, where it is released into maternal circulation. It is released in response to breast stimulation, sensory stimulation of the lower genital tract, and cervical stretching. Oxytocin released in response to vaginal and cervical stretching results in uterine contractions. Synthetic oxytocin is chemically and physiologically identical to endogenous oxytocin.

Oxytocin circulates in the blood as a free peptide and has a molecular weight of 1007 d (Zeeman et al., 1997). Volume of distribution is estimated to be 305 ± 46 mL/kg; thus, oxytocin is distributed into both the intravascular and extravascular compartments (Zeeman et al., 1997). Plasma clearance of oxytocin is through the maternal kidneys and liver by the enzyme oxytocinase, with only a small amount excreted unchanged in the urine. Maternal metabolic clearance rate of oxytocin at term is 19–21 mL/kg/min and is unaffected by pregnancy (Zeeman et al., 1997).

During the first stage of spontaneous labor, maternal circulating concentrations of endogenous oxytocin are approximately that which would be achieved with a continuous infusion of exogenous oxytocin at 2–4 mU/min (Dawood et al., 1979). The fetus is thought to secrete oxytocin during labor at a level similar to an infusion of oxytocin at approximately 3 mU/min (Dawood et al., 1978). Thus, the combined effects of maternal–fetal contributions to maternal plasma oxytocin concentration is equivalent to a range of about 5–7 mU/min (Shyken & Petrie, 1995a).

Although there are considerable variations in reports of the biologic half-life of oxytocin, it is now generally agreed that the half-life is between 10 and 12 minutes (Dawood, 1995a; Arias, 2000). Early data based on in vitro studies estimated a plasma half-life of 3–4 minutes, but Seitchik, Amico, Robinson, and Castillo (1984) used in vivo methods to study oxytocin pharmacokinetics and found half-life was probably closer to 10–15 minutes.

Oxytocin concentration and saturation follow first-order kinetics with a progressive, linear, stepwise increase with each increase in the infusion rate (Arias, 2000; Brindley & Sokol, 1988). Three to four half-lives of oxytocin are generally needed to reach a steady-state plasma concentration (Stringer, 1996). Uterine response to oxytocin usually occurs within 3–5 minutes of IV administration. There is an incremental phase of uterine activity when oxytocin is initiated during which contractions progressively increase in frequency and strength, followed by a stable phase, during which time any further increase in oxytocin will not lead to further normal changes in uterine contractions (Dawood, 1995b; Phaneuf, Rodriguez, Tamby-Raja, MacKenzie, & Lopez-Bernal, 2000). Instead, abnormal uterine activity such as frequent low intensity contractions, coupling or tripling of contractions, or uterine hyperstimulation may be produced with further increases in oxytocin rates. There has long been a myth that these types of abnormal uterine activity patterns are best treated with oxytocin rate increases (ie, "pit through the pattern"); however, an understanding of their genesis (excessive oxytocin and oxytocin receptor site desensitization) should guide clinicians to reduce the rate or discontinue oxytocin until uterine activity returns to normal. Often a 30- to 60-minute rest period along with an IV fluid bolus of lactated Ringer's solution will allow oxytocin receptors to be sensitive to artificial oxytocin and produce uterine contractions that will result in normal uterine activity and labor progress (Dawood, 1995b; Phaneuf et al., 2000; Zeeman et al., 1997).

Continued increases in oxytocin rates over a prolonged period can result in oxytocin receptor desensitization or down-regulation, making oxytocin less effective in producing normal uterine contractions and having the opposite than intended result. Several studies have shown a direct inverse relationship between the duration and dosage of oxytocin and the number of oxytocin receptor sites available for oxytocin uptake during labor (Phaneuf et al., 1998, Phaneuf et al., 2000, Robinson, Schumann, Zhang, & Young, 2003). Prolonged oxytocin infusion at higher than appropriate doses can result in oxytocin side effects such as dysfunctional uterine activity patterns and uterine hyperstimulation (Dawood, 1995b; Phaneuf et al., 2000). Once active labor is established, oxytocin rates should be discontinued to avoid receptor down-regulation, especially in cases of long labor induction (Smith & Merrill, 2006). Prolonged high-dose oxytocin infusions are counter-productive to the augmentation of established labor (Robinson et al., 2003).

Hyperstimulation is the most concerning side-effect of oxytocin. Normal uterine contractions produce intermittent diminution of blood flow to the intervillous space where oxygen exchange occurs. The decreased intervillous blood flow associated with hyperstimulation ultimately leads to decreased oxygen transfer to the fetus (Sanchez-Ramos, 2005). When fetal oxygenation is sufficiently impaired to produce fetal metabolic acidosis from anaerobic glycolysis, direct myocardial depression occurs and the FHR pattern becomes nonreassuring (ACOG & AAP, 2003). When the intermittent interruption in blood flow caused by excessive uterine activity exceeds a critical level, the fetus responds with evolving hypoxia, acidosis, and ultimately asphyxia if the situation is prolonged (ACOG & AAP, 2003). Therefore, every effort should be made to avoid hyperstimulation and treat it appropriately when identified. Waiting until the FHR is nonreassuring to treat hyperstimulation is not consistent with fetal safety. See Display 7–10 for a suggested protocol for treatment of hyperstimulation.

Oxytocin following preinduction cervical ripening prostaglandin agents appears to be more efficacious than oxytocin alone as a method of induction (Kelly & Tan, 2001). When the Bishop score is less than 6, the likelihood of success of induction of labor is significantly increased compared to women with an unfavorable cervix (Vrouenraets et al., 2005). Therefore, cervical ripening for women with a Bishop score less than 6 is recommended if possible (Tenore, 2003).

DOSAGE AND RATE INCREASE INTERVALS

Based on physiologic and pharmacokinetic principles, Seitchik et al. (1984) recommended at least a 40-minute interval between oxytocin dosage increases because the full effect of oxytocin on the uterine response to increases in dosage cannot be evaluated until steady-state concentration has been achieved. Seitchik et al. (1984) used a sensitive oxytocin radioimmonoassay to show that approximately 40 minutes was required to reach steady state plasma concentration. Their data suggested that increasing the infusion rate before steady-state concentrations were achieved resulted in laboring women receiving higher doses of oxytocin than necessary. The works of Seitchik and Castillo (1982; 1983) and Seitchik et al. (1984) were the basis of oxytocin protocols with intervals in oxytocin dosage increases between 30 and 60 minutes.

Suggested Clinical Protocol for Oxytocin-Induced Uterine Hyperstimulation

OXYTOCIN-INDUCED HYPERSTIMULATION (REASSURING FHR)

- Maternal repositioning
- IV fluid bolus of lactated Ringer's solution
- If uterine activity has not returned to normal after 10 minutes, decrease oxytocin rate by at least half; if uterine activity has not returned to normal after 10 more minutes, discontinue oxytocin until uterine activity is fewer than five contractions in 10 minutes.
- Resumption of oxytocin after resolution of hyperstimulation: If oxytocin has been discontinued for less than 20–30 minutes; the FHR is reassuring; and the contraction frequency, intensity, and duration are normal, resume oxytocin at no more than half the rate that caused the hyperstimulation and gradually increase the rate as appropriate based on unit protocol and maternal–fetal status. If the oxytocin is discontinued for more than 30–40 minutes, resume oxytocin at the initial dose ordered.

OXYTOCIN-INDUCED HYPERSTIMULATION (NONREASSURING FHR)

- Discontinue oxytocin
- Maternal repositioning
- IV fluid bolus of lactated Ringer's solution
- Consider oxygen at 10 L/min via nonrebreather facemask
- If no response, consider 0.25 mg terbutaline SQ
- Resumption of oxytocin after resolution of hyperstimulation: If oxytocin has been discontinued for less than 20–30 minutes; the FHR is reassuring; and contraction frequency, intensity, and duration are normal, resume oxytocin at no more than half the rate that caused the hyperstimulation and gradually increase the rate as appropriate based on unit protocol and maternal–fetal status. If the oxytocin is discontinued for more than 30–40 minutes, resume oxytocin at the initial dose ordered.

Considerable controversy exists about dosage and rate increase intervals when oxytocin is used for induction of labor. There is no consensus in the literature on the ideal oxytocin dosage regimen, although available data support a lower dosage rate of infusion (Arias, 2000; Brindley & Sokol, 1988; Crane & Young, 1998; Sanchez-Ramos, 2005; Shyken & Petrie, 1995a; SOGC, 2001). The most commonly used regime in the United States includes starting at 0.5–2 mU/min with incremental doses of 1–2 mU/min every 40 minutes (Sanchez-Ramos, 2005). Those researchers whose opinions are based on the work of Seitchik et al. (1984) advocate a *physiologic* approach to oxytocin dosage and rate increase intervals. Others support a *pharmacologic* approach based in part on the results from early studies about more aggressive high-dose oxytocin protocols, sometimes referred to as active management of labor (O'Driscoll, Foley, & MacDonald, 1984; O'Driscoll, Jackson, & Gallagher, 1969). It is important to note that high-dose oxytocin is only one component of the active management protocol, which was originally used for augmentation (not induction) among nulliparous women (not multiparous women) in spontaneous active labor (Pates & Satin, 2005).

There have been numerous studies comparing low-dose and high-dose oxytocin dosage protocols as well as 10- to 15-minute versus 30- to 60-minute interval protocols for induction of labor, with varying results (Blakemore, Qin, Petrie, & Paine, 1990; Chua, Arulkumaran, Kurup, Tay, & Ratnam, 1991; Crane & Young, 1998; Goni, Sawhney, & Gopalan, 1995; Hourvitz et al., 1996; Lazor, Philpson, Ingardia, Kobetitsch, & Curry, 1993; Mercer, Pilgrim, & Sibai, 1991; Merrill & Zlatnik, 1999; Muller, Stubbs, & Laurent, 1992; Orhue, 1993a, 1993b; Orhue, 1994; Satin, Leveno, Sherman, Brewster, & Cunningham, 1992; Satin, Leveno, Sherman, & McIntire, 1994; Wein, 1989). Most researchers noted that higher doses and shorter dose increase intervals led to more uterine hyperstimulation and nonreassuring FHR patterns and did not result in a clinically significant decrease in length of labor (Crane & Young, 1998; Sanchez-Ramos, 2005).

Several reviews of available data about oxytocin pharmacokinetics and dosage administration protocols have been reported (Arias, 2000; Brindley & Sokol, 1988; Crane & Young, 1998; Sanchez-Ramos, 2005; Shyken & Petrie, 1995a). These reviews concluded that the evidence to date supported a low-dose (ie, physiologic) approach to oxytocin administration for labor induction. A physiologic approach to oxytocin administration has the benefits of a lower total dose of oxytocin and a lower incidence of hyperstimulation, which can result from increasing the dose before steady-state has been reached (Sanchez-Ramos, 2005). "The current data overwhelmingly indicate that oxytocin should be started at a low dose (0.5–1 mU/min) with a slow arithmetical increase every 30 to 60 minutes" (Brindley & Sokol, 1988, p. 730). According to Brindley and Sokol (1988), the risks of nonreassuring FHR patterns and uterine hyperstimulation were not outweighed by the slight— if any—decrease in the duration of the interval from induction to birth. Shyken and Petrie (1995a) advocated using the lowest possible doses of oxytocin to affect a clinical response. "Current evidence supports using oxytocin in the physiologic range. Adequate uterine activity will occur in a reasonable amount of time, but without the troublesome uterine hypercontractility"

(Shyken & Petrie, 1995a, p. 236). These authors felt the low dose and longer intervals between dosage increases ensured sufficient time to reach physiologic steady-state and avoid uterine hyperstimulation and risks of nonreassuring fetal status (Shyken & Petrie, 1995a, 1995b). A meta-analysis of low-dose versus high-dose oxytocin for labor induction by Crane and Young (1998 p. 1215) found "low-dose protocols resulted in fewer episodes of excessive uterine activity, fewer operative vaginal births, a higher rate of spontaneous vaginal birth and a trend toward a lower rate of cesarean birth." Based on these results, Crane and Young (1998, p. 1215) concluded, "Induction of labor with the minimum dose of oxytocin to achieve active labor and increasing intervals no more than every 30 minutes is appropriate." According to Arias (2000, p. 458), "It is unnecessary and potentially harmful to adopt intervals of less than 30 minutes to increase the amount of oxytocin during induction and augmentation of labor." Shorter intervals are more likely to be associated with hyperstimulation and nonreassuring fetal status (Arias, 2000).

A cervical dilation rate of 0.5–1 cm/hr in the active phase of labor indicates that labor is progressing sufficiently and that oxytocin administration is adequate, especially in nulliparous women (Simon & Grobman, 2005; Vahratian et al., 2005; Zhang et al., 2002). Traditional definitions of prolonged latent phase do not apply to induced labor, in which a latent phase exceeding 18 hours is common (Simon & Grobman, 2005; Vahratian et al., 2005). High-dose oxytocin and shorter intervals between rate increases tend to have fewer adverse effects on maternal–fetal status during labor augmentation than during labor induction (Crane & Young, 1998). This result may be due in part to the fact that in spontaneous active labor, the unripe cervix is not a significant factor, and oxytocin receptor sites are thought to be increased in number and sensitivity (Carbillon, Seince, & Uzan, 2001; Dawood, 1995a).

Other factors that may influence the dose response to oxytocin include maternal body surface area, parity, week of pregnancy duration, and cervical status (Dawood, 1995a). Although these factors may be significant, to date there are no practical predictive models for determining the required oxytocin dosage for successful labor induction. Until more is known about the pharmacokinetics of oxytocin, each pregnant woman receiving oxytocin will continue to represent an individual bioassay.

Generally, starting doses of 0.5–2 mU/min with increases in 1–2-mU/min increments every 30–60 minutes are most appropriate and commonly used (ACOG, 1999b; SOGC, 2001) (see Appendix 7–D for a sample oxytocin policy). Shorter intervals between dosage increases are associated with a greater risk of hyperstimulation, somewhat shorter duration of labor, and no reduction in the cesarean birth rate (Arias,

2000; Crane & Young, 1998). Multiple clinical studies and current data based on physiologic and pharmacologic principles have shown that 90% of pregnant women at term will have labor successfully induced with 6 mU/min or less of oxytocin (Dawood, 1995a, 1995b; Seitchik et al., 1984). There appears to be no advantage to continuing oxytocin once active labor is established. Reducing or discontinuing oxytocin may result in an equal or shorter length of labor compared to labor of women for whom oxytocin is continued or incrementally increased after active labor is achieved (Daniel-Spiegel et al., 2005).

Although higher doses of oxytocin and short intervals between dosage increments have generally not been found to be beneficial (Crane & Young, 1998), some providers intuitively believe that this approach is better. According to ACOG (1999b), protocols that involve high-dose oxytocin are acceptable; however, ACOG cautions that high-dose oxytocin is associated with more uterine hyperstimulation. Conversely, SOGC (2001) recommends using the minimum dose to achieve active labor, increasing the dosage no more frequently than every 30 minutes, and reevaluating the clinical situation if the oxytocin dosage rate reaches 20 mU/min.

ADMINISTRATION

Oxytocin is administered intravenously and piggybacked into the mainline solution at the port most proximal to the venous site (see Table 7–4 for a summary of oxytocin administration). There are many variations in the dilution rate. Some protocols suggest adding 10 units of oxytocin to 1,000 mL of an isotonic electrolyte IV solution, resulting in an infusion dosage rate of 1 mU/min = 6 mL/hr. However, other commonly reported dilutions are 20 units of oxytocin to 1,000 mL IV fluid (1 mU/min = 3 mL/hr) and 30 units of oxytocin to 500 ml IV fluid or 60 units of oxytocin to 1,000 mL IV fluid (1 mU/min = 1 mL/hr). One advantage to the dilution rates of 30 units of oxytocin to 500 mL IV fluid or 60 units of oxytocin to 1,000 mL IV fluid is that they result in a 1:1 solution (1 mU/min = 1 mL/hr), therefore there are no calculations needed for the dosage increases, an important consideration for medication safety. The key issues are knowledge of how many milliunits per minute are administered and consistency in clinical practice within each institution. To enhance communication among members of the perinatal healthcare team and to avoid confusion, oxytocin administration rates should always be ordered by the physician or CNM as milliunits per minute and documented in the medical record as milliunits per minute.

Nursing responsibility during oxytocin infusion involves careful titration of the drug to the maternal–fetal response. The titration process includes decreasing the dosage rate or discontinuing the medication when contractions are too frequent, discontinuing the medication when fetal status is nonreassuring, and increasing the dosage rate when uterine activity and labor progress are inadequate (Arias, 2000; Clayworth, 2000; Norwitz et al., 2002). Often during oxytocin infusion, physicians and nurses are focused on the rate increase section of the protocol while ignoring the clinical criteria for dosage increases. For example, if cervical effacement is occurring or if the woman is progressing in labor at approximately 0.5–1 cm/hr, there is no need to increase the oxytocin rate, even if contractions appear to be mild and infrequent. Labor progress and maternal–fetal response to the medication should be the primary considerations.

When uterine hyperstimulation occurs or fetal status is such that oxytocin is discontinued, data are limited to guide the decision about the timing and dosage of subsequent IV oxytocin administration. Physiologic and pharmacologic principles may be used to determine the most appropriate dosage. If oxytocin has been discontinued for less than 20–30 minutes, the FHR is reassuring and contraction frequency, intensity, and duration are normal, a suggested protocol may include restarting oxytocin at least at a lower rate of infusion than before the hyperstimulation occurred. In this clinical situation, many practitioners restart the infusion at half the rate that caused the hyperstimulation and gradually increase the rate as appropriate based on unit protocol and maternal–fetal status. However, if the oxytocin is discontinued for more than 30–40 minutes, most of the exogenous oxytocin is metabolized and plasma levels are similar to that of a woman who has not received IV oxytocin. In this clinical situation, a suggested protocol may include restarting the oxytocin at or near the initial dose ordered. There are individual differences in myometrial sensitivity and the response to oxytocin during labor (Arias, 2000; Smith & Merrill, 2006; Ulstem, 1997). It may be necessary to use a lower dose and increase the interval between dosages when there is evidence of the patient's previous sensitivity to the drug. See Display 7–10 for a suggested protocol for managing oxytocin infusion during hyperstimulation with and without a nonreassuring FHR pattern.

Misoprostol

Misoprostol is also used for induction and augmentation of labor. See the section "Cervical Ripening" for a full discussion of misoprostol.

Augmentation of Labor

For some women, labor progresses more slowly than expected. The terms *dystocia* and *failure to progress* are sometimes used to characterize an abnormally long labor. However, this diagnosis is often made mistakenly before the woman has entered the active phase of labor

and, therefore, before an adequate trial of labor has been achieved (ACOG, 2003a; Simon & Grobman, 2005). Often, women have a cesarean birth because of "failure to progress in labor" when, according to ACOG (2003a) criteria for the diagnosis of lack of labor progress, active labor has not begun or labor has not been abnormally long (Gifford et al., 2000; Lin & Rouse, 2006; Ness et al., 2005; Simon & Grobman, 2005, Zhang et al., 2002). *Cephalopelvic disproportion* is another common term used when labor has not progressed. This condition can rarely be diagnosed with certainty and is usually related to malposition of the fetal head. According to the latest data, dystocia remains the most common reason for primary cesarean birth in the United States, significantly higher than nonreassuring fetal status or malpresentation (Gifford et al., 2000; Martin et al., 2006). ACOG (2003a) recommends two practical classifications for labor abnormalities: slower than normal labor (protraction disorders) and complete cessation of contractions (arrest disorders). These disorders require that the woman be in the active phase of labor; thus, a prolonged latent phase is not indicative of dystocia, and this diagnosis cannot be made in the latent phase of labor (ACOG, 2003a).

Wide variations in labor progress and duration exist among childbearing women (see the section on duration of labor). There is no consensus among perinatal experts on appropriate length of labor and the relationship to risks of adverse maternal–fetal outcomes. Undoubtedly, some believe there is benefit to decreasing the length of labor, as evidenced by the popularity of active management of labor protocols and other high-dose oxytocin protocols in some institutions. It is unclear, however, who, if anyone, benefits most from a shorter labor: the fetus, the mother, the caregivers, the institution, or a combination of all of these (Keirse, 1993; Olah & Gee, 1996; Rothman, 1993). Multiple factors, including timing and dosage of regional analgesia, fetal size, and position and maternal pelvic structure influence, the progress of labor (ACOG, 2003a). Instead of arbitrary time frames, maternal–fetal status and individual clinical situations provide the best data on which to base labor management decisions.

From a physiologic and pharmacologic standpoint, less oxytocin is needed for labor augmentation than for labor induction, but most studies and clinical protocols report higher doses of oxytocin administration during augmentation of labor (Keirse, 1993). For women in spontaneous active labor, cervical resistance is less than in women who have not yet experienced cervical effacement and dilation. The response to oxytocin seems to depend on preexisting uterine activity and sensitivity rather than the amount given (Arias, 2000; Brindley & Sokol, 1988). It is unclear why the disparity between scientific evidence and clinical practice occurs. Many research studies about labor augmentation in the past decade have focused on variations in the active management of labor, which may account for the overrepresentation of studies of high doses of oxytocin in the literature.

Active Management of Labor

Principles of active management of labor (AMOL) were developed by O'Driscoll et al., in 1969. These researchers were faced with limited space in their maternity unit in Dublin, Ireland, and an increasing volume of women in labor. The protocol was initially implemented as a method of shortening labor with a goal of achieving more effective use of space and resources. They discovered that this method of augmentation not only shortened labor for most women, but also significantly decreased the cesarean birth rate at their institution (O'Driscoll, Jackson, & Gallagher, 1970). The protocol was designed to be used for *nulliparous women in spontaneous, active labor*. The Dublin active management of labor protocol is precise:

- Candidates include only nulliparous women in spontaneous, active labor with a singleton pregnancy, cephalic presentation, and no evidence of fetal compromise.
- To exclude false and prodromal labor, true labor is specifically defined as contractions with either bloody show, spontaneous rupture of membranes, or complete (100%) cervical effacement.
- Once labor is diagnosed, the woman receives continuous 1:1 labor support from a birth attendant (midwife or labor nurse)
- Amniotomy is performed if membranes have not ruptured spontaneously within 1 hour after labor has been diagnosed.
- If cervical dilation does not progress at least 1 cm/hr, oxytocin augmentation is initiated beginning at 6 mU/min increasing by 6 mU/min every 15 minutes until adequate labor is established, up to a maximum dose of 40 mU/min.
- Hyperstimulation of uterine activity is defined as more than seven contractions in 15 minutes.

This protocol has been rigorously evaluated in three major randomized controlled studies in the United States (Frigoletto et al.,1995; Lopez-Zeno, Peaceman, Adashek, & Socol, 1992; Rogers et al., 1997). Although all of the studies demonstrated a significant difference in length of labor, none found a significant difference in the cesarean birth rate. All of the studies used protocols very similar to the O'Driscoll et al. (1970) protocol.

The logistics of providing nursing care to two women requiring increases in oxytocin every 15 minutes and accomplishing adequate maternal–fetal assessments and documentation according to published guidelines and standards of care (ACOG, 1999b; AAP & ACOG, 2002; Simpson, 2002) warrant careful consideration before implementing this type of protocol in clinical practice. The studies that demonstrated this approach was safe for mothers and babies used a nurse-to-patient ratio of 1:1. The economic and practical implications of dedicating one nurse to each woman in labor while implementing a high-dose oxytocin protocol may outweigh any possible benefits of a slightly shorter labor. The principles of active management of labor as a method to decrease cesarean birth rates have not been shown to be successful when applied to labor and birth in the United States. A physiologic dosage regimen for labor induction or augmentation has been suggested as the best approach for most women because of the risks associated with higher doses and increasing the dose at more frequent intervals (such as uterine hyperstimulation and cesarean birth for nonreassuring fetal status) (Arias, 2000; Crane & Young, 1998; Sanchez-Ramos, 2005).

Some practitioners have selected various components of the original AMOL protocol for use in isolation (usually high-dose oxytocin) with varying results (Pates & Satin, 2005). The protocol was found to be safe (although not efficacious in decreasing risk of cesarean birth) when used *in total* for appropriate patients (nulliparous women in spontaneous active labor), with appropriate staffing (1:1 nursing care), with oxytocin initiated only after cervical changes at less than 1 cm/hr following amniotomy and observation, and with a definition of hyperstimulation of more than seven contractions in 15 minutes that did not include a nonreassuring FHR pattern before intervening (Pates & Satin, 2005). Misapplication of the AMOL protocol using aggressive oxytocin induction regimes as the sole component from the original research is inappropriate (Pates & Satin, 2005). Some have termed this practice the "active mismanagement of labor" (Olah & Gee, 1996), and it is not supported by the original AMOL research team (O'Driscoll, 1996).

Induction for Women Attempting Vaginal Birth After Cesarean Birth

Awaiting the onset of spontaneous labor, thus avoiding pharmacologic agents for cervical ripening or induction, appears to significantly decrease the risk of uterine rupture for women attempting VBAC (ACOG, 2006c). ACOG (2004c; 2006c) recommends that if induction of labor is necessary for a clear and compelling clinical indication, the potential increased risk of uterine rupture should be discussed with the patient and documented in the medical record. Among women who have had a previous cesarean birth, the use of prostaglandins and oxytocin increases the risk for rupture when compared with awaiting the onset of spontaneous labor or elective repeat cesarean birth (ACOG, 2006c). It has been theorized that prostaglandins induce local biochemical modifications that weaken the prior uterine scar, thus predisposing it to rupture (Murphy, 2006). Because of the risk of uterine rupture when misoprostol is used for cervical ripening or induction, ACOG (2004c, 2006c) does not recommend misoprostol for women attempting VBAC. The manufacturer of Cervidil (Forest Pharmaceuticals) lists history of a prior uterine scar as a contraindication to its use. ACOG (2006c) does not recommend the use of Cervidil or Prepidil or any prostaglandin agent for women attempting VBAC.

Although oxytocin administration increases the risk of uterine rupture for women attempting VBAC as compared to women who have a repeat cesarean birth or await spontaneous labor, the risk with oxytocin is significantly less than that associated with the use of prostaglandins (Lydon-Rochelle et al., 2001b). If there is a compelling reason for labor induction for women with a history or a uterine scar or prior cesarean birth, ACOG recommends using an appropriate dose of oxytocin and close monitoring of maternal and fetal status during labor and birth (ACOG, 2006c).

Clinical Implications of Labor Induction

Multiple methods of cervical ripening, labor induction, and labor augmentation are currently in use in the United States and Canada. Each method has pros and cons, as well as risks and benefits to the mother and fetus. Clearly, the state of the cervix is an important clinical indicator for likelihood of induction success. There is enough evidence to suggest that cervical ripening can increase the chances of success if the indication for induction allows time for cervical ripening. Oxytocin has been used for many years and has proven safe and effective for induction and augmentation. A physiologic dosage regimen for labor induction appears to be the best approach for most women, because the risks of higher doses and increasing the doses at more frequent intervals (such as uterine hyperstimulation and cesarean birth for nonreassuring fetal status) do not outweigh the benefits (if any) of a slightly shorter labor. Misoprostol is becoming more widely used for cervical ripening and labor induction. Uterine hyperstimulation and nonreassuring FHR patterns related to hyperstimulation are more common with misoprostol than with oxytocin. Lower doses of misoprostol and increased intervals between doses will decrease risk to the mother and fetus. Women who are attempting VBAC are at increased risk for uterine rupture with subsequent catastrophic results for both the mother and fetus if pharmacologic agents are used for cervical ripening or labor induction.

The increase in the elective induction rate over the past decade has profoundly changed the practice of perinatal nursing. Instead of predominately caring for patients who present in spontaneous active labor, many labor nurses spend a significant portion of their time titrating an oxytocin infusion and managing the side-effects of oxytocin. Nurses often are pressured by physician colleagues to increase the oxytocin rate to "keep labor on track" and speed the labor process when labor is otherwise proceeding normally at 1 cm/hr and/or there is evidence of excessive uterine activity (Simpson, James, & Knox, 2006). Although nurses report that they usually resist these types of requests for patient safety reasons, these ongoing clinical conflicts are a source of dissatisfaction for both nurses and physicians (Simpson et al., 2006). Oxytocin mismanagement has become a significant factor in perinatal liability (ACOG, 2004a; Simpson, 2004a). The increase in cesarean birth rate, in part the result of wide-spread elective labor induction of nulliparous women, is changing mother–baby units into surgical units where nearly one-third of patients are recovering from major surgery. These shifts in obstetrical practice have affected staffing requirements, length of stay, and costs of healthcare for childbearing women and their babies.

There are clinical practices based on the best available evidence that promote the safest care possible for mothers and babies during labor induction. These include, but are not limited to the following:

- No elective labor inductions before 39 completed weeks of gestation
- Cervical readiness before labor induction
- Standard oxytocin protocol including a standard concentration and standard dosing regime (start at 1 mU/min and increase by 1–2 mU/min at intervals no more frequent than every 30 minutes)
- Agreed upon definition of hyperstimulation (more than five contractions in 10 minutes, contractions lasting 2 minutes or more, or contractions of normal duration occurring within 1 minute of each other)
- Rare cases of uterine hyperstimulation and, when it occurs, appropriate and timely interventions (ie, treatment is not delayed until the FHR is nonreassuring)
- Minimum of 1:2 nursing care
- Common understanding among members of the perinatal team regarding how labor induction will be conducted and an agreement that all team members will participate

Much work lies ahead to provide education to pregnant women so they have enough information to make an informed decision about labor induction. Multiple factors contribute to the steady increase in the rate of induction of labor in the United States (Rayburn & Zhang, 2002). This is a complex issue that involves all participating parties: the pregnant woman, her family, her obstetrician or CNM or both, the institution, and the intrapartum nurse. More data are needed to fully evaluate the risks and benefits of induction and stimulation of labor. On the basis of what is known, a cautious process that allows for individualization to each clinical situation should be outlined by each institution to ensure the best outcomes for mothers and babies. A major step forward would be the adoption of policies and procedures based on the ACOG Practice Bulletin *Induction of Labor* (1999a) and the ACOG and ASA (2001 [reaffirmed in 2004]) Committee Opinion *Optimal Goals for Anesthesia Care in Obstetrics* in all institutions. Documentation of indications for induction and augmentation in the medical record with analysis of outcomes in each institution would provide valuable information about the implications of these practices. Use of a form to record these data, such as that presented in Appendix 7–C, works well. Only through a rigorous evaluation of common procedures such as induction and augmentation of labor can we be assured that we are providing the best care possible for mothers and babies. Evidence-based perinatal care is an achievable goal. Evidence in this area could provide direction for establishing protocols and clinical practice guidelines that support high-quality perinatal care.

Operative Vaginal Birth

The rate of operative vaginal birth has slowly decreased over the recent years from 9% of all births in 1989 (the first year these data were collected from certificates of live births) to 5.2% in 2004 (Martin et al., 2006). Vacuum-assisted births reached a peak at 6.2% in 1997, decreasing to 4.1% in 2004. Forceps-assisted births were at 5.6% in 1989, but were only 1.1% of all births in 2004 (Martin et al., 2006). Approximately 5.2 % of births in 2004 included forceps or vacuum devices (Martin et al., 2006). Nonoperative interventions such as one-to-one support, monitoring labor progress, and using oxytocin when labor is not progressing adequately decrease the need for operative vaginal birth (SOGC, 2004). Flexibility in the management of second stage including upright positioning, adequate anesthesia, and delaying pushing until the woman has the urge to push also are beneficial in reducing risk of operative vaginal birth (SOGC, 2004). The rate of operative vaginal birth is reduced when the arbitrary time limit of 2 hours for second stage is abandoned if progress is being made (Fraser, Marcoux et al., 2000; SOGC, 2004).

While no indications are absolute, according to ACOG (2000b) indications for operative vaginal birth when the fetal head is engaged and the cervix is fully dilated include prolonged second stage, suspicion of immediate or potential compromise, or shortening of the second stage for maternal benefit. ACOG (2000b) defines prolonged second stage for nulliparous women as lack of continuing progress for 3 hours with regional anesthesia or 2 hours without regional anesthesia and for multiparous women as lack of continuing progress for 2 hours with regional anesthesia or 1 hour without regional anesthesia.

Although sometimes necessary, operative vaginal birth is not without complications for the woman and baby. Perineal trauma is the main injury risk for women including vaginal and perineal lacerations, extension of the episiotomy, hematoma, and anal sphincter disruption (Aukee, Sundstrom, & Kairaluoma, 2006; Caughey et al., 2005; Dandolu et al., 2005; FitzGerald et al., 2007; Kudish et al., 2006). Among women with operative vaginal birth, there are significant risks for rehospitalization for postpartum hemorrhage, perineal wound infection complications, and pelvic injuries when compared to women who had spontaneous vaginal birth (Liu et al., 2005; Lydon-Rochelle, Holt, Martin, & Easterling, 2000). The most common reason for rehospitalization for women after operative vaginal birth is perineal wound infection (Lydon-Rochelle et al., 2000). Maternal injuries appear to be more common with forceps as compared to vacuums, whereas fetal injuries are more common with vacuums as compared to forceps (Johnson, Figueroa, Garry, Elimian, & Maulik, 2004; Mollberg, Hagberg, Bager, Lilja, & Ladfors, 2005). Babies delivered with forceps have more facial injuries, while babies born with vacuums have more cephalohematomas (Johnson et al., 2004). Increased risks to the fetus are associated with sequential application of devices (Castro, Hoey, & Towner, 2003; Towner, Castro, Eby-Wilkens, & Gilbert, 1999; Vacca, 2002). Generally when there is a failed trial of one instrument, use of another is not recommended unless there is a compelling and justifiable reason (ACOG, 2000b; Castro et al., 2003). Fetal complications are described in the section on forceps and vacuum devices.

Forceps

Forceps are used to assist delivery of the fetal head when birth must be facilitated for the health of the mother or fetus. Piper forceps are sometimes used during breech births to assist in delivery of the fetal head after the body has been delivered. According to the latest data, 1.1% of births in the United States involve the use of forceps (Martin et al., 2006). Maternal conditions that may necessitate use of forceps are medical complications such as cardiac or pulmonary disease, maternal exhaustion, or high level of regional analgesia that diminishes the woman's expulsive efforts. Factors associated with use of forceps are birthweight greater than 4,000 g, an OP position, epidural anesthesia, maternal age over 35 years, and a prolonged first- or second-stage labor (Mazouni et al., 2006). The fetus may demonstrate signs of compromise via EFM or FHR auscultation during second-stage labor, such as bradycardia, tachycardia, or late, variable or prolonged decelerations, suggesting attempts at assisted birth may be warranted.

Forceps should not be considered unless the cervix is completely dilated, membranes are ruptured, the head is engaged, and the woman has adequate anesthesia. The woman's bladder should be emptied prior to application (Norwitz, Robinson, & Repke, 2002). Classification of forceps procedures is listed in Table 7–5. All perinatal nurses should be familiar with this classification so that documentation of the procedure is accurate if they are entering these data in the medical record. Consultation with the provider who applied the forceps before medical record documentation is appropriate to ensure accuracy. The number of forceps applications and attempts with traction are usually documented. Ultimately, the responsibility for complete documentation of the operative birth procedure rests with the provider who performed the procedure.

Use of forceps are associated with pain, vaginal and cervical lacerations, extension of the episiotomy, anal sphincter injuries, perineal wound infection, uterine rupture, bladder trauma, fracture of the coccyx, hemorrhage, increased vaginal bleeding, uterine atony, and anemia (Benavides, Wu, Hundley, Ivester, & Visco, 2005; Caughey et al., 2005; Christianson, Bovbjerg, McDavitt, & Hullfish, 2003; FitzGerald et al., 2007; Hudelist et al., 2005; Johnson et al., 2004). Newborns delivered by forceps are at risk for skin markings, lacerations, bruising, nerve injuries, skull fractures, cephalohematoma, ocular trauma, and intracranial hemorrhage (Doumouchtsis & Arulkumaran, 2006; Dupuis et al., 2005; Towner et al., 1999; Uhing, 2005) and should be observed closely in the immediate newborn period. The incidence of subarachnoid hermorrhage after forceps is estimated to be 3.3 per 10,000 forceps-assisted births and subdural hemorrhage 9.8 per 10,000 forceps-assisted birth (Towner et al., 1999). The condition of the mother and newborn at birth should be documented in the medical record.

Vacuum Extraction

Some physicians use vacuum extraction in lieu of forceps, usually dependent on their education, experience, and privileges. According to the most recently available data, 4.1% of births in the United States involve the use of a vacuum device (Martin et al., 2006). A vacuum extractor consists of a soft or rigid cup available in various sizes that has a suction device attached. The cup is placed on the fetal head, and suction is increased gradually until a seal is formed. Gentle traction is then applied to deliver the fetal head. Indications and prerequisites for vacuum extraction or for the use of forceps are generally the same; however, most experts agree that rotation is not appropriate via vacuum extraction (Bofill, Martin, & Morrison, 1998). Proponents of vacuum extraction feel that its advantages include easier application, less force applied to the fetal head, less anesthesia needed, less maternal soft tissue injury, fewer fetal injuries, and fewer parental concerns (ACOG, 2000b; Caughey et al., 2005).

Complications from both vacuum extraction and forceps use are dependant primarily on skill of the practitioner. Approximately 14% to 16% of fetuses delivered with vacuum extractors will develop a cephalohematoma (ACOG, 2000b); however, when the duration of vacuum application at maximum pressure exceeds 5 minutes, this incidence increases to 28% (Bofill et al., 1997a). The incidence of subarachnoid hermorrhage after vacuum is estimated to be 2.2 per 10,000 vacuum-assisted births; subdural hemorrhage 8.0 per 10,000 vacuum-assisted births; and subgaleal hemorrhage 59 per 10,000 vacuum-assisted births (Doumouchtsis & Arulkumaran, 2006; Towner et al., 1999). The incidence of scalp abrasions and lacerations with vacuum use is approximately 10% (Doumouchtsis & Arulkumaran, 2006). Other common newborn outcomes with

TABLE 7–5 ■ CRITERIA OF FORCEPS DELIVERIES ACCORDING TO STATION AND ROTATION

Types of Procedure	Criteria
Outlet forceps	1. Scalp is visible at the introitus without separating the labia. 2. Fetal skull has reached the pelvic floor. 3. Sagittal suture is in the anteroposterior diameter or right or left occiput anterior or posterior position. 4. Fetal head is at or on the perineum. 5. Rotation does not exceed 45 degrees.
Low forceps	Leading point of the fetal skull is at station ≥ +2 cm and not on the pelvic floor. a. Rotation ≤ 45 degrees (left or right occiput anterior to occiput anterior, or left or right occiput posterior to occiput posterior) b. Rotation > 45 degrees
Midforceps	Station above +2 cm but head engaged
High	Not included in classification

From American College of Obstetricians and Gynecologists. (2000c). *Operative vaginal delivery.* (Practice Bulletin No. 17). Washington, DC: Author. Reprinted by permission. Copyright 2000 by American College of Obstetricians and Gynecologists.

vacuum-assisted birth include a chignon, discoloration and bruising of the scalp, blisters and superficial scalp abrasions, and retinal hemorrhage (Vacca, 2002; Uhing, 2005). More serious complications for the baby include extensive or deep scalp lacerations, subgaleal (subaponeurotic) hemorrhage, intracranial hemorrhage, and skull fracture (Vacca, 2002; Uhing, 2005).

There have been reports of neonatal subgaleal hematoma and intracranial hemorrhage after the vacuum extractor has been used. The FDA issued a warning letter to providers in 1998 alerting them to these risks (FDA, 1998). Subgaleal hematoma occurs when emissary veins are damaged and blood accumulates in the potential space between the galea aponeurotica (epicranial aponeurosis) and the periosteum of the skull (pericraniaum). Because the subaponeurotic space has neither containing membranes nor boundaries, the subgaleal hematoma may extend from the orbital ridges to the nape of the neck. This condition is dangerous because of the large potential space for blood accumulation and the possibility of life-threatening hemmorhage (FDA, 1998). Signs and symptoms of subgaleal hematoma include diffuse swelling of the fetal head and evidence of hypovolemic shock (eg, pallor, hypotension, tachycardia, and increased respiration rate). These signs and symptoms may be present immediately after birth or may not become clinically apparent until several hours or up to a few days after birth (FDA, 1998). The swelling is usually diffuse, shifts when the newborn's head is repositioned, and indents easily on palpation. In some cases, the swelling is difficult to distinguish from edema of the scalp. On occasion, the hypotension and pallor are the dominant signs while the cranial signs are unremarkable (FDA, 1998). Intracranial hemorrhage includes subdural, subarachnoid, intraventricular, and/or intraparenchymal hemorrhage. Signs and symptoms of intracranial hemorrhage include indications of cerebral irritation such as seizures, lethargy, obtundation, apnea, bulging fontanelle, poor feeding, increased irritability, bradycardia, and/or shock. These signs and symptoms are sometimes delayed until several hours after birth (FDA, 1998). Mortality with subgaleal hemorrhage approaches 25% (Doumouchtsis & Arulkumaran, 2006). A decrease in hematocrit that is greater than 25% of the baseline value at birth in association with significant birth asphyxia are the most important risk factors for newborn mortality (Doumouchtsis & Arulkumaran, 2006).

Maternal complications associated with the use of vacuum devices include pain, vaginal, and cervical lacerations; extension of the episiotomy; anal sphincter injuries; perineal wound infection; bladder trauma; hemorrhage; increased vaginal bleeding; uterine atony; and anemia (ACOG, 2000b; Aukee at al., 2006; Caughey et al., 2005 Dandolu et al., 2005; Johnson et al., 2004). Careful assessment following vacuum-assisted birth is necessary to identify maternal complications and initiate appropriate treatment.

There is a lack of consensus about the number of pulls required to effect birth, the maximum number of cup detachments (pop-offs) that can be tolerated, and the total duration of the procedure (ACOG, 2000b). The concept of the "three pull rule" has become widely accepted as a safety measure for limiting the amount of traction on the fetal head (Vacca, 2002), but what constitutes a safe number of pulls has never been empirically established. However, there is evidence to suggest that using no more than 600 mm Hg pressure, and abandoning the procedure after three pop-offs and/or 15 to 20 minutes maximum total time of application, is consistent with safe care and a decreased risk of fetal injuries (Bofill et al. 1996; Bofill, 1998; O'Grady, Gimovsky, & McIllHargie, 1995; Mollberg et al., 2005; Vacca, 2002).

Cup detachment (pop-off) should not be regarded as a normal event or safety feature of using a vacuum (Vacca, 2002). The rapid decompression resulting from a sudden loss of vacuum when the cup detaches completely has been associated with injury to the scalp and its blood vessels (Vacca, 2002). Pop-offs are a warning sign that too much ineffective force is being exerted on the fetal head (Castro et al., 2003; Vacca, 2002). Safety is promoted when maximum time of application of the vacuum is 15 minutes and vacuum extraction beyond 20 minutes should be rare (Vacca, 2002, 2006). The recommendations of the manufacturer of the vacuum extractor device being used should be followed. The vacuum pressure should not exceed 500–600 mm Hg, the traction force should not exceed 11.5 kg, and the pressure should be released as soon as the contraction ends and the woman stops pushing (Brumfield, Gilstrap, O'Grady, Ross & Schifrin, 1999; Vacca, 2006). As a general guideline, progress in descent should accompany each traction attempt and no more than three pulls should be attempted (Bofill et al., 1996; Bofill et al., 1998; Brumfield et al., 1999; Vacca, 2006). Traction is used only when the woman is actively pushing.

The vacuum procedure should be timed from the moment of insertion of the cup into the vagina until birth and should not be on the fetal head for longer than 20–30 minutes (Bofill et al., 1998; Brumfield et al., 1999). When the cup has been applied at maximum pressure for more than 10 minutes, the rate of fetal injuries increase (Brumfield et al., 1999); thus, while total time of cup application can be 20 minutes, the time of maximum pressure force should not exceed 10 minutes (Puluska, 1997). As with forceps, there should be a willingness to abandon attempts at a vacuum-assisted birth if satisfactory progress is not made (ACOG, 2000b; SOGC, 2004). If the 20-minute time limit is reached, the vacuum cup is removed and the procedure is considered a failed vacuum procedure (Bofill et al, 1998; Vacca, 2002). Three pop-offs, evidence of fetal scalp trauma, and/or no descent with appropriate application and traction should warrant abandoning the vacuum procedure (Bofill et al., 1998). A unit policy about the use of vacuum devices and forceps, including a list of those credentialed in these procedures, facilitates safe maternal–fetal care and avoids clinical controversies at the bedside if there is disagreement between healthcare professionals regarding amount of pressure, length of application, number of pop-offs and pull attempts, and the need to abandon the procedure. Documentation of fetal station, the duration of application, pressure, number of pulls, and number of pop-offs should be included in the medical record.

Nurses have a role in educating and reassuring the woman when an assisted vaginal birth is anticipated. Maternal comfort level should be assessed prior to the application of forceps or vacuum extractor. If a nonreassuring FHR pattern is the indication for the immediate birth, then the nurse must be prepared for newborn resuscitation ensuring that appropriate equipment, supplies, and personnel are available. Nurses should also be aware of potential complications related to use of forceps and vacuums and observe both the mother and baby for associated signs and symptoms. Some complications may be life threatening for the mother and baby, so prompt identification and initiation of appropriate treatment is necessary. Parents should be prepared and shown any forceps or vacuum extraction marks on their baby and reassured that they should disappear in a few days.

Complete and accurate medical record documentation of any adverse effects of operative vaginal birth is required. Responsibility for documentation of station, position prior to application of the vacuum or forceps, and the complete procedure rests with the provider who conducts the operative birth. Nurses may enter duplicate data in the medical record after consultation with the provider; however, this is not necessary or required.

Amnioinfusion

Amnioinfusion is sometimes used to attempt to resolve variable FHR decelerations during the first stage of labor by alleviating umbilical cord compression as a result of oligohydramnios. Amnioinfusion has been found to significantly resolve patterns of variable decelerations but does not affect late decelerations or patterns with minimal to absent variability (Mino, Puerta, Miranda, & Herruzo, 1999; Miyazaki & Naravez, 1985). Prophylactic amnioinfusion for oligohydramnios is not necessary and does not seem to prevent the development of variable decelerations (Hofmeyr, 2003). Because of its efficacy in resolving

variable decelerations, risk of cesarean birth related to a nonreassuring FHR pattern may be decreased with amnioinfusion (Hofmeyr, 2004). Amnioinfusion appears to be safe for women who are attempting a vaginal birth after a previous cesarean birth (Hicks, 2005; Ouzounian, Miller, & Paul, 1996). There is preliminary evidence that amnioinfusion may decrease risk of puerpal infection (Hofmeyer, 2004).

Although amnioinfusion has been shown to dilute thick meconium-stained amniotic fluid and decrease the incidence of meconium below the newborn's vocal cords, (Klingner & Kruse, 1999; Pierce, Gaudier, & Sanchez-Ramos, 2000), in a recent large international study of 1,998 women in term labor, amnioinfusion did not reduce risk of moderate or severe meconium aspiration syndrome or perinatal death (Fraser et al., 2005). Based on available evidence, amnioinfusion should be limited to the treatment of variable decelerations (ACOG, 2006a). Contraindications may include vaginal bleeding, uterine anomalies, and active infection such as HIV and herpes (Feinstein, Torgersen, & Atterbury, 2003).

The amnioinfusion procedure and the indication should be explained to the woman and her support persons prior to initiation. During amnioinfusion, room temperature–normal saline or lactated Ringer's solution is infused into the uterus transcervically via an intrauterine pressure catheter. The initial bolus is usually 250–500 mL given over a 20- to 30-minute period using either an infusion pump or gravity flow. Both methods are appropriate and seem to be equally efficacious (ACOG, 2006a). Some protocols allow for a continuous infusion of 2–3 mL/min (120–180 mL/hr) after the bolus until resolution of the variable decelerations (Feinstein et al., 2003; Tucker, 2004). Usually the maximum amount of fluid infused is 1,000 mL (Tucker, 2004). If variable decelerations have not resolved after infusion of 800–1,000 mL, the infusion may be discontinued and alternative approaches used (Tucker, 2004).

During bolus of the infusion and maintenance rate, approximate amount of fluid returning should be noted and recorded to avoid iatrogenic polyhydramnios. Iatrogenic polyhydramnios can lead to an overdistended uterus and pressure on the diaphragm potentially causing maternal discomfort, shortness of breath, hypotension, or tachycardia (Tucker, 2004). Assessment of fluid return can be accomplished by weighing the underpads (1 mL of fluid equals approximately 1 g of weight) (Tucker, 2004). As a general consideration, if 250 mL has infused with no return, the amnioinfusion is discontinued until the fluid has returned. Over-distension is more likely when the presenting part obstructs flow, thus releasing the fluid by gently elevating the presenting part may be a successful intervention (Feinstein et al., 2003). A dual-lumen intrauterine catheter is preferred so that estimate of uterine resting tone can be assessed during the infusion. Uterine resting tone may appear higher than normal during the procedure (from 25–40 mm Hg). If there is a concern about an elevated uterine resting tone (>40 mm Hg), temporarily discontinue the infusion to attempt a more accurate assessment. If the uterine resting tone exceeds 25 mm Hg while the infusion is temporarily discontinued for assessment of uterine resting tone, consider discontinuing the infusion. Contraction intensity and frequency should be continually assessed during the procedure.

Fetal bradycardia may occur if the solution is colder than room temperature and/or is infused too rapidly (Tucker, 2004). Some providers prefer to warm the solution to body temperature, especially if the fetus is preterm. If the solution is warmed, acceptable temperatures are 93° to 96° F (34° to 37° C) (Feinstein et al., 2003). The safest method to warm the solution is by use of an electronic blood/fluid warmer (Feinstein et al., 2003). Microwaves and other types of warming techniques should not be used to heat the solution.

VAGINAL BIRTH

Although cesarean birth is at an all-time high in the United States, for most (70%) women labor results in vaginal birth (Martin et al., 2006). Traditionally, in the medical intervention model of the hospital, vaginal birth occurred in a sterile "green-walled" surgical environment with drapes, stirrups, and high lights. Today, instead of transfer to the delivery room for birth, nearly all vaginal births in the United States occur in the more relaxed setting of the labor-delivery-recovery (LDR) room. Recently, most providers have abandoned the practice of complete draping and stirrups, instead using towels on the maternal abdomen as needed and foot rests. "Mini-preps" or shaving the perineal area have become a thing of the past in the United States, as there are no data that this procedure decreases risk of infection or promotes healing of perineal lacerations or episiotomies (Chen & Wang, 2006; Kitzinger et al., 2006; Klein et al., 2006). Enemas in early labor to prevent fecal contamination of the birth field or newborn have been virtually eliminated in the United States because of a lack of supportive evidence (Cuervo et al., Kitzinger et al., 2006; Klein et al., 2006; Rogers, 1993, Romney & Gordon, 1981). Routine episiotomy is no longer recommended as a result of the evidence of risks of perineal trauma and its associated sequelae, and its use has greatly decreased over the past decade (ACOG, 2006b, DeFrances & Podgornik, 2006).

Healthy women should be allowed and encouraged to give birth in an upright (rather than supine lithotomy) position with minimal intervention (Kitzinger et al., 2006; Klein et al., 2006). Perineal massage or stretching is not necessary, nor does it enhance or speed the birth process (Stamp et al, 2001). The woman should be allowed and encouraged to have family and support persons at her birth as per her desire in the context of space limitations and clinical conditions (AAP & ACOG, 2002). The birth process should be conducted as a celebration of a natural life event rather than a medical intervention as much as possible based on the clinical situation. At least one registered nurse should be in attendance at every birth to assist the birth attendant and assess maternal-fetal-newborn status. There should be another person attending the birth whose sole responsibility is neonatal resuscitation in case resuscitation is required (AAP & American Heart Association [AHA], 2006) (see the section on perioperative standards and guidelines for cesarean birth for a more complete discussion of requirements for neonatal resuscitation). A comprehensive discussion of the newborn's transition to extrauterine life is presented in Chapter 11.

CESAREAN BIRTH

Incidence

According to the latest data available from the National Center for Health Statistics, the rate of cesarean birth increased 4% between 2004 and 2005 in the United States (from 29.1% to 30.2%). The latest natality data can be accessed at http://www.cdc.gov/nchs/births.htm. This was the highest cesarean birth rate ever recorded in the United States (Hamilton, Martin, & Ventura, 2006). The rate declined somewhat in the early and mid-1990s, but has risen 46% since 1996 (Hamilton et al., 2006). During the mid-90s there was an upward trend in the number VBACs (50% increase from 1989 to 1996), but since 1996, the VBAC rate has fallen significantly (Martin et al., 2006; Menacker, 2005). Based on the most recent data, once a woman has a cesarean birth, there is more than a 90% chance that subsequent births also will be by cesarean (Martin et al., 2006). "Once a cesarean, always a cesarean" has again become the norm.

The most common indications for cesarean birth noted on birth certificates is maternal medical complications and complications of labor such as dystocia, breech/malpresentation, cephalopelvic disproportion, nonreassuring fetal status, and placenta previa (Martin et al., 2006). Cesarean birth for nonreassuring fetal status has increased 1.5- to 5-fold over the past 10 years (Hendrix & Chauhan, 2005). Cesarean birth is often performed for lack of progress in labor when the woman is still in the latent phase of labor or when the second stage of labor is not prolonged (Gifford et al., 2000; Lin & Rouse, 2006). The rising rate of artificial labor induction is one factor that has had a direct influence on the increase in cesarean births. There is a cumulative body of evidence that elective induction of labor for nulliparous women is associated with a risk of cesarean birth twice that of nulliparous women who have spontaneous labor (Moore & Rayburn, 2006; Simpson & Atterbury, 2003).

There are significant risks of maternal and newborn complications with cesarean birth (Kolas, Saugstad, Daltveit, Nilsen, & Olan, 2006; MacDorman, Declercq, Menacker, & Malloy, 2006; Sakala & Mayberry, 2006). Babies born via cesarean are at significantly increased risk for respiratory complications and admission to the NICU (Jain & Dudell, 2006; Kolas et al., 2006; Manacker et al., 2006; Signore, Hemachanda, & Klebanoff, 2006). Approximately 1.1% of babies born via cesarean suffer injuries such as skin laceration, abrasion, abnormal bruising, subconjunctival hemorrhage, cephalohematoma, clavicular fracture, facial nerve injury, brachial plexus injury, skull fracture, long bone fracture, and intracranial hemorrhage (Alexander et al. 2006). Duration of the skin incision-to-birth interval, type of incision, and indication for the surgery are influencing factors in fetal injury with cesarean birth (Alexander et al., 2006). Babies born less than 5 minutes after the incision time have a higher injury rate than babies born more than 5 minutes after the incision time (Alexander et al., 2006). Low vertical incisions are associated with the lowest risk of fetal injury while "T" or "J" incisions have a higher risk (Alexander et al. 2006). Cesarean birth after a failed forceps or vacuum attempt as an indication has the highest risk of fetal injury, followed by a nonreassuring FHR pattern, abnormal presentation, and labor dystocia (Alexander et al., 2006). Because presumed fetal compromise is often a reason for an expedited cesarean with a short interval from incision to birth, risk of injuries are increased with these fetuses.

A cesarean first birth is associated with a higher risk of placenta previa, placental abruption, uterine scar dehiscence, and uterine rupture in the second pregnancy (Getahun et al., 2006; Gilliam, 2006; Lydon-Rochelle, 2001a). There is a dose-response pattern in the risk of placenta previa, with increasing numbers of previous cesareans increasing the risk (Getahun et al., 2006). Women who have a cesarean birth have a significantly increased risk of rehospitalization for uterine infection, surgical wound infection, complications from surgical wound, and cardiopulmonary and thromboembolic complications (Liu et al., 2002; Lyndon-Rochelle et al., 2000). They are 30 times more likely to have a surgical wound infection than women who have a vaginal birth; however, the rate of rehospitalization for wound infection after cesarean birth is relatively low, at only about 4 per 1,000 births (Lydon-Rochelle et al, 2000).

Although the risk of blood transfusion also is overall low with cesarean birth, when compared to vaginal birth, women who have primary and repeat cesarean birth are 4 times and 7 times respectively more likely to require blood transfusion (Rouse et al., 2006). Risk of maternal mortality after cesarean birth from anesthesia complications, puerperal infection, and venous thromboembolism is 3.6 times higher for women who have cesarean birth prior to labor and after failed labor when compared to vaginal birth (Deneux-Tharaux et al., 2006). The average length of inpatient stay for cesarean birth is 3.7 days, as compared to 2.2 days for vaginal birth (Kozak, Lees, & DeFrances, 2006). Cesarean birth after labor in the first pregnancy is associated with increased cumulative healthcare costs compared with vaginal birth, regardless of the number or type of subsequent births (Allen et al., 2006a; Druzin & El-Sayed, 2006).

Cesarean Birth Without a Medical Indication

Cesarean birth on maternal request (CDMR) has received much attention recently, although there are limited data on actual numbers of these types of births. Approximately one-half of physicians who responded to a February 2006 survey of ACOG members indicated that they had performed at least one CDMR, and a similar number believed that women have the right to CDMR (Bettes et al., 2007). Nearly 60% indicated that they have experienced an increased in these types of requests, yet most of their practices did not have a policy on CDMR (Bettes et al., 2007). Female obstetricians who responded to the survey were more negative toward CDMR than male obstetricians and noted more risks and fewer benefits (Bettes et al., 2007).

Based on birth certificate data, the number of cesarean births without an indicated risk has increased over the past several years. However, these data do not include information regarding whether the mother requested a cesarean birth absent any risks or whether the decision was made by the provider (Menacker, Declercq, & Macdorman, 2006). Birth certificate data does not include CDMR information (Kirby & Hamsiu, 2006). There have been attempts to estimate CDMR through use of diagnostic codes from the International Classification of Diseases, Ninth Revision, Clinical Modification (ICD-9-CM). These processes are based on exclusion of codes for cesarean births for other reasons because there is not an ICD-9-CM code for CDMR. Even if there were an associated code, there may be resistance to universal use of a CDMR code by both physicians and patients because of concerns about reimbursement (Gossman, Joesch, & Tanfer, 2006). Based on these issues and with current limitations in natality data collection, the ability to accurately measure the rate of CDMR is not possible at this time and may not be possible for the foreseeable future. Although there is evidence that medical risk factors and complications of labor and delivery are significantly underreported on birth certificates, this limitation alone does not account for the rise in cesarean births without an indicated risk. It is plausible that some of the cesarean births without an indicated risk were as a result of maternal request (NIH, 2006; Menacker et al., 2006). Estimates of CDMR vary from 0.08% to 2.6% of all births (Declercq, Sakala, Corry, & Applebaum, 2006; HealthGrades, 2005; Gossman et al, 2006; NIH, 2006).

There is limited evidence upon which to develop national policy and clinical practice related to CDMR (Lavender, Hofmeyr, Neilson, Kingdon, & Gyte, 2006). A review of available evidence up to March 2006 is presented here based on the findings of the *State of the Science Conference on Cesarean Delivery on Maternal Request*, sponsored by the NIH (2006). Two maternal outcomes are significantly in favor of vaginal birth over cesarean birth. These include risk of postpartum hemorrhage and an increased maternal hospital length of stay. Other maternal outcomes with weaker evidence that favor vaginal birth are an increased risk of infections, anesthesia complications, subsequent placenta previa, and delayed or impaired breast-feeding. There are no maternal outcomes with strong evidence that favor cesarean birth over vaginal birth. Maternal outcomes with weak evidence to favor cesarean birth are a decreased risk of urinary incontinence and surgical and traumatic complications. For women who have cesarean birth with future pregnancies after a prior cesarean birth, there is weak evidence of less risk of uterine rupture and cesarean hysterectomy. These women may have decreased fertility after cesarean birth. Maternal outcomes with equivocal evidence include anorectal function, sexual function, pelvic organ prolapse, subsequent stillbirth, and mortality.

A neonatal outcome with strong evidence that favors vaginal birth over cesarean birth is decreased risk of respiratory morbidity. Other neonatal outcomes with weak evidence supporting vaginal birth include risk of iatrogenic prematurity and an increased length of stay. There are no neonatal outcomes with strong evidence that favor cesarean birth over vaginal birth. Neonatal outcomes with weak evidence that favor cesarean birth are fetal mortality, intracranial hemorrhage, neonatal asphyxia, encephalopathy, birth injury, laceration, and neonatal infection.

The following conclusions and recommendations resulted from the NIH (2006) *State of the Science Conference on Cesarean Delivery on Maternal Request*:

- The incidence of cesarean birth without medical or obstetric indication is increasing in the United States, and a component of this increase is CDMR. Given the tools available, the magnitude of this component is difficult to quantify.
- There is insufficient evidence to evaluate fully the benefits and risk of CDMR as compared to planned vaginal birth; more research is needed.
- Until quality evidence becomes available, any decision to perform a CDMR should be carefully individualized and consistent with ethical principles.
- Given that the risks of placenta previa and accreta rise with each cesarean birth, CDMR is not recommended for women desiring more children.
- CDMR should not be performed prior to 39 weeks of gestation or without verification of lung maturity, because of the significant danger of respiratory complications.
- CDMR should not be motivated by unavailability of effective pain management. Efforts must be made to ensure availability of pain management services for all women.
- NIH or appropriate federal-level agencies should establish and maintain a Web site to provide up-to-date information on the benefits and risks of all modes of birth.

Since the NIH (2006) *State of the Science Conference on Cesarean Delivery on Maternal Request*, several studies have been published confirming risks of cesarean birth to mothers and babies, including twice the risk of respiratory complications and NICU admissions (Dudell & Jain, 2006; Jain & Dudell, 2006; Kolas et al., 2006; MacDorman et al., 2006; Visco et al., 2006), an increased risk of endometritis and cystitis (Wax, 2006), and increased risk of placenta previa, placental abruption, uterine scar dehiscence, and uterine rupture in the second pregnancy (Getahun et al., 2006; Gilliam, 2006). While there have been incidental reports of gynecologic benefits of CDMR over vaginal birth, there is no consistent evidence from adequately powered, rigorously designed studies that risks of sexual dysfunction (Handa, 2006), anal incontinence (Fenner, 2006), urinary incontinence (Nygaard, 2006), and pelvic organ prolapse (Richter, 2006) can be diminished or prevented by CDMR. Adverse fetal/neonatal outcomes occur after both vaginal and cesarean birth. Based on estimates of the incidence and prevalence of neonatal encephalopathy, intrauterine fetal demise, shoulder dystocia, and trauma to the baby as a result of operative vaginal birth, even a universal policy of cesarean birth for all women at 39 weeks of gestation would theoretically only decrease, but not eliminate, these types of adverse outcomes (Hankins, Clark, & Munn, 2006). Women have a low tolerance for fetal risk associated with vaginal birth, and many would choose cesarean birth over labor and vaginal birth if they were presented information that vaginal birth in their clinical situation was risky for the fetus (Walker et al., 2007).

Although supportive evidence for CDMR is lacking, a number of women may request a cesarean birth absent medical or obstetric indications (Bettes et al., 2007). According to ACOG (2003b, 2004b), the physician should counsel the woman within the framework of the ethical principles of autonomy, beneficence, non-maleficence, veracity, and justice using the opportunity to explore the woman's concerns with the goal of reaching a mutually acceptable decision. These same principles apply to nurses caring for women who choose CDMR (Carlton, Callister, & Stoneman, 2005). Beneficence-based clinical judgment favors vaginal birth (Minkoff, Powderly, Chervenak, & McCullough, 2004). Offering or performing CDMR is not consistent with substantive justice–based considerations, and there is no autonomy-based obligation to offer cesarean birth in an ethically and legally appropriate informed consent process (Minkoff et al., 2004). Promotion of CDMR as a standard of care or mandated part of patient counseling is highly questionable in light of finite healthcare resources in the United States (Druzin & El-Sayed, 2006).

Physicians should respond to patient-initiated requests for cesarean birth with a thorough informed consent process (including potential risks and benefits to the mother and fetus in the current pregnancy and implications for risks in future pregnancies) and request that the woman reconsider to ensure her autonomy is meaningfully exercised (Hankins et al., 2006; Minkoff et al., 2004). Discussing options, attempting to dissuade women, but ultimately acquiescing to their judgment is not incompatible with obstetrical ethics (Minkoff, 2006). If an acceptable balance cannot be reached by the woman and her physician, she may choose to continue care with another provider (ACOG, 2004b). Limited available data suggest that interventions to dissuade women from CDMR have not been effective (Horey, Weaver, & Russell, 2004); however, lack of compelling supportive evidence for vaginal birth over cesarean birth has hampered these types of intervention processes. With the level of interest in this topic, it is likely that more rigorous research will be conducted and disseminated. As the body of knowledge on CDMR evolves, it is important to develop plans to promulgate this information to healthcare providers, women, and their families so they are able to make an informed decision in their best interests and the best interests of their baby (Sakala & Mayberry, 2006).

Perioperative Standards and Guidelines for Cesarean Birth

Perioperative perinatal nursing incorporates the skills of the specialties of obstetrics, surgery, and postanesthesia care to provide comprehensive care to women who have a cesarean birth. Patients with the same health status and condition should receive a comparable level of quality care regardless of where that care is provided (JCAHO, 2007a). This standard ensures that obstetrical patients receiving general and regional anesthesia and having surgery are provided consistent perioperative care. Therefore, perinatal units should maintain comparable care standards as the main hospital surgical suites/postanesthesia care unit (PACU) (ASA, 2003, 2006; JCAHO, 2007a). It is important to distinguish between the concepts of comparable care and equivalent care. Comparable care to that which is provided in the main hospital surgical department is recommended by ASA (2006) and JCAHO (2007a); however, equivalent care is not required. The special needs of obstetrical patients, their babies, and their families must be considered when planning care and designing protocols and clinical practices. For example, care during cesarean birth should include the patient's support person and family. In the main hospital surgical suite, family members are rarely allowed to be with patients during surgery. However, women having cesarean birth should be allowed to have a support person with them prior to and during the procedure and the recovery period. Some institutions allow more than one support person. Patient desires and patient safety should guide practice. During the recovery period, the newborn should be allowed to stay with the mother as long as the condition of the mother and baby are stable. Support should be provided so that breastfeeding can be initiated as soon as possible if the woman has chosen to breastfeed.

When unplanned cesarean birth occurs, and the decision is made to proceed, the surgical team should be notified so they can begin preparations. In some hospitals this will involve calling in a surgical team whose members are not in-house, while other hospitals maintain a full surgical team around the clock. A full surgical team includes a surgeon, anesthesia provider, surgical first assistant, scrub tech, circulating nurse, and person whose sole responsibility is for potential neonatal resuscitation. All hospitals offering labor and birth services should be equipped to perform an emergent cesarean birth (AAP & ACOG, 2002; ACOG & ASA, 2001). In general, the consensus has been that hospitals should have the capacity of beginning a cesarean birth within 30 minutes of the decision to do so (AAP & ACOG, 2002). Some indications for cesarean birth can be appropriately accommodated in greater than 30 minutes (AAP & ACOG, 2002); for example, "failure to progress in labor" or admission of a woman at term with spontaneous rupture of membranes who had a repeat cesarean birth scheduled in the next week, as long as there is evidence of reassuring fetal and maternal status. On the other hand, some clinical situations require more expeditious birth because they can directly or indirectly cause fetal death or other adverse maternal–fetal outcomes. These include hemorrhage from placenta previa, abruptio placenta, umbilical cord prolapse, and uterine rupture (AAP & ACOG, 2002; Silver, 2007). Sterile materials and supplies needed for emergent cesarean birth should be kept sealed but properly arranged and available so that the instrument table can be made ready at once for an obstetric emergency (AAP & ACOG, 2002). Whenever possible, a surgical suite should be kept available for emergent cases. If keeping at least one surgical suite continuously available to handle emergencies is not possible, at a minimum elective or nonemergent cases should be staggered to allow rapid readiness if an emergency occurs that requires expeditious cesarean birth.

Plans should be in place for calling in back-up team members such as surgeons and anesthesia providers when those who are primarily responsible for covering the service for obstetrical emergencies are occupied with other procedures that would preclude their ready availability. A list of those in-house and on-call who are responsible for responding to obstetric emergencies should be available at all times to the labor and delivery charge nurse. This list should include current telephone numbers of the quickest method to reach these professionals. Access to direct telephone numbers of those on-call is more likely to result in the fastest communication rather than beepers, which require additional time to send the signal and await response. Most professionals have cellular telephones that can be used while they are on-call. If the attending physician is notified of an obstetric emergency likely to require emergent cesarean birth while not in-house, including but not limited to, fetal bradycardia, umbilical cord prolapse, significant bleeding, suspected placental abruption, or uterine rupture, and he or she orders preparations for the surgery, hospital policy should allow preparations to begin prior to arrival of the attending physician. Hospital policies requiring that the physician be in-house to order preparations for emergent cesarean birth can delay the process and potentially contribute to an adverse maternal or fetal outcome.

In July 2004, JCAHO's Sentinel Event Alert *Preventing Infant Death and Injury During Delivery* recommended conducting periodic drills for emergent cesarean birth (JCAHO, 2004b). Because emergent cesarean birth is a common event in most labor and delivery units, there is the perception by some providers that emergent cesarean birth drills are redundant and unnecessary (Simpson, 2005a). Although there are few data supporting improved outcomes in units where emergent cesarean birth drills are routine, it would seem likely that when all members of the perinatal team have practiced what to do and know their roles and responsibilities, the location of key equipment and whom to call, the chances of the chaotic environment often associated with a "crash" cesarean birth would be minimized. In one study, researchers found that a structured process with clearly delineated roles of all team members and 24-hour availability of a surgical team resulted in improved outcomes after emergent cesarean birth (Roemer & Heger-Romermann, 1993). Another study's findings indicated that teamwork training involving all members of the interdisciplinary perinatal team was associated with a shorter decision to incision time (33.3 minutes vs. 21.2 minutes) for cesarean birth compared to perinatal teams that had not participated in teamwork training (Nielsen et al., 2007).

To prepare for a drill, develop a list of roles and responsibilities for each team member (Simpson, 2005a). For example, after an emergent cesarean birth is ordered, the charge nurse ensures that all members of the surgical team have been notified and are en route. The first person to arrive in the surgical suite is responsible for opening the instruments and preparing the field. The second person to arrive assembles the equipment necessary for neonatal resuscitation and makes sure the neonatal team is notified and on their way. The primary nurse caring for the patient when the emergency develops ensures that the patient is prepped and the Foley catheter is in place before the surgery begins. Some have found it helpful to use a scribe or videorecording of the drill so that the organization of events and interventions can be analyzed retrospectively and plans developed for improvement as appropriate. Using a volunteer staff member as a surrogate for the patient can make the drill seem more realistic.

During surgery, the minimum nurse-to-patient ratio is 1:1 (Association of periOperative Registered Nurses [AORN], 2007). This standard is met by the registered nurse acting in the role of the surgical circulating nurse. During cesarean birth, at least one additional person should be present to care for the baby and whose sole responsibility is management of the newborn in case the baby's condition necessitates resuscitation (AAP & AHA, 2006). Either this person or someone else who is immediately available should have the skills required to perform a complete resuscitation, including endotracheal intubation and administration of medications (AAP & AHA, 2006). It is not sufficient to have someone on-call (either at home or in a remote area of the hospital) for newborn resuscitation at birth (AAP & AHA, 2006). When resuscitation is needed, it must be initiated without delay (AAP & AHA, 2006). Although more than 90% of babies make the transition to extrauterine life smoothly with little to no assistance required, some babies need assistance to begin breathing at birth; about 1% of babies need extensive resuscitation to survive (AAP & AHA, 2006). If the birth is high risk and thus more complex resuscitation is anticipated, additional personnel should be in attendance (AAP & AHA, 2006). In this high-risk situation, at least two persons should be present solely to manage the baby (one with complete resuscitation skills and one or more to assist) (AAP & AHA, 2006). All the equipment necessary for complete resuscitation must be in the room where birth occurs and be fully operational (AAP & AHA, 2006). When birth of a high-risk newborn is expected, appropriate equipment should be ready to use (AAP & AHA, 2006).

Perioperative assessments for women having cesarean birth should be comparable to those used in the main hospital surgical suite and PACU for patients having similar surgery. Cardiac monitoring of women post-cesarean birth is not required by ASA (2000, 2002; Luppi, 2002); however, if similar types of patients in the main hospital PACU are receiving cardiac monitoring, obstetrical patients may also. Remote cardiac monitoring is one option that provides a competent individual to assess cardiac data on an ongoing basis without requiring obstetrical nurses to do so. Usually the period of cardiac monitoring post-cesarean birth is brief, so this option works well for some institutions. When obstetrical nurses are required to interpret findings from cardiac monitoring, adequate education and competence validation processes should be developed. Completion of an advanced cardiac life support course is not required for obstetrical nurses providing perioperative care as long as a team with these skills is available to respond to provide emergent care for an obstetrical patient if needed within a timely manner. The time frame for response is usually defined by what is expected for code team response time in other departments in the hospital. Display 7–11 lists suggested guidelines for perioperative care for cesarean birth.

A method should be in place to ensure that equipment is available for PACU care and maintained according to manufacturer specifications (American Society of Perianesthesia Nurses [ASPAN], 2006). Equipment must be available to administer oxygen; provide suction; maintain IV access; and monitor postoperative cardiac status, including BP, heart rhythm and rate, and SpO2 (ASPAN, 2006). Emergency equipment, an emergency communication system, and knowledgeable emergency assistive personnel should be readily available. Emergency equipment and supplies should include a defibrillator, medications, oxygen, a positive-pressure breathing device, suction equipment, and appropriate nasal and oral airways (ASPAN, 2006).

Every effort should be made to avoid hypothermia, beginning in the preoperative phase and continuing into the postoperative phase of perioperative care. Ensuring normal body temperature during the perioperative period has a significant influence on the patient's risk for surgical site infection, surgical bleeding, and patient discomfort (AORN, 2007). When the woman is anesthetized for cesarean birth, she loses heat intraoperatively and is unable to restore body heat through the normal mechanism of shivering or increased muscle activity (AORN, 2007). Several factors contribute to perioperative hypothermia. They include decreased metabolic heat production, increased environment heat loss, redistribution of heat within the body, induced inhibition of thermoregulation during the cesarean birth, age, physical status, body fat, and length of procedure (AORN, 2007). The nurse can prevent or decrease risk of hypothermia by applying warm blankets upon arrival in the surgical suite and after sterile drapes are removed, limiting the amount of skin surface exposed, limiting time between prepping of the skin and draping, preventing surgical drapes from becoming wet, adjusting the room temperature, warming irrigation or infusion solutions, and using warming devices (AORN, 2007).

Phase I postanesthesia recovery focuses on providing a transition from a totally anesthetized state to one requiring less acute interventions (ASPAN, 2006). The purpose of this phase is for patients to regain physiologic homeostasis and receive appropriate nursing interventions as needed (ASPAN, 2006). It is important to consider that phase I postanesthesia recovery is a level of care, rather than a location or time frame. During postoperative recovery, the nurse-to-patient ratio on the perinatal unit should be comparable to that of the main hospital PACU. Phase I recovery for general surgical patients usually occurs in the PACU; however, obstetrical patients may be cared for during phase I in an LDR or a labor/delivery/recovery/postpartum room (LDRP) if there is the availability of continuous one-to-one nursing care. When phase I recovery care occurs in an obstetric PACU, the nurse may be able to care for more than one patient after the newborn is transferred to the nursery. Most women recovering from cesarean birth after regional anesthesia meet ASPAN criteria for patients who are appropriate for 1:2 nursing care during phase I; however, when the recovery nurse also is responsible for the newborn, the 1:2 care limit is met. If the woman has had general anesthesia, once the airway is removed and the patient is conscious and breathing on her own, she meets criteria for phase I recovery criteria for patients who are appropriate for 1:2 nursing care. Like care for the women after regional anesthesia, when the recovery nurse caring for women after general anesthesia also is responsible for the newborn, the 1:2 care limit is met.

In settings where the postoperative patient returns to an LDR or an LDRP immediately after surgery, the perinatal nurse remains at the bedside until cardiac monitoring is discontinued (if applicable), the patient is stable, and the patient is discharged from postanesthesia care. Postoperative patients may be discharged from postanesthesia phase I care status when the following criteria are met: (a) vital signs are stabilized for at least three consecutive readings with intervals of 15 minutes;

DISPLAY 7-11

Perioperative Cesarean Birth Care

PREOPERATIVE CARE

- Admission assessment comparable to that for all women admitted for labor and birth.
- Obtain a 20- to 30-minute baseline fetal heart rate (FHR) tracing by electronic fetal monitoring (EFM). If the woman is not in active labor and the FHR is reassuring, EFM may be discontinued after this initial assessment.
- Provide a thorough explanation of what to expect in preparation for, during, and after the surgery to the woman and her support person.
- Ensure that the woman has maintained no oral intake (NPO) according to the institutional protocol.
- Initiate intravenous fluids.
- Witness informed consent signature for cesarean birth.
- Obtain surgical laboratory blood specimens if not done prior to admission.
- Prepare the abdomen.
- Insert a Foley catheter; note the amount and color of urine; delay until after epidural catheter is placed and dosed if possible.
- Administer preoperative medications according to the physician order.
- If woman is in labor, periodic assessments of maternal–fetal status should continue according to the institutional protocol.
- Transport the woman to the surgical suite or operating room.

INTRAOPERATIVE CARE

- Position the woman on the surgical table with a hip wedge in place.
- If EFM is used, continue monitoring until the abdominal prep is initiated.
- If a fetal scalp electrode is in place, EFM continues until the abdominal prep is completed. The electrode should be removed before birth.
- Prepare abdomen for surgery as per institutional protocol.
- Apply grounding device according to manufacturer's instructions.
- Note maternal vital signs, FHR, condition of the skin before the incision, and the woman's emotional status.
- Assist the support person to a position at the head of the surgical table according to the institutional protocol.
- Ensure that newborn resuscitation equipment is assembled and ready and personnel responsible are in attendance. Responsibility for resuscitation and stabilization of the healthy, full-term newborn differs by institution and could include an additional staff nurse, pediatrician, or neonatal nurse practitioner.
- Perform the duties of a circulating nurse according to the institutional protocol.
- Ensure that the sponge, needle, and equipment counts are correct according to the institutional protocol.
- Assist with application of abdominal dressing.
- Note maternal and newborn status before transport to the postanesthesia care unit (PACU).
- Assist with transport.

POSTANESTHESIA RECOVERY CARE

- Postoperative assessments are performed according to PACU protocols and should be comparable to care provided in the main hospital PACU.
- Initial and ongoing assessments include review of intraoperative course, including medications and intravenous fluids received:
    Respiratory assessment
        Airway patency
        Oxygen needs
        Rate, quality, and depth of respirations
        Auscultation of breath sounds
        Arterial oxygen saturation via pulse oximetry
    Circulation assessment
        Blood pressure
        Pulse
        Electrocardiogram (if applicable)
        Color
    Level of consciousness
        Orientation
        Response to verbal, tactile, and painful stimulation
    Obstetric status
        Uterine fundus position and contraction
        Abdominal dressing
        Maternal–newborn attachment
        Lochia amount and color
        Newborn condition
        Breastfeeding desires
    Intake and output
        Intravenous fluids
        Urinary output by Foley catheter
    Pain or comfort level
        Patient desires
        Medications given
- Discharge from PACU care occurs after the recovery period and when the woman is stable as determined by PACU discharge criteria. A scoring system including the following parameters is useful to assess readiness for discharge:
    Level of consciousness
    Neuromuscular activity
    Level of sensation
    Circulation
    Respiration
    Color
    (Fig. 7–10 provides a sample PACU discharge scoring tool; using this system, the patient's score must be at least 10 before discharge.)
- Additional assessment before PACU discharge:
    Vital signs
    Urinary output by Foley catheter
    Uterine fundus position and contraction
    Abdominal dressing
    Intravenous fluids or oral intake
    Pain or comfort level
    Lochia amount and color
    Maternal–newborn attachment
The anesthesia provider is involved in the decision to discharge from PACU care.
If responsibility for care is transferred to another nurse after discharge, a complete report of intraoperative and postanesthesia course is vital.

POST ANESTHESIA RECOVERY SCORE			
	CRITERIA	SCORE	DISCHARGE
CONSCIOUSNESS	Fully awake Arousable on calling Not responding	2 1 0	
NEUROMUSCULAR ACTIVITY	Move 4 extremities Move 2 extremities Move 0 extremities	2 1 0	
SENSATION	Normal None below pubis None below xiphoid	2 1 0	
CIRCULATION	B/P 10–20 mmHg ± admission B/P 10–50 mmHg ± admission B/P >51 mmHg ± admission	2 1 0	
RESPIRATION	Deep breathing or cough Dyspnea Apnea	2 1 0	
COLOR	Pink Pale, blotchy, jaundiced, other Cyanotic	2 1 0	
	Total		
Signature:	Date:	Time	

FIGURE 7–10. PACU discharge scoring tool.

(b) the airway is clear and the danger of vomiting and aspiration has passed; (c) patients recovering from general anesthesia must have regained consciousness and be oriented to time, place, person, or equivalent preoperative level of orientation; and (d) patients who have received spinal or epidural anesthesia must have progressive increase in movement of extremities.

A PACU discharge scoring tool as shown in Figure 7–10 is helpful in conducting a systematic assessment and determining readiness for discharge from postanesthesia care. See Display 7–12 for critical components of obstetric postanesthesia nursing. Whenever a patient is transferred from one level of care to another level of care requiring a change in caregivers, communicate all pertinent information to the next caregiver. Transfers or patient hand-offs present a risk of missing key information with the potential to adversely affect patient status, thus development of a checklist for important clinical content to be included in the hand-off report can be beneficial (Simpson, 2005b). Suggested components of a comprehensive transfer report are included in Display 7–13. These components may vary based on the type of care model in place. In some perinatal units, discharge from postanesthesia care will not result in the physical transfer of the patient; rather, care will continue in the same room. Transfer of care from one caregiver to another may or may not occur at this time. In other units, discharge from postanesthesia care will result in a physical transfer of the patient from the OB PACU to the mother–baby unit and care will be transferred to another nurse. Standards and guidelines for perioperative care are available from AORN www.aorn.org, ASPAN www.aspan.org, the ASA www.asahq.org, and JCAHO www.jcaho.org.

Perioperative Patient Safety

Patient safety goals from JCAHO (2007b) include strategies to decrease risk of potentially preventable surgical errors and perioperative harm. A recent closed-claims review of 444 surgical errors revealed that most (75%) errors occur during the intraoperative period, 25% during preoperative care, 35% during postoperative care, with approximately 33% occurring during multiple phases of care and approximately 66% involving more than one clinician (Rogers et al., 2006). Patients having cesarean birth are particularly susceptible to two types of adverse surgical events: anesthesia awareness and retained foreign bodies, such as instruments, sponges, or needles.

Risk of a retained instrument or sponge is significantly increased with emergency surgery, unplanned changes in procedure, not counting sponges or instruments, and higher body mass (Gawande, Studdart, Orav, Brennan, & Zinner, 2003). Cesarean birth is often emergent, at times proceeding without a complete count. A cesarean birth can develop into a significant postpartum hemorrhage and/or a cesarean

DISPLAY 7-12

Critical Components of Obstetric Postanesthesia Nursing

1. Women in the obstetric postanesthesia period after major regional or general anesthetic shall receive care comparable to that available in the surgical postanesthesia care unit (PACU).
2. The anesthesiologist or nurse anesthetist is responsible for determining whether the condition of the women warrants PACU or routine obstetric postpartum recovery care.
3. If the woman is admitted to obstetric PACU care, surgical PACU standards shall be followed until PACU discharge criteria are met and routine postpartum recovery care ensues.
4. Before patient arrival, the obstetric postanesthesia recovery area shall have required equipment in place. Otherwise, the woman should remain monitored by the anesthesiologist or nurse anesthetist until the recovery area is appropriately equipped to ensure patient safety.
5. A woman transported to the obstetric PACU shall be accompanied by a member of the anesthesia care team, who shall provide a verbal report to the responsible obstetric PACU nurse and remain in the obstetric PACU nurse accepts responsibility for the nursing care of the patient.
6. After the woman is admitted to obstetric PACU care, she shall be continually observed and monitored by methods appropriate to her medical condition. Particular attention should be given to monitoring oxygenation, ventilation, circulation, and temperature. Additional staff may be needed to interact with family members and the newborn infant. After PACU discharge criteria are met, postpartum care should continue per obstetric standards.
7. Each hospital is responsible for developing guidelines, policies, and procedures collaboratively among the obstetric department, anesthesia department, and surgical PACU (eg, assessment criteria, PACU discharge criteria, documentation, malignant hypothermia, crisis management, medications and equipment, staff education and qualifications, staffing requirements).
8. Each hospital shall ensure that advanced cardiac life support (ACLS) care (eg, code team) is readily available at all times. ACLS certification is not required for obstetric nurses providing postanesthesia care.

hysterectomy. In some institutions, a cesarean hysterectomy may involve the addition of other experts to the original surgical team to assist with the procedure. Pregnant patients have higher body mass than the general population. Obesity and a higher body mass index predispose obstetrical patients to an increased risk of

retained foreign bodies and anesthesia adverse events (Gawande et al., 2003; Ross, 2003). Every effort should be made to obtain a complete count of instruments, sponges, and needles prior to beginning cesarean birth (AORN, 2007). However, if a count is not possible due to emergent conditions, an x-ray following the surgery

DISPLAY 7-13

Suggested Components of Communication Between Care Providers During Transfer from Postanesthesia Care to Postpartum Care for Women After Cesarean Birth

- Vital signs
- Level of consciousness
- Muscular strength and ability to move lower extremities
- Allergies
- Condition of the operative site and dressing
- Fundal height
- Lochia characteristics and amount
- Condition of the perineum if vaginal birth was attempted
- Location and patency of any tubes and/or drains including indwelling urinary catheter
- Intake and output (eg, IV fluids, oral fluids, estimated blood loss, urinary output)

- Medications given and response to those medications
- Pain level, interventions for pain, and response to those interventions
- Nausea and vomiting
- Tests ordered with pertinent results, if available
- Initiation of breastfeeding and quality of first breastfeeding experience (eg, successful latch-on; mother's confidence), if applicable
- Status of the baby (eg, admitted to special care nursery or NICU and preliminary diagnosis)
- Psychosocial status
- Involvement of the significant other and family
- Plans for immediate care of the baby (eg, rooming-in if support person will be continuously available to assist the mother)
- If the baby is being relinquished for adoption, the mother's wishes for handling newborn care
- If the mother does not want any publicity or it to be known that she is a patient at the hospital or has given birth
- Discharge orders
- Attending physician
- Attending pediatrician

while the patient is still on the surgical table is a reasonable option to decrease the likelihood of a retained instrument, sponge, or needle (Gawande et al., 2003). This option has merit for selected high-risk cases even when the counts are believed to be correct, because in the overwhelming majority of cases of retained instruments, sponges, or needles, the final count is recorded as correct (Gawande et al., 2003). A unit policy should be in place to guide practice for surgical situations involving a high risk of retained foreign bodies.

Anesthesia awareness occurs under general anesthesia when a patient becomes cognizant of some or all of the events during surgery and has direct recall of those events (JCAHO, 2004a). Because of the routine use of neuromuscular blocking agents (also known as paralytics) during general anesthesia, the patient is often unable to communicate with the surgical team when this occurs (JCAHO, 2004a). Women having cesarean birth are at risk for anesthesia awareness because anesthesia providers usually give the mother light anesthesia to avoid causing depression in the newborn (Spitellie, Holmes, & Domino, 2002). The most common patient perceptions of awareness are sounds and conversations, sensation of paralysis, anxiety and panic, helplessness and powerlessness, and pain. Least common are visual perceptions, feeling the intubation or tube and feeling the operation without pain, although some patients do feel significant pain (Spitellie et al., 2002). The exact incidence of anesthesia awareness with recall in the United States is unknown but is estimated to be approximately 0.24% or 26,000 cases per year based on 20 million general anesthetics per year (Sebel et al., 2004). Many patients who experience anesthesia awareness are adversely affected long after the surgery (JCAHO, 2004a; Spitellie et al., 2002). The psychological sequelae of anesthesia awareness includes sleep disturbances, nightmares, anxiety and panic attacks, flashbacks, avoidance of medical care, and post-traumatic stress disorder (PTSD) (Spitellie et al., 2002). Most patients who develop PTSD recover in a few months to a few years; however, it is estimated that 10% to 25% of patient who experience PTSD as a result of anesthesia awareness suffer from chronic PTSD. Implementing the JCAHO (2004a) recommendations for preventing and managing anesthesia awareness may decrease risk to the woman having cesarean birth.

The term *wrong-site surgery* often is used to refer to any surgical procedure performed on the wrong patient, wrong body part, wrong side of the body, or at the wrong level of the correctly identified anatomic site (ACOG, 2006d). The following definitions are useful to describe potential surgical errors (ACOG, 2006d). *Wrong-side surgery* indicates a surgical procedure performed on the wrong extremity or side of the patient's body (eg, the left ovary rather than the right ovary). *Wrong-patient surgery* describes a surgical procedure performed on a different person than the one intended to receive the operation (eg, circumcision of a baby whose parents did not intend or consent to circumcise or a tubal ligation performed during cesarean birth of a woman who did not consent to tubal ligation). *Wrong-level surgery* and *wrong-part surgery* are used to indicate surgical procedures that are performed at the correct operative site, but at the wrong level or part of the operative field or patient's anatomy.

The following are factors that may contribute to an increased risk of surgical errors (JCAHO, 2006; Rogers et al.): emergent cases, multiple surgeons involved in the case, multiple procedures during a single surgical visit, changes in members of the surgical team during the procedure, unusual time pressures to start or complete the procedure, and unusual physical characteristics, including morbid obesity or physical deformity. Some of these factors apply to obstetrical patients having cesarean birth. A common theme in cases of surgical errors involves failed communication between the surgeon or surgeons, nurses, other members of the healthcare team, and the patient (ACOG, 2006d; Rogers et al., 2006). Communication is crucial throughout the surgical process, particularly during the preoperative assessment of the patient and the procedures used to verify the planned procedure. Effective preoperative patient assessment includes a review of the medical record or imaging studies immediately before starting surgery. To facilitate this step, all relevant information sources, verified by a predetermined checklist, should be available in the operating room and rechecked by the entire surgical team before the operation begins (ACOG, 2006d). A formal procedure for final confirmation of the correct patient and surgical procedure (a "time out") that requires the participation of all members of the surgical team is helpful (JCAHO, 2003, 2007a, 2007b). It is inappropriate to place total reliance on the surgeon or to assume that the surgeon should never be questioned (ACOG, 2006d). The risk of error may be reduced by involving the entire surgical team in the verification process and encouraging any member of that team to point out a possible error without fear of ridicule or reprimand (ACOG, 2006d).

Beepers, radios, telephone calls, and other potential distractions in the surgical environment should be kept to a minimum, if allowed at all, especially during critical stages of the operation such as the birth and surgical counts (ACOG, 2006d). Nonessential conversation should be postponed until surgery is finished (ACOG, 2006d). Appropriate nurse staffing during cesarean birth is essential for patient safety. A circulating nurse and another person whose sole responsibility is the baby in case neonatal resuscitation is necessary are minimally required in addition to the other members of the surgical team (AORN, 2007; AAP & AHA, 2006).

Because of the potential for serious harm from surgical errors, vigorous efforts are required to eliminate or reduce their frequency (ACOG, 2006d). Preventing these types of errors requires a team effort by all individuals participating in the surgical process. Although all members of the surgical team share in this responsibility, ACOG (2006d) recommends that the primary surgeon should oversee these efforts. The circulating nurse partners with the surgeon in ensuring that the process is as safe as it can be for mothers and babies during cesarean birth (Simpson, 2004c). This may present a challenge to the circulating nurse if all members of the surgical team do not value or actively participate in perioperative safety procedures (Simpson, 2004c). Often there is pressure to proceed with the case prior to completing all of the components of perioperative safety protocol, including reviewing the preoperative checklist, patient history, reason for surgery and time-out. While these pressures may occur in the face of an emergency, often they are the result of the desire by some members of the surgical team to complete the case as soon as possible for their convenience. Support from the perinatal leadership team is essential to promote universal active participation by all members of the surgical team with appropriate actionable follow-up for those who do not comply. Rarely is there an emergency during which the time-out process and all surgical counts cannot be safely implemented. In nearly all cases, there is time to conduct the surgical counting process, make sure it is the right patient, the right procedure, and the right site, and that documented consent has been procured (Simpson, 2004c).

In 2003, JCAHO published the *Universal Protocol for Preventing Wrong Site, Wrong Procedure, and Wrong Person Surgery*. The universal protocol is based on three levels of activity before initiation of any surgical procedure:

1. *Preoperative verification process*
   The healthcare team ensures that all relevant documents and studies are available before the procedure starts and that the documents have been reviewed and are consistent with each other, with the patient's expectations, and with the team's understanding of the intended patient, procedure, site, and, as applicable, any implants. The team must address missing information or discrepancies before starting the procedure.
2. *Marking of the operative site*
   The healthcare team, including the patient (if possible), identifies unambiguously the intended site of incision or insertion by marking all operative sites involving laterality, multiple structures, or multiple levels. The site for cesarean birth is not included as part of this process.

3. *"Time out" before starting the procedure*
   The operative team conducts a final verification of the correct patient, procedure, site, and, as applicable, implants. A relatively new but essential element of this overall process is the formal enlistment of active involvement by the patient to avert errors in the operative arena. Involving the patient in this manner requires personal effort by the surgeon to educate the patient during the preoperative evaluation process. The patient, who has the greatest stake in avoiding errors, thus becomes integrally involved in helping ensure that errors are avoided.

Supporting Mother–Baby Attachment After Cesarean Birth

Whether anticipated or unexpected, the need for surgical birth increases the families' anxiety, places additional strain on the maternal–newborn relationship, makes postpartum recovery more difficult for the woman and family, and creates a need for accepting the altered birth experience. Women who give birth via cesarean have special needs for information, presence of the partner throughout cesarean birth, and sustained contact with their newborn (Fig. 7–11). An unplanned emergent cesarean birth can result in significant stress for the new mother (Ryding, Wijma, & Wijma, 1997). Continuity in caregivers, choice where possible, and control over specific aspects of care can reduce stress (Hundley et al., 1997). In order to facilitate a positive birth experience and attachment to the newborn, consideration should be given to ongoing attention of the family's understanding of cesarean birth, ways to maintain the father or support person's presence throughout the birth experience, and early and sustained contact with the newborn (Fig. 7–12).

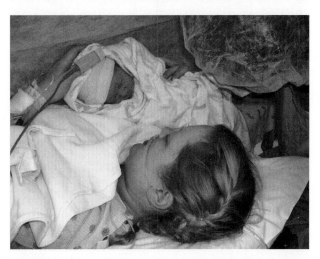

FIGURE 7–11. Promoting mother–baby attachment during cesarean birth.

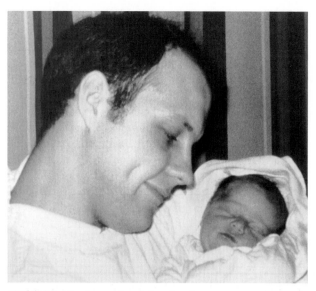

FIGURE 7–12. Promoting father involvement.

Encouraging sibling interaction promotes attachment and integration of the baby into the family (Fig. 7–13).

If the mother who has had a cesarean birth requests rooming-in with her newborn in the immediate postoperative period, it is important that a support person be available to assist her with newborn care. Women in the immediate postoperative period are likely receiving

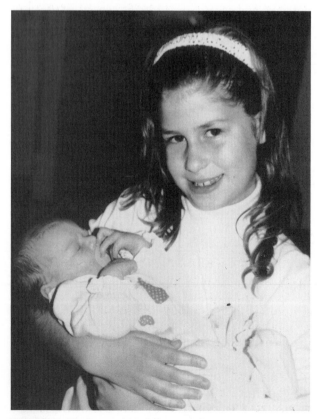

FIGURE 7–13. Promoting sibling attachment.

parental or regional pain medications and may inadvertently fall asleep while holding their baby, thus increasing risk of injuries to the baby. Women recovering from cesarean birth have limited mobility and may be unsteady on their feet the first few times getting out of bed after surgery. They are at risk of falling when ambulating unassisted to care for their baby in the early recovery period. A policy requiring rooming-in for post-cesarean birth mothers is not appropriate for safety reasons; unit policies and practice should be based on individual patient condition and availability of a support person for assistance.

Vaginal Birth After Cesarean

The VBAC rate has fallen 67% since 1996, after increasing during the mid-1990s (Martin et al, 2006). The steep decline in the VBAC rate corresponds with an increasing repeat cesarean birth rate now and in the future. Based on current data, once a woman has a cesarean birth, there is more than a 90% chance that subsequent births also will be by cesarean (Martin et al., 2006). This significant decrease in VBAC may be related to reports of associate risks, physician or maternal preference, more conservative practice guidelines such as the requirement for immediate availability of a surgical team during a trial of labor of women attempting VBAC, legal pressures, as well as the continuing debate regarding the potential risks and benefits of vaginal birth compared to cesarean birth (Martin et al., 2006). A VBAC is associated with a small but significant risk of uterine rupture with poor maternal–fetal outcomes (ACOG, 2004c). A thorough discussion between the primary care provider and the woman and her family that includes individual risks and benefits of VBAC is recommended by ACOG (2004c) before a decision about a trial of labor is made. Selection criteria for identifying women who are candidates for VBAC include (ACOG, 2004c) all of the following:

- One previous low-transverse cesarean birth
- Clinically adequate pelvis
- No other uterine scars or previous rupture
- Physician immediately available throughout active labor capable of monitoring labor and performing an emergent cesarean birth
- Availability of anesthesia and surgical team for emergent cesarean birth

Contraindications for a trial of labor include women at high risk for uterine rupture. Circumstances under which a trial of labor should not be attempted are as follows (ACOG, 2004c):

- Prior classical or T-shaped incision or extensive transfundal uterine surgery
- Contracted pelvis

- Medical or obstetric complication that preclude vaginal birth
- Inability to perform an emergent cesarean birth because of unavailable surgeon, unavailable anesthesia provider, or insufficient personnel or facility
- Two prior uterine scars and no vaginal births

Predictors of success for VBAC include a favorable cervix, no need for induction, no use of cervical ripening or induction agents, previous vaginal birth including a previous VBAC, body mass index <30, no history of labor dystocia with previous cesarean birth, and same or smaller birth weight than a baby born by previous cesarean birth (Bujold, Hammoud, Schild, Krapp, & Baumann, 2005; Cahill et al., 2006; Durnwald & Mercer, 2004; Landon et al., 2005; Macones, Cahill et al., 2005; Peaceman et al., 2006). Outcomes of a trial of labor for women with preterm pregnancy are comparable to women who attempt VBAC at term (Durnwald et al., 2006).

Benefits of VBAC are the shorter recovery period and inpatient stay following a vaginal birth. Overall morbidity, mortality, and rehospitalization are lower with vaginal births compared with surgical births (Lydon-Rochelle et al., 2000). Women who have an unsuccessful trial of labor are at greater risk of postpartum fever and infection, other morbidity, and rehospitalization (ACOG, 2004c; Clark et al., 2000; Durnwald & Mercer, 2004; Lydon-Rochelle et al., 2000). Major maternal complications such as hemorrhage, uterine rupture, hysterectomy, and operative injury are more likely for women who have a trial of labor as compared to women who have a repeat cesarean birth (ACOG, 2004c; Clark et al., 2000). Neonatal morbidity also is increased with an unsuccessful trial of labor, as evidenced by the increased incidence of arterial umbilical cord blood pH levels below 7, 5-minute Apgar scores below 7, and infection (ACOG, 2004c; Durnwald & Mercer, 2004).

Uterine Rupture

Risk of uterine rupture during a trial of labor for women attempting VBAC is generally acknowledged to be approximately 1% (ACOG, 2004c; Hibbard et al., 2001; Landon et al., 2004; Shipp, 2004), although absolute risk varies based on type of previous uterine scar, number of prior cesarean births, whether the mother had a prior vaginal birth, whether labor was spontaneous or induced, the cervical ripening/induction agent, a history of postpartum fever after a previous cesarean birth, a previous preterm cesarean birth, a single-layer uterine closure, interval between pregnancies of less than 24 months, and maternal age over 30 years (ACOG, 2004c; Buold, Bujold, Hamilton, Harel, & Gauthier, 2002; Buold, Mehta, Bujold, & Gauthier

2002; Bujold et al., 2004; Hendler & Bujold, 2004; Hoffman, Sciscione, Srinivasana, Shackelford, & Ekbladh, 2004; Landon et al., 2005; Lieberman, 2001; Lydon-Rochelle et al., 2001b; Macones, Cahill et al., 2005; Macones, Peipert et al., 2005; O'Brien-Abel, 2003; Rochelson et al., 2005; Shipp et al., 2002; Smith, Pell, Pasupathy, & Dobbie, 2004). Inconsistencies in definitions of uterine rupture and scar dehiscence in the literature to date have made it difficult to determine with complete accuracy an incidence rate of uterine rupture for women who attempt VBAC (ACOG, 2004c; Guise et al., 2004).

Waiting for spontaneous labor, thus avoiding cervical ripening agents and oxytocin, appears to significantly decrease the risk of uterine rupture for women attempting VBAC (ACOG, 2004c, 2006c; Asian, Unlu, Agar, & Ceylan, 2004; Durnwald & Mercer, 2004; Landon et al., 2005; Mauldin & Newman, 2006; Zelop, Shipp, Cohen, Repke, & Leiberman, 2000). There are enough data to suggest that prostaglandins and high rates of oxytocin infusion increase the risk for rupture (ACOG, 2006c; Asian et al., 2004; Lieberman, 2001; Durnwald & Mercer, 2004; Lydon-Rochelle et al., 2001b). Uterine ruptures at the scar site and remote from the previous scar site have been reported with high doses of oxytocin (Murphy, 2006). It has been theorized that prostaglandins induce local biochemical modifications that weaken the prior uterine scar, thus predisposing it to rupture (Murphy, 2006). Due to the risk of uterine rupture with the use of misoprostol or any prostaglandin agent for cervical ripening or induction, ACOG (2004b, 2006c) does not recommend prostaglandins for women attempting VBAC.

Women undergoing a trial of labor require comprehensive care by an interdisciplinary perinatal team (Murphy, 2006). The patient and family need additional reassurance and support. Maternal–fetal status, including uterine activity, should be observed closely (O'Brien-Abel, 2003). Most experts recommend continuous EFM during the trial of labor (ACOG, 2004c). IV access is a reasonable precaution because of the risk of uterine rupture, which would require administration of rapid volume expanders and blood products. Rate of cervical dilation and fetal descent should be assessed frequently and abnormal labor progress reported to the primary care provider. Close attention should be given to any complaints of severe pain in the area of the prior incision. The onset of abdominal pain is classically suprabubic and "stabbing" (Raskin, Dachauer, Doeden, & Rayburn, 1999). Epidural anesthesia may be used during a trial of labor because it rarely masks the signs and symptoms of uterine rupture (ACOG, 2004c: Johnson, Oriol, & Flood, 1992). Additional maternal clinical signs of uterine rupture include vaginal bleeding, blood-tinged urine, ascending of station of the fetal presenting part, and hypovolemia (Mastrobattista, 1999).

Impending rupture may be preceded by increasing uterine hypertonus or hyperstimulation (Sheiner et al., 2004). Contrary to earlier reports, *usually* there is no decrease in uterine tone or cessation of contractions prior to or during uterine rupture (ACOG, 2006c; Leung, Leung et al., 1993), although this finding has been reported by some researchers (Sheiner et al., 2004). Nonreassuring changes in the FHR pattern may be early signs of impending or evolving uterine rupture (Ayres, Johnson, & Hayashi, 2001; Sheiner et al., 2004). The FHR pattern prior to rupture may demonstrate minimal to absent variability, recurrent variable, prolonged, or late decelerations followed by bradycardia, or fetal bradycardia may be sudden onset (Ayres et al., 2001; Leung, Leung et al., 1993; Menihan, 1999, Ridgeway, Weyrich & Benedetti, 2004; Sheiner et al., 2004; Yap, Kim, & Laros, 2001). The most consistent nonreassuring FHR patterns noted with uterine rupture are recurrent late decelerations and fetal bradycardia (Ayres et al., 2001; Ridgeway et al., 2004). If the uterine rupture is preceded by late decelerations, the fetus will tolerate a shorter period of prolonged decelerations (Leung, Leung et al., 1993). Significant neonatal morbidity has been reported when the time between onset of prolonged decelerations and birth is equal to or greater than 18 minutes (Leung, Leung et al., 1993). Kirkendall et al. (2000) reported a significant risk of brain damage, intrapartum death, and death within one year of life for infants who were partially or completely extruded into the maternal abdomen during uterine rupture.

Because uterine rupture may be catastrophic, VBAC should only be attempted in institutions equipped to respond to emergencies with physicians immediately available to provide emergency care (ACOG, 2004c). A physician should be immediately available throughout active labor that is capable of monitoring labor and performing an emergent cesarean birth (ACOG, 2004b). An anesthesia provider and other personnel who complete the surgical team should be immediately available as well (ACOG, 2004c). In essence, a full surgical team (surgeon, anesthesia provider, surgical first assistant, scrub tech, circulating nurse, and person whose sole responsibility is for potential neonatal resuscitation) should be immediately available (in-house or on campus and not engaged in any activity that would preclude leaving immediately to attend to a potential VBAC emergency, such as scrubbed in for another surgery) during the labor of a woman attempting VBAC. There is often much discussion about the meaning of "immediately" available as required in the ACOG (2004c) Practice Bulletin *Vaginal Birth After Cesarean Delivery*. In lay terms, immediately is defined as at once, right now, without delay, instantly.

Common sequelae associated with uterine rupture include excessive hemorrhage requiring surgical exploration; need for hysterectomy; need for blood product transfusion; hypovolemia; hypovolemic shock; injury to the bladder or ureters; bowel laceration; extrusion of any part of the fetus, cord, or placenta through the disruption; emergent cesarean birth for suspected rupture; emergent cesarean birth for nonreassuring fetal status; and general anesthesia (Guise et al., 2004; Hibbard et al., 2001; Kirkendall et al, 2000; Landon et al., 2004; Pare, Quinones, & Macones, 2006; Shipp, 2004). Many women with uterine rupture experience more than one of these complications (Landon et al., 2004).

Complete or partial placental abruption usually occurs concurrently with rupture (84%), and in many cases (60%), the placenta may be at the site of the rupture (Jauregui, Kirkendall, Ahn, & Phelan, 2000). It is possible that the placenta may play a part in uterine rupture; however, more data are needed about the relationship between placental implantation/abruption and the process of uterine rupture. Maternal death is a rare complication (Chauhan, Martin, Henrichs, Morrison, & Magann, 2003; Guise et al., 2004; Landon et al., 2004).

Although the actual numbers of adverse fetal or neonatal outcomes are low with VBAC, risks to the baby associated with uterine rupture are significant and can be catastrophic. They include hypoxemia, neurologic depression, pathologic fetal acidosis, seizures, asphyxia, hypoxic ischemic encephalopathy, cerebral palsy, and death (Chauhan et al., 2003; Guise et al., 2004; Landon et al., 2004; Smith, Pell, Cameron, & Dobbie, 2006; Yap et al., 2001).

Rupture of the uterus is a perinatal emergency. Maternal–fetal survival depends on prompt identification and surgical intervention. Rapid volume expanders, blood, and blood products should be readily available. Policies, procedures, and protocols should be written and evaluated to ensure optimum care for women who are having a trial of labor after a previous cesarean birth. If the primary care provider is a family practitioner or CNM without privileges or ability to perform an emergent cesarean birth, clear policies and protocols should be in place to ensure appropriate and timely surgical coverage in case of maternal complications.

Safe care during a trial of labor to attempt VBAC is resource intensive. Many obstetrical units do not have the financial and personnel resources to provide in-house anesthesia and a surgical team for the course of VBAC labor. Approximately 50% of hospitals providing perinatal services have fewer than 500 births per year (ACOG & AAP, 2001). These hospitals and others without around the clock anesthesia and surgical team support may find it challenging to supply the resources to meet the full scope of the ACOG (2004) recommendations during VBAC labor. Not all obstetricians have the desire or ability to devote the time to remain in-house during VBAC labor. The decision to offer a trial of labor for women attempting VBAC should be based on commitment of resources and agreement of providers to be in-house during the course of labor. If this commitment cannot be made for whatever reason, the hospital should not offer VBAC care. Alternatives are repeat cesarean birth or patient referral to another hospital with resources consistent with the ACOG (2004b) recommendations.

SUMMARY

Nurses who care for women during the intrapartum period require knowledge of the labor process and a thorough understanding of techniques and interventions that enhance safe labor and birth. The woman's desires about her labor and birth experience should guide care. We should consider ourselves supportive guests at the woman's momentous life event rather than routine interventionists. A philosophy that labor and birth are normal processes will facilitate appropriate care and avoid unnecessary interventions that can lead to iatrogenic maternal–fetal injuries.

Some of the age-old nursing traditions surrounding birth have not been found to be based on sound scientific evidence. Positioning for labor and birth has evolved from supine lithotomy to positions that are more woman- and fetus-oriented. For most women, fasting during labor is not necessary to avoid adverse outcomes. Aggressive coached closed-glottis, second-stage pushing techniques should be abandoned in favor of second-stage care practices that are more mother- and baby-friendly. Routine episiotomy should become a thing of the past. Nurses can influence changes related to routine childbirth practices by keeping abreast of current research in perinatal nursing and using this knowledge in caring for laboring women. There are many opportunities for nursing research to evaluate efficacy and effects of routine interventions during labor and birth.

Cervical ripening procedures, labor induction/augmentation, and operative births are necessary interventions for some women to promote optimal maternal and fetal outcome, but the least invasive approach should be the first considered. Nurses must also have expertise in perioperative standards for women experiencing cesarean births. This chapter has presented an overview of nursing considerations for clinical practice during childbirth. Perinatal care based on national standards, current research, and principles of patient safety will enhance quality outcomes for women and newborns. The nurse has an important role in facilitating a positive childbirth experience (Figure 7–14). Attending the birth of a healthy newborn and sharing the joy with the new mother is one of the most rewarding experiences in perinatal nursing practice.

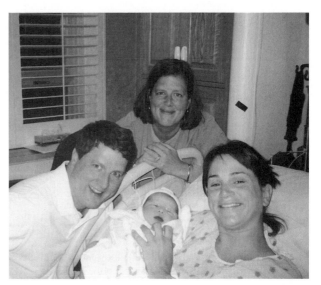

FIGURE 7–14. The nurse and the new family.

REFERENCES

Aikens-Murphy, P., & Feinland, J. B. (1998). Perineal outcomes in a home birth setting. *Birth: Issues in Perinatal Care and Education, 25*(4), 226–234.

Akhan, S. E., Iyibozkurt, A. C., & Turfanda, A. (2001). Unscarred uterine rupture after induction of labor with misoprostol: A case report. *Clinical and Experimental Obstetrics and Gynecology, 28*(2), 118–120.

Albers, L. L. (1999). The duration of labor in healthy women. *Journal of Perinatology, 19*(2), 114–119.

Albers, L. L., Anderson, D., Cragin, L., Daniels, S. M., Hunter, C., Sedler, K. D. & Teaf, D. (1997). The relationship of ambulation in labor to operative delivery. *Journal of Nurse Midwifery, 42*(1), 4–8.

Albers, L. L., Schiff, M., & Gorwoda, J. G., (1996). The length of active labor in normal pregnancies. *Obstetrics and Gynecology, 87*(3), 355–359.

Albers, L. L., Sedler, K. D., Bedrick, E. J., Teaf, D.. & Peralta, P. (2005). Midwifery care measures in the second stage of labor and reduction of genital tract trauma at birth: A randomized trial. *Journal of Midwifery and Women's Health, 50*(5), 365–372.

Albers, L. L., Sedler, K. D., Bedrick, E. J., Teaf, D., & Peralta, P. (2006). Factors related to genital tract trauma in normal spontaneous vaginal births. *Birth, 33*(2), 94–100.

Albrecht, L. (1997, September). Therapy options for pre-induction cervical ripening. *U.S. Pharmacist,* HS13–HS24.

Aldrich, C. J., D'Antona, D., Spencer, J. A. D., Wyatt, J. S., Peebles, D. M., Delpy, D. T., et al. (1995). The effect of maternal pushing on cerebral oxygenation and blood volume during the second stage of labour. *British Journal of Obstetrics and Gynecology, 102*(6), 448–453.

Alexander, J. M., Leveno, K. J., Hauth, J., Landon, M. B., Thom, E., Spong, C. Y., et al. (2006). Fetal injury associated with cesarean delivery. *Obstetrics and Gynecology, 108*(4), 885–890.

Alexander, J. M., Sharma, S. K., McIntire, D. D., & Leveno, K. J. (2002). Epidural anesthesia lengthens the Friedman active phase of labor. *Obstetrics and Gynecology, 100*(1), 46–50.

Alfirevic, Z., & Weeks, A. (2006). Oral misoprostol for induction of labour. *Cochrane Database of Systematic Reviews, 19*(2), CD001338

Allen, V. M., O'Connell, C. M., & Baskett, T. F. (2006a). Maternal morbidity associated with cesarean delivery without labor compared with induction of labor at term. *Obstetrics and Gynecology, 108*(2), 286–294.

Allen, V. M., O'Connell, C. M., & Baskett, T. F. (2006b). Cumulative economic implications of initial method of delivery. *Obstetrics and Gynecology, 108*(3), 549–555.

American Academy of Pediatrics & American College of Obstetricians and Gynecologists. (2002). *Guidelines for perinatal care* (5th ed.). Elk Grove Village, IL: Author.

American Academy of Pediatrics & American Heart Association. (2006). *Textbook of neonatal resuscitation* (5th ed.). Elk Grove Village, IL: Author.

American College of Nurse Midwives (2000). *Intrapartum nutrition* (Clinical Bulletin No 3). Washington, DC: Author.

American College of Obstetricians and Gynecologists. (1995). *Shoulder dystocia* (Video). Washington, DC: Author.

American College of Obstetricians and Gynecologists. (1999a). *Antepartum fetal surveillance* (Practice Bulletin No. 9), Washington, DC: Author.

American College of Obstetricians and Gynecologists. (1999b). *Induction of labor* (Practice Bulletin No. 10), Washington, DC: Author.

American College of Obstetricians and Gynecologists. (1999c). *Induction of labor with misoprostol* (Committee Opinion No. 228; Reaffirmed 2003), Washington, DC: Author.

American College of Obstetricians and Gynecologists. (2000a). *Fetal macrosomia* (Practice Bulletin No. 22). Washington, DC: Author.

American College of Obstetricians and Gynecologists. (2000b). *Operative vaginal delivery* (Practice Bulletin No. 17). Washington, DC: Author.

American College of Obstetricians and Gynecologists. (2000c). *Response to Searle's drug warning on misoprostol* (Committee Opinion No. 248). Washington, DC: Author.

American College of Obstetricians and Gynecologists. (2002a). *Obstetric analgesia and anesthesia* (Practice Bulletin No. 40). Washington, DC: Author.

American College of Obstetricians and Gynecologists. (2002b). *Shoulder dystocia* (Practice Bulletin No. 40). Washington, DC: Author.

American College of Obstetricians and Gynecologists. (2003a). *Dystocia and augmentation of labor* (Practice Bulletin No. 49). Washington, DC: Author.

American College of Obstetricians and Gynecologists. (2003b). *Surgery and patient choice: The ethics of decision making* (Committee Opinion No. 289). Washington, DC: Author.

American College of Obstetricians and Gynecologists. (2004a). *2003 ACOG survey of professional liability.* Washington, DC: Author.

American College of Obstetricians and Gynecologists. (2004b). Surgery and patient choice. In: *Ethics in obstetrics and gynecology.* Washington, DC: Author.

American College of Obstetricians and Gynecologists. (2004c). *Vaginal birth after cesarean delivery* (Practice Bulletin No. 54). Washington, DC: Author.

American College of Obstetricians and Gynecologists. (2005). *Intrapartum fetal heart rate monitoring* (Practice Bulletin No. 70). Washington, DC: Author.

American College of Obstetricians and Gynecologists. (2006a). *Amnioinfusion does not prevent meconium aspiration syndrome* (Committee Opinion No. 346). Washington, DC: Author.

American College of Obstetricians and Gynecologists. (2006b). *Episiotomy* (Practice Bulletin No. 71). Washington, DC: Author.

American College of Obstetricians and Gynecologists. (2006c). *Induction of labor for vaginal birth after cesarean delivery* (Committee Opinion No. 342). Washington, DC: Author.

American College of Obstetricians and Gynecologists. (2006d). *Patient safety in the surgical environment* (Committee Opinion No. 328). Washington, DC: Author.

American College of Obstetricians and Gynecologists & American Academy of Pediatrics. (2003). *Neonatal encephalopathy and cerebral palsy: Defining the pathogenesis and pathophysiology.* Washington, DC: Author.

American College of Obstetricians and Gynecologists & American Society of Anesthesiologists. (2001). *Optimal Goals for Anesthesia Care in Obstetrics* (Committee Opinion No. 256; Reaffirmed 2004). Washington, DC: Author.

American Society of Anesthesiologists. (2000). *Guidelines for regional anesthesia in obstetrics:* Park Ridge, IL: Author.

American Society of Anesthesiologists. (2002). *Practice guidelines for management of the difficult airway: An updated report from the American Society of Anesthesiologists Task Force on Management of the Difficult Airway.* Park Ridge, IL: Author.

American Society of Anesthesiologists. (2003). *Practice guidelines for postanesthesia care: A report by the American Society of Anesthesiologists Task Force on Postanesthesia Care.* Park Ridge, IL: Author.

American Society of Anesthesiologists. (2006). *Practice guidelines for obstetrical anesthesia: An updated report by the American Society of Anesthesiologists Task Force on Obstetrical Anesthesia.* Park Ridge, IL: Author.

American Society of Perianesthesia Nurses. (2006). *Standards of perianesthesia nursing practice 2006–2008.* Cherry Hill, NJ: Author.

Amiel-Tison, C., Sureau, C., & Shnider, S. M. (1988). Cerebral handicap in full-term neonates related to the mechanical forces of labour. *Baillieres Clinical Obstetrics and Gynaecology, 2*(1), 145–165.

Anderson, G. C., Moore, E., Hepworth, J., & Bergman, N. (2003). Early skin-to-skin contact for mothers and their healthy newborn infants. *Cochrane Database of Systematic Reviews, 2,* CD003519.

Andrews, V., Sultan, A. H., Thakar, R., & Jones, P. W. (2006). Risk factors for obstetric anal sphincter injury: A prospective study. *Birth, 33*(2), 117–122.

Arias, F. (2000). Pharmacology of oxytocin and prostaglandins. *Clinical Obstetrics and Gynecology, 43*(3), 455–468.

Asian, H., Uniu, E., Agar, M., & Ceylan, Y. (2004). Uterine rupture associated with misoprostol labor induction in women with a previous cesarean delivery. *European Journal of Obstetrics, Gynecology, and Reproductive Biology, 113*(1), 45–48.

Association of periOperative Registered Nurses. (2007). *Standards, recommended practices, and guidelines.* Denver, CO: Author.

Association of Women's Health, Obstetric and Neonatal Nurses. (2000). *Nursing management of the second stage of labor.* (Evidence-Based Clinical Practice Guideline). Washington, DC: Author.

Association of Women's Health, Obstetric and Neonatal Nurses. (2001). *Nursing care of the woman receiving regional analgesia/anesthesia in labor* (Evidence-Based Clinical Practice Guideline). Washington, DC: Author.

Association of Women's Health, Obstetric and Neonatal Nurses. (2004). *Second stage labor support.* (High touch nursing care during labor: Video Series). Longmont, CO: Injoy Birth and Parenting Videos.

Association of Women's Health, Obstetric and Neonatal Nurses. (2006). *Amniotomy and placement of internal fetal spiral electrode through intact membranes.* (Clinical Position Statement). Washington, DC: Author.

Aukee, P., Sundstrom, H., & Kairaiuoma, M. V. (2006). The role of mediolateral episiotomy during labour: Analysis of risk factors for obstetric anal sphincter tears. *Acta Obstetricia et Gynecologica Scandinavica, 85*(7), 856–860.

Ayres, A. W., Johnson, T. R., & Hayashi, R. (2001). Characteristics of fetal heart rate tracings prior to uterine rupture. *International Journal of Gynaecology and Obstetrics, 74*(3), 235–240.

Baacke, K. A., & Edwards, R. K. (2006). Preinduction cervical assessment. *Clinical Obstetrics and Gynecology, 49*(3), 564–572.

Bahar, A. M. (1996). Risk factors and fetal outcome in cases of shoulder dystocia compared with normal deliveries of a similar birthweight. *British Journal of Obstetrics and Gynaecology, 103*(9), 868–872.

Barnett, M. M., & Humenick, S. S. (1982). Infant outcome in relation to second stage labor pushing method. *Birth and the Family Journal, 9*(4)221–229.

Bassell, G. M., Humayun, S. G., & Marx, G. F. (1980). Maternal bearing down efforts: Another fetal risk. *Obstetrics and Gynecology, 56*(1), 39–41.

Beall, M. H., Spong, C. Y., & Ross, M. G. (2003). A randomized controlled trial of prophylactic maneuvers to reduce head-to-body delivery time in patients at risk for shoulder dystocia. *Obstetrics and Gynecology, 102*(1), 31–35.

Beckmann, M. M., & Garrett, A. J. (2006). Antenatal perineal massage for reducing perineal trauma. *Birth, 33*(2), 159.

Benavides, L., Wu, J. M., Hundley, A. F., Ivester, T. S., & Visco, A. G. (2005). The impact of occiput posterior fetal head position on the risk of anal sphincter injury in forceps-assisted vaginal deliveries. *American Journal of Obstetrics and Gynecology, 192*(5), 1702–1706.

Benedetti, T. J. (1995). Shoulder dystocia. *Contemporary OB/GYN, 40*(3), 39–43.

Bennett, B. B. (1997). Uterine rupture during induction of labor at term with intravaginal misoprostol. *Obstetrics and Gynecology, 89*(5, Pt. 1), 832–833.

Bennett, K. A., Butt, K., Crane, J. M. G., Hutchens, D., & Young, D. C. (1998). A masked randomized comparison of oral and vaginal misoprostol for labor induction. *Obstetrics and Gynecology, 92*(4, Pt. 1), 481–486.

Bernal, A. L. (2003). Mechanisms of labour: Biochemical aspects. *British Journal of Obstetrics and Gynaecology, 110*(Suppl. 20), 39–45.

Bettes, B. A., Coleman, V. H., Zinberg, S., Spong, C. Y., Portnoy, B., DeVoto, E., & Schulkin, J. (2007). Cesarean delivery on maternal request: Obstetrician-gynecologist' knowledge, perception, and practice patterns. *Obstetrics and Gynecology, 109*(1), 57–66.

Bishop, E. H. (1964). Pelvic scoring for elective induction. *Obstetrics and Gynecology, 24*, 266–268.

Blakemore, K. J., Qin, N. G., Petrie, R. H., & Paine, L. L. (1990). A prospective comparison of hourly and quarter-hourly oxytocin dose increase intervals for the induction of labor at term. *Obstetrics and Gynecology, 75*(5), 757–761.

Bloom, S. L., Casey, B. M., Schaffer, J. I., McIntire, D. D., & Leveno, K. J. (2006). A randomized trial of coached versus uncoached maternal pushing during the second stage of labor. *American Journal of Obstetrics and Gynecology, 194*(1), 10–13.

Bloom, S. L., McIntire, D. D., Kelly, M. A., Beimer, H. L., Burpo, R. H., Garcia, M. A., & Leveno, K. J. (1998). Lack of effect of walking on labor and delivery. *New England Journal of Medicine, 339*(2), 76–79.

Bodner-Adler, B., Bodner, K., Kimberger, O., Lozanov, P., Hussiein, P., & Mayerhofer, K. (2003). Women's position during labour: Influence on maternal and neonatal outcome. *Wiener Klinische Wochenschrift, 115*(19-20), 720–723.

Bofill, J. A., Martin, J. N. Jr.. & Morrison, J. C. (1998). The Mississippi operative vaginal delivery trial: Lessons learned. *Contemporary OB/GYN, 48*(10), 60–79.

Bofill, J. A., Rust, O. A., & Schorr, S. J. (1996). A randomized prospective trial of the obstetric forceps versus the M-cup vacuum extractor. *American Journal of Obstetrics and Gynecology, 175*(5), 1325–1330.

Bofill, J. A., Rust, O. A., Devidas, M., Roberts, W. E., Morrison, J. C., & Martin, J. N. Jr. (1997a). Neonatal cephalohematoma from vacuum extraction. *Journal of Reproductive Medicine, 42*(9), 565–569.

Bofill, J. A., Rust, O. A., Devidas, M., Roberts, W. E., Morrison, J. C., & Martin, J. N. Jr. (1997b). Shoulder dystocia and operative vaginal delivery. *Journal of Maternal Fetal Medicine, 6*(4), 220–204.

Boulvain, M., Kelly, A., Lohse, C., Stan, C., & Irion, O. (2001). Mechanical methods for induction of labour. *Cochrane Database of Systematic Reviews, 4*, CD001233.

Boulvain, M., Stan, C., & Irion, O. (2005). Membrane sweeping for induction of labour. *Cochrane Database of Systematic Reviews, 1*, CD000451.

Bricker, L., & Luckas, M. (2000). Amniotomy alone for labor induction. *Cochrane Database of Systematic Reviews, 4*, CD002862.

Brindley, B. A., & Sokol, R. J. (1988). Induction and augmentation of labor: Basis and methods for practice. *Obstetrical and Gynecological Survey, 43*(12), 730–743.

Britton, G. R. (1980). Early mother-infant contact and infant temperature stabilization. *Journal of Obstetric, Gynecologic and Neonatal Nursing, 9*(2), 84–86.

Brown, M. A., Reiter, L., Smith, B., Buddle, M. L., Morries, R., & Whiteworth, J. A. (1994). Measuring blood pressure in pregnant women: A comparison of direct and indirect methods. *American Journal of Obstetrics and Gynecology, 171*(3), 661–667.

Brumfield, C., Gilstrap, L. C., O'Grady, J. P., Ross, M. G., & Schifrin, B. S. (1999). Cutting your legal risks with vacuum-assisted deliveries. *OBG Management, 3*, 2–6.

Bruner, J. P., Drummond, S. B., Meenan, A. L., & Gaskin, I. M. (1998). All-fours maneuver for reducing shoulder dystocia during labor. *Journal of Reproductive Medicine, 43*(5), 439–443.

Bujold, E., Bujold, C., Hamilton, E. F., Harel, F., & Gauthier, R. J. (2002). The impact of single-layer or double-layer closure on uterine rupture. *American Journal of Obstetrics and Gynecology, 186*(6), 1326–1330.

Bujold, E., Hammoud, A. O., Hendler, I., Berman, S., Blackwell, S. C., Duperron, L., & Gauthier, R. J., (2004). Trial of labor in patients with a previous cesarean section: Does maternal age influence the outcome? *American Journal of Obstetrics and Gynecology, 190*(4), 1113–1118.

Bujold, E., Hammoud, A., Schild, C., Krapp, M., & Baumann, P. (2005). The role of maternal body mass index in outcomes of vaginal births after cesarean. *American Journal of Obstetrics and Gynecology, 193*(4), 1517–1521.

Bujold, E., Mehta, S. H., Bujold, C., & Gauthier, R. J. (2002). Inter-delivery interval and uterine rupture. *American Journal of Obstetrics and Gynecology, 187*(5), 1199–1202.

Buser, D., Mora, G., & Arias, F. (1997). A randomized comparison between misoprostol and dinoprostone for cervical ripening and labor induction in patients with unfavorable cervices. *Obstetrics and Gynecology, 89*(4), 581–585.

Bystrova, K., Widstrom, A. M., Matthiesen, A. S., Ransjo-Arvidson, A. B., Welles-Nystrom, B., Wassberg, C., et al. (2003). Skin-to-skin contact may reduce negative consequences of "the stress of being born": A study on temperature in newborn infants subjected to different ward routines in St. Petersberg. *Acta Paediatrica, 92*(3), 320–326.

Cahill, A. G., Stamillo, D. M., Odibo, A. O., Peipert, J. F., Ratcliffe, S. J., Stevens, E. J., et al. (2006). Is vaginal birth after cesarean (VBAC) or elective repeat cesarean safer in women with a prior vaginal delivery? *American Journal of Obstetrics and Gynecology, 195*(4), 1143–1147.

Caldeyro-Barcia, R. (1979). The influence of maternal bearing-down efforts during second stage on fetal wellbeing. *Birth and the Family Journal, 6*, 17–21.

Caldeyro-Barcia, R., & Poseiro, J. J. (1960). Physiology of the uterine contraction. *Clinical Obstetrics and Gynecology, 3*, 386–408.

Caldeyro-Barcia, R., Giussi, G., Storch, E., Poseiro, J. J., Kettenhuber, K., & Ballejo, G. (1981). The bearing down efforts and their effects on fetal heart rate, oxygenation, and acid-base balance. *Journal of Perinatal Medicine, 9*(Suppl. 1), 63–67.

Campbell, D. A., Lake, M. F., Falk, M., & Backstrand, J. R. (2006). A randomized control trial of continuous support in labor by a lay doula. *Journal of Obstetric, Gynecologic and Neonatal Nursing, 35*(4), 456–464.

Carbillon, L., Seince, N., & Uzan, M. (2001). Myometrial maturation and labour. *Annals of Medicine, 33*, 571–578.

Carfoot, S., Williamson, P., & Dickson, R. (2005). A randomised controlled trial in the north of England examining the effects of skin-to-skin care on breast feeding. *Midwifery, 21*(1), 71–79.

Carlton, T., Callister, L. C., & Stoneman, E. (2005). Decision making in laboring women: Ethical issues for perinatal nurses. *Journal of Perinatal and Neonatal Nursing, 19*(2), 145–154.

Carmen, S. (1986). Neonatal hypoglycemia in response to maternal glucose infusion before delivery. *Journal of Obstetric, Gynecologic and Neonatal Nursing, 15*(4), 319–322.

Carroli, G., & Belizan, J. (2000). Episiotomy for vaginal birth. *Cochrane Database of Systematic Reviews, 2*, CD000081.

Castro, M. A., Hoey, S. D., & Towner, D. (2003). Controversies in the use of the vacuum extractor. *Seminars in Perinatology, 27*(1), 46–53.

Catanzarite, V., Cousins, L., Dowling, D., & Daneshmand, S. (2006). Oxytocin-associated rupture of an unscarred uterus in a primagravida. *Obstetrics and Gynecology, 108*(3, Pt. 1), 723–725.

Caughey, A. B., Sandberg, P. L., Zlatnik, M. G., Thiet, M., Parer, J. T., & Laros, R. K. (2005). Forceps compared with vacuum: Rates of neonatal and maternal morbidity. *Obstetrics and Gynecology, 106*(5, Pt. 1), 908–912.

Cerri, V., Tarantini, M., Zuliani, G., Schena, V., Redaelli, C., & Niconlini, U. (2000). Intravenous glucose infusion in labor does not affect maternal and fetal acid base status. *Journal of Maternal-Fetal Medicine, 9*(4), 204–208.

Chalfen, M. F. (1993). Obstetric-Gynecologic care and survivors of childhood sexual abuse. *AWHONN'S Clinical Issues in Perinatal and Women's Health Nursing, 4*(2), 191–195.

Chauhan, S. P., Grobman, W. A., Gherman, R. A., Chauhan, V. B., Chang, G., Magann, E. F., & Hendrix, N. W. (2005). Suspicion and treatment of the macrosomic fetus: A review. *American Journal of Obstetrics and Gynecology, 193*(2), 332–346.

Chauhan, S. P., Martin, J. N. Jr., Hendricks, C. E., & Morrison, J. C. (2003). Maternal and perinatal complications with uterine rupture in 142,075 patients who attempted vaginal birth after cesarean delivery: A review of the literature. *American Journal of Obstetrics and Gynecology, 189*(2), 408–417.

Chen, C. Y., & Wang, K. G. (2006). Are routine interventions necessary in normal birth? *Taiwan Journal of Obstetrics and Gynecology, 45*(4), 302–306.

Cheng, Y. W., Hopkins, L. M., & Caughey, A. B. (2004). How long is too long: Does a prolonged second stage of labor in nulliparous women affect maternal and neonatal outcomes? *American Journal of Obstetrics and Gynecologists, 191*(3), 933–938.

Cheng, Y. W., Shaffer, B. L., & Caughey, A. B. (2006). The association between persistent occiput posterior position and neonatal outcomes. *Obstetrics and Gynecology, 107*(4), 837–844.

Christianson, L. M., Bovbjerg, V. E., McDavitt, E. C., & Hullfish, K. L. (2003). Risk factors for perineal injury during delivery. *American Journal of Obstetrics and Gynecologists, 189*(1), 255–260.

Chua, S., Arulkumaran, S., Kurup, A., Tay, D., & Ratnam. S. S. (1991). Oxytocin titration for induction of labour: A prospective randomized study of 15 versus 30-minute dose increment schedules. *Australian New Zealand Journal of Obstetrics and Gynaecology, 31*(2), 134–137.

Clark, S. L., Scott, J. R., Porter, T. F., Schlappy, D. A., McClellan, V., & Burton, D. A. (2000). Is vaginal birth after cesarean delivery less expensive than repeat cesarean delivery? *American Journal of Obstetrics and Gynecology, 182*(2), 599–602.

Clayworth, S. (2000). The nurse's role during oxytocin administration. *MCN The American Journal of Maternal Child Nursing, 25*(2), 80–85.

Clemons, J. L., Towers, G. D., McClure, G. B., & O'Boyle, A. L. (2005). Decreased anal sphincter lacerations associated with restrictive episiotomy use. *American Journal of Obstetrics and Gynecologists, 192*(5), 1620–1625.

Cohen, S. E., Yeh, J. Y., Riley, E. T., & Vogel, T. M. (2000). Walking with labor epidural analgesia: The impact of bupivacaine concentration and a lidocaine-epinephrine test dose. *Anesthesiology, 92*(2), 387–392.

Cohen, W. R. (1977). Influence of the duration of second stage labor on perinatal outcome and puerperal morbidity. *Obstetrics and Gynecology, 49*(3), 266–269.

Colachis, S. C., Pease, W. S., & Johnson, E. W. (1994). A preventable cause of foot drop during childbirth. *American Journal of Obstetrics and Gynecology, 171*(1), 270–272.

Collis, R. E., Harding, S. A., & Morgan, B. M. (1999). Effect of maternal ambulation on labour with low-dose combined spinal-epidural analgesia. *Anaesthesia, 54*(6), 535–539.

Cosner, K. R. (1996). Use of fundal pressure during second-stage labor: A pilot study. *Journal of Nurse Midwifery, 41*(4), 334–337.

Cosner, K. R., & deJong, E. (1993). Physiologic second-stage labor. *MCN The American Journal of Maternal Child Nursing, 18*(1), 38–43.

Crane, J. M. (2006). Factors predicting labor induction success: A critical analysis. *Clinical Obstetrics and Gynecology, 49*(3), 573–584.

Crane, J. M., & Young, D. C. (1998). Meta-analysis of low-dose versus high-dose oxytocin for labour induction. *Journal of the Society of Obstetricians and Gynaecologists of Canada, 20*(13), 1215–1223.

Crane, J. M., Young, D. C., Butt, K. D., Bennett, K. A., & Hutchens, D. (2001). Excessive uterine activity accompanying induced labor. *American Journal of Obstetrics and Gynecology, 97*(6), 926–931.

Cuervo, L. G., Bernal Mdel, P., & Mendoza, N. (2006). Effects of high volume saline enemas vs no enema during labour: The N-MA randomized controlled trial. *BMC Pregnancy and Childbirth, 19*, 6–8.

Cuervo, L. G., Rodriguez, M. N., & Delgado, M. B. (2000). Enemas during labor. *Cochrane Database of Systematic Reviews, 2*, CD00330.

Dandolu, V., Chatwani, A., Harmanli, O., Floro, C., Gaaughan, J. P., & Hernandez, E. (2005). Risk factors for obstetrical anal sphincter lacerations. *International Urogynecology Journal and Pelvic Floor Dysfunction, 16*(4), 304–307.

Daniel-Spiegel, E., Weiner, Z., Ben-Shlomo, I., & Shalev, E. (2004). For how long should oxytocin be continued during induction of labour? *British Journal of Obstetrics and Gynaecology, 111*(4), 331–334.

Dawood, M. Y. (1995a). Novel approach to oxytocin induction-augmentation of labor: Application of oxytocin physiology during pregnancy. *Advances in Experimental Medicine and Biology, 395*, 585–594.

Dawood, M. Y. (1995b). Pharmacologic stimulation of uterine contractions. *Seminars in Perinatology, 19*(1), 73–83.

Dawood, M. Y., Wang, C. F., Gupta, R., & Fuchs, F. (1978). Fetal contribution to oxytocin in human labor. *Obstetrics and Gynecology, 52*(2), 205–209.

Dawood, M. Y., Ylikorkala, O., Trivedi, D., & Fuchs, F. (1979). Oxytocin in maternal circulation and amniotic fluid during pregnancy. *Journal of Clinical Endocrinology and Metabolism, 49*(3), 429–434.

de Chateau, P., & Wiberg, B. (1984). Long-term effect on mother-infant behavior of extra contact during the first hour post partum. III: Follow-up at one year. *Scandinavian Journal of Social Medicine, 12*(2), 91–103.

Declercq, E. R., Sakala, C., Corry, M. P., & Applebaum, S. (2006). *Listening to mothers: Report of the second national US survey of women's childbearing experiences.* New York: Childbirth Connections.

DeFrances, C. J., & Podgornik, M. N. (2006). 2004 National hospital discharge survey. *Vital and Health Statistics, 371,* 1–20.

de Jong, P. R., Johanson, R. B., Baxen, P., Adrians, V. D., van der Westhuisen, S., & Jones, P. W. (1997). Randomised trial comparing the upright and supine positions for the second stage of labour. *British Journal of Obstetrics and Gynaecology, 104*(5), 567–571.

DelGiudice, G. T. (1986). The relationship between sibling jealousy and presence at a sibling's birth. *Birth, 13*(4), 250–254.

Deneux-Tharaux, C., Carmona, E., Bouvier-Colle, M. H., & Breart, G. (2006). Postpartum maternal mortality and cesarean delivery. *Obstetrics and Gynecology, 108*(3), 541–548.

Derham, R. J., Crowhurst, J., & Crowther, C. (1991). The second stage of labor: Durational dilemmas. *Australian New Zealand Journal of Obstetrics and Gynaecology, 31*(1), 31–36.

Devine, J. B., Ostergard, D. R., & Noblett, K. L. (1999). Long-term complications of the second stage of labor. *Contemporary OB/GYN, 49*(6), 119–126.

Dilbaz, B., Ozturkoglu, E., Dilbaz, S., Ozturk, N., Sivaslioglu, A. A., & Haberal, A. (2006). Risk factors and perinatal outcomes associated with umbilical cord prolapse. *Archives of Gynecology and Obstetrics, 274*(2), 104–107.

Doumouchtsis, S. K., & Arulkumaran, S. (2006). Head injuries after instrumental vaginal deliveries. *Current Opinion in Obstetrics and Gynecology, 18*(2), 129–134

Downe, S., Gerrett, D., Renfrew, M. J. (2004). A prospective randomised trial on the effect of position in the passive second stage of labour on birth outcome in nulliparous women using epidural analgesia, *Midwifery, 20*(2), 157–168.

Dudell, G. G., & Jain, L. (2006). Hypoxic respiratory failure in the late preterm infant. *Clinics in Perinatology, 33*(4), 803–830.

Dupuis, O., Silveira, R., Dupong, C., Mottolese, C., Kahn, P., Dittmar, A., & Rudigoz, R. C. (2005). Comparison of "instrumented-associated" and "spontaneous" obstetric depressed skull fractures in a cohort of 68 neonates. *American Journal of Obstetrics and Gynecology, 192*(1), 165–170.

Durnwald, C., & Mercer, B. (2004). Vaginal birth after cesarean delivery: Predicting success, risks of failure. *Journal of Maternal-Fetal and Neonatal Medicine, 15*(6), 388–393.

Durnwald, C. P., Rouse, D. J., Leveno, K. J., Spong, C. Y., MacPherson, C., & Varner, M. W. (2006). The Maternal-Fetal Medicine Units Cesarean Registry: Safety and efficacy of a trial of labor in preterm pregnancy after a prior cesarean delivery. *American Journal of Obstetrics and Gynecology, 195*(4), 1119–1126.

Driver, I., Popham, P., Glazebrook, C., & Palmer, C. (1996). Epidural bupivacaine/fentanyl infusions vs intermittent top-ups: A retrospective study of the effects on mode of delivery in primparous women. *European Journal of Anaesthesiology, 13*(5), 515–520.

Druzin, M. L., & El-Sayed, Y. Y. (2006). Cesarean delivery on maternal request: Wise use of finite resources? A view from the trenches. *Seminars in Perinatology, 30*(5), 305–308.

Eason, E., Labrecque, M., Wells, G., & Feldman, P. (2000). Preventing perineal trauma during childbirth: A systematic review. *Obstetrics and Gynecology, 95*(3), 464–471.

Eason, E., & Feldman, P. (2000). Much ado about a little cut: Is episiotomy worthwhile? *Obstetrics and Gynecology, 95*(4), 616–618.

Edwards, H., Grotegut, C., Harmanli, O. H., Rapkin, D., & Dandolu, V. (2006). Is severe perineal damage increased in women with prior anal sphincter injury? *Journal of Maternal-Fetal and Neonatal Medicine, 19*(11), 723–737.

Engelman, G. J. (1884). *Labor among primitive peoples* (3rd ed.). St. Louis, MO: J. H. Chambers.

Eogan, M., Daly, L., & O'Herlihy, C. (2006). The effect of regular antenatal perineal massage on postnatal pain and anal sphincter injury: A prospective observational study. *Journal of Maternal-Fetal and Neonatal Medicine, 19*(4), 225–229.

Esiamian, L., Marsoosi, V., & Pakneeyat, Y. (2006). Increased intravenous fluid intake and the course of labor in nulliparous women. *European Journal of Obstetrics and Gynecology, 93*(2), 102–105

Farah, L. A., Sanchez-Ramos, L., Del Valle, G. O., Gaudier, F. L., Delke, I., & Kaunitz, A. M. (1997). Randomized trial of two doses of the prostaglandin E1 analog misoprostol for labor induction. *American Journal of Obstetrics and Gynecology, 177*(2), 364–369.

Feinstein, N. F., Sprague, A., & Trepanier, M. J. (2000). *Fetal heart rate auscultation.* (Symposium). Washington, DC: Association of Women's Health, Obstetric, and Neonatal Nurses.

Feinstein, N., Torgersen, K. L., & Atterbury, J, (Eds.). (2003). *Fetal heart monitoring principles and practices* (3rd ed.). Washington, DC: Association of Women's Health, Obstetric and Neonatal Nurses.

Fenner, D. (2006), Anal incontinence: Relationship to pregnancy, vaginal delivery, and cesarean section. *Seminars in Perinatology, 30*(5), 261–266.

Ferguson, J. K. W. (1941). Study of motility of intact uterus at term. *Surgery, Gynecology and Obstetrics, 73,* 359–366.

FitzGerald, M. P., Weber, A. M., Howden, N., Cundiff, G. W., & Brown, M. B. for the Pelvic Floor Disorders Network. (2007). Risk factors for anal sphincter tear during vaginal delivery. *Obstetrics and Gynecology, 109*(1), 29–34.

Fleming, N., Newton, E. R., & Roberts, J. (2003). Changes in postpartum perineal muscle function in women with and without episiotomies. *Journal of Midwifery and Women's Health, 48*(1), 53–59.

Flynn, P., Franiek, J., Janssen, P., Hannah, W. J., & Klein, M. C, (1997). How can second stage management prevent perineal trauma? *Canadian Journal of Family Practice, 43*(1), 73–84.

Food and Drug Administration. (1998). *Need for caution when using vacuum assisted delivery devices.* (FDA Public Health Advisory), Washington, DC: Author.

Food and Drug Administration (2002) *FDA approves new labeling information for Cytotec (misoprostol).* http://www.fda.gov/cder (Accessed January 2007).

Forest Pharmaceuticals, Inc. (1995). *Cervidil prescribing information.* St. Louis, MO: Author.

Fransson, A. L., Karlsson, H., & Nilsson, K. (2005). Temperature variation in newborn babies: Importance of physical contact with the mother. *Archives of Disease in Childhood. Fetal and Neonatal Edition, 90*(6), F500–F504.

Franx, A., van der Post, J. A. M., Elfering, I. M., Veerman, D. P., Merkus, H. M. W. M., Boer, K., & van Montfrans, G. A. (1994). Validation of automatic blood pressure recording in pregnancy. *British Journal of Obstetrics and Gynaecology, 101*(10), 66–69.

Fraser, W. D., Hofmeyr, J., Lede, R., Faron, G., Alexander, S., Goffinet, F., et al. for the Amnioinfusion Trial Group. (2005). Amnioinfusion for the prevention of the meconium aspiration syndrome. *New England Journal of Medicine, 353*(9), 909–917.

Fraser, W. D., Marcoux, S., Krauss, I., Douglas, J., Goulet, C., & Boulvain, M. for the PEOPLE (Pushing Early or Pushing Late with Epidurals) Study Group. (2000). Multicenter randomized controlled trial of delayed pushing for nulliparous women in the second stage of labor with continuous epidural analgesia. *American Journal of Obstetrics and Gynecology, 182*(5), 1165–1172.

Fraser, W. D., Turcot, L., Krauss, I., & Brisson-Carrol, G. (2000). Amniotomy for shortening spontaneous labor. *Cochrane Database of Systematic Reviews, 2,* CD000015.

Freeman, R. K., Garite, T. J., & Nageotte, M. P. (2003). *Fetal heart rate monitoring* (3rd ed.). Philadelphia: Lippincott Williams & Wilkins.

Friedman, E. A. (1955). Primigravid labor: A graphicostatistical analysis. *Obstetrics and Gynecology, 6,* 567–589.

Friedman, E. A. (1978). *Labor: Clinical evaluation of management* (2nd ed.). New York: Appleton-Century-Crofts.

Friedman, E. A., Niswander, K. R., Bayonet-Rivera, N. P., & Sachtleben, M. R. (1966). Relationship of prelabor evaluation to induciblity and the course of labor. *Obstetrics and Gynecology, 28*, 495–501.

Frigoletto, F. D. Jr., Lieberman, E., Lang, J. M., Cohen, A., Barss, V., Ringer, S., & Datta, S. (1995). A clinical trial of active management of labor. *New England Journal of Medicine, 333*(12), 745–750.

Fuchs, A. R., Fuchs, F., Husslein, P., & Soloff, M. S. (1984). Oxytocin receptors in the human uterus during pregnancy and parturition. *American Journal of Obstetrics and Gynecology, 150*(12), 734–741.

Fuchs, A. R., Husslein, P., & Fuchs, F. (1981). Oxytocin and the initiation of human parturition. II: Stimulation of prostaglandin production in the human decidua by oxytocin. *American Journal of Obstetrics and Gynecology, 141*(6), 694–699.

Fuchs, A. R., Romero, R., Keefe, D., Parra, M., Oyarzun, E., & Behnke, E. (1991). *American Journal of Obstetrics and Gynecology, 165*(5, Pt. 1), 1515–1523.

Gannon, J.M. (1992). Delivery on the hands and knees: A case study approach. *Journal of Nurse-Midwifery, 37*(1), 48–52.

Garite, T. J., Porto, M., Carlson, N. J., Rumney, P. J., & Reimbold, P. A. (1993). The influence of elective amniotomy on fetal heart rate patterns and the course of labor in term patients: A randomized study. *American Journal of Obstetrics and Gynecology, 168*(6, Pt. 1), 1827–1831.

Garite, T. J., Weeks, M. D., & Peters-Phair, K. (2000). A randomized trial on the influence of increased intravenous hydration on the course of nulliparous labor. *American Journal of Obstetrics and Gynecology, 182*(1, Pt. 2), S37.

Gawande, A. A., Studdert, D. M., Orav, E. J., Brennad, T. A., & Zinner, M. J. (2003). Risk factors for retained instruments and sponges after surgery. *New England Journal of Medicine, 348*(3), 229–235.

Gelber, S., & Sciscione, A. (2006). Mechanical methods of cervical ripening and labor induction. *Clinical Obstetrics and Gynecology, 49*(3), 642–657.

Getahun, D., Oyelese, Y., Salihu, H. M., & Ananth, C. V. (2006). Previous cesarean delivery and risks of placenta previa and placental abruption. *Obstetrics and Gynecology, 107*(4), 771–778.

Gherman, R. B. (2002). Shoulder dystocia: An evidence-based evaluation of the obstetric nightmare. *Clinical Obstetrics and Gynecology, 45*(2), 345–362.

Gherman, R. B., Chauhan, S., Ouzounian, J. G., Lerner, H., Gonik, B., & Goodwin, M. (2006). Shoulder dystocia: The unpreventable obstetric emergency with empiric management guidelines. *American Journal of Obstetrics and Gynecology, 195*(3), 657–672.

Gherman, R. B., Tramont, J., Muffley, P., & Goodwin, T. M. (2000). Analysis of McRoberts' maneuver by x-ray pelvimetry. *Obstetrics and Gynecology, 95*(1), 43–47.

Gifford, D. S., Morton, S. C., Fiske, M., Keesey, J., Keeler, E., & Kahn, K. L. (2000). Lack of progress as a reason for cesarean. *Obstetrics and Gynecology, 95*(4), 589–595.

Gilder, K., Mayberry, L. J., Gennaro, S., & Clemmens, D. (2002). Maternal positioning in labor with epidural analgesia: Results from a multi-site survey. *AWHONN Lifelines, 6*(1), 40–45.

Gilliam, M. (2006). Cesarean delivery on request: Reproductive consequences. *Seminars in Perinatology, 30*(5), 257–260

Glantz, J. C. (2005). Elective induction vs spontaneous labor: Associations and outcomes. *Journal of Reproductive Medicine, 50*(4), 235–240.

Goffinet, F., Fraser, W., Marcoux, S., Breart, G., Moutquin, J. M., & Darvis, M. (1997). Early amniotomy increases the frequency of fetal heart rate abnormalities: Amniotomy Study Group. *British Journal of Obstetrics and Gynaecology, 104* (5), 548–553.

Golay, J., Vedam, S., & Sorger, L. (1993). The squatting position for the second stage of labor: Effects on labor and on maternal and fetal well being. *Birth: Issues in Perinatal Care and Education 20*(2), 73–78.

Goldberg, A. B., Greenberg, M. B., & Darney, P. D. (2001). Misoprostol and pregnancy. *New England Journal of Medicine, 344*(1), 38–47.

Goni, S., Sawhney, H., & Gopalan, S. (1995). Oxytocin induction of labor: A comparison of 20- and 60-min dose increment levels. *International Journal of Gynaecology and Obstetrics, 48*(1), 31–36.

Green, L. A., & Froman, R. D. (1996). Blood pressure measurements during pregnancy: Auscultatory versus oscillatory methods. *Journal of Obstetric, Gynecologic and Neonatal Nursing, 25*(2), 155–159.

Gross, S. J., Shime, J., & Farine, D. (1987). Shoulder dystocia: Predictors and outcome. A five year review. *American Journal of Obstetrics and Gynecology, 156*(2), 334–336.

Grossman, G. L., Joesch, J. M., & Tanfer, K. (2006). Trends in maternal request cesarean delivery from 1991 to 2004. *Obstetrics and Gynecology, 108*(6), 1506–1516.

Grylack, L. J., Chu, S. S., & Scanlon, J. W. (1984). Use of intravenous fluids before cesarean section: Effects on perinatal glucose, insulin, and sodium homeostasis. *Obstetrics and Gynecology, 63*(5), 654–658.

Guise, J. M., Berlin, M., McDonagh, M., Osterwell, P., Chan, B., & Helfand, M. (2004). Safety of vaginal birth after cesarean: A systematic review. *Obstetrics and Gynecology, 103*(3), 420–429.

Gupta, J. K., & Hofmeyr, G. J. (2004). Position for women during second stage labour. *Cochrane Database of Systematic Reviews, 2*, CD002006.

Hadi, H. (2000). Cervical ripening and labor induction: Clinical guidelines. *Clinical Obstetrics and Gynecology, 43*(3),524–536.

Hagelin, A., & Leyon, J. (1998). The effect of labor on the acid-base status of the newborn. *Acta Obstetricia et Gynecologica Scandinavica, 77*(8), 841–844.

Halpern, S. H., Leighton, B. L., Ohlsson, A., Barrett, J. F., & Rice, A. (1998). Effect of epidural vs opioid analgesia on the progress of labor: A meta-analysis. *Journal of the American Medical Association, 280*(24), 2105–2110

Hamilton, B. E., Martin, J. A., & Ventura, S. J. (2006). Births: Preliminary data for 2005. *National Center for Health Statistics.* Retrieved December 24, 2006, from http://www.cdc.gov.nchs/products/pubs/pubd/hestats/prelimbirths05/prelimbirths05.html

Handa, V. L. (2006). Sexual function and childbirth. *Seminars in Perinatology, 30*(5), 253–256.

Handa, V. L., Harris, T. A., & Ostergard, D. R. (1996). Protecting the pelvic floor: Obstetric management to prevent incontinence and pelvic organ prolapse. *Obstetrics and Gynecology, 88*(3), 470–478.

Hankins, G. D. V. (1998). Lower thoracic spinal cord injury: A severe complication of shoulder dystocia. *American Journal of Perinatology, 15*(7), 443–444.

Hankins, G. D. V. (2006). Cesarean section on request at 39 weeks: Impact on shoulder dystocia, fetal trauma, neonatal encephalopathy, and intrauterine fetal demise. *Seminars in Perinatology, 30*(5), 276–287

Hansen, S. L., Clark, S. L., & Foster, J. C. (2002). Active pushing versus passive fetal descent in the second stage of labor: A randomized controlled trial. *Obstetrics and Gynecology, 99*(1), 29–34.

Hartmann, K., Viswanathan, M., Palmieri, R., Gartiehner, G., Thorp, J. Jr., & Lohr, K. N. (2005). Outcomes of routine episiotomy. *Journal of the American Medical Association, 293*(17), 2141–2148.

Hasan, M. A., Thomas, T. A., & Prys-Roberts, C. (1993). Comparison of automatic oscillometric arterial pressure measurement with conventional auscultatory measurement in the labour ward. *British Journal of Anaesthesia, 70*(2), 141–144.

Hawkins, J. L. (2003). Anesthesia-related mortality. *Clinical Obstetrics and Gynecology, 46*(3), 679–687.

HealthGrades. (2005). *Third annual report on "patient-choice" cesarean section rates in the United States*. Golden, CO: Author.

Heimstad, R., Dahloe, R., Laache, I., Skogvoll, E., & Schel, B. (2006). Fear of childbirth and history of abuse: Implications for labor and delivery. *Acta Obstetricia et Gynecologica Scandinavica, 85*(4), 435–440.

Hellman, L. M., & Prystowsky, H. (1952). The duration of the second stage of labor. *American Journal of Obstetrics and Gynecology, 63*(6), 1223–1233.

Hendler, I., & Bujold, E. (2004). Effect of prior vaginal delivery or prior vaginal birth after cesarean delivery on obstetric outcomes in women undergoing trial of labor. *Obstetrics and Gynecology, 104*(2), 2004.

Hendrix, N. W., & Chauhan, S. P. (2005). Cesarean delivery for nonreassuring fetal heart rate tracing. *Obstetrics and Gynecology Clinics of North America, 32*(4), 273–286.

Heritage, C. (1998). Working with childhood sexual abuse survivors during pregnancy, labor, and birth. *Journal of Obstetric, Gynecologic and Neonatal Nursing, 27*(6), 671–677.

Hibbard, J. U., Ismail, M. A., Wang, Y., Te, C., Karrison, T., & Ismail, M. A. (2001). Failed vaginal birth after cesarean section: How risky is it? I. Maternal morbidity. *American Journal of Obstetrics and Gynecology, 184*(7), 1365–1371.

Hicks, P. (2005). Systematic review of the risk of uterine rupture with the use of amnioinfusion after previous cesarean delivery, *Southern Medical Journal, 98*(4), 458–461.

Hobbins, D. (2004). Survivors of childhood sexual abuse: Implications for perinatal nursing care. *Journal of Obstetric, Gynecologic and Neonatal Nursing, 33*(4), 485–497.

Hodnett, E. D. (2002). Pain and women's satisfaction with the experience of childbirth: A systematic review. *American Journal of Obstetrics and Gynecology, 186*(5, Suppl.), S160–S172.

Hodnett, E. D., Gates, S., Hofmeyr, G. J., & Sakala, C. (2003). Continuous support for women during childbirth. *Cochrane Database of Systematic Reviews, 3*, CD003766.

Hodnett, E. D., Lowe, N. K., Hannah, M. E., Willan, A. R., Stevens, B., Weston, J. A. et al. for the Nursing Supportive Care in Labor Trial Group. (2002). Effectiveness of nurse providers of birth labor support in North American hospitals: A randomized controlled trial. *Journal of the American Medical Association, 288*(11), 1373–1281.

Hoffman, M. K., Sciscione, A., Srinivasana, J., Shackelford, P. D., & Ekbladh, L. (2004). Uterine rupture in patients with a prior cesarean delivery: The impact of cervical ripening. *American Journal of Obstetrics and Gynecology, 21*(4), 217–222.

Hoffman, M. K., Vahratian, A., Sciscione, A. C., Troendle, J. F., & Zhang, J. (2006). Comparison of labor progression between induced and noninduced multiparous women. *Obstetrics and Gynecology, 107*(5), 1029–1034.

Hofmeyr, G. J. (2003). Amnioinfusion for potential of suspected umbilical cord compression in labour. *Cochrane Database of Systematic Reviews, 2*, CD000013.

Hofmeyr, G. J. (2004). Prophylactic versus therapeutic amnioinfusion for oligohydramnios in labour. *Cochrane Database of Systematic Reviews, 2*, CD000176.

Hofmeyr, G. J., & Gulmezoglu, A. M. (2003). Vaginal misoprostol for cervical ripening and induction of labour. *Cochrane Database of Systematic Reviews, 1*, CD000941.

Horey, D., Weaver, J., & Russell, H. (2004). Information for pregnant women about caesarean birth. *Cochrane Database of Systematic Reviews 1*, CD003858.

Hourvitz, A., Alcalay, M., Korach, J., Lusky, A., Barkai, G., & Seidman, D.S. (1996). A prospective study of high- versus low-dose oxytocin for induction of labor. *Acta Obstetricia et Gynecologica Scandinavica, 75*(7), 636–641.

Hudelist, G., Gelle'n, J., Singer, C., Ruecklinger, E., Czerwenka, K., Kandolf, O., & Keckstein, J. (2005). Factors predicting severe perineal trauma during childbirth: Role of forceps delivery routinely combined with mediolateral episiotomy. *American Journal of Obstetrics and Gynecology, 192*(3), 875–881.

Hundley, V. A., Milne, J. M., Glazener, C. M. A., & Mollison, J. (1997). Satisfaction and the three C's: Continuity, choice and control: Women's views from a randomised controlled trial of midwife-led care. *British Journal of Obstetrics and Gynaecology, 104*(11), 1273–1280

Husslein, P., Fuchs, A. R., & Fuchs, F. (1981). Oxytocin and the initiation of human parturition 1, prostaglandin release during induction of labor by oxytocin. *American Journal of Obstetrics and Gynecology, 141*(6), 688–693.

Ifnan, F., & Jameel, M. B. (2006). Ripening of cervix for induction of labour by hydrostatic sweeping of the membranes versus Foley's catheter ballooning alone. *Journal of the College of Physicians and Surgeons—Pakistan, 16*(5), 347–350.

Jain, L., & Dudell, G. G. (2006). Respiratory transition in infants delivered by cesarean section. *Seminars in Perinatology, 30*(5), 296–304.

Janni, W., Schiessl, B., Peschers, U., Huber, S., Strobl, B., Hantschmann, P., et al. (2002). The prognostic impact of a prolonged second stage of labor on maternal and fetal outcome. *Acta Obstetricia et Gynecologica Scandinavica, 81*(3), 214–221.

Jauregui, I., Kirkendall, C., Ahn, M. O., & Phelan, J. (2000). Uterine rupture: A placentally mediated event? *Obstetrics and Gynecology, 95*(4 Suppl. 1), S75.

Johnson, C., Oriol, N., & Flood, K. (1991). Trial of labor: A study of 110 patients. *Journal of Clinical Anesthesiology, 3*(3), 216–218.

Johnson, J. H., Figueroa, R., Garry, D., Elimian, A., & Maulik, D. (2004). Immediate maternal and neonatal effects of forceps and vacuum-assisted deliveries. *Obstetrics and Gynecology, 103*(3), 513–518.

Joint Commission on Accreditation of Healthcare Organizations (2003). *Universal protocol for preventing wrong site, wrong procedure, and wrong persons surgery*. Oakbrook Terrace, IL: Author.

Joint Commission on Accreditation of Healthcare Organizations (2004a). *Preventing and managing the impact of anesthesia awareness* (Sentinel Alert No. 32). Oakbrook Terrace, IL: Author.

Joint Commission on Accreditation of Healthcare Organizations. (2004b). *Preventing infant death and injury during delivery* (Sentinel Event Alert No. 30). Oakbrook Terrace, IL: Author.

Joint Commission on Accreditation of Healthcare Organizations (2007a). *Comprehensive accreditation manual for hospitals*. Oakbrook Terrace, IL: Author.

Joint Commission on Accreditation of Healthcare Organizations (2007b). *Patient safety goals*. Oakbrook Terrace, IL: Author.

Kashanian, M., Akbarian, A., Baradaran, H., & Samiee, M. M. (2006). Effect of membrane sweeping at term pregnancy on duration of pregnancy and labor induction: A randomized trial. *Gynecologic and Obstetric Investigation, 62*(1), 41–44.

Kaul, B., Vallejo, M. C., Ramanathan, S., Mandell, G., Phelps, A. L., & Daftary, A. R. (2004). Induction of labor with oxytocin increases cesarean section rate as compared with oxytocin for augmentation of spontaneous labor in nulliparous parturients controlled for lumbar epidural analgesia. *Journal of Clinical Anesthesia, 16*(6), 411–414.

Kazandi, M., Sendag, R., Akercan, F., Terek, M. C., & Gundem, G. (2003). Different type of variable decelerations and their effects to neonatal outcomes. *Singapore Medical Journal, 44*(5), 243–247.

Keirse, M. J. (1993). A final comment. Managing the uterus, the woman or whom? *Birth, 20*(3), 159–161.

Keirse, M. J. N. C. (2006). Natural prostaglandins for induction of labor and preinduction cervical ripening. *Clinical Obstetrics and Gynecology, 49*(3), 609–626.

Kelly, A. J., Kavanagh, J., & Thomas, J. (2001). Castor oil, bath and/or enema for cervical ripening and induction of labor. *Cochrane Database of Systematic Reviews, 2*, CD003099.

Kelly, A. J., & Tan, B. (2001). Intravenous oxytocin alone for cervical ripening and induction of labour. *Cochrane Database of Systematic Reviews, 3*, CD003246.

Keppler, A. B. (1988). The use of intravenous fluids during labor. *Birth, 15*(2), 75–79.

Khabbaz, A. Y., Usta, I. M., El-Hajj, M. I., Abu-Musa, A., Seoud, M., & Nassar, A. H. (2001). Rupture of an unscarred uterus with misoprostol induction: Case report and review of the literature. *Journal of Maternal-Fetal and Neonatal Medicine, 10*(2), 141–145.

Kirby, R. S. (2004). Trends in labor induction in the United States: Is it true that what goes up must come down? *Birth, 31*(2), 148–151.

Kirby, R. S., & Hamisu, M. S. (2006). Back to the future? A critical commentary on the 2003 U.S. national standard certificate of live birth. *Birth, 33*(3), 238–244.

Kirkendall, C., Jauregui, I., Kim, J. O., & Phelan, J. (2000). Catastrophic uterine rupture: Maternal and fetal characteristics. *Obstetrics and Gynecology, 95*(4 Suppl.), S74.

Kitzinger, J. (1990). Recalling the pain: Medical procedures can bring back memories of sexual violence. *Nursing Times, 86*(3), 8–40.

Kitzinger, S., Green, J. M., Chalmers, B., Keirse, M., Lindstrom, K., & Hemminki, E. (2006). Why do women go along with this stuff? *Birth, 33*(2), 154–158.

Klaus, M. H., Kennel, J. H., McGrath, S., Robertson S. S., & Hinkley, C. (1988). Medical intervention: The effect of social support during labor. *Pediatric Research, 23*(4), 211A. (Part 2 abstract).

Klaus, M. H., Kennel, J. H., Robertson, S. S., & Sosa, R. (1986). Effects of social support during parturition and maternal and infant morbidity. *British Medical Journal, 293*(6547), 585–587.

Klein, M. C., Sakala, C., Simkin, P., Davis-Floyd, R., Rooks, J. P., & Pincus, J. (2006). Why do women go along with this stuff? *Birth, 33*(3), 245–250.

Klingner, M. C., & Kruse, J. (1999). Meconium aspiration syndrome: Pathophysiology and prevention. *Journal of the American Board of Family Practice, 12*(6), 450–466.

Koger, K., Shatney, Hodge, K., & McClenathan, J. (1993). Surgical scar endometrioma. *Surgery, Gynecology, and Obstetrics, 177*(3), 243–246.

Kolas, T., Suagstad, O. D., Daltveit, A. K., Nilsen, S. T., & Oian, P. (2006). Planned cesarean versus planned vaginal delivery at term: Comparison of newborn infant outcomes. *American Journal of Obstetrics and Gynecology, 195*(6), 1538–1543.

Kozak, L. J., Lees, K. A., & DeFrances, C. J. (2006). National hospital discharge survey: 2003 annual summary with detailed diagnoses and hospital procedure data. *Vital Health Statistics, 13*(160), 1–215.

Kudish, B., Blackwell, S., Mcneely, S. G., Bujold, E., Kruger, M., Hendrix, S. L., & Sokol, R. (2006). Operative vaginal delivery and midline episiotomy: A bad combination for the perineum. *American Journal of Obstetrics and Gynecology, 195*(3), 749–754.

Kwek, K., & Yeo, G. S. H. (2006). Shoulder dystocia and injuries: Prevention and management. *Current Opinion in Obstetrics and Gynecology, 18*(2), 123–128.

Labrecque, M., Eason, E., Marcoux, S., Lemieux, F., Pinault, J. J., Feldman, P., & Laperriere, L. (1999). Randomized controlled trial of prevention of perineal trauma by perineal massage during pregnancy. *American Journal of Obstetrics and Gynecology, 180*(3, Pt. 1), 593–600.

Labrecque, M., Eason, E., & Marcoux, S. (2000). Randomized trial of perineal massage during pregnancy: Perineal symptoms three months after delivery. *American Journal of Obstetrics and Gynecology, 182*(1, Pt. 1), 76–80.

Landon, M. B., Hauth, J. C., Leveno, K. J., Spong, C. Y., Leindecker, S., Varner, M. W., et al. (2004). Maternal and perinatal outcomes associated with a trial of labor after prior cesarean delivery. *New England Journal of Medicine, 351*(25), 2581–2589.

Landon, M. B., Leindecker, S., Spong, C. Y., Hauth, J. C., Bloom, S., Varner, M. W., et al. (2005). The MFMU cesarean delivery registry: Factors affecting the success of a trial of labor after previous cesarean delivery. *American Journal of Obstetrics and Gynecology, 193*(3, Pt. 2), 1016–1023.

Langer, B., Carbonne, B., Goffinet, F., Le Goueff, F., Berkane, N., & Laville, M. (1997). Fetal pulse oximetry and fetal heart rate monitoring during stage II of labour. *European Journal of Obstetrics and Gynecology, 72*(Suppl. 1), S57–S61.

Lavender, T., Hofmeyr, G. J., Neilson, J. P., Kingdom, C., & Gyte, G. M. (2006). Caesarean section for non-medical reasons at term. *Cochrane Database of Systematic Reviews, 19*(3), CD004660

Lazor, L. Z., Philipson, E. H., Ingardia, C. J., Kobetitsch, E. S., & Curry, S. L. (1993). A randomized comparison of 15- and 40-minute dosing protocols for labor augmentation and induction. *Obstetrics and Gynecology, 82*(6), 1009–1012.

Lederman, R. P., Lederman, E., Work, B., & McCann, D. S. (1985). Anxiety and epinephrine in multiparous women in labor: Relationship to duration of labor and fetal heart rate pattern. *American Journal of Obstetrics and Gynecology, 153*(8), 870–877.

Lee, W. K., Baggish, M. S., & Lashgari, M. (1978). Acute inversion of the uterus. *Obstetrics and Gynecology, 51*(2), 144–147.

Leung, A., Farmer, R. M., Leung, E. K., Medearis, A. L., & Paul, R. H. (1993). Risk factors associated with uterine rupture during trial of labor after cesarean birth: A case control study. *American Journal of Obstetrics and Gynecology, 168*(5), 1358–1363.

Leung, A., Leung, E., & Paul, R. (1993). Uterine rupture after previous cesarean delivery: Maternal and fetal consequences. *American Journal of Obstetrics and Gynecology, 169*(4), 945–950.

Liao, J. B., Buhimschi, C. S., & Norwitz, E. R. (2005). Normal labor: Mechanism and duration. *Obstetrics and Gynecology Clinics of North America, 32*(2), 145–164.

Lieberman, E. (2001). Risk factors for uterine rupture during a trial of labor after cesarean. *Clinical Obstetrics and Gynecology, 44*(3), 609–621.

Lin, M. G., & Rouse, D. J. (2006). What is a failed labor induction? *Clinical Obstetrics and Gynecology, 49*(3), 585–593.

Liu, S., Heaman, M., Joseph, K. S., Liston, R. M., Huang, L., Sauve, R., et al. (2005). Risk of maternal postpartum readmission associated with mode of delivery. *Obstetrics and Gynecology, 105*(4), 836–842.

Liu, S., Heaman, M., Kramer, M. S., Demissie, K., Wen, S. W., & Marcoux, S. (2002). *American Journal of Obstetrics and Gynecology, 187*(3), 681–687.

Liu, Y. C. (1989). The effects of the upright position during childbirth. *Image, The Journal of Nursing Scholarship, 21*(1), 14–18.

Lopez-Zeno, J. A., Peaceman, A. M., Adashek, J. A., & Socol, M. L. (1992). A controlled trial of a program for the active management of labor. *New England Journal of Medicine, 326*(7), 450–454.

Lothian, J. (2006). Birth plans: The good, the bad, and the future. *Journal of Obstetric, Gynecologic and Neonatal Nursing, 35*(2), 295–303.

Low, L, K., Seng, J. S., Murtland, T. L., & Oakley, D. (2000). Clinician-specific episiotomy rates: Impacts on perineal outcomes. *Journal of Nurse Midwifery and Women's Health, 43*(2), 87–93.

Ludka, L., & Roberts, C. (1993). Eating and drinking in labor: A literature review. *Journal of Nurse Midwifery, 38*(4), 199–207.

Lupe, P. J., & Gross, T. L. (1986). Maternal upright posture and mobility in labor: A review. *Obstetrics and Gynecology, 67*(5), 727–734.

Luppi, C. J. (2002). Should ECG monitoring during the postanesthesia period be the standard of care for all women who have cesarean birth? *MCN The American Journal of Maternal Child Nursing, 27*(4), 218.

Lydon-Rochelle, M., Holt, V. L., Easterling, T. R., & Martin, D. P. (2001). Risk of uterine rupture during labor among women with a prior cesarean delivery. *New England Journal of Medicine, 345*(1), 3–8.

Lydon-Rochelle, M., Holt, V. L., Easterling, T. R., & Martin, D. P. (2001). First-birth cesarean and placental abruption or previa at second birth. *Obstetrics and Gynecology, 97*(5, Pt. 1), 765–769.

Lydon-Rochelle, M., Holt, V. L., Martin, D. P., & Easterling, T. R. (2000). Association between method of delivery and maternal rehospitalization. *Journal of the American Medical Association, 283*(18), 2411–2416.

Macarthur, A. J., & Macarthur, C. (2004). Incidence, severity, and determinants of perineal pain after vaginal delivery: A prospective cohort study. *American Journal of Obstetrics and Gynecology, 191*(4), 1199–1204.

MacDorman, M. F., Declercq, E., Menacker, F., & Malloy, M. H. (2006). Infant and neonatal mortality for primary cesarean and vaginal births to women with "no indicated risk", United States, 1998-2001 birth cohorts. *Birth, 33*(3), 175–182.

MacKinnon, K., McIntyre, M., & Quance, M. (2005). The meaning of the nurse's presence during childbirth. *Journal of Obstetric, Gynecologic and Neonatal Nursing, 34*(1), 28–36.

Macones, G. A., Cahill, A., Pare, E., Stamilio, D. M., Ratcliffe, S., Stevens, E., et al. (2005). Obstetric outcomes in women after two prior cesarean deliveries: Is vaginal birth after cesarean delivery a viable option? *American Journal of Obstetrics and Gynecology, 192*(4), 1223–1229.

Macones, G. A., Peipert, J., Nelson, D. B., Odibo, A., Stevens, E., Stamilio, D., et al. (2005). Maternal complications after vaginal birth after cesarean delivery: A multicenter study. *American Journal of Obstetrics and Gynecology, 193*(5), 1656–1662.

Malone, F., Geary, M., Chelmow, D., Stronge, J., Boylan, P., & D'Alton, M. E. (1996). Prolonged labor in nulliparas. Lessons from the active management of labor. *Obstetrics and Gynecology. 88*(2), 211–215.

Manning, J. (1996). Intrathecal narcotic: New approach for labor analgesia. *Journal of Obstetric, Gynecologic, and Neonatal Nursing, 25*(3), 221–224.

Maresh, M., Choong, K. H., & Bead, R. W. (1983). Delayed pushing with lumbar epidural analgesia in labour. *British Journal of Obstetrics and Gynaecology, 90*(7), 623–627.

Martin, J. A., Hamilton, B. E., Sutton, P. D., Ventura, S. J., Menacker, F., & Kirmeyer, S. (2006). Births: Final data for 2004. *National Vital Statistics Reports, 55*(1), 1–102.

Marx, G. F., Schwalbe, S. S., Cho, E., & Whitty, J. E. (1993). Automatic blood pressure measurements in laboring women: Are they reliable? *American Journal of Obstetrics and Gynecology, 168*(3, Pt. 1), 796–798.

Mastrobattista, J. M. (1999). Vaginal birth after cesarean delivery. *Obstetrics and Gynecology Clinics of North America, 26*(2), 295–304.

Matthews, R., & Callister, L. C. (2004). Childbearing women's perceptions of nursing care that promotes dignity. *Journal of Obstetric, Gynecologic and Neonatal Nursing, 33*(4), 498–507.

Maul, H., Macray, L., & Garfield, R. E. (2006). Cervical ripening: Biochemical, molecular, and clinical considerations. *Clinical Obstetrics and Gynecology, 49*(3), 551–563.

Mauldin, J. G., & Newman, R. B. (2006). Prior cesarean: A contraindication to labor induction? *Clinical Obstetrics and Gynecology, 49*(3), 684–697.

Mayberry, L. J., Hammer, R., Kelly, C., True-Driver, B., & De, A. (1999). Use of delayed pushing with epidural anesthesia: Findings from a randomized controlled trial. *Journal of Perinatology, 19*(1), 26–30.

Mayberry, L. J., Strange, L. B., Suplee, P. D., & Gennaro, S. (2003). Use of upright positioning with epidural analgesia: Findings from

an observational study. *MCN The American Journal of Maternal Child Nursing, 28*(3), 152–159.

Mayerhofer, K., Bodner-Adler, B., Bodner, K., Rabl, M., Kaider, A., Wagenbichler, P., et al. (2002). Traditional care of the perineum during birth: A prospective, randomized, multicenter study of 1,076 women. *Journal of Reproductive Medicine, 47*(6), 477–482.

Mazzone, M. E., & Woolever, J. (2006). Uterine rupture in a patient with an unscarred uterus: A case study. *Wisconsin Medical Journal, 105*(2), 64–66.

Mazzouni, C., Porcu, G., Bretell, F., Loundou, A., Heckenroth, H., & Gamerre, M. (2006). Risk factors for forceps delivery in nulliparous patients. *Acta Obstetricia et Gynecologica Scandinavica, 85*(3), 298–301.

McGuinness, M., Norr, K., & Nacion, K. (1991). Comparison between different perineal outcomes on tissue healing. *Journal of Nurse-Midwifery, 36*(3), 192–198.

McKay, S., & Smith, S.Y. (1983). What are they talking about? Is something wrong? Information sharing during the second stage of labor. *Birth: Issues in Perinatal Care and Education, 20*(3), 142–147.

Mendiola, J., Grylack, L. J., & Scanton, J. W., (1982). Effects of intrapartum maternal glucose infusion on the normal fetus and newborn. *Anesthesia and Analgesia, 61*(1), 32–35.

Menacker, F. (2005). Trends in cesarean rates for first births and repeat cesarean rates for low-risk women: United States, 1990-2003. *National Vital Statistics Reports, 54*(2), 1–9

Menacker, F., Declercq, E., & Macdorman, M. F. (2006). Cesarean delivery: Background, trends, and epidemiology. *Seminars in Perinatology, 30*(5), 235–241.

Mendelson, C. L. (1946). The aspiration of stomach contents into the lungs during obstetric anesthesia. *American Journal of Obstetrics and Gynecology, 52*, 191–205.

Mengert, W., & Murphy, D. (1933). Intra-abdominal pressures created by voluntary muscular effort. *Surgery and Gynecologic Obstetrics, 57*, 745–751.

Menihan, C. A. (1999). The effect of uterine rupture on fetal heart rate patterns. *Journal of Nurse Midwifery, 44*(1), 40–46.

Mercer, B., Pilgrim, P., & Sibai, B. (1991). Labor induction with continuous low-dose oxytocin infusion: A randomized trial. *Obstetrics and Gynecology, 77*(5), 659–663.

Merhi, Z. O., & Awonuga, A. O. (2005). The role of uterine fundal pressure in the management of the second stage of labor: A reappraisal. *Obstetrical and Gynecological Survey, 60*(9), 559–603.

Merrill, D. C., & Zlatnik, F. J. (1999). Randomized, double-masked comparison of oxytocin dosage in induction and augmentation of labor. *Obstetrics and Gynecology, 94*(3), 455–463.

Menticoglou, S. M., Manning, F., Harman, C., & Morrison, I. (1995). Perinatal outcome in relation to second-stage duration. *American Journal of Obstetrics and Gynecology, 173*(3), 906–912.

Mikiel-Kostyra, K., Boltruszko, I., Mazur, J., & Sielenska, M. (2001). Skin-to-skin contact after birth as a factor determining breastfeeding duration. *Medycyna Wieku Rozwojowego, 5*(2), 179–189.

Mikiel-Kostyra, K., Mazur, J., & Boltruszko, I. (2002). Effect of early skin-to-skin contact after delivery on duration of breastfeeding: A prospective cohort study. *Acta Paediatrica, 91*(12), 1301–1306.

Minkoff, H. (2006). The ethics of cesarean section by choice. *Seminars in Perinatology, 30*(5), 309–312.

Minkoff, H., Powederly, K. R., Chervenak, F., & McCullough, L. B. (2004), Ethical dimensions of elective primary cesarean delivery. *Obstetrics and Gynecology, 103*(2), 387–392.

Mino, M., Puertas, A., Miranda, J. A., & Herruzo, A. J. (1999). Amnioinfusion in term labor with low amniotic fluid due to rupture of membranes: A new indication. *European Journal of Obstetrics, Gynecology, and Reproductive Biology, 82*(1), 29–34.

Mitchell, M. D., Flint, A. P., Bibby, J., Brunt, J., Arnold, J. M., Anderson, A. B., et al. (1977). Rapid increases in plasma prostaglandin concentrations after vaginal examinations and amniotomy. *British Medical Journal, 2*(6096), 1183–1185.

Miyazaki, F. (1985). Saline amnioinfusion for relief of repetitive variable decelerations: A prospective randomized study. *American Journal of Obstetrics and Gynecology, 153*(3), 301–306.

Mizuno, K., Mizuno, N., Shinohara, T., & Noda, M. (2004). Mother-infant skin-to-skin contact after delivery results in early recognition of own mother's mild odor. *Acta Paediatrica, 93*(12), 1640–1645.

Mollberg, M., Hagberg, H., Bager, B., Lilja, H., & Ladfors, L. (2005). Risk factors for obstetric brachial palsy among neonates delivered by vacuum extraction. *Obstetrics and Gynecology, 106*(5, Pt. 1), 913–918.

Moon, J. M., Smith, C. V., & Rayburn, W. F. (1990). Perinatal outcome after a prolonged second stage of labor. *Journal of Reproductive Medicine, 35*(3), 229–231.

Moore, L. E., & Rayburn, W. F. (2006). Elective induction of labor. *Clinical Obstetrics and Gynecology, 49*(3), 698–704.

Muller, P. R., Stubbs, T. M., & Laurent, S. L. (1992). A prospective randomized clinical trial comparing two oxytocin induction protocols. *American Journal of Obstetrics and Gynecology, 167*(2), 373–380.

Murphy, D. J. (2006). Uterine rupture. *Current Opinion in Obstetrics and Gynecology, 18*(2), 135–140.

Murray, M. M. (2004). Maternal or fetal heart rate? Avoiding intrapartum misidentification. *Journal of Obstetric, Gynecologic, and Neonatal Nursing, 33*(1), 93–104.

Myles, T. D., & Santolaya, J. (2003). Maternal and neonatal outcomes in patients with a prolonged second stage labor. *Obstetrics and Gynecology, 102*(1), 52–58.

Mynaugh, P. A. (1991). A randomized study of two methods of teaching perineal massage: Effects on practice rates, episiotomy rates, and lacerations. *Birth: Issues in Perinatal Care and Education, 18*(3), 153–159.

Mzurek, T., Mikieil-Kostyra, K., Mazur, J., & Wieczorek, P. (1999). Influence of immediate newborn care on infant adaptation to the environment. *Medycyna Wieku Rozwojowego, 3*(2), 215–224.

Natarajan, P., Shennan, A. H., Penny, J., Halligan, A. W., de Swiet, M., & Anthony, J. (1999). Comparison of auscultatory and oscillometric automatic blood pressure monitors in the setting of preeclampsia. *American Journal of Obstetrics and Gynecology, 181*(5, Pt. 1), 1203–1210.

Nathanielsz, P. W. (1998). Comparison studies on the initiation of labor. *European Journal of Obstetrics, Gynecology and Reproductive Biology, 78*(2), 127–132.

National Institute of Child Health and Human Development. (2005). *Optimizing care and long-term outcomes of near-term pregnancy and near-term newborn infants.* Bethesda, MD: Author.

National Institutes of Health. (2006). *State of the science conference statement: Cesarean delivery on maternal request.* Bethesda, MD: Author.

Nesbitt, T. S., Gilbert, W. M., & Herrchen, B. (1998). Shoulder dystocia and associated risk factors with macrosomic infants born in California. *American Journal of Obstetrics and Gynecology, 179*(2), 476–480.

Ness, A., Goldberg, J., & Berghella, V. (2005). Abnormalities of the first and second stages of labor. *Obstetrics and Gynecology Clinics of North America, 32*(2), 201–220.

Newman, R. B. (2005). Uterine contraction assessment. *Obstetrics and Gynecology Clinics of North America, 32*(3), 341–367.

Nielsen, P. E., Goldman, M. B., Mann, S., Shapiro, D. E., Marcus, R. G., Pratt, S. D., et al. (2007). Effects of teamwork training on adverse outcomes and process of care in labor and delivery: A randomized controlled trial. *Obstetrics and Gynecology, 109*(1), 48–55.

Noble, E. (1981). Controversies in maternal effort during labor and delivery. *Journal of Nurse Midwifery, 26*(2), 13–22.

Norbeck, J. S., & Anderson, N. J. (1989). Psychosocial predictors of pregnancy outcomes in low-income black, hispanic, and white women. *Nursing Research, 38*(4), 204–209.

Norwitz, E. R., Robinson, J. N., & Repke, J. T. (2002). Labor and birth. In S. G. Gabbe, J. J. R. Niebyl, & J. L. Simpson (Eds.), *Obstetrics: Normal and problem pregnancies* (4th ed., pp. 353–394). New York: Churchill Livingstone.

Nygaard, I. (2006). Urinary incontinence: Is cesarean delivery protective? *Seminars in Perinatology, 30*(5), 267–271.

O'Brien-Abel, N. (2003). Uterine rupture during VBAC trial of labor: Risk factors and fetal response. *Journal of Midwifery and Women's Health, 48*(4), 249–257.

O'Driscoll, K. (1996). Active management of labor: True purpose has been misunderstood. *British Medical Journal, 309*(6960), 1015.

O'Driscoll, K., Foley, M., & MacDonald, D. (1984). Active management of labor as an alternative to cesarean section for dystocia. *Obstetrics and Gynecology, 63*(4), 485–490.

O'Driscoll, K., Jackson, R. J., & Gallagher, J. T. (1969). Prevention of prolonged labour. *British Medical Journal, 2*(655), 477–480.

O'Driscoll, K., Jackson, R. J., & Gallagher, J. T. (1970). Active management of labour and cephalopelvic disproportion. *Journal of Obstetrics and Gynaecology of the British Commonwealth, 77*(5), 385–389.

O'Grady, J. P., Gimovsky, M. L., & McIlhargie, C. J. (1995). *Vacuum extraction in modern obstetric practice.* New York: The Parthenon Publishing Group.

Ogunyemi, G., Manigat, B., Marquis, J., & Bazargan, M. (2006). Demographic variations and clinical associations of episiotomy and severe perineal lacerations in vaginal delivery. *Journal of the National Medical Association, 98*(11), 1874–1881.

Olah, K.S., & Gee, H. (1996). The active mismanagement of labour. *British Journal of Obstetrics and Gynaecology, 103*(8), 729–731.

Olofsson, C., Ekblom, A., Ekman-Ordeberg, G., & Irestedt, L. (1998). Obstetric outcome following epidural analgesia with bupivacaine-adrenaline 0.25% or bupivacaine 0.125% with sufentanil: A prospective randomized controlled study in 1000 parturients. *Acta Anaesthesiologica Scandanavia, 42*(3), 284–292.

Orhue, A. A. (1993a). A randomized trial of 30-min and 15 min oxytocin infusion regime for induction of labor at term for women of low parity. *International Journal of Gynaecology and Obstetrics, 40*(3), 219–225.

Orhue, A. A. (1993b). A randomized trial of 45-minutes and 15 minutes incremental oxytocin infusion regimes for the induction of labour in women of high parity. *British Journal of Obstetrics and Gynaecology, 100*(1), 126–129.

Orhue, A. A. (1994). Incremental increases in oxytocin infusion regimens for induction of labor at term in primigravidas: A randomized controlled trial. *Obstetrics and Gynecology, 83*(2), 229–233.

Ouzounian, J. G., Korst, L. M., Ahn, M. O., & Phelan, J. P. (1998). Shoulder dystocia and neonatal brain injury: Significance of the head –shoulder interval. *American Journal of Obstetrics and Gynecology, 178*(Suppl. 1), S76.

Ouzounian, J. G., Miller, D. A., & Paul, R. H. (1996). Amnioinfusion in women with previous cesarean births: A preliminary report. *American Journal of Obstetrics and Gynecology, 174*(2), 783–786.

Paluska, S. A. (1997). Vacuum-assisted vaginal delivery. *American Family Physician, 55*(6), 2197–2203.

Pare, E., Quinones, J. N., & Macones, G. A. (2006). Vaginal birth after cesarean section versus elective repeat cesarean section: Assessment of maternal downstream health outcomes. *British Journal of Obstetrics and Gynaecology, 113*(1), 75–85.

Parer, J. T., King, T., Flanders, S., Fox, M., & Kilpatrick, S. J. (2006). Fetal acidemia and electronic fetal heart rate patterns: Is there evidence of an association? *Journal of Maternal-Fetal and Neonatal Medicine, 19*(5), 289–294.

Parnell, C., Langhoff-Roos, J., Iverson, R., & Damgaard, P. (1993). Pushing method in the explusive phase of labor: A randomized trial. *Acta Obstetricia et Gynecologica Scandinavica, 72*(1), 31–35.

Parsons, M., Bidewell, J., & Nagy, S. (2006). Natural eating behavior in latent labor and its effect on outcomes in active labor. *Journal of Midwifery and Women's Health, 51*(1), e1–e6.

Pascoe, J. M. (1993). Social support during labor and duration of labor: A community based study. *Public Health Nursing, 10*(2), 97–99.

Paterson, C. M., Saunders, N. S., & Wadsworth, J. (1992). The characteristics of the second stage of labor in 25,069 singleton deliveries in the North West Thames Health Region, 1988. *British Journal of Obstetrics and Gynaecology, 99*(5), 377–380.

Pates, J. A., & Satin, A. J. (2005). Active management of labor. *Obstetrics and Gynecology Clinics of North America, 32*(2), 221–230.

Peaceman, A. M., Gersnoviez, R., Landon, M. B., Spong, C. Y., Leveno, K. J., Varner, M. W., et al. (2006). The MFMU cesarean registry: Impact of fetal size on trial of labor success for patients with previous cesarean for dystocia. *American Journal of Obstetrics and Gynecology, 195*(4), 1127–1131.

Peleg, D., Kennedy, C. M., Merrill, D., & Zlatnik, F. J. (1999). Risk of repetition of a severe perineal laceration. *Obstetrics and Gynecology, 93*(6), 1021–1024.

Perez, P. G. (2005). Birth plans: Are they really necessary? *MCN The American Journal of Maternal Child Nursing, 30*(5), 288.

Phelan, J. P., Ouzounian, J. G., Gherman, R. B., Korst, L. M., & Goodwin, M. (1997). Shoulder dystocia and permanent Erb's palsy: The role of fundal pressure. *American Journal of Obstetrics and Gynecology, 176*(Suppl. 1), S138.

Phaneuf, S., Asboth, G., Carrasco, M. P., Rodriguez Linares, B., Kimura, T., Harris, A., & Lopez-Bernal, A. (1998). Desensitization of oxytocin receptors in human myometrium. *Human Reproduction Update, 4*(5), 625–633.

Phaneuf, S., Rodriguez Linares, B., Tambyraja R. L., MacKenzie, I. Z., & Lopez Bernal, A. (2000). Loss of myometrial oxytocin receptors during oxytocin-induced and oxytocin-augmented labour. *Journal of Reproduction and Fertility, 120*(1), 91–97.

Philipson, E. H., Kalihan, S. C., Riha, M. M., & Pimental, R. (1987). Effects of maternal glucose infusion on fetal acid-base status in human pregnancy. *American Journal of Obstetrics and Gynecology, 157*(4, Pt. 1), 866–873.

Phillips, K. C., & Thomas, T. A. (1983). Second stage of labour with or without extradural analgesia. *Anaesthesia, 38*(10), 972–976.

Pierce, J., Gaudier, F. L., & Sanchez-Ramos, L. (2000). Intrapartum amnioinfusion for meconium-stained fluid: Meta-analysis of prospective clinical trials. *Obstetrics and Gynecology, 95*(6, Pt. 2), 1051–1556.

Piquard, F., Schaefer, A., Hsiung, R., Dellenbach, P., & Haberey, P. (1989). Are there two biological parts in the second stage of labor? *Acta Obstetricia et Gynecologica Scandinavica, 68*(8), 713–718.

Pomini, F., Scavo, M., Ferrazzani, S., DeCarolis, S., Caruso, A., & Mancuso, S. (2001). There is poor agreement between manual auscultatory and automatic oscillometric methods for the measurement of blood pressure in normotensive pregnant women. *Journal of Maternal-Fetal Medicine. 10*(6), 398–403.

Raja, T. N. K., Higgins, R. D., Stark, A. R., & Leveno, K. J. (2006). Optimizing care and outcomes for late preterm (near-term) infants: A summary of the workshop sponsored by the National Institute of Child Health and Human Development. *Pediatrics, 118*(3), 1207–1214.

Ragnar, I., Altman, D., Tyden, T., & Olsson, S. E. (2006). Comparison of the maternal experience and duration of labour in two upright delivery positions: A randomised controlled trial. *British Journal of Obstetrics and Gynaecology, 113*(2), 165–170.

Ramsey, P. S., Ramin, K. D., & Ramin, S. M. (2000). Labor induction. *Current Opinion in Obstetrics and Gynecology, 12*(6), 463–473.

Raskin, K. S., Dachauer, J. D., Doeden, A. L., & Rayburn, W. F. (1999). Uterine rupture after use of a prostaglandin E2 vaginal insert during vaginal birth after cesarean. *Journal of Reproductive Medicine, 44*(6), 571–574.

Rayburn, W. F., Records, J., & Swanson, K. (1996, November). Prelabor cervical ripening with Prostaglandin E₂ gel and other agents. *Hospital Pharmacist Report* (Suppl.), 1–12.

Rayburn, W. F., Tassone, S., & Pearman, C. (2000). Is Cervidil appropriate for outpatient cervical ripening? *Obstetrics and Gynecology, 95*(Suppl. 4), S63.

Rayburn, W. F., & Zhang, J. (2002). Rising rates of labor induction: Present concerns and future strategies. *Obstetrics and Gynecology, 100*(1), 164–167.

Renfrew, M. J., Hannah, W., Albers, L., & Floyd, E. (1998). Practices that minimize trauma to the genital tract in childbirth: A systematic review of the literature. *Birth: Issues in Perinatal Care and Education, 25*(3), 143–160.

Renfrew, M. J., Lang, S., & Woolbridge, M. W. (2000). Early versus delayed initiation of breastfeeding. *Cochrane Database of Systematic Reviews, 2,* CD000043.

Rhodes, N., & Hutchinson, S. (1984). Labor experiences of childhood sexual abuse survivors. *Birth, 21*(4), 213–220.

Richter, H. E. (2006). Cesarean delivery on maternal request versus planned vaginal delivery: Impact on development of pelvic organ prolapse. *Seminars in Perinatology, 30*(5), 272–275.

Ridgeway, J. J., Weyrich, D. L., & Benedetti, T. J. (2004). Fetal heart rate changes associated with uterine rupture. *Obstetrics and Gynecology, 103*(3), 506–512.

Roberts, C. L., Algert, C. S., Cameron, C. A., & Torvaldsen, S. (2005). A meta-analysis of upright positions in the second stage of labor to reduce instrumental deliveries in women with epidural anesthesia. *Acta Obstetricia et Gynecologica Scandinavica, 84*(8), 794–798.

Roberts, C. L., Torvaldsen, S., Cameron, C. A., & Olive, E. (2004). Delayed versus early pushing in women with epidural analgesia: A systematic review and meta-analysis. British *Journal of Obstetrics and Gynaecology, 111*(12), 1333–1340.

Roberts, J. E. (2002). The "push" for evidence: Management of the second stage. *Journal of Midwifery and Women's Health, 47*(1), 2–15.

Roberts, J. E. (2003). A new understanding of the second stage of labor: Implications for nursing care. *Journal of Obstetric, Gynecologic, and Neonatal Nursing, 32*(6), 794–801.

Roberts, J. E., Goldstein, S. A., Gruener, J. S., Maggio, M., & Mendez-Bauer, C. (1987). A descriptive analysis of involuntary bearing-down efforts during the expulsive phase of labor. *Journal of Obstetric, Gynecologic, and Neonatal Nursing, 16*(1), 48–55.

Roberts, J., & Woolley, D. (1996). A second look at the second stage of labor. *Journal of Obstetric, Gynecologic, and Neonatal Nursing, 25*(5), 415–423.

Robinson, C., Schumann, R., Zhang, P., & Young, R. C. (2003). Oxytocin-induced desensitization of the oxytocin receptor. *American Journal of Obstetrics and Gynecology, 188*(2), 497–502.

Rochelson, B., Pagano, M., Conetta, L., Goldman, B., Vohra, N., Frey, M., et al. (2005). Previous preterm cesarean delivery: Identification of a new risk factor for uterine rupture in VBAC candidates. *Journal of Maternal-Fetal and Neonatal Medicine, 18*(5), 339–342.

Roemer, V. M., & Heger-Romermann, G. (1993). Clinic structure and timely management of emergency cesarean section—reference values and recommendations. *Zeitschrift fur Geburtshilfe und Perinatologie, 197*(4), 153–161.

Rogers, R., Gilson, G. J., Miller, A. C., Izquierdo, L. E, Curet, L. B., & Qualls, C. R. (1997). Active management of labor: Does it make a difference? *American Journal of Obstetrics and Gynecology, 177*(3), 599–605.

Rogers, S. O. Jr., Gawande, A. A., Kwaan, M., Puopolo, A. L., Yoon, C., Brennan, T. A., et al. (2006). Analysis of surgical errors in closed malpractice claims at 4 liability insurers. *Surgery, 140*(1), 26–33.

Rojansky, N., Tanos, V., Reubinoff, B., Shapira, S., & Weinstein, D. (1997). Effect of epidural analgesia on duration and outcome of induced labor. *International Journal of Obstetrics and Gynecology and Reproductive Biology, 56*(3), 153–158.

Rommal, C. (1996). Risk management issues in the perinatal setting. *Journal of Perinatal and Neonatal Nursing, 10*(3), 1–31.

Rommal, C. (1999). *Nursing policy on fundal pressure.* Los Angeles, CA: Farmers Insurance Group, Healthcare Professional Liability Division.

Romney, M. L., & Gordon, H. (1981). Is your enema really necessary? *British Medical Journal (Clinical Research Ed.) 282*(6272), 1269–1271.

Ross, B. K. (2003). ASA closed claims in obstetrics: Lessons learned. *Anesthesiology, 21*(1), 183–197.

Rothman, B. K. (1993). The active management of physicians. *Birth, 20*(3), 158–159.

Rouse, D. J., MacPherson, C., Landon, M., Varner, M. V., Leveno, K. J., Moawad, A. H., et al. (2006). Blood transfusion and cesarean delivery. *Obstetrics and Gynecology, 108*(4), 891–897.

Rouse, D. J., Owen, J., Savage, K. G., & Hauth, J. C. (2001). Active phase labor arrest: Revisiting the 2-hour minimum. *Obstetrics and Gynecology, 98*(4), 550–554.

Roussillon, J. A. (1998). Adult survivors of childhood sexual abuse: Suggestions for perinatal caregivers. *Clinical Excellence for Nurse Practitioners: The International Journal of NPACE, 2*(6), 329–327.

Royal College of Obstetricians and Gynaecologists. (2001). *Induction of labour* (Evidence-Based Clinical Guideline No. 9). London: Author.

Rozenberg, P., Goffinet, F., & Hessabi, M. (2000). Comparison of the Bishop score, ultrasonographically measured cervical length, and fetal fibronectin assay in predicting time until birth and type of birth at term. *American Journal of Obstetrics and Gynecology, 182*(1, Pt. 1), 108–113.

Rutgers, S. (1993). Hot, high and horrible: Should routine enemas still be given to women in labour? *Central African Journal of Medicine, 39*(6), 117–120.

Ryding, E. L., Wijma, B., & Wijma, K. (1997). Posttraumatic stress reactions after emergency cesarean section. *Acta Obstetricia et Gynecologica Scandinavica, 76*(9), 856–861.

Sakala, C., & Mayberry, L. J. (2006). Vaginal or cesarean birth: Application of an advocacy organization-driven research translational model. *Nursing Research, 55*(2 Suppl.), S68–S74.

Sampselle, C. M., & Hines, S. (1999). Spontaneous pushing during birth—relationship to perineal outcomes. *Journal of Nurse Midwifery, 44* (1), 36–39.

Sampselle, C. M., Miller, J. M., Luecha, Y., Fischer, K., & Rosen, L. (2005). Provider support of spontaneous second stage pushing during the second stage of labor. *Journal of Obstetric, Gynecologic, and Neonatal Nursing, 34*(6), 695–702.

Sanchez-Ramos, L. (2005). Induction of labor. *Obstetrics and Gynecology Clinics of North America, 32*(2), 181–200.

Sanchez-Ramos, L., & Kaunitz, A.M. (2000). Misoprostol for cervical ripening and labor induction: A systematic review of the literature. *Clinical Obstetrics and Gynecology, 43*(3), 475–488.

Sandberg, E. C. (1999). The Zavanelli maneuver: 12 years of recorded experience. *Obstetrics and Gynecology, 93*(2), 312–317.

Satin, A. J., Leveno, K. J., Sherman, M. L., Brewster, D. S., & Cunningham, F. G. (1992). High-versus low-dose oxytocin for labor stimulation. *Obstetrics and Gynecology, 80*(1), 111–116.

Satin, A. J., Leveno, K. J., Sherman, M. L., & McIntire, D. (1994). High-dose oxytocin: 20- versus 40-minute dosage interval. *Obstetrics and Gynecology, 83*(2), 234–238.

Sauls, D. J. (2002). Effects of labor support on mothers, babies, and birth outcomes. *Journal of Obstetric, Gynecologic and Neonatal Nursing, 31*(6), 733–741.

Schaffer, J. I., Bloom, S. L., Casey, B. M., McIntire, D. D., Nihira, M. A., & Leveno, K. J. (2005). A randomized trial of the effects of coached vs uncoached maternal pushing during the second stage of labor on postpartum pelvic floor structure and function. *American Journal of Obstetrics and Gynecology, 192*(5), 1692–1696.

Schiessl, B., Janni, W., Jundt, K., Rammel, G., Peschers, U., & Kainer, F. (2005). Obstetrical procedures influencing the duration of the second stage of labor. *European Journal of Obstetrics, Gynecology, and Reproductive Biology, 118*(1), 17–20.

Scott, J. R. (2005). Episiotomy and vaginal trauma. *Obstetrics and Gynecology Clinics of North America, 32*(2), 307–321.

Sebel, P. S., Bowdle, T. A., Ghoneim, M. M., Rampil, I. J., Padilla, R. E., Gan, T. J., et al. (2004). The incidence of awareness during anesthesia: A multicenter United States study. *Anesthesia and Analgesia, 99*(3), 833–839.

Segel, D., Sheiner, E., Yohai, D., Sholam-Vardi, I., & Katz, M. (1999). Early amniotomy: High risk for cesarean birth. *European Journal of Obstetrics, Gynecology and Reproductive Biology, 86*(2), 145–149.

Seitchik, J., Amico, J., Robinson, A. G., & Castillo, M. (1984). Oxytocin augmentation of dysfunctional labor. IV Oxytocin pharmacokinetics. *American Journal of Obstetrics and Gynecology, 150*(3), 225–228.

Seitchik, J., & Castillo, M. (1982). Oxytocin augmentation of dysfunctional labor: I. Clinical data. *American Journal of Obstetrics and Gynecology, 144*(8), 899–905.

Seitchik, J., & Castillo, M. (1983). Oxytocin augmentation of dysfunctional labor: III. Multiparous patients. *American Journal of Obstetrics and Gynecology, 145*(7), 777–780.

Sellers, S. M., Hodgson, H. T., Mitchell, M. D., Anderson, A. B. M., & Turnbull, A. C. (1980). Release of prostaglandins after amniotomy is not mediated by oxytocin. *British Journal of Obstetrics and Gynaecology, 87*(1), 43–46.

Sheehan, P. M. (2006). A possible role for progesterone metabolites in human parturition. *Australian and New Zealand Journal of Obstetrics and Gynaecology, 46*(2), 159–163.

Sheiner, E., Levy, A., Ofir, K., Hadar, A., Shoham-Verdi, I., Hallak, M., et al. (2004). Changes in fetal heart rate and uterine patterns associated with uterine rupture. *Journal of Reproductive Medicine, 49*(5), 373–378.

Sheiner, E., Segal, D., Shoham-Vardi, I., Ben-Tov, J., Katz, M., & Mazor, M. (2000) The impact of early amniotomy on mode of delivery and pregnancy outcomes. *Archives of Gynecology and Obstetrics, 264*(2), 63–67.

Sheiner, E., Walfisch, A., Hallak, M., Marley, S., Mazor, M., & Shoham-Vardi, I. (2006). Length of second stage labor as a predictor of perineal outcome after vaginal delivery. *Journal of Reproductive Medicine, 51*(2), 115–119.

Shermer R. H., & Raines, D. A. (1997). Positioning during the second stage of labor: Moving back to the basics. *Journal of Obstetric, Gynecologic, and Neonatal Nursing, 26*(6), 727–734.

Shifrin, B. S., & Ater, S. (2006). Fetal hypoxic and ischemic injuries. *Current Opinion in Obstetrics and Gynecology, 18*(2), 112–122.

Shin, K. S., Brubaker, K. L., & Ackerson, L. M. (2004). Risk of cesarean delivery in nulliparous women at greater than 41 weeks gestational age with an unengaged vertex. *American Journal of Obstetrics and Gynecology, 190*(1), 129–134.

Shipman, M. K., Boniface, D. R., Tefft, M. E., & McCloghery, F. (1997). Antenatal perineal massage and subsequent perineal outcomes: A randomized controlled trial. *British Journal of Obstetrics and Gynaecology, 104*(7), 787–791.

Shipp, T. D. (2004). Trial of labor after cesarean: So, what are the risks? *Clinical Obstetrics and Gynecology, 47*(2), 365–377.

Shipp, T. D., Zelop, C., Repke, J. T., Cohen, A., Caughey, A. B., & Lieberman, E. (2002). The association of maternal age and symptomatic uterine rupture during a trial of labor after prior cesarean delivery. *Obstetrics and Gynecology, 99*(4), 585–588.

Shyken, J. M., & Petrie, R. H. (1995a). Oxytocin to induce labor. *Clinical Obstetrics and Gynecology, 38*(2), 232–245.

Shyken, J. M., & Petrie, R. H. (1995b). The use of oxytocin. *Clinics in Perinatology, 22*(4), 907–931.

Signore, C., Hemachandra, A., & Klebanoff, M. (2006). Neonatal morbidity and morbidity after elective cesarean delivery versus routine expectant management: A decision analysis. *Seminars in Perinatology, 30*(5), 288–295.

Silbar, E. L. (1986). Factors related to the increasing cesarean section rates for cephalopelvic disproportion. *American Journal of Obstetrics and Gynecology, 154*(5), 1095–1098.

Silver, R. M. (2007). Fetal death. *Obstetrics and Gynecology, 109*(1), 153–167.

Simon, C. E., & Grobman, W. A. (2005). When has an induction failed? *Obstetrics and Gynecology, 105*(4), 705–709.

Simpson, K. R. (1999). Shoulder dystocia: Nursing interventions and risk management strategies. *MCN The American Journal of Maternal Child Nursing, 24*(6), 305–311.

Simpson, K. R. (2002). *Cervical ripening and induction and augmentation of labor.* (Practice Monograph). Washington, DC: Association of Women's Health, Obstetric and Neonatal Nurses.

Simpson, K. R. (2004a). Management of oxytocin for labor induction and augmentation. *MCN The American Journal of Maternal Child Nursing, 29*(2), 136.

Simpson, K. R. (2004b). Second-stage labor care. *MCN The American Journal of Maternal Child Nursing, 29*(6), 416.

Simpson, K. R. (2004c). Time out: It's time well spent. *MCN The American Journal of Maternal Child Nursing, 29*(4), 272.

Simpson, K. R. (2005a). Emergency drills in obstetrics. *MCN The American Journal of Maternal Child Nursing, 30*(2), 220.

Simpson, K. R. (2005b). Handling handoffs safely. *MCN The American Journal of Maternal Child Nursing, 30*(2), 76.

Simpson, K. R. (2006). When to push and how to push: Providing the most current information about second stage labor to women during childbirth education. *Journal of Perinatal Education, 15*(4), 4–9.

Simpson, K. R. (2007). Intrauterine resuscitation during labor: Review of current practice and supportive evidence. *Journal of Midwifery and Women's Health, 52*(3), 229–237.

Simpson, K. R., & Atterbury, J. (2003). Labor induction in the United States: Trends and issues for clinical practice. *Journal of Obstetric, Gynecologic and Neonatal Nursing, 32*(6), 767–779.

Simpson, K. R., & James, D. C. (2005a). Effects of immediate versus delayed pushing during second stage labor on fetal wellbeing. *Nursing Research, 54*(3), 149–157.

Simpson, K. R., & James, D. C. (2005b). Efficacy of intrauterine resuscitation techniques in improving fetal oxygen status during labor. *Obstetrics and Gynecology, 105*(6), 1362–1368.

Simpson, K. R., James, D. C., & Knox, G. E. (2006). Nurse-physician communication during labor and birth: Implications for patient safety. *Journal of Obstetric, Gynecologic and Neonatal Nursing, 35*(4), 547–556.

Simpson, K. R., & Knox, G. E. (2001). Fundal pressure during the second stage of labor: Clinical issues and risk management perspectives. *MCN The American Journal of Maternal Child Nursing, 26*(2), 64–70.

Singhi, S. (1988). Effect of maternal intrapartum glucose therapy on neonatal blood glucose levels and neurobehavioral status of hypoglycemic term infants. *Journal of Perinatal Medicine, 16*(3), 217–224.

Slater, D. M., Zervou, S., & Thorton, S. (2002). Prostaglandins and prostanoid receptors in human pregnancy and parturition. *Journal of the Society for Gynecologic Investigation, 9*(3), 118–124.

Sleutel, M., & Golden, S. S. (1999). Fasting in labor: Relic or requirement. *Journal of Obstetric, Gynecologic and Neonatal Nursing, 28*(5), 507–512.

Smith, G. C. S., Pell, J. P., Cameron, A. D., & Dobbie, R. (2002). Risk of perinatal death associated with labor after previous cesarean delivery in uncomplicated term pregnancies. *Journal of the American Medial Association, 287*(20), 2684–2690.

Smith, G. C. S., Pell, J. P., Pasupathy, D., & Dobbie, R. (2004). Factors predisposing to perinatal death related to uterine rupture during attempted vaginal birth after cesarean: Retrospective cohort study. *British Medical Journal, 329*(7462), 375–379.

Smith, J. G., & Merrill, D. C. (2006). Oxytocin for induction of labor. *Clinical Obstetrics and Gynecology, 49*(3), 594–608.

Society of Obstetricians and Gynaecologists of Canada. (2001). *Induction of labour at term.* (Clinical Practice Guideline No. 107). Ottawa, Canada: Author.

Society of Obstetricians and Gynaecologists of Canada. (2004). *Guidelines for operative vaginalbirth.* (Clinical Practice Guideline No. 148). Ottawa, Canada: Author.

Sommer, P. A., Norr, K., & Roberts, J. (2000). Clinical decision-making regarding intravenous hydration in normal labor in a birth center setting. *Journal of Midwifery and Women's Health, 45*(2), 114–121.

Song, J. (2000). Use of misoprostol in obstetrics and gynecology. *Obstetrical and Gynecological Survey, 55*(8), 503–510.

Spitellie, P. H., Holmes, M. A., & Domino, K. B. (2002). Awareness during anesthesia. *Anesthesiology Clinics of North America, 20*(3), 555–570.

Spong, C. Y., Beall, M., Rodrigues, D., & Ross, M. G. (1995). An objective definition of shoulder dystocia: Prolonged head-to-body delivery intervals and/or the use of ancillary obstetric maneuvers. *Obstetrics and Gynecology, 86*(3), 433–436.

Spydslaug, A., Trogstad, L. I., Skrondal, A., & Eskild, A. (2005). Recurrent risk of anal sphincter laceration among women with vaginal deliveries. *Obstetrics and Gynecology, 105*(2), 307–313.

Stamp, G. E. (1997). Care of the perineum in the second stage of labour: A study of the views and practices of Australian midwives. *Midwifery, 13*(2), 100–104.

Stamp, G., Kruzins, G., & Crowther, C. (2001). Perineal massage in labour and prevention of perineal trauma: Randomised controlled trial. *British Medical Journal, 322*(7297), 1277–1280.

Stremler, R., Hodnett, E., Petryshen, P., Stevens, B., Weston, J., & Willan, A. R. (2005). Randomized controlled trial of hands-and-knees positioning for occipitoposterior position in labor. *Birth, 32*(4), 243–251.

Stringer, J. L. (1996). *Basic concepts in pharmacology.* St. Louis, MO: McGraw-Hill.

Sultatos, L. G. (1997). Mechanisms of drugs that affect uterine motility. *Journal of Nurse Midwifery, 42*(2), 367–370.

Summers, L. (1997). Methods of cervical ripening and labor induction. *Journal of Nurse Midwifery, 42*(2), 71–85.

Tan, P. C., Jacob, R., & Omar, S. Z. (2006). Membrane sweeping at initiation of formal labor induction: A randomized controlled trial. *Obstetrics and Gynecology, 107*(3), 569–577.

Tenore, J. L. (2003). Methods for cervical ripening and induction of labor. *American FamilyPhysician, 67*(10), 2123–2128.

Terry, R. R., Westcott, J., O'Shea, L., & Kelly, F. (2006). Postpartum outcomes in supine delivery by physicians vs nonsupine delivery by midwives. *Journal of the American Osteopathic Association, 106*(4), 199–202.

Thomson, A. M. (1993). Pushing techniques in the second stage of labour. *Journal of Advanced Nursing, 18*(2), 171–177.

Thomson, A. M. (1995). Maternal behaviour during spontaneous and directed pushing in the second stage of labour. *Journal of Advanced Nursing, 22*(6), 1027–1034.

Torvaldsen, S., Roberts, C. L., Bell, J. C., & Raynes-Greenow, C. H. (2004). Discontinuation of epidural analgesia late in labour for reducing the adverse delivery outcomes associated with epidural analgesia. *Cochrane Database of Systematic Reviews, 18*(4), CD004457.

Towner, D., Castro, M. A., Eby-Wilkens, E., & Gilbert W. M. (1999). Effect of mode of delivery in nulliparous women on neonatal intracranial injury. *New England Journal of Medicine, 341*(23), 1709–1704.

Tucker, S. M. (2004). *Fetal monitoring and assessment* (5th ed.). St. Louis, MO: Mosby.

Tubridy, N., & Redmond, J. M. T. (1996). Neurological symptoms attributed to epidural analgesia in labour: An observational study of seven cases. *British Journal of Obstetrics and Gynaecology, 103*(8), 832–833.

Tumblin, A., & Simkin, P. (2001). Pregnant women's perceptions of their nurse's role during labor and delivery. *Birth, 28*(1), 52–56.

Uhing, M. R. (2005). Management of birth injuries. *Clinics in Perinatology, 32*(1), 19–38.

Ulmsten, U. (1997). Onset and forces of term labor. *Acta Obstetricia et Gynecologica Scandinavica, 76*(6), 499–514.

Usta, I. M., Mercer, B. M., & Sibai, B. M. (1999). Current obstetrical practice and umbilical cord prolapse. *American Journal of Perinatology, 16*(9), 479–484.

Vacca, A. (2002). Vacuum-assisted delivery. *Best Practice & Research: Clinical Obstetrics and Gynaecology, 16*(1), 17–30.

Vacca, A. (2006). Vacuum-assisted delivery: An analysis of traction forces and maternal and neonatal outcomes. *Australian and New Zealand Journal of Obstetrics and Gynaecology, 46*(2), 124–127.

Vahratian, A., Hoffman, M. K., Troendle, J. F., & Zhang, J. (2006). The impact of parity on course of labor in a contemporary population. *Birth, 33*(1), 12–17.

Vahratian, A., Zhang, J., Troendle, J. F., Sciscione, A. C., & Hoffman, M. K. (2005). Labor progression and risk of cesarean delivery in electively induced nulliparas. *Obstetrics and Gynecology, 105*(4), 698–704.

van Gemund, N., Hardeman, A., Scherjon, S. A., & Kanhai, H. H. (2003). Intervention rates after elective induction of labor compared to labor with a spontaneous onset: A matched cohort study. *Gynecologic and Obstetric Investigation, 56*(3), 133–138.

Vaughn, K. O. (1937). *Safe childbirth: The three essentials.* London: Ballière, Tindall, and Cox.

Vause, S., Congdon, H. M., & Thornton, J. G. (1998). Immediate and delayed pushing in the second stage of labour for nulliparous women with epidural analgesia: A randomized controlled trial. *British Journal of Obstetrics and Gynaecology, 105*(2), 186–188.

Visco, A. G., Viswanathan, M., Lohr, K. N., Wechter, M. E., Gartlehner, G., Wu, J. M., et al. (2006). Cesarean delivery on maternal request: Maternal and neonatal outcomes. *Obstetrics and Gynecology, 108*(6), 1517–1529.

Vrouenraets, F. P. J. M., Roumen, F. J. M. E., Dehing, C. J. G., van den Akker, E. S. A., Aarts, M. J. B., & Scheve, E. J. T. (2005). Bishop score and risk of cesarean delivery after induction of labor in nulliparous women. *Obstetrics and Gynecology, 105*(4), 690–697.

Walker, S. P., McCarthy, E. A., Ugoni, A., Lee, A., Lim, S., & Permezel, M. (2007). Cesarean delivery or vaginal birth: A survey of patient and clinician thresholds. *Obstetrics and Gynecology, 109*(1), 67–72.

Wasserstrum, N. (1992). Issues in fluid management during labor: General considerations. *Clinics in Obstetrics and Gynecology, 35*(3), 505–513.

Wax, J. R. (2006). Maternal request cesarean versus planned spontaneous vaginal delivery: Maternal morbidity and short term outcomes. *Seminars in Perinatology, 30*(5), 247–252.

Wein, P. (1989). Efficacy of different starting doses of oxytocin for induction of labor. *Obstetrics and Gynecology, 74*(6), 863–868.

Wiberg, B., Humble, K., & de Chateau, P. (1989). Long term effect on mother-infant behavior of extra contact during the first hour post partum. V: Follow-up at three years. *Scandinavian Journal of Social Medicine, 17*(2), 181–191.

Williams, M. K., & Chames, M. C. (2006). Risk factors for the breakdown of perineal laceration repair after vaginal delivery. *American Journal of Obstetrics and Gynecology, 195*(3), 755–759.

Wing, D. A., & Lyons, C. A. (2006). Vaginal misoprostol administration for cervical ripening and labor induction. *Clinical Obstetrics and Gynecology, 49*(3), 627–641.

Winkler, M., & Rath, W. (1999). A risk-benefit assessment of oxytocics in obstetric practice. *Drug Safety, 20* (4), 323–345.

Witter, F. R. (2000). Prostaglandin E_2 preparations for preinduction cervical ripening. *Clinical Obstetrics and Gynecology, 43*(3), 469–474.

Wong, S. F., Hui, S. K., Choi, H., & Ho, L. C. (2002). Does sweeping of membranes beyond 40 weeks reduce the need for formal induction of labour? *British Medical Journal, 109*(6), 632–636.

Wood, C., Ng, K., Hounslow, D., & Benning, H. (1973). The influences of different birth times upon fetal condition in normal deliveries. *Journal of Obstetrics and Gynaecology of the British Commonwealth, 80*(4), 289–294.

Yap, O. W., Kim, E. S., & Laros, R. K. Jr. (2001). Maternal and neonatal outcomes after uterine rupture in labor. *American Journal of Obstetrics and Gynecology, 184*(7), 1576–1581.

Young, T. K., & Woodmansee, B. (2002). Factors that are associated with cesarean delivery in a large private practice: The importance of prepregnancy body mass index and weight gain. *American Journal of Obstetrics and Gynecology, 184*(2), 312–331.

Zeeman, G. G., Khan-Dawood, F. S., & Dawood, M. Y. (1997). Oxytocin and its receptor in pregnancy and parturition: Current concepts and clinical implications. *Obstetrics and Gynecology, 89*(5, Pt. 2), 873–883.

Zeiman, M., Fong, S. K., Benowitz, N. L., Banskter, D., & Darney, P. D. (1997). Absorption kinetics of misoprostol with oral and vaginal administration. *Obstetrics and Gynecology, 90*(1), 88–92.

Zelop, C. M., Shipp, T. D., Repke, J. T., Cohen, A., & Lieberman, E. (2000). Effect of previous vaginal delivery on the risk of uterine rupture during a subsequent trial of labor. *American Journal of Obstetrics and Gynecology, 183*(5), 1184–1186.

Zetterstrom, J., Lopez, A., Anzen, B., Norman, M., Holmstrom, B., & Mellgren, A. (1999). Anal sphincter tears at vaginal delivery: Risk factors and clinical outcomes of primary repair. *Obstetrics and Gynecology, 94*(1), 21–28.

Zhang, J., Troendle, J. F., & Yancey, M. K. (2002). Reassessing the labor curve in multiparous women. *American Journal of Obstetrics and Gynecology, 187*(4), 824–828.

Zhang, J., Yancey, M. K., & Henderson, C. E. (2002). U. S. National trends in labor induction, 1989-1998. *Journal of Reproductive Medicine, 47*(2), 120–124.

Sample Intrapartum Admission Assessment

PT. NAME: _____ **AGE:** _____ **OBSTETRICIAN:** _____

ADMIT DATE/TIME: _____ **PEDIATRICIAN:** _____

EDC	LMP	Weeks of Gestation	Gravida	Para	Term	Preterm	Spontaneous Abortion	Elective Abortion	Living	Stillborn	C-Section	VBAC

T	P	R	BP	Height	Weight	Pre-Pregnant Weight	Weight Gain	How Admitted		Accompanied By	

Date/Time Physician Notified	Date/Time Seen By Physician/CNM	Reason for Admission	Date/Time EFM Applied

FHR:

Presentation:

Onset of Labor		Contraction Frequency (Min)	

Dilatation (cm)	Effacement (%)		Station

Contraction Duration (Sec)	Contraction Quality	
	None Mild Moderate Strong	

Pelvic Exam By:

Pain Level Assessment: *Pain Scale 0 - 10*

Admission Membranes: Intact Ruptured Bulging Unknown

Fern: N/A Negative Positive Equivocal

AROM/SROM (Date/Time):

Amniotic Fluid:
Amount: None N/A Copious Large Moderate Small Scant

Color: N/A Clear Bloody Meconium Heavy Light Particulate

Odor: None N/A Normal Foul

Amniotic Fluid Comments:

Vaginal Bleeding: None Normal Show Frank Bleeding
Describe Vaginal Bleeding:

Mental Status: Alert Anxious Confused

Feeding Preference: Breast Bottle Breast/Bottle Undecided

Support Person: None Husband Partner Other
Support Person(s) Name:

Anesthesia Plans: None Local Epidural Spinal General Pudendal
Paracervical
Anesthesia Plans Other:

Anesthesia Class: Yes   No   Yes, Previous Pregnancy

Attended Prenatal Class: Yes No Yes, Previous Pregnancy

Labor Teaching Initiated: Yes No N/A

 Fetal Well-being   Yes No N/A
 Labor Progress   Yes No N/A
 Pain Relief Measures   Yes No N/A
 Other _____

Nutritional Screen:
[ ] N/A
[ ] History of Diabetes / Gestational Diabetes
[ ] History of Eating Disorder
[ ] Multiple Pregnancy
[ ] Special Diet / Vegetarian Diet
[ ] Pt. is 18 Years Old or Younger
[ ] Failure to Gain at Least 1/2 lb. per Wks. of Gestation
[ ] Food Allergies
[ ] Other _____

Describe Last Solid Intake (Include Date/Time):

Describe Last Fluid Intake (Include Date/Time):

In-Pt. Dietary Referral Entered in Computer: Yes No N/A	Out-Pt. Dietary Referral Entered in Computer: Yes No N/A

Medication Allergy: Yes No
Medication Allergy Detail:

Food Allergies: Yes No
Food Allergy Detail:

Latex Allergy: Yes No

REACTIONS	Denies	Swelling	Runny Nose	Itching	Tearing	Sneezing
Blowing Up Balloons						
Dental Exam						
Rectal/Vaginal Exam						
Diaphragm or Condom						
Rubber Gloves or Products						
Foods (Banana, Kiwi, Water Chestnuts, Avocado)						

Describe Latex Reaction(s):

Allergy Sticker On Chart: Yes N/A	Allergy Band on Patient: Yes N/A

Prenatal Vitamins This Pregnancy: Yes No	Anticoagulants This Pregnancy: Yes No	Describe:

For current prescription/over the counter medications taken during pregnancy see Home Medication Order Sheet.

Prescription/over the counter medications previously taken during pregnancy:

Addressograph

PERINATAL UNIT ADMISSION RECORD

ST. JOHN'S MERCY MEDICAL CENTER, ST. LOUIS, MO

Page 1

PT. NAME: _____

| GBS Tested: | Yes No | Results: | Negative Positive Unknown | Results Date: | | |

| Blood Type/Rh: | Rhogam | This Pregnancy: | N/A   Yes   No   No Record |

| Rubella: | Immune Non-Immune Unknown | HBsAg: | Negative Positive Unknown | RPR: | Non-Reactive Reactive Unknown |

| Hemaglobin = _____ g/dl Initials: _____ Reference Range: 11-14 g/dl (pregnancy) | HIV | Non-Reactive Reactive |

Heart Disease:	Yes No	Hypertension:	Yes No
MVP:	Yes No	Diabetes:	Yes No
Asthma:	Yes No	DVT:	Yes No

Blood Transfusion: Yes   No

Blood Transfusion Reason/Yr:

| Sexually Transmitted Diseases: | Denies   Chlamydia   Syphilis   Gonorrhea HIV   HPV/Genital Warts   Herpes Other _____ |

| Exposure to Infectious Disease This Pregnancy: | Denies   Measles   Mumps   HIV/AIDS Chicken Pox   TB   Hepatitis Other _____ |

| Cervical Procedures: | Denies   D & C   LEEP   Cervical Biopsy Laser   Cryo/Cautery Other _____ |

History of Major Illness or Surgery:

Patient History Detail:

| Past Pregnancy Complications: | None   PIH   Cystitis   Pyelitis   Preterm Labor Preterm Birth   Anemia   Rh Sensitization Positive GBS   Other _____ |

Comments:

| Complications Current Pregnancy: | None   PIH   Cystitis   Pyelitis   Preterm Labor Preterm Birth   Anemia   Rh Sensitization Other _____ |

Comments:

| Fetal Assessments Done This Pregnancy: | None   Non-Stress Test   OCT CVS   BPP   US   Amnio |

Previous Labor Durations:

Sibling History:

| Family History: | N/A   Adopted   Heart Disease   HTN   Diabetes   Cancer Bleeding Disorder   Other _____ |

Family History Comments:

| Smoke Use/Frequency: Denies   <5 per day   5-10 per day >10 per day   >20 per day | Alcohol Use: | Denies Occasional 3-5 Drinks/Week 6 or More Drinks/Week |

Morse Fall Scale Score:
[ ] < 45, low fall risk; initiate appropriate interventions
[ ] > 50, high fall risk; initiate appropriate interventions
[ ] ≥ 4 medications associated with increased fall risk; high fall risk; initiate appropriate interventions

Initiate Care Plan if:
[ ] Anticipated physiological fall risk
[ ] Unanticipated physiological fall risk
[ ] Accidental fall risk

Immunization History
Vaccines:	Influenza	Yes	No	Date:_____
	Pneumonia	Yes	No	Date:_____
	Tetanus	Yes	No	Date:_____
	PPD	Yes	No	Date:_____

Nursing Assessment Summary: _____

Drug Use: Denies   Yes   *If Yes, Describe*

Drug Use Comments:

Contact Lenses: Yes   No   Soft Lenses   Hard Lenses   Lenses In   Lenses Out

| Glasses: Yes   No | Dentures: Yes   No |

| Body Piercing: Yes   No | Body Piercing Location/Removed: |

Support System After Birth: Family   Friends   Community   None
If None, Social Service Referral Entered in Computer: Yes   No   N/A

History of Abuse: Denies   Emotional   Physical   Sexual   *If Other,*
Other _____   *Describe*
Social Service Referral Entered in Computer: Yes   No   N/A

Special Needs: None   Spiritual   Cultural   Emotional   *If Other,*
Other _____   Hearing/Vision Impaired: Yes   No   *Describe*

| Social Service Referral Entered in Computer: Yes   No   N/A | Pastoral Service Referral Entered in Computer: Yes   No   N/A |

Interpreter needed?   Yes   No   Primary language: _____

| Discharge Planning Risk Assessment: | Single Teen Mother Keeping Baby   History of Drug Abuse Possible Adoption   No Prenatal Care |

| Referral for Social Service Needed at This Time Per Discharge Screen: | Yes No | If Yes, Referral Entered In Computer: | Yes No |

Psychosocial Comments:

Mother - Baby Discharge Teaching Initiated: Yes   No   N/A

| Functional Status: | Pt. able to function independently Pt. unable to function independently |

Functional Status Discussed With Physician: Yes   No   N/A

Date/Time Functional Status Discussed With Physician:

| PT/OT Referral Indicated: | No referral needed at this time Yes, referral needed due to functional status change |

Referral Entered in Computer: Yes   No   N/A

Room Orientation: EFM   Bed   Phone   Call Light   Visitors   Computer

Does The Patient Have an Advance Directive?

| Yes | If Yes, is copy in Chart? | Yes No | If No Copy on Chart, Remind Pt. to Have Family Member Bring Copy AND Send Advance Directive Referral to Pastoral Services | Referral Entered in Computer: | Yes No |

| No | If No, Does Pt. Want Additional Information or Assistance? | Yes No | If Yes, Was Referral Sent to Pastoral Care? | Yes No | Referral Entered in Computer: | Yes No |

| Disposition of Valuables: | Sent Home   Kept with Pt.   Valuables in Security Office Pt. Encouraged to Take Valuables Home   Other _____ |

Valuables Comments:

Pt. Wants Other Physician or Family Notified: Yes   No

Other Physician/Family Notified:

Requests cord blood baking: Y N
Cord blood banking type: ☐ NA
☐ St. Louis Cord Blood Bank
☐ Private card blood bank

PERINATAL UNIT ADMISSION RECORD
ST. JOHN'S MERCY MEDICAL CENTER, ST. LOUIS, MO

Addressograph

Signature(s)

Labor Flow Sheet and Immediate Postpartum Recovery

INTAKE	00	2	4	6	8	10	12	14	16	18	20	22	24
IV													
Oxytocin 30 units in 500ml L/R via infusion pump													
Magnesium Sulfate 20 grams in 500ml W via infusion pump													
IV													
PO													
8° TOTAL IN													

OUTPUT	00	2	4	6	8	10	12	14	16	18	20	22	24
Urine/voided													
Urine/catheter													
Emesis													
8° TOTAL OUT													

24° TOTALS	PO INTAKE	IV INTAKE	URINE OUTPUT	OTHER OUTPUT

PROCEDURES	DATE	TIME	INITIALS
SROM			
AROM by			
Amniotic Fluid — Amount / Color			
FSE by			
IUPC by			
Epidural			
Amnioinfusion			
Other			
IV started			
Needle size/length	Site		
Tolerated well ❑ Yes ❑ No	Labeled ❑ Tubing ❑ Site		

SPECIMEN COLLECTED	
Date/Time	Specimen / Lab Test

INITIALS	SIGNATURE

Morse Fall Scale Score daily
[ ] < 45, low fall risk; initiate appropriate interventions
[ ] > 50, high fall risk; initiate appropriate interventions
[ ] ≥ 4 medications associated with increased fall risk; high fall risk; initiate appropriate interventions

CERVICAL DILATION Cm (Ο) — 10 9 8 7 6 5 4 3 2 1 Effacement

STATION (X) — −3 −2 −1 0 +1 +2 +3 +4 +5

Hour of Labor — 1 2 3 4 5 6 7 8 9 10 11 12 13 14 15 16 17 18 19 20 21

TIME→ _____

Weekly Weight q Wednesday _____ B/ R (circle)

ADDRESSOGRAPH

LABOR FLOW SHEET

ST. JOHN'S MERCY MEDICAL CENTER/ST. LOUIS, MO

PT. NAME:											PHYSICIAN:						
Date/Time:																	
VITAL SIGNS																	
Temperature																	
Pulse																	
Respirations																	
Blood Pressure																	
Maternal SpO2																	
FETAL ASSESSMENT																	
Monitor Mode																	
Baseline FHR																	
Baseline Variability																	
FHR Pattern																	
FSpO2																	
UTERINE ACTIVITY																	
Frequency Contractions (min)																	
Duration of Contractions (sec)																	
Intensity of Contractions (palp)																	
Intensity of Contractions (mmHg)																	
Uterine Resting Tone																	
Oxytocin (milliunits/min)																	
CERVICAL STATUS																	
Vaginal Exam By																	
Dilatation (cm)																	
Effacement (%)																	
Station																	
ASSESSMENTS/INTERVENTIONS																	
Position																	
Activity																	
Response to Labor																	
Affect																	
Comfort Measures																	
Oxygen Amount (liters/min)																	
Magnesium Sulfate (grams/hr)																	
Pain Assessment																	
IV Assessment																	

ALLERGIES:

MEDICATION/PATIENT'S RESPONSE

NURSE INITIALS

Addressograph

PT. NAME:_____ **PHYSICIAN:**_____

Date/Time:													
VITAL SIGNS													
Temperature													
Pulse													
Respirations													
Blood Pressure													
Maternal SpO2													
FETAL ASSESSMENT													
Monitor Mode													
Baseline FHR													
Baseline Variability													
FHR Pattern													
FSpO2													
UTERINE ACTIVITY													
Frequency Contractions (min)													
Duration of Contractions (sec)													
Intensity of Contractions (palp)													
Intensity of Contractions (mmHg)													
Uterine Resting Tone													
Oxytocin (milliunits/min)													
CERVICAL STATUS													
Vaginal Exam By													
Dilatation (cm)													
Effacement (%)													
Station													
ASSESSMENTS/INTERVENTIONS													
Position													
Activity													
Response to Labor													
Affect													
Comfort Measures													
Oxygen Amount (liters/min)													
Magnesium Sulfate (grams/hr)													
Pain Assessment													
IV Assessment													
MEDICATION/PATIENT'S RESPONSE													
NURSE INITIALS													

Monitor Mode
Ext = External US
FSE = Fetal Scalp Electrode

Baseline Variability
Ab = Absent
Min = > Ab - " 5
Mod = 6-25 bpm
Mark = > 25 bpm

FHR Pattern
L = Late
V = Variable
E = Early
P = Prolonged
A = Accelerations

Frequency of Contractions
Ø = None
I = Irregular

Intensity of Contractions
M = Mild
Mod = Moderate
S = Strong

Position
R = Right Lateral
L = Left Lateral
T = Trendelenberg
SF = Semi Fowlers
C = Chair
HF = High Fowlers

Activity
S = Sleeping
TV = Watching TV
T = Talking
BP = on Bedpan
Amb = Ambulate
B = Bedrest
BR = Bathroom

Response to Labor
Ø = Unaware of Contractions
T = Talking Through Contractions
BW = Breathing Well With Contractions
CN = Coaching Necessary to Maintain Controlled Breathing
UP = Urge to Push
PC = Pushing With Contractions
LD = Laboring Down

Affect
R = Relaxed
A = Apprehensive
F = Fatigued

Comfort Measures
R = Reassurance and Encouragement Given
P = Pericare
CP = Counter Pressure
H2O = Shower/Tub
BB = Birthing Ball
RT = Relaxation Techniques

Pain Assessment
0 = None
3 = Mild
5 = Tolerable
7 = Moderate
10 = Severe

IV Assessment
P = Patent
R = Redness
I = Infiltrated

Addressograph

Date _____

Postpartum Observation

Time	Temp	B / P	Pulse	Resp.	SpO₂	Pain Scale	Fundus	Lochia	Epis: Dressing	Intake	Output	Initials

POST ANESTHESIA RECOVERY SCORE

	CRITERIA	SCORE	DISCHARGE
CONSCIOUSNESS	Fully awake	2	
	Arousable on calling	1	
	Not responding	0	
NEUROMUSCULAR ACTIVITY	Move 4 extremities	2	
	Move 2 extremities	1	
	Move 0 extremities	0	
SENSATION	Normal	2	
	None below pubis	1	
	None below xiphoid	0	
CIRCULATION	B/P 10-20mmHg ± admission	2	
	B/P 10-50mmHg ± admission	1	
	B/P > 51mmHg ± admission	0	
RESPIRATION	Deep breathing or cough	2	
	Dyspnea	1	
	Apnea	0	
COLOR	Pink	2	
	Pale, blotchy, jaundiced, other	1	
	Cyanotic	0	
Signature: Date:		Total Time	

MEDICATIONS

Time	Drug / Dose / Route	Initials

Morse Fall Scale Score:
[ ] < 45, low fall risk; initiate appropriate interventions
[ ] > 50, high fall risk; initiate appropriate interventions
[ ] ≥ 4 medications associated with increased fall risk; high fall risk; initiate appropriate interventions

Transfer to PP Room Notes: Room # _____

Discharge Nurse _____   Nurse Receiving Report _____

Transported by: w/c or cart   Mobility _____   Time of report _____

Birth certificate / papers given _____   Call light in reach _____   Side rails up x2 _____

Addressograph

Care and Instructions: Initial if done

Bath; pericare done _____   Tucks applied _____   Spray applied _____

Ice pack applied: perineum / abdomen   Informed re: ask for help up x2 _____

IV site assessed _____   IV dc'd _____   Encouraged to TCDB _____

Foley patent and taped to ❑ Left ❑ Right leg   Other: _____

Cervical Ripening and Induction of Labor Analysis

Patient Name_____ Date_____

Please place a "P" by primary reason - check all other reasons

A. INDICATIONS BASED ON GESTATION

___40 0/7 wks-40 6/7 wks ___41 0/7 wks-41 6/7 wks ___>42 /0/7 wks Gestational age at start of induction_____

B. INDICATIONS BASED ON FETAL CONDITION (Please complete Fetal Maturity Criteria for indications with an asterisk*)

___Unstable fetal lie*   ___Fetal demise
___Postdates   ___Fetal anomaly (list)_____
___Isoimmunization
___Severe intrauterine growth retardation (estimated fetal weight falls below 10th percentile for gestational age)
___Other (list)_____

C. INDICATIONS BASED ON ANTEPARTAL FETAL TESTING

___Nonreactive nonstress test   ___Decreased variability
___Positive oxytocin challenge stress test   ___Absence of accelerations, nonreactive fetus
___Positive breast stimulation contraction test   ___Spontaneous variable or prolonged decelerations
___Biophysical profile score of_____
___Other (list)_____

D. INDICATIONS BASED ON MATERNAL CONDITION (Please complete Fetal Maturity Criteria for indications with an asterisk*)

___Cervical dilatation > 4 cms*   ___Pregnancy induced hypertension
___Chorioamnionitis   ___Diabetes mellitus
___Other (list)_____

E. INDICATIONS BASED ON MEMBRANES/AMNIOTIC FLUID STATUS

___Ruptured membranes for_____hours   ___Oligohydramnios
___Decreased amniotic fluid volume   ___Polyhydramnios

F. INDICATIONS BASED ON LOGISTIC/OTHER FACTORS (Please complete Fetal Maturity Criteria for indications with an asterisk*)

___History of rapid labor*   ___Distance from hospital*
___Psychosocial (list)*_____

*FETAL MATURITY CRITERIA (Please complete for indications with an asterisk.)

___Fetal heart tones have been documented for 20 weeks by nonelectronic fetoscope or for 30 weeks by Doppler.
___36 weeks have passed since a positive serum or urine HCG pregnancy test was performed by a reliable method.
___An US measurement of the crown-rump length, obtained at 6-12 weeks, supports a gestational age of 39 weeks or more.
___An US scan, obtained at 13-20 weeks, confirms a gestational age of 39 weeks or more determined by clinic hx and physical exam.

BISHOP SCORE The state of cervix is related to the success of labor induction. When the total cervical score exceeds 8, the likelihood of vaginal birth subsequent to labor induction is similar to that of spontaneous labor. Induction of labor with a poor cervical score has been associated with failure of induction, prolonged labor, and a high cesarean birth rate.

	Factor	0	1	2	3	
Circle	Dilatation	Closed	1-2	3-4	>5	
factors	Effacement	0 - 30%	40 - 50%	60 - 70%	>80%	
present	Station	-3	-2	-1/0	+1/+2	
at start of	Consistency	Firm	Medium	Soft	- - - -	Total score at start
induction	Cervical position	Posterior	Mid-position	Anterior	- - - -	of induction_____

INFORMED CONSENT

I have discussed the indications, methods, agents, risks, benefits and alternative approaches for cervical ripening and/or labor induction including the possibility of repeat induction or cesarean birth with

_____ and she has agreed to proceed. _____Date_____
Patient Name   Physician Signature

Induction/Augmentation of Labor with Oxytocin

PURPOSE

To promote safe and effective use of oxytocin for induction and/or augmentation of labor.

POLICY

Physician/Nurse Responsibilities

Responsibility for the decision to use oxytocin for labor induction or labor augmentation rests with the attending obstetrician. Family practice physicians and certified nurse midwives may order oxytocin for labor induction or labor augmentation in consultation with the attending obstetrician.

Labor nurses may refuse to administer oxytocin if in their best judgment it is contraindicated, or if the needs of the service make it difficult or impossible to adequately monitor maternal–fetal status.

GUIDELINES FOR PRACTICE

Before Oxytocin Administration

Verify that the provider has discussed the indications and potential risks and benefits of induction or augmentation of labor with the pregnant woman.

Verify that the indication for induction is documented in the medical record.

Follow routine admission procedure and perform vaginal examination to evaluate cervical status and fetal station and presentation. Document Bishop's score in the medical record (see below).

Assist the woman to a position of comfort, preferably an upright or left or right lateral position.

Apply electronic fetal monitor and record fetal heart rate (FHR) for at least 15 minutes prior to initiation of oxytocin infusion. Before oxytocin is administered, the FHR should be reassuring. Notify physician if the FHR is nonreassuring.

Oxytocin Dosage and Administration

Pre-mixed solution of 30 units in 500 mL of lactated Ringer's solution (1 milliunit per minute [mU/min] = 1 milliliter per hour [mL/hr]).

Start oxytocin at 1 mU/min and gradually increase by 1 to 2mU/min q 30 to 60 minutes until adequate progress of labor is established and/or contractions are q 2 to 3 minutes. Labor progress may be 0.5 to 1 centimeters of cervical dilation per hour during labor induction, particularly for nulliparous women.

Once adequate labor is established, maintain or decrease oxytocin to baseline rate necessary for continued labor progress.

Decrease or discontinue oxytocin infusion during the second stage of labor to approximate physiologic second stage contraction pattern.

May increase oxytocin infusion to 20mU/min per this protocol at the discretion of the nurse.

A bedside evaluation by the attending physician is needed to increase beyond 20 mU/minute. This should be considered only in unusual clinical situations.

Maternal–Fetal Assessment and Documentation

Assessment of maternal–fetal status described below should occur every 15 minutes during oxytocin administration. The following documentation in the medical record is required each time oxytocin dosage rate is increased or decreased (or at least every 30 minutes if the dosage is unchanged):

Fetal Heart Rate: baseline rate, baseline variability, presence or absence of FHR accelerations, presence or absence of FHR decelerations, and nursing interventions as appropriate.

BISHOP SCORING SYSTEM (BISHOP, 1964)					
Score	Dilatation (cm)	Effacement (%)	Station	Consistency	Position of Cervix
0	Closed	0–30	−3	Firm	Posterior
1	1–2	40–50	−2	Medium	Midpostion
2	3–4	60–70	−1, 0	Soft	Anterior
3	≥ 5	≥ 80	+1, +2		

Uterine Activity: contraction frequency, duration, intensity, and uterine resting tone by palpation or IUPC.

Maternal Response to Labor: the woman's response to the contractions (ie, not feeling contractions, using breathing techniques with contractions, requires intense labor coaching with contractions, comfortable with contractions with epidural analgesia, etc.)

If a registered nurse is not available to clinically evaluate the effects of the oxytocin infusion at least every 15 minutes, the infusion should be discontinued until that level of nursing care is available (AAP & ACOG, 2002; AWHONN, 2002). *The attending physician will be notified.*

Maternal Activity

Encourage the woman to try alternatives to bedrest such as ambulating in the LDR room or hall or using the rocking chair. Other labor support techniques for women who wish to be out of bed include use of the birthing ball and a warm shower. When the woman is out of bed during oxytocin infusion, use EFM telemetry unit to monitor FHR and uterine activity.

Hyperstimulation

Hyperstimulation is defined as:

- More than 5 contractions in 10 minutes
- Contractions lasting 2 minutes or more
- Contractions of normal duration occurring within 1 minute of each other
- Insufficient return of uterine resting tone between contractions via palpation, or
- Intraamniotic pressure above 25 mm Hg between contractions via IUPC.

If hyperstimulation develops, reposition the mother and decrease oxytocin rate at least by half until hyperstimulation resolves. An IV fluid bolus of 500 mL of lactated Ringer's solution may be given. Oxytocin may be discontinued if hyperstimulation does not resolve. In selected cases, where hyperstimulation persists despite discontinuation of oxytocin, an IV fluid bolus and position change, and the FHR is nonreassuring, consider administration of terbutaline .25 mg SQ.

Nonreassuring Fetal Status

If the FHR is nonreassuring during oxytocin administration, discontinue oxytocin.

Assess maternal blood pressure. An IV fluid bolus of at least 500 mL of lactated Ringer's solution may be given at the discretion of the nurse. If the woman is hypotensive and has regional analgesia/anesthesia, notify the anesthesia provider.

Maternal oxygen administration at 10 L/min per nonrebreather facemask may be indicated in some clinical situations such as recurrent variable or late decelerations of the FHR and/or minimal to absent baseline FHR variability and will be given at the discretion of the nurse.

Maternal position change may be indicated. A right or left lateral position is preferred. Identification of persistently nonreassuring fetal status that does not resolve with the usual intrauterine resuscitation techniques requires notification of the physician and documentation in the medical record of the content of the conversation and interventions to resolve the clinical situation.

Epidural Analgesia/Anesthesia

Women receiving oxytocin who have epidural analgesia/anesthesia should have pelvic examinations periodically as clinically indicated to assess labor progress.

Internal Monitoring

Internal monitoring may be appropriate based on the individual clinical situation. If unable to record an interpretable FHR tracing and/or uterine activity tracing, women receiving oxytocin may have fetal scalp electrode and/or IUPC placed, if indicated. The cervix must be at least 2 to 3 cm dilated before the nurse can insert a FSE or IUPC.

Insertion of a FSE or IUPC requires a physician order. Oxytocin is not in itself an indication for internal monitoring if external monitoring produces an interpretable tracing and there is not a clinical need for more accurate data about intrauterine pressure.

If unable to insert internal monitors and/or the FHR and/or uterine activity continues to be unable to be recorded, the oxytocin infusion should be discontinued until an interpretable FHR pattern and uterine activity pattern can be recorded. The physician who ordered the oxytocin should be notified.

Resumption of Oxytocin Administration After Discontinuation Due to Nonreassuring FHR and/or Uterine Activity Hyperstimulation

If the infusion has been discontinued for less than 20 to 30 minutes and the FHR is reassuring and uterine activity has returned to normal, oxytocin may be restarted at no more than one-half of the rate that resulted in the nonreassuring FHR and/or uterine hyperstimulation and then increased at 1 to 2 m/U per minute every 30 to 60 minutes as per protocol.

If the infusion has been discontinued for more than 30 to 40 minutes and the FHR is reassuring and uterine activity has returned to normal, oxytocin may be restarted at no more than 1m/U per minute and increased by 1 to 2 m/U per minute every 30 to 60 minutes as per protocol.

REFERENCES

American Academy of Pediatrics and American College of Obstetricians and Gynecologists (2002). *Guidelines for perinatal care.* Elk Grove Village, IL: Author.

American College of Obstetricians and Gynecologists (2005). *Intrapartum fetal heart rate monitoring.* (ACOG Practice Bulletin No. 62). Washington, DC: Author.

American College of Obstetricians and Gynecologists (2003). *Dystocia and augmentation of labor.* (ACOG Practice Bulletin No. 49). Washington, DC: Author.

American College of Obstetricians and Gynecologists (1999). *Induction of labor* (ACOG Practice Bulletin No. 10). Washington, DC: Author.

Simpson, K. R. (2002). *Cervical ripening, induction and augmentation of labor:* (AWHONN Practice Monograph). Washington, DC: Association of Women's Health, Obstetric and Neonatal Nurses.

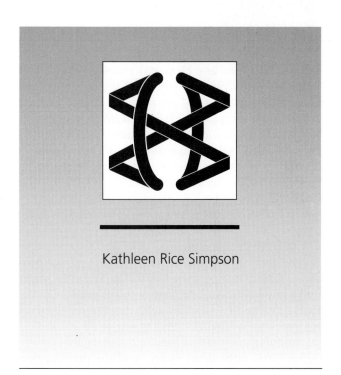

CHAPTER **8**

Fetal Assessment During Labor

Kathleen Rice Simpson

INTRODUCTION

The introduction of electronic fetal monitoring (EFM) in the late 1960s has had a far-reaching impact on perinatal care and the practice of nursing, midwifery, and medicine. Despite debate about advantages and limitations, effects on perinatal morbidity and mortality, and role in healthcare costs and malpractice litigation, EFM is used in the majority of labor and birth units in the United States and Canada today. This chapter discusses the physiologic basis for fetal heart rate (FHR) monitoring, defines FHR patterns, and reviews intrapartum management of FHR patterns.

HISTORICAL PERSPECTIVES

The discovery of fetal heart tones in 1821 marked the beginning of modern obstetric practice (Sureau, 1996; Goodlin, 1979). Jean Alexandre Le jumeau, Vicomte de Kergaradec used a stethoscope hoping to hear the noise of the water in the uterus. Although he probably was not the first person to identify fetal heart tones, he was the first person astute enough to suggest in print potential clinical uses for FHR auscultation (Sureau, 1996). In the early 1800s, researchers working independently in Switzerland, Ireland, Germany, France, and the United States described fetal heart tones, and in 1833 the British obstetrician William Kennedy published the first descriptions of "fetal distress," by describing a late deceleration and associating it with poor prognosis (Kennedy, 1833). In 1858, Schwartz of Germany suggested that the FHR be counted often during labor, both

between and during contractions, to promote improved outcomes. Schwartz described the association between fetal bradycardia and decreased uteroplacental blood flow during contractions. In 1849, Killian proposed forceps-assisted birth for an FHR of fewer than 100 beats per minute (bpm) or greater than 180 bpm (Goodlin, 1979). Soon after, Winckel described specific FHR criteria to be used for the diagnosis of fetal distress via auscultation (Goodlin, 1979). After invention of the fetoscope in the early 1900s, fetal heart sounds were commonly assessed in order to document fetal viability during the prenatal period. Winckel's criteria were used in clinical practice until the 1950s when Hon raised concern about the subjectivity of counting heartbeats during labor.

Although interest in continuous recording of fetal heart tones by various methods dates to the later years of the 19th century, the major development of modern clinical EFM occurred during the 1960s. In 1906, Cramer produced the first electrocardiographic (ECG) recording of the fetal heartbeat (Cramer, 1906). Research using abdominal leads to obtain the fetal ECG continued but remained impractical for clinical use until the mid 1960s, when techniques capable of excluding the maternal ECG from the recording became available. By the 1950s, research on electronic methods of FHR monitoring escalated. In 1958, Hon published the first report of continuous fetal electrocardiographic monitoring using a device placed on the maternal abdomen. By the 1960s, Hon, Caldeyro-Barcia, and Hammacher were reporting successful attempts at developing an electronic FHR monitor that could continuously record FHR data (Caldeyro-Barcia, Mendez-Bauer, & Poseiro, 1966; Hammacher, 1969;

Hon, 1963). Although many others have contributed to what is known about fetal assessment during labor, EFM as it is used today is largely the result of the work of these three investigators working independently on separate continents. In 1968, the first commercially available electronic fetal monitors were introduced.

Coinciding with the development of EFM technology was the emergence of data that refuted the effectiveness of intermittent auscultation with Delee or Pinard fetoscopes. The Benson, Shubeck, Deutschberger, Weiss, & Berendes (1968) study of more than 24,000 births, called the Collaborative Perinatal Project, concluded that FHR auscultation during labor was unreliable in determining fetal distress except in extreme cases of terminal bradycardias. Based on this report and rapid technologic advances, intermittent auscultation of the FHR between contractions was rapidly replaced with continuous EFM during the 1970s. Over the next three decades, EFM became the preferred method of fetal surveillance during the intrapartum period in the United States and Canada.

During the 1980s and 1990s, several randomized trials that compared intermittent auscultation to continuous EFM were conducted (MacDonald, Grant, Sheridan-Pereira, Boylan, & Chalmers, 1985; Thacker, Stroup, & Peterson, 1995; Vintzileos et al., 1993). Disappointingly, EFM did not decrease perinatal mortality or prevent cerebral palsy. Equally important, the women in EFM groups experienced a four-fold increase in operative birth (Thacker et al., 1995). The potential reasons why EFM did not demonstrate efficacy in the randomized trials are methodological flaws, inconsistent criteria and terminology to describe fetal status and the use of outcome variables for which there were insufficient sample sizes to determine a significant difference between intermittent auscultation and continuous EFM.

The demonstrated increase in cesarean birth rates fueled reexamination of all aspects of EFM use. In 1997, the National Institute of Child Health and Human Development (NICHD) of the National Institutes of Health convened a panel of FHR monitoring experts. This expert group proposed detailed, quantitative, standardized definitions of FHR patterns, which serve as a basis for interdisciplinary research, communication, and medical record documentation concerning fetal status (NICHD, 1997) (see Table 8–1). Since the proceedings of the NICHD Research Planning Workshop were published, there has been a gradual adoption of the proposed standardized FHR pattern definitions in clinical practice in the United States. In July 2004, the Joint Commission on Accreditation of Healthcare Organizations (JCAHO) recommended use of a standard language for communication and documentation of FHR patterns. In May 2005, the Association of Women's Health, Obstetric and Neonatal Nurses (AWHONN) and the American College of Obstetricians and Gynecologists (ACOG) supported adoption of the NICHD definitions for FHR patterns. These definitions have been incorporated into the AWHONN Fetal Monitoring Program and are used in the interdisciplinary electronic fetal monitoring certification examination produced by the National Certification Corporation.

Currently, clinical reliance on EFM remains high, despite the lack of positive results from published research. To date, it is the primary screening technique for the clinical determination of the adequacy of fetal oxygenation during labor. This paradox is better understood following a review of the physiology of the fetal heart and its adaptations during labor. The current feelings of many clinicians about EFM versus intermittent auscultation were summarized by Cibils in 1996: "It is difficult to understand the premise that the intermittent recording (by a crude method) of a given biologic variable [the FHR] will be better to make a clinical decision affecting the mother and fetus than the continuous, precise recording of the same variable."

Hence, although confirmatory data about improved outcomes when EFM is used during labor are lacking, most clinicians prefer EFM as the intrapartum method of fetal assessment, and it is recommended by ACOG (2005b) and the Society of Obstetricians and Gynaecologists of Canada (SOGC) (2002) for high-risk maternal–fetal conditions during labor.

DEFINITIONS AND APPROPRIATE USE OF TERMS DESCRIBING FETAL HEART RATE PATTERNS

Appropriate clinical management of variant FHR patterns depends on the use of standardized definitions that convey agreed-upon meanings among the members of the healthcare team. Adoption of a common language for FHR pattern definitions and medical record documentation that is mutually agreed upon and routinely used by all providers enhances interdisciplinary communication and, therefore, maternal–fetal safety (JCAHO, 2004). Both oral communication and written documentation must accurately convey the exact level of concern and/or record the presumed diagnosis. The chances of miscommunication between care providers, especially during telephone conversations about fetal status, are decreased when everyone is speaking the same language (Simpson & Knox, 2006). Timely intervention during nonreassuring FHR patterns is dependent on clear communication between providers sharing care of an individual patient (Fox, Kilpatrick, King, & Parer, 2000; Miller, 2005). The

TABLE 8–1 ■ FETAL HEART RATE CHARACTERISTICS AND PATTERNS

Term	Definition
Baseline rate	Approximate mean FHR rounded to increments of 5 bpm during a 10-min segment, excluding periodic or episodic changes, periods of marked variability and segments of baseline that differ by >25 bpm. During any 10-min window, the minimum baseline duration must be at least 2 min or the baseline for that period is indeterminate. In this case, one may need to refer to the previous 10-min segment for determination of the baseline.
Bradycardia	Baseline rate of <110 bpm.
Tachycardia	Baseline rate of >160 bpm.
Baseline variability	Fluctuations in the baseline FHR of 2 cycles/min or greater. These fluctuations are irregular in amplitude and frequency and are visually quantified as the amplitude of the peak to trough in bpm.
• Absent variability	Amplitude range undetectable.
• Minimal variability	Amplitude range > undetectable and ≤5 bpm.
• Moderate variability	Amplitude range 6–25 bpm.
• Marked variability	Amplitude range >25 bpm.
Acceleration	Visually apparent *abrupt* increase (onset to peak is <30 sec) in FHR above baseline. The increase is calculated from the most recently determined portion of the baseline. Acme is ≥15 bpm above the baseline and lasts ≥15 sec and <2 min from the onset to return to baseline. Before 32 weeks of gestation, an acme ≥10 bpm above the baseline and duration of ≥10 sec is an acceleration.
Prolonged acceleration	Acceleration ≥2-min and <10-min duration.
Early deceleration	Visually apparent *gradual* (onset to nadir is ≥30 sec) decrease of the FHR and return to base line associated with a uterine contraction. This decrease is calculated from the most recently determined portion of the baseline. It is coincident in timing, with the nadir of deceleration occurring at the same time as the peak of the contraction. In most cases, the onset, nadir, and recovery of the deceleration are coincident with the beginning, peak, and ending of the contraction, respectively.
Late deceleration	Visually apparent *gradual* (onset to nadir is ≥30 sec) decrease of the FHR and return to base line associated with a uterine contraction. This decrease is calculated from the most recently determined portion of the baseline. It is delayed in timing, with the nadir of deceleration occurring after the peak of the contraction. In most cases, the onset, nadir, and recovery of the deceleration occur after the onset, peak, and ending of the contraction, respectively.
Variable deceleration	Visually apparent *abrupt* (onset to beginning of nadir is <30 sec) decrease in FHR below base line. The decrease is calculated from the most recently determined portion of the baseline. Decrease is ≥15 bpm, lasting ≥15 sec and <2 min from onset to return to baseline. When variable decelerations are associated with uterine contractions, their onset, depth, and duration vary with successive uterine contractions.
Prolonged deceleration	Visually apparent decrease in FHR below baseline. The decrease is calculated from the most recently determined portion of the baseline. Decrease is ≥15 bpm, lasting ≥2 min but <10 min from onset to return to baseline.
Recurrent decelerations	Occurring with ≥50% of uterine contractions during any 20-minute segment.

From National Institute of Child Health and Human Development Research Planning Workshop. (1997). Electronic fetal heart rate monitoring: Research guidelines for interpretation. *American Journal of Obstetrics and Gynecology 177*(6), 1385–1390 and *Journal of Obstetric, Gynecologic and Neonatal Nursing, 26*(6) 635–640.

NICHD (1997) nomenclature is the basis for the pattern descriptions in this chapter.

The purpose of the NICHD *Research Planning Workshop* (1997) was to define and describe specific FHR patterns rather that assigning diagnostic or prognostic value to any one FHR characteristic or combination of characteristics. Therefore, the terms *reassuring* and *nonreassuring* were not used in the workshop proceedings. Nevertheless, these terms are frequently used by clinicians to describe FHR patterns and will be used in this chapter.

There is little controversy concerning what constitutes a reassuring FHR pattern. Most clinicians agree on the definition of a reassuring (normal) FHR tracing (ie, baseline rate within 110 to 160 bpm, moderate FHR variability, presence of accelerations, and absence of decelerations). There is general agreement that there is good evidence that this type of FHR tracing confers an extremely high predictability of a normally oxygenated fetus when it is obtained (NICHD, 1997).

At the other end of the spectrum from normality, several patterns are likely predictive of current or impending fetal asphyxia so severe that the fetus is at risk for neurologic and other fetal damage, or death (NICHD, 1997). According to the expert participants in the NICHD workshop, these patterns include recurrent late or variable decelerations or "substantial" bradycardia, with absent FHR variability. A recent review of the published literature to date on the association between FHR patterns and fetal acidemia found moderate FHR variability was strongly (98%) associated with an umbilical pH >7.15 or newborn vigor (5-minute Apgar score ≥7); absent or minimal FHR variability with late or variable decelerations was the most consistent predictor of newborn acidemia (although the association was only 23%), there was a positive relationship between the degree of acidemia and the depth of decelerations or bradycardia, and except for a sudden profound bradycardia, newborn acidemia with decreasing variability in combination with decelerations develops over a period of time approaching 1 hour (Parer, King, Flanders, Fox, & Kilpatrick, 2006). Thus, there is supportive evidence for the association between the types of FHR patterns mentioned in the NICHD workshop proceedings as likely predictive of current or impending severe fetal asphyxia and abnormal fetal acid-base status.

Many fetuses have FHR tracings that are intermediate between these two extremes, and there is no consensus on their presumed condition or clinical management. However, most clinicians do not wait until the FHR pattern is at the extreme end of abnormality before intervening to attempt to improve fetal status via one or more intrauterine resuscitation techniques (Simpson, 2007). Ideally, members of the perinatal team have a shared method of interpreting FHR patterns and an agreed-upon management guideline for specific FHR patterns (Fox et al., 2000).

Terms such as *stress* and *distress* lack the precise meaning needed to discriminate levels of concern. In 1998, ACOG recommended that *nonreassuring fetal status* replace the term *fetal distress* in its committee opinion *Inappropriate Use of the Terms Fetal Distress and Birth Asphyxia*. This committee opinion was reaffirmed in 2005 (ACOG, 2005a). The term *fetal distress* has a low positive predictive value, even in high-risk populations, and is associated often with an infant who is in good condition at birth as determined by the Apgar score or umbilical cord blood gas analysis or both. Communication between clinicians caring for the woman and those caring for her baby is best served by using nonreassuring fetal status, followed by a further description of findings (eg, recurrent variable decelerations, fetal tachycardia or bradycardia, late decelerations, or low biophysical profile score) (ACOG, 2005a). Whereas in the past, the term *fetal distress* generally referred to an ill fetus, *nonreassuring fetal status* describes the clinician's interpretation of data regarding fetal status (ie, the clinician is not reassured by the findings). This term acknowledges the imprecision inherent in the interpretation of the data. Therefore, the diagnosis of nonreassuring fetal status can be consistent with the birth of a vigorous baby (ACOG, 2005a).

Another problematic issue is use of *asphyxia* and or *acidosis* when making a presumptive diagnosis of intrapartum hypoxia. *Asphyxia* means insufficiency or absence of exchange of respiratory gases. The pathologic consequence of asphyxia is injury to the fetal tissues, primarily the brain, with subsequent neurologic impairment. However, asphyxia is a continuum of oxygen deficit that moves from hypoxemia (decreased oxygen content in blood) to acidemia (increased hydrogen ion concentration in blood), then acidosis (increased hydrogen ion concentration in the tissue) (King & Parer, 2000). Hypoxemia and acidosis are detectable via pH measurements of fetal scalp blood or umbilical cord blood at birth. These values reveal the acid-base balance within blood but not within tissue and therefore cannot directly reveal the extent or duration of metabolic acidosis or level of asphyxia in tissue. Thus, the use of terms like *asphyxia* and *acidosis* in communication and medical record documentation about characteristics of the FHR and fetal and/or newborn status is both inappropriate and confusing (Fahey & King, 2005). Imprecise and inaccurate terminology used in medical record documentation can be challenging to defend if litigation follows an unpreventable adverse outcome. Communication and documentation of intrapartum events should be descriptive and avoid the use of terms that have diagnostic meaning.

TECHNIQUES OF FETAL HEART RATE MONITORING

Assessment of Uterine Activity

During the intrapartum period, the FHR is interpreted relative to uterine activity. Therefore, interpretation of FHR patterns includes a complete assessment of four components of the uterine contractions: (a) frequency, (b) duration, (c) intensity, and (d) the uterine resting tone between contractions. These assessments can be made by either palpation, external tocodynamometer (*tokos* is Greek for *childbirth*), or the use of an intrauterine pressure catheter (IUPC).

Assessment of uterine activity begins with palpation. Contraction frequency is measured from the beginning of one contraction to the beginning of the next and is described in minutes. Duration is the length of the contraction and is described in seconds. Intensity refers to the strength of the contraction and is described as mild, moderate, or strong by palpation, or in millimeters of mercury (mm Hg) if an IUPC is used. Uterine resting tone is assessed in the absence of contractions or between contractions. By direct palpation, resting tone is described as soft or hard and via IUPC in terms of mm Hg. As with any procedure, the least invasive approach is preferred unless maternal–fetal status indicates need for more objective data.

Each technique has some limitation. Intensity cannot be determined with a tocodynamometer. The tocodynamometer detects pressure changes from the tightening of the fundus during contractions through the maternal abdomen. This technique gives a relatively accurate reading of the duration and frequency of contractions but is unable to assess intensity or resting tone. With an IUPC, the peak of the contraction as indicated on the fetal monitor tracing depicts the actual strength of the contraction measured in mm Hg pressure within the amniotic fluid. The IUPC is most accurate because direct measurement of intra-amniotic pressure is recorded, but it requires ruptured membranes for insertion.

Once the frequency, duration, intensity, and resting tone have been determined, one can assess the adequacy of the uterine activity. Normal contraction frequency in the active phase of labor is every 2–3 minutes. Some uterine activity patterns are dysfunctional or inadequate for generating progress in labor. (See Fig. 8–1 A–C.)

Various definitions of hyperstimulation have been described in the literature. For the purposes of this chapter, it is defined as a persistent pattern of more than five contractions in 10 minutes, contractions lasting 2 minutes or longer, or contractions of normal duration occurring within 1 minute of each other (ACOG, 1999b; 2003; 2005b; Simpson, 2002). While hyperstimulation can be spontaneous as a result of endogenous maternal oxytocin or prostaglandins, it is more often seen during exogenous stimulation with agents used in cervical ripening and induction and augmentation of labor (Crane, Young, Butt, Bennett, & Hutchens, 2001).

Hyperstimulation can cause a decrease in uteroplacental blood flow and precipitate FHR decelerations. If hyperstimulation occurs during oxytocin administration, the infusion should be decreased or discontinued until the uterine contraction pattern returns to normal to avoid progression to nonreassuring fetal status. If a nonreassuring FHR pattern occurs during oxytocin administration, the infusion should be discontinued until the FHR and uterine contraction pattern return to normal. Once FHR pattern characteristics indicate fetal recovery, resuming the oxytocin at a lower rate of infusion may be the only intervention necessary. If oxytocin has been discontinued for 20–30 minutes; the FHR is reassuring; and contraction frequency, intensity, and duration are normal, a suggested protocol may include restarting oxytocin at half the rate that caused the hyperstimulation and gradually increasing the rate as appropriate based on unit protocol and maternal–fetal status. However, if the oxytocin is discontinued for more than 30–40 minutes, most of the exogenous oxytocin is metabolized and plasma levels are similar to that of a woman who has not received intravenous (IV) oxytocin (Simpson, 2002). In this clinical situation, a suggested protocol may include restarting the oxytocin at the initial dose ordered. If a similar adverse clinical situation occurs with the use of other pharmacologic agents used to ripen the cervix or stimulate contractions that may require repeated dosing (eg, Cervidil, Prepidil, or misoprostol), delay the next dose until the FHR is reassuring and the uterine contraction pattern returns to normal frequency, duration, and resting tone.

Coupling or *tripling* refers to a pattern of two or three contractions with little or no interval followed by a regular interval of approximately 2–5 minutes. This pattern may be indicative of a dysfunctional labor process and saturation or down-regulation of uterine oxytocin receptor sites (Dawood, 1995; Phaneuf, Rodriguez-Linares, TambyRaja, MacKenzie, & Lopez-Bernal, 2000; Zeeman, Khan-Dawood, & Dawood, 1997). If coupling or tripling occurs, a suggested intervention to promote normal uterine activity is temporary discontinuation of oxytocin, maternal repositioning, and an IV fluid bolus of lactated Ringer's solution with resumption of oxytocin after 30–60 minutes.

External Doppler Versus Fetal Scalp Electrode

The FHR can be detected via a Doppler ultrasound transducer or fetal electrode. Leopold's maneuvers are

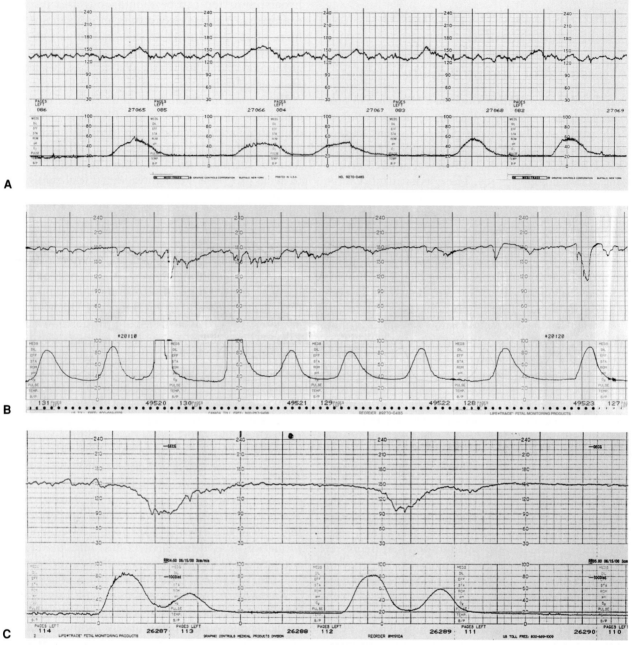

FIGURE 8–1. Three types of uterine contractions. **A,** Normal contraction frequency, duration and intensity, and uterine resting tone. **B,** Hyperstimulation of uterine activity. **C,** Coupling of contractions.

used to determine the fetal position prior to applying the Doppler transducer (see Chapter 7). The Doppler transducer is applied to the maternal abdomen over the fetal back or chest and transmits a high frequency ultrasound. Gel is applied to the transducer to help eliminate air between the transducer and maternal abdomen. The ultrasound wave will not conduct to the fetus if there is air between the emission of the wave and the object it is reflecting off. The transducer detects the ultrasound wave that is bounced back off the fetal heart and then counts the FHR by measuring

the change in ultrasound wave frequency that occurs when the waveform is reflected off the moving heart (see Fig. 8–2).

The monitor counts the time interval between each beat detected, calculates a rate based on that interval, and then plots each calculated rate on the paper that is moving at 3 cm/min. The monitor recounts the FHR every one to two beats. Because there is variability in the time interval between each beat in a normally oxygenated fetus, the line produced over time has a jagged appearance that results from the different rates

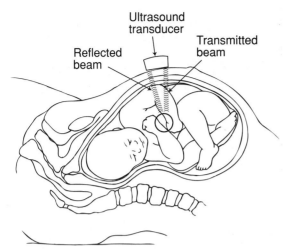

FIGURE 8–2. The Doppler ultrasound device for detecting cardiac activity. The frequency of the reflected beam is changed when it is reflected from a moving structure. (Adapted from Parer, J. T. [1997]. *Handbook of fetal heart rate monitoring* [2nd ed., p. 104]. Philadelphia: W.B. Saunders. Used with permission.)

recorded. Early Doppler technology tended to exaggerate the FHR variability, but improvements in technology have resulted in a Doppler recording that sufficiently reflects the true variability in the FHR under observation. Although the Doppler is easy to apply, maternal or fetal movement, uterine contractions, or maternal positions can interrupt a continuous recording. In cases where the mother is significantly overweight, a continuous recording via external monitoring may be challenging.

The direct fetal scalp electrode (FSE) is the most accurate way to assess the FHR but cannot be used unless the cervix is at least 2–3 cm dilated and the membranes have ruptured. The electrode has three leads, which detect the PQRST complex. The filter within the electronics of the machine removes all components except the R wave. The R wave then triggers the machine to count; it waits for a second complex, filters all but the R wave, and then calculates how much time elapsed from the first to the second R wave in a fashion similar to the technique used by Doppler machines. The elapsed time between R intervals is converted into beats per minute, and the pen records that rate on the paper. The process repeats itself for every R wave, and the variability that is recorded is slightly, but not significantly, more accurate than the variability that is recorded via Doppler.

Doppler and/or fetal scalp electrodes can produce FHR recordings that are inadequate for interpretation. Use of EFM during labor requires knowledge of sources of artifact and solutions for resolution. Many times the problem is secondary to equipment malfunction

and can be remedied easily. The most common reasons why FHR tracings do not record accurately, the FHR tracing that is produced, and the solution to the problem, are listed in Table 8–2.

Application of an FSE is invasive and increases risk of maternal–fetal infection. Therefore, it should be used only when continuous recordings are indicated and are unable to be obtained with external monitoring. If the recording obtained via external EFM is continuous, there is no need for an FSE in order to obtain a better display of FHR variability. There is evidence to suggest that application of a direct electrode could enhance maternal–fetal transmission of HIV when used in women who are HIV-seropositive (Maiques, Garcia-Tejedor, Perales, & Navarro, 1999; Stein, Handelsman, & Matthews, 2000); therefore, use of an FSE is contraindicated in women who are known to be HIV-seropositive. Other relative contraindications to the application of a direct fetal lead include women who have active or chronic hepatitis and those who have herpes simplex virus or other known and non-treated sexually transmitted diseases. Current recommendations are to avoid techniques that result in a break in the skin when there is the presence of these infectious agents (Maiques et al., 1999; Parer & Nageotte, 2004). Application of a direct fetal lead also may be deferred for women who are known hemophilia carriers when the sex of their fetus is unknown.

Intermittent Auscultation

Prior to the introduction of Doppler technology, intermittent auscultation of the FHR was accomplished with a Pinard or DeLee stethoscope between contractions. A baseline FHR can be obtained, and the presence or absence of some decelerations can be noted without determination of variability or the type of deceleration with this technique. Auscultation with a non-Doppler stethoscope is no longer common practice in the United States. Today, when the FHR is assessed during labor via an intermittent auscultation (IA) protocol, a handheld Doppler unit is used that can detect the FHR during a contraction (Display 8–1).

Current recommendations for using auscultation during the intrapartum period are outlined by the AWHONN symposium *Fetal Heart Rate Auscultation* (Feinstein, Sprague, & Trepanier, 2000), the ACOG (2005b) Practice Bulletin, *Intrapartum Fetal Heart Rate Monitoring*, the SOCG (2002) Clinical Practice Guidelines, *Fetal Health Surveillance in Labour*, and in the *Guidelines for Perinatal Care* (American Academy of Pediatrics [AAP] & ACOG, 2002). However, there are inconsistencies in the recommendations from AAP, ACOG, AWHONN, and SOGC for patients for whom IA is appropriate and the frequency of assessment when using IA. Because there is limited evidence

TABLE 8–2 ■ SOURCES OF ARTIFACT OR ERROR IN FETAL HEART RATE RECORDINGS

	Recording Produced	Solution
Signal Errors		
Faulty leg plate, electrode, or monitor	No recording	Replace equipment
Transducer does not detect fetal heart consistently	Intermittent recording	Move transducer
• Maternal muscle movements		
• Uterine contractions		
• Maternal positioning		
• Maternal obesity		
Interference by maternal signal	Recording will be maternal heart rate	Recognize maternal heart beat and use alternative method or adjust placement of transducer
Limitation of Machinery		
Counting process omits FHR that is >30 bpm different from preceding beat	Arrhythmia will be audible but does not appear on record	Use fetal EKG if improved recording needed. Arrhythmias tend to be regular and artifact tends to be irregular. Auscultate to determine correct rate
Halving or doubling of audible FHR	Very slow rates may be doubled and very fast rates (>240 bpm) may be halved	
Interpretive Errors		
Maternal heart rate recorded	Rate recorded will equal maternal pulse EFM may provide electronic cues that recording is maternal in nature.	Compare with maternal pulse. Palpate maternal pulse.
• Fetal death		
• Electrode on cervix		
Scaling Error	Two paper speeds are possible on some machines (1 and 3 cm/min). FHR pattern will change at slower speed, exaggerating variability.	Assure paper speed of 3 ms/min prior to applying transducers

Adapted with permission from Parer, J. T. (1997). *Handbook of fetal heart rate monitoring* (2nd ed.), Philadelphia: W. B. Saunders.

D I S P L A Y   8 - 1

Capabilities of Auscultation Devices

FETOSCOPE

- Detect FHR baseline
- Detect FHR rhythm
- Verify the presence of an arrhythmia
- Detect increases and decreases from FHR baseline
- Clarify double or half counting by EFM

DOPPLER

- Detect FHR baseline
- Detect FHR rhythm
- Detect increases and decreases from FHR baseline

EFM, electronic fetal monitoring; FHR, fetal heart rate.
From Association of Women's Health, Obstetric and Neonatal Nurses. (2000). *Symposium fetal heart rate auscultation* (p. 16). Washington, DC: Author.

to suggest improved outcomes for fetuses of women assessed via IA as compared to EFM, traditionally the recommendations have been as follows: in the absence of identified risk factors, auscultation of the FHR every 30 minutes in the active phase of the first stage of labor and every 15 minutes in the second stage of labor is suggested; when risk factors have been identified, assessment frequency is increased to every 15 minutes in the active phase of the first stage of labor and every 5 minutes in the second stage (AAP & ACOG, 2002; AWHONN, 2000a). However, both ACOG (2005b) and SOGC (2002) have recently recommended that IA be reserved for low-risk women and continuous EFM be used for high-risk women. Labor induction and augmentation are identified as additional criteria for continuous EFM by SOGC (2002). ACOG's (2005b) recommended assessment frequency for IA is every 15 minutes in the active phase of first stage labor and every 5 minutes during second-stage labor, while SOGC's (2002) recommended assessment frequency for IA is for 1 minute immediately after a contraction every 15 to 30 minutes in the active phase of first-stage labor and every 5 minutes during second-stage labor. No clinical trials have examined methods of fetal assessment during the latent phase of labor. Therefore, clinical judgment and unit policy should guide decisions when deciding the method and frequency of fetal assessment. When auscultation is used as the primary method of fetal surveillance during labor, a 1:1 nurse–fetus ratio is required (AWHONN, 2000a).

The decision to use IA or EFM rests with the healthcare provider but is made in collaboration with the laboring woman. The decision is based on many factors, including patient history, fetal condition, risk classification, hospital policies and procedures, and the standard of practice. As with EFM, there are benefits and limitations to the use of IA (Display 8–2). Both IA and EFM are effective in fetal evaluation when used appropriately (AAP & ACOG, 2002; ACOG, 2005b; AWHONN, 2000a; SOGC, 2002).

PHYSIOLOGIC BASIS FOR FETAL HEART RATE MONITORING

Electronic fetal monitoring is a technique for fetal assessment based on the premise that the FHR reflects fetal oxygenation. Although a FHR with a normal baseline, moderate variability, and accelerations is a good predictor of a fetus without hypoxemia, the reverse is not true. Variant FHR patterns occur in up to 80% of all fetal heart tracings obtained during labor; however, the majority do not indicate fetal hypoxemia (Berkus, Langer, Samueloff, Xernaxis, & Field, 1999; Goldaber, Gilstrap, Leveno, Dax, & McIntire, 1991; Helwig, Parer, Kilpatrick, & Laros, 1996; Herbst, Wolner-Hanssen, & Ingemarsson 1997). Because the high rate of false-positive FHR tracings has many origins and several clinical implications, a working knowledge of FHR physiology can aid clinical interpretation of FHR patterns during labor. The following section reviews oxygen and carbon dioxide transfer in the fetus, intrinsic control of the FHR, and the characteristics of the normal FHR.

Maternal Oxygen Status

The fetus is dependent on well-oxygenated maternal blood flow to the placenta. The hemoglobin concentration or oxygen carrying capacity of maternal blood must be adequate to promote fetal oxygenation. Oxygen tension in maternal arterial blood depends on adequate ventilation and pulmonary integrity and is a determinant of fetal oxygenation (Parer, 1997). Most pregnant women do not have alterations in pulmonary function and do have adequate oxygen saturation.

DISPLAY 8-2

Benefits and Limitations of Auscultation

BENEFITS

- Neonatal outcomes are comparable to those with EFM based on current RCTs.
- Lower cesarean birth rates have been associated with auscultation than with EFM in some RCTs.
- The technique is less invasive.
- The patient's freedom of movement is increased.
- The technology allows for fetal heart assessment if the patient is immersed in water.
- The equipment is less costly than EFM equipment.
- Auscultation is not automatically documented on paper (often a source of debate in legal situations).
- A caregiver must be present at the bedside to provide the 1:1 nurse-to-patient ratio that is recommended based on RCTs comparing auscultation and EFM.

LIMITATIONS

- Use of a fetoscope may limit the ability to hear the FHR (eg, in cases of maternal obesity or increased amniotic fluid volume).
- Certain FHR characteristics associated with EFM (eg, variability and types of decelerations) cannot be detected.
- Some patients may feel that auscultation is more intrusive.
- Auscultation is not automatically documented on paper (as EFM is, which is perceived as an important piece of documentation by many practitioners).
- There is a potential need to increase or realign staff to meet the 1:1 nurse-to-patient ratio that is recommended based on RCTs comparing auscultation and EFM.

EFM, electronic fetal monitoring; FHR, fetal heart rate.
From Association of Women's Health, Obstetric and Neonatal Nurses. (2000). *Symposium fetal heart rate auscultation* (p. 19). Washington, DC: Author.

However, maternal conditions such as asthma, congenital heart defects, congestive heart failure, lung disease, seizures, or severe anemia can result in impaired oxygen delivery to the fetus.

Uterine, Placental, and Umbilical Blood Flow

At term, approximately 10%–15% of maternal cardiac output, or 600–750 cc of blood volume, perfuses the uterus each minute. Oxygenated blood from the mother is delivered to the intervillous space in the placenta via the uterine arteries. Blood enters the intervillous space under positive arterial pressure from the maximally dilated uterine spiral arterioles, surrounds the villi that fill the intervillous space, and then drains back to the uterine veins. Fetal deoxygenated blood is carried to the placental villi via the two umbilical arteries. Maternal–fetal exchange of oxygen, carbon dioxide, nutrients, waste products, water, and heat occurs in the intervillous space across the membranes that separate fetal and maternal circulations. Oxygen is exchanged through passive diffusion from an area of high concentration (maternal side) to an area of low concentration (fetal side). Other nutrients are exchanged via active transport, facilitated diffusion, hydrostatic pressure, and pinocytosis (Fig. 8–3).

Oxygen and carbon dioxide diffuse across membranes rapidly and efficiently. Therefore, effective transfer of oxygen and carbon dioxide between the fetal and maternal blood streams is dependent on (a) adequate uterine blood flow, (b) sufficient placental area, and (c) an unconstrained umbilical cord. Uterine blood flow into the intervillous space can be impeded by hypertension (higher pressures decrease the time available for adequate exchange) or hypotension (inadequate perfusion of the intervillous space). A placenta with inadequate diffusing capacity can

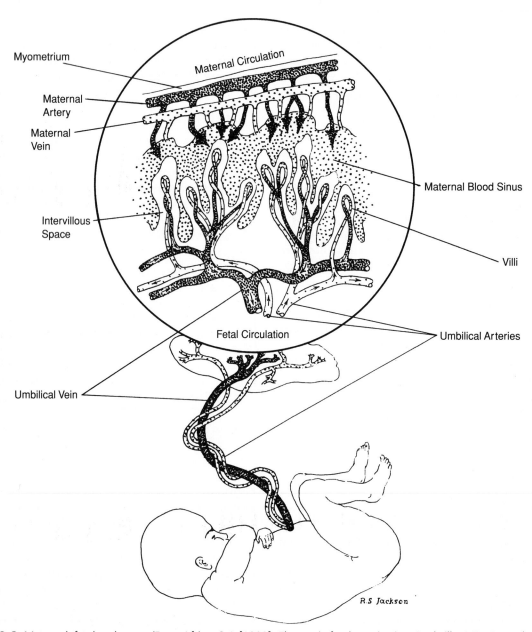

FIGURE 8–3. Maternal–fetal exchange. (From Afriat, C. I. [1989]. *Electronic fetal monitoring.* Rockville, MD: Aspen.)

develop in women who have hypertension or preeclampsia or, in those who may have had an in-utero infection such as toxoplasmosis. In addition, intrauterine growth restriction (IUGR) may be secondary to decreased placental area or diffusing capacity. Umbilical blood flow is about 360 mL/min, or 120 mL/min/kg, in an undisturbed fetus at term (Gill, Trudinger, Garrett, Kossoff, & Warren, 1981). Umbilical blood flow is most commonly impeded by acute cord compression, which can cause partial or, rarely, complete occlusion.

In summary, because poor maternal oxygenation is rare and because oxygen diffuses quite rapidly across most membranes, the significant factors affecting placental exchange of gases and nutrients for the fetus are uterine blood flow, umbilical blood flow, and the amount of placental area available for exchange. See Display 8–3 for a complete list of factors determining maternal–fetal oxygen transfer. The FHR patterns during labor reflect the function of these components of placental function and maternal oxygen status. Before discussing nursing interventions that support these physiologic mechanisms, a review of the physiology of the FHR is presented.

DISPLAY 8-3

Factors Determining Maternal-Fetal Oxygen Transfer

Intervillous blood flow

Fetal placental blood flow

Oxygen tension in maternal arterial blood

Oxygen tension in fetal arterial blood

Oxygen affinity of maternal blood

Oxygen affinity of fetal blood

Hemoglobin concentration or oxygen capacity of maternal blood

Hemoglobin concentration or oxygen capacity of fetal blood

Maternal and fetal blood pH and partial pressure of carbon dioxide

Placental diffusing capacity

Placental vascular geometry

Ratio of maternal to fetal blood flow in exchanging areas

Shunting around exchange sites

Placental oxygen consumption

From Parer, J. T. (1997). *Handbook of fetal heart rate monitoring* (2nd ed.). Philadelphia: W. B. Saunders.

Physiology of the Fetal Heart Rate

Several factors influence the FHR (Display 8–4). Interplay between the two components of the autonomic nervous system (sympathetic and parasympathetic), higher cortical functions in the brain, and chemoreceptors and baroreceptors are all reflected in the baseline rate and, in part, make up the FHR variability seen on the recording from a FHR monitor.

The parasympathetic nervous system influences the heart via the vagus nerve. Parasympathetic nerve fibers in the vagus nerve that control heart rate originate in the medulla oblongata of the brain and terminate in the sinoatrial and atrioventricular nodes within the heart. Stimulation of these fibers slow the heart rate by controlling or overriding the intrinsic rate generated within this node (Dalton, Phill, Dawes, & Patrick, 1983). The sympathetic nervous system has fibers that terminate in the muscle of the heart. Stimulation of these nerves causes an increase in heart rate and stroke volume, which then increases cardiac output (Parer & Nageotte, 2004). During gestation, the parasympathetic nervous system matures during the second trimester and the vagus nerve gradually becomes dominant over sympathetic stimulation, which explains the slow drop in normal baseline rate as the fetus matures.

The vagus nerve is subject to influences from other parts of the central nervous system. The respiratory center is geographically close to the cardio-regulatory centers in the medulla oblongata and the FHR may increase with inspiratory movement and decrease with expiratory movement. Fetal sleep is associated with decreased variability, and gross body movements are associated with accelerations (Parer & Nageotte, 2004; Dalton et al., 1983).

Chemoreceptors and baroreceptors participate in two feedback loops that decrease the heart rate as part of the normal fetal response to transient hypoxemia. Chemoreceptors found in the aortic arch and central nervous system are sensitive to changes in oxygen and carbon dioxide content within the blood. When uteroplacental blood flow falls below the threshold needed for normal gas exchange, increased carbon dioxide tension in fetal vessels causes the chemoreceptors to stimulate the vagus nerve and slow the FHR. The effect of this bradycardia is decreased cardiac metabolism and decreased oxygen consumption. Baroreceptors are found in the aortic and carotid arches, where they detect changes in pressure very quickly. When umbilical blood flow is impeded, fetal blood pressure rises and a quick reflex occurs (via the vagal nerve) to slow the heart rate rapidly, which decreases blood pressure. In addition to bradycardia, blood is redistributed to vital organs (eg, the brain, heart, and adrenal glands) and is shunted away from non-vital organs (eg, gut, spleen, kidneys, and limbs) during fetal hypoxemia

DISPLAY 8 – 4

Regulatory Control of the Heart Rate

FACTORS REGULATING FETAL HEART RATE	LOCATION
Parasympathetic division of autonomic nervous system	Vagus nerve fibers supply sinoatrial (SA) and atrioventricular (AV) node
Sympathetic division of autonomic nervous system	Nerves widely distributed in myocardium
Baroreceptors	Stretch receptors in aortic arch and carotid sinus at the junction of the internal and external carotid arteries
Chemoreceptors	Peripheral—in carotid and aortic bodies
	Central—in medulla oblongata
Central nervous system	Cerebral cortex
	Hypothalamus
	Medulla oblongata
Hormonal regulation	Adrenal medulla
	Adrenal cortex
	Vasopressin (plasma catecholamine)
Blood volume or capillary fluid shift	Fluid shift between capillaries and interstitial spaces
Intraplacental pressures	Intervillous space
Frank-Starling mechanism	Based on stretching of myocardium by increased inflow of venous blood into right atrium

From Tucker, S.M. (2004). *Fetal monitoring and assessment.* St. Louis: Mosby.

ACTION	EFFECT
Stimulation causes release of acetylcholine at myoneural synapse	Decreases heart rate Maintains beat-to-beat variability
Stimulation causes release of norepinephrine at synapse	Increases fetal heart rate (FHR) Increases strength of myocardial contraction Increases cardiac output
Responds to increase in blood pressure by stimulating stretch receptors to send impulses by the vagus or glossopharyngeal nerve to the midbrain, producing vagal response and slowing heart activity	Decreases FHR Decreases blood pressure Decreases cardiac output
Responds to a marked peripheral decrease in O_2 and increase in CO_2	Produces bradycardia sometimes with increased variability
Central chemoceptors respond to decreases in O_2 tension and increases in CO_2 tension in blood and/or cerebrospinal fluid	Produces tachycardia and increase in blood pressure with decrease in variability
Responds to fetal movement	Increases variability
Responds to fetal sleep	Decreases variability
Regulates and coordinates autonomic activities (sympathetic and parasympathetic)	
Mediates cardiac and vasomotor reflex center by controlling heart action and blood vessel diameter	Maintains balance between cardioacceleration and cardiodeceleration
Releases epinephrine and norepinephrine with severe fetal hypoxia, producing sympathetic response	Increases FHR Increases strength of myocardial contraction and blood pressure Increases cardiac output Maintains homeostasis of blood volume
Low fetal blood pressure stimulates release of aldosterone, decreases sodium output, increases water retention, which increases circulating blood volume	
Produces vasoconstriction of nonvital vascular beds in the asphyxiated fetus to increase blood pressure	Distributes blood flow to maintain FHR and variability
Responds to elevated blood pressure by causing fluid to move out of capillaries and into interstitial spaces	Decreases blood volume and blood pressure
Responds to low blood pressure by causing fluid to move out of interstitial space into capillaries	Increases blood volume and blood pressure
Fluid shift between fetal and maternal blood is based on osmotic and blood pressure gradients; maternal blood pressure is about 100 mmHg and fetal blood pressure about 55 mmHg; balance is probably maintained by some compensatory factor.	Regulates blood volume and blood pressure
In the adult, the myocardium is stretched by an increased inflow of blood, causing the heart to contract with greater force than before and pump out more blood; the adult then is able to increase cardiac output by increasing heart rate and stroke volume; this mechanism is not well developed in the fetus.	Cardiac output depends on heart rate in the fetus: $\downarrow$ FHR = $\downarrow$ cardiac output $\uparrow$ FHR = $\uparrow$ cardiac output

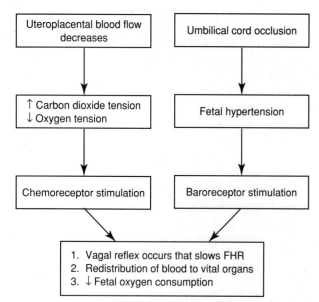

FIGURE 8-4. Fetal response to hypoxemia.

(King & Parer, 2000) (Fig. 8–4). Thus, the medulla oblongata cardio-regulatory center (via the vagus nerve) controls heart rate variability via mediation of input from several sources including the (a) central nervous system, (b) chemoreceptors and baroreceptors, and (c) respiratory center.

CHARACTERISTICS OF THE NORMAL FETAL HEART RATE

FHR pattern interpretation involves assessment of five components of the FHR: (a) baseline rate, (b) presence or absence of accelerations, (c) variability, (d) periodic and/or episodic changes, and (e) evolution over time (NICHD, 1997). Baseline changes are those that occur for 10 minutes or more. Bradycardia and tachycardia are the two alterations in baseline rate of clinical importance. Periodic changes in FHR occur in response to uterine activity. Episodic patterns are not associated with uterine activity and may occur randomly. Early decelerations, late decelerations, prolonged decelerations, and variable decelerations are the periodic or episodic patterns that can develop. In addition, there are a few unusual patterns, such as sinusoidal heart rate, arrhythmias, and marked variability (previously termed *saltatory*), that will be mentioned briefly. This section reviews the characteristics of the normal FHR, and the next section will review the etiology and management of the most common periodic and episodic changes.

Baseline Rate

The baseline FHR is the approximate mean FHR rounded to increments of 5 bpm during a 10-minute segment, excluding periodic or episodic changes, periods of marked FHR variability, and segments of the baseline that differ by >25 bpm (NICHD, 1997). During any 10-minute window, the minimum baseline duration must be at least 2 minutes or the baseline for that period is indeterminate. In this case, one may need to refer to the previous 10-minute segment(s) for determination of the baseline. The normal baseline FHR range is 110 to 160 bpm (NICHD 1997). The average FHR of the term fetus before labor is 140 bpm (Parer & Nageotte, 2004). Early in pregnancy the FHR is slightly higher. If the baseline FHR is <110 bpm, it is termed *bradycardia*; if the baseline FHR is >160 bpm, it is termed *tachycardia* (NICHD, 1997)

Variability

The FHR of the healthy fetus is displayed as an irregular line on the monitor tracing. These irregularities demonstrate the FHR variability previously described, which reflects the slight difference in time interval between each beat. If all time intervals between heartbeats were identical, the line would be flat or smooth. Baseline FHR rate variability is defined as fluctuations in the baseline FHR of 2 cycles per minute or greater. These fluctuations are irregular in amplitude and frequency and are visually quantitated as the amplitude of the peak-to-trough in bpm as follows:

Amplitude range undetectable: absent FHR variability
Amplitude range > undetectable <5 bpm: minimal FHR variability
Amplitude range 6 to 25 bpm: moderate FHR variability
Amplitude range >25 bpm: marked FHR variability

Clinically variability is visually determined as a unit without deliberately separating short- and long-term components (NICHD, 1997). Variability is assessed during the baseline of the FHR rate, not during periodic changes such as a deceleration or accelerations.

Accelerations

Accelerations are a visually apparent abrupt increase (defined as onset of acceleration to peak in <30 seconds) in FHR above the baseline (Fig. 8–5). The increase is calculated from the most recently determined portion of the baseline. The acme is 15 bpm above the baseline, and the acceleration lasts at least 15 seconds, but less than 2 minutes, from the onset to return to baseline. Before 32 weeks of gestation, accelerations are defined as having an acme of at least 10 bpm above the baseline and duration of at least 10 seconds. Like moderate variability, the presence of accelerations indicates central oxygenation and predicts the absence of fetal acidosis (Clark, Gimovsky, & Miller, 1984). Accelerations can occur as periodic or episodic changes in the FHR.

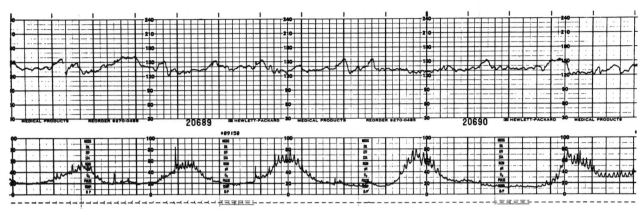

FIGURE 8–5. Accelerations of the fetal heart rate.

In summary, a normal baseline rate with moderate variability, accelerations, and no periodic changes is highly predictive of a well-oxygenated, non-acidotic fetus. (Krebs, Petres, Dunn, Jordaan, & Segreti, 1979; Krebs, Petres, & Dunn, 1981; Berkus et al., 1999; Low, Victory, & Derrick, 1999). In addition, there is a close association between the presence of accelerations and normal FHR variability. It has been well established that EFM's greatest contribution to fetal healthcare is the ability to predict normal outcomes. A reassuring fetal tracing virtually assures the perinatal team that, barring unforeseen acute insults such as abruptio placentae, uterine rupture, rupture of a vasa previa, or umbilical cord prolapse, a well-oxygenated infant will be born.

INTERVENTIONS FOR NONREASSURING FETAL HEART RATE PATTERNS

Before discussing the etiology and individual management of periodic or episodic changes in the FHR, a general review of the initial assessment and interventions used to maximize fetal oxygenation in the presence of variant FHR patterns is warranted. When a nonreassuring FHR pattern is identified, initial assessment may include a cervical exam to rule out umbilical cord prolapse, rapid cervical dilation, or rapid descent of the fetal head; a review of uterine activity to rule out uterine hyperstimulation; and an evaluation of maternal vital signs, in particular temperature and blood pressure, to rule out maternal fever or maternal hypotension (ACOG, 2005b). These assessment data can guide appropriate treatment to attempt to resolve the pattern. *Intrauterine resuscitation* refers to a series of interventions to promote fetal well-being that include a change in maternal position, a decrease in uterine activity or uterine contraction frequency, administration of IV

fluids, and administration of oxygen (Simpson, 2007). Other resuscitative techniques include correction of maternal hypotension, amnioinfusion, and alteration in second-stage labor pushing efforts (Simpson, 2007). The type of resuscitative technique is based on the specific characteristics of the nonreassuring FHR pattern. In some cases, a combination of techniques will be required to resolve the pattern. A summary of the goals and techniques for intrauterine resuscitation are presented in Table 8–3. It is generally believed that these interventions improve maternal blood flow to the placenta and oxygen delivery to the fetus. There are data to suggest that these techniques can improve fetal oxygen status, but it is important to remember that there is no evidence that these techniques will reverse asphyxia. If the clinical characteristics of the FHR patterns are thought to represent a serious risk for acidemia, these measures should be initiated only if doing so does not delay the move toward expeditious birth.

Position Change

Changing maternal position alters the relationship between the umbilical cord and fetal parts or the uterine wall and is usually done to minimize or correct cord compression and decrease the frequency of uterine contractions (Clark et al., 1991). Position change can resolve or decrease the severity of prolonged decelerations and/or variable decelerations. Position change may also modify late decelerations if the etiology of this pattern is decreased uterine blood flow (usually secondary to supine positioning and inferior vena caval compression). Generally, the supine position should be avoided in order to prevent compression of the vena cava and supine hypotensive syndrome. Several studies have compared the effects of right lateral, left lateral, and supine maternal positions on fetal oxygen status, and the findings of each suggest that lateral positioning is more favorable for enhancing fetus oxygenation when compared to a supine position (Aldrich

TABLE 8–3 ■ INTRAUTERINE RESUSCITATION

Goal	Techniques/Methods
Promote fetal oxygenation	Lateral positioning (either left or right) Oxygen administration at 10 L/min via nonrebreather facemask IV fluid bolus of at least 500 mL of lactated Ringer's solution Discontinuation of oxytocin/removal of Cervidil/withholding next dose of Cytotec Stopping pushing temporarily or pushing with every other, or every third contraction (during second-stage labor)
Reduce uterine activity	Discontinuation of oxytocin/removal of Cervidil/withhold next dose of Cytotec IV fluid bolus of at least 500 mL of lactated Ringer's solution Lateral positioning (either left or right) If no response, consider terbutaline 0.25 mg subcutaneously
Alleviate umbilical cord compression	Repositioning Amnioinfusion (during first-stage labor) Stopping pushing temporarily or pushing with every other, or every third, contraction (during second-stage labor)
Correct maternal hypotension	Lateral positioning (either left or right) IV fluid bolus of at least 500 mL of lactated Ringer's solution If no response, consider ephedrine 5 to 10 mg IV push

et al., 1995; Carbonne, Benachi, Leveque, Cabrol, & Papiernik, 1996; Simpson & James, 2005b).

Reduction of Uterine Activity

When uterine contractions are too frequent, there may be insufficient time for blood flow through the intervillous space. If FHR decelerations occur with hyperstimulation, reduction of contraction activity will optimize fetal oxygenation (Freeman, Garite, & Nageotte, 2003). Reduction of uterine activity can occur either by reducing oxytocin dosage or discontinuing oxytocin administration, which will decrease contraction frequency, or by having a mother assume the lateral position. If the FHR is nonreassuring, oxytocin should be discontinued. The next dose of pharmacologic agents used to ripen the cervix or stimulate contractions should be delayed until uterine activity returns to normal and the FHR is reassuring. Administration of tocolytics is another option occasionally used as a temporary measure to provide intrauterine resuscitation for a prolonged deceleration or other nonreassuring FHR patterns secondary to hyperstimulation by reducing uterine activity. A subcutaneous dose of terbutaline 0.25 mg is often used for this purpose. If the pattern does not resolve, preparations for birth are warranted.

IV Fluid Administration

It is believed that administration of fluids maximizes maternal intravascular volume and is therefore protective against decreases in uteroplacental perfusion. A reduction in uterine blood flow can occur following administration of regional anesthesia because the sympathectomy causes dilation of peripheral vessels, lower peripheral resistance, and a potential drop in uteroplacental blood flow. There are limited data to suggest that increasing IV fluids will positively affect uterine blood flow and, thus, fetal oxygenation, even in women who are normotensive and well-hydrated. A recent study found fetal oxygen saturation was significantly increased after at least a 500-mL bolus of lactated Ringer's solution over 20 minutes in normotensive women who were otherwise receiving lactated Ringer's solution at 125 mL per hour (Simpson & James, 2005b). The increase in fetal oxygen saturation was greatest with a 1000 mL IV fluid bolus. The positive effects on fetal oxygen status continued for more than 30 minutes after the IV fluid bolus (Simpson & James, 2005b). Thus, an IV fluid bolus of 500–1,000 mL may be useful as an intrauterine resuscitation technique. However, caution should be used when increasing IV fluids or giving repeated IV fluid boluses. It is important to remember that some clinical situations, such as preeclampsia, preterm labor treated with magnesium sulfate, or preterm labor treated with corticosteroids and beta-sympathomimetic drugs, carry an increased risk for pulmonary edema that might necessitate fluid restriction. Oxytocin has an antidiuretic effect, so prolonged use of oxytocin can also lead to fluid overload if IV fluids are used too liberally. An extreme effect of fluid overload related to excessive use of oxytocin is water intoxication.

Oxygen Administration

Maternal oxygen therapy is commonly used for intrauterine resuscitation and appears to be beneficial in improving fetal oxygen status during labor. In a classic study about the effects of maternal oxygen administration on the fetus, 100% oxygen via facemask corrected nonreassuring FHR patterns by decreasing the baseline FHR during fetal tachycardia and reducing or eliminating late decelerations (Althabe, Schwarcz, Pose, Escarcena, & Caldeyro-Barcia, 1967). There is evidence that fetal oxygen saturation ($FSpO_2$) will increase as a result of maternal oxygen administration of at least 10 L per minute via nonrebreather facemask (Aldrich, Wyatt, Spencer, Reynolds, & Delpy, 1994; Bartnicki & Saling, 1994; Haydon et al., 2006; McNamara, Johnson, & Lilford, 1993; Simpson & James, 2005b). Fetuses with lower oxygen saturation appear to benefit most from maternal oxygen administration (Haydon et al., 2006; Simpson & James, 2005b).

Even though healthy women in labor have nearly 100% SpO_2 (usually between 96% and 99%), increasing inspired oxygen increases blood oxygen tension and results in more oxygen delivered to the fetus (McNamara et al., 1993). There is a more rapid increase in $FSpO_2$ when oxygen is given as compared to the decrease in $FSpO_2$ when it is discontinued, suggesting that the fetus responds to the new placental oxygen gradient by accepting oxygen more rapidly than it gives it up. In one study, $FSpO_2$ levels higher than those pre-oxygen administration to the mother persisted 30 minutes after the oxygen was discontinued (Simpson & James, 2005b). Fetal hemoglobin has a higher affinity for oxygen than adult hemoglobin, and fetal hematocrit is higher than adults. These physiologic factors allow for a steeper increase in fetal oxygen concentration and $FSpO_2$ during maternal oxygen therapy.

When administering oxygen to the mother, use the method that provides the highest fraction of inspired oxygen (FiO_2). The nonrebreather facemask works best because the FiO_2 at 10 L per minute is approximately 80% to 100%, as compared to a simple facemask (FiO_2 27% to 40%) or nasal cannula (FiO_2 31%) (Simpson & James, 2005b). There is inconsistent evidence concerning how long maternal oxygen therapy should be continued and its effects on fetal acid-base status. One study found a deterioration in umbilical cord blood values when maternal oxygen was administered for more than 10 minutes during second-stage labor (Thorp, Trobough, Evans, Hedrick, & Yeast, 2005), while others found no change in acid-base status as measured by umbilical cord gases when maternal oxygen was administered from 15 to 60 minutes during second-stage labor or prior to cesarean birth (Haruta, Funato, Sumida, & Shinkai, 1984; Jozwik et al., 2000). Maternal oxygen therapy as an intrauterine resuscitation technique for 15 to 30 minutes appears to be reasonable, based on the fetal response as noted by the FHR pattern (Haydon et al., 2006; Jozwik et al., 2000; Simpson & James, 2005b). More data are needed on the effects of longer periods of maternal oxygen administration.

Treatment for Anesthesia-Related Hypotension

Conduction anesthetics increase the risk of decreased placental blood flow secondary to maternal hypotension due to sympathetic blockade. If maternal repositioning and IV fluid bolus are not successful in resolving the nonreassuring FHR pattern, ephedrine may be given to increase maternal blood pressure. Ephedrine is the recommended agent because it is least likely to reduce uterine blood flow (Freeman et al., 2003).

Amnioinfusion

Amnioinfusion has been used to attempt to resolve variable FHR decelerations by correcting umbilical cord compression as a result of oligohydramnios. During amnioinfusion, normal saline or lactated Ringer's solution is introduced transcervically via a double lumen intrauterine pressure catheter into the uterus either by gravity flow or through an infusion pump. Amnioinfusion has been found to significantly resolve patterns of "moderate to severe" variable decelerations but does not affect late decelerations or patterns with absent variability (Mino, Puerta, Miranda, & Herruzo, 1999; Miyazaki & Naravez, 1985).

Although amnioinfusion has been shown to dilute thick, meconium-stained amniotic fluid and decrease the incidence of meconium below the newborn's vocal cords (Klingner & Kruse, 1999; Pierce, Gaudier, & Sanchez-Ramos, 2000), in a recent large international study of 1,998 women in term labor, amnioinfusion did not reduce risk of moderate or severe meconium aspiration syndrome or perinatal death (Fraser et al., 2005). Amnioinfusion is no longer recommended as a treatment for meconium-stained fluid (ACOG, 2006a). The procedure does not seem to affect the length of labor (Strong, 1997) and appears to be safe for women who are attempting a vaginal birth after a previous cesarean birth (Ouzounian, Miller, & Paul, 1996). Based on available evidence, amnioinfusion should be limited to the treatment of variable decelerations. Careful monitoring and documentation of fluid infused is important to avoid iatrogenic polyhydramnios. See Chapter 7 for a comprehensive discussion of the technique for amnioinfusion.

Alteration in Pushing Efforts

When the FHR is nonreassuring during second-stage pushing, stopping pushing temporarily or pushing with every other or every third contraction based on the fetal response can be effective in allowing the fetus to recover. As a potential preventive measure, delaying active pushing until the woman feels the urge to push can minimize fetal stress (Simpson & James, 2005a). See Chapter 7 for a comprehensive discussion of nursing care during second-stage labor.

FETAL HEART RATE PATTERNS

Alterations in Baseline Rate

Changes in baseline rate that can occur are (a) tachycardia (a rate greater than 160 bpm), and (b) bradycardia (a rate below 110 bpm) (NICHD, 1997).

Tachycardia

A baseline tachycardia (FHR >160 bpm for 10 minutes or more) may be caused by fetal conditions such as infection, hypoxemia, anemia, prematurity (<26–28 weeks' gestation), supraventricular tachycardia, and congenital anomalies; maternal conditions such as fever, dehydration, and infection; or medical problems such as hyperthyroidism. Beta sympathomimetic drugs such as terbutaline and ritodrine may also cause both maternal and fetal tachycardia. Tachycardia represents increased sympathetic and/or decreased parasympathetic autonomic tone. There are a number of causes of tachycardia that do not reflect a risk of acidemia. The most common of these is an elevation in maternal temperature, although medications administered to the mother and extreme prematurity are other potential factors.

Fetal tachycardia in the presence of chorioamnionitis may be secondary to the maternal fever, an indication of fetal infection, or both. Thus, the determination of risk for acidemia in a fetus with tachycardia is especially difficult. Tachycardia with moderate variability in the absence of FHR decelerations rarely represents fetal acidemia (Krebs, Petres, Dunn, Jordaan, & Segreti, 1979; Tejani, Mann, Bhakthavathsalan, & Weiss, 1975; Low et al., 1999). In the presence of normal FHR variability and no periodic changes, the tachycardia must be assumed to be due to some cause other than oxygen deprivation in the fetus. Tachycardia is sometimes seen during recovery from asphyxia and, as previously discussed, probably represents catecholamine activity following sympathetic nervous or adrenal medullary activity in response to acute non-repetitive asphyxial stress. Fetal tachycardia without FHR variability signifies a significant risk for fetal acidemia.

Nursing interventions for tachycardia include assessment of maternal temperature and hydration. Elevated maternal temperature is the most common etiology of fetal tachycardia in the intrapartum period. Nursing interventions include notification of the physician or midwife, assisting the woman to a lateral position, an infusion of IV fluids and administration of oxygen at 10 L/min via nonrebreather facemask. If the fetal tachycardia is associated with absent variability, late decelerations, or variable decelerations, bedside evaluation by a physician is necessary. If maternal fever has been ruled out as the etiology of the tachycardia, oxytocin infusion should be decreased, or discontinued if infusing, or the next dose of Cervidil, Prepidil, or misoprostol delayed until fetal status is reassuring.

Bradycardia

A baseline bradycardia (FHR <110 bpm for 10 minutes or more) may be caused by fetal conditions such as hypoxemia secondary to an acute decrease in oxygen flow to the fetus, vagal stimulation, and, rarely, cardiac anomalies such as complete heart block or hypothermia. Bradycardias may cause hypoxemia or may be the result of hypoxemia. The depth, duration, and presence or absence of variability are critical components in making a clinical association between the bradycardia seen and the presence or absence of fetal hypoxemia.

A sudden, profound bradycardia is a medical emergency that may signal uterine rupture, prolapsed umbilical cord, rupture of a vasa previa. or placental abruption (Fig. 8–6). This pattern, sometimes called "terminal" bradycardia, may precede death in utero if birth does not occur rapidly. The onset of a fetal bradycardia when a woman is laboring after a prior cesarean birth should cause concern for the onset of uterine rupture, signaling provider attendance at the bedside and preparation for an emergent cesarean birth. Terminal bradycardias are the most common FHR pattern that develops during uterine rupture (Menihan, 1998; Leung, Leung, & Paul, 1993; Ridgeway, Weyrich, & Benedetti, 2004). Leung et al. (1993) evaluated the fetal consequences of catastrophic uterine rupture when the diagnosis was made at the onset of a fetal bradycardia. All infants with a previously normal FHR pattern born within 17 minutes following the onset of a prolonged deceleration survived without significant perinatal morbidity (Leung et al., 1993). However, if "severe" late and variable decelerations are present prior to the onset of bradycardia, the fetus will tolerate a shorter period of prolonged FHR deceleration and there is significantly increased risk for metabolic acidosis (Leung et al., 1993). When "severe" late and variable decelerations precede the onset of a prolonged deceleration associated with uterine rupture, perinatal asphyxia can occur as early as 10 minutes after the onset of a prolonged deceleration (Leung et al., 1993). See Chapter 7 for a discussion of uterine rupture associated with women attempting a trial of labor after a previous cesarean birth.

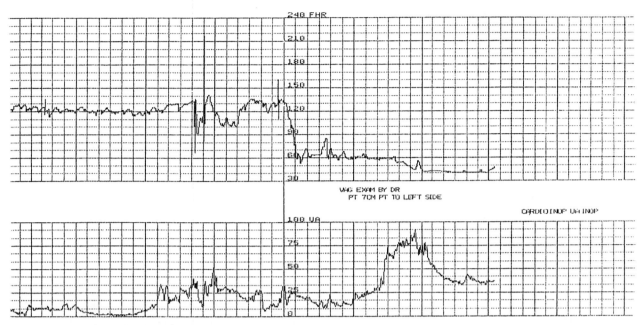

FIGURE 8–6. Terminal bradycardia.

Bradycardias that occur during the second stage of labor following a previously normal FHR pattern may be less concerning. These may be due to increased vagal tone (head compression) (Parer & Nageotte, 2004) or occasionally umbilical cord occlusion. If the variability remains moderate or minimal and the FHR does not fall below 80–90 bpm, expediting birth is not warranted (Gull et al., 1996). However, efforts should be made to alter maternal pushing to allow the fetus to recover.

During a second-stage bradycardia, the woman should be encouraged to push while in either right or left lateral position, avoiding the supine position. If possible, she should push with every other, or every third, contraction to allow the fetus to gain a few added minutes of improved blood flow (Freeman et al., 2003). Coaching a laboring woman to push with every other contraction may be difficult if she has no anesthesia, so this strategy may only be possible with regional anesthesia in place. If the woman has a regional anesthetic, another option would be to allow the fetus to descend passively with the uterine contractions without the woman exerting expulsive efforts if the contractions are of sufficient strength See Chapter 7 for a discussion about nursing interventions during the second stage of labor.

Rarely, sustained fetal bradycardia is caused by complete atrioventricular (AV) heart block associated with congenital malformations or clinical or serologic evidence of maternal collagen vascular disease, especially systemic lupus erythematosus (Hohn & Stanton, 1992). In a fetus with complete AV heart block, a FHR between 50 and 60 bpm without variability may be present (Parer & Nageotte, 2004). Interventions during the intrapartum period are usually not warranted; however, the neonatal team should be notified about the impending birth. The newborn may require a pacemaker insertion after birth.

Several clinical factors affect the potential impact of bradycardia on fetal outcome. Studies that have compared the decision to incision times for emergency cesarean section have shown that there is a time-dependent relationship between the onset of the bradycardia, the depth of the bradycardia, the presence or absence of variability, and the development of metabolic acidosis (Korhonen & Karinem, 1994). If the bradycardia is between 80 and 100 bpm and variability is maintained, the fetus will generally stay well oxygenated centrally and can tolerate these rates for an indefinite time (Gull et al., 1996). Bradycardias with rates of less than 60 bpm, those associated with late or variable decelerations, and those with minimal or absent variability are most often associated with adverse outcome (Beard, Filshie, Knight, & Roberts, 1971; Berkus et al., 1999; Low et al., 1999; Dellinger, Boehm, & Crane, 2000).

In the case of a fetal demise, both the external ultrasound transducer and the direct fetal electrode can record maternal heart rate, which will appear the same as a bradycardic FHR. The external transducer can record maternal heart rate from the aorta, and the direct lead will record maternal heart rate conducted through the dead fetal tissue. If there is any question about the origin of a bradycardia, documentation of the maternal pulse should be one of the initial nursing assessments. This assessment can be accomplished by palpating the maternal pulse. Some fetal monitors provide cues that the heart rate being detected is maternal rather than fetal. If these cues are displayed, confirm that FHR is the source of the tracing.

Nursing interventions for bradycardia include notifying the physician or midwife with a request for bedside evaluation, a vaginal exam to rule out a prolapsed umbilical cord, assisting the woman to a lateral position, administering an infusion of IV fluids, oxygen at 10 L/min via a nonrebreather facemask, and discontinuing oxytocin if infusing. If the bradycardia persists, preparations for an operative birth may be warranted.

Alterations in Variability

Fetal heart rate variability is described as absent, minimal, moderate, or marked (NICHD, 1997) (see Fig. 8–7). Moderate variability complexes are the result of the parasympathetic and sympathetic stimuli, fetal states,

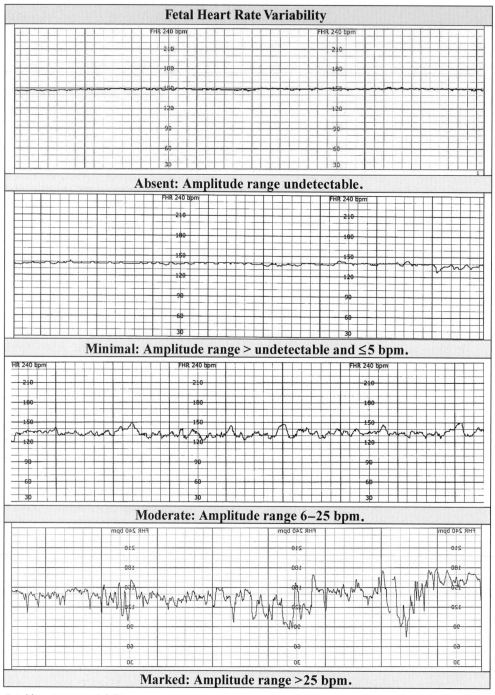

FIGURE 8–7. Fetal heart rate variability.

higher cortical centers, chemoreceptors, baroreceptors, and the cardiac conductions system, and therefore reflect adequate cerebral oxygenation more than any other component of the FHR (Parer & Nageotte, 2004). The most common causes of a decrease in variability not associated with a risk for acidemia are centrally acting drugs such as narcotics, tranquilizers, magnesium sulfate, and other analgesics administered to women during labor. Minimal (but not absent) variability is also seen in premature gestations and during fetal sleep cycles. Minimal variability without concomitant decelerations is almost always unrelated to fetal acidemia (Parer & Livingston, 1990). A fetus with a defective cardiac conduction system, anencephaly, or congenital neurologic deficit may present with minimal or absent variability, and in the case of congenital neurologic impairment, this FHR pattern may actually represent an asphyxial insult that occurred during the antepartum period (MacLennan, 1999).

Conversely, absent variability is seen in cases where the fetus has cerebral asphyxia and therefore experiences loss of either fine-tuning within the cardioregulatory center in the brain or direct myocardial depression. Loss of variability especially in the presence of other periodic patterns during labor is the most sensitive indicator of metabolic acidemia in a fetus (Beard et al., 1971; Clark et al., 1984; Low et al., 1999). Nursing interventions for absent variability include notifying the physician or midwife with a request for bedside evaluation, repositioning the woman to a lateral position, administering IV fluids and oxygen at 10 L/min via nonrebreather facemask. Oxytocin infusion should be discontinued if infusing or the next dose of pharmacologic agents used to ripen the cervix or stimulate contractions should be delayed until the FHR is reassuring. Fetal stimulation may be used to attempt to elicit an acceleration. Because absent variability is a hallmark sign of deep central asphyxia, it warrants immediate evaluation when detected.

Marked variability (previously termed *salutatory pattern*) is less common. The etiology of marked variability is uncertain, but it may be similar to that of the increase in variability noted in animal experiments when brief and acute hypoxia in the previously normally oxygenated fetus were studied (Westgate, Bennet, & Gunn, 1999). The increase in variability is presumed to result from an increase in alpha-adrenergic activity, which causes selective vasoconstriction of certain vascular beds. Two clinical situations during labor may result in marked variability: uterine hyperstimulation and ephedrine administration in total doses of 30 mg or more (O'Brien-Abel & Benedetti, 1992). Some authors believe marked variability is a fetal response to hypoxia that takes a different form than the usual progression from moderate to minimal then absent variability (Westgate et al., 1999). Because the fetus with marked variability (salutatory pattern) is hemodynamically compensated (although it may be mildly hypoxemic), interventions to resolve the pattern, such as maternal position change, avoidance of maternal hypotension, avoidance of uterine hyperstimulation, and perhaps administration of oxygen at 10 L/min via nonrebreather mask, are warranted (Parer & Nageotte, 2004). In the absence of abnormal FHR heart rate changes, marked variability is not associated with severe or progressive hypoxia (O'Brien-Abel & Benedetti, 1992; Parer & Nageotte, 2004, Westgate et al., 1999).

Periodic and Episodic Changes in Fetal Heart Rate

Periodic changes in heart rate are transient and last anywhere from a few seconds to 1 or 2 minutes or more, as compared to baseline changes in the heart rate, which must last a minimum of 10 minutes. The four types of FHR decelerations are early, late, variable, and prolonged decelerations (see Fig. 8–8 A–D). Decelerations are defined as recurrent if they occur with ≥50% of uterine contractions in any 20-minute segment. Periodic changes in FHR are usually identified and defined within the context of uterine contractions, while episodic FHR changes appear to have no relationship to uterine contractions.

Early Decelerations

Early deceleration of the FHR is a visually apparent *gradual* (defined as onset of deceleration to nadir ≥30 seconds) decrease and return to baseline FHR associated with a uterine contraction (NICHD,1997). The decrease is calculated from the most recently determined portion of the baseline. It is coincident in timing, with the nadir of the deceleration occurring at the same time as the peak of the contraction. In most cases, the onset, nadir, and recovery of the deceleration are coincident with the beginning, peak, and ending of the contraction, respectively (NICHD, 1997).

Early decelerations are presumed to be initiated by fetal head compression. Altered cerebral blood flow causes the decrease in heart rate through a vagal reflex. When the contraction occurs, the fetal head is subjected to pressure, which stimulates the vagus nerve. The heart rate begins to drop at the onset of the contraction, when the head compression begins and returns to the baseline rate at the end of the contraction when the head is no longer compressed. Early decelerations are often said to mirror the contraction causing them. They are benign decelerations, requiring no intervention or treatment and are not associated with fetal hypoxia or low Apgar scores. The key to assessment of early decelerations is to make sure one distinguishes them from late decelerations. The presence of variability is a key

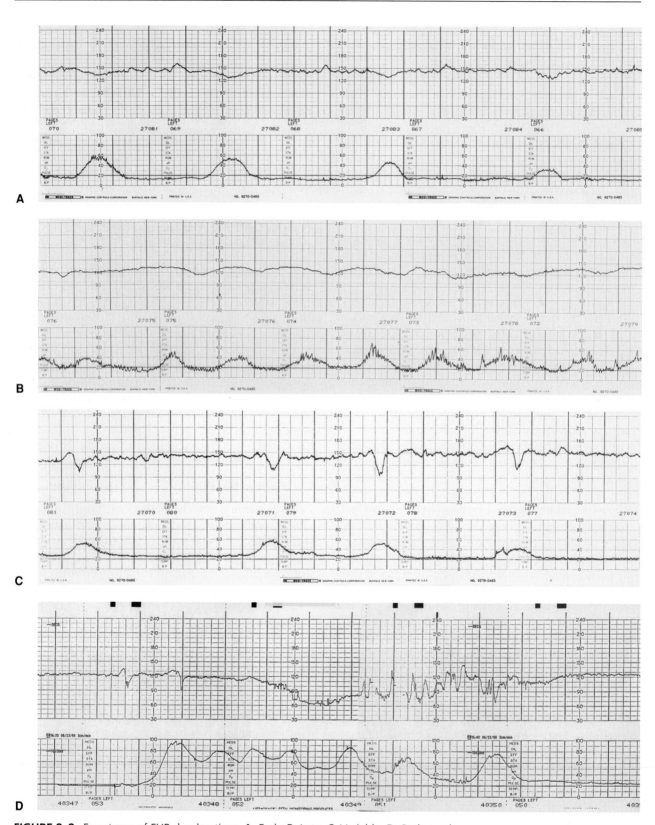

FIGURE 8–8. Four types of FHR decelerations. **A,** Early. **B,** Late. **C,** Variable. **D,** Prolonged.

clinical factor. Vagal stimulation occurs as a result of head compression, not secondary to hypoxia and will not result in a decrease in variability.

Late Decelerations

Late deceleration of the FHR is a visually apparent *gradual* (defined as onset of deceleration to nadir ≥30 seconds) decrease and return to baseline FHR associated with a uterine contraction (NICHD, 1997). The decrease is calculated from the most recently determined portion of the baseline. The deceleration is delayed in timing, with the nadir of the deceleration occurring after the peak of the contraction. In most cases, the onset, nadir, and recovery of the deceleration occur after the beginning, peak, and ending of the contraction, respectively.

Originally, all late decelerations were thought to represent uteroplacental insufficiency. More recent research has identified an additional mechanism. "Reflex" lates or late decelerations with retained variability are neurogenic in origin (Parer & Nageotte, 2004). Early decelerations may be a variant of this pattern, and some believe they are seen more frequently in fetuses in an occiput posterior position and/or during periods of rapid descent (see Figure 8–9A–B).

When a well-oxygenated fetus experiences a transient reduction in oxygenation during a contraction, chemoreceptors detect the hypoxemia and initiate the vagal bradycardic response. Once the contraction recedes, the fetus resumes normal metabolism and the bradycardia resolves. It takes a short time for hypoxemia to develop in this setting; thus, the chemoreceptor reflex occurs as the hypoxemia is detected. The nadir of the deceleration is late relative to the peak of the contraction because there is a lag in time between the detection of hypoxemia and the FHR response. The FHR pattern with both early decelerations and reflex late decelerations have retained variability, and neither is associated with significant acidemia.

Late decelerations with concomitant minimal or absent variability are possibly secondary to fetal asphyxia (Beard et al., 1971; Clark et al., 1984; Berkus et al., 1999). This type of periodic change occurs when there is insufficient oxygen for myocardial metabolism and/or normal cerebral function. These FHR patterns are likely to occur when there is chronic placental insufficiency that cannot support the transient hypoxia episodes that occur during normal labor. Late declarations with absent variability may evolve following a prolonged period of variable decelerations, bradycardia, tachycardia, or other periodic pattern that with sufficient repetition or duration interrupts normal fetal respiration.

Late decelerations should be evaluated in the context of FHR variability. For example, late decelerations with

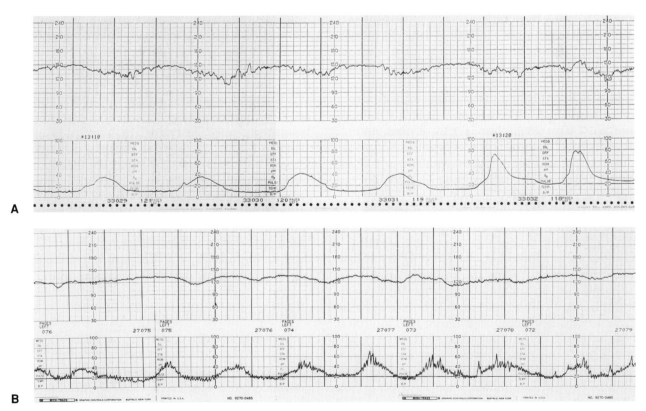

FIGURE 8–9. A, Reflex late decelerations. **B,** Non-reflex late decelerations.

moderate baseline variability and a stable rate with accelerations warrant less concern than late decelerations in the presence of an abnormal baseline rate, minimal variability, and absence of accelerations. If the FHR pattern had been reassuring prior to the onset of decelerations, an iatrogenic cause, such as maternal hypotension, frequently can be determined. Maternal history for risk factors for uteroplacental insufficiency and evaluation of the uterine activity pattern is essential.

Nursing interventions for late decelerations focus on maximizing placental function, thus improving uteroplacental exchange by maintaining a lateral maternal position, increasing IV fluids to correct dehydration or volume depletion, discontinuing oxytocin, and administering oxygen at 10 L/min via nonrebreather facemask. The next dose should be delayed of pharmacologic agents used to ripen the cervix or stimulate contractions until uterine activity returns to normal and the FHR is reassuring. The physician or midwife should be notified. If the late decelerations do not resolve after these interventions, a request for bedside evaluation by the physician or midwife is warranted. In addition, iatrogenic insults that may further compromise maternal–fetal exchange, such as hyperstimulation with oxytocin or maternal hypotension secondary to maternal supine position should be avoided. If there are late decelerations during second-stage labor, coached pushing efforts should be modified based on the fetal response.

Variable Decelerations

Variable deceleration of the FHR is defined as a visually apparent *abrupt* (defined as onset of deceleration to beginning of nadir <30 seconds) decrease in FHR below the baseline (NICHD, 1997). The decrease is calculated from the most recently determined portion of the baseline. The decrease in FHR below the baseline is ≥15 beats/min, lasting ≥15 seconds, and <2 minutes from onset to return to baseline. When variable decelerations are associated with uterine contractions, their onset, depth, and duration commonly vary with successive uterine contractions.

Variable decelerations are the most frequently seen FHR deceleration pattern in labor (Freeman et al., 2003). The initial rapid deceleration of the FHR is a response to vagal stimulation resulting from umbilical cord compression. When the umbilical arteries are occluded, there is a sudden increase in total fetal peripheral resistance resulting from the cutoff of the low resistance fetal placental circulation (Freeman et al., 2003). This increase in peripheral resistance in the fetal circulation causes sudden fetal hypertension. Stimulation of baroreceptors occurs instantly and results in a parasympathetic outflow that produces a sudden slowing of the FHR. With the release of the cord occlusion, the FHR usually returns to predeceleration values. Variable decelerations are called "variables" because they may

vary in their timing, shape, depth, and duration. Some last for brief seconds; others have very slow recoveries to the baseline rate. They may be caused by a uterine contraction pressing the cord against the fetus or by a short or nuchal cord. When variable decelerations occur during the second stage of labor, they may also be caused by the marked head compression and resultant intense vagal stimulation that occurs during rapid descent. When there is oligohydramnios, the cord is more vulnerable to compression because of the lack of cushioning provided by the amniotic fluid (Galvin, Van Mullem, & Broekhuizen, 1989). In this case, the variable decelerations may occur in response to fetal movement or uterine contractions, and they may be frequent or occasional. Therefore, variables have multiple appearances in all aspects except one: the initial FHR drop is abrupt.

Nursing interventions to correct variable decelerations focus on alleviating the cord compression and begin with assisting the woman to a lateral, knee-chest, or even supine position to release the cord from where it is entrapped. A vaginal examination may be done to palpate for an umbilical cord prolapse. If there are recurrent variable decelerations during second-stage labor, coached pushing efforts should be modified based on the fetal response. Pushing with every other, or every third, contraction may allow more blood flow to the fetus and the fetus to recover between contractions (Freeman et al., 2003). When variable decelerations continue despite modified pushing efforts, it may be necessary to stop pushing temporarily. Women without regional analgesia/anesthesia may have difficulty controlling their urge to push and may need significant encouragement to not push while the fetus recovers. If oxytocin is infusing, it should be discontinued until fetal status is reassuring. If another pharmacologic agent to ripen the cervix or stimulate contractions is being used, the next dose should be delayed until uterine activity returns to normal and the FHR is reassuring. Oxygen may be given at 10 L/min via nonrebreather facemask, and IV fluids may be increased. If position changes do not result in resolution of the variable decelerations, notification of the physician or midwife is warranted and a request for bedside evaluation may be indicated based on the clinical situation. When variable decelerations occur during first stage labor, amnioinfusion may be considered (Parer & Nageotte, 2004).

Prolonged Decelerations

Prolonged deceleration of the FHR is a visually apparent decrease in FHR below the baseline (NICHD, 1997). The decrease is calculated from the most recently determined portion of the baseline. The decrease from the baseline is ≥15 beats/min, lasting ≥2 minutes, but <10 minutes from onset to return to baseline. Prolonged deceleration of ≥10 minutes is a baseline change.

During a prolonged deceleration, the heart rate drops abruptly and stays down for several minutes and is usually an isolated occurrence. It may occur in the presence or absence of contractions and may have either an abrupt or slow return to the baseline rate. Prolonged decelerations may be the result of an isolated episode of cord compression, maternal hypotension, excessive uterine activity, vagal stimulation, uterine rupture, vasa previa rupture, or, rarely, maternal seizures or maternal respiratory or cardiac arrest.

During the first stage of labor, transient bradycardias or prolonged decelerations with moderate variability are frequently associated with an occiput posterior position or transverse position and are probably the result of increased vagal tone that is secondary to pressure on the fetal skull (Freeman et al., 2003). These types of bradycardias are also seen when there is a transient decrease in uteroplacental blood flow in a previously well-functioning maternal–fetal unit. This occasionally occurs during the administration of regional anesthesia and/or when the patient is in a supine position. Nonrecurrent prolonged decelerations that are preceded and followed by a FHR that has a normal baseline and moderate to minimal variability are not associated with fetal hypoxemia of clinical significance.

Nursing interventions for prolonged decelerations include discontinuing oxytocin if infusing, increasing IV fluids, administering oxygen at 10 L/min via nonrebreather facemask, a vaginal exam to rule out prolapsed cord, and repositioning the woman to remove pressure from the umbilical cord. The next dose of pharmacologic agents used to ripen the cervix or stimulate contractions should be delayed until uterine activity returns to normal and the FHR is reassuring. The physician or midwife should be notified and a bedside evaluation requested. A tocolytic agent may also be administered to decrease uterine activity. If there are prolonged decelerations during second-stage labor, modify coached pushing efforts based on the fetal response. When a prolonged deceleration occurs during antepartum testing, an ultrasound measurement of amniotic fluid volume should be done. A summary of the interventions for fetal heart rate changes is in Table 8–4.

TABLE 8–4 ■ MANAGEMENT OF VARIANT FETAL HEART RATE PATTERNS

FHR Pattern	Diagnosis	Action
Normal rate, moderate variability, ± accelerations, no periodic or episodic decelerations	The baby is well oxygenated	None
Normal rate, moderate variability, ± accelerations, variant pattern (eg, bradycardia, LD, VD)	The baby is still well oxygenated centrally	Conservative in-utero treatment Expect abolition of variant pattern if cause reversed.
Normal rate, moderate variability, ± accelerations, moderate/severe variant pattern (eg, bradycardia, recurrent LD, VD)	The baby is still well oxygenated centrally, but the FHR pattern suggests reductions in O_2, which may result in accumulation of fetal O_2 debt	Conservative in-utero treatment, ± amnioinfusion, ± stimulation testing Check ability to deliver rapidly in case pattern worsens
Normal rate, decreasing variability, ± accelerations, moderate/severe variant patterns (eg, bradycardia, recurrent LD, VD)	The baby may be on the verge of decompensation	Operative birth if spontaneous birth remote, or if ancillary testing (stimulation and/or blood sampling) supports diagnosis of decompensation Normal testing results may allow time to await a vaginal birth
Variability absent or minimal, no accelerations, moderate/severe variant patterns (eg, bradycardia, recurrent LD, VD)	The baby has evidence of actual or impending damaging asphyxia	Operative birth May attempt further evaluation or in-utero treatment if it does not unduly delay birth

Adapted with permission from Parer, J. T. & King, T. L. (1999). Whither fetal heart rate monitoring. *Obstetrics, Gynecology and Fertility,* *22*(5), 149–192.

LD, late decelerations; VD, variable decelerations; Conservative in-utero treatment may include maternal position change IV fluid bolus of at least 500 mL of lactated Ringer's solution; oxygen at 10 L/min via nonrebreather facemask; discontinuation of oxytocin if infusing; removal of Cervidil insert; withholding next dose of Cytotec; subcutaneous terbutaline 0.25 mg; amnioinfusion (first-stage labor), temporary discontinuation of pushing or pushing with every other, or every third, contraction (second-stage labor); correction of maternal hypotension; ephedrine 5 to 10 mg IV push.

Unusual Fetal Heart Rate Patterns

As a general caveat, whenever an unusual tracing is observed from the beginning of electronic monitoring tracing, consider the possibility of a fetus with a congenital anomaly. Hydrocephalic and anencephalic fetuses may present with unusual FHR patterns that do not fit any category or definition. If possible, an ultrasound examination may be performed to rule out gross anomalies as the cause of the pattern, even though the results of the ultrasound examination may be inconclusive. An anomaly that affects the fetal central nervous system most likely will have an impact on the variability and/or the fetal cardiac system's ability to accelerate and decelerate. Unusual decelerations with a flat, fixed rate may be seen.

Sinusoidal Heart Rate Pattern

The sinusoidal FHR pattern is a rare occurrence (Modanlou & Murata, 2004). In a true sinusoidal pattern, there is a stable baseline FHR of 110 to 160 bpm, amplitude of 5 to 15 bpm (rarely greater), frequency of 2 to 5 cycles per minute, absent variability, oscillation of the sinusoidal wave from above and below the baseline, and no areas of normal FHR variability or reactivity (Modanlou & Freeman, 1982). There is an absence of accelerations and no response to uterine contractions, fetal movement, or stimulation (Modanlou

& Freeman, 1982). The sinusoidal heart rate pattern was first identified in the early 1970s during observation of Rhesus factor (Rh)–sensitized fetuses (Rochard et al., 1976). As severe fetal anemia developed, the FHR tracing became persistently rhythmic in an undulating fashion (Fig. 8–10) and remained so. The etiology of the sinusoidal heart rate includes severe fetal anemia as a result of maternal–fetal hemorrhage, placental abruption, or Rh isoimmunization. In some clinical situations, fetal anemia can be treated with a fetal transfusion, which, if successful, will result in resolution of the sinusoidal heart rate pattern. Other fetal conditions that have been reported to be associated with sinusoidal heart rate patterns include fetal hypoxia/asphyxia, fetal infection, and fetal cardiac anomalies (Modanlou & Murata, 2004). Whatever the pathogenesis, a true sinusoidal heart rate pattern is an extremely significant finding that implies fetal jeopardy and impending fetal death.

A sinusoidal-appearing FHR pattern has been noted to follow the maternal administration of some narcotics especially butorphanol (Stadol) and fentanyl. This type of sinusoidal heart rate resolves as the drug is excreted, thus giving it the name of "pseudosinusoidal" or "drug-induced" sinusoidal. The characteristics differ from a true sinusoidal heart rate pattern in that there are fewer uniform oscillations, periods of moderate variability, and the presence of accelerations. No treatment is indicated.

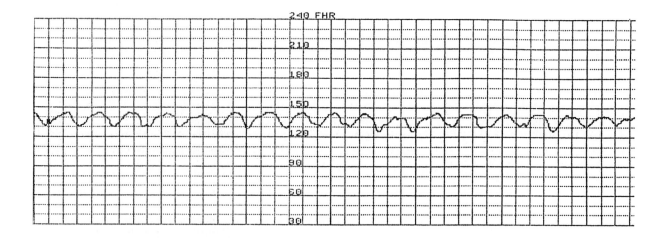

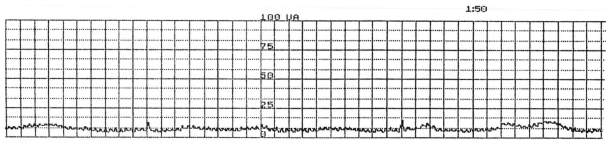

FIGURE 8–10. Sinusoidal fetal heart rate pattern.

Fetal Arrhythmias

During the past decade, fetal cardiac arrhythmias have been recognized with increasing frequency at routine prenatal visits (Fig. 8–11). The most common finding is the impression that the fetal heart is intermittently skipping beats. In most cases, the skipping actually represents either a pause following an extrasystole or an extrasystole occurring early in the cardiac cycle to result in a stroke volume that is inadequate to produce a detectable Doppler signal (Kleinman & Nehgme, 2004). While the extrasystoles may be a source of anxiety for the parents, they usually resolve spontaneously later during pregnancy or during the first few days after birth, and only rarely do they precipitate persistent tachyarrhythmias requiring further evaluation. In some instances, the neonatal resuscitation team may be requested to attend the birth.

Sustained fetal tachyarrhythmias or bradyarrhythmias are rare. However, when detected during routine prenatal visits, they require echocardiography to assess cardiac anatomy and function. The most common tachyarrhythmias are supraventricular tachycardia (SVT) and atrial flutter. Typically, SVT occurs at a rate of about 240 bpm with minimal or absent variability, while in atrial flutter, fetal atrial rates may reach 450 bpm with a 3 to 1 block, resulting in a ventricular rate of 150 bpm (Copel, Friedman, & Kleinman, 1997).

Because sustained fetal tachyarrhythmia may cause the development of hydrops fetalis, which can result in fetal death, antiarrhythmic drug therapy, administered via maternal ingestion, may be attempted using agents such as digoxin, propranolol, flecainide, sotalol, and/or amiodarone. Continuous bedside monitoring of FHR and maternal ECG must be considered throughout treatment with any of the antiarrhythmic agents (Kleinman & Nehgme, 2004).

The most important sustained bradyarrhythmia is complete heart block, in which the ventricular rate ranges 40–80 bpm. Echocardiography is used to analyze fetal cardiac anatomy and function. Approximately half of the fetuses have structurally normal hearts in early embryonic development that become damaged due to the transplacental passage of maternal antibodies. Mothers of these fetuses often have symptoms consistent with Sjogren's syndrome and usually have high titers of anti-SS-A (anti-Ro) or anti-SS-B (anti-La) (Kleinman & Nehgme, 2004). The antibodies cross the placenta and cause immune-related damage to the His-Purkinje fibers of the conduction system, causing fetal heart block around 18 to 20 weeks' gestation (Copel et al., 1997). The other half of the fetuses with complete heart block have underlying complex congenital heart malformations, usually involving the atrioventricular junction. The prognosis for these fetuses, especially if hydrops fetalis develops, is quite poor.

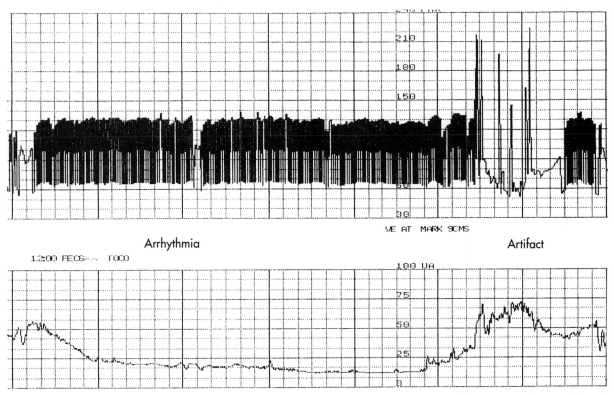

FIGURE 8–11. Arrhythmia. This tracing demonstrates fetal arrhythmia and artifact. Notice the randomness of the artifactual information compared with the organization of the arrhythmia.

Assessment of fetal well-being may be difficult in the presence of an arrhythmia because of the inability to see a consistent baseline or evaluate variability. Auscultating the FHR and listening for the irregularity may verify the presence of an arrhythmia. The fetal heart rate may appear normal on the external heart rate tracing, but if an irregularity is auscultated and a direct electrode applied, the arrhythmia will be accurately recorded.

If the heart rate is regular to auscultation, yet there are unusual excursions tracing on the fetal heart monitor strip, the most likely explanation is that it is artifactual information. Artifact may be caused by the FSE having a poor attachment to the fetal presenting part or equipment problems. Attempts to correct the problem include changing the cable or fetal monitor and/or replacing the direct electrode (see Table 8–2).

CLINICAL IMPLICATIONS FOR MONITORING THE PRETERM FETUS DURING LABOR

While the principles of EFM are the same for the preterm fetus as for the term fetus, there are differences in FHR patterns of preterm fetuses when compared to those in term labor, and there are unique clinical implications for obtaining and interpreting EFM data during preterm labor. Perinatal complications such as preeclampsia, intraamniotic infection, oligohydramnios, umbilical cord compression, placental abruption, intrauterine growth restriction, uteroplacental insufficiency, and multiple gestation are more common during preterm labor. These complications are often associated with nonreassuring FHR patterns. There is evidence to suggest that nonreassuring FHR patterns have greater significance for outcomes for the preterm fetus (Matsuda, Maeda, & Kouno, 2003). At term, approximately only 20% of infants with nonreassuring FHR patterns will be neurologically depressed; however, in preterm infants less than 33 weeks' gestation, approximately 70% to 80% of nonreassuring FHR patterns will result in the birth of a neurologically depressed, hypoxemic, or acidemic infant (Freeman et al., 2003).

The preterm fetus is more susceptible to hypoxic insults and more likely to develop and die from complications of prematurity if born depressed, hypoxemic, or acidemic (Freeman et al., 2003). An abnormal or nonreassuring FHR pattern (eg, minimal to absent variability, late decelerations, recurrent variable decelerations, tachycardia) is predictive of perinatal asphyxia and long-term neurological outcome for the preterm fetus (Braithwaite, Milligan, & Shennan, 1986; Douvas, Meeks, Graves, Walsh, & Morrison, 1984; Low et al., 1992; Low, Killen, & Derrick, 2002; Shy et al., 1990; Matsuda et al., 2003; Westgren, Malcus, & Svenningsen, 1986). Compared to the term fetus, the progression from reassuring to nonreassuring status occurs more often and more quickly (Freeman et al., 2003). Thus, timeliness of identification and initiation of interventions for nonreassuring FHR patterns is more critical and of more lasting consequences when the fetus is preterm.

Baseline Rate

The baseline rate decreases over the course of gestation as the fetus matures (Kisilevsky, Hains, & Low, 2001). In the preterm fetus, the rate is likely to be in the higher range, up to 160 bpm. An FHR greater than 160 bpm may indicate evolving fetal hypoxemia, maternal fever, intraamniotic infection, or the side effects of terbutaline administration. Development of tachycardia (baseline rate >160 bpm) is more common in the preterm fetus (Westgren, Holmquist, Svenningsen, & Ingemarsson, 1982). In one study, 78% of fetuses less than 33 weeks' gestation had periods of tachycardia, as compared to only 20% of fetuses greater than 33 weeks' gestation (Westgren, Holmquist, Ingemarsson, & Svenningsen, 1984). The presence of fetal tachycardia is more predictive of acidemia, low Apgar scores, and adverse neonatal outcomes in the preterm fetus compared to the term fetus (Burrus, O'Shea, Veille, & Mueller-Heubach, 1994; Westgren et al., 1982). Therefore, baseline rate as well as other features of the FHR merit special attention by the nurse responsible for monitoring the labor of a woman with a preterm pregnancy.

Variability

Minimal to absent FHR variability is more common in the preterm fetus (To & Leung, 1998). Loss of variability is significant when the fetus is preterm because this FHR change is more predictive of hypoxemia and academia as compared to the term fetus (Douvus et al., 1984; Freeman et al., 2003). If the FHR is tachycardic, variability may be decreased secondary to the tachycardia (Freeman et al., 2003); however, frequently in the preterm fetus, minimal to absent variability is indicative of progressive hypoxemia and acidemia (Zanini, Paul, & Huey, 1980). The combination of tachycardia and loss of variability is more often associated with low Apgar scores and acidemia in the preterm fetus (Freeman et al., 2003).

Preterm labor and birth may be indicated for women with preeclampsia. These patients receive IV magnesium sulfate as seizure prophylaxis. Preterm labor often proceeds during and despite IV magnesium sulfate tocolysis. The variability of the FHR pattern may decrease during magnesium sulfate administration, although this change is not usually clinically significant (Atkinson, Belfort, Saade, & Moise, 1994; Hiett, Devoe, Brown, & Watson, 1995; Wright, Ridgway, Wright, Covington, & Bobbitt, 1996). Antenatal steroids are indicated when there is a risk that preterm contractions will lead to active labor and preterm birth. Both betamethasone and dexamethasone cause a transient increase in baseline variability for about 24 hours, followed by a suppression of variability up to 96 hours after administration; however, these changes are not indicative of deterioration in fetal status (Rotmensch et al., 1999; Subtil et al., 2003). IV or intramuscular (IM) pain medications may result in minimal variability. It is important to know the duration of the effects of any pain medication given to be able to accurately distinguish between expected FHR side effects and evolving fetal hypoxemia.

Accelerations

Accelerations of the preterm FHR are generally lower in amplitude and less frequent than those of the term fetus, although most preterm fetuses, even at 24 to 26 weeks' gestation and beyond, will have accelerations of at least 15 bpm lasting 15 seconds (Freeman et al., 2003). The number and amplitude of accelerations increase over the course of gestation as the fetus matures (Kisilevsky et al., 2001). An acceleration of the FHR of at least 10 bpm lasting 10 seconds is considered reassuring in fetuses less than 32 weeks (NICHD, 1997).

If the woman is receiving magnesium sulfate, there may be fewer accelerations of the FHR of 10 to 15 bpm. These changes are not usually clinically significant (Atkinson et al., 1994; Hiett et al., 1995; Wright et al., 1996). Antenatal steroids may result in a transient increase in fetal movement and FHR accelerations within the first 24 hours after administration, followed by a reduction in fetal movement and FHR accelerations for the next 96 hours; however, these changes are not nonreassuring findings (Rotmensch et al., 1999; Subtil et al., 2003; van Iddekinge, Hofmeyr, & Buchmann, 2003). Pain medication given IV or IM may temporarily depress the fetal neurological system, resulting in fewer FHR accelerations and/or FHR accelerations of lower amplitude.

Decelerations

Variable decelerations are more common in preterm fetuses during the antepartum period (Sorokin et al., 1982) and labor (Freeman et al., 2003). Approximately 70% to 75% of preterm fetuses will have variable decelerations, compared to about 30% to 50% of fetuses at term (Westgren et al., 1982). Variable decelerations during preterm labor are associated with a

higher rate of hypoxemia, acidemia, neurological abnormalities, and adverse long-term outcomes (Holmes, Oppenheimer, Gravelle, Walker, & Blayney, 2001; Westgren et al., 1982). There is evidence to suggest variable decelerations are associated with intraventricular hemorrhage through a mechanism independent of fetal acidemia (Holmes et al., 2001).

Although there does not appear to be an increased incidence in late decelerations during preterm labor, the conditions that are more likely to result in late decelerations are more common (Freeman et al., 2003). These include uteroplacental insufficiency, intraamniotic infection, preeclampsia, intrauterine growth restriction, and placenta abruption. Late decelerations have more significance for the preterm fetus because there is an association between late decelerations during preterm labor and adverse outcomes such as hypoxemia, academia, and long-term neurological abnormalities (Westgren et al., 1984; Zanini et al., 1980). Prolonged decelerations occur at a similar frequency for the preterm and term fetus (Freeman et al., 2003).

Monitoring Preterm Multiple Gestations

When monitoring more than one fetus, it is important to maintain two distinct FHRs. Erroneously monitoring the same fetus results in loss of ability to detect evolving problems in the unmonitored fetus (Ramsey & Repke, 2003). Newer-generation monitors have the ability to indicate when the FHRs appear to be from the same fetus. These system cues can be helpful, but do not replace careful nursing assessment of each FHR pattern. The mother may be able to provide assistance in determining the position of each baby by indicating where she feels fetal movement.

Although some fetuses, particularly monoamniotic/monochorionic twins, may have synchronous FHR patterns at times, most fetuses in multiple gestations will not have completely synchronous FHR patterns during labor (see Fig. 8–12 A–B) (Eganhouse, 1992). Some twin fetuses will have asynchronous FHR patterns over the course of labor, especially if there are differences in fetal well-being. Accelerations and decelerations usually occur within the same time frame, but will not be identical in duration or excursion from the baseline (Gallagher, Costigan, & Johnson, 1992). Tactile communication occurs between twins in utero, and these movements often result in simultaneous accelerations of the FHR during nonstress testing (Sherer, Nawrocki, Peco, Metlay, & Woods, 1990). Periods of reactivity and nonreactivity of the FHR also are similar during nonstress testing (Sherer, Amico, Cox, Metlay, & Woods, 1994). The assumption can be made that these conditions and FHR reactions would apply to the intrapartum period, but there have been no confirmatory

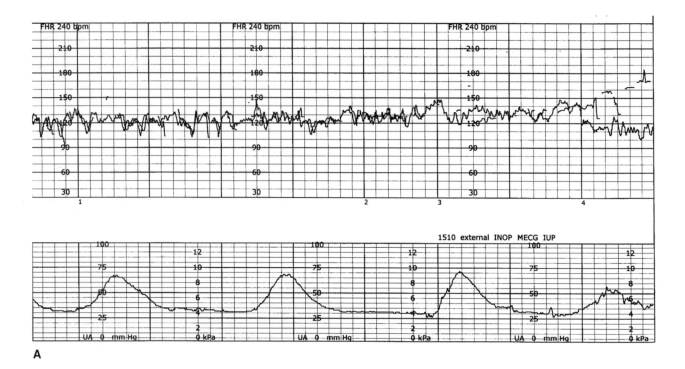

A

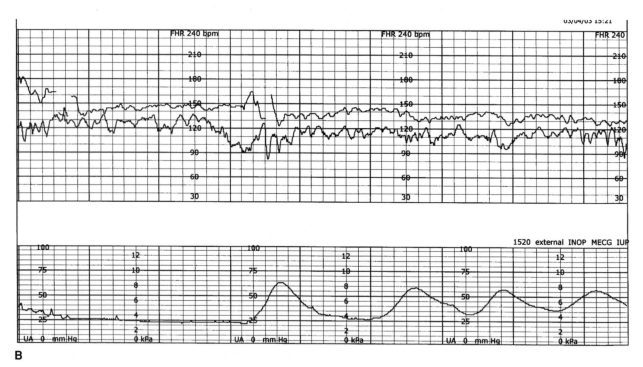

B

FIGURE 8–12. A, Synchronous fetal heart rate patterns of twins. **B,** Asynchronous fetal heart rate patterns of twins.

studies. The published data are limited to FHR patterns of twins during antepartum testing, although authors mentioned incidental data. There were no studies found about intrapartum FHR patterns of triplets and higher order multiples, presumably because these pregnancies almost always result in cesarean birth without labor. However, in selected cases when fetal status is reassuring and fetal presentation is favorable, women with triplets can labor and give birth vaginally.

ASSESSMENT OF PATTERN EVOLUTION

In clinical practice, interpretation of the FHR is an ongoing assessment that includes multiple perinatal factors, specific FHR characteristics, and, most important, the evolution of the FHR pattern as labor progresses (see Fig. 8–13). A nonreassuring FHR can suddenly develop spontaneously, but usually the evolution from reassuring to nonreassuring follows a typical pattern over time. Fetal heart rate patterns that result from an acute event such as umbilical cord prolapse, uterine rupture, or placental abruption are typically noted immediately and acted on in a timely manner by the perinatal team. However, when fetal deterioration occurs progressively over a long period, the clinical symptoms may not be fully appreciated by all members of the perinatal team. A loss of situational awareness can occur and, as a result, timely interventions may be delayed. When the FHR evolves from a baseline within

normal limits, moderate variability, and accelerations to tachycardia, minimal to absent variability and recurrent late, variable or prolonged decelerations, risk of fetal deterioration to hypoxemia and eventually acidemia is significant (Freeman et al., 2003). Oxytocin-induced hyperstimulation can exacerbate the situation, so it is essential to carefully titrate the oxytocin infusion based on contraction frequency and the fetal response (Freeman et al., 2003). If the usual intrauterine resuscitation techniques do not result in pattern resolution, consider expeditious birth. A request for bedside evaluation by the primary provider is warranted so that plans can be made and implemented for fetal rescue in a timely manner.

FHR patterns that occur during the second stage of labor are another example of how pattern evolution from moderate to minimal or absent variability reflects an increasing risk of fetal hypoxemia and acidemia. One way to minimize fetal risk during the second stage is to allow the fetus to descend passively and to delay pushing until the woman feels the urge. The active pushing phase of the second stage is the most physiologically stressful part of labor for the fetus (Roberts, 2002). Shortening the active pushing phase by allowing passive fetal descent can minimize the decrease in fetal oxygen status that is associated with maternal pushing efforts (Simpson & James, 2005a). It is common during the second stage of labor for the FHR to develop variable decelerations that become progressively more severe as the woman pushes with contractions and the fetus descends. In this scenario, if the

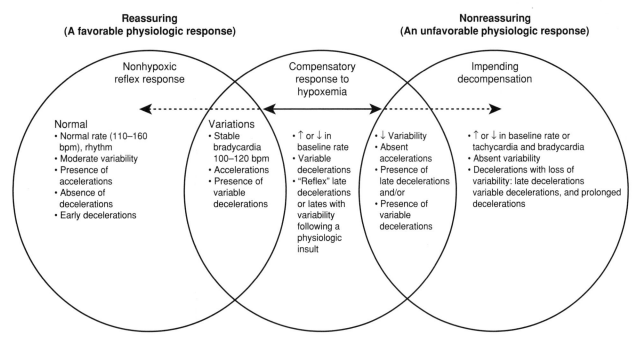

FIGURE 8–13. Alterations of fetal heart rate patterns by physiologic response. (Adapted from AWHONN. [2003]. *Principles & practice,* p. 54.)

contractions are of normal frequency and the pattern is secondary to vagal stimulation during head compression, the FHR will maintain variability because the decelerations are not caused by hypoxia (Parer & Nageotte, 2004). These decelerations can resolve intermittently as the vertex adjusts to pelvic diameters and may resolve completely when the vertex crowns. If the etiology of this pattern is cord occlusion that is worsening as the fetus descends, the decelerations may become more severe and develop a concomitant loss of variability as the fetus develops a hypoxemia.

When oxytocin is continued during second-stage pushing, it is important to avoid hyperstimulation. Normally during the second stage, contractions tend to become slightly less frequent, which may allow the fetus to tolerate the stress of maternal pushing efforts, umbilical cord compression, and vagal stimulation. When contractions are too frequent over a prolonged period, the fetus may not be able to tolerate this physiologic stress (ACOG & AAP, 2003).

Interventions for variable decelerations during the second stage should also include assessment of the pushing technique used. When recurrent variable decelerations during the second stage are associated with coached closed-glottis pushing, the most appropriate approach is to encourage the woman to push with every other, or every third, contraction (Freeman et al., 2003). In some cases, pushing may need to be temporarily discontinued to allow the fetus to recover. These techniques can be attempted for all women, but are most effective for women who have regional analgesia/ anesthesia. Open-glottis pushing with the woman bearing down for no more than 6–8 seconds per pushing effort will have less negative effect on fetal status than repetitive close-glottis pushing (AWHONN, 2000b; Simpson & James, 2005a) (see Fig. 8–14 A–B). Encouraging the woman to bear down as long as she can is more favorable for fetal well-being than telling the woman to take a deep breath and hold it for 10 seconds without making a sound (Simpson & James, 2005a). Counting to 10 with each pushing effort to encourage pushing efforts lasting 10 seconds or more is no longer considered the most appropriate method of second-stage labor coaching (Roberts, 2002). Three to four

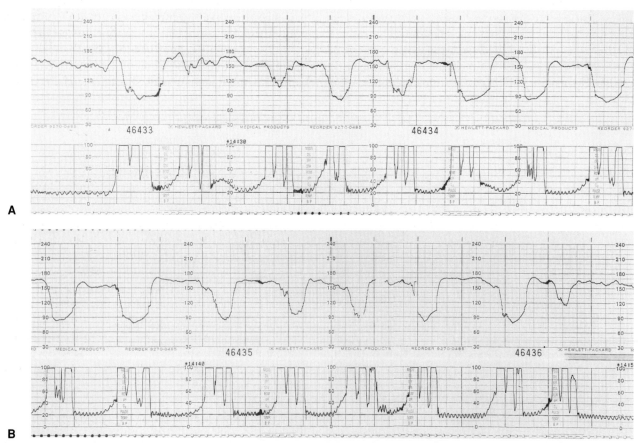

FIGURE 8–14. Iatrogenic nonreassuring fetal heart rate pattern as a result of coached closed-glottis pushing during the second stage of labor.

pushing efforts per contraction will minimize risk of fetal compromise and promote adequate fetal descent (AWHONN, 2000b). The provider should assess variable decelerations that evolve into deeper decelerations with tachycardia and/or loss of variability and intervene to minimize additional stress, such as discontinuation of oxytocin, repositioning, or emergent birth (Freeman et al., 2003). Appropriate care during the second stage of labor can prevent iatrogenic fetal stress and the birth of a depressed baby.

The end-stage bradycardia that retains mild to moderate variability is another version of head compression during rapid descent. If moderate variability is retained and the rate remains above 80 to 90 bpm, this pattern should be watched but considered a benign variant. Conversely, a bradycardia that slopes down over several minutes and loses variability within the first 4 minutes of descent is another pattern evolution that signals fetal decompensation and warrants rapid intervention (Gull et al., 1996).

It is extremely important to recognize a FHR pattern that precedes death. In any stage of labor, bradycardias that are preceded by a period of late or variable decelerations and bradycardias that are associated with minimal to absent variability are associated with metabolic acidosis in the fetus (Beard et al., 1971; Berkus et al., 1999; Low et al., 1999; Dellinger et al., 2000; Clark et al., 1984) (see Fig. 8–6). In either situation, if the problem causing fetal hypoxia is not corrected, the FHR eventually becomes a flat, fixed pattern with absent variability prior to death. Scalp stimulation elicits no response. By auscultation, a regular rate well within the normal range could be heard, thus providing false reassurance.

Retrospective studies have been published during which the authors reviewed FHR tracings from children with known central nervous system neurologic impairments. Of note in the majority of these children, the FHR tracing obtained either at admission or that developed during the intrapartum period was a pattern that was either persistently nonreactive or had minimal to absent variability and FHR decelerations (Phelan & Ahn, 1994). Therefore, if at first presentation to the hospital or office, the FHR tracing is at a persistent rate with decreased variability with or without decelerations and shows no accelerations in response to stimulation, that fetus needs to be evaluated for acidemia. Although neurologic damage diagnosed at birth is quite rare, this type of tracing may be an indication that neurologic damage has already occurred prior to admission.

Multiple authors have reviewed the relationship between FHR patterns and neonatal outcomes. The presence of baseline variability most reliably indicates adequate oxygenation to the brain. A normal baseline

TABLE 8–5 ■ FETAL HEART RATE PATTERNS ASSOCIATED WITH SIGNIFICANT RISK FOR FETAL ACIDEMIA

Absent Variability With:	Minimal Variability With:
Tachycardia	Tachycardia with variable or late decelerations
Bradycardia <80 bpm	Bradycardia with variable or late decelerations
Recurrent late decelerations	Recurrent late decelerations
Recurrent variable decelerations of increasing depth and duration	Recurrent variable decelerations of increasing depth and duration
Sinusoidal heart rate pattern	Sinusoidal heart rate pattern

rate with moderate variability and absence of periodic or episodic patterns conveys a high level of security that the fetus is both well oxygenated and not experiencing asphyxial stress in response to labor progress (ACOG & AAP, 2003). Most FHR tracings include some variant pattern, and the majority of these fetuses are also well oxygenated. The FHR patterns listed in Table 8–5 are those that have consistently been associated with fetal acidosis, low Apgar scores, or umbilical artery pH values in the acidotic range. Nurses caring for women during labor should recognize these patterns as ominous and request immediate medical consultation.

ANCILLARY TESTS OF FETAL WELL-BEING

Because most variant FHR tracings are not associated with an underlying fetal hypoxemia, it is occasionally helpful to employ ancillary testing that can discriminate between the fetus with hypoxemia and the fetus that is centrally well oxygenated. This discrimination can potentially avoid unnecessary interventions if the results of the test are reassuring. Scalp stimulation and fetal scalp blood sampling are the current techniques available for this purpose, although fetal scalp blood sampling is not available in all centers and is less commonly used.

Fetal Scalp and Acoustic Stimulation

Fetal scalp stimulation involves placing firm, digital pressure on the fetal scalp during a vaginal examination.

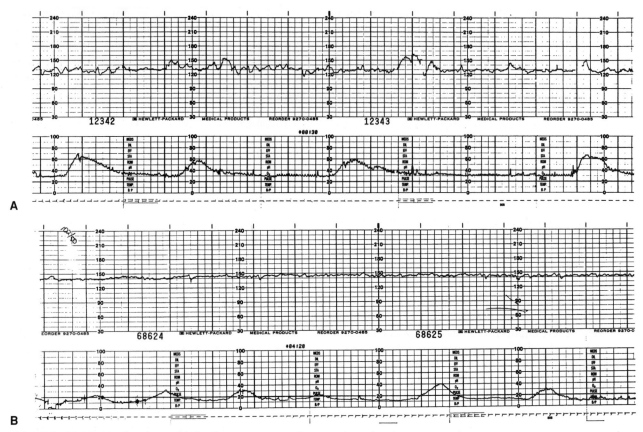

FIGURE 8–15. A, Accelerations with fetal movement. **B,** Absence of accelerations.

In response to scalp stimulation, a well-oxygenated fetus will respond by having an acceleration of the FHR that is greater than 15 bpm above the baseline, lasting greater than 15 seconds (Fig. 8–15 A–B). Research has indicated that this type of acceleration in response to scalp stimulation correlates highly with a fetal blood pH >7.19 (Clark et al., 1984). There is a similar correlation between fetal acceleration in response to sound stimulation (Freeman et al., 2003). To perform acoustic stimulation, an artificial larynx is positioned on the maternal abdomen and a stimulus of 1–2 seconds is applied (ACOG, 1999a). This may be repeated up to three times for progressively longer durations up to 3 seconds to elicit FHR accelerations (ACOG, 1999a). Although acoustic stimulation is usually used during nonstress testing, it can be used during labor if there is concern about the FHR pattern and scalp stimulation or fetal scalp blood sampling cannot be performed (Freeman et al., 2003). The absence of an acceleration does not diagnose acidemia or predict fetal compromise; however, approximately 50% of fetuses who do not respond with an acceleration to either of these stimuli will show acidemia on a simultaneously obtained fetal scalp blood sample (Freeman et al.,

2003). It is inappropriate to use scalp stimulation or vibroacoustic stimulation during a deceleration (Freeman et al., 2003). The value of these techniques is when the stimulation occurs during a time when the FHR is at its baseline rate and the acceleration can be evoked above the baseline (Freeman et al., 2003). If the FHR fails to respond to scalp stimulation, a fetal scalp sample for blood gas analysis from the presenting part may then be obtained if the technology is available in the institution. If not, plans for expeditious birth are usually made. Performing fetal scalp or vibroacoustic stimulation when concerned about the well-being of the fetus, may negate fetal scalp sampling or an unnecessary cesarean birth for nonreassuring fetal status (Elimian, Figueroa, & Tejani, 1997; Goodwin, Milner-Masterson, & Paul, 1994).

Fetal Blood Sampling

If the response to fetal stimulation is not reassuring, fetal scalp blood may be obtained for blood gas analysis. The blood gas analysis consists of all of the parameters used in adult blood gas analysis; however, generally only the pH and base excess are used to evaluate fetal status (Modanlou, 1991). If the pH is less than 7.15 to 7 and the base excess is less than –7 to –10, emergency birth is usually instituted. Both false-normal and false abnormal results may occur secondary to prolonged exposure of the sample to air, protracted sampling time, inadequate temperature control, laboratory technique, timing of sampling relating to contractions, presence of caput succedaneum, or maternal factors such as fever, hypertension, acidemia, or the supine position. If a fetal blood sampling (FBS) result seems incongruent with the EFM tracing interpretation, the FBS may be in error and must be repeated.

Although FBS provides an adjunct measure to determine fetal status when a nonreassuring FHR is noted, thereby in theory eliminating the need for cesarean birth if the result obtained indicates a well-oxygenated fetus, there has been a trend away from use of FBS. Widespread use of FBS in tertiary centers in the late 1980s did not result in a significant decrease in the rate of cesarean births (Goodwin et al., 1994). The role of FBS in clinical practice has been questioned because it is technically difficult to perform and associated with multiple possibilities for false results. Because scalp stimulation is easy to perform and is a good indicator of fetal well-being, many perinatal centers in the United States no longer use FBS or use it infrequently.

Umbilical Cord Blood Gases

Umbilical cord blood gases drawn at birth provide the most objective evidence confirming or refuting the presence of intrapartum acidemia at the moment of birth (ACOG, 2006b). Risk of moderate and severe newborn encephalopathy, respiratory, and other complications increase with umbilical arterial base deficit of 12–16 mmol/L. Moderate or severe newborn complications occur in 10% of babies who have this level of acidemia, and the rate increases when the umbilical arterial base deficit is greater than 16 mmol/L (ACOG, 2006b). Umbilical cord blood gases are not technically an ancillary method used for the purpose of clinical decision making during labor, but are included here because of the impact this information has in ruling out intrapartum asphyxia when the newborn is ill. Results may assist in guiding treatment for the newborn, especially if available in a timely manner.

Umbilical cord blood gases are useful for the infant born with low Apgar scores, severe intrauterine growth restriction, nonreassuring FHR patterns, or a sentinel clinical event (such as an umbilical cord prolapse, uterine rupture, or placental abruption); meconium-stained fluid and postterm births;

as well as in complicated births such as vaginal breech birth or twins (Gibbs, Rosenberg, Warren, Galan, & Rumack, 2004). Recent recommendations from ACOG (2006b) include attempting to obtain arterial and venous cord blood samples in the following clinical situations: cesarean birth for fetal compromise, low 5-minute Apgar score, severe growth restriction, abnormal FHR tracing, maternal thyroid disease, intrapartum fever or multifetal gestation. Immediately after birth, a segment of the umbilical cord should be double-clamped, divided, and placed on the delivery table pending assignment of the 5-minute Apgar score (ACOG, 2006b). A clamped segment of the umbilical cord is stable for pH and blood gas assessment for at least 60 minutes, and a cord blood sample in a syringe flushed with heparin is stable for up to 60 minutes (Gibbs et al., 2004). Umbilical arterial blood analysis is the basis of determining fetal acid-base status; however, umbilical venous blood analysis may also be helpful when there is a maternal or uteroplacental complication (Gibbs et al., 2004). Umbilical cord gas analysis can diagnose hypoxemia and the presence or absence of metabolic acidosis in blood samples but does not give an indication of the duration of the hypoxemia. Thus, umbilical cord results are an indirect measure of the acid base status in tissue at the time of birth and do not reveal the duration of the insult or the actual level of asphyxia in tissue (see Table 8–6).

NURSING ASSESSMENT AND MANAGEMENT STRATEGIES

Patient Education about Fetal Heart Rate Monitoring

Preparation for the application of the monitoring equipment requires an explanation of EFM and time for answering the woman's questions. Most women know prior to labor that some form of EFM may be used. Ideally, objections or concerns regarding EFM will have been discussed between the woman and perinatal healthcare provider prior to admission. However, if the woman does decline EFM, the nurse should follow institutional procedure for any patient refusing medical treatment. A positive attitude in discussing the rationale for EFM is most effective. One approach is to explain to the woman and support person that the fetal monitor can provide reassurance of fetal well-being. Most women will agree to an initial period of EFM to establish fetal well-being. Other options for ongoing fetal assessment include intermittent EFM and intermittent auscultation.

TABLE 8–6 ■ MEAN BLOOD GAS VALUES IN NONPREGNANT AND PREGNANT ADULTS VERSUS UMBILICAL ARTERIAL (UA) AND UMBILICAL VENOUS (UV) CORD BLOOD IN FETUSES WITH APGAR SCORE ≥7 AT 5 MINUTES

| | | | Term Fetus with Apgar ≥7 at 5 min | |
	Non-Pregnant Adults	Pregnant Adults	*UA*	*UV*
pH	7.40	7.40	7.26	7.34
PCO$_2$	40.00	34.00	53.00	41.00
PO$_2$	98.00	106.00	17.00	29.00
Base Excess	0	−4	−4	−3

Adapted with permission from Parer, J. T. (1997). *Handbook of fetal heart rate monitoring* (2nd ed.). Philadelphia: W. B. Saunders.

Nursing Assessment of the Fetal Heart Rate

A systematic, organized approach to interpreting FHR patterns prevents misinterpretation and confusion. The deceleration in the middle of the tracing is eye catching and anxiety producing, but it may not be the most important aspect of the tracing. Assessment of the entire FHR tracing, including uterine contractions and all procedures that transpired prior to the deceleration, is required. Review of the maternal medical record is of critical importance. Assessment should include the following (a) maternal–fetal risk for uteroplacental insufficiency, (b) administration of regional analgesia/anesthesia, (c) administration of medications or maternal drug use, and (d) pharmacologic agents used for cervical ripening and labor induction/augmentation.

Physical assessment should include maternal vital signs, hydration status, and position, as these factors can have an influence on fetal status. For example, maternal fever can cause fetal tachycardia, whereas supine positioning or hypotension can cause fetal bradycardia.

Experienced perinatal nurses assess FHR patterns for evidence of fetal well-being very quickly. They use a mental checklist that includes the following questions (Simpson, 2006):

- What is the baseline FHR?
- Is it within normal limits for this fetus?
- If not, what clinical factors could be contributing to this baseline rate?
- Is there evidence of baseline variability?
- If not, does external or fetal scalp stimulation elicit an acceleration of the FHR appropriate for gestational age?
- What clinical factors could be contributing to this baseline variability?
- Are there periodic or episodic FHR patterns?

- If so, what are they and what are the appropriate interventions (if any)?
- Does the FHR pattern suggest a chronic or acute maternal–fetal condition?
- Is uterine activity normal in frequency, duration, intensity, and resting tone?
- What is the relationship between the FHR and uterine activity?
- If the FHR pattern is nonreassuring, do the appropriate interventions resolve the situation?
- If not, are further interventions needed?
- Is the FHR pattern such that notification of the physician or midwife is warranted?

Nurses who are learning the principles of EFM may require more time to complete an assessment of fetal status; however, the essential components of a comprehensive assessment remain the same. It is helpful to devise a systematic method for FHR assessment and related appropriate interventions and consistently use that method in clinical practice to enhance optimal maternal–fetal outcomes.

After collecting all pertinent data, the following characteristics of the FHR tracing are interpreted and documented in the medical record: (a) uterine activity: frequency, duration, intensity, and resting tone; (b) baseline rate and variability; (c) presence or absence of accelerations; and (d) presence or absence of decelerations (Display 8–5). There is no need to further describe FHR decelerations in medical record documentation other than identifying them by name. In the past, some clinician were taught to describe decelerations by depth, duration, and return to baseline rate (ie, deceleration down to 60 bpm for 90 seconds with a slow return to baseline). However, this type of description is not necessary and may increase professional liability if the case should be reviewed after an adverse outcome and the medical record documentation concerning the decelerations does not match exactly with the decelerations as noted on the

DISPLAY 8-5

Essential Components of Documentation of FHR Patterns

1. Baseline rate
2. Baseline variability
3. Presence or absence of accelerations
4. Periodic or episodic decelerations
5. Changes of trends of FHR patterns over time.

Adapted from National Institute of Child Health and Human Development Research Planning Workshop. (1997). Electronic fetal heart rate monitoring: Research guidelines for interpretation. *American Journal of Obstetrics and Gynecology 177*(6), 1385–1390, and *Journal of Obstetric Gynecology and Neonatal Nursing, 26*(6), 635–640.

FHR tracing. Identification of the deceleration as early, late, variable, or prolonged implies that the deceleration meets criteria for these types of decelerations as defined by NICHD (1997). During interdisciplinary communication regarding FHR patterns, descriptions may be requested and may be appropriate for clarification and appreciation of the need for immediacy of intervention.

If the FHR pattern is nonreassuring, nursing intervention is based first on identification of the precipitating event if possible and then prioritized based on the level of concern. Eliminating the cause (eg, uterine hyperstimulation or maternal hypotension) and/or instituting interventions that provide intrauterine resuscitation may be all that is necessary for the resumption of a reassuring FHR pattern (see Table 8–3). Conversely, the presence of one of the five FHR patterns listed in Table 8–5 warrants immediate bedside evaluation by a physician who can initiate a cesarean birth. Depending on the clinical situation, there may be a decision for operative birth.

Interdisciplinary Communication

It is not unusual for disagreements in the interpretation of FHR patterns to exist between different members of the perinatal healthcare team (Beckman, Van Mullem, Beckman, & Brokhuizen, 1997; Paneth, Bommarito, & Strickler, 1993; Simpson, James, & Knox, 2006). Intrapartum fetal assessment is one of the most important clinical situations in which nurses, physicians, and midwives need to work together and trust each other's judgment (Fox et al., 2000; Simpson & Knox, 2006). Much of the

communication about ongoing maternal–fetal status during labor occurs while the nurse is at the bedside and the physician is in the office or at home (Simpson et al., 2006). If the nurse determines that the FHR pattern is nonreassuring, the physician or midwife should be notified. Nurses should describe their concerns and observations so that a clear plan of management can collaboratively be determined. Requests for orders for interventions and a bedside evaluation if necessary should be clearly stated. "Please come in to review the FHR pattern" is more effective in obtaining a bedside evaluation than "I'm worried about the fetus." If the situation is acute, "I need you to come now" is a clear, concise request for immediate action. Communication regarding nonreassuring FHR patterns should include characteristics of the pattern (baseline rate, variability, and presence or absence of accelerations and decelerations), pattern evolution (ie, how long this FHR pattern has been developing), the clinical context (eg, bleeding, hyperstimulation, hypotension), what intrauterine resuscitation techniques have been implemented and the fetal response, and request for further interventions and evaluation (eg, amnioinfusion, ephedrine, terbutaline, internal monitoring, bedside evaluation as soon as possible, immediate bedside evaluation, preparations for emergent cesarean birth) (Fox et al., 2000). The general content of this conversation, including the provider's response, should be documented in the medical record. If the discussion results in a clinical disagreement that cannot be resolved by the direct care providers, nurses should follow institutional policy about resolution of clinical disagreements. This type of policy is usually known as the chain of command. See Chapter 1 for a discussion of the chain of command.

Physicians, midwives, and nurses are responsible for maintaining competence in FHR pattern interpretation and appropriate interventions based on their interpretation. One way to both maintain competence and promote interdisciplinary collaboration is participation in EFM education programs that include physicians, midwives, and nurses. A group process can be used to review EFM strips, expected responses, appropriate interpretations, and related interventions. Interdisciplinary team discussions can lead to an increased knowledge of EFM principles for everyone involved. Developing case studies containing clinical ambiguity is an ideal avenue for clarifying ongoing clinical issues where interpretation and expectations of all provider groups are not in sync (Miller, 2005). Educational collaboration between nurses, midwives, and physicians who are jointly responsible for FHR pattern interpretation and clinical interventions enhances collaboration in everyday clinical interactions and thus promotes maternal–fetal safety (JCACHO, 2004).

Certification in EFM is another option to promote interdisciplinary knowledge related to fetal assessment. When all members of the team hold certification in EFM, there is recognition that everyone has the same level of EFM knowledge and skill and that this knowledge and these skills are not discipline-specific. Preparing for the certification exam as a group can enhance interdisciplinary team collegiality and effective communication when there is a question concerning fetal status based on the FHR pattern.

ISSUES IN THE USE OF FETAL HEART RATE MONITORING DURING LABOR

Efficacy of Electronic Fetal Heart Rate Monitoring

When EFM was developed and introduced into clinical practice, the hope was that this technique for fetal assessment would lead to a reduction in the overall incidence of cerebral palsy and intrapartum stillbirth (ACOG & AAP, 2003). This expectation was due in part to the opinion of experts in the 1960s and 1970s that most cases of cerebral palsy and other neurological morbidity were the result of asphyxia during labor and birth. The randomized trials conducted during the 1980s failed to show a decrease in the incidence of cerebral palsy among infants who were monitored during labor (Shy et al., 1990). Yet the incidence of cesarean birth and assisted operative birth in the cohorts monitored increased four-fold (Thacker et al., 1995). These results have led many to the conclusion that EFM is not efficacious (Freeman, 1990). More recent reviews of the methodology used in the randomized trials in combination with newer information on the genesis of cerebral palsy have brought to light some of the reasons why FHR monitoring did poorly in the randomized trials that were conducted (ACOG & AAP, 2003; Parer & King, 2000). Because this controversy remains unresolved, it is worth reviewing in the context of this text.

Fetal Heart Rate Monitoring and Cerebral Palsy

EFM has been in wide use for more than 30 years with no change in the incidence of cerebral palsy (2 per 1,000 live births) (ACOG & AAP, 2003; Penning & Garite, 1999). Thus, the original hope that EFM would predict and therefore prevent fetal asphyxia, which would in turn prevent cerebral palsy, has not come to pass. The majority of cases of infant and childhood cerebral palsy are related to prenatal events rather than the labor and birth process. Most cases of

cerebral palsy are associated with prematurity, disorders of coagulation, and intrauterine exposure to maternal infections (Grether & Nelson, 1997). Interruption of the oxygen supply to the fetus contributes to approximately 6% of cases of cerebral palsy (Nelson & Grether, 1999), and most experts believe that no more than 2% to 20% of cases of cerebral palsy are due to intrapartum events of any cause (ACOG & AAP, 2003; MacDonald, 1996; Nelson, 1988). These wide-ranging estimates are the result of imprecise interpretation of EFM data during labor as well as variations in diagnostic classification of the severity and type of cerebral palsy (Lent, 1999). In addition, the dramatically improved survival rates of extremely preterm infants have the potential to actually increase the incidence of cerebral palsy, and advances in neonatal care may also improve the survival rate of asphyxiated infants of any gestational age. These factors may obscure any effect that EFM has had on the incidence of cerebral palsy. In 1999, an international panel composed of specialists and researchers in perinatology, neonatology, midwifery, science, and epidemiology reviewed the literature on the causation of cerebral palsy (MacLennan, 1999). The *International Consensus Statement* published by this group lists clinical and biochemical factors that define the criteria that would implicate an acute intrapartum event as the etiology of cerebral palsy. These recommendations were recently modified and adopted by ACOG & AAP (2003) (see Display 8–6).

Specificity, Sensitivity, and Reliability of Electronic Fetal Monitoring

Approximately 30% of fetuses will demonstrate a non-reassuring FHR pattern at some time during labor (Garite et al., 2000). However, it is estimated that even the most ominous FHR patterns are associated with at most a 50% to 65% incidence of neonatal depression (Martin, 1998). Overall, EFM can have up to a 99.8% false-positive rate for term fetuses (Nelson, Dambrosia, Ting, & Grether, 1996). Conversely, when the FHR is reassuring, there is a very high probability (>99.9%) that the fetus is doing well and is adequately oxygenated (Garite et al., 2000). Thus, EFM sensitivity (the ability to detect a healthy fetus when it is indeed healthy) is high, while specificity (the ability to detect a compromised fetus when it is compromised and not include healthy fetuses in the criteria) is low (Simpson & Knox, 2000). The specificity and sensitivity limitations of EFM are related to its inability to directly evaluate fetal oxygen status.

Further complicating the issue is the fact that both inter- and intra-observer reliability in interpreting EFM data is inconsistent (Paneth et al., 1993; Martin, 1998). Not only do experienced clinicians differ in

DISPLAY 8-6

Criteria to Define an Acute Intrapartum Hypoxic Event as Sufficient to Cause Cerebral Palsy

1.1: Essential criteria (must meet all four)

1. Evidence of a metabolic acidosis in fetal umbilical cord arterial blood obtained at birth (pH <7 and base deficit ≥12 mmol/L)
2. Early onset of severe or moderate neonatal encephalopathy in infants born at 34 or more weeks of gestation
3. Cerebral palsy of the spastic quadriplegic or dyskinetic type*
4. Exclusion of other identifiable etiologies, such as trauma, coagulation disorders, infectious conditions, or genetic disorders

1.2: Criteria that collectively suggest an intrapartum timing (within close proximity to labor and birth [eg, 0–48 hours]) but are nonspecific to asphyxial insults

1. A sentinel (signal) hypoxic event occurring immediately before or during labor
2. A sudden and sustained fetal bradycardia or the absence of fetal heart rate variability in the presence of recurrent, late, or variable decelerations, usually after a hypoxic sentinel event when the pattern was previously normal
3. Apgar scores of 0–3 beyond 5 minutes
4. Onset of multisystem involvement within 72 hours of birth
5. Early imaging study showing evidence of acute nonfocal cerebral abnormality

---

*Spastic quadriplegia and, less commonly, dyskinetic cerebral palsy are the only types of cerebral palsy associated with acute hypoxic intrapartum events. Spastic quadriplegia is not specific to intrapartum hypoxia. Hemiparetic cerebral palsy, hemiplegic cerebral palsy, spastic diplegia, and ataxia are unlikely to result from acute intrapartum hypoxia.

Nelson, K. B., & Grether, J. K. (1998). Potentially asphyxiating conditions and spastic cerebral palsy in infants of normal birth weight. *American Journal of Obstetricians and Gynecologists, 179*(2), 507–513.

Modified from MacLennan, A. (1999). A template for defining a causal relation between acute intrapartum events and cerebral palsy: International consensus statement. *British Medical Journal, 319*(7216),1054–1059.

Knox, 2000). By contrast, diagnosis of fetal well-being (adequate fetal oxygenation) has much higher inter- and intra-observer reliability. Therefore, communication issues and professional disagreements regarding EFM interpretation are much more likely to occur when attempting to assign a diagnosis of fetal compromise than that of fetal well-being.

The differential predictability between specificity and sensitivity and lack reliability between different providers is the basis of the fundamental issue confounding the use of EFM (Simpson & Knox, 2000). The lack of common understanding by all involved professionals about how FHR monitoring can be relied upon when determining fetal status undermines the ability of this technique to guide clinical management (Fox et al., 2000). If the FHR pattern has a normal baseline rate, moderate variability, and no nonreassuring periodic or episodic changes, there is little disagreement about the prediction of fetal well-being. Similarly, patterns with absent variability and either bradycardia, tachycardia, or variable or late decelerations, generate significant agreement. These patterns clearly suggest the fetus is at risk for acidosis. However, the majority of FHR patterns are between these two extremes. When different members of the care team simultaneously make different assumptions concerning EFM data, communication between the involved professionals is compromised (Fox et al., 2000). Therefore, interdisciplinary processes that promote common understanding of EFM principles are highly recommended to promote the safest care possible for the mother and fetus.

SUMMARY

Monitoring and interpretation of the FHR are critical elements of intrapartum care (see Fig. 8–16). Standardized terms and definitions must be routinely used by all members of the perinatal healthcare team (JCAHO, 2004). Knowledge of the physiology underlying specific FHR patterns has increased over time. Nurses, midwives, and physicians must keep abreast of evolving knowledge in order to provide the best care for mothers and babies during labor. An appreciation of FHR pattern evolution and the use of variability in determining the risk for fetal acidemia is critical. Clinicians caring for women in labor should be able to rapidly identify FHR patterns that truly reflect the absence of fetal acidemia and those that consistently indicate a significant risk for fetal acidemia (Parer et al., 2006). Finally, an interdisciplinary team approach in which there exists mutual respect and true collaboration between nurses, midwives, and physicians will create a clinical environment that enhances safe and effective intrapartum care.

interpretations when evaluating a specific FHR pattern (Chez et al., 1990, Nelson et al., 1996), but they also disagree with their own interpretation when asked to review the same FHR strip months later (Barrett et al., 1990). This phenomenon particularly affects interpretations suggesting fetal compromise (Simpson &

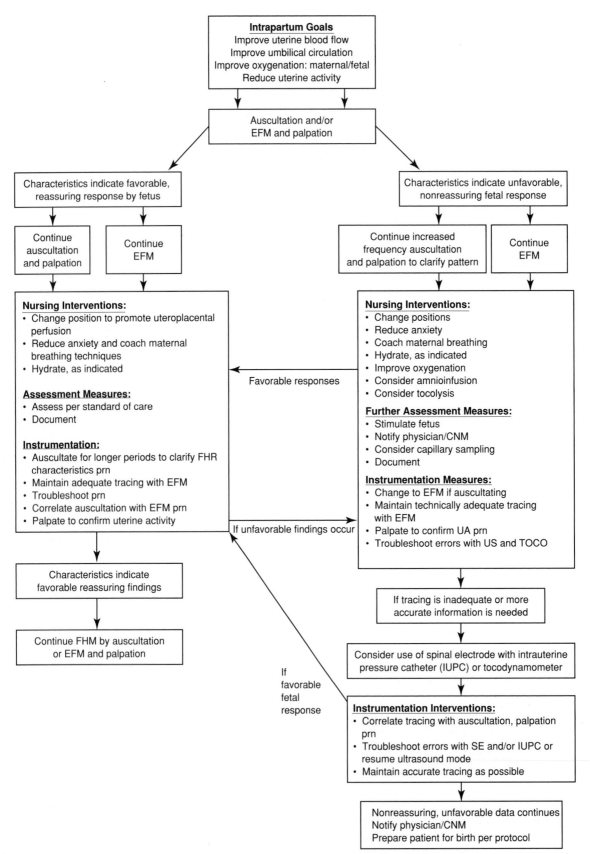

FIGURE 8–16. Decision tree for fetal heart rate monitoring. (From Feinstein, N., Torgersen, K., & Atterbury, J. [2003]. *Principles & practices*, p. 107.)

REFERENCES

Afriat, C. I. (1989). *Electronic fetal monitoring.* Rockville, MD: Aspen.

Aldrich, C. J., D'Antona, D., Spencer, J. A., Wyatt, J. S., Peebles, D. M., Delpy, D. T., et al. (1995). The effect of maternal posture on fetal cerebral oxygenation during labour. *British Journal of Obstetrics and Gynaecology, 102*(1), 14–19.

Aldrich, C. J., Wyatt, J. S., Spencer, J. A., Reynolds, E. O., & Delpy, D. T. (1994). The effect of maternal oxygen administration on human fetal cerebral oxygenation measured during labour by near infrared spectroscopy. *British Journal of Obstetrics and Gynaecology, 101*(6), 509–513.

Althabe Jr., O., Schwarcz, R. L., Pose, S. V., Escarcena, L., & Caldeyro-Barcia. R. (1967). Effects on fetal heart rate and fetal pO2 of oxygen administration to the mother. *American Journal of Obstetrics and Gynecology, 98,* 858–870.

American Academy of Pediatrics & American College of Obstetricians and Gynecologists. (2002). *Guidelines for perinatal care* (5th ed.). Washington, DC: Author.

American College of Obstetricians and Gynecologists. (1998). *Inappropriate use of the terms fetal distress and birth asphyxia.* (Committee Opinion No. 197). Washington, DC: Author.

American College of Obstetricians and Gynecologists. (1999a). *Antepartum fetal surveillance.* (Practice Bulletin No. 9). Washington, DC: Author.

American College of Obstetricians and Gynecologists. (1999b). *Induction of labor.* (Practice Bulletin No. 10). Washington, DC: Author.

American College of Obstetricians and Gynecologists. (2003). *Dystocia and the augmentation of labor.* (Practice No. 49). Washington, DC: Author.

American College of Obstetricians and Gynecologists. (2005a). *Inappropriate use of the terms fetal distress and birth asphyxia.* (Committee Opinion No. 326). Washington, DC: Author.

American College of Obstetricians and Gynecologists. (2005b). *Intrapartum fetal heart rate monitoring.* (Practice Bulletin No. 62). Washington, DC: Author.

American College of Obstetricians and Gynecologists. (2006a). *Amnioinfusion does not prevent meconium aspiration syndrome.* (Committee Opinion No. 364). Washington, DC: Author.

American College of Obstetricians and Gynecologists. (2006b). *Umbilical cord blood gas and acid-base analysis.* (Committee Opinion No. 368). Washington, DC: Author.

American College of Obstetricians and Gynecologists & American Academy of Pediatrics. (2003). *Neonatal encephalopathy and cerebral palsy: Defining the pathogenesis and pathophysiology.* Washington, DC: Author.

Association of Women's Health, Obstetric and Neonatal Nurses. (2000a). *Fetal assessment.* (Position Statement). Washington, D.C: Author.

Association of Women's Health, Obstetric and Neonatal Nurses. (2000b). *Nursing management of the second stage of labor.* (Evidence-based clinical practice guideline). Washington, DC: Author.

Association of Women's Health, Obstetric and Neonatal Nurses. (2005). *NICHD Transitional teaching guide.* (Fetal Heart Monitoring Program). Washington, DC: Author.

Atkinson, M. W., Belfort, M. A., Saade, G. R., & Moise, K. J. Jr. (1994). The relationship between magnesium sulfate therapy and fetal heart rate variability. *Obstetrics and Gynecology, 83*(6), 967–970.

Barrett, J. F., Jarvis, G. J., Macdonald, H. N., Buchan, P. C., Tyrrell, S. N., & Lilford, R. J. (1990). Inconsistencies in clinical decisions in obstetrics. *Lancet, 336*(8714), 549–551.

Bartnicki, J., & Saling, E. (1994). The influence of maternal oxygen administration on the fetus. *International Journal of Gynaecology and Obstetrics, 45*(2), 87–95.

Beard, R. W., Filshie, G. M., Knight, C. A., & Roberts, G. M. (1971). The significance of the changes in the continuous fetal heart rate in the first stage of labour. *Journal of Obstetrics and Gynaecology of the British Commonwealth, 78*(10), 865–881.

Beckmann, C. A., Van Mullem, C., Beckmann C. R., & Broekhuizen, F. F. (1997). Interpreting fetal heart rate tracings: Is there a difference between labor and delivery nurses and obstetricians? *Journal of Reproductive Medicine, 42*(10), 647–650.

Benson, R. C., Schubeck, F., Deutschberger, J., Weiss, W., & Berendes, H. (1968). Fetal heart rate as a predictor of fetal distress: A report from the collaborative project. *Obstetrics and Gynecology, 32*(2), 259–266.

Berkus, M. D., Langer, O., Samueloff, A., Xernaxis, E. M., & Field, N. T. (1999). Electronic fetal monitoring: what's reassuring? *Acta Obstetricia et Gynecologica Scandinavica, 78*(1), 15–21.

Braithwaite, N. D., Milligan, J. E., & Shennan, A. T. (1986). Fetal heart rate monitoring and neonatal mortality in the very preterm infant. *American Journal of Obstetrics and Gynecology, 154*(2), 250–254.

Burrus, D. R., O'Shea, T. M. Jr., Veille, J. C., & Mueller-Heubach, E. (1994). The predictive value of intrapartum fetal heart rate abnormalities in the extremely premature infant. *American Journal of Obstetrics and Gynecology, 171*(4), 1128–1132.

Calderyo-Barcia, R., Mendez-Bauer, E., & Poseiro, J. (1966). Control of human fetal heart rate during labor. In D. E. Cassels (Ed.), *The heart and circulation in the newborn and infant: Symposium on the heart and circulation in the newborn and infant* (pp. 7), New York: Grune and Stratton.

Carbonne, B., Benachi, A., Leveque, M. L., Cabrol, D., & Papiernik, E. (1996). Maternal position during labor: Effects on fetal oxygen saturation measured by pulse oximetry. *Obstetrics and Gynecology, 88*(5), 797–800.

Chez, B. F., Skurnick, J. H., Chez, R. A., Verklan, M. T., Biggs, S., & Hage, M. L. (1990). Interpretation of nonstress tests by obstetric nurses. *Journal of Obstetric, Gynecologic and Neonatal Nursing, 19*(3), 227–232.

Cibils, L. A., (1996). On intrapartum fetal monitoring. *American Journal of Obstetrics and Gynecology, 174*(4), 1382–1389.

Clark, S. L., Gimovsky, M. L., & Miller, F. C. (1984) The scalp stimulation test: A clinical alternative to fetal scalp blood sampling. *American Journal of Obstetrics and Gynecology, 148*(3), 274–277.

Clark, S. L., Cotton, D. B., Pivarnik, J. M., Lee, W., Hankins, G. D., Benedetti, T. J., et al. (1991). Position change and central hemodynamic profile during normal third trimester pregnancy and post partum. *American Journal of Obstetrics and Gynecology, 164*(3), 883–887.

Copel, J. A., Friedman, A. H., & Kleinman, C. S. (1997). Management of fetal cardiac arrhythmias. *Fetal Diagnosis and Therapy, 24*(1), 201–221.

Cramer, M. V., (1906). Ueber die dierkte ableitung der akionsstrome des menschlchen hersens vom oesophagus und uber das elektrokardiogramm des fotus. *Muenchener Medizinische Wochenschrift, 53,* 811–813.

Crane, J. M., Young, D. C., Butt, K. D., Bennett, K. A., & Hutchens, D. (2001). Excessive uterine activity accompanying induced labor. *Obstetrics and Gynecology, 97,* 926–931.

Dalton, K. J., Phill, D., Dawes, G. S., & Patrick, J. E. (1983). The autonomic nervous system and fetal heart rate variability. *American Journal of Obstetrics and Gynecology, 146*(4), 456–462.

Dawood, M. Y. (1995). Pharmacologic stimulation of uterine contractions. *Seminars in Perinatology, 19*(1), 73–83.

Dellinger, E. H., Boehm, F. H., & Crane, M. M. (2000). Electronic fetal heart rate monitoring: Early neonatal outcomes associated with normal rate, fetal stress and fetal distress. *American Journal of Obstetrics and Gynecology 182*(1, Pt. 1), 214–220.

Douvas, S. G., Meeks, G. R., Graves, G., Walsh, D. A., & Morrison, J. C. (1984). Intrapartum fetal heart rate monitoring as a predictor of fetal distress and immediate neonatal condition in low-birth weight (less than 1800 grams) infants. *American Journal of Obstetrics and Gynecology, 148*(3), 300–302.

Eganhouse, D. J. (1992). Fetal monitoring of twins. *Journal of Obstetric, Gynecologic and Neonatal Nursing, 21*(1), 17–27.

Elimian, A., Figueroa, R., & Tejani, N. (1997). Intrapartum assessment of fetal well-being: A comparison of scalp stimulation with scalp blood pH sampling. *Obstetrics and Gynecology, 89*(3), 373–376.

Fahey, J., & King, T. L. (2005). Intrauterine asphyxia: Clinical implications for providers of intrapartum care. *Journal of Midwifery and Women's Health, 50*(6), 498–506.

Feinstein, N., Sprague, A., & Trepenier, M. J. (2000). *Fetal heart rate auscultation.* (Symposium). Washington, DC: Association of Woman's Health, Obstetric, and Gynecologic Nurses.

Feinstein, N., Torgersen, K., & Atterbury, J. (2003). *Fetal heart rate monitoring: Principles and practices.* Washington, DC: Association of Women's Health, Obstetric, and Neonatal Nurses.

Fox, M., Kilpatrick, S., King, T., & Parer, J. T. (2000). Fetal heart rate monitoring: Interpretation and collaborative management. *Journal of Midwifery and Women's Health. 45*(6), 498–507.

Fraser, W. D., Hofmeyr, J., Lede, R., Faron, G., Alexander, S., Goffinet, F., et al. for the Amnioinfusion Trial Group. (2005). Amnioinfusion for the prevention of the meconium aspiration syndrome. *New England Journal of Medicine, 353*(9), 909–917.

Freeman, R. (1990). Intrapartum fetal monitoring: A disappointing story. *New England Journal of Medicine, 322*(9), 624–626.

Freeman, R. K., Garite, T. J., & Nageotte, M. P. (2003). *Fetal heart rate monitoring* (3rd ed.). Philadelphia, MD: Lippincott Williams & Wilkins.

Gallagher, M. W., Costigan, K., & Johnson, T. R. (1992). Fetal heart rate accelerations, fetal movement and fetal behavioral patterns in twin gestations. *American Journal of Obstetrics and Gynecology, 167*(4, Pt. 1), 1140–1144.

Galvan, B. J., Van Mullem, C., & Broekhuizen, F. F. (1989). Using amnioinfusion for the relief of repetitive variable decelerations during labor. *Journal of Obstetric, Gynecologic, and Neonatal Nursing, 18*(3), 222–229.

Garite, T. J., Dildy, G., McNamara, H., Nageotte, M. P., Boehm, F. H., Dellinger, E. H., et al. and the Mallinckrodt (Nellcor) Fetal Oximetry Research Group (2000). A multicenter controlled trial of fetal pulse oximetry in the intrapartum management of nonreassuring fetal heart rate patterns. *American Journal of Obstetrics and Gynecology, 183*(5), 1049–1058.

Gibbs, R. J., Rosenberg, A. R., Warren, C. J., Galan, H. L., & Rumack, C. M. (2004). Suggestions for practice to accompany neonatal encephalopathy and cerebral palsy. *Obstetrics and Gynecology, 103*(4), 778–779.

Gill, R. W., Trudinger, B. J., Garrett, W. J., Kossoff, G., & Warren, P. S. (1981). Fetal umbilical venous blood flow measured in utero by pulsed Doppler and B-mode ultrasound in normal pregnancies. *American Journal of Obstetrics and Gynecology, 139*(6), 720–725.

Goldaber, K. G., Gilstrap, L. C. III, Leveno, K. J., Dax, J. S., & McIntire, D. D. (1991) Pathologic fetal acidemia. *Obstetrics and Gynecology, 78*(6), 1103–1107.

Goodlin, R. C. (1979). History of fetal monitoring. *American Journal of Obstetrics and Gynecology, 133*(3), 323–352.

Goodwin, T. M., Milner-Masterson, L., & Paul, R. H. (1994). Elimination of fetal scalp blood sampling on a large clinical service. *Obstetrics and Gynecology, 83*(6), 971–974.

Grether, J. K., & Nelson, K. B. (1997). Maternal infection and cerebral palsy in infants of normal birth weight. *Journal of the American Medical Association, 278*(3), 207–211.

Gull, I., Jaffa, A. J., Oren, M., Grisaru, D., Peyser, M. R., & Lessing, J. P. (1996). Acid accumulation during end stage bradycardia: How long is too long? *British Journal of Obstetrics and Gynaecology, 103*(11), 1096–1101.

Hammacher, K. (1969). The clinical significance of cardiotocography. In P. Huntingford, K. Huter & E. Salez (Eds.), *Perinatal medicine, 1st European Congress, Berlin* (p. 81). New York: Academic Press.

Haruta, M., Funato, T., Sumida, T., & Shinkai, T. (1984). The influence of maternal oxygen inhalation for 30 to 60 minutes on fetal oxygenation. *Nippon Sanka Fujinka Gakka Zasshi, 36*(10), 1921–1929.

Haydon, M. L., Gorenberg, D. M., Nageotte, M. P., Ghamsary, M., Rumney, P. J., Patillo, C., et al. (2006). The effect of maternal oxygen administration on fetal pulse oximetry during labor in fetuses with nonreassuring fetal heart rate patterns. *American Journal of Obstetrics and Gynecology, 195*(3), 735–738.

Helwig, J. T., Parer, J. T., Kilpatrick, S. J., & Laros, R. K. Jr. (1996). Umbilical cord blood acid base state: What is normal? *American Journal of Obstetrics and Gynecology, 174*(6), 1807–1814.

Herbst, A., Wolner-Hanssen, P., & Ingelmarsson I. (1997). Risk factors for acidemia at birth. *Obstetrics and Gynecology 90*(1), 125–130.

Hiett, A. K., Devoe, L. D., Brown, H. L., & Watson, J. (1995). Effects of magnesium on fetal heart rate variability using computer analysis. *American Journal of Perinatology, 12*(4), 259–261.

Holmes, P., Oppenheimer, L. W., Gravelle, A., Walker, M., & Blayney, M. (2001). The effect of variable heart rate decelerations on intraventricular hemorrhage and other perinatal outcomes in preterm infants. *Journal of Maternal Fetal Medicine, 10*(4), 264–268.

Hohn, A., & Stanton, R. (1992). The cardiovascular system. In A. A. Fanaroff & R. J. Martin (Eds.), *Neonatal perinatal medicine: Diseases of the fetus and infant* (5th ed., pp. 883–940). St. Louis, MO: Mosby–Year Book.

Hon, E. H. (1958). The electronic evaluation of the fetal heart rate: Preliminary report. *American Journal of Obstetrics and Gynecology, 75*(6), 1215–1230.

Hon, E. (1963). The classification of fetal heart rate I: A revised working classification. *Obstetrics and Gynecology, 22*, 137–146.

Joint Commission on Accreditation of Healthcare Organizations. (2004). *Preventing infant death and injury during delivery.* (Sentinel Event Alert No. 30). Oak Brook, IL: Author.

Jozwik, M., Sledziewski, A., Klubowicz, S., Zak, J., Sajewska, G., & Pietrzycki, B. (2000). Use of oxygen therapy during labour and acid-base status in the newborn. *Medycyna wieku rozwojowego, 4*(4), 403–411.

Kennedy, E. (1833) *Observations of obstetrical auscultation* (p. 311). Dublin: Hodges and Smith.

King, T. L., & Parer, J. T. (2000). The physiology of fetal heart rate patterns and perinatal asphyxia. *Journal of Perinatal and Neonatal Nursing, 14*(3), 19–39.

Kisilevsky, B. S., Hains, S. M., & Low, J. A. (2001). Maturation of the fetal heart rate and body movements in 24–33 week old fetuses threatening to deliver prematurely. *Developmental Psychobiology, 38*(1), 78–86.

Kleinman, C. S., & Nehgme, R. A. (2004). Cardiac arrhythmias in the human fetus. *Pediatric Cardiology, 25*(3), 234–251.

Klingner, M. C., & Kruse, J. (1999). Meconium aspiration syndrome: Pathophysiology and prevention. *Journal of the American Board of Family Practice, 12*(6), 450–466.

Korhonen, J., & Kariniemi, V. (1994). Emergency cesarean section: The effect of delay on umbilical arterial gas balance and Apgar scores. *Acta Obstetricia et Gynecologica Scandinavica, 73*(10), 782–786.

Krebs, H. B., Petres, R. E., Dunn, L. J., Jordaan, H. V., & Segreti, A. (1979). Intrapartum fetal heart rate monitoring. I. Classification and prognosis of fetal heart rate patterns. *American Journal of Obstetrics and Gynecology, 133*(7), 762–772.

Krebs, H. B., Petres, R. E., & Dunn, L. J. (1981). Intrapartum fetal heart rate monitoring. V. Fetal heart rate patterns in the second stage of labor. *American Journal of Obstetrics and Gynecology, 140*(4), 435–439.

Lent, M. (1999). The medical and legal risks of the electronic fetal monitor. *Stanford Law Review, 51*(4), 807–837.

Leung, A. S., Leung, E. K., & Paul, R. H. (1993). Uterine rupture after previous cesarean delivery: maternal and fetal consequences. *American Journal of Obstetrics and Gynecology, 169*(4), 945–950.

Low, J. A., Galbraith, R. S., Muir, D. W., Killen, H. L., Pater, E. A., & Karchmar, E. J. (1992). Mortality and morbidity after intrapartum asphyxia in the preterm fetus. *Obstetrics and Gynecology, 80*(1), 57–61.

Low, J. A., Killen, H., & Derrick, E. J. (2002). The prediction and prevention of intrapartum fetal asphyxia in preterm pregnancies. *American Journal of Obstetrics and Gynecology, 186*(2), 270–282.

Low, J. A., Victory, R., & Derrick, E. J. (1999). Predictive value of electronic fetal monitoring for intrapartum fetal asphyxia with metabolic acidosis. *Obstetrics and Gynecology, 93*(2), 285–291.

MacDonald, D., Grant A., Sheridan-Pereira M., Boylan, P., & Chalmers, I. (1985). The Dublin randomized controlled trial of intrapartum fetal heart rate monitoring. *American Journal of Obstetrics and Gynecology, 152*(5), 524–539.

MacDonald, D. (1996). Cerebral palsy and intrapartum fetal monitoring. *New England Journal of Medicine, 334*(6), 659–660.

MacLennan, A. H. (1999). A template for defining a causal relationship between acute intrapartum events and cerebral palsy: International consensus statement. *British Medical Journal, 319*(7216), 1054–1059.

Maiques, V., Garcia-Tejedor, A., Perales, A., & Navarro, C. (1999). Intrapartum fetal invasive procedures and perinatal transmission of HIV. *European Journal of Obstetrics and Gynecology and Reproductive Biology, 87*(1), 63–67.

McNamara, H., Johnson, N., & Lilford, R. (1993). The effect on fetal arteriolar oxygen saturation resulting from giving oxygen to the mother measured by pulse oximetry. *British Journal of Obstetrics and Gynaecology, 100*(5), 446–449.

Martin C. B. Jr. (1998). Electronic fetal monitoring: A brief summary of its development, problems and prospects. *European Journal of Obstetrics and Gynecology and Reproductive Biology, 78*(2), 133–140.

Matsuda, Y., Maeda, T., & Kouno, S. (2003). The critical period of non-reassuring fetal heart rate patterns in preterm gestation. *European Journal of Gynecology and Reproductive Biology, 106*(1), 36–39.

Menihan, C. A. (1998). Uterine rupture in women attempting a vaginal birth following prior cesarean birth. *Journal of Perinatology, 18*(6, Pt. 1), 440–443.

Miller, L. A. (2005). System errors in intrapartum fetal monitoring: A case study. *Journal of Midwifery and Women's Health, 50*(6), 507–516.

Mino, M., Puertas, A., Miranda, J. A., & Herruzo, A. J. (1999). Amnioinfusion in term labor with low amniotic fluid due to rupture of the membranes: A new indication. *European Journal of Obstetrics, Gynecology, and Reproductive Biology, 82*(1), 29–34.

Miyazaki, F. S., & Nevarez, F. (1985). Saline amnioinfusion for relief of repetitive variable decelerations: A prospective randomized study. *American Journal of Obstetrics and Gynecology, 153*(3), 301–306.

Modanlou, H. D. (1991). Uses of biochemical profile of the fetus. *Contemporary Obstetrics and Gynecology, 36*(9) 69–85.

Modanlou, H. D., & Freeman, R. K. (1982). Sinusoidal fetal heart rate pattern: Its definition and clinical significance. *American Journal of Obstetrics and Gynecology, 142*(8), 1033–1038.

Modanlou, H. D., & Murata, Y. (2004). Sinusoidal fetal heart rate pattern: Reappraisal of its definition and clinical significance. *Journal of Obstetrics and Gynaecology Research, 30*(3), 169–180.

National Institute of Child Health and Human Development Research Planning Workshop. (1997). Electronic fetal heart rate monitoring: Research guidelines for interpretation. *American Journal of Obstetrics and Gynecology 177*(6), 1385–1390, and *Journal of Obstetric Gynecology and Neonatal Nursing, 26*(6), 635–640.

Nelson, K. B. (1988). What proportion of cerebral palsy is related to birth asphyxia? *Journal of Pediatrics, 112*(4), 572–574.

Nelson, K. B., Dambrosia, J. M., Ting, T. Y., & Grether, J. K. (1996). Uncertain value of electronic fetal monitoring in predicting cerebral palsy. *New England Journal of Medicine, 334*(10), 613–618.

Nelson, K. B., & Grether, J. K. (1998). Potentially asphyxiating conditions and spastic cerebral palsy in infants of normal birth weight. *American Journal of Obstetricians and Gynecologists, 179*(2), 507–513.

Nelson, K. B., & Grether, J. K. (1999). Causes of cerebral palsy. *Current Opinions in Pediatrics, 11*(6), 487–491.

O'Brien-Abel, N. E., & Benedetti, T. J. (1992). Saltatory fetal heart rate pattern. *Journal of Perinatology, 12*(1), 13–17.

Ouzounian, J. G., Miller, D. A., & Paul, R. H. (1996). Amnioinfusion in women with previous cesarean births: A preliminary report. *American Journal of Obstetrics and Gynecology, 174*(2), 783–786.

Paneth, N., Bommarito, M., & Stricker, J. (1993). Electronic fetal monitoring and later outcome. *Clinical and Investigative Medicine, 16*(2), 159–165.

Parer, J. T. (1997). *Handbook of fetal heart rate monitoring* (2nd Ed.). Philadelphia, PA: W. B. Saunders Company.

Parer, J. T., & King, T. L. (1999). Whither fetal heart rate Monitoring. *Obstetrics, Gynecology and Fertility, 22*(5), 149–192.

Parer, J. T., & King T. L. (2000). Fetal heart rate monitoring: Is it Salvageable? *American Journal of Obstetrics and Gynecology 182*(4), 982–987.

Parer, J. T, King, T. L., Flanders, S., Fox, M., & Kilpatrick, S. J. (2006). Fetal acidemia and electronic fetal heart rate patterns: Is there an association? *Journal of Maternal-Fetal and Neonatal Medicine, 19*(5), 289–294.

Parer, J. T., & Livingston, E. G. (1990). What is fetal distress? *American Journal of Obstetrics and Gynecology, 162*(6), 1421–1425; discussion 1475–1427.

Parer, J. T., & Nageotte, M. P. (2004). Intrapartum fetal surveillance. In R. K. Creasy & R. Resnick (Eds.), *Maternal-Fetal Medicine* (5th ed., pp. 403–427). Philadelphia, PA: W. B. Saunders Company.

Penning, S., & Garite, T. (1999). Management of fetal distress. *Obstetrics and Gynecology Clinics of North America, 26*(2), 259–274.

Phaneuf, S., Rodriguez-Linares, B., TambyRaja, R. L., MacKenzie, I. Z., & Lopez-Bernal, A. (2000). Loss of myometrial oxytocin receptors during oxytocin-induced and oxytocin-augmented labor. *Journal of Reproduction and Fertility, 120*(1), 91–97.

Phelan, J. P., & Ahn, M. O. (1994). Perinatal observations in forty-eight neurologically impaired term infants. *American Journal of Obstetrics and Gynecology, 171*(2), 424–431.

Pierce, J., Gaudier, F. L., & Sanchez-Ramos, L. (2000). Intrapartum amnioinfusion for meconium-stained fluid: Meta-analysis of prospective clinical trials. *Obstetrics and Gynecology, 95*(6, Pt. 2), 1051–1056.

Ramsey, P. S., & Repke, J. T. (2003). Intrapartum management of mutifetal pregnancies. *Seminars in Perinatology, 27*(1), 54–72.

Ridgeway, J. J., Weyrich, D. L., & Benedetti, T. J. (2004). Fetal heart rate changes associated with uterine rupture. *Obstetrics and Gynecology, 103*(3), 506–512.

Roberts, J. E. (2002). The "push" for evidence: Management of the second stage. *Journal of Midwifery and Women's Health, 47*(1), 2–15.

Rochard, F., Schifrin, B. S., Goupil, F., Legrand, H., Blottiere, J., & Sureau, C. (1976). Nonstressed fetal heart monitoring in the antepartum period. *American Journal of Obstetrics and Gynecology, 126*(6), 699–706.

Rotmensch, S., Liberati, M., Vishene, T. H., Celentano, C., Ben-Rafael, Z., & Bellati, U. (1999). The effect of betamethasone and dexamethasone on fetal heart rate patterns and biophysical activities: A prospective randomized trial. *Acta Obstetricia et Gynecologica Scandinavica, 78*(6), 493–500.

Sherer, D. M., Amico, M. L., Cox, C., Metlay, L. A., & Woods, J. R. Jr. (1994). Association of in utero behavioral patterns of twins with each other as indicated by fetal heart rate reactivity and nonreactivity. *American Journal of Perinatology, 11*(3), 208–212.

Sherer, D. M., Nawrocki, M. N., Peco, N. E., Metlay, L. A., & Woods, J. R. Jr. (1990). The occurrence of simultaneous fetal heart rate accelerations in twins during nonstress testing. *Obstetrics and Gynecology, 76*(5), 817–821.

Shy, K. K., Luthy, D. A., Bennett, F. C., Whitfield, M., Larson, E. B., van Belle, G., et al. (1990). Effects of electronic fetal heart rate monitoring, as compared with periodic auscultation, on the neurologic development of premature infants. *New England Journal of Medicine, 322*(9), 588–593.

Simpson, K. R. (2002). *Cervical ripening, induction and augmentation of labor.* (Practice Monograph). Washington, DC: Association of Women's Health, Obstetric, and Neonatal Nurses.

Simpson, K. R. (2006). Critical illness during pregnancy: Considerations for evaluation and treatment of the fetus as the second patient. *Critical Care Nursing Quarterly, 29*(1), 19–31.

Simpson, K. R. (2007). Intrauterine resuscitation during labor: Review of current methods and supportive evidence. *Journal of Midwifery and Women's Health, 52*(3), 229–237.

Simpson, K. R., & James, D. C. (2005a). Effects of immediate versus delayed pushing during second stage labor on fetal wellbeing: A randomized clinical trial. *Nursing Research, 54*(3), 149–157.

Simpson, K. R., & James, D. C. (2005b). Efficacy of intrauterine resuscitation techniques in improving fetal oxygen status during labor. *Obstetrics and Gynecology, 105*(6), 1362–1368.

Simpson, K. R., James, D. C., & Knox, G. E. (2006). Nurse-physician communication during labor and birth: Implications for patient safety. *Journal of Obstetric, Gynecologic and Neonatal Nursing, 35*(4), 547–556.

Simpson, K. R., & Knox, G. E. (2000). Risk management and EFM: Decreasing risk of adverse outcomes and liability exposure. *Journal of Perinatal and Neonatal Nursing, 14*(3), 43–58.

Simpson, K. R., & Knox, G. E. (2006). Perinatal patient safety: Essential criteria for safe care for mothers and babies during labor and birth. *AWHONN Lifelines, 9*(6), 478–483.

Society of Obstetricians and Gynaecologists of Canada. (2002). Fetal health surveillance in labour, Part I. (Clinical Practice Guidelines). *Journal of the Society of Obstetricians and Gynaecologists of Canada, 24*(3), 250–276.

Sorokin, Y., Dierker, L. J., Pillay, S. K., Zador, I. E., Schreiner, M. L., & Rosen, M. G. (1982). The association between fetal heart rate patterns and fetal movements in pregnancies between 20 and 30 weeks gestation. *American Journal of Obstetrics and Gynecology, 143*(3), 243–249.

Stein, E., Handelsman, E., & Matthews, R. (2000). Reducing perinatal transmission of HIV: Early diagnosis and interventions during pregnancy. *Journal of Midwifery and Women's Health, 45*(2), 122–129.

Strong, T. H. Jr. (1997). The effect of amnioinfusion on the duration of labor. *Obstetrics and Gynecology, 89*(6), 1044–1046.

Subtil, D., Tiberghien, P., Devos, P., Therby, D., Leclerc, G., Vaast, P., et al. (2003). Immediate and delayed effects of antenatal corticosteroids on fetal heart rate: A randomized trial that compares betamethasone acetate and phosphate, betamethasone phosphate, and dexamethasone. *American Journal of Obstetrics and Gynecology, 188*(2), 524–531.

Sureau, C. (1996). Historical perspectives: Forgotten past, unpredictable future. *Baillieres Clinical Obstetrics and Gynaecology, 10*(2), 167–184.

Tejani, N., Mann, L. I., Bhakthavathsalan, A., & Weiss, R. R. (1975). Correlation of fetal heart rate–uterine contraction patterns with fetal scalp blood pH. *Obstetrics and Gynecology, 46*(4), 392–396.

Thacker, S. B., Stroup, D. F., & Peterson, H. B. (1995). Efficacy and safety of intrapartum electronic fetal monitoring: An update. *Obstetrics and Gynecology, 86*(4, Pt. 1), 613–620.

Thorp, J. A., Trobough, T., Evans, R., Hedrick, J., & Yeast, J. D. (1995) The effect of maternal oxygen administration during the second stage of labor on umbilical cord blood gas values: A randomized controlled prospective trial. *American Journal of Obstetrics and Gynecology, 172*(2 Pt. 1), 465–474.

To, W. W., & Leung, W. C. (1998). The incidence of abnormal findings from intrapartum cardiotocogram monitoring in term and preterm labor. *Australian New Zealand Obstetrics and Gynecology, 38*(3), 258–261.

Tucker, S. M. (2004). *Pocket guide to fetal monitoring* (5th ed.). St. Louis, MO: Mosby.

van Iddekinge, B., Hofmeyr, G. J., & Buchmann, E. (2003). Visual interpretation of the effect of maternal betamethasone administration on the fetal heart rate pattern. *Journal of Obstetrics and Gynaecology, 23*(4), 360–363.

Vintzileos, A. M., Antsaklis, A., Varvarigos, I., Papas, C., Sofatzis, I., & Montgomery, J. T. (1993). A randomized trial of intrapartum electronic fetal heart rate monitoring versus intermittent auscultation. *Obstetrics and Gynecology, 81*(6), 899–907.

Westgate, J. A., Bennet, L., & Gunn, A. J. (1999). Fetal heart rate variability during brief repeated umbilical cord occlusion in near term fetal sheep. *British Journal of Obstetrics and Gynecology 106*(7), 664–671.

Westgren, M., Holmquist, P., Svenningsen, N., & Ingemarsson, I. (1982). Intrapartum fetal monitoring in preterm deliveries: Prospective study. *Obstetrics and Gynecology, 60*(1), 99–106.

Westgren, M., Holmquist, P., Ingemarsson, I., & Svenningsen, N. (1984). Intrapartum fetal acidosis in preterm infants: Fetal monitoring and long-term morbidity. *Obstetrics and Gynecology, 63*(3), 355–359.

Westgren, L. M., Malcus, P., & Svenningsen, N. W. (1986). Intrauterine asphyxia and long-term outcome in preterm fetuses. *Obstetrics and Gynecology, 67*(4), 512–516.

Wright, J. W., Ridgway, L. E., Wright, B. D., Covington, D. L., & Bobbitt, J. R. (1996). Effect of MgSO4 on heart rate monitoring in the preterm fetus. *Journal of Reproductive Medicine, 41*(8), 605–608.

Zanini, B., Paul, R. H., & Huey, J. R. (1980). Intrapartum fetal heart rate: Correlation with scalp pH in the preterm fetus. *American Journal of Obstetrics and Gynecology, 136*(1), 43–47.

Zeeman, G. G., Khan-Dawood, F. S., & Dawood, M. Y. (1997). Oxytocin and its receptor in pregnancy and parturition: Current concepts and clinical implications. *Obstetrics and Gynecology, 89*, 873–883.

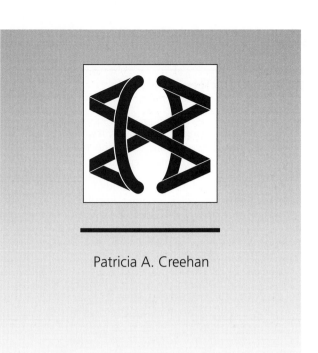

Patricia A. Creehan

CHAPTER 9

Pain Relief and Comfort Measures in Labor

MOST pregnant women have concerns about their ability to handle painful contractions during labor. Nearly every woman in labor experiences some degree of discomfort. Perception of pain is highly individual, even when two people experience the same stimuli. An appreciation of each woman's unique experience of pain is possible when perinatal nurses understand the physiologic basis of pain, physiologic responses to pain, and psychosocial factors influencing pain perception.

Many women experience intense pain in labor. Childbirth pain is one of the most severe types of pain a woman will experience in her lifetime (Camann, 2005). When the McGill Pain Questionnaire was used to compare reports of intensity of pain for a variety of clinical experiences (e.g., chronic back pain, nonterminal cancer pain, phantom limb pain, sprains, fractures), only the pain associated with accidental amputation of a digit and causalgia pain caused more discomfort than labor (Niven & Gijsbers, 1989). In a committee opinion, *Pain Relief During Labor*, the American College of Obstetricians and Gynecologists (ACOG) (2004) acknowledged that labor may result in severe pain for women and that, in the absence of any medical contraindications, pain management should be provided.

During labor, responsibility for managing pain and providing comfort is shared by the laboring woman, nurses, physicians, certified nurse midwives (CNMs), and labor-support persons. Interventions exist along a continuum, from noninvasive to invasive and from nonpharmacologic to pharmacologic. As healthcare professionals move along this continuum, the potential for complications and side effects increases. The goal of pain management during labor is to control pain without interrupting labor or doing harm to the woman or her fetus or newborn.

This chapter discusses the physiologic basis for pain along with the psychosocial factors influencing pain perception. Nonpharmacologic interventions are presented first because, in clinical practice, these are usually used before pharmacologic interventions.

PHYSIOLOGIC BASIS OF LABOR PAIN

Most pain during childbirth results from normal physiologic events. During the first stage of labor, uterine muscle hypoxia; lactic acid accumulation; cervical and lower uterine segment stretching; traction on ovaries, fallopian tubes, and uterine ligaments; and pressure on the bony pelvis cause afferent pain impulses to be carried along sympathetic nerve fibers entering the neuraxis between the 10th and 12th thoracic and first lumbar spinal segments. During the second stage of labor, distention of pelvic floor muscles, vagina, perineum, and vulva and pressure on the urethra, bladder, and rectum cause afferent pain impulses to be carried along sympathetic nerve fibers entering the neuraxis between the second and fourth sacral spinal segments (Birnbach & Browne, 2005). Some women in labor experience continuous low-back pain that is distinct from uterine contractions. This pain may be related to pressure from the fetal occipital bone on the neural plexus and bony structures of the maternal spine and pelvis.

TABLE 9–1 ■ DESCRIPTIONS OF PAIN DURING LABOR AND BIRTH

Sensory	Affective
First Stage of Labor Cramping, pulling, aching, heavy, sharp, stabbing, cutting, intermittent, localized, global, sore, heavy, throbbing	Exciting, intense, tiring, exhausting, scary, frightening, bearable or unbearable, distressing, horrible, agonizing, indescribable, overwhelming, engulfing
Second Stage of Labor Painful pressure, burning, ripping, tearing, piercing, explosive, localized	Exhausting, overwhelming, out-of-body feeling, inner focused or tunnel vision, exciting, horrible, excruciating, terrifying, less intense

Labor pain is an example of acute pain. It has a high degree of variability among individuals and at different points in labor. In a study of primiparous women during the first stage of labor, 60% described the pain during first stage of labor as unbearable, intolerable, extremely severe, and excruciating (Melzack, 1984). Obstetric factors that contribute to the pain of labor include rate of cervical dilatation, perineal distention, intensity and duration of contractions, and fetal position and size. As pain intensity increases, women experience decreased pain tolerance (Faure, 1991). Sleep deprivation and exhaustion from a long labor may alter the perception of pain (Youngstrom, Baker, & Miller, 1996). Age and parity may also influence an individual's perception of pain (Lowe, 1996). Descriptions of pain during the first and second stage of labor vary (Table 9–1). Some women describe a decrease in intensity during the second stage, probably because of maternal focus on pushing. Others experience more painful sensations, possibly because of the position of the fetus descending through the birth canal.

Events During Labor Affect the Experience of Pain

Unique circumstances of every labor influence the experience of pain. Responsiveness of the cervix to uterine contractions is influenced by prior surgical or diagnostic procedures that compromise the integrity of the cervix. Prior surgical procedures may result in an incompetent cervix and shorter labor or cause scarring and adhesions, resulting in failure to dilate and longer labor. Some medical and nursing procedures are uncomfortable. Interventions such as pharmacologic agents used for induction and augmentation of labor, vaginal examinations performed in the supine position, bed rest, amniotomy, tight external electronic fetal monitor (EFM) belts, and enemas may change the character of labor contractions and increase discomfort. Length of labor does not necessarily correlate directly with a woman's perception of pain. Women with short labors may experience very intense contractions. Women with a fetus in a persistent posterior position report severe pain during and between uterine contractions.

As duration of intense pain increases, discouragement and fatigue increase, decreasing the woman's ability to cope effectively with contractions. Fatigue may occur with a prolonged latent phase, as experienced by the woman who reports on admission that she has not slept for 2 days.

PHYSIOLOGIC RESPONSES TO PAIN

In addition to obvious physical discomfort, there are physiologic responses to pain over which women have little control. These physiologic responses may have a negative impact on the fetus and the labor process over time or in the context of other maternal or fetal conditions. Pain during labor may result in anxiety. Unrelieved anxiety causes increased production of cortisol, glucagon, and catecholamines, which increase metabolism and oxygen consumption. Increased levels of catecholamines have been shown to cause uterine hypoperfusion and decreased blood flow to the placenta, resulting in uterine irritability, preterm labor, dystocia, and fetal asphyxia (Britt & Pasero, 1999). Excessive catecholamines influence the labor process by reducing strength, duration, and coordination of uterine contractions, and they influence the fetus, as demonstrated by nonreassuring changes in the fetal heart rate (FHR) pattern (Lederman, Lederman, Work, & McCann, 1985).

PSYCHOSOCIAL FACTORS INFLUENCING PAIN PERCEPTION

In addition to the physiologic factors that influence the perception of pain, psychosocial factors influence an individual's experience. These factors include labor support, childbirth preparation, and medical and nursing interventions, including those that are medically indicated and those that reflect the culture of the organization and individual pain tolerance.

Labor Support

Labor support includes providing physical comfort, emotional support, continuous presence, information, assistance communicating with the healthcare team, and guidance and support for the husband or partner (Simkin & O'Hara, 2002). Providing for physical comfort includes offering a variety of nonpharmacologic and pharmacologic interventions. Emotional support includes behaviors such as giving praise, encouragement, and reassurance; being positive; appearing calm and confident; assisting with breathing and relaxation; providing explanations about labor progress; identifying ways to include family members in the experience; and treating women with respect (Bryanton, Fraser-Davey, & Sullivan, 1994; Sleutel, 2000). Women identify support, information, interventions, decision-making, control, and pain relief as contributing to a positive labor experience (Lavender, Walkinshaw, & Walton, 1999).

Labor support ideally is provided by a variety of individuals. The registered nurse who understands the physiologic events of labor and has been educated about supportive care in labor should take the lead in providing labor support and role model labor support behaviors for others present during labor and birth. The husband or significant other, family members and friends, or a professional or lay labor-support person (doula) should also be welcomed and encouraged to provide labor support. The presence of one or all of these additional individuals does not decrease the ultimate responsibility of the perinatal nurse.

Labor support, whether offered by a partner, family members, friends, or nursing personnel, affects a woman's perception of labor (Lowe, 2002; Wright, McCrea, Stringer, & Murphy-Black, 2002). Qualitative research has demonstrated that one of the most significant aspects of the experience of labor for women is the presence of one or more support persons (Lavender et al., 1999). In a meta-analysis of 14 clinical trials, continuous support from a nurse, CNM, or lay person resulted in decreased operative vaginal birth, cesarean birth, 5-minute Apgar scores less than 7, and use of medication for pain relief (Hodnett, 2000). In a systematic review of the literature, Hodnett (2000) determined that the attitudes and behaviors of caregivers are a stronger influence on satisfaction with childbirth than many other factors. A Cochrane Review demonstrated that women who received continuous support during labor are less likely to request intrapartum analgesia, require an operative birth, or report dissatisfaction with their childbirth experience; greatest benefits were achieved when the support person was not a member of the hospital staff (Hodnett, Gates, Hofmeyr, & Sakala, 2003). Examples of activities supportive of women in labor are outlined in Display 9–1.

Registered Nurse

It is the position of the Association of Woman's Health, Obstetric and Neonatal Nurses (AWHONN) that supporting and caring for women during labor is best performed by a registered nurse (Display 9–2). Comprehensive nursing education, clinical patient-management skills, and previous experience make the registered nurse uniquely qualified to provide skilled technical care and complex emotional care women and families need during labor and birth (AWHONN, 2000).

DISPLAY 9 - 1

Labor Support

EMOTIONAL SUPPORT

Companionship
Eye contact
Encouragement
Distraction
Reassurance

PHYSICAL COMFORT

Touch
Nourishment
Personal hygiene
Applications of heat or cold
Massage

Hydrotherapy
Position change

INFORMATION

Providing information
Offering advice
Coaching in breathing, relaxation techniques
Interpreting medical jargon

ADVOCACY

Supporting the woman's decisions
Translating the woman's wishes to others

SUPPORT FOR FAMILY MEMBERS

Role model labor support
Providing opportunity for breaks
Encouragement

DISPLAY 9-2

Professional Nursing Support of Laboring Women

AWHONN maintains that continuously available labor support by a professional registered nurse is a critical component of achieving improved birth outcomes. The childbirth experience is an intensely physical and emotional event with lifelong implications. AWHONN views labor care and labor support as powerful nursing functions and believes it is incumbent on healthcare facilities to provide an environment that encourages the unique patient–nurse relationship during childbirth. Only the registered nurse combines adequate formal nursing education and clinical patient management skills with experience in providing physical, psychological, and sociocultural care to laboring women.

Because of their comprehensive education and experience, registered nurses are capable of providing highly skilled technical and complex emotional care. The registered nurse facilitates the childbirth process in collaboration with the laboring woman. The nurse's expertise and therapeutic presence influence patient and family satisfaction with the labor and delivery experience. Women who are provided with continuously available support during labor experience improved labor and delivery outcomes compared with those who labor without a skilled support person. Such care can lead to the following:

- Shorter labors
- Decreased use of analgesia or anesthesia
- Decreased operative vaginal delivery or cesarean section
- Decreased need for oxytocin
- Increased satisfaction with the childbirth experience

Professional registered nurses draw on a deep and broad base of nursing knowledge and clinical expertise to provide a level of care and support beyond that of lay personnel. They can effectively implement patient management strategies for low- and high-risk patients. The registered nurse can assess, plan, implement, and evaluate an individualized plan of care based on each woman's physical, psychological, and sociocultural needs, including desires and expectations of the laboring process. The support provided by the professional registered nurse should include the following:

- Assessment and management of the physiologic and psychologic processes of labor
- Provision of emotional support and physical comfort measures
- Evaluation of fetal well-being during labor
- Instruction regarding the labor process
- Patient advocacy—the clinical assessment and evaluation that results from collaboration among professional members of the healthcare team
- Role modeling to facilitate family participation during labor and birth
- Direct collaboration with other members of the healthcare team to coordinate patient care

In today's healthcare environment, numerous factors may influence the nurse's ability to provide bedside labor care:

- A limited number of available experienced registered nurses
- Limited financial resources
- Rigid organizational processes and structures
- Cumbersome documentation requirements
- Decreasing reimbursement by third-party payers in the United States

AWHONN challenges healthcare facilities to continuously evaluate the impact of patient–nurse ratios on resource use, overall operating expenses, patient outcomes, and patient satisfaction. AWHONN also supports evaluation models that can measure the impact a registered professional nurse has on indirect cost savings, such as savings resulting from lower cesarean section rates, shorter labors, and fewer technologic interventions.

AWHONN encourages women and families to request labor support from a professional registered nurse or advanced practice nurse (eg, clinical nurse specialist, CNM, or nurse practitioner) for labor and birth.

Studies on professional nursing care for laboring women are in progress. AWHONN supports continued research efforts to document the essential role of professional nursing labor support on maternal–newborn outcomes and the potential financial benefits of such support for the healthcare system.

From Association of Women's Health, Obstetric and Neonatal Nurses. (2000). *Professional nursing support of laboring women.* Washington, DC: Author.

Nurses may spend anywhere from 12.4% (Gale, Fothergill-Bourbonnais, & Chamberlain, 2001) to 58% (Miltner, 2002) of their time providing supportive care to patients, usually doing so in conjunction with some technical activity. Factors that have contributed to individual nurses spending less time with women include increased technology associated with giving birth, increased requests for epidural anesthesia, and institutional staffing patterns. As use of technology has expanded in obstetrics, the perinatal nurse has moved from providing hands-on comfort to monitoring the equipment and relying on pharmacologic interventions. Technology, especially when coupled with epidural analgesia or anesthesia, makes it easy for nurses to focus on machines and assume that, because labor is no longer painful, their presence is not needed.

Epidural anesthesia has become more available, as women have come to expect this as the standard of care. When staffing patterns require nurses to care for more than one woman in labor, it is impossible to provide continuous one-to-one attention.

No published research supports the positive influence that one-to-one nursing care can have on labor and birth outcomes. In one study, use of one-to-one nursing care, defined as individual nurses spending up to 90% of their time at the bedside providing physical and emotional support, did not achieve statistically significant results (Gagnon & Waghorn, 1999). In a large multicenter, randomized clinical trial evaluating the effects of one-to-one nursing care during labor, while the women who participated reported preferring the one-to-one nursing care, both the control and experimental groups had identical cesarean section rates, and no statistical difference were identified in morbidity for either the women or their newborns (Hodnett et al., 2002).

Husband or Significant Other

Postpartum women report that one of the things contributing to a positive labor experience was the presence of a family member or friend in the room even if "they just sit there" (Lavender et al., 1999). At the time of admission, the laboring woman should identify family members or friends who will act as labor-support persons.

Fathers have an important role in providing physical and emotional support during childbirth. Chapman (1992) described three roles assumed by expectant fathers during labor without epidural analgesia or anesthesia:

- *Coaches* actively assisted their partners during and after labor contractions with breathing and relaxation techniques. Coaches led or directed their partners through labor and birth and viewed themselves as managers or directors of the experience.
- *Teammates* assisted their partners throughout the experience of labor and birth by responding to requests for physical or emotional support or both. They sometimes led their partners, but their usual role was that of follower or helper.
- *Witnesses* viewed themselves primarily as companions who were there to provide emotional and moral support. They were present during labor and birth to observe the process and to witness the birth of their child.

These roles were identified by organizing behaviors that partners were observed performing during labor or behaviors women described in interviews after birth. Most men in the study adopted the role of witness rather than teammate or coach (Chapman, 1992).

Chandler and Field (1997) report that witnessing their partners in severe pain caused men to feel helpless and fearful. They became discouraged when the comfort measures they tried did not help their partners. Ultimately, they felt they had failed in their role. These results contrast with the intentions of childbirth educators, who perceive themselves as preparing coaches and teammates for laboring women, and with perinatal nurses, who expect fathers and other family members to take a more active role in labor support.

The experience of husbands when their partners received epidural analgesia or anesthesia was explored, resulting in the grounded theory called "cruising through labor" (Chapman, 2000) (Display 9–3). During labor, critical experiences for men occurred at two points. In the *holding-out phase* of labor, before making the decision to receive an epidural, men experienced a sense of "losing her." As pain became more severe, women underwent personality changes, becoming frustrated, irritable, exhausted, and panicky. These personality changes may be totally unfamiliar qualities that the men had never seen their partners demonstrate or demonstrate to the degree that they do while in labor. Women also gradually turn inward as they attempt to cope with the pain. Withdrawing into

DISPLAY 9-3

Grounded Theory of the Expectant Father's Epidural Labor Experience

Holding-Out Phase: During labor, when couples are planning to avoid an epidural or seeing how far they can get in labor without needing an epidural.

Surrendering Phase: The point at which the decision is made to receive an epidural, which is described as yielding to the need for an epidural, giving up, feeling they have experienced all the pain they can handle and done everything they can to avoid an epidural.

Waiting Phase: Period of time after making the decision to receive an epidural until the anesthesia care provider arrives.

Getting Phase: Period of time when the anesthesia provider is present, making assessments, preparing equipment, and placing the epidural.

Cruising Phase: The time after the epidural has provided pain relief. Couples' focus changes to rest and relaxation. Labor has gone from a stressful process to a calm experience. Both may fall asleep, due to exhaustion from the stress of coping with the pain of labor.

Chapman, L. L. (2000). Expectant fathers and labor epidurals. *MCN The American Journal of Maternal Child Nursing, 25*(3), 133–139.

themselves causes women to be unable to communicate their needs and to become unresponsive to their partners' attempts at labor support. Men feel increased levels of anxiety, helplessness, frustration, and emotional pain (Chapman, 2000). These findings are consistent with the work of Somers-Smith (1999), who found that fathers experience childbirth as a stressful event.

The second and most dramatic phase for men sharing the experience of labor is during the *cruising phase*. After the epidural has provided relief from the pain of labor, men describe a sensation of "she's back." The laboring woman again is aware of her surroundings and interacting with those around her. From a man's perspective, labor has gone from a stressful event to a calm experience. Rather than describing their experience in terms of the role they assumed during labor and the frustration and disconnected feelings they had as labor intensified and women's behavior changed (Chapman, 1991, 1992), these men described their experience by the degree of frustration they felt before the epidural and the degree of enjoyment after the epidural (Chapman, 2000). It is important that childbirth educators present this content, discuss this process, and teach men in their classes about the emotions they can expect to witness and experience during labor. Perinatal nurses should remain at the bedside when women are experiencing severe pain. This allows the nurse to provide support to the laboring woman and her partner. According to Chapman (2000), nurses who remained at the bedside, explained what was occurring with the labor, and included the expectant father were viewed by those fathers as providing the most support.

Doula

There is increased interest in the role of the professional or lay labor-support person, who is present during labor in addition to the perinatal nurse. The movement toward professional or lay labor support is a result of the inability of perinatal nurses to provide women with the support they want during labor and the recognition that husbands or significant others do not always make the best coaches during labor. Being in a hospital and seeing one's wife in labor may be very stressful for some fathers (Klaus, Kennell, & Klaus, 2002). Childbirth education programs have traditional provided training labor-support persons. However, the assumption that the husband or significant other makes the best coach may not be accurate (Chapman, 1992). It is important for the father of the baby to be present during the labor and birth, but the presence of a doula may be what the laboring woman needs.

Labor-support persons, or doulas, with a variety of credentials and levels of education, are assisting women and their partners during pregnancy, birth, and the postpartum period. "A doula is a supportive companion (other than a friend or loved one) who is professionally trained to provide labor support" (Gilliland, 2002, p. 762). Most often seen during labor, their main goal is to ensure that the woman feels safe and confident (Ballen & Fulcher, 2006). A doula remains continuously at the side of the woman to provide emotional support and physical comfort (Klaus et al., 2002). While not provided by all programs, a unique aspect of the doula role occurs during postpartum, usually after discharge from the hospital. During a home visit, the doula is able to make time to review with the new mother her labor and birth experience with the goal of creating a satisfying birth experience. "The doula allows the woman to reflect on her experience, fills in gaps in her memory, praises her, and sometimes helps reframe upsetting or difficult aspects of the birth" (Ballen & Fulcher, 2006, p. 305). Table 9–2 contrasts the role of a doula with that of the perinatal nurse.

In a meta-analysis of 11 clinical trials in which continuous support by a doula was compared with traditional intermittent support of a labor and delivery nurse, continuous support was associated with significantly shorter labors; decreased use of analgesia, oxytocin, and forceps; and decreased cesarean births (Scott, Berkowitz, & Klaus, 1999). In a culture in which women experience traditional labor without their husband, those accompanied by a female support person had significantly shorter labors, less use of analgesia and oxytocin, and fewer admissions to the neonatal intensive care unit (NICU) (Mosallam, Rizk, Thomas, & Ezimokhai, 2004). Women who had the benefit of a doula during labor expressed significantly less emotional distress and had higher self-esteem at 4 months postpartum than women who had attended a traditional Lamaze class (Manning-Orenstein, 1998). When low-income pregnant women were randomized to be accompanied in labor by their family and a trained doula or just family members, those in the experimental group had significantly shorter labors and greater cervical dilation at the time of epidural anesthesia (Campbell, Lake, Falk, & Backstrand, 2006).

Doulas may be volunteers or paid and are available through a variety of programs, either hospital based, community based, or as a private, contracted service. Hospital- and community-based programs are often available to underserved populations, women who may be newly emigrating, or women who might be alone during childbirth (eg, adolescents or incarcerated women). Individual hospitals or community-based healthcare agencies may be involved in training doulas, or there are national organizations where training and certification is available (Display 9–4). Services of a doula are generally arranged by the expectant couple or presented as an available option by a healthcare agency before labor.

TABLE 9–2 ■ DIFFERENTIATING THE ROLES OF THE NURSE AND THE DOULA

Registered Nurse	Doula
Meets the woman for the first time during labor	Usually meets and begins to form a relationship with the woman during her pregnancy to try to understand her expectations, needs, fears, and concerns
Performs clinical tasks within the scope of practice of the registered nurse	Supportive role; performs no clinical tasks
Consults with the obstetrical care provider	Has no direct communication responsibility to the obstetrical care provider
Provides intermittent labor support; presence in the LDR/LDRP is not continuous; may be caring for more than one patient; depending on the length of labor, more than one nurse may care for the woman	Provides continuous labor support; leaves the LDR/LDRP only for bathroom breaks; stays with the woman throughout her labor and birth and into the early postpartum period
Keeps patient informed of labor progress: what is normal and what to expect	Keeps patient informed of labor progress in lay terms: what is normal and what to expect
Advocates for the patient by communicating her needs and desires to the obstetrical care provider	Assists the patient to formulate and articulate her questions and concerns to the nurse and the obstetrical care provider
Responsible for documenting assessments in medical record	May document events of the labor and birth to share and review with the patient later to ensure positive memories
Has a legal accountability and responsibility for his/her actions	Has prepared to be a doula through a formal education program; may be certified
May have minimal or no contact with the patient after the birth	Some type of follow-up visit or visits is usually part of the program

DISPLAY 9-4

Associations That Train and Certify Doulas

ALACE (Association of Labor Assistants & Childbirth Educators)
www.alace.org

CAPPA (Childbirth and Postpartum Professional Association)
www.cappa.net

DONA (Doulas of North America International)
www.dona.org

ICEA (International Childbirth Education Association)
www.icea.org

Lamaze International
www.lamaze.org

Adapted from Ballen, L. E., & Fulcher, A. J. (2006). Nurses and doulas: Complementary roles to provide optimal maternity care. *Journal of Obstetric, Gynecologic, and Neonatal Nursing, 35*(2), 304–311.

Childbirth Preparation

There is a relationship between women's expectation of labor and their actual experience of labor (Green, 1993). Women who expect breathing and relaxation techniques to work are more likely to find them helpful. Women who wish to avoid medications can be successful with the help of their support system and perinatal nurses.

The basis of childbirth preparation is the belief that pain during childbirth leads to fear and tension, which increases the experience of pain. As fear and anxiety heighten, muscle tension increases, inhibiting the effectiveness of contractions, increasing discomfort, and further heightening fear and anxiety. The goal of childbirth education is to interrupt this cycle intellectually, with an understanding of what is occurring, and physiologically, with nonpharmacologic and pharmacologic pain-management strategies. Nonpharmacologic and pharmacologic pain-management strategies provide women with specific techniques they can use to cope with the discomfort of labor, thereby increasing their feelings of control. An awareness of the childbirth preparation and skills that the woman and her partner are prepared to use is helpful when planning nursing support strategies during labor.

Labor admission assessment should include questions related to the type and amount of childbirth preparation (eg, classes, reading, or video tape viewing). As part of the admission assessment, the nurse should ask about the couple's plans for pain management during labor and whether this subject was discussed with the physician or CNM. Asking about their plans and goals validates their efforts to prepare for labor and birth. Nurses should assure them that they understand the couple's goals and that they will do what they can to help them achieve those goals. Nurses have a responsibility whenever possible to facilitate an experience for each couple that matches their expectations. Knowledge and skills learned in childbirth-preparation classes are enhanced when the nurse present during labor and birth believes in and actively supports the couple as they apply these principles.

Healthcare Environment

Every perinatal unit takes a unique approach to caring for laboring women. A culture develops that, over time, is accepted by most of those working within the department and is a reflection of their values and beliefs. Cultural differences may be as significant as the availability of labor, delivery, recovery, and postpartum rooms (LDRPs) or as subtle as the routine initiation of (IV) fluids on admission. These practices reflect the evolution of intrapartum care within a particular institution. Unit culture extends to treatment of pain and influences the woman's perception of pain. Nurses who value nonpharmacologic approaches to pain management use these techniques in clinical practice.

Pain Tolerance

Pain is a culturally bound phenomenon. When a patient expresses pain, the form that expression takes is related to what her culture has taught her is appropriate. *Pain tolerance* may be defined as the level of stimuli at which the laboring woman asks to have the stimulation stopped. In labor, it is the point at which a woman requests pharmacologic pain relief or increased comfort measures. Descriptive words such as mild, moderate, and severe do not provide a measure of pain tolerance, because laboring women may describe pain as severe but not request pain medication. A woman's pain tolerance or the length of time she is able to go without medication may be increased by the use of nonpharmacologic pain management techniques.

Most hospitals have adapted one of the many standardized pain assessment tools that are available. Those used in adult populations for the most part require that the patient identify the intensity of pain they are experiencing. They are useful because there is some objectivity added to assessing and documenting phenomena that are very subjective. What these simplistic tools cannot tell the nurse is how the pain is being interpreted or translated by the woman in labor. What is her perception of the pain and how much is she suffering during labor? Only by being present, really listening, observing, and empathizing with a woman during labor can the nurse begin to understand what the experience of pain is for her and what interventions might be helpful and provide some relief (King & McCool, 2004).

NONPHARMACOLOGIC PAIN MANAGEMENT STRATEGIES

Nursing expertise in a variety of pain-management strategies is important. Not all nurses believe in or use nonpharmacologic approaches to pain relief when caring for laboring women. Possible reasons are a lack of familiarity with these techniques, routine practices that tend to be pharmacologic, or the fact that caring for a woman with an epidural is less physically and emotionally draining for the nurse than caring for a woman who is planning not to use an epidural. With the increased popularity of epidural anesthesia, many nurses new to the specialty have not had the opportunity to learn about or use nonpharmacologic measures. The choice of pain-management strategies by nurses is based on what they have observed to work in practice, are personally comfortable with, or have used during their own labors.

Women choose pain-management strategies based on their previous experience with pain, what they learned in prenatal classes, primary healthcare providers' recommendations, and listening to what worked for family members and friends. The advantage of nonpharmacologic pain management strategies is their simplicity and relative ease to initiate, the sense of control women receive when they actively manage their pain, the lack of serious side effects, and the fact that they do not generally add additional cost to the birth process (Simkin & O'Hara, 2002). Also, nonpharmacologic interventions do not require additional medical interventions and provide women the opportunity involve and share with significant people their birth experience.

Although few randomized, controlled clinical trials exist supporting the effectiveness of specific nonpharmacologic techniques during labor, suggestion and initiation of any of these techniques are within the scope of perinatal nursing practice. For most women, multiple pain-management strategies are necessary during the course of labor. Habituation may occur as the continued use of one technique becomes monotonous or offers insufficient stimuli to interfere with pain perception. As any technique becomes less of a distraction and therefore less effective, perception of pain increases (Bird & Waugaman, 1999).

TABLE 9–3 ■ CLASSIFICATION OF NONPHARMACOLOGIC STRATEGIES TO CONTROL PAIN

Technique	Examples
Cutaneous techniques to relieve painful stimuli	Massage Touch Back rub Counterpressure Movement and positioning Application of heat or cold Acupuncture Hydrotherapy
Auditory or visual techniques to block the transmission of painful stimuli	Focal point Breathing techniques Attention focusing Distraction Hypnosis Music
Cognitive processes to control the degree to which a sensation is interpreted as painful	Prenatal education Relaxation Labor support Imagery

Perinatal nurses should develop expertise in a variety of pain-management strategies. There are three classifications of nonpharmacologic methods or comfort measures that can be used to decrease or alter painful sensations associated with labor and birth: measures to reduce painful stimuli, methods that activate peripheral sensory receptors and inhibit pain awareness, and cognitive techniques that enhance descending inhibitory neural pathways, thereby reducing a woman's negative psychological reaction to pain (Table 9–3).

The effectiveness of nonpharmacologic pain-management strategies can be explained by Melzack & Wall's (1965) early work on the gate-control and the processes responsible for the transmission of pain. The first process is explained by the structure of the central nervous system, which is composed of large and small sensory nerve fibers. Impulses are carried by the spinal cord from the site of the stimuli to the cerebral cortex, where impulses are interpreted. Small, thinly myelinated or unmyelinated fibers transport impulses such as pressure and pain from the uterus, cervix, and pelvic joints. Large myelinated fibers transport impulses from the skin. Because passage along large fibers occurs more quickly, it is possible for cutaneous stimulation to block or alter painful impulses. Based on this premise, tactile stimulation in the form of touch or massage is often used effectively during labor. The second process is stimulation of the reticular activating system in the brain stem. The reticular activating system interprets auditory, visual, and painful sensory stimuli. When the cerebral cortex focuses on auditory or visual stimulation, painful stimulation is less able to pass through the "gate." Many forms of distraction are used during labor to decrease pain perception.

In recent years, Melzack has reevaluated the Gate Control Theory adding to it the possibility of multiple influences within the brain, a neuromatrix that is responsible ultimately for how each individual perceives pain (1999). These other influences include past experiences, cultural conditioning, emotional state, level of anxiety, understanding of the labor process, and the meaning that the current situation has for the individual are used by the cerebral cortex to interpret a sensation as painful. Just as thoughts and emotions can increase pain, they can also increase feelings of confidence and control, decreasing painful sensations. Prenatal education and labor support are effective pain-management strategies because they enhance maternal confidence and a sense of control.

Unfortunately, because limited research has been conducted using nonpharmacologic interventions, little is understood about how or whether these strategies work. It is inaccurate to use terms such as *pain relief* when referring to these interventions. Some interventions, such as positioning, counterpressure, heat and cold, touch, massage, effleurage, and injections of sterile water, may decrease pain. Other interventions, such as relaxation, imagery, focusing, breathing techniques, and music, more likely benefit a woman by decreasing anxiety, improving overall mood, and increasing the individual's sense of control in a painful situation (McCaffery & Pasero, 1999).

Cutaneous Pain Relief Techniques
Maternal Position and Movement

Women naturally choose positions of comfort and are more likely to change position during early labor. Modern technology (eg, EFM, IV lines, automatic blood pressure monitors, fetal scalp electrodes) may interfere with a woman's ability to find a comfortable position and frequently restricts her to bed. Many nurses and physicians encourage bed rest for labor because it helps them feel more in control of the situation, and they believe it may be safer for the woman and fetus. However, it is possible to use most of the technology available in obstetrics without maintaining continuous bed rest. An upright position can be accomplished in a recliner, rocking chair, or birthing bed adjusted to a chair position. EFM telemetry units, transducers that can be submerged in water, or intermittent auscultation of the FHR can be used to evaluate fetal response to labor while women are out of bed, ambulating, or using hydrotherapy. Women should be encouraged to change their position frequently during labor. Changing position alters the relationship between the fetus and pelvis and the efficiency of uterine contractions (Roberts, Mendez-Bauer, & Wodell, 1983). Table 9–4 lists a variety of positions available to women in labor along with the benefits of each.

Maintaining a horizontal position during labor is associated with decreased blood flow and may increase uterine muscle hypoxia, resulting in the increased perception of pain associated with uterine contractions (Mayberry et al., 2000). Women in an upright position during the second stage of labor report less pain than women in a semi-Fowler's or semi-recumbent position (deJong et al., 1997). Women may initially resist suggestions to change position or may find new positions

TABLE 9–4 ■ LABOR POSITIONS

Positions	Effect of Positions
Standing or any upright position	Takes advantage of gravity during and between contractions Contractions less painful and more productive Fetus well aligned with angle of pelvis May speed labor if woman has been recumbent May increase urge to push in second stage
Walking	Movement causes changes in pelvic joints, encouraging rotation and descent
Standing and leaning forward on person or object (eg, partner, bed, or birth ball)	May relieve backache; good position for back rub More restful than standing Can maintain continuous electronic fetal monitor
Slow dancing (mother embraces partner around neck, rests head on his/her chest or shoulder; with partner's arms around mother's trunk, inter-locking fingers at her low back, she can drop her arms and rests against her partner to increase relaxation)	Swaying movements to music may causes changes in pelvic joints, encouraging rotation and descent Rhythm and music add comfort Being embraced by loved one increases sense of well-being Position permits partner to give back pressure to relieve back pain
Sitting upright	Resting position More gravity advantage then supine
Rocking in chair	Rocking movement is relaxing and increases comfort Using foot stool decreases tension in lower extremities
Sitting on toilet or commode	May help relax perineum for effective bearing down
Hands and knees (can achieve this position by kneeling on bed with head raised, kneeling on floor while leaning on a chair or birthing ball)	Helps relieve backache from occipitoposterior Assists rotation of baby from occipitoposterior Allows freedom of movement for pelvic rocking Vaginal examinations possible Takes pressure off hemorrhoids
Sidelying	Helps lower elevated blood pressure; increases perfusion of blood to the placenta and fetus Takes pressure off hemorrhoids Easier to relax between pushing efforts Effective position for pushing during second stage
Squatting while supporting herself on object like side of the bed or chair	Takes advantage of gravity Widens pelvic outlet; may enhance rotation and descent of the fetus
Supported squat: mother leans with back against standing partner who holds her under the arms and takes all her weight during contraction	Makes bearing down efforts more spontaneous Helpful if mother does not feel an urge to push
Supported squat: partner sits on high bed or counter with feet supported on chairs or foot stool; with thighs spread, mother backs between legs and places flexed arms over thighs; partner grips woman's sides with his thighs; she lowers herself, allowing partner to support her full weight	Mechanical advantage during second stage as upper trunk presses on uterine fundus Lengthens mother's trunk, allowing more room for asynclitic fetus to maneuver into position Eliminates restriction of pelvic joint mobility that can be caused by external pressure from bed or chair

Adapted from Simkin, P. (1995). Reducing pain and enhancing progress in labor: A guide to nonpharmacologic methods for maternity caregivers. *Birth, 22*(3), 161–171.

uncomfortable. When encouraging a woman to change position, the nurse should provide extra support and encouragement and suggest that she remain in the new position through several contractions before deciding whether it is comfortable.

Pillows should be used generously to maintain positions and support extremities. When a sidelying position is used, pillows can be placed behind the back and between the knees. In a semi-Fowler's position, pillows can be placed under knees or arms. Shorter women sitting in a chair may find that a pillow or stool under their feet decreases stretching of leg muscles. Women who labor with the baby's head in an occipitoposterior position report significantly less back pain when using hands-and-knees positioning (Stremler et al., 2005).

Localized Pressure to Reduce Back Labor

Interventions can be used by the perinatal nurse or other labor-support person to relieve back labor. These techniques include counterpressure, bilateral hip pressure (eg, double-hip squeeze), and the knee press (Simkin, 1995). These maneuvers are performed by applying localized pressure to reduce sacroiliac pain resulting from strain on sacroiliac ligaments caused by mechanisms of labor. Counterpressure requires application of enough force to meet the intensity of pressure from the fetal occipital bone against the sacrum (Fig. 9–1). Steady pressure from the heel of a support person's hand or another firm object counteracts the strain against the sacroiliac ligaments caused by the fetal occiput (Simkin, 1995).

Hydrotherapy

Heat and cold may be provided during labor in the way of a hot water bottle, moist towel, electric heating

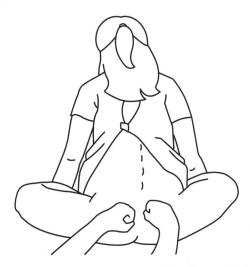

FIGURE 9–1. Firm counterpressure of the fists on the lower back.

unit, shower, whirlpool tub, ice pack, or chemical cooling unit. When commercial heating products are used, take care to ensure that the patient can tolerate the temperature and that the temperature will not cause harm. Labor activities may alter the perception of temperature. The nurse must be alert to the potential for injury and follow manufacturer recommendations and hospital-established policies when using heating or cooling equipment.

In an attempt to provide a more home-like atmosphere, many hospitals constructing new perinatal departments or renovating existing units will include spa-like amenities such as whirlpool tubs. Use of a standard or whirlpool tub during labor has been found to increase relaxation (Cammu, Clasen, Van Wettere, & Derde, 1994), decrease the need for pharmacologic agents during labor (Aird, Luckas, Buckett, & Bousfield, 1997; Rush et al., 1996), and increase maternal satisfaction (Cammu et al., 1994).

The benefits of immersion in water during labor are based on the principles of buoyancy, hydrostatic pressure, and heat (Harris, 1999):

- Buoyancy creates hydrodynamic lift. The loss of gravitational pull allows the body to float.
- Hydrostatic pressure equalizes the pressure exerted on all parts of the body below the water surface. Together, buoyancy and hydrostatic pressure provide greater support and comfort during labor because muscle tension is decreased and pressure is dispersed over the whole body.
- Heat of the water relaxes muscles that have become tense as a result of stress associated with the discomfort of labor. It is theorized that transmission of temperature sensations occurs along the same small, unmyelinated nerve fibers as painful stimuli, causing perception of pain to be interrupted. (Simkin & O'Hara, 2002).

Rush et al. (1996), in a randomized controlled trial, demonstrated a statistically significant increase in length of labor for women using whirlpool tubs; however, the study did not control for parity. The point during labor that a woman goes into a tub or whirlpool may influence the ultimate length of labor. Women who used a tub prior to dilating 5 cm were more likely to have longer labors then women who waited until they were dilated 5 cm (Eriksson, Ladfors, Mattsson, & Fall, 1996). A possible explanation for an increase length of labor may be the fact that hydrostatic pressure from immersion in water causes interstitial fluid to move into the intravascular space (Benfield, 2002). The resulting increased blood volume in the thorax may trigger the release of atrial natriuretic factor (ANF) by the heart. ANF suppresses production of various hormones, including oxytocin, from the pituitary gland (Gutkowska, Antunes-Rodrigues, & McCann, 1997).

Uterine contraction may be slowed or stop completely when use of tub or whirlpool occurs before active labor is established (Simpkin & O'Hara, 2002).

Despite a concern for potential maternal or neonatal morbidity or mortality, research findings have repeatedly demonstrated no increase risk of chorioamnionitis or postpartum endometritis for women who use a tub or whirlpool during labor regardless of whether their membrane status (Andersen, Gyhagen, & Nielsen, 1996; Cammu et al., 1994; Eriksson et al., 1996; Robertson, Huang, Croughan-Minihane, & Kilpatrick, 1998; Rush et al., 1996). Ohlsson et al. (2001), in a randomized clinical trial, found no significant difference in admissions to NICU, Apgar scores <7 at 5 minutes, transient tachypnea, third- or fourth-degree lacerations, cesarean birth, or length of postpartum stay.

Hydrotherapy may produce weakness, dizziness, nausea, maternal or fetal tachycardia, or maternal hypotension. Side effects such as these usually are related to an increase in body temperature or dehydration, both of which may be prevented by appropriate nursing inter- ventions. Nursing considerations when using hydrotherapy are outlined in Table 9–5. Women may at first be reluctant, embarrassed, or express some inhibition about laboring in a shower or tub; however, they quickly appreciate the relaxing qualities of warm water. Each perinatal department in conjunction with the organization's infection control department needs to develop a strict protocol for cleaning tubs or whirlpools. Protocols should be based on manufacturer recommendations and state and local boards of health requirements.

Using a shower may eliminate the potential for infection acquired from a tub or whirlpool. Although the effects of buoyancy and hydrostatic pressure are lacking, there is the benefit of heat. As in a tub or whirlpool, care should be taken to ensure that the water is not too hot and that the maternal temperature does not rise too high. Hand-held shower heads can be used to direct the spray of water to where it is most beneficial to the laboring woman. Holding the shower wand allows expectant fathers or coaches to participate and feel as though they are making their partner

TABLE 9–5 ■ PROTOCOL FOR USING A TUB OR SHOWER DURING LABOR

Nursing Intervention	Rationale
Establish fetal and maternal well-being by conducting a thorough assessment before using a tub or shower.	Stable maternal vital signs and reassuring fetal status are necessary before suggesting women labor in a tub or shower.
Use continuous or intermittent fetal monitoring or intermittent auscultation of the FHR while in the tub or shower.	Frequency of fetal monitoring should be consistent with recognized standards of care and institutional policies and based on the stage of labor.
Encourage oral fluids.	Prevent dehydration.
Maintain water temperature between 36°C to 37°C.	Water temperature above maternal body temperature may cause peripheral vasodilatation and redistribution of blood volume away from the fetus and uterus.
Water in the tub should cover the maternal abdomen.	The benefit of buoyancy and hydrostatic pressure can be obtained with the abdomen submerged; water covering the shoulders may not allow enough skin exposed for dissipation of excess body heat. Using a tub or shower is not contraindicated in the presence of ruptured membranes. Contraindications include thick meconium, oxytocin infusion, bleeding or large bloody show, epidural analgesia or anesthesia, and nonreassuring fetal status. If an IV line or heparin lock is in place, it can be covered with plastic.
Support person or member of the nursing staff should be present at all times. Shower seat should be available in the shower for the laboring woman as well as a seat outside of the shower or tub for their support person.	Warm water may cause dizziness.
Evaluate maternal vital signs according to hospital policy.	When evaluating maternal temperature, keep in mind that core temperature is 0.5–1 degree above oral temperature and that core temperature may more accurately reflect the fetal environmental. Even slight increases in maternal temperature may increase fetal temperature.

feel more comfortable. Perinatal nurses often share anecdotal reports of women who labored quite successfully for long periods in the shower. Women progress through labor more rapidly and report being more comfortable. Women become so comfortable that it may be difficult to entice them out of the tub or shower.

Some women in labor find relief from the application of cold in the form of ice packs, frozen gel packs, cold towels, or other cold objects. A cold washcloth applied to the face or neck is refreshing. Because cold is especially helpful for the relief of musculoskeletal pain, this is an appropriate intervention to suggest when a women experiences back labor. The numbing effect of cold is thought to slow the transmission of impulses over sensory neurons, decreasing the sensation of pain (Simkin, 1995).

Massage

Studies have shown that, although nurses touch women often during labor, it is mostly for clinical purposes, such as taking a pulse or attaching and inserting devices (McNiven, Hodnett, & O'Brien-Pallas, 1992). There is evidence to suggest that nonclinical touch (eg, hand holding, stroking a brow, patting the back) can reduce a woman's systolic blood pressure and pulse rate while increasing her comfort level and ability to cope (McNiven et al., 1992). Perinatal nurses and others who provide support during labor use touch consciously and unconsciously throughout labor to communicate their support and presence, to relieve muscle tension, and to decrease the pain of labor. Cultural norms are an important influence on how much touching (other than to perform clinical procedures) nurses are comfortable providing and women are comfortable receiving (Simkin & O'Hara, 2002).

Purposeful use of massage is employed during labor as a relaxation and stress-reduction technique. This technique is effective for reducing pain because it functions as a distraction, may stimulate cutaneous nerve fibers that block painful impulses, and stimulates the local release of endorphins (Huntley, Coon, & Ernst, 2004). In two randomized controlled trials, where the experimental group received several massages during labor, self reports of anxiety levels were the same in both groups while nurses reported observing significantly less behavioral manifestation of pain (Chang, Wang, & Chen, 2002) and pain scores were significantly less during early and active labor (Chang, Chen, & Huang, 2006).

All forms of massage are accomplished with moderate pressure, activating large myelinated nerve fibers. Because habituation can occur, decreasing the beneficial effects of massage, the type of stroke and location should vary during labor. In a randomized controlled trial during which partners provided massage during labor,

women reported significant less pain and anxiety (Field, Hemandez-Reif, Taylor, Quintino, & Burman, 1997).

Intradermal Injections of Sterile Water

Intradermal injections of sterile water (IISW) to control the pain of labor was first introduced in obstetric literature in the late 1980s. Although this technique is not widely used, it has been reported to relieve the severe, continuous discomfort of back labor that occurs when the fetal occiput is in a posterior position. Back labor is thought to complicate about 30% of labors (Reynolds, 1994).

Four small intradermal injections of 0.1 mL of sterile water are placed over the sacrum of a woman's back, leaving a temporary fluid-filled papule similar to that for a tuberculosis test (Fig. 9–2). Although it is not totally understood how this technique relieves the lower back pain associated with the first stage of labor, the Gate Control Theory is a plausible explanation. Sterile water causes distension of the skin, which irritates nerve endings, blocking other painful sensations (Huntley et al., 2004).

One hour after women with lower back pain were given IISW, they reported less (Martensson & Wallin, 1999) or no pain (Lytzen, Cederberg, & Moller-Nielsen, 1989). In randomized controlled clinical trials, when the effect of IISW was compared with injections of normal saline, women receiving the sterile water reported less pain at 45 minutes (Bahasadri, Ahmadi-Abhari, Dehghani-Nik, & Habibi, 2006), 1 hour (Trolle, Moller, Kronborg, & Thomsen, 1991),

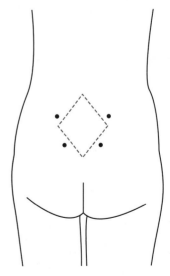

FIGURE 9–2. Location of injection sites in relation to the Michaelis' rhomboid for intradermal injections of sterile water. (From: Martensson, L. & Wallin, G. [1999]. Labor pain treated with cutaneous injections of sterile water: A randomized controlled trial. *British Journal of Obstetrics and Gynecology, 106*[7], p. 634.)

and 2 hours after the injections were given (Wiruch-pongsanon, 2006). When IISW was compared with transcutaneous electrical nerve stimulation (TENS) or standard care such as back massage, whirlpool bath, or position change, women receiving IISW reported less pain than those using TENS or receiving standard care (Labrecque, Nouwen, Bergeron, & Rancourt, 1999). Although the studies included random assignment of participants to a treatment or control group, a major limitation of all studies of TENS and IISW was inadequate sample size to detect significant differences.

The advantages of IISW include the following:

- Can be performed by a registered nurse
- Is not a technically difficult procedure
- Provides one more strategy for pain control
- Can be repeated as often as needed

The only side effect associated with the procedure is intense stinging pain at the time of injection that lasts about 30 seconds and a hyperemic zone around the papule that lasts for several hours after injection (Lytzen et al., 1989). The major disadvantage of this intervention is that it is relatively short-acting, necessitating repeated injections that women may find displeasing, depending on how uncomfortable it was to receive the intradermal injections.

Cognitive Techniques Altering Pain Perception

Relaxation

Achieving a state of relaxation is the basis of all non-pharmacologic interventions during labor. Women benefit from a state of relaxation because it conserves energy rather than creating fatigue from the prolonged tension of voluntary muscles. Relaxation enhances the effectiveness of nonpharmacologic and pharmacologic pain-management strategies. Relaxation is a skill and a physical state. The degree of relaxation a woman can achieve will influence the amount of anxiety she feels. Many women are first introduced to these skills during childbirth classes. How well they learn and are able to use these skills depends on quality of instruction, the amount of time they practice, and their belief that this technique can be beneficial. Relaxation is as contagious as panic, tension, and feelings of being overwhelmed. Relaxation skills cannot be taught during active labor, but an environment that promotes relaxation can be created by the perinatal nurse (Display 9–5). When actually faced with the forces of labor, women who learned relaxation techniques during childbirth classes will need the presence of an informed perinatal nurse to reinforce and encourage the use of these techniques during labor.

DISPLAY 9-5

Creating a Relaxed Environment During Labor

- Control the amount of light, noise, and interruptions.
- Maintain an unhurried demeanor.
- Use a calm, soft, slow voice.
- Recognize the signs of tension:
  - Changes in voice
  - Frowning
  - Clenched fists
  - Stiff, straight posture
  - Tense arms or legs
  - Stiff, raised shoulders
- Maintain eye contact.
- Use touch or massage if this is acceptable to the woman.
- Sit, rather than stand, next to the woman.

Imagery

Imagery is simple daydreaming. Childbirth educators teach imagery as a skill, encouraging expectant women to focus on pleasant scenes or experiences to increase their level of relaxation. Nurses encourage women to use imagery by making statements such as "think of the baby moving through the birth canal," "think of the baby moving down and out," and "think about the cervix dilating." Imagery is used to keep women focused and to encourage them to work with their contractions.

Auditory or Visual Techniques to Block Transmission of Pain

Attention Focusing and Distraction

During early labor, distraction is an effective strategy. Distraction is the process by which stimuli from the environment draw a woman's attention away from her pain. Walking in the hallway, sitting in a chair, talking with visitors, watching television, playing cards, and using the telephone keep laboring women occupied. Most women reach a point during labor when they no longer are able to talk comfortably through contractions. Labor is hard work that requires intense concentration to maintain a sense of control. Women are helped to concentrate by focusing on an object in the room or a support person's face or eyes. Attention focusing involves deliberate, intentional activities on the part of the laboring woman. These activities include patterned breathing and visualization or imagery.

Patterned Breathing

Breathing techniques are usually taught in prenatal classes and are used as a distraction during labor to decrease pain and promote relaxation. On admission, the perinatal nurse reviews with the woman and her support person the specific techniques they were taught in prenatal class. If a woman has not attended class, early labor is the time to discuss and practice a slow, controlled breathing pattern.

Most women are taught to take a deep breath at the beginning of a contraction. This breath ensures oxygen to the mother and baby, signals to people in the room that a contraction is beginning, and stretches and tenses respiratory muscles. Exhaling this breath relaxes respiratory muscles and voluntary muscles. At some point during labor, perinatal nurses may find it necessary to breathe synchronously with a couple through several contractions. Women are encouraged to breathe slowly. However, as labor pain increases, women may need to use a lighter, more accelerated breathing (ie, no more than two times their normal rate). Alternatively, a pant–blow method of breathing, in which a woman takes three to four light panting breaths, followed by an exhale (ie, blow), may be used. When attempting to control the urge to push, a rapid and shallow breathing pattern may be helpful.

Music

Music can be used during labor as a distraction and to provide a focus. Evidence suggests that the perception and response to pain and music travel through the same neural pathways in the limbic system and that use of particular types of music perceived as relaxing may decrease anxiety associated with the perception of pain (Browning, 2000). Familiar music associated with restful or pleasant recollections may be an adjunct to relaxation and imagery to manage the pain of labor.

Music creates an atmosphere in the birthing room that also may change the approach of healthcare professionals to laboring women. Perinatal nurses and physicians become more relaxed, slow their activities, and respond with increased respect for the unique personal event in progress (DiFranco, 2000). When women use earphones or headsets to listen to music, an auditory sensation is created that is difficult to ignore (Bird & Waugaman, 1999).

During the late 1960s and into the 1980s, several studies were conducted to determine whether music during labor facilitated relaxation and reduced pain. Methodologically, these studies were not well designed, sample sizes were small, and results were inconsistent and contradictory.

Wiand (1997) conducted an experimental study using biofeedback modalities to determine whether listening to Baroque or New Age music or to ocean sounds improved relaxation compared with a progressive relaxation exercise. Thirty-six subjects acted as their own controls. Relaxation levels were significantly improved when Baroque or New Age music or ocean sounds were played compared with progressive relaxation exercise alone.

A major limitation of all nonpharmacologic methods of pain relief during labor is the lack of large randomized controlled trials supporting their effectiveness. However, anecdotal reports and expert opinions exist regarding their usefulness. Nurses should encourage women in labor to try a variety of techniques to decrease the discomfort. Ultimately, we must listen to and honor the request of the laboring woman about the effectiveness of nonpharmacologic techniques during her labor.

PHARMACOLOGIC PAIN MANAGEMENT STRATEGIES

The perinatal nurse assesses preferences for pain management on admission and conducts ongoing assessments of factors influencing pain perception throughout labor. There will always be laboring women who need or desire pharmacologic agents. ACOG and the American Society of Anesthesiologists (ASA) published a joint statement in which both organizations reinforce a woman's right to adequate pain relief in labor:

> Labor causes severe pain for many women. There is no other circumstance where it is considered acceptable to an individual to experience untreated severe pain, amenable to safe intervention, while under a physician's care. In the absence of a medical contraindication, maternal request is a sufficient medical indication for pain relief during labor. (ACOG, 2004)

The ASA has conducted series of surveys over the past 20 years. The most recent survey, in 2001, revealed an overall increase in the use of regional analgesia and a decrease in the percentage of women receiving either parenteral or no analgesia during labor in all hospitals regardless of volume of births (Bucklin, Hawkins, Anderson, & Ullrich, 2005).

Pharmacologic pain management strategies used during labor include sedatives and hypnotics, parenteral analgesia, local anesthesia, and neuraxial analgesia. Using pain medications during labor brings with it unique concerns that are not faced in other clinical areas. These include concerns about the effects medications may have on the course and outcome of labor and the fetus or newborn. Controversy exists among professionals and consumers about the appropriateness and consequences of relieving labor pain, which is considered by some a normal experience (Cohen, 1997). The decision to use medication should be made in collaboration with the woman and her physician or CNM. Ideally, the laboring woman should clearly understand the benefits and potential maternal–fetal side effects. This information is best introduced during the prenatal period, rather than during the stress of labor.

Sedatives and Hypnotics

The term *sedative–hypnotic* describes the effect this group of medications has on the individual; it is not a classification of drug. The effects of these drugs are dose related. In low doses, they cause sedation, and higher doses cause a hypnotic effect. Two classifications of drugs used in labor to provide sedative–hypnotic effects are barbiturates and H$_1$-receptor antagonists (ie, antihistamines).

Barbiturates such as secobarbital sodium (Seconal) and pentobarbital (Nembutal) do not relieve pain. Usually given orally or as an intramuscular injection to induce sleep, during labor they depress the central nervous system and decrease anxiety (Faucher & Brucker, 2000). Women experiencing prolonged early labor may benefit from the brief period of therapeutic rest or sleep that usually follows administration of barbiturates. After a rest period, there usually is a more coordinated, effective contraction pattern. Because sedatives have a long half-life and cross the placenta, they may affect the neonatal central nervous system in the way of decreased responsiveness and inability to suck. Use of barbiturates is reserved for early labor, when birth is unlikely for 12 to 24 hours (Huffnagle & Huffnagle, 1999).

H$_1$-receptor antagonists include promethazine hydrochloride (Phenergan), hydroxyzine hydrochloride (Vistaril), and propiomazine (Largon). These medications are frequently administered with narcotics during labor to relieve anxiety, increase sedation, and decrease nausea and vomiting. They traditionally have been thought to potentate the effects of narcotics; however, there is no objective evidence to support this belief (Wakefield, 1999). Promethazine hydrochloride is frequently used with meperidine to decrease the nausea and vomiting associated with this drug. Although all H$_1$-receptor antagonists have a sedative effect on the woman in labor, and they do cross the placenta, they do not appear to increase neonatal depression (Althaus & Wax, 2005). Routes of administration and side effects are similar for all the medications in this class. Exceptions are promethazine hydrochloride, which can cause respiratory depression, and hydroxyzine, which is limited to intramuscular use.

Parenteral Analgesia

There are three types of drugs most commonly administered parenterally during labor: opioids (morphine and meperidine), synthetic opioids (fentanyl), and opioid agonist-antagonists (butorphanol and nalbuphine). These drugs bind to one of four receptor sites (mu, kappa, sigma, or delta) on nerve cells located in the brain and spinal cord. Individual drugs have an affinity for one or more receptor sites, which accounts for differences in pharmacodynamics and side effects. Examples are morphine and meperidine, which have a strong affinity for mu receptors, resulting in effective analgesia and dose-dependent respiratory depression. Butorphanol (Stadol) and nalbuphine (Nubaine), with affinity for the kappa and sigma receptors, provide effective analgesia with less respiratory depression. Table 9–6 highlights the most commonly used opioids and their receptor-binding patterns.

Depending on the dose, route of administration, and stage of labor, parenteral analgesia does not eliminate pain, but instead causes a blunting effect, decreasing the perception of pain and allowing women to relax and rest between contractions. Table 9–7 lists the most commonly used parenteral analgesia in labor and their dose, route of administration, onset of action, time of peak effect, and duration of action. After administration of these medications, the frequency and duration of contractions and FHR variability may decrease (Althaus & Wax, 2005). For this reason, parenteral analgesia may not be administered until a labor pattern is well established. The exception to this is morphine, which may be used during a prolonged period of early labor to allow a woman to sleep in preparation for active labor.

When given during labor, these medications often cause women to fall asleep or doze off between contractions. Some women, however, experience a short period of decreased uterine activity followed by an increase in uterine activity. Both effects may be the result of decreased anxiety and serum concentrations of catecholamines (Mussell, 1998). If medication administration does result in dozing, coaching by a support person or nurse is important to help the woman anticipate and recognize the beginning of a contraction rather than have her startled awake at the peak of a contraction.

All of the medications used as parenteral analgesia may cause maternal respiratory depression. The advantage of the agonist-antagonists is the "ceiling effect" related to maternal respiratory depression. Opioids can have a cumulative effect, increasing the potential for maternal respiratory depression as the

TABLE 9–6 ■ PARENTERAL ANALGESIC AGENTS USED IN LABOR AND THEIR RECEPTOR-BINDING RELATIONSHIPS

Receptor	Receptor Properties	Medication
Mu	Supraspinal analgesia Respiratory depression Euphoria Physical dependence	Morphine Meperidine Butorphanol (weak) Fentanyl Sufentanil Alfentanil
Kappa	Spinal analgesia Miosis Sedation Slight respiratory depression	Morphine (weak) Butorphanol Nalbuphine
Sigma	Dysphoria Hallucinations Respiratory and vasomotor stimulation May not mediate analgesia	Butorphanol (partial) Nalbuphine Fentanyl (partial)
Delta	Spinal analgesia and smooth muscle relaxation	Morphine (weak) Codeine (weak)

Adapted from Faucher, M. A., & Brucker, M. C. (2000). Intrapartum pain: Pharmacologic management. *Journal of Obstetric, Gynecologic, and Neonatal Nursing, 29*(2), 169–180.

patient receives more medication. Agonist-antagonists have limited effect on maternal respiratory depression, regardless of the number of doses (Althaus & Wax, 2005). An advantage of the synthetic opioid fentanyl is that it does not cause as much sedation, nausea, and emesis as patients experienced with opioids (Rayburn, Smith, Parriott, & Woods, 1989). All the medications used as parenteral analgesia can cause temporary decrease in FHR variability (Giannina et al., 1995; Smith, Rayburn, Allen, Bane, & Livezey, 1996). IV butophanol during labor has been associated with transient sinusoidal FHR patterns (Hatjis & Meis, 1986). Because it can increase blood pressure, butorphanol should be avoided if the woman has hypertension or preeclampsia (ACOG, 2002).

Parenteral analgesia can be administered every 3 to 4 hours. When given intravenously, the onset of action is quicker; however, medication effects do not last as long. IV push medications are given slowly during a contraction to decrease transfer of the medication to the fetus. During the peak of a contraction, blood supply to the placenta essentially ceases. Administering the medication at this time allows rapid distribution of the drug and decreased maternal plasma concentration to the placenta when circulation resumes (Spielman, 1987). In obstetrics, meperidine has historically been preferred over morphine because of its quicker onset and shorter duration of action.

Neonatal side effects are related to dosage and timing of administration. Because of the potential for

TABLE 9–7 ■ PARENTERAL ANALGESICS

Drug	Dose	Route	Onset of Action (min)	Peak Effect (min)	Duration of Action (hr)
Meperidine (Demerol)	50–100 mg	IM	50	40–50	2–4
	25–50 mg	IV	10	5–10	2–4
Morphine	5–10 mg	IM	10–20	60–90	4–6
	1–2 mg	IV	3–5	20	4–6
Butorphanol (Stadol)	2–4 mg	IM	10–30	30–60	3–4
	1–2 mg	IV	1–2	2–3	3–4
Nalbuphine (Nubain)	0.2 mg/kg	IM	15	60	3–6
	0.1–0.2 mg/kg	IV	2–3	30	3–6
Fentanyl (Sublimaze)	50–100 μg	IM	7–15	20–30	1–2
	25–50 μg	V	2–3	3–5	0.5–1

neonatal respiratory depression, the timing of administration relative to birth of the newborn is important. Ideally, birth should occur within 1 hour or after 4 hours following administration (Althaus & Wax, 2005). A major disadvantages of meperidine are its long half-life and the fact that it metabolizes to normeperidine, leading to neonatal neurobehavioral depression lasting for several days (Briggs & Wan, 2005). This has led many hospitals to abandon the use of this medication during labor. Kuhnert, Linn, and Kuhnert (1985) found that newborn behavioral responses were altered for several days when their mothers received meperidine during labor. Effects include decreased muscle tone and social responsiveness, ineffective suck, problems initiating breastfeeding, and abnormal reflexes.

Naloxone hydrochloride (Narcan), a narcotic antagonist, reverses the respiratory depression caused by parenteral narcotics received by the mother within the past 4 hours. It is administered to the newborn who continues to experience respiratory depression after positive pressure ventilation has restored a normal heart rate (American Heart Association & American Academy of Pediatrics [AAP], 2006). In a randomized controlled trial comparing neonatal outcomes using meperidine and fentanyl during labor, significantly fewer neonates required resuscitation and nalonxone hydrochloride in the group whose mothers received fentanyl (Rayburn et al., 1989). Naloxone should not be given to infants of mothers who are addicted or suspected of being addicted to narcotics or who are in a methadone treatment program. In these infants, naloxone can cause neonatal seizures.

Local Anesthetic

During the second stage of labor, lidocaine hydrochloride or chloroprocaine hydrochloride, local anesthetics, may be injected into the perineum and posterior vagina before performing an episiotomy. The duration of action is approximately 20–40 minutes for these medications (Briggs & Wan, 2005). This area may be reinjected after delivery of the placenta in preparation for perineal repair.

Pudendal Block

A pudendal block during the second stage of labor using lidocaine hydrochloride or chloroprocaine hydrochloride anesthetizes the lower vagina, vulva, and perineum. An anesthetic is injected through the lateral vaginal walls into the area of the pudendal nerve (Fig. 9–3). This technique provides adequate anesthesia for vaginal birth, application of outlet forceps, and perineal repair. Because it is possible for a pudendal block to be ineffective, it is frequently combined with local infiltration of the perineum.

Complications such as seizures, hypotension, and cardiac arrhythmias can result from a local anesthetic being injected into a vein. Hematoma and infection are potential complications from pudendal block (Briggs & Wan, 2005).

Neuraxial Analgesia Techniques

Of the various pharmacologic methods available for use during labor, neuraxial analgesia techniques (epidural, spinal, and combined spinal–epidural) are the most flexible and effective, and they result in the least central nervous system depression of the mother and neonate (ACOG, 2004). Because parenteral analgesia has limited effectiveness and a greater potential for neonatal toxicity, most women in labor receive regional analgesia (Briggs & Wan, 2005). The ACOG Committee on Obstetrical Practice and the ASA Committee on Obstetric Anesthesia collaborated to

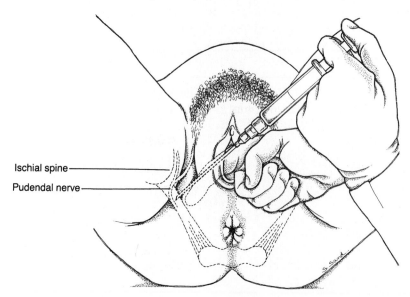

Ischial spine

Pudendal nerve

FIGURE 9–3. Procedure for administration of a pudendal block.

DISPLAY 9-6

Optimal Goals for Anesthesia Care in Obstetrics

I. Availability of a licensed practitioner who is credentialed to administer an appropriate anesthetic whenever necessary. For many women, regional anesthesia (epidural, spinal, or combined spinal epidural) will be the most appropriate anesthetic.

II. Availability of a licensed practitioner who is credentialed to maintain support of vital functions during any obstetric emergency.

III. Availability of anesthesia and surgical personnel to permit the start of a cesarean delivery within 30 minutes of the decision to perform the procedure; in cases of Vaginal Birth After Cesarean (VBAC), appropriate facilities and personnel, including obstetric anesthesia, nursing personnel, and a physician capable of monitoring labor and performing cesarean delivery, immediately available during active labor to perform emergency cesarean delivery. The definition of immediate availability of personnel and facilities remains a local decision, based on each institution's available resources and geographic location.

IV. Appointment of a qualified anesthesiologist to be responsible for all anesthetics administered. There are obstetric units where obstetricians or obstetrician-supervised nurse anesthetists administer anesthetics. The administration of general or regional anesthesia requires both medical judgment and technical skills. Thus, a physician with privileges in anesthesiology should be readily available.

Persons administering or supervising obstetric anesthesia should be qualified to manage the infrequent but occasionally life-threatening complications of major regional anesthesia, such as respiratory and cardiovascular failure, toxic local anesthetic convulsions, or vomiting and aspiration. Mastering and retaining the skills and knowledge necessary to manage these complications require adequate training and frequent application.

To ensure the safest and most effective anesthesia for obstetric patients, the director of anesthesia services, with the approval of the medical staff, should develop and enforce written policies regarding provision of obstetric anesthesia such as the following:

I. Availability of a qualified physician with obstetrical privileges to perform operative vaginal or cesarean delivery during administration of anesthesia. Regional and/or general anesthesia should not be administered until the patient has been examined and the fetal status and progress of labor evaluated by a qualified individual. A physician with obstetrical privileges who has knowledge of the maternal and fetal status and the progress of labor, and who approves the initiation of labor anesthesia, should be readily available to deal with any obstetric complications that may arise.

II. Availability of equipment, facilities, and support personnel equal to that provided in the surgical suite. This should include the availability of a properly equipped and staffed recovery room capable of receiving and caring for all patients recovering from major regional or general anesthesia. Birthing facilities, when used for analgesia or anesthesia, must be appropriately equipped to provide safe anesthetic care during labor and delivery or post-anesthesia recovery care.

III. Personnel other than the surgical team should be immediately available to assume responsibility for resuscitation of a depressed newborn. The surgeon and anesthesiologist are responsible for the mother and may not be able to leave her care for the newborn, even when a regional anesthetic is functioning adequately. Individuals qualified to perform neonatal resuscitation should demonstrate the following:

   A. Proficiency in rapid and accurate evaluation of the newborn condition, including Apgar scoring.
   B. Knowledge of the pathogenesis of a depressed newborn (acidosis, drugs, hypovolemia, trauma, anomalies, and infection), as well as specific indications for resuscitation.
   C. Proficiency in newborn airway management, laryngoscopy, endotracheal intubations, suctioning of airways, artificial ventilation, cardiac massage, and maintenance of thermal stability.

In larger maternity units and those functioning as high-risk centers, 24-hour in-house anesthesia, obstetric, and neonatal specialists are usually necessary. Preferably, the obstetric anesthesia services should be directed by an anesthesiologist with special training or experience in obstetric anesthesia. These units will also frequently require the availability of more sophisticated monitoring equipment and specially trained nursing personnel.

A survey jointly sponsored by the ASA and ACOG found that many hospitals in the United States have not yet achieved the above goals. Deficiencies were most evident in smaller delivery units, which are typical in some geographic locations. Currently, approximately 50% of hospitals providing obstetric care have fewer than 500 deliveries per year. Providing comprehensive care for obstetric patients in these small units is extremely inefficient, not cost-effective, and frequently impossible. Thus, the following recommendations are made:

1. Whenever possible, consolidate small units.
2. When geographic factors require the existence of smaller units, these units should be part of a well-established regional perinatal system.

The availability of the appropriate personnel to assist in the management of a variety of obstetric problems is a necessary feature of good obstetric care. The presence of a pediatrician or other trained physician at a high-risk cesarean delivery to care for the newborn or the availability of an anesthesiologist during active labor and delivery

(continued)

when VBAC is attempted, and at a breech or twin delivery are examples. Frequently, these professionals spend a considerable amount of time standing by for the possibility that their services may be needed emergently, but may ultimately not be required to perform the tasks for which they are present. Reasonable compensation for these standby services is justifiable and necessary.

A variety of other mechanisms have been suggested to increase the availability and quality of anesthesia services in obstetrics. Improved hospital design to place labor and delivery suites closer to the operating rooms would allow for more efficient supervision of nurse anesthetists. Anesthesia equipment in the labor and delivery area must be comparable to that in the operating room.

Finally, good interpersonal relations between obstetricians and anesthesiologists are important. Encourage joint meetings between the two departments. Anesthesiologists should recognize the special needs and concerns of the obstetrician, and obstetricians should recognize the anesthesiologist as a consultant in the management of pain and life-support measures. Both should recognize the need to provide high-quality care for all patients.

American College of Obstetricians and Gynecologists. (2001). *Optimal goals for anesthesia care in obstetrics.* (Committee Opinion No. 256). Washington, DC: Author.

develop a position statement on the optimal goals for anesthesia care in obstetrics (Display 9–6).

For many years, epidural anesthesia was limited to local anesthetics such as lidocaine (Xylocaine) and chloroprocaine (Nesacaine). These drugs act on nerve fibers as they cross the epidural space, causing sensory blockade. To obtain a therapeutic level of pain relief, the dose of local anesthetic resulted in loss of motor function. With the introduction of bupivacaine (Marcaine), practitioners found a longer duration of action, minimal motor blockade, and lack of neonatal neurobehavioral effects (Cohen, 1997). Ropivacaine (Naropin) has properties similar to those of bupivacaine, but this local anesthetic causes less motor block (Merson, 2001) and less cardiotoxic effects (Althaus & Wax, 2005).

The goal of neuraxial analgesia techniques during labor is to provide sufficient analgesia effect with as little motor block as possible. With the discovery of spinal cord opioid receptors in the late 1970s and the use of spinal and epidural opioids, pain management in labor was transformed from anesthesia to analgesia. Lower concentrations of local anesthetic, in combination with narcotics such as fentanyl (Sublimaze), sufentanil (Sufenta), alfentanil (Alfenta), and remifentanil, result in increased pain relief without significant motor block (ASA, 2006). Epidural narcotics act by crossing the dura into the cerebral spinal fluid and binding to opiate receptors in the dorsal horn of the spinal cord. Adding a narcotic to the local anesthetic lessens the risk of toxicity by decreasing the amount of local anesthetic needed, reducing the motor blockade, increasing the duration of pain relief, and improving the quality of pain relief (ASA, 2006). There was no difference in incidence of side effects (eg, nausea and hypotension), increased duration of labor, or adverse neonatal outcomes when epidural local anesthetics with opioids were compared with epidural local anesthetics without opioids (ASA, 2006). Opioid in the epidural infusion may cause pruritus, which for most women will last approximately 45 minutes after the initial loading dose (Russell & Reynolds, 1996). Adding a small amount of epinephrine decreases the amount of narcotic needed to obtain satisfactory pain relief (Armstrong et al., 2002; Polley, Columb, Naughton, Wagner, & van de Ven, 2002). Medications commonly used for neuraxial analgesia as well as their side effects are described in Table 9–8.

The anesthesiologist or certified registered nurse anesthetist (CRNA) is responsible for identifying women with contraindications to the procedure (Display 9–7). During this meeting, the procedure and potential complications are discussed and questions answered. Some institutions provide the opportunity for women to meet with an anesthesia provider before admission. Without this type of preparation, obtaining true informed consent from a woman in active labor is practically impossible. The advantages of spinal or epidural analgesia or anesthesia are outlined in Display 9–8.

Use of neuraxial analgesia techniques is not contraindicated in the presence of a nonreassuring FHR pattern (Vincent & Chestnut, 1998). However, it should be used judiciously when nonreassuring FHR or conditions associated with uteroplacental insufficiency exist (Thorp, 1999). Some practitioners believe that early placement of an epidural catheter permits rapid extension of the block in case cesarean birth for nonreassuring fetal status becomes necessary, and in the presence of complications such as twin gestation, maternal hypertension, or difficult airway, lessens the risk of needing to use general anesthesia (ASA, 2006). Obese patients present unique challenges for the anesthesia care provider in terms of positioning, identification of anatomical landmarks, and the midline and location of the epidural space (Saravanakumar, Rao, & Cooper, 2006). Placing the catheter during early labor, when the patient is still comfortable enough to fully cooperate, may make the process easier and quicker.

TABLE 9-8 ■ MEDICATIONS COMMONLY USED FOR REGIONAL ANALGESIA/ANESTHESIA DURING LABOR

Anesthesia Agents

Drug	Route	Concentration (%)	Volume (mL)	Dose (mg)	Side Effects/Adverse Reactions*	Nursing Implications
Bupivacaine	Epidural block	0.25	10–20	25–50	Hypotension[1] FHR changes[1] Dysrhythmias[2] Bronchospasm[2] Seizures[2] Respiratory arrest[2] Cardiovascular collapse[2]	Monitor maternal vital signs Monitor FHR Ensure resuscitation equipment available
		0.50	10–20	50–100		
	Intermittent infusion	0.125–0.375	5–10			
	Continuous infusion	0.0625–0.25	8–15			
	Caudal block	0.25	15–30	37.5–75		
		0.5	15–30	75–150		
	Surgical spinal	0.75 in 8.25% dextrose				
Lidocaine	Epidural block	1	25–30	250–300	Hypotension[1] FHR changes[1] Muscular twitching[2] Lightheadedness[2] Edema[2] CNS depression[2] Tinnitus[2] Coma[2] Seizures[2] Respiratory arrest[2] Cardiovascular collapse[2]	Monitor maternal vital signs Monitor FHR Ensure resuscitation equipment available
		1.5	15–20	225–300		
		2	10–15	200–300		
	Intermittent injection	0.75–1.5	5–10			
	Continuous infusion	0.5–1.0	8–15			
	Caudal block	1	20–30	200–300		
	Spinal surgical	5 in 7.5% dextrose	1.5–2.0	75–100		
Ropivacaine	Intermittent injection	0.125–0.25	5–10	20–30	Hypotension[1] FHR changes[1] Neonatal jaundice[1]	Monitor maternal vital signs Monitor FHR Ensure resuscitation equipment available
	Continuous infusion	0.125–0.25	6–12	12–28		

Narcotic Agents

Drug	Route	Concentration (mcg/mL)	Rate (mL/hr)	Side Effects/Adverse Reactions*	Nursing Implications
Fentanyl	PCEA	1–3	8–20	FHR changes[1] Hypotension[1] Nausea[1] Pruritus[1] Sedation[1] Vomiting[1] Urinary retention[1] Dysrhythmias[2] Respiratory depression[2]	Prolonged administration may ↑ risk of maternal/fetal/neonatal respiratory/CNS depression. Crosses placenta rapidly Monitor for maternal/neonatal respiratory depression Determine allergy status Ensure naloxone and resuscitation equipment available
	CSE	10–25			
Sufentanil	PCEA	0.75–1	5–15	FHR changes[1] Hypotension[1] Nausea[1] Vomiting[1] Pruritus[1] Sedation[1] Respiratory depression[2]	May improve and prolong anesthesia Monitor for maternal/neonatal respiratory depression Ensure naloxone and resuscitation equipment available
	CSE	5–11.5			

[1] Potential side effect   [2] Potential adverse reaction   * Adverse reactions are rare

DISPLAY 9-7

Contraindications to Neuraxial Analgesia

- Coagulation disorders
- Local infection at the site of injection
- Maternal hypotension and shock
- Nonreassuring FHR pattern requiring immediate birth
- Maternal inability to cooperate
- Allergy to local anesthetics
- Last dose of low-molecular-weight heparin within 12 hours

When randomized controlled clinical trials were conducted to evaluate the effect of patient-controlled epidural (PCE) with patient-controlled IV opioid analgesia (PCIA), the group using PCIA required more antiemetics, reported more sedation, and newborns required more resuscitation, received naloxone more often (Halpern et al., 2004) and had lower 1 minute Apgars (Wong et al., 2005) while the PCE group had lower pain scores (Halpern et al., 2004; Liu & Sia, 2004; Sharma, McIntire, Wiley, & Leveno, 2004; Wong et al., 2005) and higher patient satisfaction scores (Halpern et al., 2004). Several studies have demonstrated that there was no difference in the rate of cesarean section rate or instrumental vaginal birth between women receiving PCE or PCIA (Halpern et al., 2004; Liu & Sia, 2004; Sharma et al., 2004; Wong et al., 2005). When the length of labor was compared for women receiving PCE and PCIA, labor for the PCE

DISPLAY 9-8

Advantages of Neuraxial Analgesia

- It generally provides superior pain relief, and position changes are less uncomfortable.
- The method usually provides sufficient anesthesia for episiotomy and/or repair of lacerations.
- Placement of an epidural catheter in labor means that an emergency cesarean section can occur more quickly, should this become necessary.
- Patient for whom general anesthesia is a risk (eg, marked obesity, history of difficult/failed intubation, abnormalities of face, neck, spine, severe medical complications such as cardiac pulmonary or neurologic disease) may benefit from having an epidural catheter placed and functioning in early labor (AAP & ACOG, 2002).

group was longer, reaching statistical significance, but the increased length of time would probably not have any clinical significance (Halpern et al., 2004; Liu & Sia, 2004; Sharma, McIntire, Wiley, & Leveno, 2004). The timing of neuraxial analgesia, given before or after cervical dilatation reaches 5 cm, does not have an effect on cesarean section rate (Wong et al., 2005). As a result of these data, the current recommendation by ACOG is that use of neuraxial analgesia techniques and the timing of catheter placement does not influence cesarean section rate and "should not influence the method of pain relief that women can choose during labor" (ACOG, 2006).

Standard Epidural

The epidural catheter is placed in the epidural space between the fourth and fifth lumbar vertebrae. A test dose of a local anesthetic mixed with epinephrine may be injected to determine that the catheter is not in the epidural vein (Figure 9–4). Injection of epinephrine into an epidural vein causes almost immediate increased heart rate, palpitations, increased blood pressure, numbness of the tongue or around the mouth, metallic taste, tinnitus, slurred speech, jitteriness, or agitation. In some women, a test dose may not determine intravascular injection because there is existing maternal tachycardia or because the effects occur too quickly to be observed. For this reason, some practitioners prefer to place a 10-mL anesthetic dose combining bupivacaine, fentanyl, and epinephrine in 5-mL increments through the catheter. If the catheter is positioned correctly, onset of analgesia is approximately 5 minutes, and decreased sensation in lower extremities occurs within 20 minutes (Youngstrom et al., 1996). Inadvertent placement of the catheter in the subarachnoid space causes immediate upper thoracic sensory loss, initiates severe lower extremity motor blockade, and potentially causes respiratory arrest.

When the anesthesiologist or CRNA is satisfied that the catheter is properly placed, a bolus of anesthetic medication is injected. Depending on the specific medications used, women begin to feel relief in 5 to 10 minutes. A complete block usually occurs in 15 to 20 minutes. A small group of women experience what is called "windows," areas or even whole sides of their body where pain relief is not obtained. In circumstances where the patient is not satisfied with her pain relief, a bolus might be given or the catheter removed and replaced. The failure to obtain complete pain relief despite proper placement of the catheter may be due to the presence of connective tissue bands in the epidural space that limit areas of the epidural space that can be reached by the medication infused (Althaus & Wax, 2005; Savolaine, Pandya, Greenblatt, & Conover, 1988).

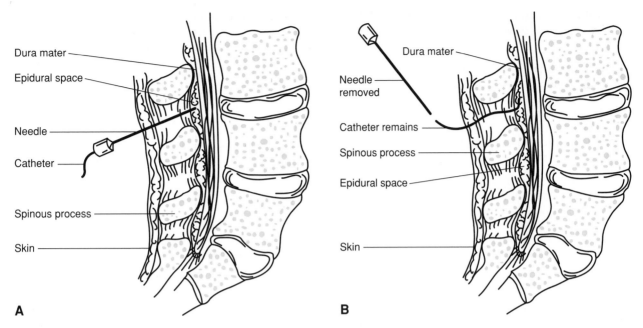

A

B

FIGURE 9–4. A, A needle is inserted into the epidural space. **B,** A catheter is threaded into the epidural space; the needle is then removed. The catheter allows medication to be administered intermittently or continuously to relieve pain during labor and childbirth.

Combined Spinal Epidural

Combined spinal epidural (CSE) is performed by first placing a 17- or 18-gauge Tuohy needle in the epidural space using the loss-of-resistance technique. After the needle is positioned in the epidural space, the smaller-gauge spinal needle is placed through the epidural needle into the subarachnoid space. An initial dose of local and opioid analgesia (25 μg of fentanyl and 2.5 mg of bupivacaine) is injected into the subarachnoid space. The spinal needle is removed, an epidural catheter is threaded through the epidural needle, the needle is removed, and the catheter is taped in place.

Advantages of CSE are the fast onset of pain relief with a small amount of medication place in the subarachnoid space and the ability to provide continuous epidural analgesia through the epidural catheter.

Regardless of the technique used, after the catheter is in place, epidural anesthesia or analgesia is administered by intermittent bolus, continuous epidural infusion, or patient-controlled epidural analgesia. Advantages of a continuous infusion include a consistent level of pain relief and prevention of hemodynamic changes associated with the repeated occurrence of pain. Continuous flow through the catheter also stabilizes the catheter, decreasing the risk of migration into an epidural vein or through the dura into the subarachnoid space. The continuous infusion may be a local anesthetic alone (bupivacaine, lidocaine, or ropivacaine) or a combination of a local and a narcotic (fentanyl or sufentanil). Women who receive local anesthetic alone need more medication to obtain satisfactory pain relief

than women who receive a combination of local and opioid (Russell & Reynolds, 1996). When a local anesthetic is combined with an opioid, there is less motor block and increased maternal satisfaction with pain management; there is no difference in rate of spontaneous deliveries or perineal pain during second-stage labor (Russell & Reynolds, 1996). Women who receive CSE analgesia or anesthesia report significantly more pruritus than women receiving standard epidural (Collis, Davies, & Aveling, 1995; Nageotte, Larson, Rumney, Sidhu, & Hollenbach, 1997). As cervical dilatation progresses, some women require an increase in the rate of the continuous infusion or a second bolus with a higher concentration of local anesthetic or narcotic.

Nursing Care

AWHONN has a clinical position statement providing guidelines for practice for nurses caring for pregnant women receiving anesthesia/anesthesia by catheter techniques (eg, epidural, intrathecal, spinal, patient-controlled epidural anesthesia catheters):

Only qualified, credentialed, licensed anesthesia care providers as described by the American Society of Anesthesiologists and the American Association of Nurse Anesthetists, and/or as authorized by state law should perform the following procedures:

- Insertion, initial injection, bolus injection, rebolus injection or initiation of a continuous infusion of catheters for analgesia/anesthesia

- Verification of correct catheter placement
- Increasing or decreasing the rate of the continuous infusion

Following stabilization of vital signs after either initial insertion, initial injection, bolus injection, rebolus injection, or initiation of continuous infusion by a licensed, credentialed anesthesia care provider, non-anesthetist registered nurses, in communication with the obstetric and anesthesia care providers, may:

- Monitor the patient's vital signs, mobility, level of consciousness, and perception of pain
- Monitor the status of the fetus
- Replace empty infusion syringes or infusion bags with new, pre-prepared solutions containing the same medication and concentration,

according to standing orders provided by the anesthesia care provider
- Stop the continuous infusion if there is a safety concern or the woman has given birth
- Remove the catheter, if educational criteria have been met and institutional policy and law allow. Removal of the catheter by a RN is contingent upon receipt of a specific order from a qualified anesthesia or physician provider.
- Initiate emergency therapeutic measures according to institutional policy and/or protocol if complications arise

Nonanesthetist registered nurses should not:

- Rebolus an epidural either by injecting medication into the catheter or increasing the rate of a continuous infusion

---

DISPLAY 9-9

Professional Organizations' Guidelines for Maternal–Fetal Assessment Frequency During Neuraxial Analgesia

MATERNAL ASSESSMENTS

Guidelines for Perinatal Care (AAP & ACOG, 2002, p. 141)

When regional anesthesia is administered during labor, the patient's vital signs should be monitored at regular intervals by a qualified member of the health care team.

Evidence-Based Clinical Practice Guideline: Nursing Care of the Woman Receiving Regional Analgesia/Anesthesia in Labor (AWHONN, 2001, p. 13)

Assess maternal blood pressure after the initiation or re-bolus of a regional block, including PCEA. Blood pressure may be assessed every 5 minutes for the first 15 minutes. More or less frequent monitoring may be indicated based on consideration of factors such as the type of analgesia/anesthesia, route and dose of medication used, the maternal–fetal response to medication, maternal–fetal condition, the stage of labor or facility protocol. The frequency of subsequent assessment should be based on consideration of the variables listed above. Assess pulse and respiratory rate consistent with the frequency of blood pressure assessment.

Guidelines for Regional Anesthesia in Obstetrics (ASA, 2006, p. 2)

Regional anesthesia for labor and/or vaginal delivery requires that the parturient's vital signs and the fetal heart rate be monitored and documented by a

qualified individual. Additional monitoring appropriate to the clinical condition of the parturient and the fetus should be employed when indicated.

FETAL ASSESSMENTS

Practice Guidelines for Obstetric Anesthesia (ASA, 2006, p. 7)

Fetal heart rate should be monitored by a qualified individual before and after administration of regional analgesia for labor. Continuous electronic recording of the fetal heart rate may not be necessary in every clinical setting and may not be possible during initiation of neuraxial anesthesia.

Evidence-Based Clinical Practice Guideline: Nursing Care of the Woman Receiving Regional Analgesia/Anesthesia in Labor (AWHONN, 2001, p. 11)

Assess the FHR tracing before initiating regional analgesia, ideally, to identify a reassuring pattern. If a non-reassuring FHR pattern is identified, initiate corrective measures as needed and notify the anesthesia/obstetric care provider.

Evidence-Based Clinical Practice Guideline: Nursing Care of the Woman Receiving Regional Analgesia/Anesthesia in Labor (AWHONN, 2001, p. 16)

Assess FHR after the initiation or re-bolus of a regional block, including PCEA. FHR may be assessed every 5 minutes for the first 15 minutes. More or less frequent monitoring may be indicated based on consideration of factors such as the type of analgesia/anesthesia, route and dose of medication used, the maternal–fetal response to medication, maternal–fetal condition, the stage of labor or facility protocol. The frequency of subsequent assessment should be based on consideration of the variables listed above. Assess FHR prior to ambulation to identify a reassuring heart rate pattern.

TABLE 9–9 ■ CARE OF PATIENTS RECEIVING NEURAXIAL ANALGESIA

Nursing Care	Rationale
Obtain a 20- to 30-minute baseline EFM strip before placement of the epidural, with continuous EFM for the duration of epidural infusion. Nurses should continue EFM during catheter placement to the best of their ability.	Maternal hypotension may decrease uteroplacental blood flow, adversely affecting fetal oxygenation, which is reflected in a nonreassuring FHR pattern.
Initiate IV access using a large-bore catheter. Infuse an IV bolus of 500–1,000 mL lactated Ringer's or normal saline solution 15–30 minutes before the procedure (Collis, Harding, & Morgan, 1999).	Because epidural anesthesia causes a sympathetic block and vasodilation, an IV bolus may decrease the risk of maternal hypotension. The ASA (2006) does not recommend any fixed volume of IV fluid prior to initiation of neuraxial analgesia. Using IV fluids containing glucose may increase insulin production in the fetus and hypoglycemia after birth. Avoid rapidly infusing IV fluids into women with cardiac disease or severe preeclampsia without direct measurement of hemodynamic status.
Ensure that necessary emergency equipment is readily available, set up, and functioning before the start of the procedure (eg, oxygen and suction, ambu bag and mask, equipment to maintain and airway and perform endotracheal intubation (laryngoscope and blades, endotracheal tubes), and resuscitation medications).	
Assist the woman to maintain a sitting or sidelying position with feet supported on a chair or stool; head flexed forward supported by herself with elbows resting on knees or leaning against the shoulder of a support person. Stress the importance of remaining still during insertion of the catheter.	Avoid severe spinal flexion, because it can decrease the epidural space and increase the possibility of puncturing the dura.
Encourage the use of breathing and relaxation techniques during the procedure.	Epidurals are most often placed once a patient has become uncomfortable due to uterine contractions. This combined with the positioning for the procedure and the need to remain still during placement of the catheter may be a challenge for some women.
After the catheter has been placed and the initial medication dose given, facilitate lateral or upright maternal position. Maintain left lateral tilt of the pelvis with a pillow, foam wedge, or rolled up blanket.	Left lateral tilt (placing a wedge under the right hip) may decrease the risk of maternal hypotension and placental insufficiency by displacing the weight of the gravid uterus away from the inferior vena cava and aorta, increasing blood flow to the right side of the maternal heart and eventually to uteroplacenta circulation.
Monitor vital signs after initiation of epidural analgesia/anesthesia according to institutional policy. If maternal hypotension occurs, initiate interventions for intrauterine resuscitation (eg, increase IV fluids, change maternal position, maintain uterine displacement, administer oxygen, stop oxytocin infusion, notify obstetrician and anesthesia care providers, prepare for the administration of medications such as ephedrine to improve maternal hypotension).	A decrease in systolic blood pressure to <100 mm Hg or below 20% from baseline can be corrected by administering ephedrine, 3–6 mg IV (Parry, Fernandez, Bawa, & Poulton, 1998). Ephedrine is a vasopressor that promotes peripheral vasoconstriction without constricting the umbilical vessels and increasing cardiac output.
Assess for symptoms of respiratory distress. Notify the anesthesia care provider and administer naloxone as ordered. Most organizations will have a standing order indicating at what respiratory rate naloxone should be administered.	Difficulty breathing may indicate migration of the catheter into the subarachnoid space.

(continued)

TABLE 9–9 ■ CARE OF PATIENTS RECEIVING NEURAXIAL ANALGESIA (Continued)

Nursing Care	Rationale
Once the patient has obtained pain relief, she should be assisted to change position at least every hour. Encourage patients to maintain a lateral rather then supine position.	Turning avoids continued pressure on one single area of the body and decreases the risk of unilateral blocks. Supine position is associated with decrease maternal cardiac output (Danilenko-Sixon, Tefft, Cohen, Haydon, & Carpenter, 1996) and lower fetal oxygen saturation measured by fetal pulse oximetry (Carbonne, Benachi, Leveque, Cabrol, & Papiernik, 1996).
Evaluate pain with each assessment of maternal vital signs or using a visual or verbal analogue scale according to institutional policy. If pain continues to be felt on one side of the body, sometimes lying on that side will achieve increased relief. Request that the anesthesia care provider reevaluate the patient as needed for further pain management.	93% of women with labor epidurals, who reported a pain score >3 using a 0–10 numeric rating scale, wanted additional medication (Beilin, Hossain, & Bodian, 2003)
Encourage the woman to void frequently during labor. If the bladder is distended and the woman experiences decreased bladder sensation or is unable to use a bed pan to void, placement of an indwelling catheter eliminates the need for repeated catheterizations.	Naloxone can also be used to reverse the effect of the medication on the bladder.
Small amounts of clear liquids may be provided to women with uncomplicated labors.	Controversy exists around oral intake during labor. The ASA (2006) recommends that solid foods be avoided in labor and that clear liquids increases maternal comfort and satisfaction and does not increase maternal complications.
Women who experience pruritus should be assured that this is usually a transitory symptom.	
Alert the nurse to prepare for an emergency cesarean section should fetal distress occur during labor with epidural analgesia/anesthesia.	

- Increase/decrease the rate of a continuous infusion
- Re-initiate an infusion once it has been stopped
- Manipulate PCEA doses or dosage intervals
- Be responsible for obtaining informed consent for analgesia/anesthesia procedures/however, the nurse may witness the patient signature for informed consent prior to analgesia/anesthesia administration. (AWHONN, 2002)

Perinatal nurses must be comfortable with the operation of additional technology, familiar with nursing care during all phases of the procedure, and able to recognize potential complications. Continuous epidural anesthesia is always delivered through an infusion pump, and continuous EFM is the most frequently used method of fetal assessment. Depending on institutional practice, women may also be monitored using a cardiac monitor, pulse oximeter, and automatic blood pressure devices. *Guidelines for Perinatal Care* (AAP & ACOG, 2002) suggest a 1:1 nurse–patient ratio for initiating epidural anesthesia.

Published statements from professional organizations and individual state nursing practice acts are inconsistent regarding the role of the nurse in caring for women in labor who receive anesthesia or analgesia and do not provide specific guidelines for how often and what type of monitoring will lead to optimal maternal–fetal outcomes. Controversy exists in the literature and in clinical practice about the frequency of maternal–fetal assessments during epidural anesthesia or analgesia for laboring women. Many perinatal units have policies that require completion of specific aspects of maternal–fetal assessment every 15 to 30 minutes for women with epidurals. There are, however, no published standards of care or practice guidelines from the ASA, American Association of Nurse Anesthetists, ACOG, or AWHONN that prescribe what the maternal–fetal assessment includes or the specific frequencies for making assessments during epidural infusion for labor and delivery. Existing published standards are general and outlined in Display 9–9. Nursing and medical textbooks may contain suggested protocols and valuable clinical information, but they do not alone define standards of care. There are no research-based data to demonstrate optimal time intervals for maternal–fetal assessments during epidural infusion. The type and amount of medication used, the level of the block given, and maternal–fetal status should be considered when determining intensity of monitoring. Perinatal nurses, in collaboration with obstetric and anesthesia providers in each institution, must develop protocols that delineate responsibilities and care for women receiving epidural anesthesia or analgesia during labor and delivery. Table 9–9 presents and overview of the nursing care to consider as policies and procedures are developed for care of the intrapartum patient receiving neuraxial analgesia.

Pharmacologic pain-management strategies represent one aspect of intrapartum pain management. They should be used for augmentation, not as a substitute for nonpharmacologic strategies. Nursing must remember that a woman who has been given IV pain medication or received epidural analgesia/anesthesia may still need, and can benefit from, all of the available nonpharmacologic nursing interventions.

Additional Techniques

Two methods of regional anesthesia, paracervical block and saddle block, were once widely accepted techniques for relief of labor pain. Paracervical block is now rarely used because of the potential for fetal bradycardia caused by rapid absorption of local anesthetic from the paracervical space. Saddle block, an injection of a local anesthetic into the subarachnoid L4–L5 space at the onset of the second stage of labor, is also used infrequently, because pain relief is generally so complete that women were unable to push effectively with their contractions, necessitating the application of forceps or a vacuum extractor. Paracervical block and saddle block are uncommon in clinical obstetric practice today because of the popularity of epidural anesthesia.

REFERENCES

Aird, I. A., Luckas, M. J., Buckett, W. M., & Bousfield, P. (1997). Effects of intrapartum hydrotherapy on labor related parameters. *Australian & New Zealand Journal of Obstetrics and Gynecology, 37*(2), 137–142.

Althaus, J., & Wax, J. (2005). Analgesia and anesthesia in labor. *Obstetrics and Gynecology Clinics of North America, 32*(2), 231–244.

American Academy of Pediatrics & American College of Obstetricians and Gynecologists. (2002). *Guidelines for perinatal care* (5th ed.). Elk Grove Village, IL: Author.

American College of Obstetricians and Gynecologists. (2001). *Optimal goals for anesthesia care in obstetrics.* (Committee Opinion No. 256), Washington, DC: Author.

American College of Obstetricians and Gynecologists. (2002). *Obstetric analgesia and anesthesia* (Practice Bulletin No. 36). Washington, DC: Author.

American College of Obstetricians and Gynecologists. (2004). *Pain relief during labor.* (Committee Opinion No. 295). Washington, DC: Author.

American College of Obstetricians and Gynecologists. (2006). *Analgesia and cesarean delivery rates.* (Committee Opinion No. 339). Washington, DC: Author.

American Heart Association & American Academy of Pediatrics. (2006). *Textbook of neonatal resuscitation* (5th ed.). Elk Grove Village, IL: American Academy of Pediatrics.

American Society of Anesthesiologists. (2006). *Practice guidelines for obstetrical anesthesia.* Park Ridge, IL: Author.

Andersen, B., Gyhagen, M., & Nielsen, T. (1996). Warm bath during labor: Effects on labor duration and maternal and fetal infectious morbidity. *Journal of Obstetrics and Gynecology, 16,* 326–330

Armstrong, K. P., Kennedy, B., Watson, J. T., Morley-Forster, P. K., Yee, I., & Butler, R. (2002). Epinephrine reduces the sedative side effects of epidural sufentanil for labor analgesia. *Canadian Journal of Anesthesia, 49*(1), 72–80.

Association of Women's Health, Obstetric and Neonatal Nurses. (2001). *Evidence-based clinical practice guideline: Nursing care of the woman receiving regional analgesia/anesthesia in labor.* Washington, DC: Author.

Association of Women's Health, Obstetric and Neonatal Nurses. (2002). *Role of the registered nurse (RN) in the management of the patient receiving analgesia by catheter techniques (epidural, intrathecal, intrapleural, or peripheral nerve catheters).* Washington, DC: Author.

Association of Women's Health, Obstetric and Neonatal Nurses. (2000). *Professional nursing support of laboring women.* (Policy Statement). Washington, DC: Author.

Bahasadri, S., Ahmadi-Abhari, S., Dehghani-Nik, M., & Habibi, G. R. (2006). Subcutaneous sterile water injections for labor pain: A randomized controlled trial. *Australia & New Zealand Journal of Obstetric & Gynecology, 46*(2), 102–106.

Ballen, L. E., & Fulcher, A. J. (2006). Nurses and doulas: Complementary roles to provide optimal maternity care. *Journal of Obstetrics, Gynecologic, and Neonatal Nursing, 35*(2), 304–311.

Beilin, Y., Hossain, S., & Bodian, A. A. (2003). The numeric rating scale and labor epidural analgesia. *Anesthesia & Analgesia, 96*(6), 1794–1798.

Benfield, R. D. (2002). Hydrotherapy in labor. *Journal of Nursing Scholarship, 34*(4), 347–352.

Bird, I. S., & Waugaman, W. (1999). In S. J. Reeder, L. L. Martin, & D. Koniak (Eds.), *Maternity nursing: Family, newborn, and women's health care* (18th ed., pp. 573–615). Philadelphia: Lippincott Williams & Wilkins.

Birnbach, D. J., & Browne, I. M. (2005). Anesthesia in Obstetrics. In R. D. Miller (Ed.), *Miller's anesthesia* (6th ed., pp. 2307–2344). Philadelphia: Elsevier Churchill Livingston.

Briggs, G. G., & Wan, S. R. (2005). Drug therapy during labor and delivery, part 2. *American Journal of Health-system Pharmacology, 63*(12). 1131–1139.

Britt, R., & Pasero, C. (1999). Pregnancy, childbirth, postpartum, and breastfeeding. In M. McCaffery & C. Pasero (Eds.), *Pain: Clinical manual* (2nd ed., pp. 608–625). St. Louis, MO: Mosby.

Browning, C. A. (2000). Using music during childbirth. *Birth, 27*(4), 272–276.

Bryanton, J., Fraser-Davey, H., & Sullivan, P. (1994). Women's perceptions of nursing support during labor. *Journal of Obstetric, Gynecologic, and Neonatal Nursing, 23*(8), 638–644.

Bucklin, B. A., Hawkins, J. L., Anderson, J. R., & Ullrich, F. A. (2005). Obstetric anesthesia workforce survey. *Anesthesiology, 103*(3), 645–653.

Camann, W. (2005). Pain relief during labor. *New England Journal of Medicine, 352*(7), 718–720.

Cammu, H., Clasen, K., Van Wettere, L., & Derde, M. (1994). To bathe or not to bathe during the first stage of labor. *Acta Obstetrics & Gynecology Scandinavica, 73*(6), 468–472

Campbell, D. A., Lake, M. F., Falk, M., & Backstrand, J. R. (2006). A randomized control trial of continuous support in labor by a lay doula. *Journal of Obstetric, Gynecologic, and Neonatal Nursing, 35*(4), 456–464.

Carbonne, B., Benachi, A., Leveque, M., Cabrol, D., & Papiernik, E. (1996). Maternal position during labor: Effects of fetal oxygen saturation measured by pulse oxymetry. *Obstetrics & Gynecology, 88*(5), 797–800.

Chandler, S., & Field, P. (1997). Becoming a father: First-time fathers' experience of labor and delivery. *Journal of Nurse-Midwifery, 42*(1), 17–24.

Chapman, L. L. (1991). Searching: Expectant fathers' experience during labor and birth. *Journal of Perinatal and Neonatal Nursing, 4*(4), 21–29.

Chapman, L. L. (1992). Expectant fathers' roles during labor and birth. *Journal of Obstetric, Gynecologic, and Neonatal Nursing, 21*(2), 114–120.

Chapman, L. L. (2000). Expectant fathers and labor epidurals. *MCN The American Journal of Maternal Child Nursing, 25*(3), 133–139.

Chang, M. Y., Chen, C. H., & Huang, K. F. (2006). A comparison of massage effects on labor pain using the McGill Pain Questionnaire. *Journal of Nursing Research, 14*(3), 190–197.

Chang, M. Y., Wang, S. Y., & Chen, C. H. (2002). Effects of massage on pain and anxiety during labor: A randomized controlled trial in Taiwan. *Journal of Advanced Nursing, 38*(1), 68–73.

Church, L. K. (1989). Water birth: One birthing center's observations. *Journal of Nurse-Midwifery, 34*(4), 165–170.

Collis, R. E., Baxandall, M. L., Srikantharajah, I. D., Edge, G., Kadim, M. Y., & Morgan, B. M. (1993). Combined spinal epidural analgesia with ability to walk throughout labor. *Lancet, 341*(8851), 767–768.

Collis, R. E., Harding, S. A., & Morgan, B. M. (1999). Effect of maternal ambulation on labor with low-dose combined spinal-epidural analgesia. *Anaesthesia, 54*(6), 535–539.

Cohen, S. (1997). Strategies for labor pain relief—past, present and future. *ACTA Anaesthesiologica Scandinavia, 110*, 17–21.

Danilenko-Dixon, D. R., Tefft, L., Cohen, R. A., Haydon, B., & Carpenter, M. W. (1996). Positional effects on maternal cardiac output during labor with epidural analgesia. *American Journal of Obstetrics & Gynecology, 175*(4 Pt. 1), 867–872.

DiFranco, J. (2000). Relaxation: Music. In F. Nichols & S. B. Humenick (Eds.), *Childbirth education: Practice, research, and theory* (pp. 201–215). Philadelphia: W. B. Saunders.

deJong, P. R., Johanson, R. B., Baxen, P., Adrians, V. D., vander Westhuisen, S., & Jones, R. W. (1997). Randomized trial comparing the upright and supine positions for the second stage of labor. *British Journal of Obstetrics and Gynecology, 104*(5), 567–571.

Eriksson, M., Ladfors, L., Mattsson, L. A., & Fall, O. (1996). Warm tub bath during labor: A study of 1385 women with prelabor rupture of the membranes after 34 weeks of gestation. *Acta Obstetricia et Gynecologica Scandinavica, 75*(7), 642–644.

Faucher, M. A., & Brucker, M. C. (2000). Intrapartum pain: Pharmacologic management. *Journal of Obstetric, Gynecologic, and Neonatal Nursing, 29*(2), 169–180.

Faure, E. A. (1991). The pain of parturition. *Seminars in Perinatology, 15*(5), 342–347.

Field, T., Hemandez-Reif, M., Taylor, S., Quintino, O., & Burman, I. (1997). Labor pain is reduced by massage therapy. *Journal of Psychosomatic Obstetrics & Gynecology, 18*(4), 286–291.

Gagnon, A. J., & Waghorn, K. (1999). One-to-one nurse labor support of nulliparous women stimulated with oxytocin. *Journal of Obstetrics, Gynecology, and Neonatal Nursing, 28*(4), 371–376.

Gale, J., Fothergill-Bourbonnais, F., & Chamberlain, M. (2001). Measuring nursing support during childbirth. *MCN The American Journal of Maternal Child Nursing, 26*(5), 264–271.

Giannina, G., Guzman, E. R., Lai, Y. L., Lake, M. F., Cernadas, M., & Vintzileos, A. M. (1995). Comparison of the effects of meperidine and nalbuphine on intrapartum fetal heart rate tracings. *Obstetrics & Gynecology, 86*(3), 441–445.

Gilliland, A. L. (2002). Beyond holding hands: The modern role of the professional doula. *Journal of Obstetric, Gynecologic, and Neonatal Nursing, 31*(6), 762–769.

Green, J. (1993). Expectations and experiences of pain in labor: Findings from a large prospective study. *Birth: Issues in Perinatal Care and Education, 20*(2), 65–72.

Gutkowska, J., Antunes-Rodrigues, J., & McCann, S. (1997). Atrial natriuretic peptide in brain and pituitary gland. *Physiology Review, 77*(2), 465–515.

Halpern, S., Muir, H., Breen, T. W., Campbell, D. C., Barrett, J., Liston, R., et al. (2004). A multicenter randomized controlled trial comparing patient-controlled epidural with intravenous analgesia for pain relief in labor. *Anesthesia & Analgesia, 99*(5), 1532–1538.

Harris, K. T. (1999). Hydrotherapy: An alternative method for relieving labor pain. *Mother-Baby Journal, 4*(5), 14–20.

Hatjis, C. G., & Meis, P. J. (1986). Sinusoidal fetal heart rate pattern associated with butorphanol administration. *Obstetrics & Gynecology, 67*(3), 377–380.

Hodnett, E. (2000). Caregiver support of women during childbirth. *Cochrane Database Systematic Review, 2*, CD000199.

Hodnett, E. D. (2002). Pain and women's satisfaction with the experience of childbirth: A systematic review. *American Journal of Obstetrics & Gynecology, 186*(5), S160–S172.

Hodnett, E. D., Gates, S., Hofmeyr, G. J., & Sakala, C. (2003). Continuous support for women during childbirth. *Cochrane Database of Systematic Review, 3*, CD003766.

Hodnett, E. D., Lowe, N. K., Hannah, M. E., Willan, A. R., Stevens, B., Weston, J. A., et al. (2002). Effectiveness of nurses as providers of birth labor support in North American hospitals: A randomized controlled trial. *Journal of the American Medical Association, 288*(11), 1373–1381.

Huffnagle, H. J., & Huffnagle, S. L. (1999). Alternatives to conduction analgesia. In M. C. Norris (Ed.), *Obstetric anesthesia* (2nd ed., pp. 282). Philadelphia: Lippincott Williams & Wilkins.

Huntley, A. L., Coon, J. T., & Ernst, E. (2004). Complementary and alternative medicine for labor pain: A systematic review. *American Journal of Obstetrics and Gynecology, 191*(1), 36–44.

King, T. L., & McCool, W. F. (2004). The definition and assessment of pain. *Journal of Midwifery & Women's Health, 49*(6), 471–472.

Klaus, M. H., Kennell, J. H., & Klaus, P. H. (2002). *The doula book: How a trained labor companion can help you have a shorter, easier, and healthier birth.* Cambridge, MA: Perseus Publishing.

Kuhnert, B. R., Linn, P. L., & Kuhnert, P. M. (1985). Obstetric medication and neonatal behavior. *Clinics in Perinatology, 12*(2), 423–440.

Labrecque, M., Nouwen, A., Bergeron, M., & Rancourt, J. F. (1999). A randomized controlled trial of nonpharmacologic approaches for relief of low back pain during labor. *Journal of Family Practice, 48*(4), 259–230.

Lavender, T., Walkinshaw, S. A., & Walton, I. (1999). A prospective study of women's views of factors contributing to a positive birth experience. *Midwifery, 15*(1), 40–46.

Lederman, R. P., Lederman, E., Work, B., & McCann, D. S. (1985). Anxiety and epinephrine in multiparous women in labor: Relationship to duration of labor and fetal heart rate pattern. *American Journal of Obstetrics and Gynecology, 153*(8), 870–871.

Lowe, N. (1996). The pain and discomfort of labor and birth. *Journal of Obstetric, Gynecologic, and Neonatal Nursing, 25*(1), 82–92.

Lowe, N. (2002). The nature of labor pain. *American Journal of Obstetrics & Gynecology, 186*(Suppl.), S16–S24.

Liu, E. H., & Sia, A. T. (2004). Rates of cesarean section and instrumental vaginal delivery in nulliparous women after low concentration epidural infusions or opioid analgesia: Systematic review. *British Medical Journal, 328*(7453), 410–415.

Lytzen, T., Cederberg, L., & Moller-Nielsen, J. (1989). Relief of low back pain in labor by using intracutaneous nerve stimulation with sterile water papules. *Acta Obstetricia et Gynecologica Scandinavica, 68*(4), 341–343.

Manning-Orenstein, G. (1998). A birth intervention: The therapeutic effects of doula support versus Lamaze preparation on first-time mother's working models of caregiving. *Alternative Therapeutic Health Medicine, 4*(4), 73–81.

Martensson, L., & Wallin, G. (1999). Labor pain treated with cutaneous injections of sterile water: A randomized controlled trial. *British Journal of Obstetrics and Gynecology, 106*(7), 633–637.

Mayberry, L. J., Wood, S. H., Strange, L. B., Lee, L., Heisler, D. R., & Nielsen-Smith, K. (2000). *Second stage labor management: Promotion of evidence-based practice and a collaborative approach to patient care.* (Symposium). Washington, DC: Author.

McCaffery, M., & Pasero, C. (1999). Practical nondrug approaches to pain. In M. McCaffery & C. Pasero (Eds.), *Pain: Clinical manual for nursing practice* (2nd ed., pp. 399–427). St Louis, MO: Mosby.

McNiven, P., Hodnett, E., & O'Brien-Pallas, L. L. (1992). Supporting women in labor: a work sampling study of the activities of labor and delivery nurses. *Birth, 91*(1), 3–8.

Melzack, R., & Wall, P. D. (1965). Pain mechanisms: A new theory. *Science, 150,* 971–979.

Melzack, R. (1984). The myth of painless childbirth. *Pain, 19*(4), 321–327.

Melzack, R. (1999). From the gate to the neuromatrix. *Pain, 82*(Suppl.), S121–126.

Merson, N. (2001). A comparison of motor block between ropivacaine and bupivacaine for continuous labor epidural analgesia. *Journal of the American Association of Nurse Anesthetists, 69*(1), 54–58.

Miltner, R. S. (2002). More than support: Nursing interventions provided to women in labor. *Journal of Obstetric, Gynecologic, and Neonatal Nursing, 31*(6), 753–761.

Mosallam, M., Rizk, D. E., Thomas, L., & Ezimokhai, M. (2004). Women's attitudes towards psychosocial support in labour in United Arab Emirates. *Archives of Gynecology and Obstetrics, 269*(3), 181–187.

Mussell, S. (1998). Narcotic analgesia during labor and birth: Maternal and newborn effects. *Mother-Baby Journal, 3*(6), 19–23.

Nageotte, M. P., Larson, D., Rumney, P. J., Sidhu, M., & Hollenbach, K. (1997). Epidural analgesia compared with combined spinal-epidural analgesia during labor in nulliparous women. *New England Journal of Medicine, 337*(24), 1715–1719.

Niven, C. A., & Gijsbers, K. J. (1989). Do low levels of labor pain reflect low sensitivity to noxious stimulation? *Social Science and Medicine, 29*(4), 585–588.

Ohlsson, G., Buchhave, P., Leandersson, U., Nordstrom, L., Rydhstrom, H., & Sjolin, I. (2001). Warm tub bathing during labor: Maternal and neonatal effects. *Acta Obstetrics & Gynecology of Scandinavica, 80*(4), 311–314.

Parry, M. G., Fernando, R., Bawa, G. P., & Poulton, B. B. (1998). Dorsal column function after epidural and spinal blockage: Implications for the safety of walking following low-dose regional analgesia for labor. *Anesthesia, 53*(4), 382–387.

Polley, L. S., Columb, M. O., Naughton, N. N., Wagner, D. S., & van de Ven, C. J. (2002). Effect of epidural epinephrine on the minimum local analgesic concentration of epidural bupivacaine in labor. *Anesthesiology, 96*(5), 1123–1128.

Rayburn, W. F., Smith, C. V., Parriott, J. E., & Woods, R. E. (1989). Randomized comparison of meperidine and fentanyl during labor. *Obstetric & Gynecology, 74*(4), 604–606.

Reynolds, J. L. (1994). Intracutaneous sterile water for back pain in labor. *Canadian Family Physician, 40,* 1785–1788, 1791–1792.

Robertson, P. A., Huang, L. J., Croughan-Minihane, M. S., & Kilpatrick, S. J. (1998). Is there an association between water baths during labor and the development of chorioamnionitis or endometritis? *American Journal of Obstetrics and Gynecology, 178*(6): 1215–1221.

Roberts, J. E., Mendez-Bauer, C., & Wodell, D. A. (1983). The effects of maternal position on uterine contractility and efficiency. *Birth 10*(4), 243–249.

Rush, J., Burlock, S., Lambert, K., Loosley-Millman, M., Hutchison, B., & Enkin, M. (1996). The effects of whirlpool baths in labor: A randomized, controlled trial. *Birth, 23*(3), 136–143.

Russell, R., & Reynolds, F. (1996). Epidural infusion of low-dose bupivacaine and opioid in labor. *Anaesthesia, 51*(3), 266–273.

Saravanakumar, K., Rao, S. G., & Cooper, G. M. (2006). The challenges of obesity and obstetric anesthesia. *Current Opinion in Obstetrics and Gynecology, 18*(6), 631–635.

Savolaine, E., Pandya, J. B., Greenblatt, S. H., & Conover, S., R. (1988). Anatomy of the human lumbar epidural space: New insights using CT epidurography. *Anesthesiology, 68*(2), 217–220.

Scott, K. D., Berkowitz, G., & Klaus, M. (1999). A comparison of intermittent and continuous support during labor: A meta-analysis. *American Journal of Obstetrics and Gynecology, 180*(5), 1054–1059.

Sharma, S. K., McIntire, D. D., Wiley, J., & Leveno, K. (2004). Labor analgesia and cesarean delivery: An individual patient meta-analysis of nulliparous women. *Anesthesiology, 100*(1), 142–148.

Simkin, P. (1995). Reducing pain and enhancing progress in labor: A guide to nonpharmacologic methods for maternity caregivers. *Birth, 22*(3), 161–171.

Simkin, P., & O'Hara, M. (2002). Nonpharmacologic relief of pain during labor: Systematic reviews of five methods. *American Journal of Obstetrics and Gynecology, 186*(5), S131–S159.

Sleutel, M. R. (2000). Climate, culture, context, or work environment: Organizational factors that influence nursing practice. *Journal of Nursing Administration, 30*(2), 53–58.

Smith, C. V., Rayburn, W. F., Allen, K. V., Bane, T., M., & Livezey, G. T. (1996). Influence of intravenous fentanyl on fetal biophysical parameters during labor. *Journal of Maternal Fetal Medicine, 5*(2), 89–92.

Somers-Smith, M. J. (2000). A place for the partner? Expectations and experiences of support during childbirth. *Midwifery, 15*(2), 101–108.

Spielman, F. J. (1987). Systemic analgesics during labor. *Clinical Obstetrics and Gynecology, 30*(3), 495–504.

Stremler, R., Hodnett, E., Petryshen, P., Stevens, B., Weston, J., & Willan, A. R. (2005). Randomized controlled trial of hand-and-knees positioning for occipitoposterior position in labor. *Birth, 32*(4), 243–251.

Thorp, J. (1999). Epidural analgesia during labor. *Clinical Obstetrics and Gynecology, 42*(4), 785–801.

Trolle, B., Moller, M., Kronborg, H., & Thomsen, S. (1991). The effect of sterile water blocks on low back labor pain. *American Journal of Obstetrics and Gynecology, 164*(5, Pt. 1), 1277–1281.

Vincent, R. D., & Chestnut, D. H. (1998). Epidural analgesia during labor. *American Family Physician, 58*(8), 1785–1792.

Wakefield, M. L. (1999). Systemic analgesia: Opioids, ketamine, and inhalational agents. In D. H. Chestnut (Ed.), *Obstetric anesthesia: Principles and practice* (pp. 340–353). St. Louis, MO: Mosby.

Wiand, N. E. (1997). Relaxation levels achieved by Lamaze-trained pregnant women listening to music and ocean sound tapes. *The Journal of Perinatal Education, 6*(4), 1–7.

Wiruchpongsanon, P. (2006). Relief of low back labor pain by using intracutaneous injections of sterile water: A randomized clinical trial. *Journal of the Medical Association of Thailand, 89*(5), 571–576.

Wong, C. A., Scavone, B. M., Peaceman, A. M., McCarthy, R. J., Sullivan, J. T., Diaz, N. T., et al. (2005). The risk of cesarean delivery with neuraxial analgesia given early versus late in labor. *New England Journal of Medicine, 352*(7), 566–665.

Wright, M., McCrea, H., Stringer, M., & Murphy-Black, T. (2000). Personal control in pain relief during labor. *Journal of Advanced Nursing, 32*(5), 1168–1177.

Youngstrom, P. C., Baker, S. W., & Miller, J. L. (1996). Epidurals redefined in analgesia and anesthesia: A distinction with a difference. *Journal of Obstetric, Gynecologic, and Neonatal Nursing, 25*(4), 350–354.

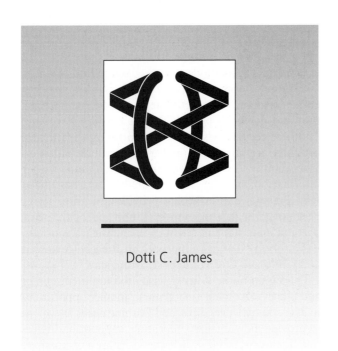

Dotti C. James

CHAPTER **10**

Postpartum Care

A woman experiences significant alterations in physical and psychosocial status after childbirth. The postpartum period is a time of transition involving physiologic changes, adaptation to the maternal role, and modification of the family system by the addition of the baby. Nurses have a unique opportunity to promote and support maternal and family adaptation. Inpatient postpartum care routines are ideally focused on the needs of the mother, baby, and family, rather than on arbitrary rules and unit traditions. Postpartum nursing care should be as individualized and flexible as needed. The perinatal nurse recognizes women and their families as integral members of the healthcare team and encourages them to enter into decision-making processes and planning of care (Association of Women's Health, Obstetric and Neonatal Nurses [AWHONN], 2003). Open visiting and family interaction with the new mother and newborn are supported. The father of the baby and other support persons should be encouraged to be present, according to the desires of the woman, and actively involved in postpartum and newborn care. Family-centered maternity care is based on the philosophy that the physical, social, psychological, and spiritual needs of the family are included in all aspects of the nursing care provided (AWHONN, 2003).

Implementation of family-centered maternity care requires collaboration among childbearing women, families, and healthcare providers. The family is defined by the woman and frequently extends beyond traditional definitions. Cultural beliefs and values of the woman and her family should be respected and accommodated. Chapter 2 and the March of Dimes Nursing Module *Cultural Competence in the Care of Childbearing Families* (Moore & Moos, 2002) provide a comprehensive review and discussion of various cultural and religious perspectives and can be helpful in developing nursing care for specific women. This chapter begins with a discussion of physiologic changes during the postpartum period and then describes the appropriate nursing assessments and interventions for healthy women and for those with common postpartum complications. Selected topics for patient education are presented. A woman experiences significant changes in physical and psychosocial status following childbirth. Nurses have a unique opportunity to promote and support maternal and family adaptation during this time.

PLANNING FOR THE TRANSITION TO PARENTHOOD

According to current trends, length of stay (LOS) for childbirth is now more realistically in line with the physical and psychosocial needs of the new mother and her family rather than with the previous arbitrary mandates from health insurance companies in an effort to control costs. However, although LOS has slightly increased over the past several years, it is still relatively short in all settings (Martell, 2000). Thus, discharge planning cannot be delayed until admission for childbirth. Women in active labor and women who have just given birth are not candidates for a discussion of learning needs or for typical classroom education about self- or infant care. The woman's focus during the intrapartum period is on safe passage through labor and on a healthy positive childbirth experience.

Rubin's (1961a) classic research suggests that during the immediate postpartum period, the new mother is not physically or emotionally ready to listen to extensive presentations of how to care for herself and her newborn. Postpartum women have transient deficits in cognition, particularly in memory function, the first day after giving birth. According to Rana, Lindheimer, Hibbard, and Pliskin (2005), normal pregnant women can temporarily develop mild cognitive defects during labor and after birth when compared with nonpregnant women. Women in their study reported problems with attention, concentration, and memory throughout pregnancy and in the early postpartum period (Rana et al., 2006). This decline was not attributed to depression, anxiety, sleep deprivation, or other physical changes associated with pregnancy. Causes suggested included the increased levels of pregnenolone and allopregnanolone that are correlated with negative effects on memory, as well as the high levels of endogenous and exogenous cortisol, which affect hippocampal integrity and therefore explicit memory (Rana et al., 2005). Oxytocin also is known for its amnestic effects. Based on available evidence, traditional discharge planning that includes verbal transmission of information or instruction in child care techniques immediately after birth or on the first postpartum day will be poorly remembered. These findings underscore the importance of providing the family with appropriate written material they can review after discharge. Priorities for most women in the first 24 hours postpartum are rest, time to touch, hold and get to know their baby, and an opportunity to review and discuss their labor and birth (Rubin, 1961a).

New mothers recognize their babies by olfactory and/or tactile cues, senses that do not primarily require cognitive function (Kaitz, Good, Rokem, & Eidelman, 1987). In a recent study, 90% of women tested identified their newborns by olfactory cues after only 10 minutes to 1 hour exposure to their babies. All of the women tested recognized their babies' odor after exposure periods greater than 1 hour (Jacob, 2006). The childbearing experience is very different today than it was nearly 50 years ago when Rubin (1961a, b) began her research. Major changes include the availability of prenatal classes, women and families as active participants in all aspects of perinatal care, fathers, siblings, and other support persons present for labor and birth, epidural anesthesia/analgesia, open visiting, single-room maternity care, couplet care models, and shorter hospitalizations. However, despite the progress made toward a healthcare environment where childbearing women have more participation and control, much of Rubin's work about the taking-in and taking-hold phases of the postpartum period is still valid today.

The discharge planning process should be ongoing during pregnancy, labor, and the postpartum period. Although education about maternal and infant care can occur during the inpatient stay, information should be offered during pregnancy and reinforced after discharge in many different settings using a variety of teaching methods. The prenatal period provides a window of opportunity to prepare families not only about pregnancy and birth but also about the postpartum and newborn periods (Martell, 2000; Zwelling, 2000). Prenatal visits to the primary healthcare provider are an ideal time for the perinatal nurse to assess family learning needs and concerns and to offer information, support, and resources in a personalized way. Prenatal classes should provide education about pregnancy, health promotion, labor and birth, postpartum, maternal and infant care, and the transition to parenthood. Critical concepts can then be reviewed and reinforced during the postpartum stay.

Follow-up home visits or visits to outpatient clinics and offices offer the perinatal nurse another opportunity to assess knowledge, skills, and learning needs as well as to provide individualized education, support, and referrals (Lieu et al., 2000). If home visits are not possible, follow-up phone calls after discharge provide the perinatal nurse an opportunity to clarify information and answer additional questions. Finally, classes and support groups for new parents are another way for families to continue learning about maternal and infant care, parenting, and how to nurture the couple relationship.

Healthcare providers continue to struggle to find innovative ways to provide safe, cost-effective, comprehensive perinatal care in response to economic pressures. Although consumer pressures resulted in state and federal laws mandating minimal LOS coverage, costs remain a very real issue for institutions and individual healthcare providers. Prenatal education in healthcare provider offices and in the classroom combined with case management and written materials and/or videos effectively are some methods that prepare women and their families for discharge (Brown, 2006; Roudebush, Kaufman, Johnson, Abraham, & Clayton, 2006).

Women feel more in control and express greater feelings of maternal confidence and competence when they have adequate knowledge about how to care for themselves and their newborns after discharge (Brown, 2006; Lieu et al., 2000; Roudebush, Kaufman, Johnson, Abraham, & Clayton, 2006). This chapter describes strategies for developing a comprehensive approach to postpartum care and discharge planning for the woman and her family. Through the use of prenatal databases, prenatal classes, case management models, clinical pathways, individualized assessment tools, postdischarge follow-up visits or phone calls, and a variety of creative and innovative teaching methods, perinatal nurses can ease the transition from hospital to home and ensure childbearing families have acquired enough information and skills to safely care for the mother and baby.

Prenatal Patient Database

Early identification and entry into the system can facilitate prenatal preparation for hospitalization and postpartum discharge. Successful programs require communication among primary healthcare providers, prenatal educators, community resources, and the perinatal center. A simple, user-friendly system that incorporates demographic data, estimated date of birth, significant clinical history, family assessment and learning needs, participation in prenatal education programs, and a mechanism to communicate all pertinent information to the inpatient unit is critical. A computerized database is ideal, but traditional file systems in addition to communication in person or by phone, facsimile (FAX), and e-mail also works well for women with access to the Internet. Healthcare providers at each institution can develop a prenatal patient database to meet specific needs. For example, when a woman registers her intent to give birth at the institution early in pregnancy, demographic and insurance data can be entered into the system. Primary healthcare providers and those in community prenatal clinics that refer women for inpatient care can be encouraged to send notification about women who have selected the institution for childbirth.

Some hospitals have developed Internet Web sites where women can register for childbirth classes, seek prenatal care information, download patient education materials, and take a virtual tour of the facilities. Summaries of the educational and clinical backgrounds, services, office hours and insurance plan participation of healthcare providers that have privileges at the institutions can offer valuable information to women who are in the process of selecting a healthcare provider and an institution for birth. Links to offices of obstetricians, family practice physicians, and nurse midwives on staff can be helpful as well. Information about financial criteria for eligibility to participate in programs such as Medicaid and the Special Supplemental Feeding Program for Women, Infants, and Children's (WIC) are useful for selected families. As more families of childbearing age gain access to the Internet, these Web sites will meet the needs of both patients and healthcare institutions.

Healthcare providers can provide mothers with a childbirth and parenting preparation book (or suggest one to be purchased) in early pregnancy, supply expectant families with information about the institution, and urge them to take a tour of the perinatal unit. Brochures describing all perinatal services available at the institution including telephone numbers are especially helpful and ideally should be available in the offices of all healthcare providers affiliated with the institution. Written materials should be available in the languages of the population served. Families should be informed about prenatal classes and encouraged to attend. Selected women and their families can be referred for case management, especially when the pregnancy and the social or economic situation are complex.

By the 36th week of pregnancy, a record of prenatal care should be sent by the primary healthcare provider to the perinatal institution to be available when the woman is admitted for labor and birth (American Academy of Pediatrics [AAP] & American College of Obstetricians and Gynecologists [ACOG], 2002). Specific individualized care plans or guides developed by the case manager, social worker, or perinatal nurse for the woman's inpatient stay also should be added to the patient database. With this type of system, when the woman is admitted for childbirth, the perinatal nurse has valuable information about current maternal–fetal health status, family learning needs, and the education programs the family attended. The quality and quantity of prenatal data about the childbearing family enhance the perinatal nurse's ability to provide individualized care and teaching.

Prenatal Classes

In the past, most prenatal classes consisted of a series lasting 6 to 8 weeks in the last trimester of pregnancy focused primarily on preparation for labor and birth and to a lesser extent on pregnancy, infant care, and the transition to parenthood. For many working couples, making the time commitment to attend a series of six classes is often difficult. Multiple factors such as perceived knowledge, support systems, transportation issues, work schedules, childcare availability, and previous newborn and childbirth experience influence the decision to attend prenatal classes. Many institutions and perinatal educators have responded to consumer needs by streamlining content to decrease program length and offering alternatives such as weekend programs, flexible hours, informative Web sites, and antepartum home visits.

Information about health promotion should be presented early in pregnancy to have the opportunity to make a difference in pregnancy outcomes. Topics of early pregnancy classes may include:

- Fetal growth and development
- Expected physical changes during pregnancy
- Normal discomforts of pregnancy
- Lifestyle modifications
- Nutrition
- Activity and exercise
- Effects of smoking cigarettes, drinking alcohol, and using illegal drugs
- The need to ask primary healthcare providers about use of over-the-counter medications and medications prescribed by other healthcare providers prior to use
- Warning signs of pregnancy complications including a comprehensive discussion about preterm labor signs and symptoms and when to call their primary healthcare provider if these signs and symptoms should occur

Many hospitals have developed courses that cover early pregnancy content and have systems in place that prompt referral to these classes when women are seen for their first prenatal visit. Close partnerships with healthcare providers who are affiliated with the institution are essential to encourage women and their partners to attend classes that focus on early pregnancy health promotion.

Traditional prepared childbirth classes are offered during the third trimester when the mother and her partner are intent on learning about how to cope with labor pain and what to expect during labor and birth. Although the process of labor and birth is valuable con-

tent, information about parenthood and infant care is also important for expectant parents (see Display 10–1 for course content for classes that include prepared childbirth and infant care information for a 6-week course). For couples unable to meet the 6-week time commitment, classes that meet less frequently can be designed. Options can include a 1-, 2-, or 3-week series covering critical content that is prioritized based on class time limitations. Display 10–2 lists sample curricula for prenatal classes based on a 1-, 2-, or 3-week

DISPLAY 10-1

Prepared Childbirth and Infant Care Class Curriculum Overview

Prepared Childbirth	*Infant Care*
Class I	
Introduction	Selecting a pediatrician
Discomforts of pregnancy	Immunizations
Preterm labor	Child care
Exercises	Baby time
Relaxation and breathing patterns	
Slow-paced breathing and progressive relaxation	
Class II	
Preview of labor	Bathing video or bathing baby demonstration
Relaxation and breathing patterns	Changing or diapering
Favorite place, slow-paced, and bridged breathing	Holding baby
Position changes for labor	
Class III	
Birth video	Breastfeeding versus bottle-feeding
Goody bag	Burping
Relaxation and breathing patterns	Sleeping patterns
Transition	Pacifiers
Class IV	
Labor, birth, and nursery tour	Newborn characteristics
Medical interventions	
Class V	
Labor rehearsal	Infant CPR
Review breathing and relaxation	Choking demonstration
Emergency childbirth	Illness and when to call pediatrician
Cesarean birth video	Parents as teachers video
Medication, analgesia, anesthesia	
Class VI	
Postpartum discussion	Safety discussion
Postpartum care	Car seat safety
Party	

Adapted from Harper, J. (2006). *Prenatal class content outline*. St. Louis: St. John's Mercy Medical Center.

DISPLAY 10-2

Sample Curricula for Prenatal Classes

CLASS CONTENT: ONE 3-HOUR PRENATAL CLASS

Essentials to bring to the hospital

Early signs of labor and when to come to the hospital

What to expect during labor and birth

Formulating a birth plan

Anesthesia and analgesia options

Visiting policies

How to anticipate length of stay (LOS), third-party payer issues, precertification, deductibles, and copayments

Choosing a pediatrician

Warning signs of pregnancy complications, including preterm labor and preeclampsia

Maternal care issues: episiotomy care, normal lochia, afterpains, incision care, breast care, nutrition, rest, "baby blues"

Newborn care issues: umbilical cord care, circumcision care, breastfeeding, formula feeding, diapering, bathing, behavioral and satiation cues, crying, comforting, car seats, sleep positioning, and other safety issues

Videotapes and booklets to reinforce class content

Parent hotline number for additional questions

Community and institutional resources

CLASS CONTENT: TWO 3-HOUR PRENATAL CLASSES

Class I

Essentials to bring to the hospital

Formulating a birth plan

Early signs of labor, relaxation, and breathing techniques

When to come to the hospital

The admission process

Ambulation in early labor

Electronic fetal monitoring and intermittent auscultation

Labor induction and augmentation

Amniotomy

Active labor

Transition

Second stage of labor

Anesthesia and analgesia options, review of pain relief and comfort measures, nonpharmacologic and pharmacologic

The unanticipated cesarean birth

Visiting policies

How to anticipate LOS, third-party payer issues, precertification, deductibles, and copayments

Warning signs of pregnancy complications, including preterm labor and preeclampsia

Class II

Choosing a pediatrician

Maternal care issues: episiotomy care, normal lochia, afterpains, incision care, breast care, nutrition, rest, baby blues, sexuality issues, contraception, and family planning

Newborn care issues: umbilical cord care, circumcision care, breastfeeding, formula feeding, diapering, bathing, behavioral and satiation cues, sleep–awake state, crying, comforting, car seats, sleep positioning, other safety issues

Videotapes and booklets to reinforce class content

Parent hotline number for additional questions

Community and institutional resources

CLASS CONTENT: THREE 3-HOUR PRENATAL CLASSES

Class I

Brief overview of fetal development

Changes during pregnancy

Nutrition and lifestyle modification

Sexuality during pregnancy

Formulating a birth plan

Relaxation and breathing techniques

Childbirth options

Visiting policies

How to anticipate LOS, third-party payer issues, precertification, deductibles, and copayments

Choosing a pediatrician

Tour of perinatal unit

Warning signs of pregnancy complications, including preterm labor and preeclampsia

Class II

Essentials to bring to the hospital

Early signs of labor and when to come to the hospital

The admission process

Ambulation in early labor

Electronic fetal monitoring and intermittent auscultation

Labor induction and augmentation

Amniotomy

Active labor

Transition

Second stage of labor

Anesthesia and analgesia options, review of pain relief and comfort measures, nonpharmacologic and pharmacologic

Reinforcement of relaxation and breathing techniques

The unanticipated cesarean birth

(continued)

Class III

Maternal care issues: episiotomy care, normal lochia, afterpains, incision care, breast care, nutrition, rest, baby blues, sexuality issues, contraception and family planning

Newborn care issues: umbilical cord care, circumcision care, breastfeeding, formula feeding, diapering,

bathing, behavioral and satiation cues, sleep–awake state, crying and comforting, car seat, sleep positioning, other safety issues

Videotapes and booklets to reinforce class content
Parent hotline number for additional questions
Community and institutional resources

series). Classes about parenting issues and infant care have been developed by many institutions. These classes are more commonly attended during pregnancy; however, some institutions have been successful in offering these classes to new parents during evening hours and inviting them to bring their newborn.

Although there is a significant need for information to assist in preparing couples for labor and birth, pregnant women and their partners can benefit from a comprehensive educational program that includes preconception health promotion, healthy behaviors during the prenatal period, breastfeeding, the postpartum period, and infant care content (see Display 10–3 for suggested course content from early pregnancy to the postpartum period).

Prenatal education classes should be designed to meet the needs of the population served, and based on the knowledge of what information and skills are useful and relevant to expectant parents, at various stages of pregnancy. Classes should be made available to a variety of women including teenagers, women who have previously given birth but desire a review class, women requesting private instruction, women who are hospitalized or on bed rest at home for much of their pregnancy, and women who speak a language other than English. Classes focusing on breastfeeding, sibling preparation, grandparents, car seat safety, exercise during pregnancy, labor preparation for women who desire a vaginal birth after a previous cesarean birth (VBAC), and families expecting more than one baby complement the core curriculum.

A comprehensive education program developed by parent and childbirth educators in partnership with healthcare providers, perinatal nurses, and parents is ideal. An education curriculum designed using a team approach ensures that educators provide families with important information about pregnancy, childbirth, infant and postpartum care, and the transition to parenthood. Parent and birth educators play a significant role in preparing families for the postpartum period. It is important that their work is valued and that there is ongoing communication between the educators and the perinatal unit staff, especially if the educators are not formally affiliated with the institution. Disappointments and unmet expectations for the labor, birth, and postpartum experience can be avoided if childbirth educators are fully familiar with the policies of the perinatal

unit. In some institutions, educators are invited to attend staff meetings and retreats and are offered the opportunity to spend time on the unit with a labor nurse periodically to maintain an awareness of the daily realities of the childbirth experience and unit routines.

Educational Methods and Materials

Whether education is provided at the bedside, in a large auditorium, or in a small classroom, the teaching method must complement the information presented and must be appropriate for the learner. Skills such as comfort measures and pain relief during labor, infant bathing, or cord care are most effectively taught by demonstration and return demonstration. Feelings and beliefs are best addressed individually or in a small group setting. Consideration needs to be given to personal learning styles and basic education level and knowledge (Zwelling, 2000). Including parents as part of the prenatal education team enhances the likelihood that topics offered will be what parents want and need to know. Some institutions periodically hold new parent focus groups or use telephone or mailed surveys to validate the content of their educational materials and classes and to make sure they are consistent with the needs of their patients.

Written materials support and reinforce interactive learning. Books, pamphlets, brochures, and other handouts must have a consistent message and support the philosophy of the perinatal institution. There are a number of excellent resources in print or the prenatal educators may develop their own education materials. Selection or development of written materials should be based on the education level of the population served and the financial resources available. The healthcare provider, educator, and representatives from the perinatal institution should collectively choose written materials and be familiar with the contents. Parents should be asked to evaluate the usefulness and helpfulness of the written materials. Providing families with standardized written materials can be a timesaving and cost-effective strategy. If the institution chooses to use materials purchased from companies that specialize in developing childbirth and parenting educational materials, it is important to thoroughly review the content for accuracy before distributing to patients. Standardized materials (either purchased or developed

Becoming Parents Course

The *Becoming Parents* course is designed to provide expectant families with the knowledge and skills needed to promote health during pregnancy and to prepare for childbirth and parenting. It reflects our philosophy that birth is one of life's most special events and that the role of family maternity education is to enhance the joy of this experience by providing families with support and education throughout the childbearing years in partnership with healthcare providers and hospital staff.

Celebrating Your Pregnancy—First Trimester

This informative and entertaining evening seminar focuses on how to grow a healthy baby and have a healthy pregnancy. You will learn about fetal growth and development, optimal lifestyle choices for pregnancy, workplace and environmental hazards to avoid, common changes in family relationships during pregnancy, how to be an informed healthcare consumer, and resources for education and support at our hospital and in the community. *2-hour seminar*

Growing the Baby of Your Dreams—Second Trimester

In the middle trimester, most families begin to imagine what their baby will look like and be like. You'll be amazed to discover the unique physical characteristics and capabilities of newborns and how able they are to respond to your love. We'll talk about what it means to be a parent and how becoming a parent affects your family relationships. You'll also learn about baby care and what supplies you'll need, and you will begin to master some of the labor coping skills such as relaxation and the first level of breathing. This series is also offered as *Christian Growing the Baby of Your Dreams*, with time to discuss the spiritual aspects of pregnancy, birth, and parenting. *Two 2-hour classes or one 4-hour class, small group*

Breastfeeding Basics—Second or Third Trimester

This class is recommended for all expectant families. You will learn about the health benefits of breastfeeding for mothers and infants, how to get off to a good start, how fathers, partners and family can support breastfeeding, and resources for support. A panel of families shares their breastfeeding experiences and valuable insights. *2-hour seminar*

Breastfeeding and the 21st Century Family: Beyond the Basics—Second or Third Trimester (can be repeated after the birth)

Expectant mothers, fathers, partners, and family are encouraged to attend this class to learn about how breastfeeding fits into a busy lifestyle. You will learn how to express or pump breast milk, which pumps are best, how to store breast milk and for how long, and how to feed your baby when mother is away or at work. Tips for working mothers are provided. Breastfeeding Basics is a prerequisite. *2-hour seminar*

Sneak Peek: A Look at Postpartum—Early Third Trimester

Take a peek at the realities of life with a newborn baby—the joys and the challenges. You will learn about physical recovery from birth and self-care to enhance healing and increase comfort. Also discussed are emotional and lifestyle changes to expect after delivery and resources to help you cope. A new-parent panel offers suggestions for a smooth transition to parenthood. *2-hour seminar*

Birth Basics—Middle to Late Third Trimester

This class prepares you for childbirth. What to expect in labor and birth, how to develop an individual approach to birth, the partner's role in labor, breathing and relaxation techniques, methods of pain management, medical procedures, common variations in childbirth, and cesarean birth will be discussed. Included in this class is a tour of the Family Maternity Center. This series is also offered as Christian, Spanish-language, and Teen Birth Basics courses. *Four 2-hour classes or two 4-hour weekend classes, small group*

OTHER CLASSES RELATED TO CHILDBIRTH AND EARLY PARENTING

During Pregnancy

Vaginal Birth After Cesarean (VBAC)
Labor and Birth Refresher
Becoming Grandparents
For Dads Only
Sibling Preparation
Car Safe Kids
Maternity Fitness and Education
Yoga for Pregnancy
Family Maternity Center Tours

After Birth

Parent–Baby Classes—a weekly class for parents and babies through the first year
Yoga for New Moms
Infant Massage
Infant and Child CPR
Early parenting seminars and series
  Guiding Children's Behavior
  Toddler Development
  Parenting with Love and Logic

(continued)

Breastfeeding the Older Baby

Starting Solids

Infant Sleep and the Conflict with American Culture

Young Moms Support Group

This Is Not What I Expected—emotional support for new families in post partum

During Pregnancy or After

IMET: Keys for Couples—a weekend seminar to strengthen couple relationships

In Special Circumstances

Private classes for childbirth preparation are available.

---

by the institution) provide a ready resource for parents at any time and potentially decrease the volume of calls to the perinatal center and to the primary healthcare provider. Written materials should be developed or chosen with consideration to the basic language level of the family and to the language they speak. Families who do not speak English should be supplied with language-appropriate materials.

Some institutions use in-hospital television channels with programs on newborn bath, cord and circumcision care, and breast- and formula feeding. Purchased videos or those produced by the institution are another method of providing important information. The videos can be given as gifts, loaned to families, or purchased in the hospital gift shop. As with written materials, television instruction and videos need to be evaluated for consistent, correct information that is learner appropriate and reflects the philosophy of the perinatal institution.

Family Preference Plan

Involving women and their families in decisions about their perinatal care increases satisfaction and promotes a collaborative relationship between healthcare providers and families. A preference plan helps to individualize the family's care (see Display 10–4). Women who are asked about care preferences feel their unique needs will be met by nurses and other healthcare providers. Advantages of methods that encourage women and their families to define their individual approach to birth such as a birth plan or a list of family preferences include validation of the family's knowledge of available labor and birth options and perinatal center policies. The family preference plan can be given to all pregnant women registered for birth or given to families during prenatal classes. The preference plan provides the healthcare provider with information about the family's special needs, concerns, and requests and allows the healthcare provider to have a meaningful discussion with the family about their expectations. This discussion should occur during the pregnancy with the primary healthcare provider and with the perinatal nurse on admission to the unit for labor and birth.

Preference plans can be helpful in clarifying unit protocols and avoiding unmet expectations when women have plans for techniques or procedures that are not available on the unit. For example, the woman may have learned about the benefits of hydrotherapy in a Jacuzzi tub and wish to labor in the tub, but the unit may not have a Jacuzzi tub available; the woman may intend to use candles for aromatherapy; however, the unit may not allow burning candles for safety reasons; or the woman may plan to use a birthing ball during labor and the unit may not have birthing balls. If these limitations are known in advance of admission, alternative plans can be made. In the examples described here, hydrotherapy can be provided in the shower, aromatherapy can be used with methods that do not include candles, and a birthing ball can be obtained on loan from a childbirth educator or purchased before admission.

The preference plan can be sent to the hospital with the prenatal care records or brought to the unit by the woman on admission for childbirth. It is important that any record-keeping process about childbirth preferences includes a system to ensure that it is available to all healthcare providers when the woman is admitted for labor and birth. The initial interaction during the admission process is used to develop rapport with the woman and her family and to get a sense of their expectations for their birth experience. Ideally, the amount of childbirth preparation and type of pain management anticipated during labor are covered prior to or during the admission assessment. A review of preferences for childbirth, including reinforcement of options that are available at the institution, works best to facilitate a positive experience. Although some nurses and physicians have negative feelings about written birth plans, a birth plan helps the nurse meet the couple's expectations and indicates that the woman has given considerable thought to how she would like labor and birth to proceed. Every effort should be made to meet the expectations and wishes of the woman. The woman's desires for positioning, ambulation, and method of fetal assessment should be honored in ways that are consistent with safe care. If maternal and/or fetal status is such that the woman's wishes cannot be met within reason, a thorough discussion with adequate explanation of the

DISPLAY 10-4

Family Preference Plan

My name: _____   My doctor's name: _____

1. I would like to have these persons visit during labor:
   _____   _____
   _____   _____

2. My main support person is:
   Relationship: _____

3. For pain control/positioning during labor and birth, I would like to:

_____ walk in room/halls		_____ listen to special music
_____ sit in recliner		_____ use special focal point
_____ use shower		_____ use my own pillows
_____ use jacuzzi		_____ use squat bar
_____ use heat/cold/massage		_____ use foot pads on bed

4. I would like to have these persons present during birth:
   _____   _____

5. I have these religious requests:
   _____ birth blessing by chaplain
   _____ eucharist or communion
   _____ have visit by my own clergy
   _____ other: _____
   _____ none

6. After birth: I would like to:
   _____ place baby skin-to-skin
   _____ wrap baby in blanket before holding
   _____ breastfeed my baby
   _____ bathe my baby
   _____ have doctor circumcise my son
   _____ have pictures taken of my baby
   _____ keep baby in my room as long as he/she is stable

7. During my hospital stay, I would like to have my support person:
   _____ put baby skin-to-skin to him or her
   _____ assist with baby care
   _____ give the baby's first bath
   _____ spend the night in my room
   _____ take pictures of birth experience

8. I plan to attend, or have already attended, these classes/services during this pregnancy:
   _____ prenatal class
   _____ hospital OB tour
   _____ sibling class
   _____ exercise sessions
   _____ Lamaze

9. Child care has been arranged for other dependent children:
   _____ during the hospital stay
   _____ after mom and baby go home
   _____ not applicable
   _____ other:

10. I plan to have my other child(ren) come to visit:
    _____ during labor
    _____ during birth
    _____ in the first 2-hour recovery time
    _____ after I arrive in my postpartum room
    _____ not at all
    _____ not applicable

(continued)

11. After going home, these persons will help out for the first two days:

_____

_____

12. Additional ideas:

_____

_____

_____

_____

_____

rationale for the decision should occur. The woman should be allowed and encouraged to ask any questions and be given appropriate answers to those questions. It may be necessary for the primary healthcare provider to talk to the woman in person or by telephone about her concerns. The nurse should acknowledge the woman's disappointment and assure her that every attempt to meet her expectations will be made if the clinical situation changes.

Arbitrary rules prohibiting more than one support person during labor and birth are contrary to the philosophy that the birth experience belongs to the woman and her family rather to those providing clinical care. Although healthcare providers are sometimes inclined to attempt to control this aspect of the birth process using various arguments for safety and convenience, when examined critically, these arguments have little scientific merit. Women should be able to choose who will be with them during this very special and unique life experience (Rouse & MacNeil, 2000). Family-centered care supports the concept that the "family" is defined by childbearing women. Families should be free to take still pictures and record video and/or audio tapes during labor and birth. Policies restricting cameras are in conflict with the philosophy that the birth experience should be what the woman and her family desire within reason. Concerns about safety, liability, privacy, and space limitations can be adequately addressed without restrictive policies about visitors and use of cameras or filming during labor and birth if care providers are committed to meeting the needs of childbearing women and their support persons.

Learning Needs Assessment

Needs-assessment tools, care paths, or teaching lists can assist nurses and families in identifying learning needs and in documentation of the type and timing of prenatal education (Brown, 2006). A learning-needs assessment can be initiated at various times during the perinatal period depending on when a woman has first contact with the hospital system. Opportunities include prenatal classes, prenatal visits, hospital tours, and telephone contact with a case manager, during admission to the hospital, following birth, and at the mother–infant follow-up visit or contact. Many families attending prenatal classes are first-time parents. A detailed assessment of individual learning needs discussed during the first prenatal class alerts prospective parents to information and skills they need to acquire by the time they are discharged from the hospital. The learning-needs assessment tool or the defined curriculum and supporting written materials document the information, instruction provided, and the skills taught. When a formal needs-assessment tool is used during pregnancy, the tool is forwarded to the perinatal unit from the prenatal instructor to be stored with the woman's prenatal data. Display 10–5 is an example of a learning-needs assessment tool used on admission (if not in active labor) and after birth to assess the woman's knowledge of self-care and baby care, and it then becomes the discharge teaching record. Content with an asterisk is reviewed with all women prior to hospital discharge. Referencing specific content to written materials provides reinforcement and promotes use of materials as a reference for both families and perinatal nurses.

For women who have not attended prenatal classes or completed a learning-needs assessment during a prenatal visit, the process begins on admission to the hospital. With the help of the labor nurse, families identify specific learning needs they want to address during the inpatient stay. Whether the needs assessment is completed prior to admission, during early labor, or after birth, the education process begins as soon as possible for each woman and family.

Primary responsibility for patient and family education varies with the institution. Patient education may be coordinated by the case manager, clinical nurse specialist, or perinatal educator; however, in any practice model, the perinatal staff nurse plays a key role. Critical concepts and essential information that families need have been identified. They are presented regardless of the family's past experience or self-assessment. Critical concepts include the following:

MATERNAL CARE

- Activity and rest
- Pain relief and comfort measures

DISPLAY 10-5

Mother–Baby Discharge Record

M = Mother
S = Significant Other

Please go through the following list and check whether you understand each topic or need to know more.

Please read ...*For Moms and Babies* booklet given to you **after** the birth of your baby.

NURSES MUST DATE & INITIAL

I know this already		Doesn't apply to me		I need to know more			Booklet page #	Mother & family reviewed/ demonstrated	
M	S	M	S	M	S			Date	Initials
						POSTPARTUM			
						Activity – how much is OK	10		*
						Care of perineum and episiotomy	7,8		*
						Postoperative C-section instructions	9		*
						Signs of postpartum complications	11		*
						Changes in vaginal bleeding, return of my period	7		
						Comfort measures for afterpains, constipation and hemorrhoids	7,9		
						Postpartum exercises for the first weeks	8		
						Postpartum "baby blues," depression, hormonal changes	9		
						How to minimize milk production if I'm not nursing			
						BABY CARE			
						What to do if baby is choking or gagging	14		*
						How to do skin care/cord care	14		*
						How to take care of the circumcision or genital area Type: Bell/Gomco	13		*
						How to know if my baby is sick and what to do	21		
						What is jaundice? What to look for: (Recieved Handout) • Increasing yellow color of baby's skin • Poor feeding/lethargy/irritability • Dark urine/light stool	15		
						Use and cleaning of bulb syringe	14,15		*
						How and when to burp baby	17		
						How to position baby after feeding	17		*
						Parents aware to never shake a baby			
						How to complete and obtain a birth certificate			
						BREASTFEEDING			
						I attended Breastfeeding class/watched Breastfeeding video ❑ YES ❑ NO			
						How to position baby for feeding	23		*
						How to get baby to latch onto my nipple properly	23		*
						Removal of baby from my nipple	24		*
						What is the supply and demand concept	23,24		
						When does breast milk come in	25		
						Implications of supplementing for breastfeeding mothers	24		
						Prevention and comfort measures for sore nipples	24		
						Prevention and comfort measures for engorgement	25		
						How to express milk by hand/breast pump	25		
						BOTTLE FEEDING			
						How and when to feed my baby a bottle	16		*
						Reasons for NOT propping bottles	17		
						What formula should my baby drink	16		

STATE LAW REQUIRES USE OF INFANT CAR SEAT. I have a baby/infant car seat and know how to use it.   ❑ YES   ❑ NO

LEARNING EVALUATION   How do you like to learn new information? Check all that may apply.
[ ] Reading material handouts   [ ] Personal demonstration   [ ] Videotapes/TV   [ ] Hearing/audiotapes

Discharge weight ____lb ___oz   Discharge Transcutaneous Bilirubin ____
State Mandated Hearing Screen: Completed___ Refusal Form Signed: ____
__ Pass ___ Fail __ Repeat

Medications:
Mother: None____ Prescriptions:_____

_____
Baby: None____ Prescriptions:_____
Discharge Instructions: _____

Follow-up doctor's appointment:
Mother: Date:_____
Baby: Date:_____ if <48 hrs of age call physician for an appt.
Please call your doctor if you have any questions or concerns.

❑ Patient has physician contact phone numbers.

My discharge instructions have been explained to me and I have received a copy.

Mother Signature:_____

Significant Other Signature (if applicable): _____

Person receiving infant: _____

Discharge Nurse:_____ Date:_____ Time:_____

MOTHER–BABY DISCHARGE RECORD
ST. JOHN'S MERCY MEDICAL CENTER/ST. LOUIS, MO

Your baby is required by law to have testing done prior to discharge from the hospital for metabolic and genetic disorders (Including: PKU/Hypo-Thyroidism/ Galactosemia/Hemoglobin abnormalities). Testing will be done at least 24 hours after the initiation of feeding and prior to discharge. Colostrum is considered to be adequate feeding. Repeat testing will be required if initial testing was collected prior to 24 hours of feeding.
Criteria met - completed Metabolic Screen on: Date_____Time_____
(Repeat Not Needed)

Initial criteria not met - Repeat needed _____
Written physician order must accompany the baby at time of repeat collection and certain insurance companies may need pre-authorization. Bring your baby to the admitting lab on 2L (next to the escalators). The repeat metabolic test will require registration which will generate a fee for the service. Appropriate insurance information is necessary. The estimated time for the process is 1 hour. No appointment is necessary. For specific hours call 569-6814.

Nurses Signature(s) and Initials	

PATIENT IDENTIFICATION

- Care of the perineum and care of lacerations or episiotomy
- Breast care for breastfeeding women and lactation suppression for women who are formula feeding
- Postoperative cesarean birth instructions
- Expected emotional adaptations
- Signs of postpartum complications to report to the nurse in the hospital or to the healthcare provider after discharge

Newborn Care

- Newborn adaptation to extrauterine life: need to be held, need for thermoregulation, need for comfort
- Newborn feeding cues
- Breastfeeding basics
- Formula feeding basics
- Care of an infant who is spitting up or choking
- Use of the bulb syringe
- Umbilical cord care
- Circumcision care and care of the uncircumcised penis
- Position for sleep: Back to Sleep campaign to reduce the risk of sudden infant death syndrome (SIDS)
- Information about immunizations and newborn screening tests
- Signs of newborn complications to report to the nurse in the hospital or to the healthcare provider after discharge and contact telephone numbers
- Safe use of infant and child car seats
- Appointment made for follow-up clinic or home visit offered by the hospital or community nursing agency
- When to schedule the first mother and newborn visits with their primary care provider

Written materials provided to the woman and her family should contain information about all critical concepts. Some institutions have adopted interactive documentation forms signed by the mother and the nurse providing the education (Brown, 2006; Roudebush, Kaufman, Johnson, Abraham, & Clayton, 2006).

Before discharge, knowledge and skills about self- and infant care are validated. Validation can be accomplished by discussion with the new mother during which understanding is verbalized or by demonstration of critical skills such as feeding, sleeping position, or umbilical cord care. No one method of validation is superior; rather, nurses in each institution can develop a system with enough flexibility to meet the needs of the population served. Validation ensures that women who indicate they need no additional information are, in reality, prepared and knowledgeable. The goal is for all women to verbalize understanding or demonstrate skills related to all critical concepts. Women with special needs, who have not demonstrated knowledge of critical concepts or have

not acquired the skills to care for themselves or their infants are referred for follow-up support and care. Referrals are made to the clinical nurse specialist, lactation consultant, social worker, dietician, and/or home care agency. Follow-up contacts to ensure that the critical concepts have been learned and to verify the woman can safely care for her infant and herself can occur at a clinic or home visit, during a phone assessment, through involvement in support groups and community programs, or at healthcare provider office visits. Assessment of maternal knowledge and skills is documented on the discharge teaching record or other appropriate medical record form.

ANATOMIC AND PHYSIOLOGIC CHANGES DURING THE POSTPARTUM PERIOD

Perinatal nurses should have knowledge of normal anatomical and physiologic changes that occur during the postpartum period in order to plan comprehensive assessments and interventions for new mothers. Many changes are apparent immediately after birth and require inpatient nursing assessment and intervention. However, over the course of the first 12 weeks postpartum, there are ongoing alterations as the woman's body returns to nearly its prepregnant state.

Uterus

Involution results from a decrease in myometrial cell size, not in the number of myometrial cells. This decrease is the result of ischemia, autolysis, and phagocytosis. Ischemia occurs when the retraction of uterine musculature necessary for hemostasis after placental separation results in decreased blood flow to the uterus. Proteolytic enzymes are released, and macrophages migrate to the uterus, resulting in autolysis or self-digestion and subsequent reduction in myometrial cell size. Some of the excess elastic and fibrous tissue is removed by phagocytosis, but the incomplete process results in a uterus that does not return to its nulliparous size. Within 24 hours, the uterus is approximately the size it was at 20 weeks' gestation (Resnik, 2004). Immediately after birth, the uterus weighs approximately 1,000 g (2 lb, 4 oz). As involution occurs, the uterine weight continues to decrease to 500 g (1 week), 300 g (2 weeks), and by 6 weeks postpartum, it weighs 100 g or less. Immediately after birth, the uterine fundus can be palpated midway between the umbilicus and symphysis pubis. During the first 12 hours after birth, the muscles relax slightly, and the fundus returns to the level of the umbilicus. Beginning on postpartum Day 2 or 3, the usual progression of uterine descent into the pelvis is 1 centimeter (cm) per day (Display 10–6).

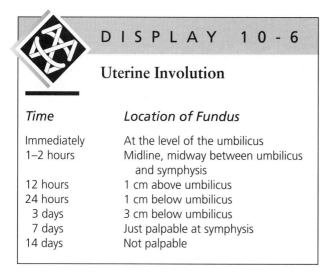

Time	Location of Fundus
Immediately	At the level of the umbilicus
1–2 hours	Midline, midway between umbilicus and symphysis
12 hours	1 cm above umbilicus
24 hours	1 cm below umbilicus
3 days	3 cm below umbilicus
7 days	Just palpable at symphysis
14 days	Not palpable

During the first few days after birth, oxytocin secretion causes strong uterine contractions and a further reduction in size, especially after breastfeeding and in multiparas. Multiparity, multiple gestation, polyhydramnios, and bladder distention can influence uterine size and the progression of uterine involution.

Placental Site and Lochia

The placenta separates spontaneously from the uterus within 15 minutes of birth in 90% of women and within 30 minutes after birth in 95% of women. Separation of the placenta and membranes includes the spongy layer of the endometrium, leaving the decidua basalis in the uterus. This remaining layer reorganizes into basal and superficial layers. The superficial layer becomes necrotic and is sloughed in the lochia, and the basal layer becomes the source of new endometrium. The endometrium is regenerated by 2 to 3 weeks after birth, except at the site of placental attachment (Blackburn, 2003; Cunningham et al.,

2005; Resnik, 2004). Immediately after delivery of the placenta, the placental site is approximately 8 to 10 cm, and by end of the second week, it is about 3 to 4 cm. Exfoliation, the process of placental site healing, occurs over the first 6 weeks after birth by necrotic sloughing of the infarcted superficial tissues. A reparative process follows in which the endometrium regenerates from the margins and base. This process prevents the formation of a fibrous scar in the decidua. At 7 to 14 days postpartum, the infarcted superficial tissue over the placental site sloughs. At this time, the woman may notice an episode of increased vaginal bleeding, which is usually self-limited. Bleeding lasting more than 1 to 2 hours should be evaluated for late postpartum hemorrhage. Ultrasonography can be useful in determining the presence of retained placental tissue (Bowes & Thorp, 2004).

Lochia is the postpartum uterine discharge. Although lochia varies in amount, the total volume lost usually is 150 to 400 mL. Initially, lochia rubra is reddish and continues 3 to 4 days. Lochia serosa, a pinkish discharge, continues from Day 4 to Day 10. Lochia alba, a yellow-white discharge, follows lochia serosa (Table 10–1). The choice of feeding method for the baby and the use of oral contraceptives do not affect duration of lochia (Cunningham et al., 2005).

Cervix, Vagina, and Pelvic Floor

The cervix and lower uterine segment are thin and flaccid immediately postpartum. Cervical lacerations can occur during any birth; however, women with precipitous labor and operative procedures are at increased risk for lacerations. At 2 to 3 days, the cervix has resumed its customary appearance but remains dilated 2 to 3 cm. By the end of the first week, the cervical os narrows to a diameter of 1 cm. The external cervical os remains wider than its pregravid state, and bilateral depressions typically are seen at the site of lacerations. Cervical edema

TABLE 10–1 ■ TYPES OF LOCHIA			
	Rubra	**Serosa**	**Alba**
Normal Color	Red	Pink, brown tinged	Yellowish-white
Normal Duration	1 to 3 days	3 to 10 days	10 to 14 days, but not abnormal to last longer
Normal Discharge	Bloody with clots; fleshing odor; increased flow on standing or breastfeeding, or during physical activity	Serosanguineous (blood and mucus) consistency; fleshy odor	Mostly mucus, no strong odor
Abnormal Discharge	Foul smell; numerous and/or large clots; quickly saturates perineal pad	Foul smell; quickly saturates perineal pad	Foul smell; saturates perineal pad; reappearance of pink or red lochia; discharge lasts far too long (past 4 weeks)

may persist for several months (Resnik, 2004; Cunningham et al., 2005). The vagina and vaginal outlet are smooth walled and may appear bruised early in the puerperium. The apparent bruising, caused by pelvic congestion, disappears quickly after birth. Rugae reappear in the distended vagina by the third week. The voluntary muscles and supports of the pelvic floor gradually regain tone during the first 6 weeks postpartum. These changes occur in response to the reduced amount of circulating progesterone. For some women, vaginal tone may be improved by perineal tightening exercises, such as Kegel exercises (Ladewig, London, & Davidson, 2006; Weber & Richter, 2005). In the lactating woman, the hypoestrogenic state resulting from ovarian suppression may cause the vagina to appear pale and without rugae. This may result in dyspareunia.

Ovarian Function and Return of Menses

Although the return of menses and ovulation vary, the first menstrual period usually occurs within 7 to 9 weeks postpartum in non-nursing mothers. There are great variations in the return of menses for women who are nursing because of depressed estrogen levels. In nursing mothers, menstruation usually returns between months 2 and 18.

Estrogen and progesterone levels decrease suddenly after placental delivery. For the first 2 to 3 weeks after birth, there is minimal gonadotropin activity, possibly because of a transient pituitary insensitivity to luteinizing hormone–releasing factor. As sensitivity returns, hormonal function returns to normal levels. The first menstrual cycle is usually anovulatory, but 25% of women may ovulate before menstruation. The mean for the return of ovulation is 10 weeks postpartum for women who are not lactating and approximately 17 weeks postpartum for women who are breastfeeding. The delay in the resumption of menses in lactating women in part may result from elevated prolactin levels (Resnik, 2004; Cunningham et al., 2005).

Metabolic Changes

Prolactin, a pituitary hormone, is responsible for stimulating and sustaining lactation. Like estrogen and progesterone, prolactin levels decrease with placental delivery, although they remain elevated over nonpregnant levels. The decrease in estrogen and progesterone stimulates the anterior pituitary to produce prolactin. Between the third and fourth week postpartum, the prolactin level returns to normal in women who formula feed their infants. For those who breastfeed, prolactin levels increase with each nursing episode (Resnik, 2004).

Thyroid function returns to prepregnant levels within 4 to 6 weeks after birth. Because immunosuppression is a normal physiologic consequence of pregnancy, there is an increased risk of developing transient autoimmune thyroiditis, followed by hypothyroidism. This depression of thyroid function may cause depression, carelessness, and impairment of memory and concentration. There is a slightly increased risk of recurrence of autoimmune hypothyroidism or hyperthyroidism postpartum (Nader, 2004; Cunningham et al., 2005).

Low levels of placental lactogen, estrogen, cortisol, growth hormone, and the placental enzyme insulinase, reduce their anti-insulin effect in the early puerperium. This results in lower glucose levels for women during this period and a reduction in insulin requirements for insulin-dependent diabetic women (Cunningham et al., 2005). Breastfeeding may precipitate hypoglycemic episodes in women with insulin-dependent diabetes. Women with gestational diabetes often have normal glucose levels immediately postpartum. Nutritional needs must be reassessed during this period. The basal metabolic rate (BMR) increases 20% to 25% during pregnancy because of fetal metabolic activity. The BMR remains elevated for 7 to 14 days after giving birth.

The first 2 hours postpartum, plasma renin and angiotensin II levels (involved in blood pressure maintenance) fall to normal, nonpregnant levels and then rise again and remain elevated for up to 14 days (Roberts, 2004). Blood pressure should remain stable during the postpartum period, but lowered vascular resistance in the pelvis may result in orthostatic hypotension when a woman moves from a supine to a sitting position. An increase in blood pressure, especially if accompanied by headaches or visual changes, may indicate postpartum preeclampsia and should be evaluated. In the past, an incremental increase of 30 mm Hg systolic or 15 mm Hg diastolic above baseline values was used as diagnostic criteria. This is no longer recommended, as research shows those women are not likely to have adverse outcomes; however, patients with blood pressure increases should be closely observed, especially if the blood pressure is above 140/90 on two or more occasions at least 6 hours apart (Roberts, 2004; Cunningham et al., 2005).

Kidneys and Bladder

Mild proteinuria (1+) may exist for 1 to 2 days after birth in 40% to 50% of women. Nonpathology can be assumed only in the absence of the symptoms of infection or preeclampsia (Atterbury, Groome, Hoff, & Yarnell, 1998).

If a urine specimen is necessary, it should be obtained through catheterization or as a clean-catch technique. These methods avoid contamination by protein-laden lochia (Gilbert & Harmon, 2005). Glycosuria of pregnancy disappears, and creatinine clearance is usually normal by 1 week postpartum. Pregnancy-induced hypotonia and dilation of the ureters and renal pelves return to the prepregnant state by 8 weeks postpartum. The catabolic process of involution causes an increase of the blood urea nitrogen (BUN). By the end of the first week postpartum, the BUN level rises to values of 20 mg/dL, compared with 15 mg/dL in the late third trimester (Resnik, 2004; Cunningham et al., 2005). Glomerular filtration rate, renal blood flow, and plasma creatinine return to normal levels by 6 weeks postpartum.

Labor may result in displacement of the urinary bladder and stretching of the urethra. Other factors that interfere with normal micturition include the numbing effect of anesthesia and the temporary neural dysfunction of the traumatized bladder. These may cause decreased sensitivity. As a result, overdistention and incomplete emptying may occur. Signs of bladder distention include uterine atony reflected in increased lochia, displacement of the uterus to the right and significantly above the umbilicus, decreased urine output compared with oral and intravenous intake, and a "soft fullness," sometimes with a palpable margin, in the suprapubic area. Normal postpartum diuresis combined with the often large amount of intravenous fluids administered during labor can result in bladder filling in a relatively short time. The woman should be encouraged to void as soon as possible after birth to avoid bladder filling, which can inhibit uterine contraction, thus predisposing to postpartum hemorrhage. Assistance to the bathroom or on a bedpan may be helpful in facilitating bladder emptying. Women may report an urge but inability to urinate. Spontaneous voiding, however, should resume by 6 to 8 hours after birth, and bladder tone usually returns to normal levels 5 to 7 days later. Each voiding should be at least 150 mL. Edema, hyperemia, and submucous extravasation of blood are frequently evident in the bladder postpartum (Resnick, 2004; Cunningham et al., 2005). The effects of trauma from labor on the bladder and urethra diminish during the first 24 hours, unless a urinary tract infection is present. Some women may require in-and-out catheterization to empty their bladder in the immediate postpartum period. Avoid rapid emptying of the bladder if catheterization is performed. No more than 800 mL of urine should be removed at one time. This can avoid a precipitous drop in intraabdominal pressure, which may result in splenetic engorgement and hypotension.

Stress Incontinence

Many women report transient stress incontinence during the first 6 weeks postpartum. Although there are conflicting data on the effect of vaginal birth on future urinary status, some researchers have estimated that two vaginal births increase the risk of developing urinary incontinence twofold, and increase the risk of surgery for pelvic organ prolapse eightfold (Schaffer et al., 2005). Other researchers have suggested that pregnancy itself may be a predisposing factor for urinary incontinence and pelvic organ prolapse, thus cesarean birth may not be protective against these conditions (Nygaard, 2006; Richter, 2006). Persistent stress incontinence may result from pregnancy, labor, operative birth, a large baby, and perineal tissue damage. The influences of obstetric factors diminish over 3 months. The length of the second stage of labor, infant head size, birth weight, and episiotomy correlate with the development of postpartum stress incontinence (Casey et al., 2005). Impairment of muscle function near and surrounding the urethra underlies stress incontinence. Prompt catheterization for urinary retention during the postpartum can prevent urinary difficulties (Cunningham et al., 2005). Schaffer et al. (2005) suggest that the pelvic floor is exposed to compression and extreme pressures during vaginal delivery and maternal expulsive efforts. Uncoached (non-Valsalva) pushing, a response to the urge to push, is characterized by several short bearing-down efforts per contraction with breath holding for 6 to 8 seconds. In contrast, coached pushing begins as soon as a contraction is noted by the coach, and the mother is urged to push for 10 seconds, take a deep breath, and push again. Therefore, coached pushing could potentially increase the pressure on the pelvic floor with subsequent deleterious effects. See Chapter 7 for a comprehensive discussion of second-stage pushing techniques that can minimize risk of injuries to the perineum and pelvic floor. Knowledge about clinical factors implicated in stress incontinence allows anticipatory guidance and interventions for women at risk.

Fluid Balance and Electrolytes

The physiologic reversal of the extracellular or interstitial fluid accumulated during a normal pregnancy begins during the immediate postpartum period. Diuresis begins within 12 hours after birth and continues up to 5 days. Diuresis occurs in response to the decrease in estrogen that stimulated fluid retention during pregnancy, the reduction of venous pressure in the lower half of the body, and the decrease in residual hypervolemia (Cunningham et al., 2005). Urine output may be 3,000 mL or more each day. Additional fluid is lost through increased perspiration. Diuresis results in a decrease in body weight of 2 to 3 kg. Electrolyte levels return to nonpregnant homeostasis by 21 days or earlier. Fluid loss is greater in women who have experienced preeclampsia or eclampsia. By the third postpartum day, resolution of the vasoconstriction and additional extracellular fluid of gestational hypertension contribute to significant expansion of the vascular volume (Cunningham et al., 2005).

Neurologic Changes

Discomfort and fatigue are common concerns after birth. Afterpains or painful uterine contractions during the first 2 to 3 days after birth; discomfort associated with episiotomy, incisions, lacerations, or tears; muscle aches; and breast engorgement may contribute to a woman's discomfort during the postpartum period. Neurologic changes related to anesthesia and analgesia are transient and, if present, require attention to ensure the woman's safety. Deep tendon reflexes remain normal. Sleep disturbances contributing to fatigue are related to discomfort and the demands of newborn care. The presence of children or a lack of social support may limit the time available for rest. Natural or pharmacologic comfort measures should be offered. Psychosocial support is necessary, and referral to home-care nursing may be appropriate.

The carpal tunnel syndrome that results from compression of the median nerve by the physiologic edema of pregnancy is relieved by postpartum diuresis. Headaches may result from fluid shifts in the first week after birth, leakage of cerebrospinal fluid into the extradural space during spinal anesthesia, fluid and electrolyte imbalance, gestational hypertension, or stress. Assessment of the quality and location of the headache and of the vital signs are necessary. Interventions such as environmental control of lighting, noise levels, and visitors and administration of analgesic medications may be effective for nonpathologic headaches. Postpartum eclampsia (ie, seizures beginning >48 hours and <4 weeks after birth) is often preceded by severe headache or visual disturbances. Women may have a postpartum eclamptic seizure without a prenatal diagnosis of preeclampsia or hypertension. Because women may experience prodromal signs and symptoms after discharge from the hospital, information should be provided about these subjective signs and symptoms, which include a severe and persistent occipital headache, scotomata (ie, spots before the eyes), blurred vision, photophobia, and epigastric or right upper-quadrant pain. Women should be encouraged to notify their primary healthcare provider if any of these symptoms develop to facilitate immediate evaluation.

Hemodynamic Changes

Changes in the cardiovascular system occur early in the postpartum period, with a variable rate of return to baseline levels that ranges from 6 to 12 weeks. Blood volume changes occur rapidly. Autotransfusion occurs as a result of elimination of blood flow to the placenta. The blood flow of 500 to 750 mL per minute, formerly flowing to the uteroplacental unit, is diverted to maternal systemic venous circulation immediately after birth. The blood loss with an uncomplicated vaginal birth is approximately 500 and 1,000 mL, or more with a cesarean birth. Plasma volume is diminished by approximately 1,000 mL as a result of blood loss and diuresis. By the third day postpartum, blood volume has decreased 16% from peak pregnancy levels and returns to nearly prepregnant levels by 1 to 2 weeks postpartum.

Cardiac output after birth depends on use and choice of anesthesia or analgesia, mode of birth, blood loss, and maternal position. Cardiac output peaks immediately after birth to approximately 80% above the prelabor value in women who have received only local anesthesia. After reaching a maximum value at 10 to 15 minutes after birth, cardiac output begins to decline, reaching prelabor values approximately 1 hour postpartum, although it remains elevated for 48 hours after birth (Blackburn, 2003; Resnick, 2004). It returns to prepregnant levels by 2 to 3 weeks after birth. Because the heart rate is stable or slightly decreased, the cardiac output is most likely caused by an increased stroke volume from venous return. Cesarean birth before labor onset avoids the hemodynamic effect of contractions but not the rise in cardiac output immediately postpartum. It is thought that epidural anesthesia during labor moderates the increase in cardiac output after birth by decreasing pain and anxiety (Cunningham et al., 2005; Resnik, 2004).

The pulse rate remains stable or decreases slightly after birth. If the pulse rate is above 100, the woman should be assessed for infection or delayed postpartum hemorrhage. Some women may exhibit puerperal bradycardia, with a pulse rate of 40 to 50 beats per minute. No conclusive proof has been given for this phenomenon. Orthostatic hypotension may occur when a woman sits up from a reclining position. Preeclampsia should be suspected if blood pressure values are 140/90 on two or more occasions at least 6 hours apart.

Hematologic and Liver Changes

The decrease in plasma volume is greater than the loss of red blood cells after birth, causing an increase in the hematocrit between day 3 and day 7. The hematocrit returns to normal levels 4 to 8 weeks later as red blood cells reach the end of their normal life span (Cunningham et al., 2005; Kilpatrick & Laros, 2004; Monga, 2004). In assessing postpartum laboratory values, a 1- to 1.5-g decrease in hemoglobin levels or 2- to 3-point decrease in the hematocrit value reflects a 500-mL blood loss. During the first 48 hours after birth, the physiologic reversal of the extracellular fluid accumulated during a normal pregnancy and intravenous fluids given during labor make accurate blood loss assessment difficult, because hemodilution occurs as this fluid enters the vascular system. This phenomenon is seen even in women who have lost 20% of their circulating blood volume during birth. Hemoconcentration may occur with minimal blood loss if a woman has preexisting polycythemia (AWHONN & Johnson and Johnson Consumer Products, 2006; Cunningham et al., 2005; Monga, 2004).

Normal serum iron levels are regained by the second week postpartum. A relative erythrocytosis is seen in women who have received iron supplementation during pregnancy and had an average blood loss during the birth process. In the absence of iron supplementation, iron deficiency develops in most women (Abrams, Minassian, & Pickett, 2004; Cunningham et al., 2005). The serum ferritin level correlates closely with the body's iron stores and is predictive of iron deficiency anemia (Abrams, Minassian, & Pickett, 2004; Cunningham et al., 2005). Changes in blood coagulation factors remain for variable periods postpartum. Plasma fibrinogen levels and sedimentation rate levels remain elevated for at least the first week.

Leukocytosis from the stress of labor and birth is seen in the postpartum period. A nonpathologic white blood cell (WBC) count may reach 25,000/μL to 30,000/μL, with the increase predominantly granulocytes. Relative lymphopenia (ie, lymphocyte deficiency) and absolute eosinopenia (ie, decreased eosinophils) may also be seen. This phenomenon, coupled with the increase in the sedimentation rate, may confuse the interpretation or assessment of infections during this period. Pathology should be suspected, and further evaluation is indicated when the WBCs increase 30% over a 6-hour period (AWHONN & Johnson and Johnson Consumer Products, 2006; Cunningham et al., 2005: Kilpatrick & Laros, 2004).

The alterations in liver enzymes and lipids that occurred in response to increased estrogen levels and hemodilution during pregnancy are reversed and returned to normal levels within 3 weeks postpartum. Elevated levels of free fatty acids, cholesterol, triglycerides, and lipoproteins seen during pregnancy return to normal levels within 10 days. Alkaline phosphatase, derived from the placenta, liver, and bone during pregnancy, may remain elevated for 6 weeks. The previously atonic gallbladder demonstrates increased contractility as progesterone levels decrease (Cunningham et al., 2005; Landon, 2004).

Respiratory and Acid–Base Changes

The respiratory system quickly returns to its prepregnant state after the birth of the baby. These changes result from the decrease in progesterone levels, the decrease in intraabdominal pressure that accompanies emptying of the uterus, and the increased excursion of the diaphragm. This reduction of diaphragmatic pressure results in the immediate return of chest wall compliance to normal levels and partially relieves the dyspnea experienced during pregnancy. Residual volume (ie, amount of air remaining in the lung after maximum expiration)

and tidal volume (ie, volume of air inhaled and exhaled during each breath) normalize soon after birth; the expiratory reserve volume (ie, maximum amount of air that can be exhaled), however, may remain in the abnormal range for several months. Vital capacity, inspiratory capacity, and maximum breathing capacity decrease after birth. The response to exercise may therefore be affected in the early postpartum weeks (Cunningham et al., 2005; Whittey & Dombrowski, 2004).

Length and severity of the second stage of labor appear to contribute to an "oxygen debt" (ie, extra oxygen required after strenuous exercise) that extends into the immediate postpartum period (Cunningham et al., 2005; Whittey & Dombrowski, 2004). The basal metabolic rate remains elevated for 7 to 14 days into the postpartum period and is attributable to mild anemia, lactation, and psychologic factors.

As progesterone levels fall, the $PaCO_2$ rises to the normal prepregnant values (35 to 40 mm Hg) within the first 2 days after birth. During the postpartum period, the PaO_2 should be normal at 95% or higher. Normal levels of pH and base excess gradually return by approximately 3 weeks postpartum.

Skin, Muscle, and Weight Changes

Overdistention of the abdominal wall as a result of pregnancy can rupture collagen fibers of the dermis, resulting in striae, which can occur also on the breasts, buttocks, and thighs. Striae eventually become irregular white lines. Diastasis (ie, separation) of the rectus muscles is common, and usually is re-approximated by the late postpartum period. Evidence of diastasis can be assessed by asking the woman to lift her head while lying in a supine position. If diastasis has occurred, a tent-like protrusion in the lower abdomen is noticeable. Abdominal binders are not recommended, and mild exercise to restore tone may be started after 1 to 2 weeks. The joint instability that occurred during pregnancy may not resolve until 6 to 8 weeks postpartum.

A woman loses an average of 12 pounds (5.5 kg) at birth. Additional weight is lost between 2 weeks and 6 months postpartum, especially if the woman is breast-feeding (Cunningham et al., 2005). Women who choose formula feeding can expect a 0.5 to 1 kg/week loss when eating a balanced diet containing slightly fewer calories than their usual daily expenditure. Weight loss occurs more rapidly in women of lower parity, age, and prepregnancy weight.

Gastrointestinal Changes

After birth, there is a decrease in gastrointestinal muscle tone and motility. When these changes are coupled with relaxation of abdominal muscles, gaseous distention can occur during the first 2 to 3 days postpartum. Decreased motility can result in postpartum ileus. Constipation may result from hemorrhoids, perineal trauma, dehydration, pain, fear of having a bowel movement, immobility, and medication (ie, magnesium sulfate antenatally for tocolysis, iron supplementation, codeine for pain, anesthetics during labor or surgery). Constipation can be minimized by encouraging the woman to drink adequate fluids and eat foods high in fiber. Hemorrhoids that develop during pregnancy may increase in size during labor and result in significant discomfort during the postpartum period. If the woman has hemorrhoids, suggesting warm or cold sitz baths and applying topical anesthetics can decrease discomfort. Stool softeners and laxatives are sometimes given. Bowel movements typically resume 2 to 3 days after birth, and normal bowel elimination patterns resume by 2 weeks postpartum.

Hernias and Perineal, Pelvic Floor and Anal Sphincter Damage

Genital hernias (eg, cystocele, rectocele, uterine prolapse, enterocele) may occur because of overstretching or tearing of the muscles or fascia during birth. There is limited evidence that women who perform perineal massage, beginning at 35 weeks' gestation, are less likely to have perineal trauma (episiotomy or tears) that requires suturing in association with vaginal birth (Beckmann & Garrett, 2006). Controversy exists regarding the use of episiotomy. Some practitioners recommend minimizing the use of midline episiotomy and using mediolateral episiotomy when the risk for extension is increased (eg, macrosomia, shallow perineal body, operative vaginal birth), but there is little supportive evidence for that practice (Christianson, et al., 2005). Episiotomy does not always prevent third- or fourth-degree lacerations. Risk factors for lacerations include nulliparity, second-stage labor arrest, persistent occiput posterior positions, forceps assistance, and use of vacuum extractors. Routine episiotomy is not recommended by ACOG (2006a; see Chapter 7 for an in-depth discussion of episiotomy).

Obstetric trauma such as injury to the sphincter muscle or damage to the innervation of the pelvic floor is a leading cause of anal incontinence in healthy women (Eason, Lebrecque, Marcoux, & Mondor, 2002; Garcia, Rogers, Kim, Hall, & Kammerer-Doak, 2005). Other associations with anal incontinence include prolonged second-stage labor, macrosomia, labor augmentation, and episiotomy (Boreham et al., 2005; Casey et al., 2005). One-half of women with third-degree tears experience anal incontinence. Abramov et al. (2005) report no increased risk for fecal or flatal incontinence in women following forceps-assisted birth. Disturbances in bowel function (ie, fecal urgency and anal incontinence of stool and flatus) from mechanical or neurologic injury to the anal sphincter during vaginal birth may also be the result of damage from the large size of the baby's head in relation to the vaginal opening. Women who experience a third- or fourth-degree perineal laceration report a greater incidence of incontinence of flatus than those without anal sphincter rupture. Women with a long second-stage of labor, a large newborn, or both have the greatest risk of nerve damage (Cunningham et al., 2005; Pollack et al., 2004).

Embarrassment may prevent women from reporting symptoms of anal sphincter damage. Symptoms may disappear or worsen with time. An accurate history is helpful so that women with major sphincter defects can be offered a cesarean birth when appropriate. Aging, menopause, progression of neuropathy, and effects of subsequent births may contribute to long-term sphincter weakness.

Fluid and Nutritional Needs

After vaginal birth, there are no dietary restrictions for women without underlying medical conditions or pregnancy-induced complications. Oral fluids or intravenous fluid administration helps restore the balance altered by fluid loss during the labor and birth process. Women should be encouraged to drink 3,000 mL of water and other liquids every 24 hours. Nurses should encourage healthy food choices with respect for ethnic and cultural preferences. Snack trays should be available for women who give birth when regular food service is unavailable. After cesarean birth, women usually receive clear liquids until bowel sounds are present and then advance to solid foods. For each 20 mL of breast milk produced, the woman must consume an additional 30 calories. This results in a dietary increase of 500 to 1,000 calories each day for women who are maintaining body weight (Lawrence & Lawrence, 2004). By 6 weeks postpartum, decreased pressure and distortion of the stomach from the gravid uterus and the normalization of lower esophageal sphincter pressure and tone resolves the heartburn experienced by many pregnant women.

Immediate Postpartum Period

During the immediate postpartum period, the perinatal nurse focuses on maternal and newborn stabilization and recovery from the birth process. Maternal–newborn attachment and breastfeeding (if the woman desires) should be promoted and encouraged (Fig. 10–1 and Fig. 10–2). Nursing assessments and interventions should occur concurrently with activities celebrating the joy of childbirth and welcoming the new baby into the family. Family and visitor interactions, including holding the new baby and taking video and still pictures of the first hours of life, should be supported as much as possible based on the condition of the mother and newborn. Every effort should be made to accommodate the wishes of the woman and her family.

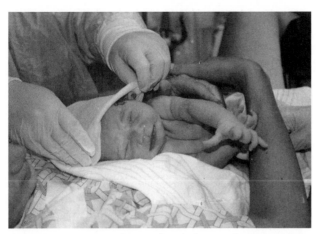

FIGURE 10–1. Promoting mother–baby attachment at birth.

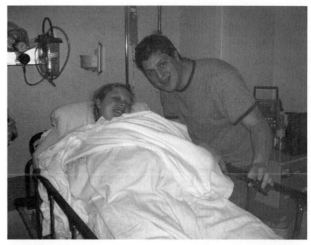

FIGURE 10–3. Support person with mother in the OB PACU.

When regional analgesia or anesthesia or general anesthesia has been used for vaginal or cesarean birth, the woman should be observed in an appropriately staffed and equipped labor–delivery–recovery room or postanesthesia care unit until she has recovered from the anesthetic (AAP & ACOG, 2002; American Society of Anesthesiologists [ASA], 2006). The patient's desires for support persons to be with her during the postanesthesia care period should be honored as much as possible. At a minimum at least one support person should be encouraged and allowed (Fig. 10–3). The woman should be discharged from postanesthesia care only at the discretion of and after communication among the attending physician or a certified nurse midwife, anesthesiologist, and certified registered nurse anesthetist (AAP & ACOG, 2002; ASA, 2006). See Chapter 7 for an in-depth discussion of postanesthesia care.

According to the wishes and condition of the woman, she and the newborn should be kept together as much as possible during the inpatient stay. Most perinatal units have models of care that support maternal–newborn

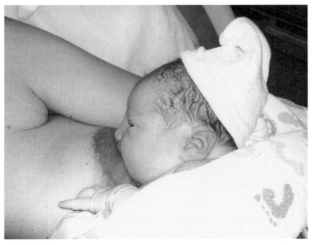

FIGURE 10–2. Promoting breastfeeding immediately after birth.

attachment. Mother–baby or couplet care in which one nurse is responsible for both patients facilitates optimal interaction between the mother and baby and coordination of appropriate nursing assessments and interventions. Opportunities for rest for the new mother should be promoted, although this may be challenging for the nurse because of the number of congratulatory telephone calls and visitors and because of the unit routines that interrupt sleep. Nursing care should be planned so that necessary interventions and medication administration (if needed) can be grouped together, minimizing the need to wake the woman during daytime naps or during the night. A plan for rest designed collaboratively with the new mother and her family works well. Ambulation as soon as the mother feels able should be encouraged, but the woman should be instructed not to get out of bed on her own without assistance the first time after birth (AAP & ACOG, 2002). In the absence of complications or surgical recovery, a regular diet should be resumed as soon as the woman desires. Education for the new mother and her family about maternal postpartum care and newborn care should focus on easing the transition from hospital to home.

During the immediate postpartum period, maternal blood pressure and pulse should be monitored at least every 15 minutes for the first hour or more often as indicated (AAP & ACOG, 2002). Most institutions have protocols that include comprehensive maternal assessments at least every 15 minutes for the first hour, then every 30 minutes for 1 hour, and then every 4 hours (or more frequently if complications are present) for 12 to 24 hours. If the mother is stable, some institutions defer the 4-hour assessments after the first 12 hours when the mother is sleeping. There are no data from prospective clinical trials to determine how often maternal status should be assessed during the postpartum period to promote safety and optimal outcomes. Each institution should develop protocols that are reasonable and based on the condition of the mother. A sample medical form for documentation of the immediate postpartum assessment is included in Chapter 7, Appendix 7B. The following clinical parameters are included in a comprehensive assessment during the immediate postpartum period:

- Assess blood pressure and pulse (AAP & ACOG, 2002).
- Assess the uterine fundus for tone and position. Uterine massage is indicated if the uterus is not firmly contracted.
- Support the lower uterine segment during massage to prevent uterine prolapse or inversion (Fig. 10–4). Uterine inversion is an obstetric emergency associated with hemorrhage and shock.
- Assess the amount of lochia on perineal pad and under buttocks.
- Assess the condition of the perineum.
- Assess the condition of episiotomy after assisting the woman into lateral position with upper leg flexed; use the acronym REEDA (*redness*, *edema*, *ecchymosis*, *discharge*, *approximation* of edges of episiotomy) to guide assessment.
- Assess the temperature at least every 4 hours (AAP & ACOG).
- Decisions about postanesthesia status and readiness for discharge from the recovery area are made at the discretion of the attending physician, nurse midwife, anesthesiologist, or certified registered nurse anesthetist (AAP & ACOG; ASA, 2006).

Pain Management

Pain during the postpartum period may be caused by the episiotomy, lacerations, perineal trauma, incisions, uterine contractions after birth, hemorrhoids, breast engorgement, and nipple tenderness. Nursing assessments, such as fundal assessment, may also result in discomfort. Some strategies can reduce the level of discomfort. After cesarean birth, pain may be related to the incision and intestinal gas. Pain causes stress and interferes with the woman's ability to interact with and care for her infant. Evidence for the effectiveness of topically applied local anesthetics for treating perineal pain is not compelling (Hedayati, Parsons, & Crowther, 2005). However, alternative methods, such as crushed ice in freezer-strength zip-lock plastic bags wrapped in a washcloth, work just as well at less cost (Simpson & Knox, 1999).

The following interventions are included in a comprehensive assessment during the immediate postpartum period:

- Ask about type and severity of pain.
- Explain rationale for uterine massage and periodic assessments. Encourage slow, deep breathing during the assessment.

- Gentle palpation with warm hands can enhance comfort and encourage participation in the procedure.
- Apply ice pack to perineum during first 24 to 48 hours to reduce edema (some women may prefer an ice pack to the perineum intermittently for more than 48 hours); apply moist heat (ie, sitz bath) after 24 hours to increase circulation and promote healing.
- Administer analgesic medication as ordered.
- Women who have cesarean birth may or may not require uterine massage to stimulate uterine contraction. If the amount of lochia indicates excessive bleeding, combine palpation and pain-management measures. If pain management is inadequate, additional pain medication, reassurance, and comfort measures may be helpful after necessary procedures.
- Gas pains can be relieved by ambulation, rocking in a rocking chair, and avoiding gas-forming foods and carbonated beverages.

Psychosocial Status

Ongoing assessment of the psychosocial status should be personalized during the postpartum period to promote the development of healthy mother–infant relationships and maternal confidence (AAP & ACOG, 2002).

The following interventions are included in a comprehensive assessment during the immediate postpartum period:

- Determine the level of emotional lability and level of social support.
- Identify actual and potential sources of support.
- Assess the fatigue level.
- Ascertain educational needs and the level of confidence.
- Assess the teaching needs based on interview and observation.
- Use interactions with mothers as potential teaching moments.
- Use assessment of the fundus as an opportunity to provide information about involution.
- During perineal care, explain cleansing the vulva from front to back to avoid contamination, changing the pad at least four times each day or after each voiding or bowel movement, and washing hands before and after changing pads.
- Use bathing of the newborn at mother's bedside as an opportunity to discuss basic techniques of newborn care such as feeding, clothing, holding, and safety.

- Assess the interaction with the newborn and attachment behaviors.
  - Note whether the mother looks directly at the infant and maintains eye contact (ie, en face position).
  - Note whether the mother touches and talks to the infant.
  - Note whether the mother interprets the infant's behaviors positively.
- Provide an early opportunity to hold infant after birth, and keep the infant with the parents as much as possible.
- Ensure flexibility in visiting policies and opportunities for privacy.
- Demonstrate acceptance of expression of maternal feelings and reinforce parenting behaviors.
- Be a role model for infant-care activities.
- Assist parents in interpreting infant cues.
- Offer appropriate educational materials (ie, consider age, educational level, and resources).
- Identify risk factors for parenting (ie, lack of economic or psychosocial resources) and assist in obtaining appropriate referrals and assistance.

Physical Status

Physical assessment is an essential component of comprehensive nursing care during the postpartum period. Changes in the breasts, uterus, lochia, bladder, abdomen, perineum, legs, and feet should be assessed periodically and appropriate nursing interventions initiated as needed. A sample medical record form for documentation of ongoing postpartum assessments is included in Appendix 10A. The following interventions are included in a comprehensive assessment during the immediate postpartum period:

- Assess breasts for redness, pain, engorgement, and if nursing, correct latch-on and removal of the newborn from the breast.
- Assess the uterus and lochia as described previously.
- Note any foul-smelling lochia.
- Assess the bladder for fullness before and after voiding.
- Measure amount of the first void (repeat if an insufficient amount).
- Assess for burning, frequency, and flank tenderness.
- Assess the abdomen for muscle tone, and check the incision site if applicable.
- Assess bowel sounds in all four quadrants.
- Assess the perineum, labia, and anus for edema, redness, pain, bruising, and hematoma.
- Assess the episiotomy or abdominal incision for approximation and drainage.

- Assess for the presence, size, and condition of hemorrhoids.
- Assess dietary intake and elimination patterns.
- Assess legs and feet for edema and varicosities.
- Assess for the Homan's sign if agency protocol requires (ie, positive if the woman reports pain in calf muscles when the foot is dorsiflexed), and measure the width of the calf if thrombophlebitis is suspected; the Homan's sign has not been found to be consistently predictive of the presence of deep vein thrombosis).
- Assess activity tolerance.
- Assess the comfort level and response to pain medication.
- Assess breath sounds if the woman has received magnesium sulfate, other tocolytics, or oxytocin; has been on bed rest; has an infection; or had a multiple birth (ie, greater risk for pulmonary edema, especially if the patient received large amounts of intravenous therapy).
- Use the acronym BUBBLERS (*b*reasts, *u*terus, *b*ladder, *b*owel, *l*ochia, *e*pisiotomy or incision, emotional *r*esponse) to guide this assessment.

Postpartum Hemorrhage

The physiologic changes that occur during pregnancy are in anticipation of natural blood loss at birth. These changes include a plasma volume increase of approximately 40% and a red cell mass increase of approximately 25% (ACOG, 2006b). Some women experience a greater than normal blood loss evolving into postpartum hemorrhage. Clinical signs and symptoms such as hypotension, dizziness, pallor, and oliguria do not occur until blood loss is substantial; approximately 10% or more of total blood volume (ACOG). Postpartum hemorrhage occurs in about 2% to 6% of women who have a vaginal birth (Cunningham et al., 2005; Dildy, 2002; Karpati et al., 2004). It can occur early (first 24 hours) or late (>24 hours and <6 weeks after birth). Early or primary postpartum hemorrhage is caused by uterine atony in 80% or more of cases (ACOG). Display 10–7 lists factors associated with postpartum hemorrhage etiology and clinical factors predisposing women to risk. The term *postpartum hemorrhage* is a description of an event, not a diagnosis. Estimates of blood loss after birth are notoriously inaccurate with significant underreporting most common (ACOG, 2006b; Cunningham et al., 2005). Postpartum hemorrhage has traditionally been defined as blood loss of 500 mL or more after completion of the third stage of labor, as more than 500 mL after vaginal birth, more than 1,000 mL during cesarean birth, or more than 1500 mL during a repeat cesarean birth. This definition is not considered reasonable or realistic because nearly half of women giving birth vaginally lose that amount or more.

DISPLAY 10-7

Factors Associated With Postpartum Hemorrhage

ETIOLOGY

Early or Primary Postpartum Hemorrhage

Uterine atony (most common)
Retained placenta
Placenta accreta
Defects in coagulation
Uterine inversion
Genital tract hematomas

Late or Secondary Postpartum Hemorrhage

Infection
Subinvolution of placental site
Retained placenta
Inherited coagulation defects

RISK FACTORS

History of uterine atony or postpartum hemorrhage
Trauma, lacerations, or hematoma of cervix and/or birth canal
Precipitous labor and birth
Prolonged labor
Induced or augmented labor
Difficult third stage (ie, use of aggressive fundal manipulation or cord traction)
Operative vaginal birth (eg, use of forceps or vacuum)
Cesarean birth
Uterine overdistention (eg, large infant, multiple gestation, polyhydramnios)
Multiparity
Sepsis
Coagulopathies
Uterine rupture
Drugs (large dosages of oxytocin, magnesium sulfate, beta-adrenergic tocolytic agents; diazoxide [potent antihypertensive agent]; calcium channel blockers, such as nifedipine; and halothane [anesthetic agent])

During birth, a normal, healthy woman tolerates blood loss equal to the volume of blood added during pregnancy without any significant decrease in the postpartum hematocrit. Hematocrit and hemoglobin levels are often used to estimate blood loss after birth; however, laboratory values may not always reflect current hematologic status, especially when blood is drawn soon after the event before equilibrium has occurred and large amounts of rapid volume expanders have been administered intravenously (ACOG, 2006b). Within the clinical context of these limitations, blood loss is often estimated at 500 mL for every 3% drop in hematocrit values when comparing the admission hematocrit with the postpartum hematocrit (Cunningham et al., 2005). For example, a decrease in hematocrit from 38% on admission to 32% postpartum would represent an approximate blood loss of 1,000 mL. Hemoglobin values can be used similarly. The hemoglobin value can be assumed to decrease 1 to 1.5 g/dL for each 500 mL of blood loss (ACOG; AWHONN & Johnson and Johnson, 2006; Cunningham et al., 2005).

The greatest risk for early postpartum hemorrhage is during the first hour after birth, because large venous areas are exposed after placental separation. According to ASA (2006), the following resources should be available in the event of an obstetric hemorrhagic emergency: large-bore intravenous catheters; intravenous fluid warmer; forced-air body warmer; an available blood blank; equipment for infusing intravenous fluids or blood products rapidly, such as hand-squeezed fluid chambers, hand-inflated pressure bags, and automatic infusion devices. The frontline treatment for the management of postpartum hemorrhage is uterotonic agents (oxytocin, methylergonovine, 15-methyl PGF$_{2\alpha}$, dinoprostone, misoprostol) when atony is the cause of the bleeding (ACOG, 2006b). If these medications fail, an exploratory laparotomy is the next step. Maintaining uterine contraction by using fundal massage (Fig. 10–4) and

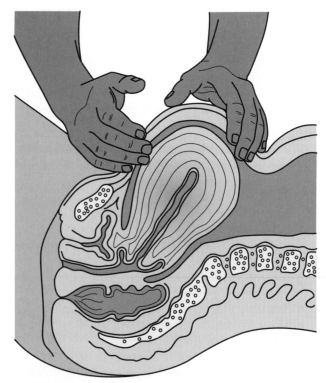

FIGURE 10–4. Fundal massage. The nurse uses two hands for fundal massage. One hand anchors the lower uterine segment just above the symphysis. The other gently massages the fundal area.

intravenous oxytocin administration (20 units (U)/L) reduces the incidence of hemorrhage from uterine atony (AAP & ACOG, 2002; ACOG, 2006b; Bowes & Thorpe, 2004; Cunningham et al., 2005). Late postpartum bleeding most commonly occurs between day 6 and day 14.

Preexisting risk factors for postpartum hemorrhage include:

- High parity
- Previous postpartum hemorrhage
- Previous uterine surgery
- Coagulation defects or medical disorders of clotting

Current pregnancy risk factors for postpartum hemorrhage include:

- Antepartal hemorrhage
- Uterine overdistention (macrosomia, multiple gestation, or polyhydramnios)
- Chorioamnionitis/intraamniotic infection
- Placental abnormality (succenturiate lobe, placenta previa, placenta accreta, abruptio placentae, hydatidiform mole)
- Fetal death

Risk factors for postpartum hemorrhage associated with labor and birth include:

- Rapid or prolonged labor
- Use of tocolytic or halogenated anesthetic agents
- Large episiotomy
- Operative vaginal birth
- Cesarean birth
- Abnormally located or attached placenta
- Inversion of uterus

When postpartum hemorrhage occurs, the perinatal team must work together to treat the underlying condition, manage the blood loss, and minimize the risk to the mother (see Display 10–8). The following assessments and interventions are included in comprehensive care during postpartum hemorrhage based on the individual clinical situation:

- Plan for care and assessment to ensure early recognition of hemorrhage.
- Packed red blood cells should be typed and cross matched if excessive blood loss is anticipated (AAP & ACOG, 2002).
- Assess blood loss.
- Weigh peripads or Chux dressing (1 g = 1 mL). (Keep a gram scale on unit.)
- Assess excessive bleeding, which is defined as one perineal pad saturated within 15 minutes.
- Look for severe loss that may occur with steady, slow seepage.
- Assess vital signs at least every 15 minutes or more often if indicated.

DISPLAY 10-8

Management of Postpartum Hemorrhage

GOALS

Stop hemorrhage
Correct hypovolemia
Return of hemostasis
Identification of risk factors
Early recognition and treatment of hemorrhage
Treatment of underlying cause of hemorrhage

MEDICAL–SURGICAL MANAGEMENT

Medications
    Oxytocin
    Ergot
    Prostaglandins (15-methyl prostaglandin $F_{2\alpha}$, prostaglandin E2, misoprostol)
Fundal massage
Bladder management
Mast trousers
Bimanual compression
Uterine packing
Curettage
Ligation of blood vessels (uterine, ovarian, hypogastric arteries)
Arterial embolization

- Mean arterial pressure (MAP), which is the mean blood pressure (BP) in arterial circulation, should be assessed because the first blood pressure response to hypovolemia may be a pulse pressure decreased to 30 mm Hg or less (Cunningham et al., 2005). MAP in nonpregnant women is normally 86.4 ± 7.5 mm Hg, with a slightly higher value for pregnant women, 90.3 ± 6 (Gonik & Foley, 2004; Cunningham et al., 2005). MAP can be calculated with this formula:

$$\text{MAP} = \text{systolic BP} + 2 \text{ (diastolic BP)}/3.$$

- Assess for tachypnea and tachycardia, which may occur while the BP is constant or slightly lowered.
- Assess for shock. Normal vital signs do not mean that the woman is not in shock. Traditional signs of hypovolemic shock are not evident until 10% to 30% of the total blood volume is lost due to the pregnancy-induced hypervolemia that accounts for the 30% to 70% increase in blood volume (an additional 1 to 2 L) that prevents symptoms with the typical 500 mL blood loss (ACOG, 2006b; Gonik & Foley, 2004; Magann & Lanneau, 2005). The initial response of vasoconstriction shunts blood to vital organs to maintain their function and viability.

- Maintain accurate measurements of intake and output.
- Ensure large-bore (14-, 16-, or 18-gauge) needle intravenous access.
- Use lactated Ringer's solution or plasma expanders to counteract hypovolemia (ie, produce at least 30 mL/hour of urine output and hematocrit values of 30%) (Cunningham et al., 2005).
- Draw blood for hemoglobin and hematocrit (compare with prenatal or admission values), type and cross-match, coagulation studies (ie, fibrinogen, prothrombin time, partial thromboplastin time, fibrin split products, and fibrin degradation products), and blood chemistry. The blood bank should be notified that transfusion may be necessary.
- The clot observation test provides a simple measure of fibrinogen. A volume of 5 mL of the patient's blood can be placed into a clean red-topped tube and observed frequently. Normally, blood will clot within 8 to 10 minutes and will remain intact. If the fibrinogen concentration is low, generally less than 150 mg/dL, the blood in the tube will not clot, or if it does, it will undergo partial or complete dissolution in 30 to 60 minutes (ACOG, 2006b).
- Arterial blood may be drawn for blood gas determinations.
- If blood transfusion is necessary, each unit of packed red blood cells (240 mL is the usual volume of 1 U) can be expected to increase hematocrit 3 percentage points and hemoglobin by 1 g/dL. Packed red blood cells contain red blood cells, white blood cells, and plasma (ACOG, 2006b).
- Transfusion can be withheld with adequate urine output and no appreciable postural hypotension or tachycardia (AAP & ACOG, 2002).
- Deficits in clotting factors may necessitate cryoprecipitate (ie, for fibrinogen deficiency), recombinant activated factor VII, or fresh-frozen plasma (ie, for decreased levels of clotting factors) AAP & ACOG, 2002; ACOG, 2006b; Bouwmeester, Jonkoff, Verheijen, & Geijn, 2003). Each unit of 50 mL of platelets can be expected to increase platelet count 5,000 to 10,000/mm^3. Platelets contain platelets, red blood cells, white blood cells, and plasma. Each unit of 250 mL of fresh frozen plasma can be expected to increase fibrinogen by 10 mg/dL. Fresh frozen plasma contains fibrinogen, antithrombin III, and factors V and VIII. Each unit of cryoprecipitate can be expected to increase fibrinogen by 10 mg/dL. Cryoprecipitate contains fibrinogen, factors VII and XIII, and von Willebrand factor (ACOG, 2006b).
- Use correct uterine massage to avoid ligament damage and potential uterine inversion (see Fig. 10-4). Place one hand pointing toward the woman's head with thumb resting on one side of the uterus and fingers along the other side. Use other hand to massage with *only the force needed to effect contraction or expulsion of clots.* Over-aggressive uterine massage may tire muscle fibers and contribute to further atony.
- Early recognition minimizes blood loss and potential sequelae such as anemia, puerperal infection, thromboembolism, and necrosis of the anterior pituitary (ie, Sheehan's syndrome).
- Anticipate pain-management needs for fundal massage and uterotonic medications for treatment of hemorrhage
- Urine should be sent to the laboratory as indicated.
- Insert a Foley catheter to empty the bladder and allow accurate measurement of output. A full bladder can impede complete uterine contraction.
- Administer prescribed medication. Labor and birth units should have the following pharmacologic agents available: oxytocin, methylergonovine, ergot alkaloids, 15-methyl-prostaglandin $F_{2\alpha}$, prostaglandin $F_{2\alpha}$, misoprostol, and dinoprostone (AAP & ACOG, 2002; ACOG, 2006b):

Oxytocin (Pitocin)	10–40 U in 500–1,000 of normal saline or lactated Ringer's solution at 50 mU/minute
	Intramuscular: 10 units
	Avoid undiluted rapid IV infusion, which causes hypotension
Methyl ergonovine (Methergine)	0.2 mg IM q 2–4 hours maleate (× 5 dose maximum)
	0.2 mg PO q 6–12 hours IV administration not recommended
	Avoid if patient is hypertensive
Ergonovine maleate	0.2 mg IM q 2–4 hours (× 5 dose maximum)
	0.2 mg PO q 6–12 hours (IV administration not recommended)
15-α-methyl-prostaglandin $F_{2\alpha}$ (Carboprost/ Hemabate)	IM 250 μg 15–90 minutes (8 doses maximum)
	Physician may administer by intramyometrial route
	Avoid in asthmatic patients; relative contraindication if patient has hepatic, renal, or cardiac disease; can cause diarrhea, fever, and tachycardia

Misoprostol (Cytotec)	800–1,000 μg rectally
Dinoprostone (Prostin E$_2$)	Suppository (vaginally or rectally) 20 μg every 2 hours
	Avoid if patient is hypotensive; fever is common; stored frozen—must be thawed to room temperature

- Apply pulse oximeter and administer oxygen according to unit protocol. This is usually accomplished with a nonrebreather facemask at 10 to 12 L/minute.
- Continuous electrocardiographic monitoring may be indicated for hypotension, continuous bleeding, tachycardia, or shock.
- Elevate the legs to a 20- to 30-degree angle to increase venous return.
- Prepare for additional interventions if the situation does not resolve. These include packing the uterus with gauze or using a balloon tamponade, dilatation and curettage, exploratory laparotomy, bilateral uterine artery ligation, arterial embolization, and other surgical techniques. In some cases, postpartum hemorrhage may require a transfer or return to the surgical suite. The surgical team should be notified that they may be needed.
- Provide emotional support and explanations for the woman and her family.

Once the patient is stable, replacement of red blood cell mass is an important clinical intervention. The patient should be instructed to continue prenatal vitamins that contain about 60 mg of elemental iron and 1 mg of folate during the hospitalization and at least until the first postpartum office visit. Additional iron should be encouraged (two tablets of 300 mg ferrous sulfate) to maximize red cell production and restoration (ACOG, 2006b).

In July 2004, the Joint Commission on Accreditation of Healthcare Organizations (JCAHO) recommended conducting periodic drills for obstetric emergencies such as postpartum hemorrhage. Although there are few data supporting improved outcomes in units where postpartum hemorrhage birth drills are routine, it would seem likely that when all members of the perinatal team know their roles and responsibilities, the location of key medications and equipment, and whom to call, the chances of the chaotic environment often associated with a significant postpartum hemorrhage would be minimized (Simpson, 2005). During postpartum hemorrhage, immediate access to required medications can be challenging. Common medications used to treat postpartum hemorrhage

such as oxytocin, methergine, prostin, and misoprostol are kept in locked drug-dispensing systems often remote from the labor room. Intravenous fluids (IV) required for rapid volume expansion also may be not be available in the labor room. Development of a clinical algorithm for interventions during postpartum hemorrhage in addition to drills to evaluate the feasibility of getting necessary medications and IV fluids quickly may be helpful. Rizvi, Mackey, Barrett, McKenna, and Geary (2004) found that clinical algorithms, drills, and perinatal team education were successful in reducing the incidence of severe postpartum hemorrhage in one obstetrical unit. To prepare for a drill, develop a list of roles and responsibilities for each team member. Some have found it helpful to use a scribe or video-recording of the drill so that the organization of events and interventions can be analyzed retrospectively. Using a volunteer staff member as a surrogate for the patient can make the drill seem more realistic.

Postpartum Infections

A puerperal infection should be suspected when a woman has an oral temperature higher than 38°C (100.4°F) on two occasions that are 6 hours apart during the first 10 days postpartum, exclusive of the first 24 hours. The nursery should be notified of these findings, although the newborn need not be separated from the mother (AAP & ACOG, 2002; Cunningham et al., 2005; Gibbs, Sweet, & Duff, 2004).

Endometritis

Postpartum endometritis occurs in 1% to 3% of vaginal births and is 10 times more common in cesarean births (Cunningham et al., 2005; French & Smaill, 2004; Gibbs, Sweet, & Duff, 2004). Postpartum uterine infections, called *endometritis* (ie, inflammation of endometrium), *endomyometritis* (ie, inflammation of endometrium and myometrium), or *endomyoparametritis* (ie, inflammation of endometrium and parametrial tissue), are the most commonly identified causes of puerperal morbidity. One of the most effective methods of prevention of infection is handwashing.

The most common cause of uterine infection tends to be polymicrobial, including aerobic and anaerobic organisms that have ascended to the uterus from the lower genital tract. Isolated organisms include streptococci A and B, enterococci, *Staphylococcus aureus*, *Gardnerella vaginalis*, *Escherichia coli*, *Enterobacter*, *Proteus mirabilis*, *Klebsiella pneumoniae*, *Bacteroides* species, *Peptostreptococcus* species, *Ureaplasma urealyticum*, *Mycoplasma hominis*, and *Chlamydia trachomatis*. *C. trachomatis* has been specifically associated with late-onset postpartum endometritis

(Cunningham et al., 2005; Gibbs, Sweet, & Duff, 2004). Blood cultures are positive in about 10% of women. Endometrial cultures may have limited value, because of cervicovaginal contamination of the specimen, yet they may provide useful information if the woman does not respond to initial antibiotic therapy (Cunningham et al., 2005; Gibbs, Sweet, & Duff, 2004).

Parenteral broad-spectrum antibiotic therapy is promptly initiated when postpartum endometritis is diagnosed. Treatment continues until the woman has been afebrile for 48 hours. A common treatment regimen is a combination of clindamycin and gentamicin, with ampicillin in refractory cases, and is cost-effective therapy. Women usually respond rapidly (48–72 hours) to antibiotic therapy. Occasional complications include pelvic abscesses, septic pelvic thrombophlebitis, persistent fever, and retained infected placenta (AAP & ACOG, 2002).

Other causes of postpartum infection include wound and urinary tract infections, pneumonia (usually related to general anesthesia), mastitis, pelvic thrombophlebitis, and necrotizing fasciitis, an uncommon but serious localized infection of the deep soft tissues.

Risk factors for endometritis are:

- Operative birth
- Prolonged labor or rupture of membranes
- Use of invasive procedures (eg, internal monitoring, amnioinfusion, fetal scalp sampling)
- Multiple pelvic examinations
- Excessive blood loss
- Pyelonephritis or diabetes
- Socioeconomic and nutritional factors compromising host defense mechanisms
- Anemia and systemic illness
- Smoking

The following assessments and interventions are included in comprehensive nursing care for postpartum infections:

- Fever occurring about the third postnatal day is the most important finding.
- Observe for tachycardia (rise of 10 beats/min for every degree Celsius).
- Determine possible causes of malaise.
- Assess lower abdominal pain.
- Assess uterine tenderness on palpation (extending laterally) and slight abdominal distention.
- Determine cause of foul-smelling lochia (if organism is anaerobic).
- Obtain urinalysis to rule out urinary tract infections (UTI).
- Assess leukocytosis (WBC count >20,000/mm^3 with increased neutrophils or polymorphonuclear leukocytes).

- Blood cultures are positive in about 10% of women.
- Endometrial cultures may have limited value because of cervicovaginal contamination of the specimen, but they may provide useful information if the woman does not respond to initial antibiotic therapy (Cunningham et al., 2005; Gibbs, Sweet, & Duff, 2004).
- Parenteral broad-spectrum antibiotic therapy is promptly initiated when postpartum endometritis is diagnosed. Treatment continues until the woman has been afebrile for 48 hours. A common treatment regimen is a combination of clindamycin and an aminoglycoside such as gentamicin, with ampicillin added in refractory cases. A protocol including activity against the Bacteroides fragilis group and other penicillin-resistant anaerobic bacteria is better than one without. No one regimen is associated with fewer side effects, with the exception of cephalosporins, which are associated with less diarrhea (French & Smaill, 2004).
- Women usually respond rapidly (48 to 72 hours) to antibiotic therapy. Occasional complications include pelvic abscesses, septic pelvic thrombophlebitis, persistent fever, and retained infected placenta (AAP & ACOG, 2002).
- Increase fluid intake, and encourage adequate nutrition.
- Encourage intake of a minimum of six to eight glasses (1,500 to 2,000 mL) of water, milk, or juices; 3,000 mL is the preferred amount.
- Encourage intake of at least 1,800 to 2,000 calories daily if lactating, and 1,500 calories if not lactating.
- Encourage the woman to eat a varied diet, with representation of foods from all food groups, that is high in protein and vitamin C to promote wound healing.
- Ensure adequate output (30 mL/hour) because renal toxicity can occur with antibiotic therapy.
- Provide comfort through meeting the woman's personal hygiene needs. Cool compresses, linen changes, massage, and positioning may enhance comfort.
- Assess vital signs every 4 hours or every 2 hours if her temperature is elevated.
- Use a semi-Fowler position, ambulation, or both to promote uterine drainage.
- Administer oxytocics as ordered to promote uterine contraction and drainage.
- Observe for signs of septic shock: tachycardia (>120 beats), hypotension, tachypnea, changes in sensorium, and decreased urine output (ie, oliguria) (Cunningham et al., 2005). If septic shock develops, increase the frequency of obtaining vital signs and other assessments, depending on the clinical situation.

Wound Infections

Wound infections can be classified as early onset (within 48 hours) or late onset (within 6 to 8 days). Early-onset wound infections are usually treated with antibiotic therapy and excision of necrotic tissue. Late-onset infections are treated with incision and drainage, and they may not require antibiotics unless there is extensive cellulitis (Cunningham et al., 2005; Gibbs, Sweet, & Duff, 2004). The following are risk factors for wound infections:

- History of chorioamnionitis or intraamniotic infection
- Hemorrhage or anemia
- Obesity
- Underlying medical problems such as diabetes and malnutrition
- Multiple vaginal examinations
- Corticosteroid therapy
- Immunosuppression
- Advancing age
- Malnutrition

The following assessments and interventions are included in comprehensive nursing care for wound infections:

- Observe for wound erythema, swelling, tenderness, and purulent discharge.
- Assess for localized pain and dysuria.
- Assess vital signs.
- Check for a low-grade temperature (101°F or 38.3°C).
- Acute cases may exhibit sudden chills and spikes in temperature to 40°C (104°F).
- The pulse usually is <100 beats/min.
- Perform cultures as ordered.
- Assist with drainage, irrigation, and occasionally, débridement procedures.
- Sitz baths are used for cleaning and promotion of increased circulation to the affected area.
- The wound may be packed. Treatment is directed toward cleaning the wound and promoting granulation.
  - Change dressings and dispose appropriately of soiled dressings.
  - Dressings may be continued after discharge. The patient and family will need instruction for dressing and wound care.
- Ensure frequent changes of peripads.
- Ensure pain management and appropriate administration of analgesia.
- Ensure adequate room ventilation prior to dressing changes.
- Continued hospitalization or readmission may be required.
- Provide explanations during this stressful period.
- Offer reassurance and encouragement.

- Encourage frequent visits by the family to help reduce anxiety.
- Assist breastfeeding women with pumping or lactation suppression.
- Administer antibiotic therapy as ordered (may be continued after discharge).
- Provide referrals for postpartum follow-up visits by home care nurses.
- Reduce anxiety and the incidence of rehospitalization by early identification and treatment of infections.

Necrotizing Fasciitis

Necrotizing fasciitis is a severe infection (polymicrobial more common) that is characterized by severe tissue necrosis, erythema, discharge, and severe pain. Partial liquefaction of fascia adjacent to the incision may also occur. Secondary healing may take 6 to 12 weeks (Cunningham et al., 2005; Gibbs, Sweet, & Duff, 2004).

Risk factors for necrotizing fasciitis include:

- Diabetes
- Obesity
- Hypertension

The following assessments and interventions are included in comprehensive nursing care for necrotizing fasciitis:

- Wound status (ie, erythema, discharge)
- Pain
- Administration of broad-spectrum antibiotics, as ordered
- Surgical débridement

Mastitis

Both congestive and infectious mastitis are more commonly seen in primigravidas and nursing mothers. Symptoms usually appear between the third and fourth week after birth and are typically unilateral. Symptoms of mastitis may include fever, chills, localized tenderness, and a palpable, hard, reddened mass. Nipple trauma has been implicated in the development of mastitis. Trauma from incorrect latch-on or removal of the newborn from the breast permits the introduction of organisms from the newborn into the mother's breast. *S. aureus* is the most common causative organism. Administration of penicillinase-resistant antibiotics such as dicloxacillin for 7 to 10 days is recommended.

If a breast abscess develops, incision and drainage may be indicated. The decision to continue breastfeeding should be made jointly by the woman and the healthcare provider. If breastfeeding is delayed while purulent drainage continues, the woman may need assistance with breast pumping to reestablish lactation. If advised to discontinue breastfeeding, emotional support, reassurance, and comfort measures are important. Lactation consultant referral is indicated as a preventive or treatment measure when these services are available.

Risk factors for mastitis include:

- Infrequent breastfeeding
- Incomplete breast emptying
- Plugged milk duct
- Cracked and bleeding nipples (may be secondary to improper latch-on and removal)

The following assessments and interventions are included in comprehensive nursing care for mastitis:

- Assess fever and chills.
- Assess localized tenderness and a palpable, hard, reddened mass.
- Assess for tachycardia.
- Assess for purulent discharge.
- Offer education about preventive measures (ie, hand washing, breast cleanliness, frequent breast-pad changes, exposure of the nipples to air, and correct infant latch-on and removal from the breast).
- Obtain a culture of the breast milk before initiating antibiotic therapy, if ordered.
- The infection usually resolves within 24 to 48 hours of antibiotic therapy.
- Suggest comfort measures, including warm or cold compresses, wearing a supportive bra, and analgesia as ordered.
- Offer education about completing the full regimen of antibiotic therapy.
- Encourage an increase in fluid intake from 2 to 2.5 L/day.
- Massage, positioning the newborn in the direction of the site, and frequent breastfeeding promote milk flow.
- Assist with the use of a breast pump or manual expression if indicated (Cunningham et al., 2005; Gibbs, Sweet, & Duff, 2004).

Urinary Tract Infections

Urinary tract infections (UTIs) are the most common medical complication occurring during pregnancy. They may be asymptomatic (eg, bacteriuria) or symptomatic (eg, cystitis, acute pyelonephritis). Asymptomatic UTIs occur in 4% to 7% of pregnant women. Diagnosis and treatment of bacteriuria can prevent the development of pyelonephritis, which places the fetus at increased risk for preterm birth or low birth weight. Women who develop UTIs during pregnancy are at increased risk for a UTI during the postpartum period (Cunningham et al., 2005; Gibbs, Sweet, & Duff, 2004).

Risk factors for UTIs include:

- A shorter urethra in women than men
- Contamination of the urethra with pathogenic bacteria from vagina and rectum
- High probability that women do not completely empty bladders
- Movement of bacteria into bladder during sexual intercourse
- Pregnancy-related changes (eg, decreased ureteric muscle tone and activity from progesterone and pressure of gravid uterus, resulting in lower rate of urine passing through urinary collecting system)
- Urinary catheterization, frequent pelvic examinations, epidural anesthesia, genital tract injury, and cesarean birth

Asymptomatic Bacteriuria

The following assessments and interventions are included in comprehensive nursing care of asymptomatic bacteriuria:

- Evaluate urinalysis for bacteriuria (presence of 10^5 or more bacterial colonies/mL of urine on two consecutive, clean-catch, midstream voided specimens).
- *E. coli* is cultured in 60% to 90% of cases. (Other pathogens include *Proteus mirabilis*, *Klebsiella pneumoniae*, group B hemolytic streptococci, and *Staphylococcus saprophyticus*)
- Educate women about the importance of repeat urinalysis to determine the effectiveness of antibiotics.
- Risk is associated with sickle cell trait, lower socioeconomic status, increased parity, and reduced availability of medical care.
- Administer or educate the woman to take antibiotics as ordered to eliminate bacteria in urine.
- Ampicillin and cephalosporins are used (no significant risk to the fetus); antibiotics are administered for 7 days.
- If continuous antimicrobial therapy is required, typically use a single daily dose of nitrofurantoin (100 mg), preferably after the evening meal (Gibbs, Sweet, & Duff, 2004).

Pyelonephritis and Cystitis

The following assessments and interventions are included in comprehensive nursing care for pyelonephritis and cystitis:

- Assess urinalysis for presence of untreated, asymptomatic bacteriuria.
  - High risk for pyelonephritis with untreated bacteriuria
  - Bacterial growth more than 100,000 colonies/mL
  - May have increased WBCs, protein, or blood in specimen
  - Most common bacteria: *E. coli* (80%), *Klebsiella*, *Enterobacter*, *Proteus*

- First choice of therapy: cephalosporins for single-agent therapy
- Assess for symptoms of cystitis.
  - Urinary urgency, frequency, dysuria
  - Suprapubic pain without fever or tenderness at the costovertebral angle
  - Gross hematuria
- Assess for symptoms of pyelonephritis.
  - Shaking chills, fever, tachycardia, flank pain, nausea, vomiting
  - Urinary frequency, urgency, dysuria, and costovertebral angle tenderness
  - Possible endotoxin-mediated tissue damage (Gibbs, Sweet, & Duff, 2004)
- Administer antibiotics as ordered.
  - Short courses (1–3 weeks) of sulfonamides, ampicillin, or nitrofurantoin recommended for pyelonephritis
  - Recommended 7-day course of antibiotics for acute cystitis in pregnant women
- Monitor intake and output.
  - Maintain adequate hydration (at least 3,000 mL/day) with water and cranberry juice.
  - Measure urinary output for adequacy (at least 30 mL/hour).
- Administer antipyretics, antispasmodics, or urinary analgesics (Pyridium) and antiemetics as ordered.
- Encourage rest.
- Monitor vital signs every 4 hours.
- Educate the woman about monitoring temperature, bladder function, appearance of urine, importance of completing antibiotic therapy, proper perineal care (eg, wiping front to back), wearing cotton underwear, adequate hydration, and balanced nutrition.

If readmission for treatment of a UTI is necessary, reassurance and family support are essential. Separation from the newborn is distressing to the mother and child. If the woman has been breastfeeding, interventions such as pumping and newborn visits can help to maintain lactation after antibiotic therapy has been initiated. If breastfeeding is temporarily contraindicated, the nurse can provide emotional support and offer strategies to maintain lactation (eg, breast pump) until breastfeeding can be resumed (Cunningham et al., 2005; Gibbs, Sweet, & Duff, 2004).

Thrombophlebitis and Thromboembolism

Thrombophlebitis (inflammation of a vein after formation of a thrombus) is classified as superficial or deep. Superficial thrombophlebitis involves the superficial veins of the saphenous system. Deep vein thrombophlebitis affects the veins of the calf, thigh, or pelvis. Stasis is the most significant predisposing event to the development of deep vein thrombosis. Diagnosis of thrombophlebitis is based on objective and subjective signs and symptoms. Septic pelvic thrombophlebitis is a condition more common in women after a cesarean birth and occurs with infections of the reproductive tract. Ascending infection within the venous system results in thrombophlebitis. This condition should be suspected when the infection does not respond to antibiotics and is accompanied by abdominal or flank pain and guarding on the second or third postpartum day.

A more serious complication occurs when a thrombus forms in any of the dilated pelvic veins. Accompanied by thrombophlebitis, these formations can be a source of potentially fatal pulmonary emboli. In those cases, the clot becomes friable, and the pieces detach from the vessel wall and travel through the heart into the pulmonary circulation. Pulmonary embolism should be treated as a life-threatening event; interruption of blood flow to the pulmonary bed can result in cardiovascular collapse and death (Cunningham et al., 2005; Laros, 2004).

Risk factors for thrombophlebitis and thromboembolism include:

- Normal changes in coagulation status during pregnancy
- History of thromboembolic disease or varicosities
- Increased parity
- Obesity
- Advanced maternal age (≥30 years)
- Immobility associated with extended antepartum bed rest
- Use of forceps
- Cesarean birth
- Blood vessel and tissue trauma
- Prolonged labor with multiple pelvic examinations
- Sepsis/trauma
- Blood type other than type O
- Dehydration

Thrombus formation can potentially be prevented by these interventions:

- Early ambulation or leg exercises for women on bed rest
- Education about correct posture
  - Avoiding crossing legs
  - Avoiding extreme flexion of legs at the groin
  - Positioning without pressure on the backs of knees
- Use of support hose by women with a history of thrombophlebitis
- Padding of pressure points during birth while in the lithotomy position

Thrombophlebitis

The following assessments and interventions are included in comprehensive nursing care of thrombophlebitis:

- Evaluate the woman's physical status.
- A superficial vein (usually varicose) is reddened, hard, and tender.
- Apply a supportive bandage or antiembolic support stockings.
- Apply a soothing agent (ie, glycerin and Ichthyol).
- Apply warm packs to the affected area.
- Slightly elevate the involved leg.
- Permit ambulation as indicated and ordered.
- Perform serial measurements of the circumferences of the calves; a circumference difference of more than 2 cm is classified as leg swelling.
- Monitor vital signs every 4 hours; there may be a slight increase in temperature.
- Compare pulses in both extremities, which may reveal decreased venous flow to the affected area.
- Heparin anticoagulation therapy may be ordered.
- If Homans' sign is part of the assessment protocol, the assessment is performed with the knee slightly flexed. The nurse abruptly and forcibly dorsiflexes the ankle, observing for pain in the calf and popliteal area. Numerous studies have questioned the accuracy and utility of Homan's sign. Accuracy estimates range from a positive result in 8% to 56% of documented cases of deep vein thrombosis (DVT) to a positive result in more than 50% of patients without DVT. "Pain from muscular causes will be absent or minimal on dorsiflexion of the ankle with the knee flexed but maximal on dorsiflexion of the ankle with the knee extended or during straight-leg raising (Homans' sign); thus, this test is unreliable for DVT" (Beers & Berkow, 2006). Therefore, most authors conclude that Homans' sign is unreliable, insensitive, and nonspecific in the diagnosis of DVT (Urbano, 2001).

Nursing interventions for DVT include all of the previously described care measures plus the following:

- Bed rest with elevation of involved extremity until swelling is reduced and anticoagulation therapy are effective (promote venous return and decreases edema).
  - As soon as symptoms allow, ambulation is encouraged as bed rest can increase venous stasis.
  - There is no evidence to support that bed rest prevents embolus detachment (Laros, 2004).
- Anticoagulation therapy with intravenous heparin, followed by oral warfarin
  - Maintenance of activated partial thromboplastin time that is prolonged by 1.5 to 2 times laboratory control value (Cunningham et al., 2005)

- Dosing regimens (Cunningham et al.):
  - 5,000-U bolus of heparin and then continuous infusion to a total 24,000 to 32,000 U/day
  - Intermittent intravenous injections of 5,000 U every 4 hours or 7,500 U every 6 hours
  - Subcutaneous heparin at dose of 10,000 U every 8 hours or 20,000 U every 12 hours
- Monitor coagulation laboratory values.
- Carefully assess unusual bleeding. Heavy vaginal bleeding, generalized petechiae, bleeding from the mucous membranes, hematuria, or oozing from venipuncture sites should be reported to the physician. The heparin antidote protamine sulfate should be readily available.
- Educate and prepare women for diagnostic testing:
  - Physical assessments look for muscle pain, palpable deep linear cord, tenderness, swelling, and dilated superficial veins.
  - Doppler ultrasonography provides more sensitivity and is more specific for the diagnosis of popliteal and femoral vein thrombosis than for calf vein thrombosis. It can evaluate venous flow and possible occlusion.
  - Venography is a more specific test, but it is invasive, expensive, and difficult to interpret. Contrast material may cause chemical phlebitis.
  - Impedance plethysmography has had little research to support its efficacy during pregnancy, but coupled with ultrasound, the reliability increases. A thigh cuff is inflated, resulting in temporary occlusion of venous return. Release results in a rapid decrease in volume as blood drains proximally. Volume changes are detected by measurement of electrical resistance in the calf.
  - Blood studies can determine the formation of intravascular fibrin; results are positive in cases of thrombosis. Results are also positive in presence of hematomas or inflammatory exudates containing fibrin.

Septic Pelvic Thrombophlebitis

The following assessments and interventions are included in comprehensive nursing care of septic pelvic thrombophlebitis:

- Assess the woman for physical symptoms:
  - Fever and tachycardia
  - Spiking fever persisting despite antibiotic therapy
  - Abdominal and flank pain (paralytic ileus may develop)
  - Prepare and support the woman during examination (ie, parametrial mass found on bimanual examination).
- Obtain appropriate laboratory testing:
  - Complete blood count
  - Blood chemistry

- Coagulation profile
- Chest radiography, computed tomography, magnetic resonance imaging
- Administer medications as ordered:
  - Heparin regimen initiated with diagnosis
  - Coumarin agent substituted and continued for total course of anticoagulation of 3 to 6 weeks

Pulmonary Embolism

The following assessments and interventions are included in comprehensive nursing care of pulmonary embolism:

- The most common signs are dyspnea, chest pain, hemoptysis, and abdominal pain.
- The most serious signs are sudden collapse, cyanosis, and hypotension.
- Prepare the woman for diagnostic testing:
  - Ventilation/perfusion (VQ) scan
  - Blood gas studies
  - Radiography
  - Pulmonary angiography
- Elevate the head of the bed to facilitate breathing.
- Administer oxygen 10 L/min using a nonrebreather facemask; use pulse oximetry.
- Maintain the PaO_2 ≥70 mm Hg.
- Monitor arterial blood gases.
- Frequently assess vital signs.
- Provide for intravenous fluids (ie, pulmonary artery catheter may be placed).
- Administer salt-poor or hypertonic intravenous fluids, as ordered.
- Administer medications as ordered to counteract symptoms:
  - Medium dose of intravenous heparin (continued subcutaneous heparin or oral anticoagulant therapy for 6 months)
  - Total daily heparin dose of 30,000 to 40,000 U (Cunningham et al., 2005)
  - Dopamine to maintain blood pressure
  - Morphine for analgesia
- Maintain adequate staffing:
  - Personnel who have completed an Advanced Cardiac Life Support (ACLS) course should be available for full resuscitation support, if needed. Care usually occurs in a medical–surgical ICU. Collaboration between the ICU staff and perinatal staff is essential. Maternal transport should be considered if the level of care and supportive staff necessary are unavailable.

Although most women have a normal postpartum course, complications can occur. Comprehensive, frequent nursing assessments contribute to early identification and prompt treatment. Collaboration between the perinatal nurse and the primary healthcare provider

DISPLAY 10-9

Clinical Signs and Symptoms to Report to the Primary Healthcare Provider

- Uterine atony or large/excessive clots; passage of placental tissue
- Excessive bleeding
- Continued bleeding in the presence of a firm uterus (suggests lacerations)
- Perineal pain greater than expected (suggests hematoma)
- Foul-smelling lochia (suggests endometritis)
- Temperature elevated to >100°F (38°C) (suggests dehydration in first 24 hours; thereafter, after 24 hours, suggests infection, ie, thrombophlebitis or systemic infection)
- Bladder distention and/or inability to void
- Diminished urinary output (<30 mL/hour)
- Enlarging hematomas
- Restlessness; pallor of skin or mucous membranes; cool, clammy skin; tachycardia; thready pulse; fearfulness; vertigo; shaking; visual disturbances; (symptoms of shock)
- Pain, redness, warmth, firm area in the calf area (although pain may be absent in DVT)
- Dyspnea, tachypnea, tachycardia, chest pain, cough, apprehension, hemoptysis, change in skin/mucous membrane color (paleness and/or cyanosis): symptoms of pulmonary embolism or amniotic fluid embolism

is essential. Display 10–9 lists the clinical signs and symptoms suggesting postpartum complications that warrant communication with the primary healthcare provider.

INDIVIDUALIZING CARE FOR WOMEN WITH SPECIAL NEEDS

Cesarean Birth

The cesarean birth rate in the United States (US) in 2005 was 30.2% and has continued to rise each year since these data began to be collected from certificates of live birth (Hamilton, Martin, & Ventura, 2006). Both the primary and the repeat cesarean birth rates have steadily increased. Elective labor induction for nulliparous women is one factor that has had an impact on the rise in primary cesarean births. As vaginal birth after cesarean birth has fallen out of favor with many providers and patients, once a woman has a cesarean birth, it is likely that she will have another with a future pregnancy. When labor ends in cesarean birth, there is risk of lowered self-esteem related to failure to achieve the planned vaginal birth. The desired outcome of birth is for each couple to verbalize a positive birth experience and to feel happiness and excitement about a healthy baby, even if labor and birth do not go as planned. Nurses can assist in achieving this outcome for women experiencing a cesarean birth by involving the couple as much as possible in the decision-making process, keeping the couple informed, supporting the coach and family, encouraging verbalization, and providing reassurance that a cesarean birth is not a failure. If the cesarean birth was unexpected and/or emergent (Fig. 10–5) with minimal time to prepare the couple, time should be allocated as soon as possible after birth to discuss what occurred and why the provider felt cesarean birth was the safest option at that time for the mother and baby. Efforts should be made to allow the father of the baby to see the baby as soon as possible if the emergent birth resulted in the baby's admission to the special care nursery (SCN) or neonatal intensive care unit (NICU); thus, the baby has been separated from the couple during postanesthesia care (Fig. 10–6). Some nurseries have cameras available to take pictures of the baby to immediately share with the mother until she is able to go to the nursery to see the baby herself.

Nurses caring for women after a cesarean birth should stress that the woman is a new mother with the same needs as other new mothers; however, she also requires supportive postoperative care. It is important to provide that extra level of care and include consideration of women in the postoperative period when planning nurse staffing. The woman who has experienced a cesarean birth usually has increased levels of fatigue, activity intolerance, and incisional pain. Women who have cesarean birth after a long labor may be especially fatigued. Women who are in the postoperative recovery period and during the first day or two postoperatively should have a support person with them to help care for

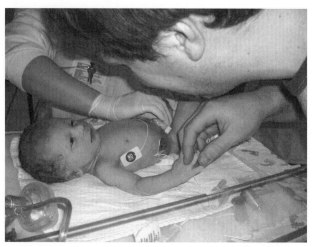

FIGURE 10–6. Promoting father visiting baby in the neonatal intensive care unit after emergent cesarean birth.

the baby if they choose rooming in with the baby (Fig. 10–7). Policies that require rooming in for these patients are not appropriate if the mother does not have a support person available to stay with her continuously until she can assume newborn care on her own. Mothers have a cesarean birth stay longer in the hospital and require more intensive nursing care than for women who have a vaginal birth. The average length of inpatient stay for cesarean birth is 3.7 days as compared to 2.2 days for vaginal birth (Kozak, DeFrances, & Hall, 2006). Chapter 7 provides a full discussion of cesarean birth and the immediate postoperative recovery period.

Antepartum Bed Rest and Postpartum Recovery

Approximately 700,000 women annually in the United States experience pregnancy complications treated with activity restrictions in the hospital (Maloni, Alexander,

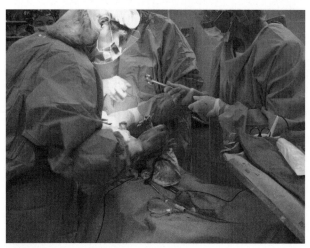

FIGURE 10–5. Emergent cesarean birth.

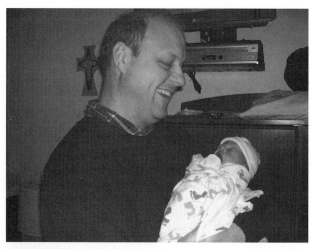

FIGURE 10–7. Support person in attendance to help mother care for baby after cesarean birth.

Schluchter, Shah, & Park, 2004; Thorman & McClean, 2006). Bed rest has not been supported as an effective treatment for preterm labor or prolonging multifetal pregnancy and is not recommended by ACOG (2003). Despite lack of evidence to support bed rest therapy as contributing to positive outcomes, it has been prescribed routinely for women with high-risk pregnancies. Bed rest of more than 3 days has been associated with increased thromboembolic complications. Women with bleeding, preterm labor, and pregnancy-induced hypertension are frequently encouraged to maintain modified or strict bed rest in the hope of prolonging the pregnancy. It has been estimated that up to 18.2% of pregnant women in the United States who give birth after 20 weeks have been prescribed at least 1 week of bed rest at some time during their pregnancy (Maloni & Kutil, 2000). Some research suggests that modified rest or some level of activity restriction at home, rather than strict bed rest, is an acceptable form of treatment for women with pregnancy-induced hypertension remote from term and women at risk for preterm labor and birth (ACOG, 2002a, 2003).

Complete bed rest causes physiologic and psychosocial changes, including cardiovascular deconditioning; muscle loss, especially in the gastrocnemius muscle (used in ambulation); diuresis with fluid, electrolyte, and weight loss; bone demineralization; increased heart rate and blood coagulation; heartburn and reflux; constipation; glucose intolerance; and sensory disturbances, including depression, fatigue, and inability to concentrate (Maloni & Kutil, 2000). Isometric and isotonic conditioning exercises, Kegel exercises, pelvic tilts, and range-of-motion exercises can be used during hospitalization for the woman on bed rest. Deep breathing and coughing are added to exercise abdominal muscles and promote venous return.

After birth, the woman requires additional time, support, and education to prepare for safe and progressive levels of activity (Maloni & Park, 2005). Postpartum recovery may be prolonged. Ambulation after prolonged bed rest requires the continued presence of the perinatal nurse. Women should be alerted to the possibility of weakness, dizziness, shortness of breath, and muscle soreness and be reassured that these are normal physiologic consequences of prolonged bed rest that will reverse over time after resumption of normal activity (Maloni & Kutil, 2000; Maloni & Park, 2005).

Planning for education during the postpartum period begins as soon as possible after inpatient admission. Ideally, women had opportunities during the prenatal period to learn about postpartum and newborn care, but this may not be true for all pregnant women because of access to care issues, complications of pregnancy, unavailability of resources, or lack of knowledge about existing programs. During shortened hospital stays, there are limited opportunities for assessment and education of new mothers. Access, availability, and acceptability must be considered when providing postpartum education. All available resources may not be able to be integrated within the shortened admission period. Closed-circuit educational television and printed materials collaboratively developed by obstetric and pediatric professionals can help new parents. Individual and group educational sessions held regularly during the postpartum period are beneficial. Newborn care, normal infant behaviors, and expected maternal physical and psychological changes should be included in the educational plans for each mother. New mothers should be aware of available community and healthcare resources (AAP & ACOG, 2002). The CDC (2006) has issued a series of recommendations for preconception health and care. Two of the four goals of these recommendations are applicable during the postpartum period. These include reducing the risks identified by a previous adverse pregnancy outcome through interventions during the interconception period. Addressing these risks can prevent or minimize health problems for a mother and her future children. The second goal focuses on reducing the disparities in adverse pregnancy outcomes (Johnson et al., 2006).

Preterm Birth

The incidence of preterm birth (birth at less than 37 completed weeks of gestation) increased to 12.7% in 2005, the highest level in 2 decades (Hamilton, Martin, & Ventura, 2006). The preterm birth rate has risen 20% since 1990 (Hamilton, Martin, & Ventura). The low-birth-weight rate (babies weighing less than 2,500 g) increased to 8.2% in 2005 and has increased more than 20% since the mid-1980s, influenced in part by the increased rate of multiple births (Hamilton, Martin, & Ventura). Women who have experienced a preterm birth may have special needs related to a long period of antepartum bed rest and/or a cesarean birth as previous described. In addition, based on the gestational age and condition of the baby, they may be worried about their baby's survival. The day-to-day fluctuations in the baby's status can be emotionally draining for the woman and her family (Vargo & Trotter, 2006). Even if the preterm baby is healthy with no apparent life-threatening conditions, the woman and her family will likely be spending time visiting the baby in the neonatal intensive care unit (NICU; Freda, 2004). Travel to and from the hospital and NICU observation can be physically exhausting. The mother is likely not to get adequate rest and nutrition for recovery. Nursing education prior to the mother's discharge should include an explanation of the importance of rest and proper diet to promote postpartum recovery. Some hospitals provide hospitality rooms for mothers and their families after discharge when the baby has to remain in the NICU. These accommodations can be helpful in avoiding maternal exhaustion and offer easy access to the baby. For a more in-depth review of nursing care for women who experience preterm birth and the implications for postpartum recovery, see Chapter 6. Additional information can be found in the March of Dimes Nursing Module *Preterm Labor: Prevention and Nursing Management* (Freda, 2004).

Multiple Birth

There has been a dramatic increase in the number of multiple births over the past 2 decades, mostly related to advances in assisted reproductive technologies and ovulation inducing drugs (Russell, Petrini, Damus, Mattison, & Schwartz, 2003). Women of advanced age, especially those aged 30 to 34, 35 to 39, and 40 to 44 had the greatest increases (62%, 81%, and 110%, respectively; Russell, et al., 2003). Women who have a multiple birth have special needs during the postpartum period for multiple reasons. They may have experienced antepartum bed rest and/or a cesarean birth and are likely to have preterm babies admitted to the NICU. As compared to singleton births, (10%), multiple birth babies are much more likely to be born preterm (twins: 57%, triplets: 93%, quadruplets: 99.9%) and are more likely to need NICU care (Keith & Oleszczuk, 2002). After the babies are discharged, mothers of multiples have additional responsibilities related to the condition and number of babies (Bowers & Gromada, 2005, 2006). Although often there are many offers of help for some families, as time goes on the burden of ongoing care falls to the mother. A recent meta-analysis of qualitative research about mothers of multiples revealed five themes that can help increase understanding of what the mother experiences caring for multiples during the first year of life (Beck, 2002). These themes include "bearing the burden," "riding an emotional roller coaster," "lifesaving support," "striving for maternal justice," and "acknowledging individuality" (Beck, 2002). The mother's experiences are helpful for nurses when reviewing realistic expectations with patients with multiple births for postpartum recovery and newborn care. For a complete discussion of the nursing care of women with multiple birth, see Chapter 6. Additional information can be found in the March of Dimes Nursing Module *Care of the Multiple-Birth Family: Pregnancy and Birth* (Bowers & Gromada, 2006).

Perinatal Loss

Not all pregnancies end in a healthy baby. Some women experience a pregnancy loss, stillbirth, or a neonatal death. Postpartum nursing care for these women can be a challenging and humbling experience. Nurses must examine their own thoughts, feelings, and assumptions about the death of a baby and the bereaved family. This self-examination covers preconceived ideas, judgments, and experiences of loss (Gemma & Arnold, 2002). To provide effective nursing care, the nurse must display an open and caring attitude expressed through appreciation and acceptance of validation of the experiences of the mother and her family (Gemma & Arnold, 2002). Sensitivity to the mother's wishes is critical. Most, but not all, women who experience a perinatal loss prefer a room on another unit away from the nursery and postpartum area. It is important to allow the woman and her family as much time as they need to be with their baby. The woman and her family's desires should guide postpartum nursing care. A comprehensive guide to caring for women who experience a perinatal loss is the March of Dimes Nursing Module *Loss and Grieving in Pregnancy and the First Year of Life: A Caring Resource for Nurses* (Gemma & Arnold, 2002).

POSTPARTUM LEARNING—NEEDS ASSESSMENT AND EDUCATION

Planning for education during the postpartum period begins as soon as possible after inpatient admission. Ideally, women have had opportunities during the prenatal period to learn about postpartum and baby care by attending classes and reading appropriate materials, but this may not be true for all pregnant women because of access to care issues, complications of pregnancy, unavailability of resources, language barriers, literacy issues, or lack of knowledge about existing programs. During the hospital stay, there are limited opportunities for assessment and education of new mothers. Access, availability, and acceptability must be considered when providing postpartum education. All available resources may not be able to be integrated within the hospital stay. Closed-circuit educational television and printed materials collaboratively developed by obstetric and pediatric professionals are helpful to new parents. Individual and group educational sessions held regularly during the postpartum period are beneficial. Baby care and normal infant behaviors, and expected maternal physical and psychological changes should be included in the educational plans for each mother. New mothers should be aware of available community and health care resources (AAP & ACOG, 2002; see earlier section on educational methods and materials). Additional topics of interest to many new mothers are presented.

Selected Postpartum Teaching Topics

Pelvic-Floor Exercises

Patient education should include pelvic muscle exercises according to the institutional protocol. Kegel exercises help the woman to regain muscle tone lost as pelvic tissues are stretched. Research suggests that few women who learn Kegel exercises perform them incorrectly and may increase their risk of later incontinence (Weber & Richter, 2005). Each contraction should be held at least 10 seconds, with a 10-second or longer rest between contractions for muscular recovery. Women with third- or fourth-degree lacerations, a long second stage of labor, a large newborn, or a combination of these factors should be taught to report potential anal sphincter symptoms, such as incontinence of flatus or stool, to the primary healthcare provider.

DISPLAY 10-10

Factors Contributing to a Decline in Sexual Interest or Activity During the Postpartum Period

- Fatigue
- Fear of not hearing the infant
- Emotional distress on a continuum from baby blues to postpartum depression
- Adjustments to role change
- Hormonal changes
- Physical discomfort related to changes of vulva, vagina, perineum, and breasts
- Breastfeeding
- Decreased sense of attractiveness

Postpartum Exercise

Exercise may begin soon after birth with simple exercises such as arm raises, leg rolls, and buttock lifts and proceed as the woman feels beneficial. Walking works well to get back to prepregnancy shape. After cesarean birth, abdominal exercises should be postponed for 4 weeks. Exercise benefits the mood, self-image, and energy level and improves or maintains muscular endurance, strength, and tone, but only if the exercise is stress-relieving rather than stress-provoking (ACOG, 2002b). Women who exercise vigorously demonstrate better scores on measures of postpartum adaptation and are more likely to engage in social activities, hobbies, and entertainment. Research suggests that postpartum exercise has the capacity to improve aerobic fitness, high-density lipoprotein–cholesterol level, insulin sensitivity, and psychological well-being; but no conclusive evidence was seen that postpartum exercise itself promotes greater body weight or body-fat loss after childbirth (Larson-Meyer, 2002). Discharge instructions should include written information regarding activity, rest, and exercise for women who have given birth vaginally or by cesarean. Women should be instructed to listen to their bodies and avoid fatigue and pain.

Sexuality

Sexuality is one of the least understood and most superficially discussed topics by healthcare providers during a woman's postpartum experience. Sexuality encompasses physical capacity for sexual arousal and pleasure (ie, libido), personalized and shared social meanings attached to sexual behavior, and formation of sexual and gender identities. Sexuality and gender attitudes and behaviors carry profound significance for women and men in every society. Sexuality is a vital component of physical and emotional well-being for men and women. Display 10–10 lists the factors contributing to decline in sexual interest during the postpartum period.

Nurses must assume responsibility for anticipatory guidance, reassurance, and counseling or referral. Research about dyspareunia (ie, painful intercourse) suggests some nontraditional forms of therapy, such as acupuncture and ultrasound, may be helpful. Information about sexuality can be provided to the couple prenatally and after birth. Knowledge about normal physiologic and emotional changes allows the couple to discuss coping mechanisms and alternate means of maintaining intimacy during this challenging period. Education about sexuality during the postpartum period should include the following information:

- Sexual intercourse may be resumed approximately 3 to 4 weeks after the birth, although this should be individualized based on the woman's condition (eg, a woman with a third- or fourth-degree laceration or other significant perineal trauma may not be comfortable resuming sexual intercourse until 6 to 8 weeks or more after birth)
- Sexual intercourse should be avoided until vaginal bleeding has stopped.
- A water-soluble gel may be necessary for additional lubrication.

Contraception

The infant feeding method and the involution process influence the woman's choice and use of postpartum contraception. Ideally, the primary healthcare provider has discussed the choice, use, advantages, and disadvantages of a variety of contraceptive methods with both partners during prenatal care. The nurse should encourage the woman to ask questions regarding contraception prior to discharge from the hospital. Although many couples wait 4 to 6 weeks after birth to resume sexual relations, some couples choose earlier resumption; thus, it is important to have this discussion while still in the hospital and not wait until the first postpartum office or clinic visit. Consideration of the couple's needs and preferences is important when selecting a contraceptive method that is acceptable and effective for their unique situation. This approach allows sharing of responsibility, an opportunity to discuss advantages and disadvantages of methods, clarification of misconceptions, and discussion of prevention of sexually transmitted diseases (STDs). Information about contraception should include effectiveness, acceptability, and safety. Some of the available options for women and their partners are described in the following sections. This list is not all-inclusive. Although it is not the responsibility of the postpartum nurse to provide in-depth counseling to women regarding contraception, some basic knowledge is necessary if women have questions and if these types of discussions are not discouraged because of the institution's religious affiliation.

Depo-Provera

- Injections are given four times each year (150 mg given intramuscularly in the deltoid or gluteus maximus).
- The effectiveness rate is 99.7%.
- Advantages include long-lasting action, unimpaired lactation, and independence from coitus.
- Disadvantages include prolonged amenorrhea or uterine bleeding, weight gain, increased risk of venous thrombosis and thromboembolism, no STD protection, need for continued injections, fluid retention or edema, abdominal discomfort, and glucose intolerance.

Implanon

- The subdermal implant is inserted surgically and provides up to 3 years of contraception.
- The effectiveness rate is 99%.
- Advantages include long-lasting and reversible action.
- Disadvantages include menstrual irregularities, need for surgical removal, headaches, weight gain,

breast pain, nervousness, nausea, skin changes, vertigo, no STD protection, and raised area on the arm.

Oral Contraceptives—Combined Estrogen–Progestin

- Dosage is 1 pill each day.
- The effectiveness rate is 96.8%.
- Advantages include coitus-independent; decreased menstrual blood loss; decreased incidence of dysmenorrhea and premenstrual syndrome; reduction in endometrial adenocarcinoma, ovarian cancer, and benign breast disease; improvement in acne; protection against development of functional ovarian cysts; and decreased risk of ectopic pregnancy (Ladewig, London, & Davidson, 2006).
- Disadvantages include contraindications for women with a history of thromboembolic disorders; cerebrovascular or coronary artery disease; breast cancer; estrogen-dependent tumors; pregnancy; impaired liver function or tumors; hypertension; or diabetes of 20 years' duration; and for women who smoke (if older than 35 years), are lactating, or have had a period of immobilization (Ladewig, London, & Davidson). The drug can cause libido changes, breast tenderness, weight gain, nausea, and a delay in return of fertility.

Oral Contraceptives—Progestin-Only

- Dosage is 1 pill each day.
- The effectiveness rate is 95%.
- In addition to the advantages of oral contraceptives listed previously, lactation is not impaired by this formulation, which is less likely to cause cardiovascular complications, headaches, or hypertension.
- In addition to the disadvantages of oral contraceptives listed previously, drug interactions are more likely, and irregular bleeding, amenorrhea, and functional ovarian cysts can occur. The pill must be taken at same time each day.

Barrier Methods

- Device must be used at the time of sexual act.
- The effectiveness rate is 78% to 86%, depending on the device.
- Advantages include prevention of pregnancy, STDs, or both (used in combination with spermicides to achieve maximal protection); newer male condoms have various lengths, shapes, and adhesives.
- Tactylon (approved by the Food and Drug Administration [FDA] in 1991) is a hypoallergenic, synthetic polymer that is impervious to sperm and virus and is not degraded by oxidation or oil-based lubricants; it is used in male and female condoms.

- Reality vaginal pouch (approved by the FDA in 1992) is a female condom with two rings connected by a polyurethane sheath. The inner ring is fitted like a diaphragm; the outer ring protects the vulva and prevents slipping. It has a 15% failure rate.
- A diaphragm covers the cervix and requires fitting by healthcare professional. Its effectiveness is increased with the use of spermicide. It must be refitted after weight loss or gain greater than 22 kg and after birth. It has an 18% failure rate.
- A male condom is a latex or synthetic sheath placed over the erect penis before coitus. It must be applied before penile–vulvar contact and removed before the penis becomes flaccid (ie, risk of sperm leakage at withdrawal). It has a 12% failure rate.

Chemical Methods (Spermicidal Creams, Jellies, Foams, Suppositories, and Vaginal Film Containing Nonoxynol 9)

- Agent must be used at the time of the sex act.
- The effectiveness rate is 50% to 95%.
- Advantages include ease of application, safety, low cost, no prescription required, and help in lubrication.
- Disadvantages include a maximum effect that lasts no longer than 1 hour, required reapplication for repeat intercourse, possibility of an allergic response or irritation, and messiness.

Intrauterine Devices (IUDs)

- No action is required at time of intercourse.
- Two types are approved for use in United States: Progestasert, which is T shaped with a progesterone reservoir in the stem and must be replaced yearly, and Copper T380, which is T shaped, wrapped with copper, and effective for 8 years.
- The effectiveness rate is 97% to 98%.
- Advantages include use for postpartum and breastfeeding women, long-term and continuous use requiring minimal effort, and no continual expense.
- Disadvantages include contraindications for women with a history of pelvic inflammatory disease or STDs; need for professional insertion; and generation of cramping, pain, and bleeding, which should be evaluated.

Postpartum Tubal Ligation/ Vasectomy (Sterilization)

- It requires no additional effort after surgical procedure.
- The effectiveness rate is 99.5% (female) to 99.9% (male).

- Advantages include no need for additional contraception (should be considered permanent although reversal is technically possible).
- Its disadvantage is no STD protection.
- Before surgery, appropriate counseling is necessary regarding risks of failure, surgical risks, and potential psychosocial reactions to the procedure. A signed consent form according to institutional protocol is required.

Natural Family Planning

- It relies on fertility awareness, observations, and abstinence during the fertile portion of a woman's menstrual cycle.
- It requires an understanding of the changes occurring in a woman's ovulatory cycle.
- The fertile period is calculated with a set formula, basal body temperature, cervical mucus assessment, symptothermal techniques (ie, combines body temperature and cervical mucus assessment), or over-the-counter ovulation test kit (ie, Creighton Model, Billings Method, or Sympto Thermal).
- Advantages include a couple-centered method, low cost, lack of harm to fertility, no side effects, usefulness in diagnosing gynecologic disorders and infertility, and use in achieving pregnancy when desired.
- Disadvantages include no STD protection, difficult application during irregular cycles postpartum, need to begin charting 3 weeks after birth, and ovulation possibly occurring before the first postpartum menses (Alliende, Cabezon, Figueroa, & Kottmann, 2005; Ladewig, London, & Davidson, 2006).

PSYCHOLOGICAL ADAPTATION TO THE POSTPARTUM PERIOD

Postpartum Mood and Anxiety Disorders

Postpartum mood disorders have finally been given the attention they deserve by healthcare providers, unfortunately because of high profile cases of both maternal and child deaths. In 2001, a woman in Chicago committed suicide by drowning in Lake Michigan after weeks of bed rest to prolong her pregnancy and after giving birth to quadruplets (while they were still in the neonatal intensive care unit). In another 2001 case, a woman in Texas drowned her five children several months after giving birth to a much-wanted daughter after four sons. Numerous women suffering from postpartum psychosis, a severe and progressive form of postpartum depression, have killed themselves and/or children before they were able to get the medical help they desperately needed. Prominent women, such as Marie Osmond and Brooke Shields, have admitted suffering from postpartum depression and written of their experience with the disorder. Some of the attention is helpful to women who have suffered in the past and are currently struggling with postpartum depression. These women know they are not alone and that the feelings they are experiencing have been experienced by other new mothers who were successfully treated. Women with postpartum depression report feeling very alone and helpless. Although family members notice abnormal changes in the woman's mood and behavior, they frequently underestimate the extent of the illness. Women are told by well-meaning others that they just have the "baby blues" and they should snap out of it and take care of their beautiful baby. Women suffering from postpartum depression wish it could be that easy. Prompt diagnosis and treatment is needed for postpartum depression. Nurses can be helpful in identifying women who could benefit from referral and treatment.

During the postpartum hospital stay, the new mother has to move quickly from self-concern to other-concern: her baby. It is important that her physical and psychological needs be met so that she will be better able to focus on her newborn's care. She may become intensely focused on the cognitive learning needs related to newborn feeding and physical care. The new mother may verbalize anxiety and concern. If so, she needs to be heard, and her concerns must be validated. The newly evolving relationship between the mother and her newborn is based on connection and care. If the woman has difficulty with these beginning skills, it may alter her self-esteem and maternal development. The nurse can assist the mother in this attachment process by establishing a responsive, nurturing environment, maximizing mother–infant contact, and assisting the mother to understand the newborn's behaviors (Karl, Beal, O'Hare, & Rissmiller, 2006). The woman brings with her many performance expectations that need to be discussed and clarified. Mercer (1986) described maternal role attainment as a process that takes a period of about 10 months to develop. During this postpartum phase, the new mother attaches to her newborn, gains competence as a mother, and should expresses gratification in the mother–baby interaction. This adaptation can be delayed or altered if the woman's health and mental status is less than optimal. The reality of the current healthcare delivery system is that much of the work of the postpartum maternal adjustment and role attainment is done after discharge. Referral to community resources and discharge planning are thus imperative in the total care plan.

Emotionally, the early days after giving birth can be disconcerting. It is supposed to be such an exciting time, but in reality the new mother may be experiencing alternating periods of crying and joy, irritability, anxiety, headaches, confusion, forgetfulness, depersonalization, and fatigue. These are characteristics of the "baby blues." It has been estimated that up to 50% of new mothers experience this transitory mood disorder (Miller, 2002). Unfortunately, this phenomenon occurs so frequently that it is often considered normal and therefore does not get the attention that it deserves. The causes of postpartum depression may be biologic, psychologic, situational, or multifactorial (Beck, 2002; Beck & Indman, 2005). It is felt that this disorder is related to the normal physiologic and psychosocial changes that occur in the process of becoming a new mother. The rapid decrease in the levels of female reproductive hormones after birth may dysregulate the complex balance of neurotransmitters, stress hormones, and reproductive hormones (Driscoll, 2006a). Having the "baby blues" can greatly affect the new mother and her family, especially if they are unaware of the possibility or what to do about it.

Women and their families need information about normal mood changes after childbirth. They should be aware that with a lot of support, reassurance, rest, and good nutrition, these labile moods usually balance out, and the woman will begin to feel better and feel more organized and confident. However, if the moods do not stabilize, referral should be made to the psychiatric/mental health team specialists in postpartum mood and anxiety disorders (Driscoll, 2006b). Inpatient perinatal nurses interact with women during the first days after birth and are in the position to make initial assessments of mother–baby interactions and mood alterations. An important aspect of this nursing assessment is determining when the mother's behaviors are beyond normal "baby blues" and pathologic such as postpartum depression (Beck, 2006). This is challenging, because alterations in mood are common during the immediate hours after labor and birth. An awareness of the risk factors for postpartum depression facilitates prompt diagnosis, treatment, and early recovery (see Display 10–11). Because most postpartum LOSs are 1 to 4 days, there is a greater likelihood of mood disorders occurring at home, rather than in the hospital environment. If a follow-up appointment with a healthcare provider occurs at 4 to 6 weeks after birth, the woman experiences these conditions alone, without medical or nursing support. Thus, women and their families need anticipatory information about postpartum mood disorders so that prompt identification and early treatment can be initiated. A heightened awareness among perinatal healthcare providers about the incidence of postpartum mood and anxiety disorders, knowledge of common signs and symptoms, and

Risk Factors for Postpartum Depression

- Prenatal depression
- Low self-esteem
- Stress of child care
- Prenatal anxiety
- Life stress
- Lack of social support
- Marital relationship problems
- History of depression
- "Difficult" infant temperament
- Postpartum blues
- Single status
- Low socioeconomic status
- Unplanned or unwanted pregnancy

Adapted from Beck, C. (2001). Predictors of postpartum depression: An update. *Nursing Research, 50*(5), 275–282; Beck, C. (2002). Revision of the Postpartum Depression Predictors Inventory. *Journal of Obstetric, Gynecologic, and Neonatal Nursing, 31*(4), 394–402.

DISPLAY 10-12

Instruments for Assessing Postpartum Depression, Mood Disorders, and Psychosis

- Edinburgh Postnatal Depression Scale (EPDS; Cox, Holden, & Sagovsky, 1987)
- Postpartum Depression Predictors Inventory (PDPI; Beck, 2001, 2002)
- Postpartum Depression Checklist (PDC; Beck, 1995, 2001, 2002)
- Hamilton Rating Scale for Depression (Thompson, Harris, Lazarus, & Richards, 1998)

the prospects for recovery can contribute to successful outcomes for affected women and their families.

Each woman should be routinely assessed for maternal mental status and adjustment, and mood disorders as a standard part of postpartum clinical nursing assessments (Driscoll, 2006a, 2006b; Logsdon, Wisner, & Pinto-Foltz, 2006). This assessment is facilitated by a professional nurse who is willing to listen to the woman's birth experience, observant of mother–baby interactions, and knowledgeable about the normal physiologic adaptations that are similar to symptoms of depression such appetite fluctuations, fatigue, and decreased libido. Prior to discharge from the hospital, the woman should be given a list of telephone numbers of her care providers as well as any emergency services that she may need. It is important to go over the key support people with the new mother and her partner during discharge teaching. When home visits by skilled perinatal nurses are available, the nurse should include a thorough assessment of the psychological adaptation of the new mother.

Psychiatric professionals have several instruments available for assessing women for postpartum depression (Display 10–12). These assessments require careful planning and knowledge about the instruments themselves, and appropriate referral options. If perinatal care providers are knowledgeable about the woman's psychological well-being, appropriate referral

and early identification of these disorders can be made, thus potentially preventing a crisis. Preparation for appropriate assessments and interventions can result from interdisciplinary efforts involving all who are involved in the care including physicians, nurse practitioners, nurse midwives, nurses, perinatal educators, lactation consultants, and support services such as social services and counselors. Educational programs sponsored by experts in postpartum mood disorders can be helpful to increase awareness and lead to appropriate, timely referral. Educational programs should also be offered within the community to increase public awareness and knowledge of available resources.

Validating the woman's experience as normal may provide needed reassurance. Talking with the woman in a familiar, comfortable environment about the stresses and challenges of new motherhood provides opportunities for early interventions, such as counseling, referrals to support services, and pharmacologic assistance. Help with infant and self-care, coupled with support from family members, promotes recovery. Providing appropriate interventions and therapy has far-reaching effects—improving the health of the women, their infants, and the family itself. These interventions become an investment in the future.

Psychosocial adaptation to pregnancy and postpartum is a dynamic process. The nurse plays a significant role in the promotion and facilitation of this experience in a healthy way. It is a time when the woman is open to great psychological growth and relies on the healthcare team for information and support. The nurse needs to be aware of the normal process in order to identify those that are abnormal. It is helpful in the assessment of mood, anxiety, and emotional states to remember three words: *frequency, duration, and intensity*. If the woman describes that she is having difficulty functioning in her activities of daily living and having a tough time coping due to emotional, mood, and/or anxiety changes, referral is necessary. The referral process needs to be managed in an empowering, supportive way. Letting her know that she is valued and her concerns and feelings are important is a way for the perinatal nurse to give the woman the message that she deserves good care. Appropriate healthcare provider attitudes support the referral process. Due to the rapid changes in the healthcare delivery system and decreasing lengths of stay, it is imperative for the perinatal nurse to actively pursue, nurture, and promote collaborative relationships with colleagues in the community. It is this active communication and relational approach to the care of this new mother and her family that will promote, facilitate, and encourage healthy maternal and paternal psychosocial adaptation and adjustment. An in-depth discussion of psychosocial adaptation to pregnancy and postpartum including postpartum mood disorders is presented in Chapter 4.

WOMEN'S PERSPECTIVES ON THE TRANSITION TO PARENTHOOD

Fatigue

The 6 weeks after giving birth are a time of change and adjustment for the woman and the family. Fatigue, stress, depression, and infection are interrelated in postpartum mothers. These variables change over time, possibly placing mothers and infants in a psychoneuroimmunologically vulnerable group (Groer et al., 2005). The variables reinforce one another and make it difficult to determine which occurs first, fatigue causing depression and stress or the reverse. Their alteration of immune function in new mothers may result in increased vulnerability to infection. In the breastfeeding woman, fatigue is associated with increased levels of melatonin in the mother's milk, which is transferred to the infant and influence the sleep–wake cycle. Fatigue affects emotional adjustment and adaptation to the maternal role, and it may cause feelings of inadequacy in meeting the needs of other family members and in assuming household responsibilities. Anticipatory guidance in identifying rest opportunities and organizing new responsibilities and tasks is important for the new mother. Education about the causes of fatigue and possible community and family resources enables the new mother to assume control and promotes problem-solving behaviors. Together, the nurse and woman can develop strategies for requesting help with newborn care, household chores, and sibling care. Listing daily and weekly tasks provides an organizational framework and may serve as a readily available wish list that can be used when family and friends offer to help. Identification of family members and friends available to help provides an initial supportive structure for the new family.

Additional Stressors

In addition to fatigue, several stressors have been identified as contributing to adaptation difficulties in the postpartum period. These stressors include physical changes and complications, role-adaptation conflicts, newborn needs, relationship changes, and possibly the return to the workplace and selecting a child-care setting.

FAMILY TRANSITION TO PARENTHOOD

After birth, the woman experiences psychological changes as well as physiologic reversal of the physical changes of pregnancy. For the woman, adoption of a maternal role begins during pregnancy as she develops an attachment to the fetus. This role evolution continues postpartum with the birth separation of the mother–infant pair, or polarization (Rubin, 1977). As the mother develops her style of parenting, she considers her behavior in relation to the infant and notices familial characteristics in the infant. These changes in the mother are referred to as maternal role attainment (Mercer, 1995). Mercer identified four stages in this process: anticipatory, formal, informal, and personal. The anticipatory stage, occurring during pregnancy, involves the observation of role models for mothering behaviors. During the formal stage, the new mother tries to perform infant care tasks as expected by others. The mother begins to make personal choices about mothering during the informal stage and attains comfort with the role during the personal stage. The final stages, informal and formal, correspond to the taking-in and taking-hold stages identified by Rubin (1961). During the taking-in phase (first 24 hours or longer), the woman relives the birth experience, clarifies her understanding of the experience, and focuses on food and sleep. The taking-hold phase (second to fourth day) centers on concern with bodily functions, and the woman focuses on regaining control over her life and succeeding in infant-care responsibilities. Rubin (1961) includes the letting-go phase to describe the new mother's letting go of who she was and full participation in the mothering role. Nurses can foster success in these processes by meeting the woman's needs during each stage and providing a supportive environment for listening and educating the new mother.

Paternal satisfaction with the birth experience and its associated stresses influences marital happiness and family life. For most women, being comfortable as a mother occurs during the first 3 to 10 months after birth. Nursing assessments about the quality of parenting behaviors during the postpartum period can guide the educational plan for the new couple. Display 10–13 lists adaptive and maladaptive parenting behaviors. Evidence of maladaptive parenting behaviors should prompt nursing communication with the primary healthcare provider and appropriate referral.

Nurses caring for women and families during the postpartum period must consider their cultural expectations and norms when planning care. This requires an open-minded, sensitive, and creative approach. Knowledge about various traditions and services within ethnic groups and a willingness to give up control demonstrate respect and encourage a collaborative approach to providing these women with a positive and satisfying birth experience (Callister, 2005).

The changes that occur within the family are not limited to the woman. The family, however it is defined, experiences changes in structure and process. Parents

---

D I S P L A Y 1 0 - 1 3

Adaptive and Maladaptive Parenting Behaviors

	ADAPTIVE	MALADAPTIVE
Feeding	Provides an appropriate amount and type of food Burps the child both during and after feeding Prepares the meal appropriately Feeds the infant regularly and as frequently as necessary	Makes inappropriate types or inadequate amounts of food available Does not burp the baby, though she or he knows it is necessary to do so Prepares the meal inappropriately Rushes or delays feeding the child
Rest	Provides a quiet and relaxed environment for the resting baby Schedules rest periods	Does not provide a quiet and relaxed environment Does not schedule rest periods
Stimulating Caring for Infant	Speaks to the child and makes other appropriate sounds Provides tactile stimulation at a variety of times and not only when the baby is hungry or in danger Provides age-appropriate toys Positions infant comfortably while holding the child The baby seems satisfied with the way it is being handled Sees that the baby is dry, warm, and not hungry Exhibits initiative in trying to find how to deal with the baby's problems	Speaks aggressively or not at all to the infant Plays aggressively with the baby or does not touch her or him Provides inappropriate toys Does not hold the baby or ignores child's discomfort when being held The baby seems frustrated with the way it is handled Does not care for the baby who is hungry, cold, or soiled Lacks initiative and does not try to meet the baby's needs
Self Perception/ Emotional State of Parent	Usually maintains a realistic perception of and realistic expectations for the baby Exhibits a realistic perception of her or his own mothering and fathering abilities Shows some interest in understanding and/or discussing the childbirth Exhibits friendly or neutral behavior with other children Appears generally satisfied to be a parent Is able or willing to turn to other people for social support when necessary	Develops distorted perceptions of and unrealistic expectations for the baby Holds unrealistic expectations of her or his own parenting abilities Is unable or unwilling to discuss the childbirth Exhibits hostility/aggression toward other children Appears dissatisfied to be a parent Is unable to provide adequately for relaxation and own emotional needs Is isolated and without adequate social support Is depressed

adapt to these changes more easily when they are involved with a support network. This network may include family, friends, and institutional components. New parents often report a change in their immediate social network. This change typically involves increased contact with other new parents or with families facing similar challenges. For new parents living without immediate access to family, referral to support groups sponsored by hospitals or community centers may provide an opening into a circle of new parents and friends. New parents may place increased importance on family and the traditions they include. For other couples, increased familial contacts may result in an increased level of stress as the new family attempts to meet the external demands placed on them by enthusiastic or demanding family members. If the new mother decides not to return to a work environment outside the home, she may face the challenge of redefining herself as a mother.

Nurses caring for families during this time can provide anticipatory guidance about possible areas of stress and options for stress reduction. Providing this information in a written format enables the couple to review the information as situations develop.

POSTPARTUM DISCHARGE FOLLOW-UP

In response to the current length of stay, many perinatal centers now offer postdischarge follow-up home visits, clinic visits, or telephone calls. The AAP *Committee on the Fetus and Newborn* (2004) recommends in-person follow-up by an experienced healthcare professional occur within 48 hours of discharge following a maternity stay of 48 hours or less. The optimal time for assessing mothers and their infants is between 3 and 4 days after birth when infections, poor infant feeding, excessive weight loss, jaundice, and other problems become evident (Brown, 2006; Roudebush, Kaufman, Johnson, Abraham, & Clayton, 2006).

In-person follow-up visits afford the perinatal nurse an opportunity to carefully assess maternal and infant well-being and provide the family with continuing education and support (Brown, 2006). In some institutions, the primary staff nurse may see the family for their follow-up visit. The family may return to the hospital and be seen in a room set aside for outpatient follow-up visits, or the primary nurse may make a follow-up visit at the family's home. In other institutions, the volume of visits is large enough to require a separate nursing staff for follow-up visits (Brown, 2006; Ladewig, London, & Davidson, 2006; Lieu et al., 2000; Roudebush, Kaufman, Johnson, Abraham, & Clayton, 2006).

Medical complications identified during the visit are immediately referred to the primary healthcare provider. Other issues or concerns are addressed during the visit or referred to an appropriate resource. This assessment visit can take place in a home or clinic setting as long as the nurse examining the infant is competent in newborn assessment and the results of the follow-up visit are reported to the infant's physician or his or her designees on the day of the visit. The visit should include:

- Infant weight, general health, hydration, and degree of jaundice (if present)
- Identification of any new problems
- Review of feeding patterns and technique, including observation of breastfeeding for adequacy of position, latch-on, and swallowing
- Historical evidence of adequate urination and defecation patterns
- Assess quality of mother–infant interaction and infant behavior
- Reinforce maternal or family education in infant care, particularly regarding infant feeding
- Review of outstanding results of laboratory tests performed before discharge
- Performance of screening tests in accordance with state regulations and other tests that are clinically indicated, such as serum bilirubin
- Verification of the plan for health care maintenance, including a method for obtaining emergency services, preventive care and immunizations, periodic evaluations and physical examinations, and necessary screenings (AAP, 2004)

When in-person follow-up visits are not offered, a postdischarge phone call gives families another opportunity to ask questions and receive important information and referrals. The perinatal nurse can use a standardized assessment tool to ask the family about infant feeding and elimination patterns, cord care, infant appearance and behavior, maternal comfort, lochia flow, perineal care, breast care, and maternal emotional well-being (Display 10–14). The nurse should ask the mother if she has any concerns about herself or her infant and reminds the mother about specific situations that would warrant a telephone call to the healthcare provider. The nurse should refer the mother to the written materials provided by the institution for further information.

Ideally, all women should receive a postdischarge visit or telephone call. If resources are limited, the following criteria define circumstances where postdischarge follow-up is essential:

- Length of stay less than 24 hours after a vaginal birth
- Length of stay less than 48 hours after a cesarean birth
- Limited or no prenatal care

DISPLAY 10-14

Early Discharge Follow-Up Telephone Call Report

Mother: Age _____   G/P _____   Vag Birth _____   C/Birth _____

Marital status: S   M   W   Discharge date: _____

Baby: Sex: M   F   Gestational age: _____

Newborn birth weight _____   Discharge weight: _____

Breast _____ Formula _____   Person making call: _____

BABY CARE	NO CONCERNS	PROBLEM IDENTIFIED	SUGGESTION MADE
Circumcision assessment			
Cord assessment			
Jaundice			
Changes in newborn:			
Behavior			
Feeding			
Temperature			
Breastfeeding:			
# wet diapers			
# & character of stools			
latch-on/positioning			
Frequency of feeding/24 hours			
Breast & nipple assessment:			
Sore nipples			
Cracked nipples			
Breast fullness			
Suck/swallow assessment			
Other concerns			
Formula Feeding:			
# wet diapers			
# & characteristics of stools			
Ounces/feedings			
Frequency of feedings			
Skin appearance			
Sleep patterns			
Ability to care for newborn			

MATERNAL CARE	NO CONCERNS	PROBLEM IDENTIFIED	SUGGESTION MADE
Lochia			
Episiotomy			
Incision			
Discomforts:			
Breast			
Perineal			
Incisional			

(continued)

MATERNAL CARE	NO CONCERNS	PROBLEM IDENTIFIED	SUGGESTION MADE
Cramping			
Calf/leg tenderness			
Hemorrhoids			
Voiding:			
Frequency			
Dysuria			
Bowel movement			
Emotional:			
Weepy			
Fatigue			
Sadness			
Onset of feelings			
Adequate rest:			
Taking naps			
Sleeps well when baby sleeps			
Other			
Ability to care for self			
REFERRALS	**DATE**	**PROBLEM IDENTIFIED**	**SUGGESTION MADE**
Lactation Consultant			
Social Services			
Physician			
Clinical Specialist			
Home Health Care			
WIC			
Other			

- Infant feeding problems identified during hospital stay
- Infant gestational age less than 37 completed weeks
- Multiple birth
- Risk factors for developing hyperbilirubinemia
- Maternal or infant health conditions putting mother or infant at risk for complications
- Lack of adequate support system
- Women who express or show they feel overwhelmed, very anxious, or depressed
- Discharge evaluation indicates need for further teaching

The nurse providing postdischarge follow-up should have access to essential patient information including maternal age, health history, birth information, newborn assessment, infant weight, method of infant feeding, and name of the infant's and mother's healthcare providers. The nurse's assessment is documented and maintained as part of the permanent medical record. Periodic reviews of accumulated assessment forms provide the institution with important data to identify common concerns and outcomes. Data can be used to revise and strengthen patient education programs and patient care provided as part of discharge planning.

EVALUATION OF POSTPARTUM SERVICES

An essential first step in program evaluation is identification of goals and expected outcomes. Primary outcome criteria include family knowledge about maternal–newborn care, ability to identify support persons and community resources, and familiarity with signs and symptoms of complications that warrant a call to the primary healthcare provider. Criteria met both at discharge and in the immediate postpartum period should be included in the evaluation process. Both quantitative and qualitative approaches to data collection are useful.

It is important that nursing care as well as patient use of services following discharge are tracked to ensure that resources are available that are beneficial for new families. These evaluations can be quantitative and qualitative. Quantitative evaluation may be a concurrent or retrospective review of medical record data, tracking readmissions, and/or keeping a log of parent phone calls to the nursery or maternity unit. Variance data provide information about maternal–newborn teaching and care completed within suggested time frames during the inpatient stay. Primary healthcare providers can participate in data collection by tracking phone calls, commonly asked questions, and nonroutine office visits. Data collected from postdischarge follow-up assessment tools can be used to identify topics of maternal and newborn care that suggest perinatal education was effective and identify areas for improvement. In addition, results of individual follow-up contacts can be compared with learning-needs assessments completed prior to discharge. If data analyses suggest specific topics should be covered in more depth in the inpatient setting, nurses can make appropriate revisions in patient teaching strategies.

Qualitative methods of evaluation such as patient interviews, focus groups, written surveys, letters or phone calls from parents who have used programs and services are additional valuable sources of data (Zwelling, 2000). Women and their families frequently identify important issues not addressed on surveys or evaluation tools. Tracking data trends and adjusting discharge plans accordingly lead to improvements in the system. For example, if analysis of the parents' phone call log indicates many calls about a particular issue such as umbilical cord care, parent teaching plans can be redesigned to include comprehensive coverage of that topic. Childbearing family surveys may suggest a need to offer more flexibility in class schedules. Prenatal class evaluations provide information about class content and teaching methods that parents find useful. Prenatal classes can be revised based on consistent themes in participant feedback.

An additional benefit of soliciting patient feedback about services provided is the ability to share with perinatal educators and staff nurses' positive remarks about their individual contributions. Often, women will take time to write lengthy comments about their prenatal educator and the nurses who cared for them during the inpatient stay or at the outpatient home or clinic visit. Although perinatal nurses many times feel rushed to accomplish all there is to do in the limited time available, it is gratifying to know we can still make a positive difference. Conversely, a complaint or criticism offered by the mother or her family about a staff member, the education program, or the hospital stay is always valuable. Complaints can increase the nurse's understanding of how the family perceived their interactions with the nurse and the care provided. With this insight, the nurse has the opportunity to make improvements in clinical or interpersonal skills. Complaints also provide the institution with an opportunity to change or revise existing programs to meet consumer expectations. A well-designed postpartum discharge-planning program can be cost effective if unnecessary calls and return visits to the healthcare provider or institution are decreased and readmissions to the hospital are decreased or stabilized. However, to demonstrate a change in readmissions or a decrease in unnecessary calls and return visits, a systematic method of data collection and analysis must be in place. As healthcare dollars become scarcer, increased sophistication in linking positive outcomes (both clinical and financial) to perinatal education and discharge planning programs will be critical.

SUMMARY

The postpartum period is a time of transition and change for the new mother and her family. Physiologic and psychologic changes occur immediately and over time, necessitating careful planning to meet the needs of the new family. Timely, frequent assessments and appropriate interventions require clinical skills and adequate knowledge about these processes. Supportive care that includes education for the woman and her family about what to expect in the first few weeks facilitates the transition from the inpatient setting to home. Being present during this period is a responsibility and a privilege that can affect society as a whole, one family at a time.

REFERENCES

Abramov, Y., Sand, P. K., Botros, S. M., Gandhi, S., Miller, J. R., Nickolov, A., & Goldberg, R. P. (2005). Risk factors for female anal incontinence: New insight through the Evanston-Northwestern twin sisters study. *Obstetrics and Gynecology, 106*(4), 726–732.

Abrams, B., Minassian, D., & Pickett, K. E. (2004). Maternal nutrition. In R. K.Creasy & R. Resnick (Eds.), *Maternal-fetal medicine: Principles and practice* (5th ed, pp.155–164). Philadelphia: Saunders.

Alliende, M. E., Cabezon, C., Figueroa, H., & Kottmann, C. (2005). Cervicovaginal fluid changes to detect ovulation accurately. *American Journal of Obstetrics and Gynecology. 193*(1), 71–75.

American Academy of Pediatrics. (2004). Hospital stay for healthy term newborns. *Pediatrics, 113*(5), 1434–1436.

American Academy of Pediatrics & American College of Obstetricians and Gynecologists. (2002). *Guidelines for perinatal care* (5th ed.). Elk Grove Village, IL: Author.

American College of Obstetricians and Gynecologists. (2002a). *Diagnosis and management of preeclampsia and eclampsia.* (Practice Bulletin No. 33). Washington, DC: Author.

American College of Obstetricians and Gynecologists. (2002b). *Exercise during pregnancy and the postpartum period.* (Committee Opinion No. 267). Washington, DC: Author.

American College of Obstetricians and Gynecologists. (2003). *Management of preterm labor.* (Practice Bulletin No. 43). Washington, DC: Author.

American College of Obstetricians and Gynecologists. (2006a). *Episiotomy.* (Practice Bulletin No. 71). Washington, DC: Author.

American College of Obstetricians and Gynecologists. (2006b). *Postpartum hemorrhage.* (Practice Bulletin No. 76). Washington, DC: Author.

American Society of Anesthesiologists. (2006). *Practice guidelines for obstetrical anesthesia: An updated report by the American Society of Anesthesiologists Task Force on Obstetrical Anesthesia.* Park Ridge, IL: Author.

Association of Women's Health, Obstetric, and Neonatal Nurses & Johnson & Johnson Consumer Products, Inc. (2005). *Compendium of postpartum care.* Washington, DC: Author.

Association of Women's Health, Obstetric and Neonatal Nurses. (2003). *Standards and guidelines for professional nursing practice in the care of women and newborns* (6th ed.). Washington, DC: Author.

Atterbury, J. L., Groome, L. J., Hoff, C., & Yarnell, J. A. (1998). Clinical presentation of women readmitted with postpartum severe preeclampsia or eclampsia. *Journal of Obstetric, Gynecologic, and Neonatal Nursing, 27*(2), 134–141.

Beck, C. T. (2001). Predictors of postpartum depression: An update. *Nursing Research, 50*(5), 275–282.

Beck, C. T. (2002). Revision of the Postpartum Depression Predictors Inventory. *Journal of Obstetric, Gynecologic, and Neonatal Nursing, 31*(4), 394–402.

Beck, C. T. (2006). Postpartum depression: It isn't just the blues. *American Journal of Nursing, 106*(5), 40–50.

Beck, C. T., & Indman, P. (2005). The many faces of postpartum depression. *Journal of Obstetric, Gynecologic, and Neonatal Nursing, 34*(5), 569–576.

Beckmann, M. M., & Garrett, A. J. (2006). Antenatal perineal massage for reducing perineal trauma. *Cochrane Database of Systematic Reviews, 1*, CD005123.

Beers, M. H., & Berkow, R. (2006). Venous thrombosis. *The Merck manual of diagnosis and therapy, (18th ed., Section 16, Ch. 212.)* Retrieved May 2, 2006, from http://www.merckshared/mmanual/section16/chapter212/212g.jsp

Blackburn, S. T. (2003). *Maternal, fetal, & neonatal physiology: A clinical perspective.* Philadelphia: Saunders.

Boreham, M. K., Richter, H. E., Kenton, K. S., Nager, C. W., Thomas, G. W., Aronson, M. P., et al. (2005). Anal incontinence in women presenting for gynecologic care: Prevalence, risk factors, and impact upon quality of life. *American Journal of Obstetrics and Gynecology, 192*(5), 1637–1642.

Bouwmeester, F. W., Jonhoff, A. R., Verheijen, R. H., & van Geijn, H. P. (2003). Successful treatment of life-threatening postpartum hemorrhage with recombinant activated factor VII. *Obstetrics and Gynecology, 101*(6), 1174–1176.

Bowers, N., & Gromada, K. K. (2006). *Care of the multiple-birth family: Pregnancy and birth.* (Nursing Module). White Plains, NY: The March of Dimes Birth Defects Foundation.

Bowes, W. A., & Thorp, J. M. (2004). Clinical aspects of normal and abnormal labor. In R. K. Creasy & R. Resnick (Eds.), *Maternal-fetal medicine: Principles and practice* (5th ed, pp. 671–705). Philadelphia: Saunders.

Brown, S. E. (2006). Tender beginnings program: An educational continuum for the maternity patient. *Journal of Perinatal and Neonatal Nursing, 20*(3), 210–219.

Callister, L. C. (2005). What has the literature taught us about culturally competent care of women and children? *MCN The American Journal of Maternal Child Nursing, 30*(6), 380–388.

Casey, B. M., Schaffer, J. I., Bloom, S. K., Heartwel, S. F., McIntire, D. D., & Leveno, K. J. (2005). Obstetric antecedents for postpartum pelvic floor dysfunction. *American Journal of Obstetrics and Gynecology, 192*(5), 1655–1662.

Christianson, L. M., Bovbjerg, V. E., McDavitt, E. C., & Hullfish, K. L. (2003). Risk factors for perineal injury during delivery. *American Journal of Obstetrics and Gynecology, 189*(1), 255–260.

Cunningham, F. G., Leveno, K. J., Bloom, S. K., Hauth, J. C., Gilstrap, L. C., & Wenstrom, K. D. (2005). The puerperium. In *Williams obstetrics* (22nd ed., pp. 693–758). New York: McGraw-Hill.

Dildy, G. A. (2002). Postpartum hemorrhage: New management options. *Clinical Obstetrics and Gynecology, 45*(2), 330–344.

Driscoll, J. W. (2006a). Postpartum depression: The state of the science. *Journal of Perinatal and Neonatal Nursing, 20*(1), 40–42.

Driscoll, J. W. (2006b). Postpartum depression: How nurses can identify and care for women grappling with this disorder. *AWHONN Lifelines, 10*(5), 401–409.

Eason, E., Lebrecque, Marcoux, S., & Mondor, M. (2002). Anal incontinence after childbirth. *Canadian Medical Association Journal, 166*(3), 326–30.

Freda, M. C. (2004). *Preterm labor: Prevention and nursing management.* (Nursing Module 3rd ed.). White Plains, NY: March of Dimes Birth Defects Foundation.

French, L. M., & Smaill, F. M. (2004). Antibiotic regimens for endometritis after delivery. *Cochrane Database of Systematic Reviews, 18*(4), CD001067.

Garcia, V., Rogers, R. G., Kim, S. S., Hall, R. J., & Kammerer-Doak D. N. (2005). Primary repair of obstetric and anal sphincter laceration: A randomized trial of two surgical techniques. *American Journal of Obstetrics and Gynecology, 192*(5), 1697–1701.

Gemma, P. B., & Arnold, J. (2002). *Loss and grieving in pregnancy and the first year of life: A caring resource for nurses.* (Nursing Module). White Plains, NY: The March of Dimes Birth Defects Foundation.

Gibbs, R. S., Sweet, R. L., & Duff, W. P. (2004). Maternal and fetal infectious disorders. In R. K. Creasy & R. Resnick (Eds.), *Maternal-fetal medicine: Principles and practice* (5th ed, pp. 741–801). Philadelphia: Saunders.

Gilbert, E. S., & Harmon, J. S. (2003). *Manual of high risk pregnancy & delivery.* St. Louis, MO: Mosby.

Gonik, B., & Foley, M. R. (2004). Intensive care monitoring of the critically ill pregnant patient. In R. K. Creasy & R. Resnick (Eds.), *Maternal-fetal medicine: Principles and practice* (5th ed, pp. 925–951). Philadelphia: Saunders.

Groer, M., Davis, M., Casey, K., Short, B., Smith, K., & Groer, S. (2005). Neuroendocrine & immune relationships in postpartum fatigue. *MCN The American Journal of Maternal/Child Nursing, 30*(2), 133–138.

Hamilton, B. E., Martin, J. A., & Ventura, S. J. (2006). Births: Preliminary data for 2005. *National Center for Health Statistics.* Retrieved January 1, 2007, from http://www.cdc.gov.nchs/products/pubs/pubd/hestats/prelimbirths05/prelimbirths05.html

Hedayati, H., Parsons, J., & Crowther, C. A. (2005). Topically applied anaesthetics for treating perineal pain after childbirth. *Cochrane Database of Systematic Reviews, 18*(2), CD004223.

Hudelist, G., Gelle'n, J., Singer, C., Ruecklinger, E., Czerwenka, K., Kandolf, O., et al. (2005). Factors predicting severe perineal trauma during childbirth: Role of forceps delivery routinely combined with mediolateral episiotomy. *American Journal of Obstetrics and Gynecology, 192*(3), 875–881.

Jacob, T. (2006). *Smell.* Retrieved January 1, 2007, from http://www.cf.ac.uk/biosi/staff/jacob/teaching/sensory/olfact1.html

Johnson, K., Posner, S. F., Biermann, J., Cordero, J. F., Atrash, H. K., Parker, C. F., et al. (2006). Recommendations to improve preconception health and health care—United States. *Morbidity and Mortality Weekly Report, 55*(RR06), 1–23.

Joint Commission on Accreditation of Healthcare Organizations. (2004). *Preventing infant death and injury during delivery.* (Sentinel Event Alert No. 30). Oakbrook Terrace, IL: Author.

Kaitz, M., Good, A., Rokem, A. M., & Eidelman, A. I. (1987). Mother's recognition of their newborns by olfactory cues. *Developmental Psychobiology, 20*(6), 587–591.

Karl, D. J., Beal, J. A., O'Hare, C. M., & Rissmiller, P. N. (2006). Reconceptualizing the nurse's role in the newborn period as an attacher. *MCN The American Journal of Maternal/Child Nursing, 31*(4), 257–262.

Karpati, P. C., Rossignol, M., Pirot, M., Cholley, B., Vicaut, E., Henry, P., et al. (2004). High incidence of myocardial ischemia during postpartum hemorrhage. *Anesthesiology, 100*(1), 30–36.

Keith, L. G., & Oleszczuk, J. J. (2002). Triplet births in the United States: An epidemic of high-risk pregnancies. *Journal of Reproductive Medicine, 47*(4), 259–265.

Kilpatrick, S. J., & Laros, R. K. (2004). Maternal hematologic disorders. In R. K.Creasy & R. Resnick (Eds.), *Maternal-fetal medicine: Principles and practice* (5th ed, pp. 975–1004). Philadelphia: Saunders.

Kozak, L. J., DeFrances, C. J., & Hall, M. J. (2004). National hospital discharge survey: 2004 Annual summary with detailed diagnosis and procedure data. *Vital Health Statistics, 13*(162), 1–218.

Ladewig, P. A., London, M. L., & Davidson, M. R. (2006). *Contemporary maternal-newborn nursing care.* Upper Saddle River, NJ: Prentice Hall.

Landon, M. B. (2004). Diseases of the liver, biliary system, & pancreas. In R. K. Creasy & R. Resnick (Eds.), *Maternal-fetal medicine: Principles and practice* (5th ed, pp. 1127–1145). Philadelphia: Saunders.

Laros, R. K. (2004). Thromboembolic disease. In R. K.Creasy & R. Resnick (Eds.), *Maternal-fetal medicine: Principles and practice* (5th ed, pp. 845–857). Philadelphia: Saunders.

Larson-Meyer, D. E. (2002). Effect of postpartum exercise on mothers and their offspring: A review of the literature. *Obesity Research, 10*(8), 841–853.

Lieu, T. A., Braveman, P. A., Escobar, G. J., Fischer, A. F., Jensvold, N. G., & Capra, A. M. (2000). A randomized comparison of home and clinic follow-up visits after early postpartum hospital discharge. *Pediatrics, 105*(5), 1058–1065.

Logsdon, M. C., Wisner, K. L., & Pinto-Foltz, M. D. (2006). The impact of postpartum depression on mothering. *Journal of Obstetric, Gynecologic, and Neonatal Nursing, 351*(5), 652–661.

Lawrence, R. M., & Lawrence, R. A. (2004). The breast and the physiology of lactation. In R. K. Creasy & R. Resnick (Eds.), *Maternal-fetal medicine: Principles and practice* (5th ed, pp. 135–153). Philadelphia: Saunders.

Magann, E. F., & Lanneau, G. S. (2005). Third stage of labor. *Obstetrics and Gynecology Clinics of North America, 32*(2005), 323–332.

Maloni J. A., Alexander G. R., Schluchter M. D., Shah D. M., & Park S. (2004). Antepartum bed rest: Maternal weight change and infant birth weight. *Biological Research for Nursing, 5*(3), 177–186.

Maloni, J. A., & Kutil, R. L. (2000). Antepartum support group for women hospitalized on bedrest. *MCN The American Journal of Maternal Child Nursing, 25*(4), 204–210.

Maloni, J. A., & Park, S. (2005). Postpartum symptoms after antepartum bedrest. *Journal of Obstetric, Gynecologic, and Neonatal Nursing, 34*(2), 163–171.

Martell, L. K. (2000). The hospital and the postpartum experience: A historical analysis. *Journal of Obstetric, Gynecologic, and Neonatal Nursing, 29*(1), 65–72.

Mercer, R. T. (1995). *Becoming a mother.* New York: Springer.

Miller, L. J. (2002). Postpartum depression. *Journal of the American Medical Association, 287*(6), 762–765.

Monga, M. (2004). Maternal cardiovascular and renal adaptation to pregnancy. In R. K.Creasy & R. Resnick (Eds.), *Maternal-fetal medicine: Principles and practice* (5th ed, pp. 111–120). Philadelphia: Saunders.

Moore, M. L., & Moos, M. K. (2002). *Cultural competence in the care of childbearing families.* (Nursing Module). White Plains, NY: The March of Dimes Birth Defects Foundation.

Nader, S. (2004). Thyroid disease and pregnancy. In R. K. Creasy & R. Resnick (Eds.), *Maternal-fetal medicine: Principles and practice* (5th ed, pp. 1063–1081). Philadelphia: Saunders.

Nygaard, I. (2006). Urinary incontinence: Is cesarean delivery protective? *Seminars in Perinatology, 30*(5), 267–271.

Pollack, J., Nordenstam, J., Brismar, S., Lopez, A., Altman, D., & Zetterstrom, J. (2004). Anal incontinence after vaginal delivery: A five-year prospective cohort study. *Obstetrics and Gynecology, 104*(6), 1397–1402.

Rana, S., Lindheimer, M., Hibbard, J., & Pliskin, N. (2006). Neuropsychological performance in normal pregnancy and preeclampsia. *American Journal of Obstetrics and Gynecology, 195*(1), 186–191.

Resnick, R. (2004). The puerperium. In R. K.Creasy & R. Resnick (Eds.), *Maternal-fetal medicine: Principles and practice* (5th ed, pp. 165–180). Philadelphia: Saunders.

Richter, H. E. (2006). Cesarean delivery on maternal request versus planned vaginal delivery: Impact on development of pelvic organ prolapse. *Seminars in Perinatology, 30*(5), 272–275.

Rizvi, F., Mackey, R., Barrett, T., McKenna, P., & Geary, M. (2004). Successful reduction of massive postpartum haemorrhage by use of guidelines and staff education. *British Journal of Obstetrics and Gynaecology, 111*(5), 495–498.

Roberts, J. M. (2004). Pregnancy-related hypertension. In R. K. Creasy & R. Resnick (Eds.), *Maternal-fetal medicine: Principles and practice* (5th ed, pp. 859–899). Philadelphia: Saunders.

Roudebush, J. R., Kaufman, J., Johnson, B. H., Abraham, M. R., & Clayton, S. P. (2006). Patient and family centered perinatal care: Partnerships with childbearing women and families. *Journal of Perinatal and Neonatal Nursing, 20*(3), 201–209.

Rouse, C. L., & MacNeil, J. (2000). Should there be policies to restrict visitors during labor and birth? *MCN The American Journal of Maternal Child Nursing, 25*(1), 8–9.

Rubin, R. (1961a). Puerperal change. *Nursing Outlook, 9, 753*–755.

Rubin, R. (1961b). Puerperal change. *Nursing Outlook, 11,* 828–831.

Rubin, R. (1977). Binding-in in the postpartum period. *Maternal-Child Nursing Journal, 6,* 67–75.

Russell, R. B., Petrini, J. R., Damus, K., Mattison, D. R., & Schwartz, R. H. (2003). The changing epidemiology of multiple births in the United States. *Obstetrics and Gynecology, 101*(1), 129–135.

Schaffer, J. I., Bloom, S. L., Casey, B. M., McIntire, D. D., Nihira, M. A., & Leveno, K. J. (2005). A randomized trial of the effects of coached vs uncoached maternal pushing during the second stage of labor on postpartum pelvic floor structure and function. *American Journal of Obstetrics and Gynecology, 192*(5), 1692–1696.

Simpson, K. R. (2005a). Emergency drills in obstetrics. *MCN The American Journal of Maternal Child Nursing, 30*(2), 220.

Simpson, K. R., & Knox, G. E. (1999). Strategies for developing an evidence-based approach to perinatal care. *MCN The American Journal of Maternal Child Nursing, 24*(3), 122–132.

Thorman, K. E., & McClean, A. (2006). While you are waiting: A family-centered antepartum support program. *Journal of Perinatal and Neonatal Nursing, 20*(3), 220–226.

Urbano, F. L. (2001). Homans' sign in the diagnosis of deep venous thrombosis. *Hospital Physician, 37*(3), 22–24.

Vargo, L. E., & Trotter, C. W. (2006). *The premature infant: Nursing assessment and management.* (Nursing Module, 2nd ed.). White Plains, NY: The March of Dimes Birth Defects Foundation.

Weber, A. M., & Richter, H. E. (2005). Pelvic organ prolapse. *Obstetrics and Gynecology, 106*(3), 615–634.

Whitty, J. E., & Dombrowski, M. P. (2004). Respiratory diseases in pregnancy. In R. K. Creasy & R. Resnick (Eds.), *Maternal-fetal medicine: Principles and practice* (5th ed, pp. 953–974). Philadelphia: Saunders.

Zwelling, E. (2000). Trendsetter: Celeste Phillips, the mother of family-centered maternity care. *Journal of Obstetric, Gynecologic, and Neonatal Nursing, 29*(1), 90–94.

Postpartum Assessment Form

Previous 24 hour I/O

I	O

Date:_____

WT _____

		2300-0659								0700-1459								1500-2259							
		23	00	01	02	03	04	05	06	07	08	09	10	11	12	13	14	15	16	17	18	19	20	21	22
VITAL SIGNS	TEMP																								
	PULSE																								
	RESP																								
	BP																								
	O2 SAT																								
	_____ LITERS O2																								
	O2 TYPE																								

INTAKE	ORAL																								
	IV																								
	NS FLUSH																								
	IVPB																								
	SHIFT TOTAL	PO =			IV =					PO =			IV =					PO =			IV =				

24 Hour Total

OUTPUT	VOID																								
	CATHETER																								
	EMESIS																								
	DRAIN																								
	SHIFT TOTAL																								
	STOOLS																								
	GUAIAC																								
	SHIFT TOTAL																								

24 Hour Total

Signature/Title   Initials   Shift

_____ _____ _____
_____ _____ _____
_____ _____ _____
_____ _____ _____
_____ _____ _____

ADDRESSOGRAPH

POSTPARTUM ASSESSMENT FORM
ST. JOHN'S MERCY MEDICAL CENTER, ST. LOUIS, MISSOURI

Date: _____

Patient's stated comfort goal/Pain Intensity Level of:_____

PAIN: Assess **minimally every 8 hours. Document "no pain" or "no complaint of pain" as "0" in Pain Scale column.** Pain intensity and quality are maintained at patient's comfort goal.

PAIN SCALES

0-10 Numeric Pain Intensity Scale

0	1	2	3	4	5	6	7	8	9	10
No Pain		Mild		Moderate		Quite a Lot		Very Bad		Worst Pain

O=Other (as described in Nurses Narrative)

NIPS (Neonatal/Infant Pain Scale)

Facial Expression
0=relaxed muscles/neutral expression
1=tight facial muscles/furrowed chin, brow
Sense of Arousal
0=sleeping/awake, quiet peaceful settled
1=fussy/alert, restless and thrashing

Cry
0=quiet, not crying
1=mild moaning, intermittent cry
2=loud scream/rising, shrill, continuous or silent cry due to intubation or trach

Arms
0=relaxed, no muscular rigidity
1=flexed/extended, tense straight arms
Legs
0=relaxed, no muscular rigidity and/or alert
1=flexed/extended, tense straight legs

Faces Pain Rating Scale

0	1-2	3-4	5-6	7-8	9-10
No Hurt	Hurts Little Bit	Hurts Little More	Hurts Even More	Hurts Whole Lot	Hurts Worst

RAMSAY SEDATION SCALE

1=Anxious and agitated or restless
2=Cooperative, oriented, tranquil
3=Responds to commands only
4=Asleep, but response to glabellar tap or loud auditory stimulus
5=Asleep, sluggish response to glabellar tap or loud auditory stimulus
6=NO RESPONSE
O=Other (as described in Nurses Narrative)

INTERVENTIONS

M=Medication *(anything except PCA or Epidural)*
CD=Cold application
CL=Child Life
EPI=Epidural
H=Heat application
MST=Massage Therapy
PCA=PCA
RLT=Relaxation Therapy
RP=Repositioning
T=TENS Unit
O=Other (as described in Nurses Narrative)

RESPONSE KEY

PGA=Pain Goal Achieved
SL=Sleeping
NV=Nausea and/or Vomiting
IT=Itching
UR=Urinary Retention
C=Constipation
SD=Sensory Deficit
NB=Numbness
MW=Muscle Weakness/ Motor Deficit
O=Other (as described in Nurses Narrative)

ASSESSMENT					INTERVENTIONS		EVALUATION						
Time	Pain Intensity Rating	Respiratory Rate	Ramsay Rating	Location/Comments	See Key Above	Initials	Time	Pain Intensity Rating	Respiratory Rate	Ramsay Rating	Other Responses/Comments	Initials

INFUSION SYSTEM

❑ Epidural   ❑ PCA

Drug Concentration: _____   Rate △ or Bolus _____ Time_____

Basal Rate: _____   Rate △ or Bolus _____ Time_____

Dose: _____ Interval: _____   Rate △ or Bolus _____ Time_____

Lockout: _____ ❑ Pt button in reach   Epidural/PCA checked by RN _____ _____ _____ (initial)

	2300-0700	0700-1500	1500-2300
PCA Attempts			
Doses Delivered			
Shift Drug Total			
Time/Initials			

Signature/Title   Initials Shift

_____ ____ ____

_____ ____ ____

_____ ____ ____

_____ ____ ____

_____ ____ ____

ADDRESSOGRAPH

Date: _____

2300 - 0700 Time:_____		0700-1500 Time:_____

POSTPARTUM:

Fundus Firm: Y ☐ N ☐   Location: _____

Lochia: Scant ☐ Small ☐ Moderate ☐

Rubra ☐ Serosa ☐

Vaginal Delivery:

Episiotomy/Perineum/Laceration Intact ☐ Bruised ☐

Edematous ☐ Hemorrhoids: Y ☐ N ☐

Cesarean Section:

Abdominal Incision/Dressing Intact Y ☐ N ☐

Drainage Y ☐   N ☐   Marked ☐

SubQ sutures ☐ Staples ☐ Steristrips ☐

Drain/Tubes N/A ☐ Type: _____ Intact _____

Compressed_____ Gravity _____ Patent _____

BREAST:

Soft ☐ Intact Nipples ☐ No Soreness ☐ Bra On ☐

Filling ☐ Full ☐ Engorged ☐

Nipples: Flat ☐ Inverted ☐ Sore ☐ Nipple Trauma ☐

Bottle Feeding: Tight Bra ☐ Ice Packs ☐

BREASTFEEDING ASSESSMENT:

Proper Latch On: Y ☐ N ☐

Appropriate Position Y ☐ N ☐

Audible Swallowing Y ☐ N ☐

Feeding Observed Y ☐ N ☐

Baby in NICU Y ☐ N ☐

Breast Pump Instructions Y ☐ N ☐

Return Demo Y ☐ N ☐

Lactation Consultant Y ☐ N ☐

NEURO/MUSCULOSKELETAL:

Alert ☐ Oriented x3 ☐ Speech Clear ☐

Moves all extremities well ☐

Full ROM, No weakness, numbness or tingling of legs ☐

See Nurses Note ☐

RESPIRATORY:

Respirations even and unlabored ☐

Lungs clear to auscultation ☐

See Nurses Note ☐   Other ☐

GENITOURINARY:

Voiding without difficulty ☐   No bladder distention ☐

Up with assist x1 void Y / N Fundus: _____

Up with assist x2 void Y / N Fundus: _____

Pericare: ☐ ☐ ☐ ☐

Catheters: Foley ☐   IN / OUT catheter ☐

Patent ☐ Color _____ Clear ☐

Burning ☐ Dysuria ☐

Foul smelling ☐ Cloudy ☐ Hematuria ☐

Foley D/C: _____ Date/Time

See Nurses Note ☐

GASTROINTESTINAL:

Abdomen soft non-tender ☐ Tolerates prescribed diet ☐

Bowel sounds all 4 quadrants ☐

No N/V, diarrhea, or constipation ☐

Passing flatus ☐

Abdomen: Firm ☐ Flat ☐ Rounded ☐ Distended ☐

Diarrhea ☐ Constipation ☐ Nausea ☐ Vomiting ☐

Bowel Sounds:

Absent ☐ Hyperactive ☐ Hypoactive ☐ ____quadrants

See Nurses Note ☐

INTEGUMENTARY:

Skin and mucous membranes intact

Skin warm and dry ☐

Pressure site: Heels without redness or evidence of skin breakdown ☐

Except as noted below ☐

Skin: Flushed ☐ Gray ☐ Pale ☐ Jaundiced ☐

Diaphoretic ☐ Cool ☐ Mottled ☐ Petechiae ☐

IV/HEPLOCK SITE: N/A ☐

No redness, swelling, drainage or pain at site ☐

Patent ☐   Dressing dry/intact ☐

Dressing Changed _____

Tubing Changed _____

IV D/C'd _____ Date/Time

IV Restart _____ Date/Time

Gauge _____ Site _____

Attempts _____

PIH ASSESSMENT:

No symptoms ☐ Hypertensive ☐ Headache ☐

Visual Disturbance ☐   Epigastric Pain ☐

Edema _____ Urine Protein _____

Hyperreflexia ☐

LABORATORY DATA:

Rubella Vaccine Given Y ☐ N ☐   N/A ☐

Rhogam Given Y ☐ N ☐ N/A ☐

Lot number _____ Expiration Date_____

Other lab work _____

_____

MATERNAL/INFANT BONDING:

Appropriate eye contact and touching ☐

See Nurses Note ☐

PSYCHOSOCIAL:

Demonstrates ability to cope with situation ☐

Support Systems Available:

Family ☐ Significant Other ☐ Friends ☐

Social Service Consult ☐

WIC ☐

See Nurses Note ☐

SPIRITUALITY:

No concerns expressed at this time ☐

Concerns/Interactions: _____

Pastoral Care ☐

See Nurses Note ☐

PATIENT/S.O. TEACHING:

Teaching Need: Postpartum ☐ Baby Care ☐

Breastfeeding ☐ Bottle Feeding ☐ Meds ☐

Nutrition ☐ Equipment ☐

Method: Verbal Instruction ☐ Demonstration ☐

Video ☐ Written Instruction ☐ Booklet/Pamphlet ☐

Patient Response: Verbalized Understanding ☐

Observed Demonstration ☐   Performed w/Assist ☐

Unable to teach due to: _____

PLAN OF CARE REVIEWED ☐

2ND ASSESSMENT/TIME _____

Unchanged ☐   See Nurses Note ☐

POSTPARTUM:

Fundus Firm: Y ☐ N ☐   Location: _____

Lochia: Scant ☐ Small ☐ Moderate ☐

Rubra ☐ Serosa ☐

Vaginal Delivery:

Episiotomy/Perineum/Laceration Intact ☐ Bruised ☐

Edematous ☐ Hemorrhoids: Y ☐ N ☐

Cesarean Section:

Abdominal Incision/Dressing Intact Y ☐ N ☐

Drainage Y ☐   N ☐   Marked ☐

SubQ sutures ☐ Staples ☐ Steristrips ☐

Drain/Tubes N/A ☐ Type: _____ Intact _____

Compressed_____ Gravity _____ Patent _____

BREAST:

Soft ☐ Intact Nipples ☐ No Soreness ☐ Bra On ☐

Filling ☐ Full ☐ Engorged ☐

Nipples: Flat ☐ Inverted ☐ Sore ☐ Nipple Trauma ☐

Bottle Feeding: Tight Bra ☐ Ice Packs ☐

BREASTFEEDING ASSESSMENT:

Proper Latch On: Y ☐ N ☐

Appropriate Position Y ☐ N ☐

Audible Swallowing Y ☐ N ☐

Feeding Observed Y ☐ N ☐

Baby in NICU Y ☐ N ☐

Breast Pump Instructions Y ☐ N ☐

Return Demo Y ☐ N ☐

Lactation Consultant Y ☐ N ☐

NEURO/MUSCULOSKELETAL:

Alert ☐ Oriented x3 ☐ Speech Clear ☐

Moves all extremities well ☐

Full ROM, No weakness, numbness or tingling of legs ☐

See Nurses Note ☐

RESPIRATORY:

Respirations even and unlabored ☐

Lungs clear to auscultation ☐

See Nurses Note ☐   Other ☐

GENITOURINARY:

Voiding without difficulty ☐   No bladder distention ☐

Up with assist x1 void Y / N Fundus: _____

Up with assist x2 void Y / N Fundus: _____

Pericare: ☐ ☐ ☐ ☐

Catheters: Foley ☐   IN / OUT catheter ☐

Patent ☐ Color _____ Clear ☐

Burning ☐ Dysuria ☐

Foul smelling ☐ Cloudy ☐ Hematuria ☐

Foley D/C: _____ Date/Time

See Nurses Note ☐

GASTROINTESTINAL:

Abdomen soft non-tender ☐ Tolerates prescribed diet ☐

Bowel sounds all 4 quadrants ☐

No N/V, diarrhea, or constipation ☐

Passing flatus ☐

Abdomen: Firm ☐ Flat ☐ Rounded ☐ Distended ☐

Diarrhea ☐ Constipation ☐ Nausea ☐ Vomiting ☐

Bowel Sounds:

Absent ☐ Hyperactive ☐ Hypoactive ☐ ____quadrants

See Nurses Note ☐

Signature/Title   Initials   Shift

_____ _____ _____

_____ _____ _____

_____ _____ _____

_____ _____ _____

_____ _____ _____

_____ _____ _____

ADDRESSOGRAPH

Date: _____

0700-1500 continued	1500 - 2300 Time: _____

INTEGUMENTARY:
Skin and mucous membranes intact
Skin warm and dry ☐
Pressure site: Heels without redness or evidence of skin breakdown ☐
Except as noted below ☐
Skin: Flushed ☐ Gray ☐ Pale ☐ Jaundiced ☐
Diaphoretic ☐ Cool ☐ Mottled ☐ Petechiae ☐

IV/HEPLOCK SITE: N/A ☐
No redness, swelling, drainage or pain at site ☐
Patent ☐ Dressing dry/intact ☐
Dressing Changed _____
Tubing Changed _____
IV D/C'd _____ Date/Time
IV Restart _____ Date/Time
Gauge _____ Site _____
Attempts _____

PIH ASSESSMENT:
No symptoms ☐ Hypertensive ☐ Headache ☐
Visual Disturbance ☐ Epigastric Pain ☐
Edema _____ Urine Protein _____
Hyperreflexia ☐

LABORATORY DATA:
Rubella Vaccine Given Y ☐ N ☐ N/A ☐
Rhogam Given Y ☐ N ☐ N/A ☐
Lot number _____ Expiration Date_____
Other lab work _____

MATERNAL/INFANT BONDING:
Appropriate eye contact and touching ☐

See Nurses Note ☐

PSYCHOSOCIAL:
Demonstrates ability to cope with situation ☐
Support Systems Available:
  Family ☐ Significant Other ☐ Friends ☐
Social Service Consult ☐
WIC ☐
See Nurses Note ☐

SPIRITUALITY:
No concerns expressed at this time ☐
Concerns/Interactions: _____

Pastoral Care ☐
See Nurses Note ☐

PATIENT/S.O. TEACHING:
Teaching Need: Postpartum ☐ Baby Care ☐
Breastfeeding ☐ Bottle Feeding ☐ Meds ☐
Nutrition ☐ Equipment ☐
Method: Verbal Instruction ☐ Demonstration ☐
Video ☐ Written Instruction ☐ Booklet/Pamphlet ☐
Patient Response: Verbalized Understanding ☐
Observed Demonstration ☐ Performed w/Assist ☐
Unable to teach due to: _____

PLAN OF CARE REVIEWED ☐

2ND ASSESSMENT/TIME _____
Unchanged ☐   See Nurses Note ☐

POSTPARTUM:
Fundus Firm: Y ☐ N ☐   Location: _____
Lochia: Scant ☐ Small ☐ Moderate ☐
           Rubra ☐ Serosa ☐
Vaginal Delivery:
Episiotomy/Perineum/Laceration Intact ☐ Bruised ☐
Edematous ☐ Hemorrhoids: Y ☐ N ☐
Cesarean Section:
Abdominal Incision/Dressing Intact Y ☐ N ☐
   Drainage Y ☐ N ☐   Marked ☐
   SubQ sutures ☐ Staples ☐ Steristrips ☐
Drain/Tubes N/A ☐ Type: _____ Intact _____
   Compressed_____ Gravity _____ Patent _____

BREAST:
Soft ☐ Intact Nipples ☐ No Soreness ☐ Bra On ☐
Filling ☐ Full ☐ Engorged ☐
Nipples: Flat ☐ Inverted ☐ Sore ☐ Nipple Trauma ☐
Bottle Feeding: Tight Bra ☐ Ice Packs ☐
BREASTFEEDING ASSESSMENT:
Proper Latch On: Y ☐ N ☐
Appropriate Position Y ☐ N ☐
Audible Swallowing Y ☐ N ☐
Feeding Observed Y ☐ N ☐
Baby in NICU Y ☐ N ☐
Breast Pump Instructions Y ☐ N ☐
Return Demo Y ☐ N ☐
Lactation Consultant Y ☐ N ☐

NEURO/MUSCULOSKELETAL:
Alert ☐ Oriented x3 ☐ Speech Clear ☐
Moves all extremities well ☐
Full ROM, No weakness, numbness or tingling of legs ☐
See Nurses Note ☐

RESPIRATORY:
Respirations even and unlabored ☐
Lungs clear to auscultation ☐
See Nurses Note ☐   Other ☐

GENITOURINARY:
Voiding without difficulty ☐ No bladder distention ☐
Up with assist x1 void Y / N Fundus: _____
Up with assist x2 void Y / N Fundus: _____
Pericare: ☐ ☐ ☐ ☐
Catheters: Foley ☐   IN / OUT catheter ☐
Patent ☐ Color _____ Clear ☐
Burning ☐ Dysuria ☐
Foul smelling ☐ Cloudy ☐ Hematuria ☐
Foley D/C: _____ Date/Time
See Nurses Note ☐

GASTROINTESTINAL:
Abdomen soft non-tender ☐ Tolerates prescribed diet ☐
Bowel sounds all 4 quadrants ☐
No N/V, diarrhea, or constipation ☐
Passing flatus ☐
Abdomen: Firm ☐ Flat ☐ Rounded ☐ Distended ☐
Diarrhea ☐ Constipation ☐ Nausea ☐ Vomiting ☐
Bowel Sounds:
Absent ☐ Hyperactive ☐ Hypoactive ☐ _____quadrants
See Nurses Note ☐

INTEGUMENTARY:
Skin and mucous membranes intact
Skin warm and dry ☐
Pressure site: Heels without redness or evidence of skin breakdown ☐
Except as noted below ☐
Skin: Flushed ☐ Gray ☐ Pale ☐ Jaundiced ☐
Diaphoretic ☐ Cool ☐ Mottled ☐ Petechiae ☐

IV/HEPLOCK SITE: N/A ☐
No redness, swelling, drainage or pain at site ☐
Patent ☐ Dressing dry/intact ☐
Dressing Changed _____
Tubing Changed _____
IV D/C'd _____ Date/Time
IV Restart _____ Date/Time
Gauge _____ Site _____
Attempts _____

PIH ASSESSMENT:
No symptoms ☐ Hypertensive ☐ Headache ☐
Visual Disturbance ☐ Epigastric Pain ☐
Edema _____ Urine Protein _____
Hyperreflexia ☐

LABORATORY DATA:
Rubella Vaccine Given Y ☐ N ☐ N/A ☐
Rhogam Given Y ☐ N ☐ N/A ☐
Lot number _____ Expiration Date_____
Other lab work _____

MATERNAL/INFANT BONDING:
Appropriate eye contact and touching ☐

See Nurses Note ☐

PSYCHOSOCIAL:
Demonstrates ability to cope with situation ☐
Support Systems Available:
  Family ☐ Significant Other ☐ Friends ☐
Social Service Consult ☐
WIC ☐
See Nurses Note ☐

SPIRITUALITY:
No concerns expressed at this time ☐
Concerns/Interactions: _____

Pastoral Care ☐
See Nurses Note ☐

PATIENT/S.O. TEACHING:
Teaching Need: Postpartum ☐ Baby Care ☐
Breastfeeding ☐ Bottle Feeding ☐ Meds ☐
Nutrition ☐ Equipment ☐
Method: Verbal Instruction ☐ Demonstration ☐
Video ☐ Written Instruction ☐ Booklet/Pamphlet ☐
Patient Response: Verbalized Understanding ☐
Observed Demonstration ☐ Performed w/Assist ☐
Unable to teach due to: _____

PLAN OF CARE REVIEWED ☐

2ND ASSESSMENT/TIME _____
Unchanged ☐   See Nurses Note ☐

Signature/Title	Initials	Shift	ADDRESSOGRAPH
_____	_____	_____	
_____	_____	_____	
_____	_____	_____	
_____	_____	_____	

Date_____

Key: ✔ = Task Performed / Intervention
     ✱ = Significant Finding Documented in Nurses Notes

Interventions

	BREAKFAST	LUNCH	DINNER	MORSE FALL INDICATORS
Nutrition	% Eaten _____ Supplement _____ % Eaten _____ Snack (type) _____ % Eaten _____ Snack (time) _____	% Eaten _____ Supplement _____ % Eaten _____ Snack (type) _____ % Eaten _____ Snack (time) _____	% Eaten _____ Supplement _____ % Eaten _____ Snack (type) _____ % Eaten _____ Snack (time) _____	1. History of Falling: No=0 Yes = 25 2. Secondary Diagnosis: No = 0 Yes = 15 3. Ambulatory Aid: None/bedrest/nurse assist = 0 Crutches/cane/walker = 15 Furniture = 30 4. IV Therapy/Heplock: No = 0 Yes = 20 5. Gait: Normal/bedrest/wheelchair = 0 Weak = 10 Impaired = 20 6. Mental Status: Oriented to own ability = 0 Overestimates/forgets limitations = 15

Morse Fall	Morse Fall Score: _____ Time: _____ Check the following classes of medications the patient has taken in the last 24 hours. ❑ Antihistimines ❑ Hypoglycemics ❑ Laxatives ❑ Narcotics ❑ Diuretics ❑ Psychotropics ❑ Sedatives/Hypnotics If patient has taken 4 or more of these classes of medications in the last 24 hours inititiate HIGH FALL RISK PRECAUTIONS ❑ Patient instructed to call for assistance when out of bed ❑	Morse Fall Score: _____ Time: _____ Check the following classes of medications the patient has taken in the last 24 hours. ❑ Antihistimines ❑ Hypoglycemics ❑ Laxatives ❑ Narcotics ❑ Diuretics ❑ Psychotropics ❑ Sedatives/Hypnotics If patient has taken 4 or more of these classes of medications in the last 24 hours inititiate HIGH FALL RISK PRECAUTIONS ❑ Patient instructed to call for assistance when out of bed ❑	≤**45;** low fall risk; initiate STANDARD FALL PRECAUTIONS ≥**50;** high fall risk; initiate HIGH FALL RISK PRECAUTIONS

Safety																									
ID Bracelet On-Name and Allergy																								
Phone/Call Light Within Reach																								
Side Rails (put x2 or x3 in box)																								
Bed in Low Position																								
Bed Brakes On																								
Verbal Safety Reminders Given																								
Night Lighting																								
Non-skid Slippers/Appropriate Footwear																								

	23	00	01	02	03	04	05	06	07	08	09	10	11	12	13	14	15	16	17	18	19	20	21	22
Routine Care — Bath/Shower																								
Oral Care																								
Other																								
Activity — Independent																								
Bedrest																								
Turned																								
Chair																								
Dangle																								
Ambulate / Distance																								
PT / OT																								
Sleeping																								
Resp. — Cough and Deep Breathe																								
Incentive Spirometer																								
Circ. — Teds/SCDs																								
Other:																								

Signature/Title   Initials   Shift

_____ _____ _____

_____ _____ _____

_____ _____ _____

_____ _____ _____

_____ _____ _____

ADDRESSOGRAPH

Date_____

Time	Focus	Nurse's Notes

LAB STICKERS   ADDRESSOGRAPH

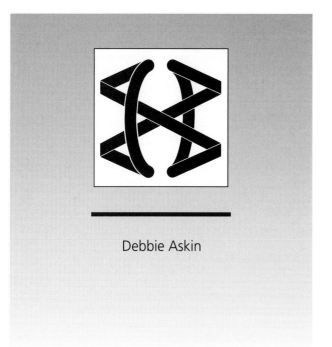

CHAPTER 11

Newborn Adaptation to Extrauterine Life

Debbie Askin

TRANSITION from fetal to newborn life is a critical period involving diverse physiologic changes. The newborn must move from an organism completely dependent on another for life-sustaining oxygen and nutrients to an independent being, a task that requires intense adjustment carried out over a period of hours to days. In addition to the normal physiologic tasks of transition, some neonates have congenital abnormalities, birth injury, or underlying disease processes. Careful assessment and nursing care is needed during the period of transition to ensure that the neonate who is experiencing problems with transition is recognized and that appropriate interventions are initiated.

This chapter focuses on those factors influencing adaptation and physiologic changes during the early newborn period. These factors include the maternal history and medical and obstetrical conditions, intrapartum status, delivery issues, and nursing assessment and interventions during transition, such as resuscitative needs and interventions facilitating maternal–newborn attachment.

MATERNAL MEDICAL AND OBSTETRIC CONDITIONS INFLUENCING NEWBORN ADAPTATION

A thorough review of the mother's prenatal and intrapartum history is essential to identify factors with the potential to compromise successful transition. Table 11–1 lists maternal risk factors and associated fetal

and neonatal complications. In addition to identification of current pregnancy complications, it is important to review prior obstetrical history. Conditions that predispose the newborn to risk may recur in subsequent pregnancies (Display 11–1). Intrapartum risk factors may also influence adaptation (Table 11–2).

Intrapartum fetal assessment provides important data about the fetal response to labor. Electronic fetal heart rate (FHR) monitoring or intermittent auscultation provides documentation of fetal well-being. Requisite perinatal nursing skills include knowledge of the physiologic basis for monitoring, an understanding of FHR patterns, and the initiation of appropriate nursing interventions based on data from the monitor or from auscultation. The FHR reflects the fetal response to labor. The perinatal nurse focuses on discriminating between reassuring and nonreassuring patterns. If the FHR pattern is nonreassuring, intrauterine resuscitation procedures such as maternal position change, oxygen therapy, and intravenous fluids are initiated. Oxytocin should be decreased or discontinued if infusing, or the next dose of Prepidil, Cervidil, or Cytotec should be delayed. Safe passage through the labor and birth process sets the stage for successful transition to extrauterine life.

UNIQUE MECHANISMS OF NEWBORN PHYSIOLOGIC ADAPTATION

The respiratory, cardiovascular, thermoregulatory, and immunologic systems undergo significant physiologic changes and adaptations during transition from fetal

TABLE 11–1 ■ MATERNAL RISK FACTORS AND POTENTIAL FETAL AND NEONATAL COMPLICATIONS

Risk Factors	Potential Complications
Maternal Substance Abuse	
Drug addiction	Small for gestational age (SGA); neonatal abstinence syndrome; neonatal human immunodeficiency virus (HIV); hepatitis B and C
Alcoholism	Fetal alcohol syndrome
Smoking	SGA; polycythemia
Maternal nutritional status	
Maternal weight <100 lb	SGA
Maternal weight >200 lb	SGA; large for gestational age (LGA)
Maternal Medical Complication	
Hereditary CNS disorders	Inherited central nervous system (CNS) disorder
Seizure disorders requiring medication	Congenital anomalies (eg, result of medication [Dilantin] use)
Chronic hypertension	Intrauterine growth restriction (IUGR); asphyxia; SGA
Congenital heart disease with congestive heart failure	Preterm birth; inherited cardiac defects
Anemia <10 g	Preterm birth; low birth weight
Sickle cell disease	IUGR; fetal demise
Hemoglobinopathies	IUGR; inherited hemoglobinopathies
Idiopathic thrombocytopenic purpura	Transient ITP purpura (ITP)
Chronic glomerulonephritis, renal insufficiency	IUGR; SGA; preterm birth; asphyxia
Recurrent urinary tract infection	Preterm birth
Uterine malformation	Preterm birth; fetal malposition
Cervical incompetence	Preterm birth
Diabetes	LGA; hypoglycemia & hypocalcemia; anomalies; respiratory distress syndrome
Thyroid disease	Hypothyroidism; CNS defects; hyperthyroidism; goiter
Current Pregnancy Complications	
Pregnancy-induced hypertension	IUGR; SGA
TORCH infections	IUGR; SGA; active infection; anomalies
Sexually transmitted diseases	Ophthalmia neonatorum; congenital syphilis
Hepatitis	Hepatitis
AIDS or HIV seropositive	Neonatal HIV
Multiple gestation	Preterm birth; asphyxia; IUGR; SGA, twin-to-twin transfusion
Fetal malposition	Prolapsed cord; asphyxia; birth trauma
Maternal blood group antibodies	Anemia, hyperbilirubinemia, immune-mediated hydrops fetalis
Prolonged pregnancy	Postmaturity; meconium aspiration; IUGR; asphyxia
Intraamniotic infection	Newborn sepsis; preterm birth
Group B streptococcal infection	Newborn sepsis; preterm birth

to neonatal life. Successful transition requires a complex interaction among these systems.

Respiratory Adaptations

Critical to the neonate's transition to extrauterine life is the ability to clear fetal lung fluid and the establishment of respiration allowing the lungs to become the organ of gas exchange after separation from maternal uteroplacental circulation. Pulmonary fluid, secreted by the lung epithelium, is essential to the normal growth and development of alveoli (Strang, 1991). Toward the end of gestation, production of lung fluid gradually diminishes. The catecholamine surge that occurs just before the onset of labor has been shown to correspond to a more rapid drop in fetal lung fluid levels (Pfister et al., 2001). Those infants who do not experience labor, those born by elective cesarean section, are more likely to develop transient tachypnea of the newborn (TTN) because of lower levels of serum catecholamine (Bakewell-Sachs, Shaw, & Tashman, 1997).

Previous Pregnancy Complications That May Recur in Subsequent Pregnancies

Fetal loss beyond 28 weeks' gestation
Preterm birth
Abnormal fetal position or presentation
Previous neonate with Group B streptococcal infection
Rh sensitization
Fetal compromise of unknown origin
Birth of newborn with anomalies
Birth of newborn weighing more than 10 lb
Birth of postterm newborn
Neonatal death

Initiation of breathing is a complex process that involves the interplay of biochemical, neural, and mechanical factors, some of which have yet to be clearly identified (Alvaro & Rigatto, 2005). Pulmonary blood flow, surfactant production, and respiratory musculature also influence respiratory adaptation to extrauterine life. Establishment of independent breathing and oxygen–carbon dioxide exchange depends on these physiologic factors.

Chemical Stimuli

A number of factors have been implicated in the initiation of postnatal breathing: decreased oxygen concentration, increased carbon dioxide concentration, and a decrease in pH all of which may stimulate fetal aortic and carotid chemoreceptors, triggering the respiratory center in the medulla to initiate respiration. Some researchers have questioned the influence of these factors and suggest instead that factors secreted by the placenta may inhibit breathing, and that regular breathing is initiated with the clamping of the cord (Alvaro & Rigatto, 2005).

Mechanical Stimulation

In utero, the fetal lungs are filled with fluid. Mechanical compression of the chest during vaginal birth forces approximately one third of this fluid out of fetal lungs. As the chest is delivered through the birth canal, it re-expands, creating negative pressure and drawing air into the lungs. This passive inspiration of air replaces fluid that previously filled the alveoli. Further expansion and distribution of air throughout the alveoli occurs when the newborn cries. Crying creates positive intrathoracic pressure that keeps alveoli open and forces the remaining fetal lung fluid into pulmonary capillaries and the lymphatic circulation.

Sensory Stimuli

The newborn is exposed to numerous tactile, visual, auditory, and olfactory stimuli during and immediately after birth. Tactile stimulation begins in utero as the fetus experiences uterine contractions and descent through the pelvis and birth canal. Stimulation to initiate breathing continues after birth as the neonate is exposed to stimuli such as light, sound, touch, smell, and pain. Vigorously drying the newborn immediately after birth is a significant tactile stimulation.

Contributing Factors

Pulmonary Blood Flow

In utero, the placenta is the organ of gas exchange for the fetus. Oxygenated blood is delivered from the placenta through the umbilical vein, through the ductus venosus into the inferior vena cava, and then to the left and right side of the fetal heart for distribution to the fetal body. Oxygenated blood is diverted away from pulmonary circulation in utero and instead flows through the foramen ovale and ductus arteriosus to the fetal body.

The fluid-filled lungs of the fetus create a state of alveolar hypoxia. Fetal pulmonary arterioles, which are very sensitive to oxygen, have thick musculature because of low oxygen tension in utero (Alvaro & Rigatto, 2005). This results in constriction of pulmonary arterioles, which causes increased pulmonary vascular resistance (PVR) and decreased pulmonary blood flow. After birth, pulmonary vasodilatation occurs when oxygen enters the lungs as oxygen is a potent pulmonary vasodilator. This significantly decreases PVR. Increased pulmonary blood flow is established as PVR decreases with normal changes in arterial PO_2, alveolar PO_2, acid–base status, and absence of vasoactive substances such as prostaglandin and bradykinin. Adequate pulmonary blood flow is crucial for newborn gas exchange and successful transition. After the onset of breathing, fluid in the lungs is replaced by air.

Surfactant Production

Pulmonary surfactant is necessary to maintain expanded alveoli. Surfactant lowers surface tension, preventing alveolar collapse during inspiration and expiration. By approximately 34 to 36 weeks' gestation, there is adequate surfactant production to

TABLE 11–2 ■ INTRAPARTUM RISK FACTORS AND POTENTIAL FETAL AND NEONATAL COMPLICATIONS

Risk Factors	Potential Complications
Umbilical Cord	
Prolapsed umbilical cord	Asphyxia
True knot in cord	Asphyxia
Velamentous insertion	Intrauterine blood loss; shock; anemia
Vasa previa	Intrauterine blood loss; shock; anemia
Rupture or tearing of cord	Blood loss; shock; anemia
Membranes	
Premature rupture of membranes	Infection; respiratory distress syndrome; prolapsed cord; asphyxia
Prolonged rupture of membranes	Infection
Amnionitis	Infection
Amniotic Fluid	
Oligohydramnios	Congenital anomalies; pulmonary hypoplasia
Polyhydramnios	Congenital anomalies; prolapsed cord
Meconium-stained fluid	Asphyxia; meconium aspiration syndrome
Placenta	
Placenta previa	Preterm birth; asphyxia
Abruptio placenta	Preterm birth; asphyxia
Placental insufficiency	Intrauterine growth restriction; small for gestational age; asphyxia
Abnormal Fetal Presentations	
Breech birth	Asphyxia; birth injuries (CNS, skeletal)
Face or brow presentation	Asphyxia; facial trauma
Transverse lie	Asphyxia; birth injuries; cesarean birth; umbilical cord prolapse
Birth Complications	
Forceps-assisted birth	CNS trauma; cephalhematoma; asphyxia; facial trauma
Vacuum extraction	Cephalhematoma; subgaleal hemorrhage
Manual version or extraction	Asphyxia; birth trauma; prolapsed cord
Shoulder dystocia	Asphyxia; brachial plexus injury; fractured clavicle
Precipitous birth	Asphyxia; birth trauma (CNS)
Undiagnosed multiple gestation	Asphyxia; birth trauma
Administration of Drugs	
Oxytocin	Complications of uterine hyperstimulation (asphyxia)
Magnesium sulfate	Hypermagnesemia; CNS depression
Analgesics	CNS and respiratory depression
Anesthetics	CNS and respiratory depression; bradycardia

support respiration and protect against development of respiratory distress syndrome (Hagedorn, Gardner, & Abman, 2002). Surfactant deficiency results in atelectasis and requires greater than normal breathing efforts. Oxygen and metabolic needs increase as the newborn must use more energy to maintain respirations. Preterm newborns are at high risk for surfactant deficiency, which may significantly jeopardize respiratory adaptation to extrauterine life.

Respiratory Musculature

Intercostal muscles support the rib cage and assist with inspiration by creating negative intrathoracic pressure.

Intercostal muscles may not be fully developed at birth, increasing risk of respiratory compromise by increasing breathing effort.

Cardiovascular Adaptations

Transition from fetal to neonatal circulation is a major cardiovascular change and occurs simultaneously with respiratory system adaptation. To appreciate hemodynamic changes, an understanding of structural and blood-flow differences between fetal and neonatal circulation is necessary. Figure 11–1 illustrates fetal circulation. Also influencing the cardiovascular system

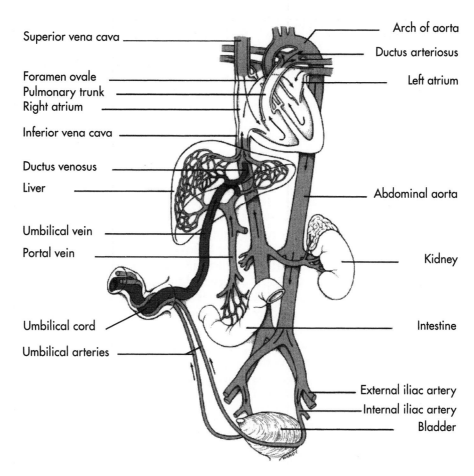

Superior vena cava

Foramen ovale
Pulmonary trunk
Right atrium

Inferior vena cava

Ductus venosus

Liver

Umbilical vein

Portal vein

Umbilical cord

Umbilical arteries

Arch of aorta

Ductus arteriosus

Left atrium

Abdominal aorta

Kidney

Intestine

External iliac artery
Internal iliac artery
Bladder

FIGURE 11–1. Fetal circulation.

are physiologic changes in the vasculature, which include decreased PVR, resulting in increased pulmonary blood flow, and increased systemic vascular resistance (SVR).

Fetal Circulation

In utero, oxygenated blood flows to the fetus from the placenta through the umbilical vein. Although a small amount of oxygenated blood is delivered to the liver, most blood bypasses the hepatic system through the ductus venosus. The ductus venosus is a vascular structure that forms a connection between the umbilical vein and the inferior vena cava. Oxygenated blood from the inferior vena cava enters the right atrium, and most of it is directed through the foramen ovale to the left atrium, then to the left ventricle, and on to the ascending aorta, where it is primarily directed to the fetal heart and brain. The foramen ovale is a flap-like structure between the right and left atria. Blood flows through the foramen ovale because pressure in the right atrium is greater than that in the left atrium. In addition, the superior vena cava drains deoxygenated blood from the head and upper extremities into the right atrium, where it mixes with oxygenated blood

from the placenta. This blood enters the right ventricle and pulmonary artery where again, increased resistance in the pulmonary vessels causes 60% of this blood to be shunted across the ductus arteriosus and into the descending aorta. This mixture of oxygenated and deoxygenated blood continues through the descending aorta, oxygenating the lower half of the fetal body and eventually draining back to the placenta through the two umbilical arteries. The remaining 40% of the blood coming from the right ventricle perfuses lung tissue to meet metabolic needs. The blood that actually reaches the lungs represents about 8% of fetal cardiac output (Blackburn, 2003; Grant, 1999).

Neonatal Circulation

During fetal life, the placenta is an organ of low vascular resistance. Clamping the umbilical cord at birth eliminates the placenta as a reservoir for blood, causing increased SVR, an increase in blood pressure, and increased pressures in the left side of the heart. Removal of the placenta also eliminates the need for blood flow through the ductus venosus, causing functional elimination of this fetal shunt. Systemic venous blood flow is then directed through the portal system for hepatic circulation. Umbilical vessels constrict, with functional closure occurring immediately. Fibrous infiltration leads to anatomic closure in the first week of life (Alvaro & Rigatto, 2005).

Several other significant events must also take place for successful transition to neonatal circulation. With the infant's first breath and exposure to increased oxygen levels, the pulmonary blood flow must increase allowing the lungs to become the organ for exchange of oxygen and carbon dioxide, the foramen ovale must close (this occurs because left atrial pressures exceed right atrial pressures due to the increased pulmonary venous return of blood flow from the lungs) (Johnson & Ades, 2005), and the ductus arteriosus must close. In utero, shunting of blood from the pulmonary artery through the ductus arteriosus to the aorta occurs as a result of high PVR. After birth, SVR rises and PVR falls, causing a reversal of blood flow through the ductus. The major contributing factor to closure of the ductus arteriosus is sensitivity to rising arterial oxygen concentrations in the blood (Clyman, 2004). As the PaO_2 level increases after birth, the ductus arteriosus begins to constrict. In utero, elevated prostaglandin levels helped maintain ductal patency. Removal of the placenta decreases prostaglandin levels, further influencing closure (Alvaro & Rigatto, 2005; Kenner 2003). Constriction of the ductus arteriosus is a gradual process, permitting bidirectional shunting of blood after birth. PVR may be higher than the SVR, allowing some degree of right-to-left shunting, until the SVR rises above PVR and blood flow is directed left to right. Most neonates have a patent ductus arteriosus in the first 8 hours of life with spontaneous closure occurring in 42% at 24 hours of age, in 90% at 48 hours of age, and in all infants at 96 hours of age (Gentile et al., 1981; Johnson & Ades, 2005). Permanent anatomic closure of the ductus arteriosus occurs within 3 weeks to 3 months of age. Any clinical situation that causes hypoxia, with pulmonary vasoconstriction and subsequent increased PVR, potentiates right-to-left shunting (Lott, 2003). Successful transition and closure of fetal shunts creates a neonatal circulation where deoxygenated blood returns to the heart through the inferior and superior vena cava. It enters the right atrium to the right ventricle and travels through the pulmonary artery to the pulmonary vascular bed. Oxygenated blood returns through pulmonary veins to the left atrium, the left ventricle, and through the aorta to systemic circulation.

Relationship Between Respiratory and Cardiovascular Adaptation

Successful initiation of respirations and transition from fetal to neonatal circulation are essential to maintain life after birth. Conditions that lead to sustained elevated PVR such as hypoxia, acidosis, sepsis, or congenital heart defects can interrupt the normal sequence of events. Closure of fetal shunts depends on oxygenation and pressure changes within the cardiovascular system as described in the previous section. Foramen ovale and ductus arteriosus closure occurs only if PVR drops with the onset of respiration and subsequent oxygenation. The pulmonary vascular bed is very reactive to low oxygen levels. If the neonate experiences significant hypoxia, PVR will remain elevated with resultant decreased pulmonary blood flow and right-to-left shunting across the foramen ovale and ductus arteriosus. These events may induce a state of hypoxia as deoxygenated blood bypasses the lungs through the patent fetal shunts to be mixed with oxygenated blood entering the systemic circulation. The result is persistent pulmonary hypertension of the newborn (PPHN) requiring aggressive cardiorespiratory support.

Thermoregulation

The newborn's ability to maintain temperature control after birth is determined by external environmental factors and internal physiologic processes. Characteristics of newborns that predispose them to heat loss include a large body surface area in relation to body mass and a limited amount of subcutaneous fat. Newborns attempt to regulate body temperature by nonshivering thermogenesis, increased metabolic rate, and increased muscle activity. Peripheral vasoconstriction also decreases heat loss to the skin surface. Mechanisms of heat loss including evaporation, conduction, convection, and radiation play an integral part in newborn adaptation to extrauterine life. Nursing care is critical in supporting thermoregulation through ongoing assessments and environmental interventions to decrease heat loss.

Mechanisms of Heat Production

Nonshivering Thermogenesis

Newborns have a limited capacity to shiver and, therefore, must generate heat through nonshivering thermogenesis. Heat is produced by metabolism of brown fat, a unique process present only in newborns. This highly vascular adipose tissue is located in the neck, scapula, axilla, and mediastinum, and around kidneys and adrenal glands. Production of brown fat begins around 26 to 28 weeks' gestation and continues for 3 to 5 weeks after birth (Blackburn, 2003). When exposed to cold stress, thermal receptors in skin transmit messages to the central nervous system, activating the sympathetic nervous system and triggering metabolism of brown fat, a process that utilizes glucose and oxygen and produces acids as a byproduct (Noerr, 2004). Once utilized, brown fat stores are not replaced (Noerr, 2004).

Voluntary Muscle Activity

Heat produced through voluntary muscle activity is minimal in the newborn. Flexion of the extremities and maintaining a fetal position decreases heat loss to the environment. Term newborns have the ability to maintain this flexed posture, whereas preterm and compromised newborns may lack the muscle tone for this posturing, making them more vulnerable to cold stress (Kenner, 2003).

Mechanisms of Heat Loss

Evaporation

Evaporation and heat loss occur as amniotic fluid on skin is converted to a vapor. Drying the newborn immediately after birth and removing wet blankets decreases evaporative losses and prevents further cooling. The amount of insensible water loss from the skin is inversely related to gestational age. Skin of a preterm newborn is more susceptible to evaporative losses, because the keratin layer of the skin has not matured. Absence or greater permeability of this skin layer allows increased heat loss (Blake & Murray, 2002; Kenner, 2003). Because the newborn's head is the largest surface area of the body, covering the head with a knit cap after birth when not under the radiant warmer greatly conserves heat. Under the radiant warmer, use of a cap prevents heat from reaching the newborn's head and may contribute to cold stress. Adding humidity to the environment may also decrease evaporative heat loss.

Conduction

Conductive heat loss occurs when two solid objects of different temperatures come in contact. Heat loss occurs if the newborn is placed in direct contact with a cold scale, mattress, x-ray plate, or blanket. Mechanisms for preventing conductive heat loss in the birthing room immediately after birth include using preheated radiant warmer, warm blankets for drying, and covering scales and x-ray plates with warm blankets. Preheating the radiant warmer is necessary, because it may take 15 to 30 minutes to warm the mattress.

Providing skin-to-skin contact between mother and newborn after birth helps prevent conductive heat loss and enhances maternal–newborn attachment (Blake & Murray, 2002; Bohnhorst, Heyne, Peter, & Poest, 2001). Newborns who experience extended periods of skin-to-skin contact beginning soon after birth demonstrate

heart rates, respiratory rates, and oxygen saturation levels within normal limits (Ludington-Hoe et al., 1993). Preterm newborns provided with opportunities for skin-to-skin contact with their mothers maintained their temperature, demonstrated normal vital signs, had increased episodes of deep sleep and alert inactivity, cried less, had no increase in infection rates, had greater weight gain, longer breastfeeding periods, and earlier discharge (Browne 2004; Ludington-Hoe, Anderson, Swinth, Thompson, & Hadeed, 2004).

Convection

Convection is the transfer of heat from a solid object to surrounding air. Heat is lost from newborn skin as cooler air passes over it. Convection heat loss depends on the amount of exposed skin surface, temperature of air, and amount of air turbulence created by drafts. Interventions that prevent convection heat loss in the newborn include clothing, eliminating source of drafts, and when necessary, providing heated, humidified oxygen through a face mask or hood (Blackburn, 2003).

Radiation

Radiation heat loss occurs when heat is transferred between two objects not in contact with each other. The newborn loses heat by radiation to nearby cooler surfaces such as those of the crib, isolette, windows, or other objects. Some of the more common and efficient methods for preventing radiant heat loss are use of a radiant warmer after birth, moving the crib or isolette away from a cold window, and use of a heat shield inside an incubator (for small, preterm newborns), creating an additional warmer barrier between skin and incubator wall.

Effects of Cold Stress

Thermal management of the newborn during the first few hours of life is critical to prevent detrimental effects of cold stress and hypothermia. Table 11–3 summarizes nursing interventions that support the newborn and prevent cold stress. Because heat production requires oxygen consumption and glucose use, persistent hypothermia may deplete these stores, leading to metabolic acidosis, hypoglycemia, decreased surfactant production, increased caloric requirements, and if chronic, impaired weight gain (Blackburn, 2003; Hackman, 2001). This process is illustrated in Figure 11–2.

Immune System Adaptation

Newborns are vulnerable to infection because of their immature immune system and lack of exposure to organisms. Neonates depend on passive immunity acquired from their mother through active transport

TABLE 11–3 ■ MECHANISMS OF HEAT LOSS AND NURSING INTERVENTIONS THAT PREVENT COLD STRESS

Type of Heat Loss	Nursing Interventions
Evaporation	Dry infant thoroughly Remove wet linen Place knit cap on infant's head when not under radiant warmer Bathe infant under radiant heat source after temperature stabilizes
Convection	Move infant away from drafts, open windows, vents, and traffic patterns When necessary, use humidified, warmed oxygen Avoid using ceiling fans in birthing room Move infant in prewarmed transport Isolette
Conduction	Preheat radiant warmer Place infant skin-to-skin with mother Use warmed blanket Warm stethoscope and your hands Place cover between newborn and metal scale or x-ray plate
Radiation	Place stabilizing unit on an interior wall of the birthing room (away from cold windows) Preheat radiant warmer or transport Isolette

via the placenta of IgG during the third trimester (Simister, 2003). Preterm newborns are at greater risk for infection because they may not have received this passive immunity and because the immaturity of the immune system is even more pronounced than in term infants (Cavaliere, 2004).

Immunity is conferred through immunoglobulins, antibodies secreted by lymphocytes, and plasma cells.

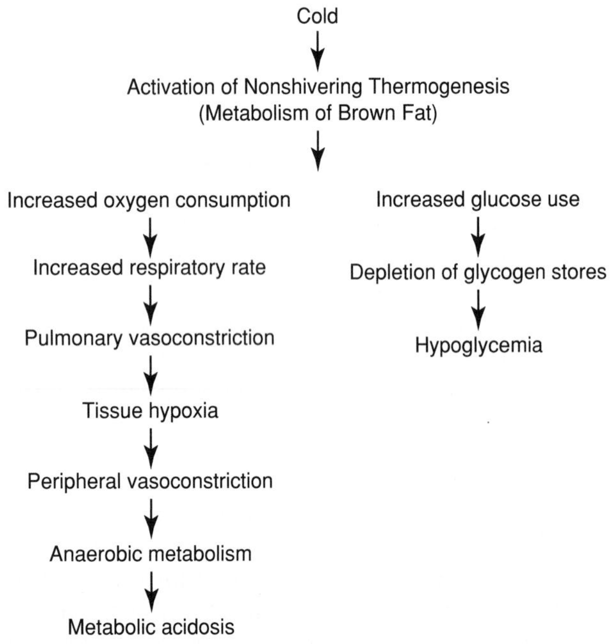

Cold
↓
Activation of Nonshivering Thermogenesis
(Metabolism of Brown Fat)
↓

Increased oxygen consumption
↓
Increased respiratory rate
↓
Pulmonary vasoconstriction
↓
Tissue hypoxia
↓
Peripheral vasoconstriction
↓
Anaerobic metabolism
↓
Metabolic acidosis

Increased glucose use
↓
Depletion of glycogen stores
↓
Hypoglycemia

FIGURE 11–2. Effects of cold stress in the newborn.

There are three main classes of immunoglobulins responsible for immunity: IgG, IgA, and IgM. Because of their small molecular size, only IgG antibodies are capable of crossing the placenta. Maternally transmitted IgG provides protection for the newborn against bacterial and viral infections for which the mother already has antibodies (eg, diphtheria, tetanus, smallpox, measles, mumps, poliomyelitis).

IgM and IgA immunoglobulins do not cross the placenta. If elevated levels of IgM are found in the newborn, it may indicate the presence of an intrauterine infection such as one organism traditionally known by the acronym TORCH (ie, *Toxoplasma gondii* [toxoplasmosis]; other agents such as *Treponema pallidum* [syphilis], varicella virus, human immunodeficiency virus, and *Chlamydia*; rubella virus; cytomegalovirus; and herpesvirus). IgA, found in colostrum, is thought to contribute to passive immunity for breast-fed newborns (Hanson, Korotkova, & Telemo, 2003).

Immature leukocyte function in the newborn inhibits the ability to destroy pathogens. Deficiency in response prevents mature processes of chemotaxis (ie, movement of leukocytes toward site of infection), opsonization (ie, altering or preparing the cells for ingestion), and phagocytosis (ie, ingestion of cells) from occurring. Low levels of immunoglobulin and complement components (ie, plasma proteins that assist the immune system) leave newborns, especially preterm newborns, vulnerable to infection (Cavaliere, 2004).

Lymphocytes are responsible for the specific response in the immune system that involves antibody production. When lymphocytes are exposed to pathogens, they become sensitized to them. If repeated exposure occurs, lymphocytes will attempt to destroy the pathogen. Because newborns lack exposure to most common organisms, any action by lymphocytes is delayed.

Weak newborn defenses against infection make it imperative for the perinatal nurse and anyone coming in contact with newborns to follow careful hand-washing practices and use of aseptic technique. Promoting skin integrity is essential for preventing neonatal infections. Newborn skin is thin and delicate, making it susceptible to alterations in integrity. Fetal scalp electrodes, fetal scalp pH sampling, and skin abrasions create portals for the entry of organisms. Umbilical cord and circumcision sites are also potential sites of infection.

Preterm newborns, with more fragile skin, are at a greater risk for infection. Invasive procedures, performed during the early hours after birth, further challenge the immune system. Treatments such as vitamin K injection, suctioning, and heel-stick blood samples predispose newborns to infection if proper aseptic technique is not maintained.

Although most births result in a healthy newborn making the transition to extrauterine life without difficulty, perinatal nurses must anticipate and prepare for complications. This includes ensuring immediate availability of functioning resuscitation equipment and knowledge of equipment operation. An International Liaison Committee on Resuscitation (ILCOR) and the American Academy of Pediatrics (AAP) recommend that someone trained in neonatal resuscitation be available for all births (Kattwinkel, 2000). Display 11–2 identifies equipment that should be available in every birthing room.

The Neonatal Resuscitation program developed by the American Heart Association and the AAP (AHA & AAP, 2006) has become the standard for educating healthcare providers involved in newborn stabilization. Figure 11–3 illustrates steps used to evaluate and establish airway, breathing, and circulation as a basis for stabilization of the newborn immediately after birth. Although most newborns respond successfully to oral suctioning and tactile stimulation, 5% to 10% may require additional interventions, including ventilation by bag and mask or endotracheal intubation, chest compressions, and administration of resuscitative medications (Kattwinkel, 2000; Zaichkin, 2002).

Good communication among health team members is essential in anticipating and preparing for high-risk births. Communicating the details of the maternal and family history that will affect the resuscitation and treatment of the newborn is particularly important. In addition to undergoing dramatic physical changes to adapt to extrauterine life, newborns must handle the events and procedures they are subjected to after birth. After airway, breathing, and circulation have been

DISPLAY 11-2

Equipment Needed For Neonatal Resuscitation

Clock with second hand
Preheated radiant warmer
Firm, padded resuscitation surface
Warmed blankets
Neonatal stethoscope
Bulb syringe
Gloves and appropriate personnel protection
Cardiac monitor and electrodes or pulse oximeter and probe (optional for delivery room)
Mechanical suction with manometer and tubing
Oxygen source, flowmeter (flow rate up to 10 L/min), tubing
Resuscitation bag capable of delivering 90%–100% oxygen and pressure gauge
Face masks (newborn and preemie size)
Laryngoscope with size 0 and 1 blades (extra batteries; extra laryngoscope bulbs)
Endotracheal tubes (sizes 2.5, 3.0, 3.5, and 4.0 mm)
CO_2 detector or capnograph
Laryngeal mask airway (optional)
Suction catheters (sizes 5 Fr, 8 Fr, 10 Fr, 12 F, or 14 F)
Meconium aspirator device
8-Fr feeding tube and 20-mL syringe
Syringes (sizes 1, 3, 5, 10, 20, and 50 mL)
Needles 25-, 21-, 18-gauge, or puncture device for needleless system
Umbilical vessel catheterization supplies
Cord clamp
Tape
Scissors
Resuscitative drugs
   Epinephrine 1:10,000 concentration
   Sodium bicarbonate (4.2%)
   Naloxone hydrochloride (1 mg/mL or 0.4 mg/mL)
   Volume expanders
      Normal saline solution
      Lactated Ringer solution 100 or 250 mL
      Dextrose 10% 250 mL
Normal saline for flushes

established, a thorough assessment of the newborn is performed. This assessment includes Apgar scoring, evaluation of vital signs, physical examination, and measurements. Ideally, all aspects of transitional assessments are performed in the presence of parents in the birthing room. Only if significant maternal or

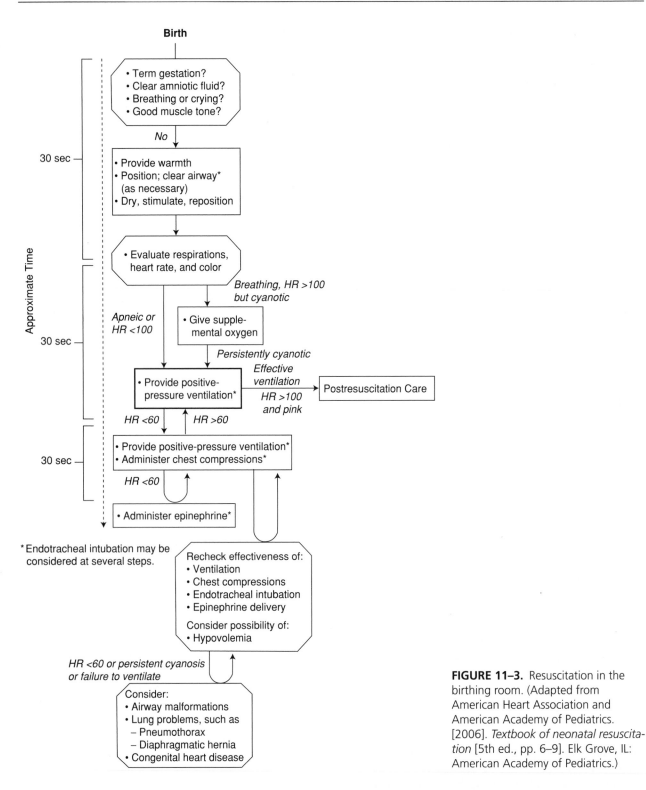

Birth

• Term gestation?
• Clear amniotic fluid?
• Breathing or crying?
• Good muscle tone?

No

• Provide warmth
• Position; clear airway*
  (as necessary)
• Dry, stimulate, reposition

• Evaluate respirations,
  heart rate, and color

Apneic or HR <100   *Breathing, HR >100 but cyanotic*

• Give supple-
  mental oxygen

Persistently cyanotic

Effective ventilation

• Provide positive-
  pressure ventilation*   Postresuscitation Care

HR >100 and pink

HR <60   *HR >60*

• Provide positive-pressure ventilation*
• Administer chest compressions*

HR <60

• Administer epinephrine*

*Endotracheal intubation may be considered at several steps.

Recheck effectiveness of:
• Ventilation
• Chest compressions
• Endotracheal intubation
• Epinephrine delivery

Consider possibility of:
• Hypovolemia

HR <60 or persistent cyanosis or failure to ventilate

Consider:
• Airway malformations
• Lung problems, such as
  – Pneumothorax
  – Diaphragmatic hernia
• Congenital heart disease

Approximate Time

30 sec

30 sec

30 sec

FIGURE 11–3. Resuscitation in the birthing room. (Adapted from American Heart Association and American Academy of Pediatrics. [2006]. *Textbook of neonatal resuscitation* [5th ed., pp. 6–9]. Elk Grove, IL: American Academy of Pediatrics.)

newborn complications occur should parents and newborns be separated.

APGAR SCORE

The Apgar score was introduced in 1952 by Dr. Virginia Apgar, an anesthesiologist. It provides a simple method to evaluate the condition of the newborn at 1 and 5 minutes after life (Apgar, 1966). Five assessment criteria (ie, heart rate, respiratory rate, muscle tone, reflex irritability, and color) are scored from 0 to 2. The highest total possible score is 10. The AAP and American College of Obstetricians and Gynecologists (AAP & ACOG, 2002) recommend continuing assessment every 5 minutes until the Apgar score is greater than 7. When used to evaluate preterm newborns, the Apgar score may have less validity. Findings common in the preterm newborn such as irregular respirations, decreased muscle tone, and decreased reflex irritability affect the overall score (Paxton & Harrell, 1991). The Apgar score should not be used as an indication for resuscitation (AHA & AAP, 2006). The Apgar score by itself is not an accurate predictor of long-term outcome (Juretschke, 2000).

PHYSICAL ASSESSMENT

A care provider skilled in newborn assessment should perform a physical assessment within the first 2 hours after birth (AAP & ACOG, 2002). This examination gives the perinatal nurse an opportunity to evaluate overall newborn well-being and transition to extrauterine life (Fig. 11–4). Chapter 12 describes a comprehensive physical examination, including normal and abnormal findings. During the initial examination in the birthing room, all systems are evaluated using inspection, auscultation, and palpation. During the transitional period after birth, temperature, heart rate, rate and character of respirations, skin color, level of consciousness, muscle tone, and activity level are evaluated and documented at least once every 30 minutes until the newborn's condition has remained stable for 2 hours (AAP & ACOG, 2002).

Skin

An overall visual assessment of the newborn is performed noting any obvious defects (eg, neural tube defects, abdominal wall defects, extra digits) or trauma (eg, bruising, petechiae, puncture wound from fetal scalp electrode). Skin is observed for color, texture, birthmarks, rashes, jaundice, and meconium staining. The newborn's back is inspected, noting a closed vertebral column or presence of abnormalities, such as masses and dimple or tuft of hair along the spine.

Head and Neck

Symmetry of the head and face is noted, as well as the presence of molding, caput succedaneum, and bruising. Fontanelles are palpated. Although it is not uncommon for eyelids to be edematous, drainage from the eye is not normal during this period. Subconjunctival hemorrhage, although not normal, is sometimes seen and resolves spontaneously. The neck is palpated for masses and full range of motion. The examiner assesses the position of the ears and looks for skin tags or evidence of a sinus on or around the ears. While assessing the mucous membrane of the mouth for a normal pink color, the lips and palate are inspected for a cleft.

Respiratory System

Inspection of the chest includes observing the shape, symmetry, and equality of chest movement. Asymmetry in chest movement may indicate pneumothorax or congenital defect. Respirations are nonlabored at a rate of 30 to 60 breaths per minute. Retractions, grunting, and nasal flaring are abnormal findings indicating respiratory distress. Breath sounds should be equal bilaterally. Initially, moist sounds may be heard as fluid is cleared from the lungs by absorption through pulmonary capillaries and by drainage through the nose and mouth. Special attention is paid to newborns when meconium-stained amniotic fluid is present. If meconium-stained amniotic fluid is noted prior to delivery, personnel capable of intubating the nonvigorous infant and clearing the trachea of meconium must be present at the delivery (AHA & AAP, 2006). Because meconium aspiration is a risk, careful assessment of the respiratory rate, quality of breath sounds, and color determines the need for interventions such as suctioning and supplemental oxygen. In the absence of meconium-stained amniotic fluid and respiratory depression, the newborn's mouth and nose are suctioned with a bulb syringe after delivery.

Cardiovascular System

Inspection of the cardiovascular system includes observation of the color of the skin and mucous membranes and location of the point of maximal impulse (PMI). Although acrocyanosis (blueness of the hands and feet) is a normal finding, central cyanosis indicates inadequate oxygenation and the need for supplemental oxygen. Heart rate, rhythm, and normal heart sounds and murmurs are best identified when auscultated using a newborn stethoscope.

Cardiovascular assessment also includes palpation for the presence and equality of femoral pulses. Pulses should be equal and nonbounding. Bounding pulses may indicate patent ductus arteriosus, whereas absent or decreased pulses may occur with coarctation of the aorta (Vargo, 2003). Depending on the condition of the newborn, a baseline blood pressure may be recorded. Taking the blood pressure in all four extremities is usually reserved for a newborn showing signs of distress. Routine blood pressure screening for newborns in the absence of risk factors and without complications is not recommended by the AAP (1993).

Abdomen

The examiner assesses the shape, symmetry, and consistency of the abdomen. The umbilical cord stump is inspected for the presence of three vessels (ie, two arteries and one vein). The umbilical cord of a newborn

INITIAL ASSESSMENT

DOB _____

TIME _____

TRANSITIONAL CARE ADMINISTERED IN:

☐ LDRP   ☐ Special Care Nursery

Initial Bath: _____
                   Time/Initials

Triple Dye to Cord _____
                        Time/Initials

Infant Removed from Radiant Warmer:

Date: _____ Time: _____

Weight: _____ gms. lbs. _____ oz. _____

Length: _____ cm. _____ in.

Head: _____ cm. _____ in.

Chest: _____ cm. _____ in.

Abdomen: _____ cm. _____ in.

Time	Radiant Warmer Temp	Temp	Pulse	Resp.	Breath Sounds	B/P	Color	Activity	Muscle Tone	SILVERMAN Upper Chest	Lower Chest	Xiphoid	Flare	Grunt	Total	Chest PT	Initials

COLOR
Pink   Plethoric
Pale   Mottled
Dusky   Cyanosis
Jaundiced   Acrocyanosis

MUSCLE TONE
Normal flexion
Flaccidity
Spasticity

ACTIVITY
Active
Active With Stimulation
Quiet, alert
Irritable
Lethargic   Hyperactive
Tremors   Sleeping

BREATH SOUNDS
Equal   Rales
Clear   Diminished
Rhonchi

✓ = chest PT

SKIN
_____ Pink _____ Acrocyanosis
_____ Central cyanosis _____ Dusky
_____ Pale _____ Plethoric
_____ Mottled _____ Jaundice
_____ Abrasions
_____ Birthmarks_____
_____ Dry _____ Meconium stained
_____ Ecchymosis _____
_____ Lacerations _____
_____ Milia _____ Peeling
_____ Mongolian spots _____
_____ Petechiae _____ Pustules
_____ Rash_____
_____ Skin tags _____
_____ Vesicles

CHEST
_____ Symmetrical _____ Asymmetrical
_____ Barrel chest
_____ Breast engorgement
_____ Supranummary nipples
_____ Breast discharge

RESPIRATIONS
_____ Normal _____ Labored
_____ Apnea _____ Grunting
Length_____

BREATH SOUNDS
_____ Equal _____ Clear
_____ Rales _____ Rhonchi

CLAVICLES
_____ Straight _____ Smooth
_____ Crepitus _____ Rt _____ Lt

REFLEXES
_____ Moro _____ Suck _____ Grasp

CRY
_____ Normal _____ Weak _____ Shrill
_____ No cry, quiet, alert

HEAD
_____ Symmetrical _____ Molding
_____ Caput
_____ Cephalohematoma _____ Lt _____ Rt
_____ Forcep marks _____
_____ Fontanels normal

FACE
_____ Symmetrical _____ Asymmetrical

EYES
_____ Clear _____ Discharge
_____ Lid edema
_____ Subconjunctival hemmorhage

NECK
_____ Full ROM _____ Limited ROM

HEART
_____ Regular _____ Irregular
_____ Murmur _____ Abnormal PMI
              Location: _____

FEMORAL PULSES
_____ Equal _____ Unequal

EXTREMITIES
_____ Symmetrical _____ Asymmetrical
_____ Normal ROM _____ Limited ROM
_____ Hipclicks _____ Rt _____ Lt
_____ Polydactylism _____ Syndactylism
_____ Abnormal foot position

FEMALE GENITALIA
_____ Normal _____ Discharge
_____ Vaginal skin tag

MALE GENITALIA
_____ Normal
_____ Epispadias
_____ Hypospadias
_____ Undecended testicle
_____ Rt _____ Lt
_____ Hydrocele

EARS
_____ Normal _____ Low set
_____ Sinus _____ Skin tags

NOSE
_____ Normal _____ Discharge

MOUTH
_____ Clear

  MUCOUS MEMBRANE
  _____ Pink_____ Cyanosis_____ Thrush
  _____ Cleft palate _____ Cleft lip
  _____ Hard _____ Soft

CORD
_____ 3 vessels _____ 2 vessels
_____ Meconium stained

ABDOMEN
_____ Symmetrical _____ Asymmetrical
_____ Flat _____ Scaphold
_____ Rounded _____ Distended
_____ Soft _____ Hard

BOWEL SOUNDS
_____ Present _____ Absent

RECTUM
_____ Patent

SPINE
_____ Closed vertebral column
_____ Asymmetry _____ Mass
_____ Dimple _____ Tuft of hair

Initials _____ Date/Time _____

PALOS COMMUNITY HOSPITAL
PALOS HEIGHTS, ILLINOIS

P-768
91480
Rev. 6/94

NEWBORN CARE RECORD

FIGURE 11–4. Documentation of initial newborn assessment.

exposed to meconium in utero for an extended period has a yellowish-brown discoloration. The abdomen is auscultated to detect bowel sounds.

Musculoskeletal System

Extremities are assessed for symmetry, range of motion, and the presence of extra or missing digits. While moving the newborn's arm, clavicles are palpated for crepitus, which may indicate a fracture. The newborn's hips are evaluated for "clunks," which may indicate dislocation. Normal muscle tone is noted during this part of the examination and while evaluating the Apgar score.

Genitalia

The presence of normal male or female genitalia is evaluated. Male newborns are assessed for location of the urethral meatus and presence of a hydrocele. The scrotum is palpated to detect the testes.

Neurological System

A complete neurological assessment is usually reserved for newborns that are born with or develop complications. A brief neurological assessment is performed by evaluating reflexes such as Moro, grasp, and suck.

In addition to ongoing physical assessments of the newborn, procedures such as newborn identification, instillation of eye prophylaxis, administration of vitamin K, and cord care are performed soon after birth. Ideally, each perinatal unit develops policies and procedures outlining expected newborn care. *Guidelines for Perinatal Care* (AAP & ACOG, 2002) is a resource for developing unit standards.

NEWBORN IDENTIFICATION

One of the first procedures after birth is newborn identification. Perinatal nurses must be meticulous when recording the identification band number and applying identification bands to mothers and newborns (AAP & ACOG, 2002). Some hospitals use a four-band system that includes a band for the support person or father of the newborn in addition to the band for the mother and two bands for the newborn, with one placed on an ankle and one on a wrist. Newborn footprinting and fingerprinting are not adequate methods of identification (AAP & ACOG). Some hospitals have abandoned these practices altogether, whereas others continue to do footprinting and fingerprinting but give the prints to the parents as a birth souvenir.

According to the National Center for Missing and Exploited Children (NCMEC, 2005), statistics for

TABLE 11–4 ■ REPORTED INFANT ABDUCTION CASES PERPETRATED BY NONFAMILY MEMBERS, 1983–2002

Year	Number of Cases	Year	Number of Cases
1983	5	1993	11
1984	7	1994	14
1985	7	1995	8
1986	11	1996	7
1987	18	1997	10
1988	14	1998	14
1989	17	1999	3
1990	15	2000	13
1991	17	2001	13
1992	10	2002	3

Burgess, A. W., & Lannin, K. V. (Eds.). (2003). *An analysis of infant abductions* (2nd ed.). Washington, DC: National Center for Missing and Exploited Children (NCMEC).

newborn abductions from hospital facilities may underrepresent the number of actual abductions from health care facilities (Table 11–4). Abductions and attempted abductions remain a significant threat to infant safety. In 2000, there were 13 hospital abductions reported. Infant abductions can be successfully prevented through a comprehensive safety program that may include alarm systems, video surveillance, and education of both staff and parents (Howard & Broughton, 2004; Shogan, 2002). NCMEC in cooperation with Mead Johnson Nutritionals and the Association of Women's Health, Obstetric and Neonatal Nurses (NCMEC, 2000) offer a prevention training program called Safeguard Their Tomorrows. This educational program includes a DVD, proactive measures healthcare agencies can take to prevent abduction, abductor profiles, case studies, statistics, safety measures for parents, and instructions for creating a crisis response plan in each hospital. NCMEC also has guidelines that healthcare professionals can use to identify and eliminate the risk of newborn abduction within their facilities. Staff education should be combined with the development and testing of critical incident response procedures including mock infant abductions as mandated by Joint Commission on Accreditation of Health Care Organizations (JCAHO, 2001).

Newborn safety and security, including unit visiting policies, should be discussed with parents and family members. Parents should be made aware of what the hospital is doing to ensure the safety of every newborn and should understand what they can do to increase safety. An important part of any newborn security program is a discussion with the parents, including directions not to leave their newborn unattended and information about identification of caregivers who

DISPLAY 11-3

Infant Safety Information

We, the nursing staff, welcome you to Palos Community Hospital and hope your family's stay here is a safe and pleasurable experience. During your stay, we ask for your cooperation to ensure your infant's safety.

1. If you are feeling weak, faint, or unsteady on your feet, do not lift your baby. Instead, call for assistance from the nurse.
2. Our birthing beds are narrower than your bed at home. We suggest that you place your baby in the crib when you become drowsy, plan on sleeping, or are using the bathroom. Please call a nurse if you need help. Never leave your newborn alone on your bed.
3. Never leave your baby alone in your room. If you walk in the halls or take a shower, please have a family member watch him or her or return your baby to the nursery.
4. Always keep an eye and hand on your infant when he or she is out of the crib.
5. When walking in the corridor, your baby should be in the crib and the crib flat.
6. Newborns possess some immunity from infections, but we still must protect them. Please ask your visitors to leave if they have any of the following: cold, diarrhea, sore that has a discharge, or contagious disease.

7. The only personnel that should be handling your baby or taking him or her from your room are employees wearing Palos Community Hospital scrubs and a picture ID tag. If you don't know the staff person, call for your nurse to help you.
8. Please call the nurse any time a situation arises with your baby that you do not feel comfortable with. We wish to give you as much teaching and information as possible to make your transition to parenthood as easy as possible.
9. Based on careful evaluation of existing data indicating an association between sudden infant death syndrome (SIDS) and prone (tummy-lying) sleeping position for infants, the American Academy of Pediatrics recommends that normal infants, when being put down for sleep, be positioned on their back. It should be stressed that the actual risk of SIDS for an infant placed on his or her stomach is still extremely low.
10. If your new baby's siblings visit, please keep a watchful eye on them so that they do not get hurt.

I understand the above information:

Date: _____

Mother's Signature: _____

Date: _____

*Significant Other: _____

*If available at the time of admission.

PALOS COMMUNITY HOSPITAL

PALOS HEIGHTS, ILLINOIS

---

may transport the newborn to and from the nursery or other hospital department. Display 11–3 is an example of information that might be reviewed with parents increasing their awareness of the need for vigilance and what they can do to support hospital systems designed to keep infants secure.

The efficacy of electronic newborn security systems in preventing newborn abductions remains controversial. No one method is superior; the key issue is that there must be some systematic newborn safety program in place known to the parents and perinatal healthcare providers to decrease the risk of newborn abduction. Nothing replaces vigilance on the part of parents, perinatal nurses, and other hospital employees.

VITAMIN K

One of the most important causes of a bleeding syndrome in an otherwise healthy newborn is hemorrhagic disease caused by vitamin K deficiency (Johnson, Rodden, & Collins, 2002). During the first week of life, newborns are at risk for bleeding disorders because of

an immature liver that is unable to produce several coagulation factors and a sterile gastrointestinal tract that has not begun producing vitamin K. Consumption of breast milk and formula causes colonization of bacteria in the gastrointestinal tract, which is necessary for vitamin K production. Vitamin K stimulates the liver to synthesize coagulation factors II, VII, IX, and X (Tsang, DeMarini, & Rath, 2003). A single dose of 0.5 mg for newborns weighing less than 1.5 kg and 1 mg for newborns weighing more than 1.5 kg is administered intramuscularly within the first hour of life (AAP Committee of the Fetus and Newborn, 2003).

EYE PROPHYLAXIS

Most states in the United States mandate that every newborn receive prophylaxis against eye infections. Erythromycin ointment is the drug of choice because of its effectiveness against gonococcal and chlamydial infections. Some evidence suggests that when the pregnant woman has received ongoing prenatal care and been screened for sexually transmitted diseases, the decision to use eye prophylaxis can be left up to parents (Bell, Grayston, Krohn, & Kronmal, 1993). After the agent for prophylaxis is chosen, care should be taken to instill the ointment throughout the conjunctival sac. Excessive medication can be wiped away with a sterile cotton ball 1 minute after instillation (AAP & ACOG, 2002).

UMBILICAL CORD CARE

As part of the initial newborn assessment in the birthing room, the umbilical cord is examined for the presence of two arteries and a vein. Because a moist cord is vulnerable to pathogens, measures should be taken to promote drying of the cord, including exposing the cord to air. Over the years a variety of methods of cord care have been used including alcohol, triple dye, and other antimicrobial agents. Research has shown that use of sterile water or air drying results in cords separating more quickly than those treated with alcohol (Dore et al., 1998; Medves & O'Brien, 1997). The cord should be observed for the presence of serous, purulent, or sanguineous drainage.

PSYCHOLOGICAL ADAPTATION

After addressing physiologic adaptation to extrauterine life, the focus of nursing interventions is psychological adaptation. Perinatal nurses are in a position to promote early maternal–newborn attachment. Early and extended contact between mother and newborn facilitates development of a positive relationship (Kennell & McGrath, 2005; Rapley, 2002). In a Cochrane review, Anderson, Moore, Hepworth, and Bergman (2003) identified positive benefits of early skin-to-skin contact on breastfeeding duration, maintenance of infant temperature, infant crying, and increased scores when maternal affectionate love and touch were measured. The perinatal nurse assists in the attachment process by encouraging parents to see, touch, and hold their newborn. Providing uninterrupted time for them to be together gives parents the opportunity to recognize and identify unique behavioral and physical characteristics of their newborn.

Practices used to promote attachment usually do not interfere with transition to extrauterine life. The perinatal nurse can make a positive contribution to enhancing the attachment process by modifying practices that separate mothers and newborns immediately after birth. Newborn treatments can be performed in the birthing room, decreasing separation time between the mother and the newborn. The mother may immediately hold the newborn if the newborn is dried and covered with a warm blanket. The newborn could also

be placed skin-to-skin with the mother. If both are covered with a blanket, neonatal thermoregulation is not interrupted. Application of ophthalmic antibiotics may safely occur within the first hour of life, enhancing maternal–newborn eye contact (AAP & ACOG, 2002). Maternal attachment is also supported when women are provided the opportunity to breast-feed immediately after birth. breastfeeding is more than a feeding method; it is an intimate relationship between a mother and her newborn. Early suckling and opportunities for uninterrupted contact between mother and newborn increases breastfeeding duration (Mizuno, Mizuno, Shinohara, & Noda, 2004; International Lactation Consultant Association, 1999).

COMPLICATIONS AFFECTING TRANSITION

Infection with group B streptococci (GBS) was one of the leading causes of morbidity and mortality in newborn infants before labor prophylaxis was instituted (Apgar, Greenberg, & Yen, 2005). It is estimated that 15% to 30% of women are GBS carriers (Askin, 2004). Before the use of prophylactic intrapartum antibiotics, newborns who survived GBS disease experienced developmental disabilities, mental retardation, and hearing and vision loss (Schrag et al., 2000). Pregnant women colonized with GBS are mostly asymptomatic but may experience urinary tract infections and amnionitis. The incidence of early-onset GBS infection is 0.6 cases per 1,000 live births when prenatal screening and a program of intrapartum antibiotic prophylaxis are in place. This represents a 65% decrease in neonatal infections between 1993 and 1998, the years that followed the introduction of the first screening and treatment guidelines (Schrag et al., 2000).

Early-onset GBS infection can occur in the first 7 days of life but most commonly manifests in the first 24 hours after delivery. Early-onset infection presents as bacteremia, meningitis, or pneumonia. The mortality rate associated with each of these presentations is 4% (Schrag et al., 2000). Risk factors for the development of GBS infection include gestational age less than 37 weeks, rupture of membranes more than 18 hours before birth, intrapartum fever of 38°C (99.4°F) or higher, a previous GBS-infected newborn, and GBS bacteriuria during pregnancy (Hager et al., 2000). Although it is unclear why, rates of GBS infection are higher among African-American women than among any other ethnic or racial groups.

Late-onset GBS infections occur between 1 week and 3 months of age. Sixty-three percent of these newborns develop bacteremia, 24% develop meningitis, and 2% develop pneumonia; the mortality rate for late-onset GBS is 2.8% (Schrag et al., 2000).

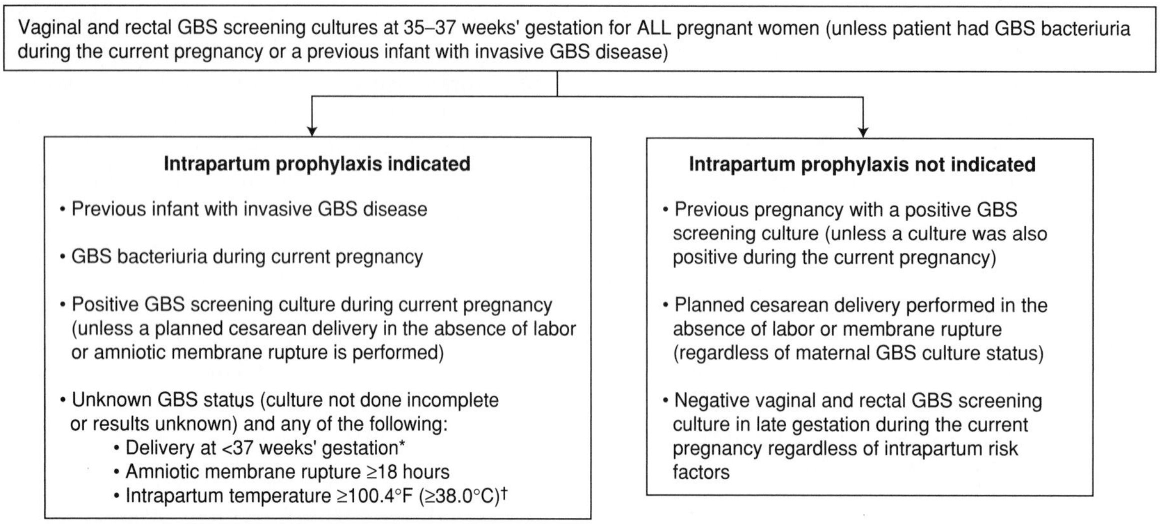

Vaginal and rectal GBS screening cultures at 35–37 weeks' gestation for ALL pregnant women (unless patient had GBS bacteriuria during the current pregnancy or a previous infant with invasive GBS disease)

Intrapartum prophylaxis indicated

• Previous infant with invasive GBS disease

• GBS bacteriuria during current pregnancy

• Positive GBS screening culture during current pregnancy (unless a planned cesarean delivery in the absence of labor or amniotic membrane rupture is performed)

• Unknown GBS status (culture not done incomplete or results unknown) and any of the following:
  • Delivery at <37 weeks' gestation*
  • Amniotic membrane rupture ≥18 hours
  • Intrapartum temperature ≥100.4°F (≥38.0°C)†

Intrapartum prophylaxis not indicated

• Previous pregnancy with a positive GBS screening culture (unless a culture was also positive during the current pregnancy)

• Planned cesarean delivery performed in the absence of labor or membrane rupture (regardless of maternal GBS culture status)

• Negative vaginal and rectal GBS screening culture in late gestation during the current pregnancy regardless of intrapartum risk factors

* If onset of labor or rupture of amniotic membranes occurs at <37 weeks' gestation and there is a significant risk for preterm delivery (as assessed by the clinician), a suggested algorithm for GBS prophylaxis management is provided (Figure 3).
† If amnionitis is suspected broad-spectrum antibiotic therapy that includes an agent known to be active against GBS should replace GBS prophylaxis.

FIGURE 11–5. Indications for antibiotic prophylaxis to prevent perinatal GBS disease. (From Schrag, S., Gorwitz, R., Fultz-Butts, K., & Schuchat, A. [2002]. Prevention of perinatal group B streptococcal disease: Revised guidelines from *CDC MMWR, 51*[RR11], 1–22.

Guidelines issued by the CDC in 1996 offered two approaches for the screening and treatment of GBS: screening cultures done at 35 to 37 weeks with treatment of positive results or consideration of risk factors with no screening cultures (CDC, 1996). Studies examining the effectiveness of this approach found that compliance rates were less than expected (Chandran et al., 2001) and that the culture only approach was over 50% more effective than the risk factor approach in preventing GBS infection in the newborn (Schrag et al., 2002). In 2002, the CDC, the American College of Obstetricians and Gynecologists (ACOG), and the American Academy of Pediatrics (AAP) issued revised guidelines for prevention of perinatal invasive group B streptococcal (GBS) disease recommending universal screening of pregnant women at 35 to 37 weeks' gestation and administering intrapartum antimicrobial prophylaxis to carriers (Fig. 11–5). This change resulted in a further decrease of early-onset GBS disease in the newborn by 31% from 2000 to 2001 (CDC, 2005a). In this survey, the incidence of late-onset disease was unchanged during the 9-year period reviewed.

Cases of early-onset GBS disease continue to occur despite the new guidelines and affected infants incur significant morbidity and mortality. Inaccurate screening results, improper implementation of IAP, or antibiotic failure all may contribute to persistent disease. This highlights the importance of continued vigilance for signs of infection in the newborn. There are no guidelines for the treatment of women having elective cesarean birth. Vertical transmission in this population is low, and antibiotic chemoprophylaxis is thought to be unnecessary (Hagar et al., 2000).

The assessment and care of a newborn after birth should be based on knowledge of maternal risk factors for GBS sepsis, maternal GBS status if known, and the timing and number of doses of antibiotic administered during labor. After delivery, it is important to evaluate the newborn for signs and symptoms of infection, including respiratory distress, apnea, tachycardia, hypotension, pallor, temperature instability, lethargy, and hypotonia. Asymptomatic newborns older than 35 weeks' gestation whose mothers received appropriate intrapartum chemoprophylaxis should be managed as healthy newborns. Symptomatic newborns should receive a diagnostic workup and prophylactic treatment with antibiotics. Figure 11–6 provides an algorithm for management of the newborn born to a GBS-colonized mother.

HEPATITIS B

Hepatitis B virus currently infects more than 400 million people worldwide (Ocama, Opio, & Lee, 2005). Universal vaccination and prenatal testing for HBV have decreased the incidence rate of acute HBV infections from more than 3/100,000 to 0.34/100,000 in all children (Slowik & Jhaveri, 2005).

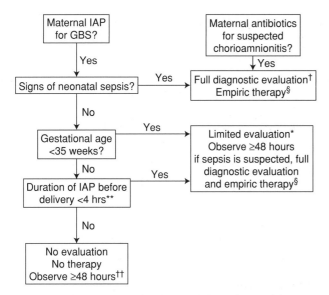

* If no maternal intrapartum prophylaxis for GBS was administered despite an indication being present, data are insufficient on which to recommend a single management strategy.

† Includes complete blood cell count and differential, blood culture, and chest radiograph if respiratory abnormalities are present. When signs of sepsis are present, a lumbar puncture, if feasible should be performed.

§ Duration of therapy varies depending on results of blood culture, cerebrospinal fluid findings, if obtained, and the clinical course of the infant. If laboratory results and clinical course do not indicate bacterial infection, duration may be as short as 48 hours.

** Applies only to penicillin, ampicillin, or cefazolin and assumes recommended dosing regimens

†† A healthy-appearing infant who was ≥38 weeks' gestation at delivery and whose mother received ≥4 hours of intrapartum prophylaxis before delivery may be discharged home after 24 hours if other discharge criteria have been met and a person able to comply fully with instructions for home observation will be present. If any one of these conditions is not met, the infant should be observed in the hospital for at least 48 hours and until criteria for discharged are achieved.

FIGURE 11–6. Management of a neonate born to a mother who received intrapartum antimicrobial prophylaxis (IAP) for prevention of early-onset group B streptococcal disease. (From Schrag, S., Gorwitz, R., Fultz-Butts, K., & Schuchat, A. [2002]. Prevention of perinatal group B streptococcal disease: Revised Guidelines from *CDC. Morbidity and Mortality Weekly Report, 51*[RR11], 1–22.

Before hepatitis B vaccination programs became routine in the United States, an estimated 30% to 40% of chronic infections are believed to have resulted from perinatal or early childhood transmission (CDC, 2005b). The spectrum of HBV infection ranges from asymptomatic seroconversion through general malaise, anorexia, nausea, and jaundice to fetal hepatitis. Development of a chronic infection is inversely proportional to the age at which the infection was acquired. Ninety percent of newborns infected in utero or at the time of birth develop chronic infection and become persistently positive for the hepatitis B surface antigen (HBsAg) (American Academy of Pedi-

atrics Committee on Infectious Diseases [AAP], 2000). In contrast, only 2% to 6% of older children, adolescents, and adults develop chronic HBV infection after acute illness (AAP, 2000). The immunologic response to infection leads to the development of cirrhosis, liver failure, or hepatocellular carcinoma (HCC) in up to 40% of patients (Wright, 2006). Routine screening of pregnant women for HBsAg should be carried out when the hepatitis status is unknown. HBsAg can be detected in individuals with acute or chronic hepatitis B viral infection.

The AAP recommends universal HBV immunization for all newborns. Newborns born to HBsAg-negative mothers should receive the first dose of vaccine at birth (before hospital discharge), with the second dose 1 to 2 months later and the third dose by 6 to 18 months of age. An alternative schedule of vaccinations gives the HBV vaccine at 2, 4, and 6 months of age concurrently with other childhood vaccines (AAP, 2000; AAP & ACOG, 2002). Babies born to HBsAg-positive mothers should receive one dose of hepatitis vaccine within 12 hours of birth, and hepatitis immunoglobulin (HBIG) should be given concurrently at a different site (AAP, 2000). HBIG provides temporary protection in postexposure situations, and HBV vaccine provides long-term protection. Newborns born to women with unknown HBsAg status should receive the first dose of HBV vaccine within 12 hours of birth (AAP & ACOG, 2002; AAP, 2000). Because the vaccine is highly effective in preventing infection in this population, further prophylaxis with HBIG can be delayed up to 7 days while awaiting maternal laboratory results.

SUMMARY

Most newborns need minimal support to make the transition to extrauterine life. Diverse and complex system adaptations make it a critical time for newborns. Strong desires to interact with their newborn make this a significant time for parents. The perinatal nurse must be knowledgeable about normal physiologic changes during the period of newborn transition from extrauterine life. Caring for newborns during this time requires the ability to recognize alterations from normal and becoming proficient at the skills necessary for conducting a newborn resuscitation.

REFERENCES

Alvaro, R. E., & Rigatto, H. (2005). Cardiorespiratory adjustments at birth. In *Avery's neonatology pathophysiology & management of the newborn* (6th ed., pp. 285–303). Philadelphia: Lippincott Williams & Wilkins.

American Academy of Pediatrics & American College of Obstetricians and Gynecologists (AAP & ACOG). (2002). *Guidelines for perinatal care* (5th ed.). Elk Grove Village, IL: American Academy of Pediatrics.

American Academy of Pediatrics Committee on Fetus and Newborn. (2003). Controversies concerning vitamin K and the newborn. *Pediatrics, 112*(1), 191–192.

American Academy of Pediatrics Committee on Fetus and Newborn. (1993). Routine evaluation of blood pressure, hematocrit, and glucose in newborns. *Pediatrics, 92*(3), 474–476.

American Academy of Pediatrics Committee on Infectious Diseases. (2000). *2000 Red book* (25th ed.). Elk Grove Village, IL: Author.

American Heart Association & American Academy of Pediatrics (AHA & AAP). (2006). *Textbook of neonatal resuscitation* (5th ed.). Elk Grove Village, IL: American Heart Association.

Anderson, G. C., Moore, E., Hepworth, J., & Bergman, N. (2003). Early skin-to-skin contact for mothers and their healthy newborn infants. *Cochrane Database of Systematic Reviews* (2), CD003519.

Apgar, B. S., Greenberg, G., & Yen, G. (2005). Prevention of group B streptococcal disease in the newborn. *American Family Physician, 71*(5), 903–910.

Apgar, V. (1966). The newborn Apgar scoring system: Reflections and advice. *Pediatric Clinics of North America, 13*(3), 645–650.

Askin, D. F. (2004). Bacterial infections. In D. F. Askin (Ed.) *Infection in the neonate. A comprehensive guide to assessment, management and nursing care* (pp. 61–82). Santa Rosa CA: NICU INK Books.

Bakewell-Sachs, S., Shaw, V. D., & Tashman, A. L. (1997). *Assessment of risk in the term newborn*. Wilkes-Barre PA: March of Dimes

Bell, T. A., Grayston, J. T., Krohn, M. A., & Kronmal, R. A. (1993). Randomized trial of silver nitrate, erythromycin, and no eye prophylaxis for the prevention of conjunctivitis among newborns not at risk for gonococcal ophthalmitis. *Pediatrics, 92*(6), 755–760.

Blackburn, S. T. (2003). *Maternal, fetal, & neonatal physiology. A clinical perspective*. Philadelphia: Saunders.

Blake, W. W., & Murray, J. A. (2002). Heat balance. In G. B. Merenstein & S. L. Gardner (Eds.), *Handbook of neonatal intensive care* (5th ed.). St. Louis: Mosby.

Bohnhorst, B., Heyne, T., Peter, C., & Poest, C. (2001). Skin-to-skin (kangaroo) care, respiratory control and thermoregulation. *Journal of Pediatrics, 138*(2), 193–197.

Browne, J. V. (2004). Early relationship environment: Physiology of skin to skin contact for parents and their preterm infants. *Clinics in Perinatology, 31*, 287–298.

Burgess, A. W., Lannin, K. V. (eds) (2003). *An analysis of infant abductions* 2nd Ed. Washington, DC. National Center for Missing and Exploited Children (NCMEC).

Cavaliere, T. (2004). The immune system. In D. F. Askin (Ed.), *Infection in the neonate. A comprehensive guide to assessment, management and nursing care* (pp. 13–36). Santa Rosa CA: NICU INK Books.

Centers for Disease Control and Prevention (CDC). (1996). Prevention of perinatal Group B streptococcal disease: A public health perspective. *Morbidity and Mortality Weekly Report, 45*(RR-7), 1–24.

Centers for Disease Control and Prevention (CDC). (2005a). Early-onset and late-onset neonatal group B streptococcal disease–United States, 1996–2004. *Morbidity and Mortality Weekly Report, 54*(47), 1205–1208.

Chandran, L., Navaie-Waliser, M., Zulqarni, N. J., Batra, S., Bayir, H., Shah, M., et al. (2001). Compliance with group B streptococcal disease prevention guidelines. *MCN: The American Journal of Maternal Child Nursing, 26*(6), 313–319.

Clyman, R. I. (2004). Mechanisms regulating closure of the ductus arteriosus. In R. A. Polin, W. W. Fox, & S. H. Abman (Eds.), *Fetal neonatal physiology*. Philadelphia: Saunders.

Dore, S., Buchan, D., Coulas, S., Hamber, L., Stewart, M., Cowan, D., et al. (1998). Alcohol versus natural drying for newborn cord care. *Journal of Obstetric, Gynecologic, and Neonatal Nursing, 27*(6), 621–627.

Gentile, R., Stevenson, G., Dooley, T., Franklin, D., Kawabori, I., & Perlman, A. et al. (1981) Pulsed Doppler echocardiographic determination of time of ductal closure in normal newborn infants. *Journal of Pediatrics, 98*, 443–448.

Grant, D. A. (1999). Ventricular constraint in the fetus and newborn. *Canadian Journal of Cardiology, 15*(1), 95–101.

Hackman, P. (2001). Recognizing and understand the cold-stressed term infant. *Neonatal Network, 20*(8), 35–41.

Hagedorn, M. I., Gardner, S. L., & Abman, S. H. (2002). Respiratory diseases. In G. B. Merenstein & S. L. Gardner (Eds.), *Handbook of neonatal intensive care* (5th ed., pp. 437–499). St. Louis: Mosby–Year Book.

Hager, W. D., Schuchat, A., Gibbs, R., Sweet, R., Mead, P., & Larsen, J. W. (2000). Prevention of perinatal group B streptococcal infection: Current controversies. *Obstetrics and Gynecology, 96*(1), 141–145.

Hanson, L. A., Korotkova, M., & Telemo, E. (2003). breastfeeding, infant formulas, and the immune system. *Annals of Allergy, Asthma and Immunology, 90*(6, Suppl. 3), 59–63.

Howard, B. J., Broughton, D. D., & Committee on Psychological Aspects of Child and Family Health. (2004). The pediatrician's role in the prevention of missing children. *Pediatrics, 114*, 1100–1105.

International Lactation Consultant Association. (1999). *Evidence-based guidelines for breastfeeding management during the first 14 days*. Raleigh, NC: Author.

Joint Commission on Accreditation of Healthcare Organizations. (2001). *Emergency management comprehensive accreditation manual for hospitals: The official handbook*. Washington DC: Author.

Johnson, B. A., & Ades, A. (2005). Delivery room and early postnatal management of neonates who have prenatally diagnosed congenital heart disease. *Clinics in Perinatology, 32*, 921–946.

Johnson, M. M., Rodden, D. J., & Collins, S. (2002). Newborn hematology. In G. B. Merenstein & S. L. Gardner (Eds.), *Handbook of neonatal intensive care* (5th ed., pp. 419–442). St. Louis: Mosby–Year Book.

Juretschke, L. J. (2000). Apgar scoring: Its use and meaning for today's newborn. *Neonatal Network, 19*(1), 17–19.

Kattwinkel, J. (Ed.). (2000). *Textbook of neonatal resuscitation* (4th ed.). Elk Grove Village, IL: American Academy of Pediatrics/American Heart Association.

Kennell, J., & McGrath, S. (2005). Starting the process of mother-infant bonding. *Acta Paediatrica, 94*(6), 775–777.

Kenner, C. (2003). Resuscitation and stabilization of the newborn. In C. Kenner & J. W. Lott (Eds.), *Comprehensive neonatal nursing: A physiologic perspective* (3rd ed., pp. 210–227). Philadelphia: Saunders.

Lott, J. W. (2003). Assessment and management of the cardiovascular system. In C. Kenner & J. W. Lott (Eds.), *Comprehensive neonatal nursing: A physiologic perspective* (3rd ed., pp. 376–408). Philadelphia: Saunders.

Ludington-Hoe, S. M., Anderson, G. C., Hollingsead, A., Argote, L. A., Medellin, G., & Rey, H. (1993). Skin-to-skin contact beginning in the delivery room for Colombian mothers and their preterm infants. *Journal of Human Lactation, 9*(4), 241–242.

Ludington-Hoe, S. M., Anderson, G. C., Swinth, J. Y., et al. (2004). Randomized controlled trial of Kangeroo care: Cardiorespiratory and thermal effects on health preterm infants. *Neonatal Network, 23*(3), 39–48.

Mast, E. E., Margolis, H. S., Fiore, A. E., Brink, E. W., Goldstein, S. T., Wang, S. A., et al. (2005b). A comprehensive immunization strategy to eliminate transmission of hepatitis B virus infection in the United States: Recommendations of the Advisory Committee on Immunization Practices (ACIP) part 1: Immunization of infants, children, and adolescents. *MMWR Recommendations and Reports, 54*(RR-16), 1–31.

Medves, J. M., & O'Brien, B. A. (1997). Cleaning solutions and bacterial colonization in promoting healing and early separation of the umbilical cord in healthy newborns. *Canadian Journal of Public Health, 88*(6), 380–382.

Mizuno, K., Mizuno, N., Shinohara, T., & Noda, M. (2004). Mother-infant skin-to-skin contact after delivery results in early recognition of own mother's milk odour. *Acta Paediatrica, 93*(12), 1640–1645.

National Center for Missing and Exploited Children (NCMEC). (2000). *Infant abduction from hospitals reduced by prevention training.* Washington, DC: Author.

Noerr, B. (2004). Thermoregulation. In T. Verklan & M. Walden (Eds.), *Core curriculum for neonatal intensive care nursing* (pp. 125–134). St. Louis: Elsevier Saunders.

Ocama, P., Opio, C. K., & Lee, W. M. (2005). Hepatitis B virus infection: Current status. *American Journal of Medicine, 118*(12), 1413.

Paxton, J. M., & Harrell, H. (1991). Delivery room management of the asphyxiated neonate. *NAACOG's Clinical Issues in Perinatal and Women's Health Nursing, 2*(1), 35–47.

Pfister, R. E., Ramsden, C. A., Neil, H. L., Kyriakides, M. A., & Berger, P. J. (2001). Volume and secretion rate of lung liquid in the final days of gestation and labour in the fetal sheep. *Journal of Physiology, 535*(3), 889–899.

Rapley, G. (2002). Keeping mothers and babies together—Breast-feeding and bonding. *RCM Midwives, 5*(10), 332–334.

Schrag, S. J., Zywicki, S., Farley, M. M., Reingold, A. L., Harrison, L. H., Lefkowitz, L. B., et al. (2000). Group B streptococcal disease in the era of intrapartum antibiotic prophylaxis. *New England Journal of Medicine, 342*(1), 15–20.

Schrag, S. J., Zell, E. R., Lynfield, R., Roome, A., Arnold, K. E., Craig, A. S., et al. (2002). A population-based comparison of strategies to prevent early-onset group B streptococcal disease in neonates. *New England Journal of Medicine, 347*(4), 233–239.

Shogan, M. (2002). Emergency management plan for newborn abduction. *Journal of Obstetric, Gynecologic and Neonatal Nursing, 31*(3), 340–346.

Simister, N. E. (2003). Placental transport of immunoglobulin G. *Vaccine, 21*(24), 3365–3369.

Slowik, M. K., & Jhaveri, R. (2005). Hepatitis B and C viruses in infants and young children. *Seminars in Pediatric Infectious Diseases, 16*(4), 296–305.

Strang, L. B. (1991). Fetal lung fluid: Secretion and reabsorption. *Physiolical Revues, 71*, 991–1016.

Tsang, R., DeMarini, S., & Rath, L. L. (2003). Fluids, electrolytes, vitamins and trace minerals. In C. Kenner & J. W. Lott (Eds.), *Comprehensive neonatal nursing: A physiologic perspective* (3rd ed., pp. 409–424). Philadelphia: Saunders.

Vargo, L. (2003). Cardiovascular assessment of the newborn. In E. P. Tappero & M. E. Honeyfield (Eds.), *Physical assessment of the newborn* (3rd ed., pp. 81–96). Petaluma, CA: NICU INK.

Wright, T. L. (2006). Introduction to chronic hepatitis B infection. *American Journal of Gastroenterology, 101*(1 Suppl.), S1-6.

Zaichkin, J., & Neonatal Resuscitation Program. (2002). Neonatal resuscitation emergencies at birth: Case reports, using NRP 2000 guidelines. *Journal of Obstetric, Gynecological and Neonatal Nursing, 31*(3),355–364.

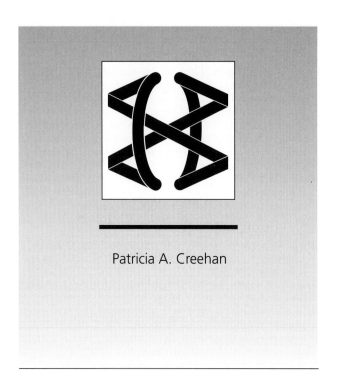

CHAPTER **12**

Newborn Physical Assessment

Patricia A. Creehan

PERINATAL nurses frequently perform the first head-to-toe physical assessment of the newborn. Ideally, this examination occurs in the presence of the parents. Conducting the examination while parents observe allows the nurse to use this time to identify and discuss normal newborn characteristics and note variations. It also provides an opportunity for parents to ask questions about the newborn's physical appearance and condition. The focus of this chapter is the physical assessment and findings that the perinatal nurse may observe during the time the newborn is in the hospital or birthing center. Home care nurses may also find the information pertinent during early postpartum home visits. Although some references are made to preterm newborns, that subject is not the intended focus of this chapter. It is also assumed that the reader has basic knowledge of physical assessment skills and terminology. Normal findings and common variations for each body system are identified in the text. Tables describe pathologic findings and their causes.

Physical assessment skills of inspection, palpation, and auscultation are used throughout the examination. When performing a physical assessment, the following equipment should be available: scale, tape measure, tongue blades, stethoscope with a neonatal diaphragm, and ophthalmoscope. The initial physical assessment may be conducted with the infant under a radiant warmer or in an open crib. Regardless of the location, attention should be given to avoiding cold stress. Adequate lighting is essential.

The sequence in which the nurse conducts the physical assessment is a matter of personal preference and depends on the cooperation of the newborn. Although we discuss the newborn assessment as a sequential examination covering one system at a time, some nurses conduct the examination in a cephalocaudal fashion, some prefer to examine the newborn system by system, and others evaluate multiple systems simultaneously.

The physical assessment usually begins by observing breathing pattern, overall skin color, general state or level of alertness, posture, and muscle tone. The newborn's *state* refers to general level of alertness and is a reflection of a group of characteristics that occur together. In the newborn, these characteristics include body activity, eye movement, facial movements, breathing pattern, and level of response to internal and external stimuli (Pearson, 1999). Understanding the differences in state provides information about how the newborn will respond to the nurse or parents and about the condition of the newborn's health, and it has implications for the education of parents. Appendix 12A describes newborn states, deep sleep, light sleep, drowsy, quiet alert, active alert, and crying and the implications these states have for caregivers.

The newborn is weighed and measured. It is normal for infants to lose up to 10% of their birth weight during the first few days of life. Figure 12–1 illustrates the technique for obtaining accurate measurements. Normal measurements are:

- Head circumference, 32 to 38 cm (13 to 15 inches)
- Chest circumference, 30 to 36 cm (12 to 14 inches)
- Length, 45 to 55 cm (18 to 22 inches)

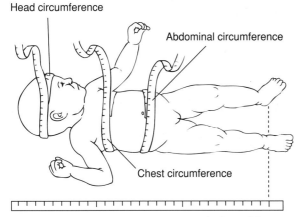

FIGURE 12–1. Newborn measurements. (Adapted from Wong, D. L. [Ed.]. [1997]. *Whaley & Wong's Nursing care of infants and children* [6th ed., p. 139]. St. Louis, MO: Mosby–Year Book.)

GESTATIONAL AGE ASSESSMENT

The American Academy of Pediatrics (AAP) and American College of Obstetricians and Gynecologists (ACOG) recommend that the gestational age of all newborns be determined after birth (AAP & ACOG, 2002). A gestational age assessment, evaluating physical and neuromuscular characteristics, is usually performed as part of the initial physical examination. Although some hospitals make gestational age assessment of all newborns a routine practice, other institutions have established criteria for performing gestational age assessment such as birth weight less than 2,500 g or more than 4,082 g, suspected intrauterine growth restriction (IUGR), gestation less than 37 weeks, and cesarean birth, and in some organizations it is not part of the nursing assessment but instead determined during the primary care provider's assessment. Identifying newborns that are preterm, term, or postterm, and those who are IUGR, small for gestational age (SGA), appropriate for gestational age (AGA), or large for gestational age (LGA) increases the likelihood of early identification and timely interventions for potential complications related to birth weight and gestational age during the immediate newborn period. Measures of gestational age are based on differences in physical and neurological maturity at different gestational ages.

The original tool, the Dubowitz Scoring System, contained 20 items combining neurological and physical parameters that successfully estimated gestational age in infants older than 34 weeks (Dubowitz, Dubowitz, & Goldberg, 1970). The tool was revised in 1999, increasing the number of items on the neurological exam. The test expanded the neurological exam to include behavior states, tone, primitive reflexes, motility, and some aspects of behavior (Dubowitz, Ricci, & Mercuri, 2005).

Most institutions use the Ballard Maturational Score (BMS), which was developed in the late 1970s (Ballard, Novak, & Driver, 1979). The original BMS contained 12 items based on the Dubowitz Scoring System. As more low-birth-weight infants were born and survived the initial neonatal period, an instrument that could accurately measure their gestational age was needed. In 1991, the BMS was reevaluated and expanded resulting in the development of a New Ballard Score (Fig. 12–2), which is what most organizations are using today. Criteria were broadened to provide greater accuracy when evaluating extremely premature neonates (Ballard et al., 1991).

The BMS is conducted by comparing the characteristics of the newborn with the pictures on the form and assigning a number for each characteristic. Appendix 12B describes each characteristic evaluated. Controversy exists about the timing of this assessment. The BMS is most accurate if performed between 10 and 36 hours of age. Assessment of newborns younger than 26 weeks' gestation is best conducted within the first 12 hours (Gagliardi, Brambilla, Bruno, Martinelli, & Console, 1993). The examination is separated into two parts: neuromuscular maturity assessment and physical maturity assessment. Scores from both sections are added together to determine gestational age.

SKIN ASSESSMENT

The newborn's entire body, as well as skin folds and scalp, should be inspected and palpated for changes in texture and the presence of masses that are not visible. Color, birth marks, rashes, skin lesions, texture, and turgor are noted. At birth, newborns are covered with vernix, an odorless, white, cheesy, protective coating produced by sebaceous glands. Vernix develops during the third trimester and increases with gestational age. At about 37 weeks, the amount of vernix begins to decrease, and at term, it is present only in the creases of the arms, legs, and neck.

Color

Skin color reflects circulation, oxygenation, and hemoglobin saturation. Color is best observed when the newborn is quiet. At birth, color ranges from pale to plethoric, depending on hematocrit and blood flow to the skin. Skin pigmentation depends on ethnic origin and deepens over time. Caucasian newborns have pinkish red skin tones a few hours after birth, and

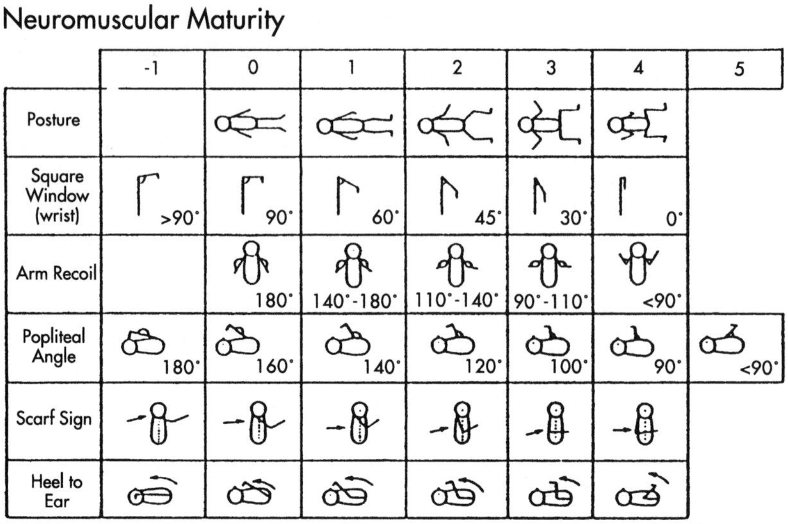

Neuromuscular Maturity

	-1	0	1	2	3	4	5
Posture							
Square Window (wrist)	>90°	90°	60°	45°	30°	0°	
Arm Recoil		180°	140°-180°	110°-140°	90°-110°	<90°	
Popliteal Angle	180°	160°	140°	120°	100°	90°	<90°
Scarf Sign							
Heel to Ear							

Physical Maturity

Skin	sticky iriable transparent	gelatinous red, translucent	smooth pink visible veins	superficial peeling &/or rash few veins	cracking pale areas rare veins	parchment deep cracking no vessels	leathery cracked wrinkled
Lanugo	none	sparse	abundant	thinning	bald areas	mostly bald	
Plantar Surface	heel-toe 40-50 mm:-1 < 40 mm:-2	>50mm no crease	faint red marks	anterior transverse crease only	creases ant. 2/3	creases over entire sole	
Breast	imperceptible	barely perceptilble	flat areola no bud	slippled areola 1-2mm bud	raised areola 3-4mm bud	full areola 5-10 mm bud	
Eye/Ear	lids fused loosely:-1 tightly:-2	lids open pinna flat stays folded	sl. curved pinna; soft; slow recoil	well-curved pinna: soft but ready recoil	formed & firm instant recoil	thick cartillage ear stiff	
Genitals male	scrotum flat, smooth	scrotum empty faint rugae	testes in upper canal rare rugae	testes descending few rugae	testes down good rugae	testes pendulous deep rugae	
Genitals female	clitoris prominent labia flat	prominent clitoris small labia minora	prominent clitoris enlarging minora	majora & minora equally prominent	majora large minora small	majora cover clitoris & minora	

Maturity Rating

score	weeks
-10	20
-5	22
-0	24
5	26
10	28
15	30
20	32
25	34
30	36
35	38
40	40
45	42
50	44

FIGURE 12–2. Gestational age assessment. (From Ballard, J. L., Khoury, J. C., Wedig, K., Wang, L., Ellers-Walsman, B. L., & Lipp, R. [1991]. New Ballard Score, expanded to include extremely premature infants. *Journal of Pediatrics, 119*[3], 417–423.)

African-American newborns have a reddish-brown skin color. Hispanic and Asian newborns have an olive or yellow skin tone. Changes in the skin color of Caucasian newborns may be the first sign of illness such as sepsis, cardiopulmonary disorders, or hematological diseases. Variations in skin color indicating illness are more difficult to evaluate in African-American and Asian newborns.

Generalized cyanosis may be seen at the time of birth as the newborn transitions from fetal to neonatal circulation. Cyanosis may be observed when the oxygen saturation in <85% (Hernandez & Glass, 2005.) Deep breaths and crying should quickly improve the newborn's color and oxygen saturation if the cause is not underlying pathology. Acrocyanosis, the blue discoloration of newborn hands and feet, is seen in the first 24 to 48 hours of life. Usually a benign condition, it is related to poor peripheral circulation and tends to worsen if the newborn becomes chilled. Persistent generalized or circumoral cyanosis (surrounding the mouth) is always abnormal outside of immediately after birth. The presence of either of these symptoms may indicate a pathologic condition and should be reported to the physician or nurse practitioner.

Jaundice

Jaundice, a bright yellow or orange discoloration of the skin, results from deposits of unconjugated bilirubin. Sixty percent of term newborns and 80% of preterm newborns develop jaundice during the first 3 to 4 days of life (Stoll & Kliegman, 2004). Jaundice results from the inability of the newborn's liver to conjugate bilirubin. A mildly elevated indirect bilirubin level is considered normal in the first few days of life. An elevated direct bilirubin level that may occur as early as 24 hours of life is never normal and suggests some pathology involving the liver. The skin color change associated with an elevated direct bilirubin is greenish or muddy yellow (Ulshen, 2000). Jaundice progresses in a cephalocaudal fashion. Seen first on the head and face, jaundice progresses downward to the truck and extremities and then to the sclera of the eye. When gentle pressure is applied to skin over cartilage or a bony prominence, skin blanches to a yellow hue on the face when bilirubin levels are 5 mg/dL, on the abdomen when levels are 15 mg/dL, and on the soles of the feet when levels reach 20 mg/dL (Stoll & Kliegman, 2004). Newborns with a positive Coombs test result almost certainly develop jaundice. In dark-skinned newborns, jaundice is more easily observed in the sclera and buccal mucosa.

Bruising

Ecchymosis may occur over the head or buttocks if forceps or a vacuum extractor was applied or after a breech or face presentation. Petechiae are common over the presenting part, especially when there has been a rapid descent during second stage of labor. Bruising may also result from a tight nuchal cord or a cord wrapped tightly around the upper body.

Variations Related to Vasomotor Instability

Cutis marmorata, mottling, or a lace-like pattern on the skin is a vasomotor response to chilling. Parents should be aware that this may continue after discharge. The harlequin sign occurs when some newborns are positioned on their sides. The dependent side of the body becomes pink, and the upper half of the body is pale. This phenomenon is considered benign. The color change lasts 1 to 30 minutes and disappears gradually when the infant is placed on the abdomen or back (Witt, 2005).

Hemangiomas

Hemangiomas are vascular skin lesions composed of dilated blood vessels. Present at birth or within the first 8 weeks of life in 8% to 12% of newborns, hemangiomas are more likely to occur in females than in males (Darmstadt & Sidbury, 2004).

Nevus Vasculosus

Nevus vasculosus, also called strawberry hemangioma, is an elevated red lesion that can occur anywhere on the body. Present at birth or developing soon after, this lesion acquired its name from the characteristic rough texture. Strawberry hemangiomas increase in size for up to 2 years and spontaneously regress over several years. Usually, no treatment is required unless the lesion bleeds, becomes infected, or interferes with breathing or eating.

Cavernous Hemangioma

Cavernous hemangioma is a soft, compressible swelling (Fig. 12–3). These lesions are present at birth but may be small and not very obvious, appearing as a blue discoloration under normal skin. As they swell and increase in size, they become more obvious and deeper red. Cavernous hemangiomas are frequently located on the head but can be found anywhere on the body and may extend deeply into skeletal muscle, joint, or bones (Brown, Friedman, & Levy, 1998). They increase in size between 6 and 12 months. Some disappear spontaneously in early childhood, but others require a multidisciplinary medical team approach to their management.

Macular Hemangioma

Commonly referred to as "stork bites," these lesions composed of dilated capillaries are macular, pink, blanch with pressure, and become darker when the newborn cries. Lesions may last 1 to 2 years or persist into adulthood. The most common newborn skin lesion, they are most often seen at the back of the neck, on the forehead, on eyelids, on the bridge of the nose, and over the base of the occipital bones. Macular hemangioma, also

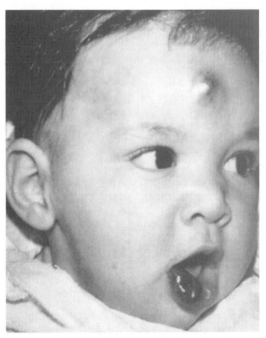

FIGURE 12–3. Hemangioma of the forehead and lip.

referred to as telangiectatic nevus, may occur on as many as 50% of newborns (Esterly, 1996).

Port Wine Stain

Port wine stains are present at birth in 0.3% to 1% of newborns (Hartley & Rasmussen, 1990). Color varies from pink in Caucasian infants to black or deep purple in newborns of African-American descent. Most often seen on the head and neck, port wine stains have discrete borders, do not blanch when pressure is applied, and do not lighten as the child ages (Darmstadt & Sidbury, 2004). These lesions composed of dilated capillaries are generally benign unless they occur along the trigeminal nerve root, in which case they may be associated with glaucoma or retinal detachment, or in the lumbosacral region, where they may be associated with spinal abnormalities (Brown, Friedman, & Levy, 1998). Certain types of lasers effectively remove port wine stains and can be used safely on infants.

Mongolian Spots

Mongolian spots are large, nonblanching, blue-gray lesions resembling a bruise most often seen over the sacrum and flanks but may be present on the posterior thighs, legs, back, and shoulders (Fig. 12–4). They occur in 70% to 90% of African-American, Asian, and Native American infants and in 5% to 13% of Caucasian infants (Darmstadt & Sidbury, 2004). Mongolian spots are caused by infiltration of melanin-forming cells into the dermal skin layer rather than the epidermis. Mongolian spots may persist into early childhood but usually fade.

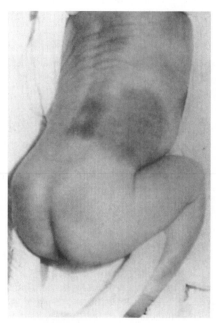

FIGURE 12–4. Mongolian spots.

Erythema Toxicum

Erythema toxicum, also called newborn rash, is benign and appears at about 24 to 48 hours of age in approximately 50% of term newborn infants (Darmstadt & Sidbury, 2004). In preterm infants, the rash may not develop for several days or weeks. Erythema toxicum is composed of small, yellow papules surrounded by an erythematous area. The rash continues to appear and disappear over various parts of the body for several days. Most commonly seen on the face, trunk, and limbs, this rash will generally resolve within 4 to 5 days (Hernandez & Glass, 2005) but may continue to appear up to 3 months of age (Witt, 2005).

Milia

Milia, clogged sebaceous glands, appears as tiny, white, 1-mm papules present at birth over the chin, cheeks, forehead, and fleshy area of the nose. They disappear during the first 2 weeks of life. Milia occur in as many as 40% of infants (Hernandez & Glass, 2005).

Texture

Skin is evaluated for texture and the presence of lanugo during the physical examination and as part of the gestational age assessment. Texture ranges from smooth to superficial peeling. Shortly after birth, most term newborns have dry, flaky skin. Peeling, leathery skin with deep cracks indicates postmaturity. Lanugo, a fine, downy hair that covers the body, begins to develop around 20 weeks' gestation (Witt, 1999). It is seen in abundance on premature infants and rarely on infants greater than 42 weeks' gestation. At term, lanugo is confined to the shoulders, ears, and forehead.

Turgor

Skin turgor is the natural rebound elasticity of the skin. It can be assessed anywhere on the body by pinching the skin between the examiners thumb and index finger and then quickly releasing it. Skin turgor is best assessed on the abdomen. Healthy, elastic tissue rapidly resumes its normal position without creases or tenting. Skin that remains tented indicates poor hydration and nutritional status. Table 12–1 identifies skin findings during the physical assessment that are abnormal and their related pathology.

HEAD ASSESSMENT

The newborn head is examined using inspection and palpation and assessed for size, shape, and symmetry. The head of a term, AGA newborn has an occipital–frontal circumference of 32 to 38 cm (12.5 to 14.5 inches).

TABLE 12–1 ■ INTEGUMENT

Assessment	Pathology
Pallor	Anemia
	Asphyxia
	Shock
	Sepsis
	Twin-to-twin transfusion
	Cardiac disease
Central cyanosis	Sepsis
	Persistent pulmonary hypertension
	Neurological disease
	Congenital heart disease
	Respiratory disorder
Plethora	Polycythemia
	Overheated
Gray color	Sepsis
Jaundice within 24 hours of birth	Liver disease
	Sepsis
	Maternal ingestion of drugs (eg, aspirin)
	Blood incompatibilities
Generalized petechiae	Clotting disorders
	Sepsis
Pustules	*Staphylococcus*
	Beta-hemolytic *Streptococcus*
	Varicella
Greenish, yellow vernix	Meconium staining
	Hemolytic disease
Generalized edema	Erythroblastosis fetalis
	Renal failure
	Turner syndrome
"Blueberry muffin" spots (purpura)	Congenital viral infection
Multiple tan or light brown macules (café au lait spots)	Neurofibromatosis
Cutis marmorata	Hypovolemia
	Sepsis
	Chromosomal abnormalities
Extensive Mongolian spots	Inborn errors of metabolism (Silengo, Battistoni, & Spada, 1999)

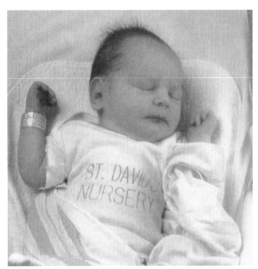

FIGURE 12–5. Molding. (From Pillitteri, A. [2003]. *Maternal and child health nursing* [4th ed., p. 644]. Philadelphia: Lippincott Williams & Wilkins.)

molding) as the fetus descends through the birth canal or as a result of the application of vacuum or forceps, giving the head an elongated, asymmetric appearance (Fig. 12–5). The overlapping cranial bones can be palpated along the suture lines. Molding may last several days and cause the head circumference to be smaller immediately after birth. The circumference returns to normal within 2 to 3 days after birth. Newborns delivered by cesarean section or in breech position have a more rounded, symmetric head.

Caput succedaneum, edema under the scalp, is caused by pressure over the presenting part of the newborn's head against the cervix during labor. Caput feels soft and spongy, crosses suture lines, and resolves within a few days. Figure 12–6 pictorially compares the location of caput succedaneum and cephalhematoma.

The newborn's head is palpated for the presence of all suture lines (Fig. 12–7). Suture lines feel like soft depressions between the cranial bones. If instead a ridge of bone is felt, the examiner should determine whether it is the result of molding or premature closure of the suture. Normal mobility of the cranial bones is determined by placing each thumb on opposite sides of the suture and alternately pushing in slightly on each side. Lack of mobility of cranial bones indicates premature closure of the sutures (ie, craniosynostosis). The incidence of craniosynostosis is 1 case per 2,000 births (McCarthy, 2004). Craniosynostosis causes an abnormally shaped head, as the contents of the cranium enlarge but the cranial bones do not. This abnormally shaped head may be apparent at birth or later in infancy.

The skull is palpated for masses and assessed for craniotabes. Craniotabes is a softening of cranial bones caused by pressure of the fetal skull against the bony pelvis. When pressure is exerted with the

To measure the newborn's head, a tape measure is placed just above the eyebrows and continues around to the occipital prominence at the back of the skull (Figure 12–1). At birth most skull deformities are the result of position in utero, decrease in space in utero due to multiple gestation, or intrapartum events (AAP, 2003a). Vaginal birth may cause the cranial bones to overlap (ie,

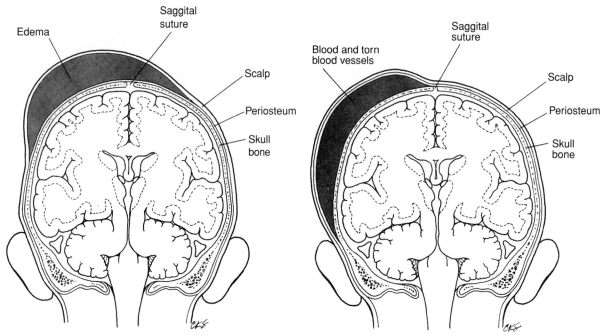

FIGURE 12–6. Comparison of caput succedaneum (*left*) and cephalhematoma (*right*).

examiner's fingers at the margins of the parietal or occipital bones, a popping sensation similar to indenting a ping-pong ball is felt. Craniotabes is primarily seen in breech presentations and usually disappears within a few weeks.

Anterior and posterior fontanelles, the soft membranous coverings where two sutures meet, are palpated and measured (Fig. 12–7). Fontanelles are measured diagonally from bone to bone rather than from suture to suture. The anterior fontanelle is diamond shaped, measuring 4 to 5 cm, and closes around 18 months of age. The posterior fontanelle is triangular, measuring 0.5 to 1 cm, and closes between 2 and 4 months. Fontanelles are best palpated when the newborn is quiet. The area is soft, is depressed slightly, and may bulge with crying. Arterial pulsations may be felt over the anterior fontanelle. Molding may make it impossible to palpate fontanelles in the first few hours of life.

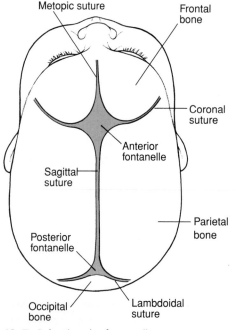

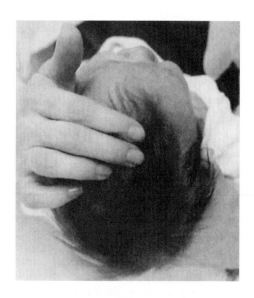

FIGURE 12–7. Palpating the fontanelles.

TABLE 12–2 ■ HEAD

Assessment	Pathology

The following assessments may indicate increased intracranial pressure:
    Sutures separated more than 1 cm
    Bulging, tense fontanelle
    Head circumference greater than 90th percentile for gestational age
	Hydrocephalus
	Hypothyroidism
	Tumor
	Meningitis

Head circumference below 10th percentile for gestational age	Genetic disorder Congenital infection Maternal drug or alcohol ingestion
Depressed fontanelle	Dehydration
Cephalhematoma: swelling due to bleeding between periosteum and skull bone; does not cross suture line; may not be evident until 1 day after birth and take several weeks to resolve (see Fig. 12–6)	Head trauma during birth
Texture of hair is fine, woolly, sparse, coarse, brittle	Prematurity Endocrine disorder Genetic disorder
Increased quantity of hair, low-set hairline	Genetic disorder
Limited forward growth of the skull; skull appears broad	Brachycephaly (fused coronal suture)
Limited lateral growth of the skull; skull appears long and narrow	Scaphocephaly (fused sagittal suture)

The scalp is examined for distribution, amount, and texture of hair. Hair is silky and may be straight, curly, or kinky, depending on ethnic origin. Bruising, lacerations, and bleeding are frequently seen as the result of the application of a scalp electrode or vacuum extractor. Table 12–2 identifies findings during the physical assessment of the head that are abnormal and their related pathology.

EYE ASSESSMENT

The newborn's eyes are assessed using inspection and an ophthalmoscope. This can be done early in the examination as part of the assessment of the head or whenever the newborn spontaneously opens his or her eyes. Eyes should be symmetric in size and shape. Lids may be edematous and puffy at birth. The distance between the eyes, measured from the inner canthus of each, is 1.5 to 2.5 cm (Hernandez & Glass, 2005). Eyes spaced closer (ie, hypotelorism) or farther apart (ie, hypertelorism) may be a variation of normal or associated with other anomalies. Eyes with small palpebral fissures (ie, eye openings) may also be normal or associated with other anomalies.

The colors of eye structures are observed. The iris is usually slate gray, brown, or dark blue. Eye color becomes permanent at about 6 months of age. The normally blue-white sclera may contain subconjunctival hemorrhages, the result of ruptured capillaries during the birth process. Subconjunctival hemorrhages usually resolve within a week. A yellow sclera indicates hyperbilirubinemia. Years ago when silver nitrate was the standard of care for prophylaxis against ophthalmia neonatorum, the conjunctiva would frequently become inflamed. Today, most hospitals are using erythromycin ointment, which usually does not cause this complication.

Tears are usually absent in the newborn until the lachrymal duct becomes fully patent at about 4 to 6 months of age. Prominent epicanthal folds (ie, Mongolian slant) is a normal finding in Asian infants but suggests Down syndrome in other ethnic groups.

Blink reflex, size, and reactivity of pupils are evaluated in a darkened room with a pen light or light from the ophthalmoscope. Pupils are equal and reactive to light (PERL). When a light is shined at an angle toward the eye, the lens should be clear. Equal color, intensity, and clarity of the red reflex in both eyes without opacities or white spots within either red reflex is considered a normal exam (AAP, 2003b). Presence of and clarity of the red reflex indicates an intact cornea and lens. Lack of a red reflex suggests congenital glaucoma or cataracts. Pale red reflexes are a normal variation in dark-skinned newborns.

Movement of the eye is observed. Strabismus, a cross-eyed appearance, is often seen in newborns because of weak eye musculature and lack of coordination. Nystagmus (ie, constant, rapid, involuntary movement of the eye) may occur and usually disappears by 4 months of age. Newborns are nearsighted at birth and respond to bright or primary colors and to

TABLE 12–3 ■ EYE

Assessment	Pathology
Persistent purulent discharge	Ophthalmia neonatorum Chlamydia conjunctivitis Blocked lachrymal duct (dacryocystitis)
Blue sclera	Osteogenesis imperfecta
Sclera visible above iris (sunset eyes)	Hydrocephalus
Black or white spots on periphery of iris (Brushfield spots)	Benign or associated with Down syndrome
Pupils not equal, nonreactive, fixed	Neurological insult
Keyhole-shaped pupil (coloboma)	Usually associated with other anomalies
Mongoloid slant of palpebral fissures (opening between eyelids)	Down syndrome

high contrast between colors such as black and white. They see objects clearly 8 to 10 inches in front of them. Table 12–3 identifies findings during the physical assessment of the eye that are abnormal and their related pathology.

EAR ASSESSMENT

The newborn ear is assessed by inspection and palpation. External structures are examined for position, presence of abnormal structures, and injury which may have occurred during the birth process. The pinna lies on or above an imaginary line drawn from the inner to the outer canthus of the eye, back toward the ear (Fig. 12–8). Low-set ears, those that fall below this line, are associated with genetic syndromes. A soft pinna lacking cartilage is seen in premature infants. Temporary asymmetry of the ears can result from intrauterine position. Folded helix may be associated with breech position in utero (Spilman, 2002). Skin tags (Fig. 12–9) and small pits (Fig. 12–10) located anterior to the ear are usually benign, may be familial, but can also be associated with other malformations or syndromes. Craniofacial anomalies including malformation of the ears may be associated with maternal diabetes or maternal history of decreased amniotic fluid as a result of oligohydramnios, leaking fluid, or prolonged or premature rupture of membranes (Ewart-Toland et al., 2000). Presence of ecchymosis, swelling, abrasions, or lacerations may be the result of pressure during the birth process, application of forceps or vacuum, or injury during cesarean section.

The ear is palpated as part of the gestational assessment to determine the presence and firmness of cartilage. By 38 to 40 weeks' gestation, the pinna is firm and well formed by cartilage, and incurving is present over two-thirds of the ear. At term, folding the pinna of the ear inward and releasing should result in brisk recoil. The more premature an infant is, the slower the pinna will be to return to its normal position. The pinna of an extremely premature infant may remain folded.

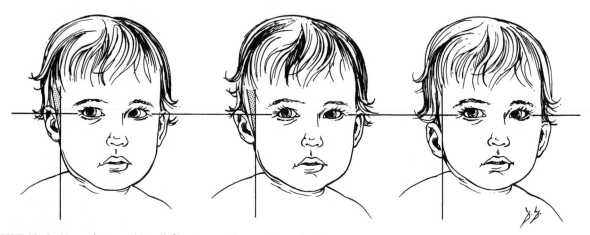

FIGURE 12–8. Normal ear position (*left*). Abnormally angled ear (*middle*). Low-set ears (*right*). (From Reeder, S. J., Martin, L. L., & Koniak-Griffin, D. [1997]. *Maternity nursing: Family, newborn and women's health* [18th ed., p. 706]. Philadelphia: Lippincott-Raven Publishers.)

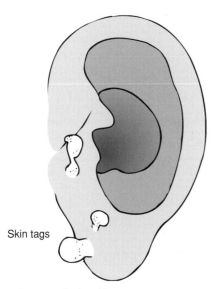

FIGURE 12–9. Preauricular skin tags.

The ear canal is inspected for patency. Use of the otoscope is limited because newborn Eustachian tubes contain vernix, mucus, and cellular debris. The ear canals clear spontaneously several days after birth. At this time, the tympanic membrane is visualized by pulling the pinna back and down. The tympanic membrane appears gray-white and highly vascular. If a neonatal infection is suspected, otoscopic examination of the ear is indicated.

Although hearing is well developed at birth, it becomes more acute as the Eustachian tubes clear. The newborn responds to high-pitched vocal sounds and the familiar voice of his or her mother and becomes quiet and relaxed when spoken to in a soft, calm manner. The incidence of hearing loss is 1 to 3 cases per 1,000 well newborns and 2 to 4 cases per 1,000 newborns admitted to intensive care nurseries (AAP, 1999). In 1994, the Joint Committee on Infant Hearing (JCIH),

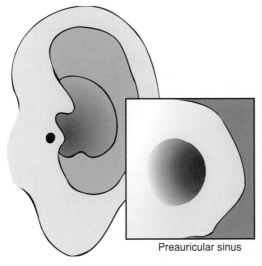

FIGURE 12–10. Preauricular sinus.

of which the AAP was a member, first proposed that there be universal hearing screening of all newborns. The AAP currently recommends that newborns receive hearing screening prior to discharge from the hospital, that when birth occurs in the home or an alternative birthing center referral for screening be made within 1 month of birth, and that newborns admitted to intensive care units receive hearing screening before discharge from the hospital (AAP, 2000). UNHS prior to 1 month of age is a goal of Healthy People 2010 (USDHHUS, 2000).

Support for UNHS is based on the premise that the first 3 years of life are the most critical period for brain development and language development whether spoken or signed. Attention to hearing deficits and loss during this period has life long implications for a child's understanding and use of language (USDHHS, 2000). Research results are mixed regarding the efficacy of UNHS to improve long-term language outcomes. Although some research indicates that when newborns are identified before 6 months of age and provided with amplification, their language skills are essentially normal at age 3 years (Mason & Herrmann, 1998; Yoshinaga-Itano, 1999). A meta-analysis, comparing the outcomes of UNHS versus using risk factors to determine what infants are screened, found that extending screening to low-risk infants resulted in detection of 1 case for every 2401 low-risk infants screened with 254 false-positives versus 48 false-positives when specific screening criteria are used (Thompson et al., 2001).

Two technologies are available for hearing screening: evoked otoacoustic emissions (EOAE) and auditory brainstem response (ABR). The sensitivity of current technology is at or near 100% (Mehl & Thompson, 1998). These methods are noninvasive, quick, and easy to perform.

EOAE evaluates hearing by measuring sound waves in the inner ear. Sound waves are created in the inner ear by the cochlea in response to clicking sounds. Small microphones placed in the newborn's ear create the clicking sounds and measure the sound waves produced in response. The disadvantage of this testing method is that debris in the ear canal such as vernix, blood, and amniotic fluid may affect the test and result in false-positive results. UNHS programs using EOAE technology result in 5% to 20% referral rates for formal audiology assessment (AAP, 1999).

ABR evaluates hearing by measuring electroencephalographic waves recorded by an electrode placed on the newborn's forehead. Electroencephalographic waves occur in response to clicks the newborn hears through small foam ear pieces. The advantage of this technology is that it is not influenced by debris in the middle or inner ear, and referral rates for formal audiology assessment are less than 3% (AAP, 1999). The challenge to using this technology is keeping the newborn in a quiet state, preferably sleeping. Table 12–4

TABLE 12–4 ■ EAR

Assessment	Pathology
Low-set ears	Genetic disorder Kidney abnormality
Poorly formed external ear	Genetic disorder
Skin tags located on the ear lobe or the skin surface surrounding the ear (Fig. 12–9)	Familial variation Alteration in normal embryologic development Genetic disorder associated with urinary tract abnormalities
Preauricular sinuses are connections between the skin surface and cysts. If they close before birth, all that is presence is a "pit" or pinpoint size indentation located in front of the ear (Fig. 12–10)	Familial variation Alteration in normal embryologic development Genetic disorder associated with deafness and renal abnormalities
Absence of Moro reflex	Hearing loss
Microtia—abnormally small external ear	Associated with inner ear malformations and hearing loss

identifies findings during the physical assessment of the ear that are abnormal and their related pathology.

NOSE ASSESSMENT

The newborn's nose is assessed using inspection. The nose should be symmetric and midline but may be misshapen at birth because of the neonate's positioning in utero. If the septum cannot be easily straightened and the nose remains asymmetric, treatment may be required. A flattened or bruised nose may result from passage through the birth canal.

Nasal stuffiness and thin, white mucus is not an uncommon finding immediately after birth. Newborns sneeze to clear the upper respiratory tract. Nasal flaring, widening of the nares, is a compensatory mechanism that decreases upper airway resistance, allowing more air to enter the nasal passages. Nasal flaring is abnormal and one of the first symptoms observed when respiratory distress occurs. Table 12–5 identifies

TABLE 12–5 ■ NOSE

Assessment	Pathology
Flat nasal bridge	Down syndrome
Pink when crying; chest retractions and cyanosis at rest; difficulty feeding	Choanal atresia
Stuffy nose and thin, watery discharge	Neonatal drug withdrawal
"Sniffles" persistent; profuse mucopurulent or bloody discharge (Green, 1998)	Congenital syphilis

findings during the physical assessment of the nose that are abnormal and their related pathology.

MOUTH ASSESSMENT

The newborn mouth is assessed using inspection and palpation. In the sequence of the total examination, this assessment is frequently left until last. If the newborn's mouth is forced open, crying may result, altering aspects of the respiratory or cardiac assessments. The lips are observed for location, color, and symmetry.

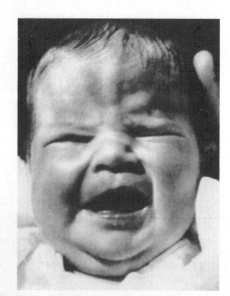

FIGURE 12–11. Facial nerve paralysis. Notice the asymmetry of the mouth during crying. (From Reeder, S. J., Martin, L. L., & Koniak-Griffin, D. [1997]. *Maternity nursing: Family, newborn and women's health* [18th ed., p. 1205]. Philadelphia: Lippincott-Raven Publishers.)

The mouth should be centrally located along the midline. At rest, the lips appear symmetric. Depending on skin color, the lips are pink or more darkly pigmented. Sucking blisters, centrally located on the upper lip, may be filled with fluid or have the consistency of a callus. Calluses may also be found on the hand as a result of vigorous sucking in utero or after birth. Muscle weakness or facial paralysis is best observed when the infant is sucking or crying; both conditions may be missed altogether if the infant is observed only in a quiet, alert state (Fig. 12–11). Rooting, suck, and gag reflexes are evaluated during this portion of the examination or during feeding.

The mucous membrane and internal structures of the mouth are inspected. If the mouth does not open spontaneously while the newborn cries, it can be gently opened by a downward pressure on the chin or with a pediatric tongue blade. In a healthy newborn, the mucous membrane is pink. Increased amounts of

mucus during the first 1 to 2 days of life are removed with a bulb syringe. This is especially common in newborns born by cesarean section, because they do not benefit from compression of the thorax through the birth canal. The tongue is mobile and prominent within the mouth. Occasionally, the frenulum is short, causing a notch at the tip of the tongue. True congenital ankyloglossia (ie, tongue tie) is rare.

Using adequate lighting, the hard and soft palates are examined. The uvula is midline and located at the posterior soft palate. Some practitioners use an index finger to palpate the hard and soft palates for the presence of clefts (Fig. 12–12). Whitish-yellow cysts (ie, Epstein's pearls) containing epithelial cells may be present on the hard palate at birth, but they disappear within a few weeks. Some newborns are born with one or two natal teeth. These immature caps of enamel and dentin have poor root formation and are usually loose. These teeth may be aspirated if dislodged and make

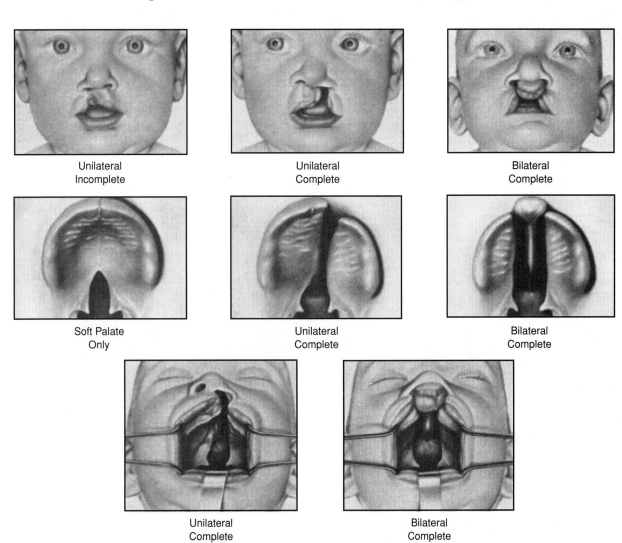

FIGURE 12–12. Cleft lip and cleft palate (redrawn from drawings by Ross Laboratories). (From Reeder, S. J., Martin, L. L., & Koniak-Griffin, D. [1997]. *Maternity nursing: Family, newborn and women's health* [18th ed., p. 1108]. Philadelphia: Lippincott-Raven Publishers.)

TABLE 12–6 ■ MOUTH

Assessment	Pathology
Mucous membranes dry	Dehydration
Cyanotic mucous membranes	Poor oxygenation
Asymmetric movement of mouth	Facial nerve injury
Cleft lip and/or palate (see Fig. 12–12)	Teratogenic injury Genetic disorder Multifactorial inheritance
Hypertrophied tongue	Down syndrome Beckwith-Wiedmann syndrome Hypothyroidism
Protrusion of tongue	Genetic disorder
Weak, uncoordinated suck and swallow	Prematurity Neuromuscular disorder Asphyxia Maternal analgesia during labor Inborn error of metabolism
Frantic sucking	Infant of drug-addicted mother
Excessive drooling and salivating; unable to pass a nasogastric tube	Esophageal atresia
Circumoral cyanosis	Respiratory distress
Thin upper lip, smooth philtrum, short palpebral fissures	Fetal alcohol syndrome
Translucent, bluish swelling on either side of the frenulum under the tongue	Mucous or salivary gland retention cyst
Bifid uvula	Genetic disorder
Small lower jaw (micrognathia)	Pierre Robin syndrome Treacher Collins syndrome De Lange syndrome
Patches of white on tongue and mucous membrane	Candida albicans

breastfeeding difficult, or cause lacerations on the mucosa, lips, or tongue. They are usually removed during the neonatal period. Table 12–6 identifies findings during the physical assessment of the mouth that are abnormal and their related pathology.

NECK ASSESSMENT

Inspection and palpation are used to assess the neck. The neck is inspected for symmetry and range of motion. Newborns have short, thick necks with multiple skin folds. A predominant fat pad in the back of the neck, redundant skin, and webbing are findings associated with genetic syndromes.

Full range of motion is present at term. The newborn's head should be able to turn completely to face each shoulder. Torticollis, contraction of the neck muscles that pulls the head toward the affected side with the chin pointing toward the opposite shoulder and side, results from injury to the sternocleidomastoid muscle. More common on the right side, this injury may be congenital or occur during the birth process. A small mass at the site of the injury is palpated along the sternocleidomastoid muscle at birth or soon after. Parents are taught to perform stretching exercises to lengthen the muscle, and the newborn is followed by a physical therapist through the first year of life. If the contracture persists after 1 year, surgery may be necessary.

Cystic hygroma is one of the most common neck lesions (Fig. 12–13). This particular cystic structure occurs at lymphatic–venous connections, most commonly in the posterior neck (Gallagher, Mahoney, & Gosche, 1999). The lesions vary in size from a few millimeters to large enough to deviate the trachea, cause respiratory distress, or interfere with feeding. A cystic hygroma requires surgical excision.

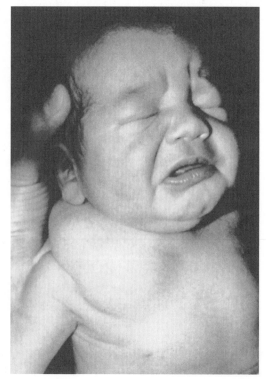

FIGURE 12–13. Cystic hygroma.

TABLE 12–7 ■ NECK

Assessment	Pathology
Multiple skin folds in the lateral, posterior region of the neck (webbing)	Down syndrome Turner syndrome
Enlarged thyroid	Hyperthyroidism Hypothyroidism
Absence of head control	Prematurity Genetic disorder Asphyxia Neuromuscular disorder
Abnormal opening along the anterior surface of the sternocleidomastoid muscle leads to a blind pouch or communicates with deeper structures	Brachial sinus
Mass high in the neck at midline extending to the base of the tongue; often appears after an upper respiratory infection	Thyroglossal duct cyst
Palpable cystic mass may open onto the skin surface or drain into the pharynx	Brachial cleft cyst

The neck is palpated along the midline for the trachea and abnormal masses. The thyroid gland is difficult to palpate unless it is enlarged, an unusual finding during the newborn period. A potential for infection exists within all the cystic structures and abnormal sinuses arising around the newborn's neck. Table 12–7 identifies additional findings during the physical assessment of the neck that are abnormal and their related pathology.

CHEST AND LUNG ASSESSMENT

Auscultation and inspection are used to assess the newborn's chest and respiratory status. The newborn's chest is cylindrical. Measured at the nipple line, its circumference is approximately 33 cm or 2 to 3 cm less than the infant's head (see Fig. 12–1). The xiphoid process is sometimes seen as a small protuberant area at the end of the sternum. Respirations are shallow and irregular. Chest movement should be symmetric and not labored. An accurate respiratory rate is obtained by counting for 1 full minute, preferably when the newborn is quiet. Newborns are obligatory nose breathers and have an average respiratory rate of 30 to 60 breaths per minute. With each respiration, synchronous abdominal movement occurs. The color of the newborn's skin and mucous membranes is evaluated simultaneously. Presence of cyanosis may be a sign of respiratory distress.

Tachypnea (ie, respiratory rate >60) may be one of the first symptoms of morbidity in the newborn. If tachypnea is present, the respiratory rate may reach 120 breaths per minute. The primary healthcare provider should be notified when respiratory rates are increased, and oral feedings should be withheld because of the risk of aspiration.

Other signs of respiratory distress include retractions, nasal flaring, and grunting. Retractions are the drawing inward or shortening of small muscles in the chest wall. Retractions occur when more energy is needed to assist respiratory effort. Retractions are seen between the ribs (intercostal), below the rib cage (subcostal), above the sternum (tracheal tug), below the xiphoid process, and surrounding the clavicles. Flaring of the nares occurs with inspiration. It is a compensatory mechanism used by the newborn in respiratory distress. Flaring of the nares widens the upper airway, decreasing airway resistance and making breathing easier. Grunting is a sound produced on expiration when air passes through a partially closed glottis. The partially closed glottis is a compensatory mechanism that traps air in the alveoli, increasing the time that gas exchange can occur. Grunting may be audible or heard only with a stethoscope. The Silverman-Anderson Index is a tool used for systematically assessing and documenting newborn respiratory effort and the presence of physical symptoms of respiratory distress (Table 12–8). A score of zero indicates no respiratory distress.

Inspection of the newborn's chest includes placement, shape, and amount of palpable breast tissue. Hypertrophy of breast tissue, with or without secretion of milky fluid, may be present by the second or third day of life because of maternal hormones (Fig. 12–14). This condition lasts approximately 1 week. Supernumerary nipples (ie, accessory nipples) are considered a benign congenital anomaly. They are often seen below and medial to the normal nipples.

Auscultation of the anterior and posterior chest proceeds in an orderly fashion from top to bottom, comparing from side to side for equality of breath sounds and the presence of abnormal sounds such as grunting and rales. The term *crackles* may be used in

TABLE 12–8 ■ SILVERMAN-ANDERSON INDEX

Score	Upper Chest	Lower Chest	Xiphoid	Nares	Grunt
0	Chest and abdomen rise together	No intercostals retractions	No xiphoid retractions	No nasal flaring	No expiratory grunt
1	Lag or minimal sinking of upper chest as abdomen rises	Minimal intercostals retractions	Minimal xiphoid retractions	Minimal nasal flaring	Expiratory grunt heard with stethoscope
2	Upper chest and abdomen move as a "see-saw"	Marked intercostals retractions	Marked xiphoid retractions	Marked nasal flaring	Audible expiratory grunt

place of the traditional term *rales* for the fine cracking, bubbling, or fine rustling noises heard when air passes fluid. Rhonchi and wheezing are less common in the newborn period. These lower-pitched sounds result from obstruction or narrowing of larger airways.

Newborns have a periodic breathing pattern resulting from the immaturity of their respiratory and central nervous systems. It is common to observe brief pauses in respiratory effort. Pauses lasting 20 seconds or longer and associated with color change or bradycardia are considered apneic periods and should be reported to the primary healthcare provider.

Apnea (ie, pauses in respirations lasting 20 seconds or longer) or other signs of respiratory distress may occur in almost all illnesses in the newborn period. The list of differential diagnoses for respiratory distress and apnea in the newborn is extensive (Table 12–9). Table 12–10 identifies findings during the respiratory assessment that are abnormal and their related pathology.

TABLE 12–9 ■ DIFFERENTIAL DIAGNOSIS OF RESPIRATORY DISTRESS IN THE NEWBORN

Respiratory	Extrapulmonary
Respiratory distress syndrome	Congenital heart disease
Transient tachypnea	Patent ductus arteriosus
Meconium aspiration	Hypothermia
Primary pulmonary hypertension	Metabolic acidosis
Pneumonia	Hypoglycemia
Pulmonary hemorrhage	Septicemia
Pneumothorax	Ventricular hemorrhage
Airway obstruction	Edema
Diaphragmatic hernia	Drugs
Hypoplastic lung	Trauma
	Hypovolemia
	Twin-to-twin transfusion

Adapted from Askin, D. F. (1997). *Acute respiratory care of the newborn* (p. 32). Petaluma, CA: NICU INK.

TABLE 12–10 ■ RESPIRATORY SYSTEM

Assessment	Pathology
Cessation of breathing for more than 20 seconds (apnea)	Hypo-/hyperthermia Infection Prematurity Respiratory disorders Cardiovascular disorders Neurological disorders Maternal medications Metabolic disorders Gastroesophageal reflux Vigorous suctioning Passage of feeding tube Airway obstruction
Tachypnea	Retained lung fluid (transient tachypnea of the newborn) Meconium aspiration Respiratory distress syndrome Pneumonia Hyperthermia Pulmonary edema Sepsis Metabolic disorders
Decreased or absent breath sounds	Meconium aspiration Atelectasis Pneumothorax Diaphragmatic hernia Hypoplastic lungs Diaphragmatic hernia
Bowel sounds heard in place of breath sounds	Diaphragmatic hernia

CARDIOVASCULAR ASSESSMENT

The cardiovascular system is assessed using inspection, auscultation, and palpation. The examination begins with inspection of the newborn's color as one indication of oxygenation and perfusion. As the newborn transitions

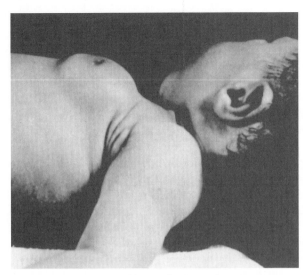

FIGURE 12–14. Neonatal breast hypertrophy.

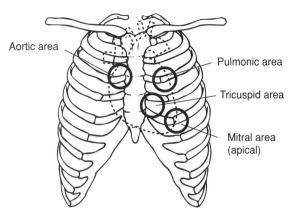

FIGURE 12–15. Ausculatory areas of the heart. (From Tappero, E. P., & Honeyfield, M. E. [Eds.]. [2003]. *Physical assessment of the newborn* [3rd ed., p. 87]. Petaluma, CA: NICU INK.

from intrauterine to extrauterine life, skin color changes occur. At birth, the infant may be pale or cyanotic, becoming pink as respirations are established, fetal circulation is reversed, and blood is oxygenated by the lungs and circulated by the strength of the heart muscle.

The precordium (ie, area on the anterior chest to the left of the sternum and above the heart) is inspected and palpated for movement. In a term newborn, very little movement should be observed in this area. The point of maximal impulse (PMI) is normally auscultated or palpated in the third to fourth intercostal space just lateral to the left midclavicular line. Displacement of the PMI can occur with cardiac enlargement, diaphragmatic hernia, dextrocardia, or pneumothorax. Increased activity, an active precordium, could indicate patent ductus arteriosus or congestive heart failure in a newborn or occur as a variation of normal in preterm or SGA newborns who are thin and have minimal subcutaneous tissue. Three additional sensations—heave, tap, and thrill—may be felt as the chest is palpated. A heave is a diffuse pulsation that can occur with ventricular volume overload. A tap is a pronounced localized pulsation of the PMI. A thrill is a palpated vibration that is associated with a murmur.

Heart rate and rhythm are best auscultated using the bell and diaphragm of a small neonatal stethoscope while the newborn remains quiet. The stethoscope should be warmed before placement so the newborn is not startled. The apical rate is counted for 1 full minute. The normal heart rate is 120 to 160 beats per minute. In deep sleep, the heart rate may be 80 to 110 beats per minute but should increase quickly if the newborn is disturbed. Auscultation begins at the mitral area (PMI) and proceeds systematically to the tricuspid, pulmonic, and aortic areas using the diaphragm of the stethoscope. The process is then repeated using the bell of the stethoscope (Fig. 12–15). Heart sounds are louder in infants because of the thin chest wall.

Heart sounds become clearer over the first few hours of life as fetal circulation is reversed. Rapid heart rates often make it difficult to auscultate specific heart sound. The first heart sound, S_1, is traditionally thought to be caused by the closure of the tricuspid and mitral valves as ventricular pressure rises during systole. It is heard best at the apex of the heart, in the fourth intercostal space. S_1 is usually loudest at birth, decreasing in intensity over 24 to 48 hours. The second heart sound, S_2, is thought to be caused by the closure of the pulmonic and aortic valves as the ventricular pressure falls during diastole. Splitting of S_2 with inspiration is common after the first few hours of life. Other forms of splitting may be considered pathologic and a sign of congenital heart disease.

Heart murmurs in newborns are common during the neonatal period. Murmurs are evaluated for loudness or intensity of sound (ie, grade), timing in the cardiac cycle (ie, systolic or diastolic), location of the murmur's maximum intensity, radiation, and pitch or quality of sound. Ninety percent of all murmurs are related to incomplete closure of the ductus arteriosus or foramen ovale and are transient in nature. These murmurs are usually grade 1 or 2 (Display 12–1). Murmurs are best

DISPLAY 12-1

Grading of Murmurs

Grade 1: Soft; requires extended listening

Grade 2: Soft; heard immediately

Grade 3: Moderate intensity; no thrill

Grade 4: Loud; often with a thrill or palpable vibration at the murmur site

Grade 5: Loud; thrill present; audible with the stethoscope partially off the chest

Grade 6: Loud; audible with the stethoscope off the chest

auscultated at the left lower sternal border in the third or fourth interspace. The diaphragm of the stethoscope can detect high-pitched murmurs, whereas the bell is better for detecting low-pitched murmurs.

Peripheral pulses (ie, brachial, radial, femoral, popliteal, and dorsalis pedis) are evaluated for presence, equality, and strength. Femoral pulses may be difficult to palpate but should be present in all infants.

Routine blood pressure screening is not recommended for all newborns (AAP & ACOG, 2002). Evaluating the blood pressure is usually reserved for newborns with signs of distress, persistent murmurs, or abnormal pulses. Blood pressure is measured in all four extremities. Blood pressure varies depending on birth weight, gestational age, cuff size, and state of alertness. Blood pressures should be taken when the infant is quiet and reserved for the end of the assessment since the pressure of the cuff inflating may cause the newborn to cry. An appropriate size of blood pressure cuff is necessary to ensure an accurate measurement. Both length and width should be considered when determining the appropriate size cuff. The width of the cuff should cover no more than 50% to 70% of the length of the extremity being tested such as 50% to 70% of the length from knee to hip, elbow to shoulder, or ankle to knee (Barryman & Glass, 2005). If cuff size is based only on the length of the extremity it does not take into account the large-for-gestational age infant with increased amount of subcutaneous fat. In these newborns, the cuff is apt to be tight and produce an abnormally low blood pressure reading. In addition to considering the length of the extremity, the width of the cuff used should be no more than 40% to 50% of the circumference of the extremity (Parks, 2002). At term, the normal blood pressure range is 65 to 95 mm Hg systolic and 30 to 60 mm Hg diastolic. Blood pressure in the lower extremities is usually higher than that in the upper extremities. Table 12–11 identifies findings during the cardiovascular assessment that are abnormal and their related pathology.

ABDOMINAL ASSESSMENT

The abdomen is assessed using inspection, auscultation, and palpation. The abdomen is inspected for size and symmetry and is normally rounded, symmetric, protuberant, and soft because of weak abdominal musculature with a slightly greater diameter above the umbilicus than below. The subcutaneous blood vessels in the abdomen may appear distended and blue (Hernandez & Glass, 2005). Abdominal movements correspond to respirations, because newborns use the muscle of the diaphragm, rather than intercostal muscles, to assist with breathing. Movement of the diaphragm causes the

abdomen to move. If abdominal distention is suspected, the circumference of the abdomen is periodically measured at the level of the umbilicus (see Fig. 12–1). The umbilical cord is examined for number of vessels, color, and condition. The cord should be opaque to white-blue and contain two arteries and one vein. Variations include a thin, dry cord associated with intrauterine growth restriction or a thick cord seen in LGA newborns. A greenish-yellow discoloration of the cord sometimes occurs with relaxation of the anal sphincter and subsequent passage of meconium. The area surrounding the umbilical cord is observed for masses or the herniation of abdominal contents (Fig. 12–16). Umbilical hernias occur when the intestinal muscle does not close completely around the umbilicus during embryologic development. They are more common in low-birth-weight, African-American, and male newborns. Some hernias are observable only when the newborn is crying. Separation of the abdominorectus muscle (ie, diastasis recti) 0.5 to 2 inches wide may occur along the midline from the xiphoid to umbilicus, occasionally extending to the symphysis pubis. Separation of this muscle is not uncommon and is the result of the newborn's weak abdominal muscles.

The perianal region is inspected for the presence of a patent anus. Most newborns pass meconium within the first 24 hours of life. Failure to pass meconium may indicate a gastrointestinal obstruction and necessitates further evaluation.

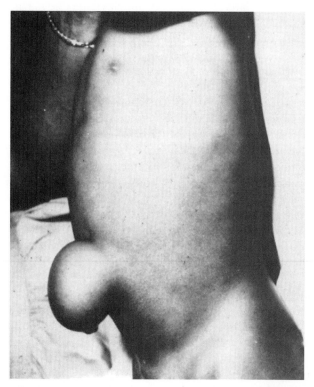

FIGURE 12–16. Umbilical hernia. (Courtesy of Dr. Mark Ravitch.)

TABLE 12–11 ■ CARDIOVASCULAR SYSTEM

Assessment	Pathology
Tachycardia >160 beats/min	Anemia Congestive heart failure Shock or hypovolemia Respiratory distress Supraventricular tachycardia Sepsis Congenital heart anomalies Hyperthermia
Persistent bradycardia <100 beats/min	Congenital heart block Sepsis Asphyxia Hypoxemia Increased intracranial pressure
Persistent murmurs	Persistent fetal circulation Congenital heart defects Peripheral pulmonic stenosis
Muffled heart sounds	Pneumothorax Pneumopericardium Diaphragmatic hernia Pneumomediastinum
Heart sound muffled on left side, loud on right side	Dextrocardia Pneumothorax with mediastinal shift
Decrease in intensity or absence of femoral pulses	Hip dysplasia Coarctation of the aorta
Bounding peripheral pulses; active precordium	Patent ductus arteriosus Fluid overload Congestive heart failure Ventricular septal defect
Difference of blood pressure >20 mm Hg between upper and lower extremities	Coarctation of aorta
Central cyanosis	Congenital heart disease Hypertension Lung disease Sepsis Persistent pulmonary hypertension
Cyanosis that does not improve with 100% oxygen	Congenital heart disease
Cyanosis that worsens with crying	Congenital heart disease

Bowel sounds are normally present within the first hour of life as the newborn swallows air with crying and the sympathetic nervous system stimulates peristalsis. Bowel sounds are auscultated in all four quadrants.

Most perinatal nurses conduct a limited assessment of the abdomen using light palpation for consistency and the presence of masses. A more detailed examination is conducted by the primary healthcare provider. The lower border of the liver is sharp, soft, and palpated in the right upper quadrant 1 to 2 cm below the costal margin. The spleen, located in the left upper quadrant, may be palpable in preterm newborns but rarely in term newborns. The spleen should not be palpated more than 1 cm below the left costal margin (Hernandez & Glass, 2005). Kidneys are 4 to 5 cm long and are usually only palpable during the first 1 to 2 days of life (Hernandez & Glass, 2005). After this time, the bowel and stomach become distended with fluid and air, making this assessment difficult. With the newborn's legs flexed against the abdomen, kidneys

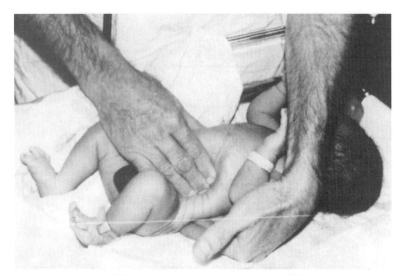

FIGURE 12–17. Examiner demonstrating technique for palpation of the left kidney.

are located using deep palpations at the level of the umbilicus, lateral to the midclavicular line. The right kidney may be lower than the left (Fig. 12–17).

Inspection and palpation of the femoral region is conducted during this portion of the examination or as part of the cardiovascular assessment. A soft, compressible swelling in the groin may indicate an inguinal hernia or undescended testes (Fig. 12–18). Bowel sounds can be auscultated in the testis if swelling is caused by herniation of the bowel. Table 12–12 identifies findings during the physical assessment of the abdomen that are abnormal and their related pathology.

GENITOURINARY SYSTEM

Assessment

The genitourinary system is assessed using inspection and palpation. External genitalia are evaluated as part of the physical examination and gestational age assess-

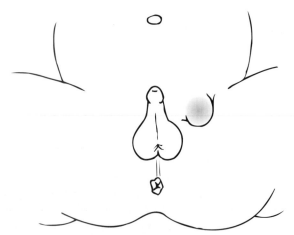

FIGURE 12–18. Left inguinal hernia producing a bulge in the groin of the affected side.

ment. Newborns should void within 24 hours of birth. A rust-colored stain on the diaper, which in some instances can be flaked off, is a normal variation caused by uric acid crystals in the urine. Bruising and edema of the genitalia and buttocks can occur in newborns that had a breech presentation.

Female Newborns

In term newborns, the clitoris and labia minora are covered by the labia majora. The urinary meatus is located beneath the clitoris. The labia majora and clitoris are enlarged because of maternal hormones circulated to the newborn in utero. In preterm newborns, the labia majora does not cover the labia minora and clitoris. Bruising and swelling of the external genitalia may be present after a vaginal birth.

In some newborns, when the introitus is gently separated, a hymenal tag is seen in the vagina. This tissue, which developed from the hymen and labia minora, disappears within a few weeks (Cavaliere, 2003). A white mucous discharge from the vagina is not uncommon during the first week of life. Pseudomenstruation, caused by withdrawal of maternal hormones, is a pink-tinged mucous discharge lasting 2 to 4 weeks.

The labia majora are palpated for masses that could indicate a hernia or ectopic glands. Palpating a suprapubic mass or mass between the labia majora suggests an imperforate hymen. An imperforate hymen causes secretions to pool within the vagina (Fig. 12–19).

Male Newborns

In term male newborns, the external genitalia are observed for a penis, with a mean length of 3.5 cm (Elder, 2000), the urethral opening located on the tip of the glans, and the glans covered by the prepuce or

TABLE 12–12 ■ ABDOMEN

Assessment	Pathology
Scaphoid	Diaphragmatic hernia Malnutrition
"Prune belly" flabby, wrinkled abdominal wall (see Fig. 12–20)	Congenital absence of abdominal musculature; associated with other gastrointestinal (GI) or genitourinary (GU) anomalies
Asymmetric abdomen	Abdominal mass GI/GU anomalies
Abdominal distention	Obstruction Masses Enlargement of abdominal organs Infection (Hernandez & Glass, 2005)
Distention in left upper quadrant	Pyloric stenosis Duodenal or jejunal obstruction
Ascites	Hydrops fetalis Viral infections (congenital)
Umbilical cord with one artery and one vein	Associated with GI/GU anomalies
Thin membrane covering herniation of abdominal contents through a defect in the umbilical ring	Omphalocele
Uncovered protrusion of abdominal contents, usually to the right of the umbilicus	Gastroschisis
Red, oozing, or foul-smelling cord	Infection (omphalitis)
Persistently moist umbilicus; clear discharge from umbilical cord stump	Granuloma of the umbilical cord (Hernandez & Glass, 2005) Umbilical urinary fistula—urachus, embryologic connection between the bladder and umbilicus remains patent Urachus cyst Omphalomesenteric duct–connection between the umbilicus and ileum (Goodwin, 2003)
Failure to pass meconium stool	Imperforate anus Meconium ileus Hirschsprung disease Meconium plug syndrome
Passage of sticky, thick, small plugs of meconium	Meconium ileus Cystic fibrosis
Bruit	Arteriovenous malformation (liver) Renal artery stenosis
Partial or complete herniation of the bladder through the abdominal wall	Bladder exstrophy—absence of muscle and connective tissue in the abdominal wall occurring during embryologic development
Hepatomegaly	Congenital heart disease Infection Hemolytic disease (Hernandez & Glass, 2005)

foreskin. The foreskin may need to be retracted slightly to accurately determine the location of the meatus. A physiologic phimosis (ie, inability to retract the prepuce or foreskin) is present at birth. By 3 years of age, the foreskin usually is able to be retracted in 90% of uncircumcised males because adhesions between the prepuce and glans lyse and the distal phimotic ring loosens (Elder, 2000). Small, white cysts filled with epithelial cells may be transiently present on the distal portion of the prepuce. Smegma, a whitish-yellow, cheesy substance from sebaceous glands, collects between the glans and the prepuce.

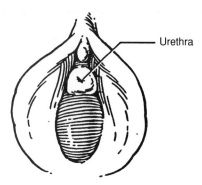

FIGURE 12–19. Imperforate hymen.

The most common genitourinary abnormality in male newborns is hypospadias, the placement of the urinary meatus on the ventral surface of the penis anywhere along a line extending from the tip of the penis, penile shaft, scrotum, or perineum. The location of the meatus along the ventral surface of the penis is used to classify the hypospadias into subgroups (Stokowski, 2004). This abnormality may be seen as frequently as 1:125 births (Elder, 2000). Because of the point in embryologic development that the defect occurs, it is usually associated with some degree of failure of the foreskin to develop completely or excessive foreskin on the dorsal surface and absent foreskin on the ventral surface, and chordee, a downward curvature of the tip of the penis. The etiology of hypospadias is thought to be multifactorial including endocrine, genetic, and environmental factors (Mason & Carr, 2003; Silver, 2004). Circumcision is delayed when an abnormally located urinary meatus is observed because if a surgery is necessary, the foreskin may be used for urethroplasty or penile shaft skin coverage. Surgical repair is an outpatient procedure that is usually performed between 4 and 8 months of age (Stokowski, 2004).

The scrotum is more darkly pigmented than the skin surrounding it. This color variation is especially prominent in African-American, Indian, and Hispanic newborns. The scrotum is palpated with the thumb and forefinger for the presence of the testes. Rugae (ie, ridges or creases) begin to appear on the surface of the scrotum around 36 weeks' gestation, and by term, the entire surface of the scrotum is covered. The scrotum may be enlarged because of the effects of maternal hormones. Rugae and a pendulous scrotum usually indicate descent of the testes. Before 28 weeks' gestation, the testes lie within the abdomen. Migration through the inguinal canal to the scrotum occurs as a result of the effect of androgen on the genitofemoral nerves. Stimulation of these nerves causes the gubernaculum testis, a fetal ligament connecting the testes to the scrotum, to move the testes into the scrotum (Ferrer & McKenna, 2000). Undescended testes (ie, cryptorchidism) may be unilateral or bilateral and occurs in about 3% of term newborns and up to 30% of preterm newborns, depending on gestational age (Elder, 2000). Undescended testes are found along the normal path of descent between the abdomen and scrotum, most often below the external inguinal ring but not in the scrotum. They can also be within the inguinal canal or still in the abdomen. If undescended at birth, the testes usually descend by 3 months of age because of the influence of rising androgen levels during infancy. It is possible for one testis or both testes to migrate to an ectopic location, away from the normal path to the scrotum, if the gubernaculum ligament is in an abnormal location. Either or both of the testes can be classified as retractile. A testis is referred to as retractile if, when stimulated by palpation or cold, the cremastic reflex causes it to move to the upper scrotum or as far as the external inguinal ring. This condition differs from the classification of undescended because gentle pressure can bring the testis completely down into the scrotum. To prevent stimulation of the cremastic reflex during examination, the index finger of the examiner's nondominant hand can be used to apply pressure to the inguinal canal to prevent the testis from slipping out of the scrotum. Surgical intervention for undescended or ectopic testes occurs when the child is 6 months to 1 year old.

An enlarged scrotum is evaluated for the presence of a hydrocele, which is an accumulation of fluid. Fluid accumulates during fetal development when sexual differentiation occurs. This fluid is usually reabsorbed in utero. If a hydrocele is present at birth, it should disappear within 3 months. The ability to transilluminate a hydrocele differentiates it from a solid or blood-filled mass. Table 12–13 identifies the findings of the physical assessment of male and female newborns that are abnormal and their related pathology.

MUSCULOSKELETAL ASSESSMENT

Inspection and palpation are used to assess the musculoskeletal system. Examination begins by observing the newborn at rest, noting position, symmetry, and presence of abnormal movements. The hands and feet are inspected for the number of digits. Nails are soft and cover the entire nail bed. In a postmature newborn, the nail may extend beyond the fingertips. Newborns exposed to meconium in utero have yellow discoloration of their nails.

Arms and legs are inspected for flexion and symmetry. Extremities should be flexed and move symmetrically through a full range of motion. Clavicles are assessed for fractures that may have occurred during the birth process. This assessment is performed by palpating along the entire length of the clavicle, feeling for a mass. The newborn's arm is moved through passive range of motion while the examiner uses her other hand

TABLE 12-13 ■ GENITOURINARY SYSTEM

Assessment	Pathology
Ambiguous genitalia	Genetic disorder
Decreased or no urination within 24 hours of birth	Urinary tract obstruction Potter syndrome Polycystic kidney Hydronephrosis Renal failure
Female	
Urinary meatus near or just inside vagina (hypospadias)	Genitourinary anomaly
Fecal discharge from vagina	Fistula between rectum and vagina
Male	
Epispadias—meatus on dorsal surface of glans	Genitourinary anomaly
Hypospadias—meatus on ventral surface of glans	Genitourinary anomaly Congenital syndromes
Scrotal mass which does not transilluminate	Inguinal hernia (Fig. 12–19)
Red to bluish-red scrotal sac; swelling or small mass palpable (Cavalieri, 2003)	Twisting of the testes and spermatic cord (testicular torsion)
Urinary stream not straight; weak urinary stream	Stenosis of the urethral meatus Urinary malformation

to palpate the newborn's clavicle on that same side. Crepitus, produced when the bone slides against itself, is felt over the clavicle if a fracture exists.

Legs appear slightly bowed with everted feet. A persistent breech presentation in utero may result in abducted hips and extended knees (Fig. 12–20). Positional deformities in the newborn period are often caused by intrauterine positioning and may continue to be present for a few days or weeks. Passive range of motion should correct positional deformities.

Hips

The newborn's hips are evaluated for developmental dysplasia. Developmental dysplasia of the hip (DDH) describes the continuum of pathologic hip disorders in the newborn traditionally referred to as congenital dislocation of the hip. This terminology has been adapted by the AAP, American Academy of Orthopaedic Surgeons, and Pediatric Orthopaedic Society of North America (French & Dietz, 1999). When 18,060 newborns were evaluated using physical assessment and ultrasonography at several points during the first 6 weeks of life, the incidence of DDH was 5 cases per 1,000 newborns (Bialik et al., 1999). The exact cause of DDH is unknown. It is probably related to a variety of factors or situations interfering with the normal development of the acetabulum. Failure of the acetabulum to develop eventually

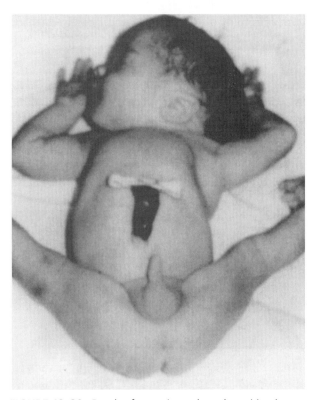

FIGURE 12–20. Result of a persistent breech position in utero. (Courtesy of Dr. David A. Clark, Louisiana State University Medical Center and Wyeth-Ayerst Laboratories, Philadelphia, PA.)

DISPLAY 12-2

Factors Associated with Developmental Dysplasia of the Hip

- Family history of developmental dysplasia of the hip
- Oligohydramnios
- Breech presentation
- Foot deformities
- Primiparity
- Female sex
- Multiple pregnancy

Barlow maneuvers. To perform the Ortolani maneuver, the examiner stabilizes one hip while the thigh of the hip being tested is abducted and gently pulled anteriorly. If the hip is dislocated, a palpable and sometimes audible "clunk" will be detected as the femoral head moves over the posterior rim of the acetabulum and back into position (Fig. 12–22). The Barlow maneuver is performed by adducting the hip while pushing the thigh posteriorly to determine whether the hip can be dislocated (Fig. 12–23). If the hip is dislocated by this maneuver, it is relocated by performing the Ortolani maneuver. An algorithm for the evaluation of a newborn hip is presented in Figure 12–24.

allows the bell-shaped femoral head to migrate completely or partially out of normal position. Because of intrauterine position, DDH is more common in the left hip (Tachdjian, 1997). Factors that put newborns at risk for DDH are listed in Display 12–2.

Evaluating the newborn's hips requires the child to be in a quiet state. Crying causes increased muscle tone that could prevent the examiner from identifying an unstable hip. Assessing the newborn for DDH begins with inspection. Position the newborn on his back, with diaper off, hips and knees flexed at 90-degree angles, and feet level (Fig. 12–21). The presence of more skin folds on the medial aspect of the thigh or one knee noticeably lower than the other knee (Galeazzi sign) may indicate the femoral head is dislocated or no longer positioned within the acetabulum.

To further determine the presence of an unstable or dislocated hip, the newborn's hips are put through three maneuvers. With the newborn's hips and knees still flexed at 90-degree angles, the hips are simultaneously abducted gently toward the examination table. Normal hips should abduct almost 90 degrees (ie, thighs resting on the table). This is followed by the Ortolani and

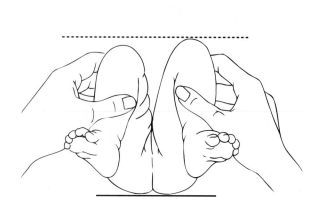

FIGURE 12–21. Asymmetry in number of thigh skin folds and uneven knee level. (Adapted from Ballock, R. T., & Richards, B. S. [1997]. Hip dysplasia: Early diagnosis makes a difference. *Contemporary Pediatrics, 14*[4], 110.)

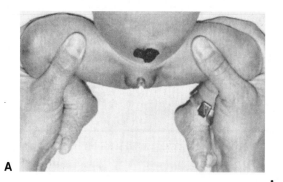

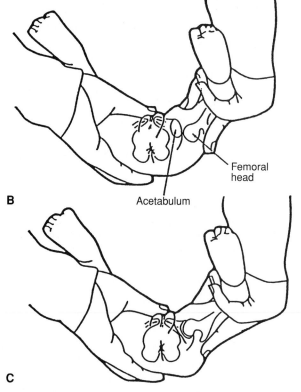

Femoral head

Acetabulum

FIGURE 12–22. Ortolani's Maneuver. **A & B,** With the newborn's legs flexed, the thumb is over the femur and the fingers are on the trocanter. The femur is lifted forward as the thighs are abducted toward the bed. **C,** A "click" is heard or felt as the head of the femur moves into the acetabulum.

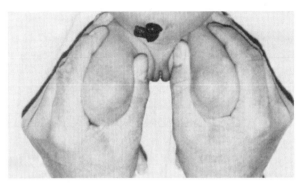

FIGURE 12–23. Barlow maneuver performed by adducting the thighs. If the head of the femur dislocates, it is felt and seen as it suddenly jerks over the acetabulum.

The continuum of DDH from dysplasia to dislocation is depicted in Figure 12–25. Only about 60% of DDH is identified clinically with initial newborn assessment (Rosenberg, Bialik, Norman, & Blazer, 1998). In combination with ultrasound evaluation when DDH is suspected, identification increases to 90% (Donaldson & Feinstein, 1997; Rosenberg, Bialik, Norman, & Blazer, 1998). Because clinical screening techniques cannot identify all newborns and because many investigators believe that undetected abnormal hips may eventually progress to dislocation, this assessment is repeated into infancy (French & Dietz, 1999). Early identification of DDH increases the possibility that conservative treatment can be initiated and surgery avoided (Ballock & Richards, 1997).

Feet

The presence of adequate amount of amniotic fluid in the second trimester of pregnancy is necessary to assure development and normal shape of the feet (Tredwell, Wilson, & Wilmink, 2001). Feet are examined to determine whether deformities are positional abnormalities versus structural malformations. Positional abnormalities are temporary, do not involve bone, and refer to alterations in shape and contour of a normally formed foot. Structural malformations are seen in about 3% of births and occur during embryologic development (Moore, Persaud, & Shiota, 2000). Feet are inspected for 10 digits.

Metatarsus adductus (ie, inward turning of the front one-third of the foot with a widening of the space between the first and second toe) is a positional abnormality occurring in utero (Fig. 12–26). Treatment depends on the severity of the abnormality, which progresses along a continuum. The least severe is a foot that returns to the midline spontaneously by stroking the lateral side and usually requires no intervention. Moderately severe is where the examiner is able to easily manipulate the foot into correct position. Exercises performed by parents will usually correct this abnormality. The most severe is the foot that resists correction by the examiner and requires serial casting during infancy.

Talipes calcaneovalgus is a positional deformity caused by the sole of the foot being positioned against the uterine wall. Dorsiflexion of the ankle causes contact between the dorsal surface of the foot and the anterior aspect of the leg (tibia). The leg and foot form the shape of a check mark (✓) rather than the shape of an "L" (Fig. 12–27).

Back

In a prone position, the newborn's back is examined for asymmetric gluteal folds, indicating the presence of

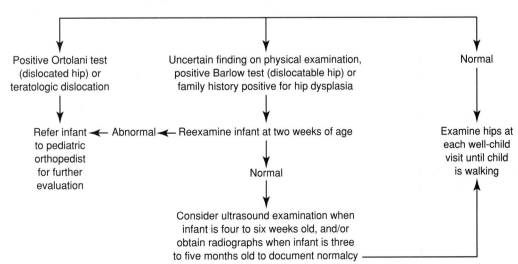

FIGURE 12–24. Algorithm for the evaluation of infants' hips. (From French, L. M. & Dietz, F. R. [1999]. Screening for developmental dysplasia of the hips. *American Family Physician, 60*[1], p. 182.)

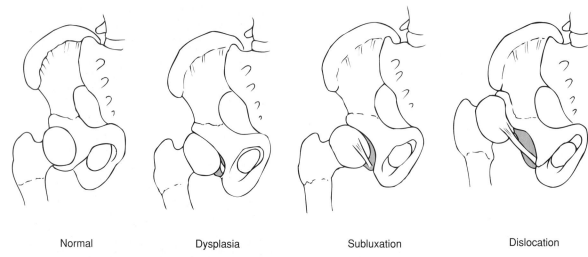

Normal   Dysplasia   Subluxation   Dislocation

FIGURE 12–25. Relationship of structures in developmental dysplasia of the hip. (Modified from Wong, D. L. [Ed.]. [1997]. *Whaley & Wong's essentials of pediatric nursing* [5th ed., p. 1137]. St. Louis: Mosby.)

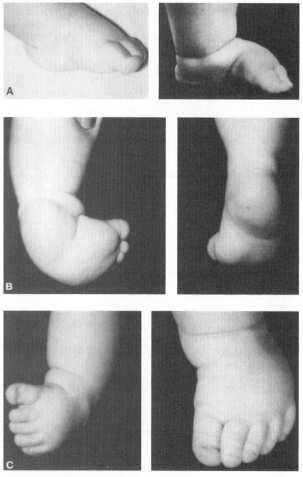

FIGURE 12–26. Comparison of clubfoot (*left*) and metatarsus adductus (*right*). **A,** Lateral view, showing the equinus (entire heel does not touch the flat surface) present only in clubfoot. **B,** Posterior view, showing the hindfoot varus in clubfoot but not in metatarsus adductus. **C,** Anterior view, showing adduction in both feet, with the varus also present in clubfoot.

a congenital hip dislocation (Fig. 12–28). During this portion of the examination, the length of the spinal column is palpated for masses and abnormal curvatures. The sacral area is inspected for the presence of a pilonidal dimple (Fig. 12–29), tuft of hair, skin lesion, or increased pigmentation that could indicate pathology. Table 12–14 identifies findings of the musculoskeletal assessment that are abnormal and their related pathology.

NEUROLOGICAL ASSESSMENT

Assessment of the central nervous system is integrated throughout the physical examination and includes evaluation of posture, cry, muscle tone, and movement; evaluation of most cranial nerves; and evaluation of all

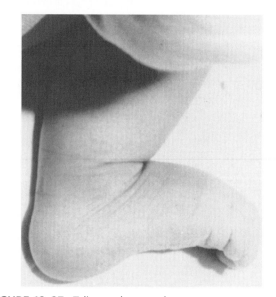

FIGURE 12–27. Talipes calcaneovalgus.

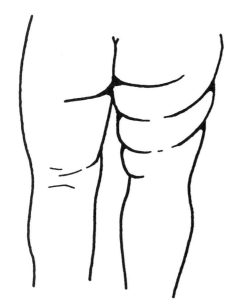

FIGURE 12–28. Asymmetric gluteal folds.

developmental reflexes. Findings during the neurological assessment are influenced by the gestational age and physical health of the newborn.

At rest, a newborn's posture is flexed, with extremities tight against the trunk. The neuromuscular portion of the gestational age assessment demonstrates the increasing muscle tone that the newborn develops as gestational age progresses. Scarf sign, popliteal

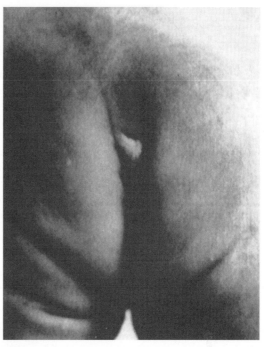

FIGURE 12–29. Pilonidal dimple. (Courtesy of Dr. David A. Clark, Louisiana State University Medical Center and Wyeth-Ayerst Laboratories, Philadelphia, PA.)

angle, and heel-to-ear movements have less range of motion as gestational age increases. Leg and arm recoil also demonstrates how muscle tone normally becomes stronger as gestational age advances.

TABLE 12–14 ■ MUSCULOSKELETAL SYSTEM

Assessment	Pathology
Weak or absent muscle tone	Neurological disorder Prematurity Genetic disorder
Extra digit (polydactyly)	Inherited as dominant trait
Partial or complete fusion of digits, more often in feet than hands (syndactyly)	Inherited as dominant trait
Short fingers, incurving of fifth finger, fusion or palmar creases (simian crease), wide space between big toe and second toe	Down syndrome
Jitteriness	Hypoglycemia Hypocalcemia
Arm extended and limp, hand rotated inward, absence of normal movement, absent Moro reflex on affected side	Brachial plexus palsy
Club foot—sole of the foot pointed medially, toes pointed downward and heel pointing upward, upper third of the foot curved downward	Environmental factors in utero which decrease the ability of the fetus to move and/or increase the size of the fetus, ie, oligohydramnios, maternal diabetes, maternal obesity, early amniocentesis Exposure to teratogens, maternal smoking Genetic (Furdon & Donlon, 2002)

TABLE 12–15 ■ ASSESSING THE INTEGRITY OF CRANIAL NERVES

Cranial Nerve	Method of Assessment
CN I, olfactory	Not assessed in the neonate
CN II, optic	Newborn follows brightly colored object or face; blinks in response to light
CN III, oculomotor CN IV, trochlear CN VI, abducens	Pupils constrict equally in response to light; as newborn's head is moved to face one side or the other, eyes move in the opposite direction (dolls' eyes maneuver)
CN V, trigeminal	Presence of rooting and sucking reflexes; biting
CN VII, facial	Symmetry of facial movement while crying or smiling
CN VIII, acoustic	Positive Moro reflex or movement in the direction of sound; quiets to voice; hearing screening using brainstem auditory evoked response (BAER)
CN IX, glossopharyngeal CN X, vagus CN XII, hypoglossal	Coordination of suck and swallow; presence of gag reflex; tongue remains midline when mouth is open
CN XI, accessory	Head turns easily to either side; newborn attempts to move head back from side to midline; height of shoulders equal

A healthy newborn's cry is strong and loud. Newborns cry for a variety of reasons. They cry in response to unpleasant environmental stimuli such as fatigue, hunger, cold, or discomfort or because they want the attention of another person. Crying helps the parents develop parenting skills as they become more alert to interpreting their newborn's needs. Responding to a newborn cry helps facilitate attachment between parent and child and increases the newborn's feeling of security. A weak cry is associated with prematurity or illness; a high-pitched cry occurs with drug withdrawal, neurological abnormalities, metabolic abnormalities, or meningitis.

All of the cranial nerves, with the exception of the olfactory nerve (CN I), should be routinely assessed in the newborn. The advent of UNHS programs has increased the sensitivity of evaluations of the acoustic nerve (CN VIII). Table 12–15 describes how to illicit a response to determine the integrity of each cranial nerve.

Reflexes are involuntary neuromuscular responses that provide protection from harm. Whether a specific reflex is present depends on the gestational age of the newborn. Newborns demonstrate two types of reflexes. The first type is protective in nature (ie, blink, cough, sneeze, and gag). The second type, which disappears during the first year of life, is a result of the neurological immaturity of newborns. These reflexes are sometimes referred to as developmental or primitive reflexes. Developmental reflexes are all present at birth in the healthy term newborn. Appendix 12C describes how to elicit these reflexes, defines normal and abnormal responses, and explains at what age they disappear. Table 12–16 identifies findings during the neurological assessment that are abnormal and their related pathology.

SUMMARY

A formal assessment of all body systems is completed by the perinatal nurse soon after birth and repeated at intervals established by institutional protocol throughout the newborn's hospitalization. Informal assessments are ongoing and occur during care-giving activities. Performing the physical assessment provides a picture of how the newborn is adapting to extrauterine life. The development of keen physical assessment skills allows the perinatal nurse to detect subtle changes in the newborn's condition, identify or anticipate the development of problems, and intervene immediately to prevent or minimize these problems.

TABLE 12–16 ■ NEUROLOGICAL SYSTEM

Assessment	Pathology
Fisting Abnormal position of hands or feet Tremors Clonus Abnormal eye movements	Brain lesions
Poor suck	Neuromuscular disorders Basal ganglia or brainstem abnormalities
Altered state of consciousness and seizures	Asphyxia Perinatal infections Inborn error of metabolism

REFERENCES

American Academy of Pediatrics. (2003a). Prevention and management of positional skull deformities in infants. *Pediatrics, 112*(1), 199–202.

American Academy of Pediatrics. (2003b). Red reflex examination in infants. *Pediatrics, 109*(5), 980–981.

American Academy of Pediatrics. (1995). Joint committee on infant hearing: 1994 position statement. *Pediatrics, 95*(1), 152–156.

American Academy of Pediatrics. (2000). Year 2000 position statement: Principles and guidelines for early hearing detection and intervention programs. *Pediatrics, 106*(4), 798–817.

American Academy of Pediatrics & American College of Obstetricians and Gynecologists (AAP & ACOG). (2002). *Guidelines for perinatal care* (5th ed.). Washington, DC: Author.

Askin, D. F. (1997). *Acute respiratory care of the newborn.* Petaluma, CA: NICU INK.

Ballard, J. L., Khoury, J. C., Wedig, K., Wang, L., Ellers-Walsman, B. L., & Lipp, R. (1991). New Ballard Score, expanded to include extremely premature infants. *Journal of Pediatrics, 119*(3), 417–423.

Ballard, J. L., Novak, K. K., & Driver, M. (1979). A simplified score for assessment of fetal maturation of newly born infants. *Journal of Pediatrics, 95*(5, Pt. 1), 769–774.

Ballock, R. T., & Richards, B. S. (1997). Hip dysplasia: Early diagnosis makes a difference. *Contemporary Pediatrics, 14*(4), 108–117.

Berryman, R. E., & Glass, S. M. (2005), Routine care. In P. J. Thureen, J. Deacon, J. Hernandez, & D. M. Hall. (Eds.), *Assessment and care of the well newborn* (pp. 198–205). Philadelphia: Saunders.

Bialik, V., Bialik, G. M., Blazer, S., Sujov, P., Wiener, F., & Berant, M. (1999). Developmental dysplasia of the hip: A new approach to incidence. *Pediatrics, 103*(1), 93–99.

Brown, T. J., Friedman, J., & Levy, M. L. (1998). The diagnosis and treatment of common birthmarks. *Clinics in Plastic Surgery, 25*(4), 509–525.

Cavaliere, T. A. (2003). Genitourinary assessment. In E. P. Tappero & M. E. Honeyfield (Eds.), *Physical assessment of the newborn: A comprehensive approach to the art of physical examination* (pp. 107–123). Petaluma, CA: NICU INK.

Darmstadt, G. L., & Sidbury, R. (2004). The skin. In R. E. Behrman, R. M. Kliegman, & H. B. Jenson (Eds.), *Nelson's textbook of pediatrics* (17th ed., pp. 2153–2250). Philadelphia: Saunders.

Dubowitz, L. M. S., Dubowitz, V., & Goldberg, C. (1970). Clinical assessment of gestational age in the newborn infant. *Journal of Pediatrics, 77*(1), 1–10.

Dubowitz, L., Ricci, D., & Mercuri, E. (2005). The Dubowitz neurological examination of the full-term newborn. *Mental Retardation and Developmental Disabilities Research Reviews, 11*, 52–60.

Donaldson, J. S., & Feinstein, K. A. (1997). Imaging of developmental dysplasia of the hip. *Pediatric Clinics of North America, 44*(3), 591–614.

Dodd, V. (1996). Gestational age assessment. *Neonatal Network, 15*(1), 27–36.

Elder, J. S. (2000). Urologic disorders in infants and children. In R. E. Behrman, R. M. Kliegman, & H. B. Jenson (Eds.), *Nelson's textbook of pediatrics* (17th ed., pp. 1783–1826). Philadelphia: Saunders.

Esterly, N. B. (1996). Cutaneous hemangiomas, vascular stains and malformations, and associated syndromes. *Current Problems in Pediatrics, 26*(1), 3–39.

Ewart-Toland, A., Yankowitz, J., Winder, A., Imagire, R., Cox, V. A., Aylsworth, A. S., et al. (2000). Oculoauriculovertebral abnormalities in children of diabetic mothers. *American Journal of Medical Genetics, 90*(4), 303–309.

Fernbach, S. A. (1998). Common orthopedic problems of the newborn. *Nursing Clinics of North America, 33*(4), 583–593.

Ferrer, F. A., & McKenna, P. H. (2000). Current approaches to the undescended testes. *Contemporary Pediatrics, 17*(1), 106–111.

French, L. M., & Dietz, F. R. (1999). Screening for developmental dysplasia of the hip. *American Family Physician, 60*(1), 177–184.

Furdon, S. A., & Donlon, C. R. (2002). Examination of the newborn foot: Positional and structural abnormalities. *Advances in Neonatal Care, 2*(5), 248–258.

Gagliardi, L., Brambilla, C., Bruno, R., Martinelli, S., & Console, V. (1993). Biased assessment of gestational age at birth when obstetric gestation is known. *Archives of Disease in Childhood, 68*(1), 32–34.

Gallagher, P. G., Mahoney, M. J., & Gosche, J. R. (1999). Cystic hygroma in the fetus and newborn. *Seminars Perinatology, 23*(4), 341–356.

Green, M. (1998). *Pediatric diagnosis: Interpretation of symptoms and signs in infants, children and adolescents* (6th ed.). Philadelphia: Saunders.

Goodwin, M. (2003). Abdomen assessment. In E. P. Tappero & M. E. Honeyfield (Eds.), *Physical assessment of the newborn: A comprehensive approach to the art of physical examination* (pp. 97–105). Petaluma, CA: NICU INK.

Hartley, A. H., & Rasmussen, J. E. (1990). Hemangiomas and spitz nevi. *Pediatric Review, 11*(9), 262–267.

Hernandez, P. W., & Glass, S. M. (2005). Physical assessment of the newborn. In P. J. Thureen, J. Deacon, P. J. Hernandez, & D. M. Hall. (Eds.), *Assessment and care of the well newborn* (pp. 119–172). Philadelphia: Saunders.

Hernandez, J. A., Zabloudil, C., & Hernandez, P. W. (1999). Adaptation to extrauterine life and management during transition. In P. J. Thureen, J. Deacon, P. O'Neill, & J. Hernandez (Eds.), *Assessment and care of the well newborn* (pp. 83–100). Philadelphia: Saunders.

Jackson, D., & Saunders, R. (1993). *Child health nursing.* Philadelphia: Lippincott.

Mason, J. A., & Herrmann, K. R. (1998). Universal infant hearing screening by automated auditory brainstem response measurement. *Pediatrics, 101*(2), 221–228.

McCarthy, P. L. (2004). The acutely ill child. In R. E. Behrman, R. M. Kliegman, & H. B. Jenson (Eds.), *Nelson's textbook of pediatrics* (17th ed., pp. 253–366). Philadelphia: Saunders.

Mehl, A. L., & Thomson, V. (1998). Newborn hearing screening: The great omission. *Pediatrics, 101*(1), 1–6.

Moore, K. L., Persaud, T. V. N., & Shiota, K. (2000). *Color atlas of clinical embryology* (2nd ed.). Philadelphia: Saunders.

Morrissy, R. T., & Weinstein, S. L. (1996). *Lovell and Winter's pediatric orthopaedics* (4th ed.). Philadelphia: Lippincott-Raven Publishers.

Parks, M. K. (2002). *Pediatric cardiology for practitioners* (4th ed.). St. Louis: Mosby–Year Book.

Pearson, J. (1999). Crying and calming: Important information and effective techniques to teach parents of full term newborns. *Mother-Baby Journal, 4*(5), 39–42.

Pressler, J. L., & Hepworth, J. T. (1997). Newborn neurologic screening using NBAS reflexes. *Neonatal Network, 16*(6), 33–46.

Rosenberg, N., Bialik, V., Norman, D., & Blazer, S. (1998). The importance of combined clinical and sonographic examination of instability of the neonatal hip. *International Orthopedics, 22*(3), 431–434.

Silengo, M., Battistoni, G., & Spada, M. (1999). Is there a relationship between extensive Mongolian spots and inform errors of metabolism? *American Journal of Medical Genetics, 87*(3), 276–277.

Spilman, L. (2002). Examination of the external ear. *Advances in Neonatal Care, 2*(2), 72–80.

Stokowski, L. A. (2004). Hypospadias in the neonate. *Advances in Neonatal Care, 4*(4), 206–215.

Stoll, B. J., & Kliegman, R. M. (2000). Noninfectious disorders. In R. E. Behrman, R. M. Kliegman, & H. B. Jenson (Eds.), *Nelson's textbook of pediatrics* (16th ed., pp. 451–553). Philadelphia: Saunders.

Tachdjian, M. O. (1997). *Clinical pediatric orthopedics: The art of diagnosis and principles of management.* Stamford, CT: Appleton & Lange.

Thompson, D. C., McPhillips, H., Davis, R. L., Lieu, T. L., Homer, C. J., Helfand, M. (2001). Universal newborn hearing screening: Summary of evidence. *Journal of the American Medical Association, 186*(16), 2000–2010.

Tredwell, S. J., Wilson, D., & Wilmink, M. A. (2001). Review of the effect of early amniocentesis on foot deformity in the neonate. *Journal of Pediatric Orthopedics, 21*(5), 636–641.

Ulshen, M. (2000). Clinical manifestations of gastrointestinal disease. In R. E. Behrman, R. M. Kliegman, & H. B. Jenson (Eds.), *Nelson's textbook of pediatrics* (16th ed., pp. 1101–1107). Philadelphia: Saunders.

United States Department of Health and Human Services (USDHHS). (2000, November). Health People 2010 (Publication No. S/N017-001-00547-9). Retrieved March 20, 2006, from Health People 2010: www.healthypeople.gov.

Versmold, H. T., Kitterman, J. A., Phibbs, R. H., Gregory, G. A., & Tooley, W. H. (1981). Aortic blood pressure during the first 12 hours of life in infants 610 to 4,220 grams. *Pediatrics, 67*(5), 703–713.

Witt, C. (2005). Skin assessment. In E. P. Tappero & M. E. Honeyfield (Eds.), *Physical assessment of the newborn: A comprehensive approach to the art of physical examination* (3rd ed., pp. 41–54). Petaluma, CA: NICU INK.

Witt, C. (1999). Neonatal dermatology. In J. Deacon & P. O'Neill (Eds.), *Core curriculum for neonatal intensive care nursing* (pp. 578–595). Philadelphia: Saunders.

Wong, D. L. (Ed.). (1998). *Whaley & Wong's nursing care of infants and children* (6th ed.). St Louis: Mosby–Year Book.

Yoshinaga-Itano, C. (1999). Benefits of early intervention for children with hearing loss. *Otolaryngology Clinics of North America, 32*(6), 1089–1102.

Characteristics of Infant State

Infant States	Body Activity	Eye Movements	Facial Movements	Breathing Pattern	Level of Response	Implications for Caregiving
Sleep States						
Deep sleep	Nearly still, except for occasional startle or twitch	None	Without facial movements, except for occasional sucking at regular intervals	Smooth and regular	Threshold to stimuli very high so that only very intense or disturbing stimuli will arouse infants	Caregivers trying to feed infants in deep sleep will probably find the experience frustrating. Infants will be unresponsive even if caregivers use disturbing stimuli (flicking feet) to arouse infants. Infants may arouse only briefly and then become unresponsive as they return to deep sleep. If caregivers wait until infants move to a higher, more responsive state, feeding or care giving will be much more pleasant.
Light sleep	Some body movements	Rapid eye movements (REM); fluttering of eyes beneath closed eyelids	May smile and make brief fussy or crying sounds	Irregular	More responsive to internal and external stimuli. When stimuli occur, infant may remain in light sleep, return to deep sleep, or arouse to drowsy.	Light sleep makes up the highest proportion of newborn sleep and usually precedes wakening. The brief fussy or crying sounds made during this state may make caregivers who are not aware that these sounds occur normally think it is time for feeding, and they may try to feed infants before they are ready to eat.

(continued)

APPENDIX **12A**

Characteristics of Infant State (*Continued*)

Infant States	Body Activity	Eye Movements	Facial Movements	Breathing Pattern	Level of Response	Implications for Caregiving
Awake States						
Drowsy	Activity level variable, with mild startles interspersed from time to time; movement usually smooth	Eyes open and close occasionally, are heavy lidded with dull, glazed appearance	Some facial movements possible	Irregular	React to sensory stimuli although responses are delayed	From the drowsy state, infants may return to sleep or awaken further. To facilitate waking, caregivers can provide something for infants to see, hear, or suck. This may arouse them to a quiet alert state, a more responsive state. Infants left alone without
Quiet alert	Minimal	Brightening and widening of eyes	Face bright, shining, sparkling	Regular	Most attentive to environment, focusing attention on any stimuli that are present	Infants in quiet, alert state provide much pleasure and positive feedback for caregivers. Providing something for infants to see, hear, or suck will often maintain this state. In the first few hours after birth, most newborns commonly experience a period of intense alertness before going into a long sleeping period.
Active alert	Much body activity; periods of fussiness possible	Eyes open with less brightening	Much facial movement; face not as bright as quiet alert state	Irregular	Increasingly sensitive to disturbing stimuli (hunger, fatigue, noise, excessive handling)	Caregivers may intervene at this stage to console and to bring infants to a lower state.

Crying	Increased motor activity, with color changes	Eyes tightly closed or open	Grimaces	More irregular	Extremely responsive to unpleasant external or internal stimuli	Crying is the infant's communication signal. It is a response to unpleasant stimuli from the environment or from within (fatigue, hunger, discomfort). Crying tells us the infant's limits have been reached. Sometimes infants can console themselves and return to lower states. At other times, they need help from caregivers.

From Pearson, J. (1999). Crying and calming: Important information and effective techniques to teach parents of full-term newborns. *Mother Baby Journal, 4*(5), 39–42.

Characteristics of the Ballard Gestation Age Assessment Tool

POSTURE

Observe the newborn lying quietly. Flexion of arms and legs increases with gestational age. The premature newborn lies with arms and legs extended. As gestational age increases, the more flexed the newborn's arms and legs are against the body.

SQUARE WINDOW (WRIST)

The angle that is created when the newborn's palm is flexed toward the forearm. A preterm newborn's wrist exhibits poor flexion and makes a 90-degree angle with the arm. An extremely preterm newborn has no flexor tone and cannot achieve even 90-degree flexion. A term newborn's wrist can flex completely against the forearm.

ARM RECOIL

After first flexing the arms at the elbows against the chest, then fully extending and releasing them, term newborns resist extension and quickly return arms to the flexed position. Very preterm newborns do not resist extension and respond with weak and delayed flexion.

POPLITEAL ANGLE

With the newborn supine and his or her pelvis flat, flex the thigh to the abdomen and hold it there while extending the leg at the knee. The angle at the knee is estimated. The preterm newborn can achieve greater extension.

SCARF SIGN

While the newborn is supine, move his or her arm across his chest toward the opposite shoulder. A term newborn's elbow does not cross midline. It is possible to bring the preterm newborn's elbow much farther.

HEEL TO EAR

Without holding the knee and thigh in place, move the newborn's foot as close to the ear as possible. A preterm newborn is able to get his or her foot closer to his or her head than a term baby.

SKIN

Assess for thickness, transparency, and texture. Preterm skin is smooth and thin with visible vessels. Extremely preterm skin is sticky and transparent. Term skin is thick, veins are difficult to see, and peeling may occur.

LANUGO

Fine hair seen over the back of premature newborns by 24 weeks' gestation. It begins to thin over the lower back first and disappears last over the shoulders.

PLANTAR CREASES

One or two creases over the pad of the foot at approximately 32 weeks' gestation. At 36 weeks, creases cover the anterior two-thirds of the foot; at term, the whole foot. At very early gestations, the length from the tip of the great toe to the back of the heel is measured.

BREAST TISSUE

Examined for visibility of nipple and areola and size of bud when grasped between thumb and forefinger. The very premature newborn does not have visible nipples or areolae. These become more defined and then raised by 34 weeks, with a small bud appearing at 36 weeks and growing to 5 to 10 mm by term.

EAR FORMATION

Lack of cartilage in earlier gestation results in the ear folding easily and retaining this fold. As gestation progresses, soft cartilage provides increasing resistance to folding and increasing recoil. The pinnae are flat in very preterm newborns. Incurving proceeds from the top, down toward the lobes as gestation advances.

GENITALIA

In males, rugae become visible at 28 weeks. By 36 weeks, the testes are in the upper scrotum, and rugae cover the anterior portion of the scrotum. At term, rugae cover the scrotum, and postterm, the testes are pendulous. In preterm females, the clitoris is prominent, and the labia minora are flat. By 36 weeks, the labia majora are larger, nearly covering the clitoris.

Developmental Reflexes

Reflex	How Elicited	Normal Response	Abnormal Response	Duration of Reflex
Rooting and sucking	Touch cheek, lip, or corner of mouth with finger or nipple.	Newborn turns head in direction of stimulus, opens mouth, and begins to suck. In the term newborn, suck is coordinated and strong.	Weak or absent response seen with prematurity, neurologic deficit, or CNS depression from maternal drug ingestion.	Rooting disappears by 3–4 months; sucking disappears by 1 year.
Swallowing	Place fluid on back.	Newborn swallows in coordination with sucking.	Gagging, coughing, or regurgitation of fluid; possibly associated with cyanosis secondary to prematurity, neurologic deficit, or injury.	Does not disappear
Extrusion	Touch tip of tongue with finger or nipple.	Newborn pushes tongue outward.	Continuous extrusion of tongue or repetitive tongue thrusting seen with CNS abnormalities or seizures.	Disappears by 6 months
Moro	Holding the newborn's head off the mattress slightly, let it drop quickly several inches into your hand.	Bilateral symmetric extension and abduction of all extremities, with thumb and forefinger forming characteristic "C," followed by adduction of extremities and return to relaxed flexion.	Asymmetric response seen with peripheral nerve injury (brachial plexus), fracture of clavicle or long bone of arm or leg, or birth trauma such as skull fracture.	Disappears by 6 months
Truck incurvature (Galant's reflex)	Use on hand to lift the prone newborn off a flat surface (ventral suspension). With a finger from the free hand, use some pressure to draw a line down the length of the back about an inch from the spinal column.	Newborn flexes pelvis toward the side stimulated.	Absence indicates spinal cord lesion or CNS depression.	Disappears by 4 months

Reflex	How Elicited	Normal Response	Abnormal Response	Duration of Reflex
Tonic neck (fencing)	Turn the newborn's head to one side when infant is resting in the supine position.	Extremity on the side to which the head is turned extends and opposite extremities flex. Response may be absent or incomplete immediately after birth.	Persistent response after 4 months may indicate neurological injury.	Diminishes by 4 months
Startle	Expose the newborn to sudden movement or loud noise.	Newborn abducts and flexes all extremities and may begin to cry.	Absence of response may indicate neurological deficit or deafness. Response may be absent or diminished during sleep.	Diminishes by 4 months
Crossed extension	Place the newborn in the supine position and extend one leg while stimulating the bottom of the foot.	Newborn's opposite leg flexes and extends rapidly as if trying to deflect stimulus to the other foot.	Weak or absent response is seen with peripheral nerve injury or fracture of a long bone.	Disappears by 6 months
Palmar grasp	Place a finger in the newborn's palm and apply slight pressure.	Newborn grasps finger; attempting to remove the finger causes newborn to tighten his grasp.	Weak or absent grasp in the presence of CNS deficit or nerve or muscle injury.	Does not disappear

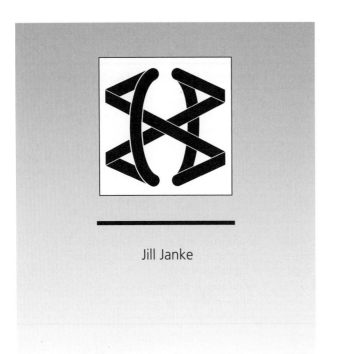

Jill Janke

CHAPTER 13

Newborn Nutrition

THE decision about what to feed a newborn is frequently made by the mother long before giving birth (Earle, 2002). Some of the factors that influence a mother's decision, include education (Callen & Pinelli, 2004; Humphreys, Thompson, & Miner 1998; Phares et al., 2004); age (Callen & Pinelli; Humphreys, et al., 1998 Meyerink & Marquis, 2002; Phares et al., 2004); previous breastfeeding experience (Humphreys et al., 1998) support from the husband, significant others (Duddridge, 2000; Earle, 2002; Meyerink & Marquis, 2002; Tarkka, Paunonen, & Laippala, 1999), or extended family (Duddridge, 2000; Meyerink & Marquis, 2002; Tarkka, Paunonen, & Laippala, 1999); prenatal breastfeeding education (Dyson, McCormick, & Renfrew, 2005; McCleod, Pullon, & Cookson, 2002; Piper & Parks, 1996); and encouragement from peers (Dennis, Hodnett, & Gallop, 2002; Schafer, Vogel, Viegas, & Hausafus, 1998; Tarkka, Paunonen, & Laippala, 1999) and professionals (Bentley et al., 1999; Guise et al., 2003; Vittoz, Labarere, Castell, Durand, & Pons, 2004). The choice of infant feeding is not always based on all available information. The mother's decision about infant feeding should not be a lifestyle choice but rather a health choice. However, a woman's choice of feeding method should be respected by all healthcare providers.

This chapter offers information and guidelines for the perinatal nurse during the initiation and early days of lactation. The chapter emphasizes that breastfeeding is the ideal method of feeding the newborn and provides helpful information for the perinatal nurse working with families who choose to formula feed their newborn.

Human milk is a dynamic food, meeting the infant's needs to construct an immune system, to grow and develop the brain, and to form attachments with other human beings. Research has produced compelling data about the advantages of breastfeeding for the mother and newborn. Exclusive use of formula is responsible for substantial expenditures of healthcare dollars during the first year of life for respiratory illness (Bachrach, Schwarz, & Bachrach, 2003; Blaymore, Oliver, Ferguson, & Vohr, 2002; Gianino et al., 2002; Oddy, Sly et al., 2003), otitis media (Aniansson, Alm, & Andersson, 1994; Daly et al., 1999), and gastrointestinal illness (Bhandari et al., 2003; Gianino et al., 2000; Kramer et al., 2003). Breastfeeding has also proven to have many economical benefits. Ball and Wright (1999) determined that, for 1,000 formula-fed babies, there was an excess of 2,033 office visits, more than 200 days of hospitalization, and more than 600 prescriptions compared with infants breastfed for at least 3 months. Wight (2001) estimated there was a cost savings of $9,998 per preterm infant when they received human milk. Finally, Weimer (2001) reported a minimum of 3.6 billion healthcare dollars (based on 1998 data) would be saved if women were breastfeeding at recommended Healthy People 2010 rates. Table 13–1 lists potential medical problems that may be associated with not breastfeeding.

INCIDENCE OF BREASTFEEDING

Given the importance of breast milk and breastfeeding to mothers, newborns, and society as a whole, experts in the United States have determined that increasing

TABLE 13–1 ■ RISK OF SPECIFIC MEDICAL CONDITIONS THAT MAY BE ASSOCIATED WITH NOT BREASTFEEDING

Disease or Condition	Study	Result
Asthma	Oddy et al. (1999)	Formula-fed infants had a 27% increase in asthma by age 6, were 44% more likely to wheeze, and 74% more likely to have sleep disturbance from wheezing.
	Oddy et al. (2002)	Children age 6 were more likely to develop asthma if they had not been breastfed exclusively for at least 4 months.
Otitis media	Aniansson et al. (1994)	Otitis media was lower in breastfed infants, and first episode occurred significantly earlier in children who were weaned before 6 months.
	Scariati et al. (1997)	Formula-fed infants had a 70% increased risk for otitis.
	Chantry, Howard, & Auinger (2002)	Infants fully breastfed for 6 months ($N = 2,277$) had twofold decrease in recurrent otitis.
Respiratory conditions	Arifeen et al. (2001)	Exclusive breastfeeding for the first months was associated with a 2.23-fold lower mortality risk due to respiratory and diarrheal diseases.
	Bulkow et al. (2002)	Breastfeeding associated with lower risk of RSV hospitalization among Alaska Native children (odds ratio 0.34).
	Chantry et al. (2002)	Infants fully breastfed for 6 months ($N = 2,277$) had significantly lower risk for respiratory infection in first 2 years when compared to 4 months of exclusive breastfeeding. Chance of contracting pneumonia reduced fivefold with 2 additional months of full breastfeeding
	Bachrach et al. (2003)	Hospitalization for severe respiratory infections was $3\times$ higher in infants who were not breastfed. Respiratory disease was reduced by 70% if exclusively breastfed for 4 months.
	Oddy et al. (2003)	Respiratory illness and infection in first year was significantly lower among babies who are predominantly breastfed.
	Martens et al. (2004)	Formula feeding associated with hospital readmission (adjusted odds ratio: 1.32).
GI disease/ diarrhea	Scariati et al. (1997)	Formula-fed babies had an 80% increased risk of diarrhea.
	Arifeen et al. (2001)	Compared with exclusive breastfeeding partial or no breastfeeding was associated with a 2.23-fold higher risk of infant deaths from respiratory illnesses and diarrhea.
	Davis, M. (2001)	Breastfeeding may protect against inflammatory bowel disease and decrease the risk of later onset of celiac disease.
	Kramer et al. (2003)	Infants exclusively breastfed for 6 months had a lower risk of GI infection.
	Klement, Cohen, Boxman, Joseph, & Reif (2004)	Breastfeeding was associated with lower risk of Crohn's disease and ulcerative colitis.
	UNICEF UK Baby Friendly Initiative (2003)	Infants breastfed exclusively for 3–6 months had a significant reduction in GI infection.
	Morrow et al. (2004)	Breastfeeding infants had lower morbidity and mortality rates resulting from diarrhea in the first few years of life.
Cognitive development	Greene, Lucas, Livingstone, Harland, & Baker (1995)	Formula-fed infants had poorer academic performance in school when compared to breastfed infants.
	Horwood & Furgusson (1998)	Formula-fed infants had up to an 8- to 10-point IQ deficit when compared to breastfed infants.
	Angelsen, Vik, Jacobsen, & Bakketeig (2001)	Longer duration of breastfeeding benefited cognitive development.

(continued)

TABLE 13–1 ■ RISK OF SPECIFIC MEDICAL CONDITIONS THAT MAY BE ASSOCIATED WITH NOT BREASTFEEDING (Continued)

Disease or Condition	Study	Result
	Bier, Oliver, Ferguson, & Vohr (2002)	Premature infants who received breast milk had higher motor and cognitive scores.
	Mortensen, Fleishcer, Sanders, & Reinisch (2002)	Significant positive association was found between durations of breastfeeding and IQ.
	Oddy et al. (2003)	Early introduction of milk was associated with reduced verbal IQ.
Obesity	Von Kries et al. (1999)	Exclusive breastfeeding for 3–5 months reduced risk of obesity by 35%. Breastfeeding for 6–12 months reduced obesity risk by 43%. Breastfeeding for >12 months reduced obesity risk by 72%.
	Gillman et al. (2001)	Infants fed breast milk more than formula, or who were breastfed longer periods, had lower risk of being overweight during older childhood and adolescence.
	Armstrong & Reilly (2002)	Breastfeeding was associated with up to a 30% reduction in risk for developing childhood obesity.
	Baker, Michaelsen, Rasmussen, & Sorensen (2005)	Decreased duration of breastfeeding and earlier food introduction were associated with increased infant weight gain.
	Grummer-Strawn & Mei (2004)	Prolonged breastfeeding was associated with reduced risk of overweight among non-Hispanic white children.
	Owens, Martin, Whincup, Smith, Cook (2005)	Initial breastfeeding protected against obesity in later life.
Diabetes	Mayer, Hamman, Gay, Lezotte, Klingensmith (1988)	Two to 26% of type 1 diabetes is attributed to not being breastfed.
	Vaarala et al. (1999)	Cow's milk may be an environmental trigger of immunity to insulin in infancy.
	Young et al. (2002)	Breastfeeding reduced the risk of type 2 diabetes among Native Canadian children.
	Taylor, Kacmar, Nothnagle, & Lawrence (2005)	Systematic review concluded that being breastfed for at least 2 months might lower the risk of diabetes in children.
Necrotizing enterocolitis	Lucas & Cole (1990)	Eighty-three percent of NEC cases may be attributed to formula feeding.
	Schanler (2001)	Compared with preterm formula, the feeding of fortified human milk may provide significant protection from infection and NEC.
	Arnold (2002)	Banked donor milk has been shown to be as effective in preventing NEC as mother's milk.
Infection	de Silva, Jones, & Spencer (2004)	Systematic review showed that prevention of infection in preterm (VLBW) infants was not proven by the existing studies due to numerous methodological flaws.
	Turck (2005)	Exclusive breastfeeding for at least 3 months was associated with a lower incidence and severity of diarrhea, otitis media, and respiratory infection.
	Martens et al. (2004)	Formula-feeding (not breastfeeding) was associated with hospital readmission (adjusted odds ratio: 1.32).
Allergies	Kull, Wickman, Lilja, Nordvall, & Pershagen (2002)	Exclusive breastfeeding had preventive effect on early development of allergic disease.
	Martin, Derkesen, Gupta (2004)	Children who were breastfed had lower blood pressure.
	Singhal, Cole, Fewtrell, & Lucas (2004)	Long-term benefits of breast-milk–feeding include lowered risk of atherosclerosis.

TABLE 13-1 ■ RISK OF SPECIFIC MEDICAL CONDITIONS THAT MAY BE ASSOCIATED WITH NOT BREASTFEEDING (Continued)

Disease or Condition	Study	Result
SIDS	McVea, Turner, & Peppler (2000)	There was an association between formula feeding and SIDS, but this may be related to confounding variables.
Cardiovascular disease	Owens, Martin, Wincup, Smith, & Cook (2005); Owens, Whincup, Odoki, Gilg, & Cook (2002)	Being breastfed as an infant was associated with lower cholesterol as an adult.
Childhood leukemia and lymphomas	Berner et al. (2001)	Those breastfed for <6 months were >2.5 times more likely to contract a lymphoid malignancy (acute lymphoblastic leukemia, Hodgkin's & non-Hodgkin's lymphoma) than children breastfed for >6 months.

the rates and duration of breastfeeding continues to be a national health goal. The Healthy People 2010 target is that 75% of women will initiate breastfeeding, 50% of women will continue exclusively breastfeeding for 6 months, and 25% will still be breastfeeding when the infant is 12 months of age (United States Department of Health & Human Services, 2000). The American Academy of Pediatrics (AAP) further recommends that women continue to breastfeed for at least a year and longer if mutually desired (2005). They maintain there is no limit to how long an infant should breastfeed. Researchers have reported no evidence of psychological or developmental harm from continued breastfeeding into the third year of life or longer. On the contrary, researchers have reported distinct benefits to extending breastfeeding past the first year. The American Academy of Family Physicians (AAFP) (2006) noted that children weaned before 2 years are at increased risk of illness; Gulick (1986) reported that toddlers between the ages of 16 and 30 months who continued to breastfeed had fewer illnesses and when they do get sick, their illness was of shorter duration when compared to non-nursing toddlers. The World Health Organization (WHO) and UNICEF both emphasized the importance of nursing up to 2 years and beyond (WHO, 2002).

Although there has been progress made toward achieving the Healthy People 2010 goals, more work is needed. According to the 2004 National Immunization Study (NIS) 70.3% of mothers in the United States initiated breastfeeding. At 6 months, 36.2% continue to do some breastfeeding, with only 14.1% breastfeeding exclusively. At 1 year, 17.8% of women were still doing some breastfeeding (Center for Disease Control [CDC], 2004). There is limited information on breastfeeding rates past 1 year. One nonscientific poll of 2,737 women who had Internet access and frequented *ParentsPlace.com* found 24% of the respondents

nursed and weaned sometime in the second year, another 6% nursed past the second year, and another 5% reported nursing past the third year (retrieved 3/21/06 from KELLYMOM.com). More research is obviously needed on the incidence of women breastfeeding beyond the first year.

Although the overall breastfeeding rates have moved toward the 2010 goals, the NIS data (CDC, 2004) report great disparity between geographic areas and various population groups. State initiation rates varied widely, from 41% to 88%. Only 14 states in 2004 achieved the national goals of a 75% initiation rate, with 10 of those states having rates that exceeded 80% (Alaska, Arizona, California, Colorado, Hawaii, Idaho, Nevada, Oregon, Utah, and Washington). Continuation of breastfeeding remains problematic; only three states met the 50% rate goal at 6 months, and five states met the 25% rate goal at 1 year (CDC, 2004). Furthermore, there is limited information on breastfeeding rates past 1 year.

The profile of women who are more likely to initiate and continue breastfeeding has not changed over the years. Women more likely to breastfeed tend to be Caucasian or Hispanic; at least 30 years of age; married; college educated; not enrolled in the Women, Infants, and Children (WIC) program; and living in the Mountain or Pacific regions of the United States. Breastfeeding continued to be lowest among women who were African-American, had less than or equal to a high school education, were younger than 20 years of age, lived in the eastern South Central region of the United States, and were enrolled in the WIC program (CDC, 2004). Display 13-1 identifies obstacles to meeting the Healthy People 2010 national goals.

The AAP Workshop on Breastfeeding (2005) maintains that, with few exceptions, human milk is preferred for all infants, including premature and sick newborns. The more common contraindications to breastfeeding include galactosemia, human T-cell lymphotropic virus type I or II infection, use of antimetabolites or chemotherapeutic agents, therapeutic doses of radioisotopes, drug of abuse, herpes simplex lesions on the breast (although feeding on the opposite breast may occur if it is lesion free), and human immunodeficiency virus (HIV) seropositivity of the mother (APA, 2005).

PHYSIOLOGY OF MILK PRODUCTION

Several hormones are responsible for the dramatic breast changes that occur during pregnancy. Estrogen causes ductular sprouting, progesterone is responsible for lobular formation, and prolactin influences lobular and alveolar development. Prolactin stimulates receptors located on the surface of alveolar cells to initiate milk secretion. Prolactin is secreted from the anterior pituitary gland and stimulates production of colostrum, which appears in the third month of gestation. During this time, prolactin is involved in cell differentiation and the formation of lactocytes (ie, mammary secretory epithelial cells) that are capable of secreting milk components. Nipple growth is also related to blood levels of prolactin. By the second trimester, placental lactogen begins to stimulate the secretion of colostrum

and is responsible for breast and areolar growth. The greatest breast growth usually occurs during the first 5 months of pregnancy. The increase in breast volume can range from 12 to 227 mL (Cox, Kent, Casey, Owens, & Hartmann, 1999). Some women, however, experience minimal breast enlargement during pregnancy, less than one cup size (Neifert, 1999). There is no relationship between breast growth during pregnancy and milk production at 1 month in mothers who breastfeed frequently (Cox, Kent, Casey, Owens, & Hartmann, 1999). Human mammary glands have the ability to increase secretory tissue during lactation in response to increased demand for milk. Women who report little to no breast growth during pregnancy need more support to breastfeed frequently during the first 2 weeks of lactation, making sure that milk transfer is taking place (Cox et al., 1999).

Between 15 to 20 weeks' gestation, lactogenesis I occurs in most mothers (Cregan & Hartmann, 1999; Riordan, 2005). This phase is the time when the breasts are capable of synthesizing the unique components of milk. Milk synthesis also requires insulin-induced cell division and the presence of cortisol.

Lactogenesis II is defined as the onset of copious milk production 48 to 72 hours after the rapid drop in blood progesterone that occurs after delivery of the placenta (Lawrence & Lawrence, 2005). Viable placental fragments retained in the uterus can delay initiation of lactation until they are removed (Neifert, McDonough, & Neville, 1981). Maternal obesity has also been associated with a lower prolactin response to suckling that may affect milk production over time (Rasmussen & Kjolhede, 2004). Copious milk production can also be delayed by 24 hours in mothers with type I diabetes mellitus. A temporary imbalance may exist between the woman's need for insulin to regulate her own glucose levels and the amount required to contribute to the initiation of lactation (Arthur, Kent, & Hartmann, 1994; Neubauer et al., 1993). The type I diabetic mother should be encouraged to put the baby to breast 12 to 14 times during each 24-hour period during the first 3 days to provide frequent, small doses of colostrum for glucose homeostasis in the infant and to stimulate milk production.

Lactogenesis III is the phase where the woman establishes a mature milk supply. This phase is also known as galactopoiesis, or more simply "lactation." It begins around day 10, at which time lactation shifts from endocrine control to autocrine control. The supply–demand of autocrine control relies on the removal of milk from the breast to facilitate ongoing milk production (Lawrence & Lawrence, 2005).

Although prolactin is necessary to maintain lactation, the concentration of blood prolactin does not regulate short-term or long-term rates of milk synthesis (Cox, Owens, & Hartmann, 1996). Prolactin levels are high during approximately the first 10 days post-partum and slowly decline over the next 6 months. Prolactin levels are also highest at night. It is thought that the frequent sucking acts as a stimulus to increase the binding capacity of prolactin receptor sites in the breast. This enhances tissue responsiveness, accounting for continued full milk production as prolactin concentrations decline over time.

For most women, milk production closely matches the needs of the newborn. The degree of breast fullness at the end of each feeding influences the short-term rate of milk synthesis. The more efficiently the newborn nurses, the faster is the rate of milk synthesis and the higher its fat content (Daly, Owens, & Hartmann, 1993). The more milk left in the breast, the slower is the rate of milk synthesis. Leaving milk in the breasts for long periods can contribute to slower and lower amounts of milk production, a process referred to as the feedback inhibitor of lactation (Wilde, Addey, Boddy, & Peaker, 1995). This mechanism works independently such that each breast can have a different rate of milk synthesis depending on the frequency and degree of drainage on each side. There is also a decrease in the rate of milk synthesis overnight, because the interval between feedings during the night is usually the longest. Although some mothers with larger storage capacities in the breasts can accommodate longer durations between breastfeeding (up to 8 to 9 hours) before milk synthesis is compromised, other mothers with smaller storage capacities could experience decreases in milk supplies sooner. Women with a large storage capacity may have greater flexibility in that their babies may not feed as often as an infant of a woman with a smaller storage capacity, even though they may be producing similar amounts of milk (Daly, Owens, & Hartmann, 1993). Infants typically remove about 76% of the available milk at a feeding (Daly, Kent, Owens, & Hartmann, 1996).

Nipple stimulation prompts oxytocin to be released from the pituitary gland in a pulsatile manner numerous times during each feeding. The sensation that accompanies the effect of oxytocin on breast tissue is referred to as the letdown reflex or the milk-ejection reflex. Some mothers feel this as a heaviness or tingling sensation in the breast. Some mothers never feel the milk let down but observe milk leaking from the other breast or the newborn swallowing milk. Oxytocin causes the network of myoepithelial cells surrounding the alveoli to contract and expel milk into the larger ductules, making it available to the newborn. This increase in pressure inside the breast overcomes the resistance to the outflow of milk and creates a pressure gradient that allows the fluid inside the breast to move from an area of high pressure to an area of low pressure inside the newborn's mouth. Oxytocin also stimulates uterine contractions that control postpartum bleeding and promote involution. Mothers, especially multiparous women, feel these "after-birth pains" during feedings for several days after the birth.

Oxytocin-producing neurons throughout the brain are thought to be associated with social behavior and attachment. In addition to being released in the maternal brain tissue, oxytocin is released into the newborn brain by means of milk transfer and is thought to modulate attachment behaviors between mother and newborn (Insel, 1997; Nelson & Panksepp, 1998). Touch, massage, and skin-to-skin contact stimulate oxytocin release. Separating mothers and newborns should be discouraged unless there is a medical indication (Uvnas-Moberg, 1997). Oxytocin also is partly responsible for the calmness women exhibit while breastfeeding and has been linked to a decreased response to stressors and pain in the breastfeeding woman (Goer, Davis, & Davis, 2002).

BIOSPECIFICITY OF HUMAN MILK

Human milk is a species-specific fluid. The composition is not static or uniform. Breast milk is designed to meet the needs of newborns to grow and develop a brain, protect the immature gut, be a substitute for an immature immune system, and assist in developing attachment behavior. The composition of human milk changes over time. Colostrum (1 to 5 days postpartum) evolves to transitional milk (6 to 13 days postpartum) and then into mature milk (14 days and beyond). Milk composition also changes during feedings, during each 24 hours, and over the course of the entire lactation. Milk of preterm mothers differs from that of term mothers. In contrast, formula is an inert medium with none of the growth factors, enzymes, hormones, live cells, and other bioactive ingredients found in breast milk.

Colostrum is present in the breast from about 12 to 16 weeks of pregnancy. This first milk is thick and has a yellowish color the result of beta-carotene. Average energy value is about 18 kcal/ounce, compared with mature milk, which contains 21 kcal/ounce (AAP Committee on Nutrition, 2003). The volume of colostrum per feeding during the first 3 days postpartum ranges from 2 to 20 mL. Compared with mature milk, colostrum is higher in protein, sodium, chloride, potassium, and fat-soluble vitamins. It is rich in antioxidants, antibodies, interferon, fibronectin, and immunoglobulins, especially secretory IgA. Secretory IgA is antigen specific. When mothers come in contact with microbes, antibodies are synthesized in her milk, targeting pathogens in the newborn's immediate environment. These antibodies are passed to the newborn. Separating the mother and newborn interferes with this defense mechanism. Colostrum begins the establishment of normal bacterial flora in the newborn's gastrointestinal tract and exerts a laxative effect that begins elimination of meconium, decreasing the potential reabsorption of bilirubin.

Nutritional Components

Water

Human milk is composed of 87.5% water, in which all other components are dissolved, dispersed, or in suspension. Infants receiving adequate amounts of breast milk do not need additional water, even in hot, arid, or humid climates (Almroth, 1978).

Fat

Fat content of human milk ranges from 3.5% to 4.5% and contributes 50% of the calories. It varies during a feeding (rising at the end), increases over the first days of lactation, and shows diurnal rhythms. Total fat content is reduced in mothers who smoke (Vio, Salazar, & Infante, 1991) and increases when women nurse more frequently. The long-chain polyunsaturated fatty acids docosahexanoic acid and arachidonic acid contained in breast milk are found in the brain, retina, and central nervous system of newborns and are necessary for the growth of these structures during the first year of life (Riordan, 2005). The absence of these fatty acids in formula is thought to contribute to differences in cognitive development (Anderson, Johnstone, & Remley, 1999).

Protein

Protein concentration is high in colostrum and settles to 0.8% to 1.0% in mature milk. The whey-to-casein ratio in human milk changes from 90:10 in the early milk, to 60:40 in mature milk, and 50:50 in late lactation (AAP Committee on Nutrition, 2003). The whey protein that predominates in human milk is acidified in the stomach, forming soft curds that are easily digested and supply the infant with most of the nutrients in human milk. One of the components of the whey protein, lactoferrin, is important in the immunologic effects of human milk. The bacteriostatic effect of lactoferrin makes iron unavailable to pathogens that require the mineral (Riordan, 2005).

Carbohydrate

The principal carbohydrate in human milk is lactose. Lactose supports the colonization of the gut with microflora that increases the acidity of the intestine, decreasing growth of pathogens; ensures a supply of galactose and glucose, which are necessary for

brain development; and enhances calcium absorption (Riordan, 2005).

Vitamins and Minerals

Breast milk contains all of the vitamins and minerals needed by most infants for about the first 6 months of life. After 6 months of exclusive breastfeeding, infants require an iron supplement (AAP Workgroup on Breastfeeding, 2005). Mothers consuming a vegan diet with no dairy products may need supplemental vitamin B_{12} or an acceptable source in their diet. Vitamin D deficiency is a risk factor for some breastfed children, and due to scattered reports of rickets in the United States, the AAP now recommends all infants receive a vitamin D supplement (Gartner & Greer, 2003).

Preterm Milk

Like milk produced by mothers of term infants, milk produced by mothers of preterm infants changes to meet the need of the growing infant. Composition differs from term milk with higher levels of immune factors, energy, lipids, protein, nitrogen, and fatty acids (Riordan, 2005). Unfortunately, initiation and duration rates of breastfeeding the preterm infant are lower than those for the term infant. It is estimated that 10% to 37% of mothers of preterm infants initiate breastfeeding. Of those, less than 50% are able to sustain breastfeeding during the infants' hospitalization (as cited in British Columbia Reproductive Care Guideline, 2001). There are many reasons for the lower breastfeeding rates among preterm infants. Nurses need to be aware that mothers of preterm infants face the same barriers as mothers of term infants. In addition, they often face using a breast pump for a prolonged period of time, limited contact with the infant, increased emotional stress, and the NICU environment, with all its machines, monitoring devices, and so forth (AAFP, 2006).

The British Columbia Reproductive Care Guidelines (2001) cite the following benefits of giving preterm infants human milk: lower rates of infection, necrotizing enterocolitis, and hospital readmissions. In addition, preterm infants who received breast milk had improved feeding tolerance, as well as enhanced neurodevelopment, and family attachment. Mothers who breastfed or provided breast milk for their preterm infants, demonstrated increased self-esteem and maternal role-attainment. Although these benefits are similar for term infants, they have far greater impact on the vulnerable preterm infant.

Nurses play a major role in promoting breastfeeding for preterm infants. Certain practices have proven helpful: early discussion of breastfeeding with written information; frequent simultaneous expression of both breasts with electric pump; breast massage; cup feeding and skin-to-skin contact (Kangaroo care), which helps with attachment, milk production, and subsequent establishment of breastfeeding (AAFP, 2006). There are several guidelines on preterm breastfeeding. For example, the British Columbia Reproductive Care Guideline: Breastfeeding the healthy preterm infant ≤37 weeks (2001) has protocols for skin-to-skin cuddling with preterm infants receiving incubator care, a cup-feeding protocol, decision guides for assisting with feeding of different gestational ages etc. This can be accessed at: http://www.rcp.gov.bc.ca/guidelines/ Master.NutritionPartII.PremBreastfeeding.October. 2001.pdf). The March of Dimes (www.modimes. org) and AWHONN (www.awhonn.org) have good resources for parents and professionals.

BREASTFEEDING PROCESS

Preparation for Breastfeeding

Physical Preparation

There is no research supporting physical preparation of the breasts during pregnancy. Prenatal nipple rolling, application of creams, and expression of colostrum have not been shown to decrease pain or nipple trauma during the postpartum period. Use of methods to improve nipple erectility, such as Hoffman's exercises and breast shells, may actually decrease a woman's desire and motivation to breastfeed by conveying the message that her nipples are inferior and need correcting (Centouri, 1999; Riordan 2005).

Prenatal Education

Women should be encouraged to attend prenatal breastfeeding classes. The current length of hospital stays puts pressure on the nurse, the mother, and the newborn to demonstrate effective breastfeeding before some mother–baby couples are ready. The fast learning pace in the inpatient setting and the mother's cognitive sluggishness for verbal instructions during the first 24 hours postpartum suggest that there could be a benefit in providing basic breastfeeding information before birth (Eidelman, Hoffman, & Kaitz, 1993). Women report that their decision to breastfeed is influenced by biases of healthcare providers, parity, plans to return to work, and maternal confidence (Balcazar, Trier, & Cobas, 1995; O'Campo, Faden, Gielen, & Wang, 1992). Prenatal breastfeeding education programs increase the knowledge levels of pregnant women and their partners, increase the support women perceive from their partners around the decision

to breastfeed, and increase breastfeeding rates and duration of breastfeeding (Guise et al., 2003; Sikorski, Renfrew, Pindoria, & Wade, 2002). In low-income populations, use of peer counselors has been shown to increase initiation, exclusivity, and duration of breastfeeding (Dyson, McCormick, & Renfrew, 2005; Kistin, Abramson, & Dublin, 1994.)

Positioning

A variety of positions are used for breastfeeding. It is important for the breastfeeding mother to assume a relaxed, comfortable position with her back and arms well supported. If she is seated in a chair, placing a footstool beneath her feet decreases strain on her back and may discourage her from leaning forward over the baby. Some mothers benefit from a pillow on the lap or use of a commercially available nursing pillow. These can be especially helpful when nursing twins. If the mother is lying on her side, place a pillow behind her back for support. Whatever position is used, instruct the mother to support her breast with her free hand, using four fingers underneath and the thumb on top of the breast in a "C hold" (Fig. 13–1).

The newborn and mother face each other while breastfeeding. The mother should not lean forward over the newborn but instead concentrate on bringing the baby toward her. The newborn should be loosely wrapped or not wrapped at all so the nurse and mother can clearly see the position. There is no need to be concerned about keeping the newborn warm because mother and baby generate body heat during breastfeeding. Skin-to-skin contact is useful for increasing a low temperature in a newborn during the transitional period. As the feeding progresses, if necessary, a light blanket may be placed over both for privacy.

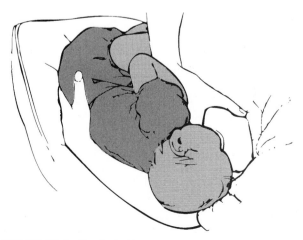

FIGURE 13–1. Cradle hold.

Cradle Hold

With the mother comfortably seated, the newborn is held in a side-lying position with its entire body completely facing the mother. Held on a slight incline, the newborn's lower arm is tucked around the outside of the breast. The newborn's body is in complete contact with the mother; the newborn's legs are wrapped around her waist. If the newborn is wrapped in a blanket, loosen it to permit the newborn to freely move its arms and legs. Avoid covering the infant's hands with the undershirt cuffs. The newborn's head rests on the mother's forearm, which along with her wrist and hands supports the baby's back and bottom (see Fig. 13–1). Specially designed L-shaped pillows fit around the mother's waist and help to elevate and support her arm. Use of this pillow has been associated with increased length of breastfeeding at 2 and 8 weeks (Humenick, Hill, & Hart, 1998). Regular bed pillows may also be used.

The cradle position can be modified by having the woman alter the position of her arms, using what is called the cross-cradle hold. This is a good position to use for preterm infants and infants with fractured clavicles. The newborn is placed in the same position as the cradle hold but held with the opposite arm such that the head is in the mother's hand and her forearm is supporting the back. This gives the mother much more control over positioning and, along with the clutch hold, may be easier to learn (Fig. 13–2).

Clutch Hold

The clutch position (ie, football hold) is useful for feeding preterm infants or twins and for mothers who have had a cesarean birth. The newborn is placed to the mother's side. Placing a pillow under the newborn raises the infant slightly and decreases the weight the mother

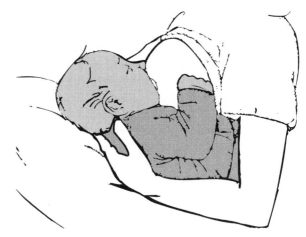

FIGURE 13-3. Clutch hold (football hold).

needs to lift. The newborn's head is in her hand, and its feet are positioned toward her back. Care should be taken to ensure that the full weight of the breast does not rest on the newborn's chest (Fig. 13–3).

Side Lying

Side-lying position works well after a cesarean birth or for a woman with a painful perineum. In this position, the newborn and mother lay on their sides facing each other. A small rolled blanket can be placed behind the newborn's back, or the mother can support the infant with her free arm (Fig. 13–4).

Supporting the Breast

Mothers are encouraged to support the breast in a C hold (see Fig. 13–1). The mother lifts her breast with her thumb on top and fingers below and against the chest wall. The thumb and fingers are away from the areola.

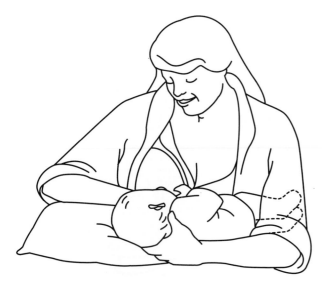

FIGURE 13–2. Modified cradle hold.

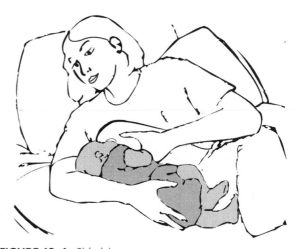

FIGURE 13–4. Side-lying.

This hold makes it easy for the mother to direct her nipple toward the center of the mouth during latch-on. Mothers are encouraged to use whichever hand is more comfortable. Pressure should not be applied to the breast with the thumb. The newborn's pug-shaped nose allows breathing through the grooves along the sides of the nares during breastfeeding, even when the nose is touching the breast. In all breastfeeding positions, pulling the newborn's buttocks closer to the mother's body or gently lifting the breast causes the newborn's head to drop back slightly, providing room for breathing.

Latch-On

Proper attachment of the newborn at the breast is necessary for pain-free and effective milk transfer. Once positioned comfortably, the mother moves the newborn's lips to the nipple; when the newborn's mouth is wide open, she draws the newborn forward toward her. The lower lip and chin contact the breast first. The newborn should grasp the nipple and about 1 to 1.5 inches of the areola, pulling it as a unit forward and deep into his mouth. The tongue is cupped and forward over the lower gum. Peristaltic ripples from the anterior tongue to the posterior tongue propel milk through the milk sinuses. When the jaw lowers and creates negative pressure, milk moves into the trough of the tongue and is channeled to the back of the mouth, where the swallow reflex is triggered. Display 13–2 lists observations made when the newborn is latched on to the breast correctly.

For women with very large breasts, a rolled receiving blanket or small towel can be placed under the breast so the baby does not drag down on the nipple.

D I S P L A Y   1 3 - 2

Observations Indicating Correct Latch-On

- Lips are rolled outward (flared).
- Clicking or smacking sounds are absent.
- Dimpled cheeks are absent.
- Muscles above and in front of the ear move.
- Both cheeks are equally close to the breast.
- Chin and nose are touching the breast.
- All of the nipple and part of the areola (at least 1 to 1.5 inches) is covered by the newborn's mouth.
- The lower lip more than the upper lip covers more of the areola.
- Angle at the corner of the mouth is wide.
- When the lower lip is gently pulled away from the breast, the tongue is visible over the lower gum line.

D I S P L A Y   1 3 - 3

Signs That Milk Transfer Is Occurring

- Proper latch-on
- Vibration on the occipital region of the head
- Deep jaw excursion
- Mother verbalizes a drawing sensation on the breast
- Absence of clicking or smacking sounds indicating that the tongue has lost contact with the nipple and areola
- Drawing inward of the areolar margins
- Evidence of swallowing (ie, puff of air from the newborn's nose or audible swallows)
- Audible swallows (usually heard after onset of copious milk production)

Care should be taken to avoid pushing the newborn's head into the breast. Pressure on the occipital region of the head causes extension of the neck. Tilting, squeezing, or distorting the nipple or areola should also be avoided, because doing so can cause pain and skin damage to the nipple or areola.

If the mother feels a pinching or biting sensation while nursing, she should be instructed to pull down gently on the newborn's chin. This causes his mouth to open wider so that more of the areola goes in his mouth. If this does not work, have the mother insert her little finger into the side of the newborn's mouth to release the suction. She should begin again to achieve a better latch-on.

Milk Transfer

When the newborn suckles effectively, the breast releases milk and milk transfer occurs. Even though a newborn may suck at the breast for 15 minutes with its jaw moving up and down, it does not mean that there has been a transfer of milk. Display 13–3 lists the signs that are observed when milk transfer occurs.

BREASTFEEDING MANAGEMENT

Getting Started

Breastfeeding, with skin-to-skin contact, should be initiated within an hour of birth. Early feedings are associated with mothers who breastfeed for a longer duration (Anderson, Moore, Hepworth, & Bergman, 2005; Ekstrom, Widstrom, & Nissen, 2003). Therefore, it is recommended that the newborn should be given the opportunity to seek and find the nipple. Nonsedated babies follow a predictable pattern of prefeeding behavior when held on the mother's chest immediately after birth that primes or imprints proper sucking mechanisms right from the start (Widstrom et al., 1987). Successful latch-on and suckling at this time greatly reduce sucking disorganization or dysfunction later on and contribute to increased breastfeeding duration (Righard & Alade, 1992). Sucking movements reach a peak 45 minutes after birth and decline until absent at 2 hours.

Some analgesics given during labor have the potential to interfere with the early development of breastfeeding behaviors (Jordan, Emery, Bradshaw, Watkins, & Friswell, 2005; Ransjo-Arvidson et al., 2001) and negatively influencing breastfeeding long term (Henderson, Dickinson, Evans, McDonald, & Paech, 2003) Newborn's whose mothers receive nalbuphine (Nubain) or butorphanol (Stadol) within an hour of birth or whose mother had no analgesia and who initiated breastfeeding within an hour of birth established effective breastfeeding significantly earlier than infants whose mothers had a longer duration of analgesia and later initiation of breastfeeding (Crowell, Hill, & Humenick, 1994). Similar results were reported with use of alphaprodine (Nisentil) (Matthews, 1989). The perinatal nurse may be able to offset some of the side effects of labor medications by helping initiate breastfeeding early, keeping the mother and newborn together, and teaching the mother to recognize hunger cues and putting the newborn to breast (Walker, 1999).

Sustained Maternal–Newborn Contact

Twenty-four-hour rooming-in supports breastfeeding and is an integral component of family-centered maternity care. However, the practice of rooming-in needs to be flexible, and its implementation needs to be respectful of the new mother. She may wish to move the newborn to the nursery in certain situations, such as fatigue or concern for newborn safety. Contact with the newborn enables a woman to recognize and respond to his needs and begin to develop confidence in her mothering role. Rooming-in provides opportunities for identifying hunger cues and to respond with a feeding (American College of Obstetricians and Gynecologists [ACOG], 2000). If the mother and newborn are together when the newborn demonstrates early hunger cues, she can begin feeding (Display 13–4). If the newborn is in a nursery, a healthcare provider witnesses the hunger cues and transports the newborn to the mother's room. During this delay, the newborn may become increasingly agitated, self-console, and return to sleep or become exhausted from crying and return to sleep. By the time the newborn reaches his mother, the infant is often sleeping or crying, and the optimal feeding opportunity is missed. Hunger

DISPLAY 13-4

Hunger Cues

- Rapid eye movements under the eyelids
- Sucking movements of the mouth and tongue
- Hand-to-mouth movements
- Body movements
- Small sounds (soft cooing or sighing sounds)
- Rooting
- Mouth opening in response to tactile stimulation
- Smacking of lips
- Restlessness

NOTE: Crying is a late feeding cue and may interfere with effective breastfeeding.

cues can be observed for up to 30 minutes before the newborn begins a sustained cry for food. Feeding is most successful if initiated while the newborn is in a quiet, alert state. Crying is a late hunger cue, and it is often necessary to console the newborn before he will settle and feed well. Feeding before the newborn begins a sustained cry reduces stress and some of the accompanying undesirable physiologic side effects such as glycogen depletion, increased intracranial pressure, resumption of fetal circulation within the heart, disorganized sucking, and poor feeding. Extended contact with the newborn may facilitate a feeding pattern that includes clustered feedings (ie, 5 to 10 feedings over 2 to 3 hours, followed by a 4- to 5-hour deep sleep).

Frequency and Duration

Historically, fixed breastfeeding schedules were thought to be more scientific, safer because the stomach had to be emptied before allowing a refill, a way to prevent sore nipples, less disruptive for the family if the newborn was on a schedule, and more efficient on a maternity unit. Current understanding of this issue is that restricting breastfeeding in the early days after birth can increase the incidence of sore nipples, engorgement, and perceived need to supplement; and more women may discontinue breastfeeding by 6 weeks postpartum (Renfrew, Lang, Martin, & Woolridge, 2000). Breastfeeding patterns, however, vary widely between mother–baby pairs, over each 24-hour period, and during the course of the lactation. When no artificial time limits are placed on breastfeeding, the number of feedings during each 24 hours ranges from 8 to 14, depending on age, physiologic capacity of the stomach, ability of the newborn, and storage capacity of the breasts.

Frequency and duration of feedings is different for breastfed and formula-fed newborns. The mean gastric half-emptying time of breast milk and formula is quite different. Formula-fed infants have a mean gastric half-emptying time of 65 minutes, with a range of 27 to 98 minutes; breastfed infants have a mean gastric half-emptying time of 47 minutes, with a range of 16 to 86 minutes (Van den Driessche et al., 1999). Newborns consuming breast milk can be hungry 30 to 60 minutes after a feeding. Newborns who frequently nurse are not using their mother as a pacifier. They are learning to feed. The amount of colostrum available meets their current physiologic stomach capacity. Providing bottles of water or formula after nursing is not based on sound scientific principles. There is no evidence in the literature to support this practice.

The newborn feeds on the first breast until he or she is satiated. The newborn is finished when he or she comes off the breast on its own after swallowing for most of the feeding. If the mother is uncertain whether the newborn is satisfied, she can use alternate massage (ie, massage and compress the breast each time there is a pause between sucking bursts). When the newborn no longer sucks and swallows when she squeezes the breast, he or she is done on that side. The mother can then burp the newborn and offer the other breast. There are no time limits on the duration of feedings. In the first days after birth, some newborns nurse only from one breast at a feeding. The other side is offered at the next feeding, usually within 1 or 2 hours. Feeding frequently encourages an abundant milk supply, minimizes engorgement and sore nipples, enhances weight gain, reduces jaundice and hypoglycemia, and increases breastfeeding duration. Display 13–5 lists behavioral signs that indicate the newborn is satiated after feeding. Observing these cues provides new parents with positive feedback that increases their confidence.

Nursing Assessment

Breastfeeding assessments may be brief or comprehensive, depending on where in the perinatal period the mother is encountered and on whether she or the newborn is having problems. The assessment should include a history of any surgery or breast trauma, as well as information about previous experiences with breastfeeding, knowledge level regarding the mechanics of breastfeeding, and finally a physical evaluation of the breast, and an observation of at least one breastfeeding episode. The breast is evaluated for protraction of the nipple. Approximately 10% of women have a truly inverted nipple (Alexander, Grant, & Campbell, 1992). A truly inverted nipple is one that retracts or dimples when gentle tactile stimulation is applied. This condition is caused by the presence of embryologic tissue behind the nipple and areola (Lawrence & Lawrence, 2005). For most women with truly inverted nipples, protraction of the nipple increases with breastfeeding and becomes more pronounced with subsequent pregnancies.

An initial assessment includes history of breastfeeding experience, problems with latch-on, sore nipples, engorgement, newborn weight gain, and amount and quality of social support. Knowing how long the mother exclusively breastfed other children, when or if she introduced pacifiers and or bottles, how satisfied she was with the feeding experience, and how long she plans to breastfeed this newborn provides insight into the mother's style and potential problem areas. Without proper evaluation, nursing interventions may be inappropriate or inadequate.

Signs of Adequate Intake

Evaluating the newborn for adequate intake is based on elimination patterns, weight gain, condition of the mucous membranes, and behavioral observations. Table 13–2 outlines elimination patterns for the early days of life. If the number of wet diapers or bowel

DISPLAY 13-5

Satiation Cues

- Gradual decrease in number of sucks over course of feeding
- Pursed lips followed by pulling away from the breast and releasing the nipple
- Relaxed body
- Legs extended
- Absence of hunger cues
- Sleep
- Small amount of milk drools from mouth
- Contented state

TABLE 13–2 ■ ELIMINATION PATTERN DURING THE FIRST WEEK OF LIFE

Age (days)	Number of Wet Diapers	Number of Bowel Movements
1	1–2	1
2	2–3	2
3	3–4	3–4
4	4–5	3–4
5	4–5	3 or more
6	6–8	3 or more
7	8 or more	3 or more

movements is below what is expected based on age, parents are instructed to notify their primary care provider. Wet diapers can be used to assess hydration, and the number of bowel movements serves as a caloric assessment. Urine should be clear and pale yellow. Because urine contains an abundance of uric acid crystals during the first week of life, occasionally a pink or rust-colored stain is apparent on the diaper. After the first week, presence of this pink stain is an indicator of insufficient intake. Super absorbent diapers make it difficult for some parents to tell when the diaper is wet. Parents can place a soft, dry paper towel, tissue, or square of toilet paper inside the diaper with each change to more easily tell when the diaper is wet. Table 13–3 describes the estimated volume of urine output over the first 2 months of life. Stools change from meconium to transitional stools to yellow, seedy liquid. Yellow stool should be present by the end of the first week. Some infants stool as frequently as every feeding for the first 4 to 6 weeks. Strang (2006) found that the more bowel movements a newborn has per day during the first 5 days of life is significantly associated with less weight loss, earlier transition to yellow bowel movements, earlier return to birth weight, and increased weight at 14 days of life.

Newborns should regain their birth weight by 2 weeks of age and continue to gain 4 to 7 ounces each week or at least a pound per month. Most experts believe that newborns should not lose more than 7% of their birth weights (Lawrence & Lawrence, 2005). Physical signs that the newborn is sufficiently hydrated include moist mucous membranes and skin that does not remain tented when pinched. The newborn should also demonstrate a range of behaviors during the day, including being alert, acting hungry, being fussy, and acting satisfied after feeding.

Assessment Tools

Common methods of documenting breastfeeding interactions do not always provide useful information. Subjective words such as well, fair, and poor do not capture the data needed to assess adequate intake or effectively identify problem areas. Similarly, the phrase "breastfeeding well" does not capture information regarding latch-on, audible swallow, time frames, or satiation. Numerous breastfeeding assessment tools assist the perinatal nurse by providing consistent guidelines for evaluating individual feeding events, ensuring continuity of care and communication between healthcare professionals, and providing a clear record in the chart of breastfeeding progress. One example of a breastfeeding assessment tool, the LATCH tool, is displayed in Table 13–4. Similar to an Apgar score, this tool assists the perinatal nurse to perform and document a thorough assessment and to identify areas where assistance and support are needed. There are other instruments being used clinically, for example, the Preterm Infant Breastfeeding Behavior Scale (PIBBS) was developed specifically for assessment of preterm infants. The instrument measures rooting, alveolar grasp, duration of latch, sucking, and swallowing (Hedberg & Ewold, 1999; Nvquist, Rubertsson, Ewald, & Sjoden, 1996). Selection of an assessment tool should be based on what it measures and whether it is appropriate for a given population. Keep in mind that many instruments need more research on their validity and reliability (Riordan & Koehn, 1997). It is important to monitor the literature, as new ones are being developed and there is ongoing refinement of existing ones.

Supplemental Feedings

Supplemental feedings for term, healthy, breastfed newborns are seldom necessary except for medical indications (AAP Committee on Nutrition, 2003). Illnesses in the mother or newborn that may require supplementation include inborn errors of metabolism, very-low-birth-weight infants, preterm infants, and certain medications being taken by the mother. Use of supplements without a medical indication is associated with earlier cessation of breastfeeding (Chezem, Friesen, Montgomery, Fortman, & Clark, 1998; Donnelly, Snowden, Renfrew, & Woolridge, 2000). Placing formula or water bottles in the bassinet or at the bedside of a breastfeeding mother sends a negative message about her ability to successfully breastfeed.

Use of Pacifiers and Artificial Nipples

Artificial nipples and pacifiers are associated with incorrect sucking techniques at the breast (Righard, 1998), decreased total duration of breastfeeding (Howard et al., 2003; Kramer et al., 2001; Nelson, Yu, & Williams, 2005), and fewer feeds in 24 hours (Aarts, Hornell, Kylberg, Hofvander, & Gebre-Medhin, 1999; Howard et al., 1999; Victora, Behague, Barros, Olinto, & Weiderpass, 1997). Pacifier and bottle use is sometimes an indicator of breastfeeding difficulties

TABLE 13–3 ■ ESTIMATED URINE VOLUME	
Age (days)	Volume (mL)
1–2	15–60
3–10	50–300
11–60	250–450

TABLE 13–4 ■ LATCH: BREASTFEEDING CHARTING SYSTEM

System Component	0	1	2
L Latch	Too sleepy or reluctant No latch achieved	Repeated attempts Hold nipple in mouth Stimulate to suck	Grasps breast Tongue down Lips flanged Rhythmic sucking
A Audible swallowing	None	A few with stimulation	Spontaneous and intermittent <24 hr old Spontaneous and frequent >24 hr old
T Type of nipple	Inverted	Flat	Everted (after stimulation)
C Comfort (breast/nipple)	Engorged Cracked, bleeding, large blisters or bruises Severe discomfort	Filling Reddened small blisters or bruises Mild or moderate discomfort	Soft Nontender
H Hold (positioning)	Full assist (staff holds infant at breast)	Minimal assist (ie, place pillows for support, elevate head of bed) Teach one side; mother does other Staff holds and then mother takes over	No assist from staff Mother able to position and hold baby

From Jensen, D., Wallace, S., & Kelsey, P. (1994). LATCH: A breastfeeding charting system and documentation tool. *Journal of Obstetric, Gynecologic, and Neonatal Nursing, 23*, 27–32.

(Benis, 2002; Kramer et al., 2001). Mothers who request bottles or pacifiers may be doing so because they lack appropriate knowledge about the effects of artificial nipples and pacifiers and confidence in their ability to successfully breastfeed. These women may benefit from contact with a skilled perinatal nurse or lactation consultant to assess the situation and provide appropriate support and education for the breastfeeding mother-infant dyad.

A Best Practice Guideline of six recently published articles reported that infants who do not use pacifiers at bedtime have a two- to fivefold increased risk for SIDS (Joanna Briggs Institute, 2005). The exact mechanism of protection is unknown, although some speculate it may be due to the pacifier protecting the airway, or perhaps it lessens the likelihood of sleep apnea. Ten additional studies were analyzed in this same guideline, and it was reported that infrequent pacifier use might not have an overall negative impact on breastfeeding outcomes. They also confirmed, however, that there was still evidence that early and regular use of a pacifier decreased breastfeeding duration. The AAP Task Force on Sudden Infant Death Syndrome (2005) says there is compelling evidence on the protective effect of pacifiers and recommends that parents consider offering a pacifier at nap and bedtime. For breastfed infants, however, pacifier introduction should be delayed until breastfeeding is well established (at least 1 month). To decrease risk of infection, pacifiers should be cleaned often and replaced regularly.

Hospital Discharge Packs

Many women in the United States come to the hospital expecting to receive some type of discharge "gift bag." The dilemma for perinatal nurses who support breastfeeding is that frequently these packs contain formula samples. Although research has not demonstrated that discharge packs with formula significantly decrease duration of breastfeeding (Bliss, Wilke, Acredolo, Berman, & Tebb, 1997; Dungy, Losch, Russell, Romitti, & Dusdieker, 1997), they are related to an increased risk that parents will introduce formula during the first 6 weeks of life, (Bliss, Wilkie, Acredolo, Berman, & Tebb, 1997; Donnelly, Snowden, Renfrew, & Woolridge, 2000). Ideally, a discharge pack given to breastfeeding women does not contain formula samples or coupons but instead has products that support breastfeeding, such as a manual pump, chemical cold packs, and breast pads.

POTENTIAL BREASTFEEDING PROBLEMS

Reluctant Nurser

Newborns are described as reluctant nursers when they latch on only after many attempts, move their head from side to side without latching on, fall asleep or aggressively push away from the breast and arch their back, have a preference for nursing only on one side, do not latch on, or latch on but feed ineffectively. Numerous factors can contribute to a newborn being reluctant to nurse (Display 13–6). Managing this situation requires that the nurse and parents be very patient and not give up on the newborn's ability to eventually latch on correctly and nurse efficiently. Table 13–5 identifies interventions that the nurse can use to encourage the newborn to latch on successfully.

Newborns should demonstrate at least one effective breastfeed before discharge. If the newborn has not latched-on at all by 24 hours, the mother should begin to express colostrum manually and feed with a syringe or cup. If the woman is unable to manually express colostrum, an electric or hand pump can be used as an alternative. These mothers should be referred to a lactation consultant for home follow-up and the primary care physician notified of the feeding difficulty.

DISPLAY 13-6

Factors Contributing to a Reluctant Nurser

- Poor position at the breast
- Interruption of the organized sequence of prefeeding behaviors immediately after birth
- Use of medications during labor that may prolong the period of state disorganization
- Hypertonia (ie, jaw clenching, pursed lips, neck and back hyperextension, and tongue retraction or elevation)
- Infrequent feeds leading to an overly hungry newborn baby
- Excessive or prolonged crying resulting in behavioral disorganization
- Interference with imprinting on the breast from separation, artificial nipples, pacifiers, or nipple shields
- Excessive pressure on the occipital region of the baby's head from pushing the head forward into the breast
- Vigorous or deep suctioning or intubation causing swelling or pain in the mouth or throat
- Ankyloglossia (tongue-tie)

Ankyloglossia (Tongue Tie)

The incidence of ankyloglossia in newborns ranges from 1.7% to 4.8%, with a male-to-female ratio of 2:1. (Ballard, Auer, & Khoury, 2002; Masaitis & Kaempf, 1996; Messner, Lalakea, Aby, Macmahon, & Blair, 2000). Untreated, it can lead to problems with latch-on and ultimately nipple pain and trauma. In one study, frenuloplasty (clipping the frenulum) of 35 infants diagnosed with ankyloglossia resulted in improved latch-on and less pain. At follow-up, 31 out of 35 of the mothers were still breastfeeding and reported satisfaction with the results (Ballard, Auer, & Khoury, 2002). Perinatal nurses should routinely assess the frenulum at birth and reassess should problems with latch-on and pain develop.

Nipple Pain

Sore nipples are common during the early days of breastfeeding. Pain or tenderness may occur in the following situations:

- When the baby first latches on, but pain disappears during the feeding after the baby starts swallowing
- Periodically during the feeding
- Throughout an entire feeding

Physical findings include vertical or horizontal red or white lines on the breast; fissures, cracks, or bleeding from the nipple; and blisters or scabs on one or both nipples. Use of formula and pacifiers in the hospital has been associated with nipple pain at the time of discharge (Centuori et al., 1999). Display 13–7 outlines factors that contribute to nipple pain. Transient nipple pain usually peaks between the third and sixth days postpartum. Prolonged or severe soreness beyond the first week requires intervention.

Various interventions can be used by the perinatal nurse to assist a woman experiencing nipple pain continuously or intermittently with feedings (Table 13–6). None of the treatments for nipple pain, including lanolin (Brent, Rudy, Redd, Rudy, & Roth, 1998; Centuori et al., 1999; Pugh et al., 1996), breast shells (Brent, Rudy, Redd, Rudy, & Roth, 1994), warm-water compresses (Buchko et al., 1994; Pugh et al., 1998), expressed breast milk (Buchko et al., 1994; Pugh et al., 1998), air-drying nipples (Buchko et al., 1994; Pugh et al., 1998, 1998), tea bags (Buchko et al., 1994), and hydrogel moist wound dressings (Brent, Rudy, Redd, Rudy, & Roth, 1998), have been shown to be more effective than any other (Morland-Schultz & Hill, 2005). With this in mind, women would probably benefit from being instructed to use the easiest and most economic treatments, which include expressing colostrum or breast milk on nipples after feedings, letting the nipples air dry, or using

TABLE 13–5 ■ TECHNIQUES TO ENCOURAGE LATCH-ON

Management	Rationale
Check positioning at the breast: • Newborn completely facing mother with head, neck, and spine aligned • Mouth directly in front of tip of nipple • Newborn brought to breast and held close • Mother does not lean forward, maneuver breast sideways, compress areola and insert it into the mouth, or tilt nipple up while attempting latch-on.	Poor positioning increases the number of latch attempts needed before obtaining milk, which can frustrate the mother and baby. Incorrect position increases the chances that the newborn will not latch correctly, leading to sore nipples, engorgement, insufficient milk production, and slow weight gain.
Position should be based on the newborn needs: • Infants who prefer the right side may need to be held in a football hold on the right breast and in a cradle or prone position for the left breast. • Some babies do better when the mother is in a side-lying position. • Breech babies may feed better sitting upright in the football hold. • Babies with birth trauma, such as a cephalohematoma, may be more comfortable and feed better when held with the affected side up. • Babies with a fractured clavicle may feed better in a football hold if the weight of the breast is kept off the chest or cradle hold with the affected side up.	Positioning in utero and events at birth may influence breastfeeding patterns. Several different positions need to be explored to find one that is satisfactory.

Keep the mother and baby together:
• After birth, allow the newborn time to seek and find the nipple before removing him from his mother's chest.
 	
• Place baby skin-to-skin on mother's chest.
• Instruct the mother to feed her baby on cue when:
  • He stirs
  • She sees rapid eye movements under the eyelids
  • She sees movements of the tongue and mouth
  • The newborn exhibits hand-to-mouth movements
  • The baby makes small sounds.
	This approach provides the opportunity for the prefeeding sequence of behaviors to occur, which increases the likelihood of proper attachment to the breasts.
	This approach reestablishes or repatterns the initial sucking sequence that may not have occurred immediately after birth.
	The mother can feel and see movements of feeding cues and place him to the breast when he is most likely to latch-on.

For a newborn making rapid side-to-side head movements: • Touch the midline of the upper lip with a dropper of colostrum. • Move him onto the breast as he follows the dropper to the nipple. • When his mouth is wide open, place a few drops of water or colostrum on his tongue to elicit sucking and swallowing.	The dropper acts to provide external control and food incentives to attach and suck at the breast.
A newborn who arches can be placed: • In the football hold • Or with the mother lying on her side.	Positioning helps the newborn to relax and flex the back and hips to avoid arching and jaw clenching.
Provide latch and sucking incentives: • A syringe placed in the side of the mouth can deliver a small amount of colostrum with each suck until the newborn demonstrates rhythmic suck and swallow at the breast. • A syringe or soft clinic dropper can be used to elicit sucking. • Butterfly tubing attached to a 10-mL syringe and taped to the breast can provide these incentives as well as a supplement if needed.	These methods help prevent baby from pulling away from the breast before he latches on or swallows. These interventions can calm the newborn and allow him to have a little food in his stomach so he is not so hungry.

(continued)

TABLE 13–5 ■ TECHNIQUES TO ENCOURAGE LATCH-ON (Continued)

Management	Rationale
After crying hard for a while, the newborn may not be able to organize himself to feed. • Allow him to suck on a finger. • Or place the tubing on a finger and allow him to suck a little colostrum by finger feeding before putting him to the breast. • If the newborn will not suck on a finger, place some colostrum in a medicine cup and have him sip from the cup until he calms down.	These interventions can calm the newborn and allow him to have a little food in his stomach so he is not so hungry.
If the newborn does not open his mouth wide enough for painless latch-on or clenches his jaw while latching-on: • Hold the jaw between your thumb and index finger • Move it gently a small amount from side to side.	This method helps inhibit jaw clenching.

warm, moist compresses to decrease discomfort. Colostrum and breast milk expressed on the nipple and areola have bacteriostatic qualities from the antibodies and anti-inflammatory factors, which assist in the healing process (Brent, Rudy, Redd, Rudy, & Roth, 1998; Pugh et al., 1996).

DISPLAY 13-7

Factors Contributing to Sore Nipples

- Transient pain while latching on may occur from lack of a keratin layer on the nipple epithelium.
- Unrelieved negative pressure is present until the milk ejection reflex occurs and is relieved by the periodic swallowing of the baby.
- Manipulation of the nipple and areola such as squeezing it, tilting or pointing it up or down, or pushing it into the mouth
- Mother leaning over to "insert" the breast into the newborn's mouth
- Nipple and areola may not be in the mouth symmetrically or far enough
- Lips curled under rather than flared out
- Tongue behind lower gum and pinching or biting of the nipple
- Breast pushed sideways into the mouth rather than centered over where the nipple points naturally
- Nipple confusion (ie, mouth configured for feeding on an artificial nipple or pacifier)
- Disorganized or dysfunctional sucking pattern
- Flat or retracted nipples
- Mouth not opened wide enough
- Ankyloglossia (tongue-tie)

Candida albicans

If the mother complains of burning pain on the nipple or burning and shooting pains in the breast, a fungal infection (ie, thrush) may be present. This is usually caused by *Candida albicans*. Predisposing factors for mothers include:

- Steroids (oral contraceptives, asthma medications)
- Broad-spectrum antibiotics
- Diabetes
- Obesity
- Poor endocrine function
- Infection in other family members or pets

Sources of *C. albicans* for newborns include:

- Vaginal canal
- Artificial bottle nipples
- Pacifiers
- Antibiotic use
- Hands of the nurse or parent
- Mechanical irritant in the mouth (ie, disruption of oral mucosa from suctioning)

During or after feedings, the mother may present with burning pain that does not improve with correct latch-on and positioning. She may have itching on the nipple or areola, with a pale or shiny spot on the areola and bright pink nipples. When *C. albicans* proliferates because of an upset in the balance of factors that normally keeps it in check, the usually noninvasive yeast can change to a fungus-like microbe that produces rhizoids. Rhizoids are long, root-like structures able to pierce duct walls and release toxins or allergens into nearby tissues, which may be responsible for the burning sensation and shooting pains deep in the breast.

TABLE 13–6 ■ INTERVENTIONS FOR SORE NIPPLES

Management	Rationale
Suggest that the mother initiate the milk ejection reflex or express drops of colostrum before latch-on.	Colostrum or milk flow prevents traumatic sucking by causing swallowing at the start of the feeding.
Review and correct positioning: • In the cradle hold, baby completely faces the mother and is held close with its legs wrapped around the mother's waist. • Four fingers are under the breast, and the thumb is on top, with all fingers off of the areola. • The baby is brought to the breast with his mouth centered over where the nipple points. • Touch the lips to the nipple. When infant's mouth opens to its widest point, the newborn is drawn the rest of the way onto the breast. • If the mouth does not open wide enough or if the nipple feels pinched, the mother can use the side of her index finger under her breast to gently pull down on the chin. This also rolls out the lower lip. • Some newborns that do not open wide enough may benefit from sucking on an adult's finger before feeds.	Proper positioning and latch techniques prevent or alleviate many of the problems with sore nipples. Proper positioning and latch-on can prevent or alleviate sore nipples. Pushing the breast sideways to the newborn may cause vertical cracks on either side of the nipple. Newborn must be brought close to the breast to facilitate enough of the areola being drawn into the mouth, rather than just the nipple tip. This technique helps draw into the mouth the portion of the breast needed to effect milk transfer without pain.
The mother can massage and compress the breast to initiate milk flow while waiting for the newborn to begin sucking. If the newborn pauses for long periods between sucking bursts, the mother can add the technique of alternate breast massage (ie, squeezing the breast when the newborn pauses).	Milk flow regulates sucking and alleviates unrelieved negative pressure when the baby is not swallowing periodically. Alternate massage provides milk incentives to start the suck and swallow sequence.
Avoid extension of the baby's back or neck; align the head and trunk. The mother can use the football hold or prone position for a high-tone newborn.	Extension causes jaw clenching, with the tongue moving behind the lower gum.
The mother should avoid the tendency to depress the top of the breast or areola under the newborn's nose to create an airway. A properly positioned baby should have the tip of the nose touching the breast and can breathe without assistance. The mother should also avoid the scissors hold on the areola, which compresses it and flattens on inverted nipple.	The incorrect method pulls the nipple and areola out of the mouth and contributes to nipple sucking and blisters.
Feedings should occur on cue 8–12 times each 24 hours. Avoid trying to lengthen time intervals between feeds or feeding a bottle at night.	Feeding frequently avoids frantic, overly hungry pulling at the breast. Full, firm breasts make latch-on more difficult and painful.
Breast milk can be applied to the nipples after feeding. Avoid creams, lotions, oils, and ointments unless medically indicated. Warm water compresses may also provide relief.	Some commercial preparations slow the healing process.
Avoid pacifiers, artificial nipples on bottles, and nipple shields. Use alternative devices for supplemental feeds if needed (eg, cup, syringe, dropper, feeding tube devices).	Some devices prevent incorrect patterning of mouth conformation. Artificial nipples do not elongate and compress like a human nipple. Their use weakens a baby's suck as the baby decreases sucking pressure to slow milk and regulate milk flow.

The newborn presents with white patches (ie, "crumbling curds") on the buccal mucosa, gums, or tongue that can travel to the hard and soft palate and down to the tonsils. It may also appear as pearly white or gray patches. If a patch is removed, a bright red base may be seen as a painfully eroded area. Most babies with thrush in the mouth also have the infection in the intestines and stools, which contributes to a *Candida*-caused diaper rash. Some newborn's mouths are colonized with *C. albicans*, but it is not clinically apparent. They may be fussy, have a poor appetite, breastfeed poorly, and experience general discomfort.

The treatment depends on the location and severity of the infection. Treatment of the mother and newborn simultaneously is important, even if only one has clinical symptoms. Topical antifungals are used to treat skin *Candida*. Antifungal topical cream or lotion can be applied to the breast and nipple before and after each feeding. They can also be applied to the diaper area of the newborn and after breastfeeding to the newborn's mouth. Gentian violet in a weak aqueous solution of 0.5% to 1% can be directly applied to the nipple and areola and to the baby's mouth once each day for 3 to 7 days. However, mothers should be forewarned that it stains the skin/mucous membranes purple. The treatment for resistant or systemic candidiasis is oral fluconazole (200 to 400 mg), followed by 100 to 200 mg/day for 14 to 21 days (Hale, 2004; Hoover, 1999).

Jaundice

Early-onset jaundice appears after 24 hours of age, peaking on the third or fourth day of life, and steadily declines through the first month to normal levels. Clinical signs of hyperbilirubinemia are present in 50% to 60% of all term newborns. Concentrations of unconjugated bilirubin can increase if production exceeds processing capabilities. Meconium is a reservoir for large amounts of unconjugated bilirubin that is reabsorbed into the circulation if there is a delay in eliminating the meconium. Failure to clear meconium quickly enhances enteric reabsorption and increases serum bilirubin levels. The laxative effect of colostrum promotes the rapid evacuation of meconium and reduces the unconjugated bilirubin available for reabsorption. Some hospital routines contribute to high bilirubin levels in breastfed newborns. Systems that do not promote rooming-in decrease the number of feedings, as do scheduled feeds. Newborns given the most sugar water have the highest bilirubin levels (Kuhr & Paneth, 1982). Dextrose (5%) water has 6 calories per ounce, and colostrum has 18 calories per ounce. For every ounce of sugar water consumed, the newborn has a deficit in two-thirds of the calories he needs to prevent intestinal reabsorption of bilirubin. Early

exaggeration of physiologic jaundice can be reduced or eliminated by effective breastfeeding management that includes 8 to 12 feedings each 24 hours. The number of effective breastfeedings per day influences the number of stools. The more stools that occur and the sooner the newborn transitions to yellow bowel movements, the less risk there is for hyperbilirubinemia (Shrago, 2006).

The technique of alternate breast massage has been used to increase milk supply when the newborn is sleepy or feeds inefficiently. When the mother notices that the newborn's rapid, shallow suckling movements decrease, she massages the base of her breast. She then alternates massaging the breast between periods of suckling.

The decision to begin phototherapy is complicated by the fact that the level of bilirubin that causes kernicterus is unknown and may differ from one newborn to another. After the first 48 hours of life, a healthy term newborn may not require phototherapy or interruption of breastfeeding until total serum bilirubin concentrations exceed 18 to 20 mg/dL. Management options when bilirubin levels go above 18 to 20 mg/dL include the following (Dixit & Gartner, 1999):

- Increasing the number of times during the day the newborn breastfeeds
- Use of alternate breast massage on each breast during feedings
- Pumping breast milk and giving it by cup as a supplement after nursing
- Phototherapy

In late-onset jaundice (ie, breastmilk jaundice), physiologic bilirubin levels decline at the end of the first week and then rise again, sometimes to much higher levels than originally. In rare situations, bilirubin levels may climb to 25 mg/dL or higher. Late-onset jaundice is thought to be caused by a component in the mother's milk that inhibits conjugation of bilirubin by the liver (Guthrie & Auerbach, 1999). Studies have demonstrated that there is a higher fat content in the milk of mothers whose newborns developed late-onset jaundice. If one infant develops late-onset jaundice, there is a high probability that subsequent infants born to the same mother will be affected. To determine whether a newborn has late-onset jaundice, a bilirubin level is assessed, and the mother is asked to formula-feed for 24 hours, after which a second bilirubin level is determined. If the bilirubin level has begun to decrease a diagnosis of late-onset or breastmilk jaundice is made. No treatment is necessary for late-onset jaundice (Gartner, 1994).

Hypoglycemia

Hypoglycemia in a term newborn usually refers to a blood glucose level below 40 mg/dL. This is a common and usually transient occurrence in the immediate newborn period. Routine monitoring of blood glucose concentration in healthy term newborns is unnecessary (AAP, 1993). Conditions that increase the risk for hypoglycemia include small for gestational age; the smaller of twins; large for gestational age; having a low birth weight or being the infant of a diabetic mother; having asphyxia, polycythemia, erythroblastosis fetalis, respiratory distress, or hypothermia; or any condition during pregnancy that contributes to under- or overnourishment in utero such as maternal hypertension, congenital defects, excessive maternal weight gain, or pre-pregnancy BMI (Johnson, 2003).

Hypoglycemia in breastfed newborns can be prevented or greatly reduced by hospital policies that support breastfeeding:

- Breastfeeding within an hour of birth
- Skin-to-skin contact between mother and newborn to prevent cold stress and use of glucose stores
- Breastfeeding 8 to 12 times per day
- Feeding in response to readiness cues, not on a schedule
- Not leaving the newborn to cry (ie, prolonged crying rapidly depletes glycogen stores and can contribute to a steep decline in blood sugar levels)
- Pump or hand expressing colostrum into a spoon or cup for the newborn reluctant to suckle at the breast and feeding the newborn colostrum every 1–2 hours until he or she is able to feed effectively at the breast

Hypoglycemia that recurs or persists longer than 48 to 72 hours of age may be caused by hyperinsulinemia, an underlying medical condition and is not related to feeding. Hypoglycemia in an asymptomatic infant that does not respond to oral feeding or in a symptomatic infant usually necessitates intravenous glucose infusions. The mother should be encouraged to hand express or pump colostrum for oral feeds (by cup or spoon if the medical condition permits) to maintain a milk supply while the newborn is not nursing.

Engorgement

Lawrence and Lawrence (2005) describe engorgement of the breast in terms of three elements: congestion and vascularity, accumulation of milk, and edema caused by the swelling and obstruction of drainage of the lymphatic system. Engorgement can involve the areola, the body of the breast, or both areas. Areolar engorgement may be caused by distended lactiferous sinuses or reflect edema from large amounts of intravenous fluids infused during labor. Some amount of engorgement is normal. No engorgement is a sign of a problem that requires close follow-up. It may be related to retained placental fragments or minimal breast tissue growth during pregnancy. If intravenous fluids cause areolar engorgement, the areola may appear puffy and is responsive to cold-pack application. If distended with milk, the areola may envelop the nipple, and the whole unit becomes difficult for the newborn to grasp. The mother should hand express some milk before putting the baby to breast to avoid tissue damage and pain (Lawrence & Lawrence, 2005).

Peripheral engorgement usually does not develop until 2 to 3 days after birth. Some swelling of the entire breast is normal, but if the breasts become hard, red, hot, shiny, and throbs, physiologic engorgement has changed to pathologic engorgement. This can be extremely painful, and the mother needs to breastfeed very frequently using gentle, alternate massage. Hand expression may provide relief, and some women are made more comfortable by using ice packs, a bag of frozen peas wrapped around the breast, or application of chilled or room-temperature cabbage leaves. It is important to nurse even when engorged because prolonged milk stasis increases the risk of mastitis, is a major cause of insufficient milk, and contributes to sore nipples, poor latch-on, reduced milk transfer, and slow weight gain by the infant. Separating mothers and babies, especially at night, giving unnecessary supplements, skipping night feedings, and long intervals between feeds exacerbates the problem of engorgement. It is vital to maintain frequent and thorough drainage of the breasts at this time. Back pressure in the ducts can lead to atrophy of the milk secreting cells.

Plugged Duct and Mastitis

Small, tender breast lumps, the size of a pea, are sometimes encountered by breastfeeding mothers. Milk stasis or a component of the milk may contribute to this. The application of hot packs and massaging the lump while the baby is sucking helps move this blockage. Some women experience repeated plugging of ducts and describes fatty strings being expressed from the breast.

Continued milk stasis increases the risk for mastitis. Mastitis is an inflammatory condition of the breast that may or may not eventually or concurrently involve an infection. Display 13–8 describes symptoms of mastitis. When symptoms become severe, most clinicians treat with antibiotics. Although antibiotics treat the infection, they do not address the underlying cause of the mastitis. Antibiotic therapy must be accompanied by interventions to identify and correct the cause. Early identification of the cause and the use of appropriate interventions may halt the inflammatory process

DISPLAY 13-8

Symptoms of Mastitis

- Fever >38°C (100.4°F)
- Flulike symptoms (eg, aching, chills)
- Feeling progressively worse
- Tenderness under the arm
- Pain or swelling at the site
- Red, hot, hard area that is often wedge shaped
- Red streaks extending from the lump toward the axilla
- Recent events that increase risk of mastitis (cracked or bleeding nipples, stress or getting run down, missed feedings, longer intervals between feedings)

and prevent progression of an infection. Pain and inflammation at this point can be treated with a nonsteroidal anti-inflammatory drug such as ibuprofen. If there is no improvement within 8 to 24 hours and the mother has signs of a bacterial infection such as a discharge of pus from the nipple, continued fever, or a sudden spike of fever, she should contact her primary care provider immediately. Because *Staphylococcus aureus* is most commonly associated with breast infections, choices of antibiotics are generally penicillinase-resistant penicillins or cephalosporins that are effective against this organism. These antibiotics are safe, and the mother should continue breastfeeding frequently from the affected side (Lawrence & Lawrence, 2005).

Insufficient Milk

Real or perceived insufficient milk supply is the most common reason for premature weaning. Qualitative research during the early postpartum period revealed that women become increasingly confident and empowered by breastfeeding or that their confidence progressively diminished as they expressed concerns about the adequacy of their breast milk. The perception of breast milk inadequacy was related to inability to quantify and visualize the amount of breast milk, anxiety about the adequacy of their own diet, inadequate and conflicting advice from healthcare professionals, and unmet needs for support and nurturing for themselves (Dykes & Williams, 1999).

A small percentage of women produce insufficient milk for psychologic, physiologic, or pathologic reasons. Psychologic, physiologic, and pathologic factors can lead to decreased production and ejection of milk (Biancuzzo, 2000). Psychological factors include stress, embarrassment, and pain, all of which may increase production of epinephrine, which causes blood vessels to constrict, and also decreases produc-

tion of oxytocin, which facilitates let-down. Physiologic factors include maternal illness, severe postpartum bleeding (Sheehan's syndrome), breast surgery (ie, reduction and augmentation), and conditions that interfere with the early, effective, and consistent stimulating of the breasts, such as restrictions on frequency and duration of feedings, more than 3 hours between feedings, skipping night feedings, and use of supplements. Pathologic factors that negatively affect milk production are related to endocrine problems. Mothers often describe perceived insufficient milk when they experience one or more of the following:

- Baby does not settle or fusses after a feeding.
- Baby wants to feed frequently (ie, growth spurt).
- Baby takes formula from a bottle directly after breastfeeding.
- Mother is unable to express much milk.
- Baby does not sleep through the night or is awake much of the day.
- Breasts are smaller and softer than they should be.
- Initial weight loss of baby after birth is a concern.

Strategies to handle real or perceived insufficient milk depend on the cause of the problem. Mismanagement of breastfeeding is the most common contributor to low milk production. This problem is usually revealed during a feeding history. Mothers should be breastfeeding 8 to 12 times each 24 hours with no supplements or pacifiers. A feeding observation is necessary to confirm whether the newborn is swallowing milk or simply engaging in nonnutritive sucking. Mothers should perform alternate massage and feed at closer intervals to increase milk production. Refer mothers to a lactation consultant for a thorough breastfeeding assessment and follow-up.

MEDICATIONS AND BREASTFEEDING

Interruption of breastfeeding for women who are taking medications is usually an unnecessary and potentially damaging recommendation. Most medications have few side effects because the dose received by the newborn is usually less than 1% of the maternal dose and may be poorly bioavailable to the newborn. Antimetabolites and therapeutic doses of radiopharmaceuticals are examples of medications that are contraindicated. If a medication is necessary for only a short time, women can be assisted to pump and dispose of their milk until it is safe for the newborn to nurse. Ideally, newborns can be syringe or cup fed during this time. There are several excellent sources providing information on the safe use of medications for breastfeeding women (Display 13–9).

DISPLAY 13-9

References for Medications and Breastfeeding

- Briggs, G. G., Freeman, R. K., & Yaffee, S. J. (Eds.). (2002). *Drugs in pregnancy and lactation* (6th ed.) Philadelphia: Lippincott Williams & Wilkins.
- American Academy of Pediatrics. (2003). *Pediatric nutrition handbook* (5th ed.). Elk Grove Village, IL: Author.
- Hale T. (2004). *Medications and mother milk: A manual of lactational pharmacology* (11th ed.). Amarillo, TX: Pharmasoft Medical Publishing.
- Lactation Fax Hotline, 24-hour fax-on-demand, registration required (806-356-9556)
- Lactation Studies Center, Rochester, NY (716-275-0088)
- Rocky Mountain Drug Consultation Center, Denver, CO (900-285-3784)
- University of California at San Diego Drug Information Service, San Diego, CA (900-288-8273)

POSTPARTUM SURGERY AND BREASTFEEDING

Occasionally, a woman needs surgery while still breastfeeding. When this occurs, she may be advised to stop breastfeeding for a variety of reasons such as the mother's condition, the mother's medications, the lack of caregiver knowledge, or the inability to room in with the infant. Ideally, everything should be done to help the woman continue breastfeeding if that is her choice. Ideally, lactating women admitted to a medical or surgical unit should be seen by a lactation consultant. The staff and the mother often need education on use of the breast pump and the recommended schedule for pumping. If the milk is still safe for the infant, additional education is needed on the storage of the milk. The perinatal nurse and lactation experts have the responsibility of letting other units and physicians know of their availability for consultation.

FORMULA FEEDING

Use of a commercially prepared, iron-fortified infant formula is another method of providing neonatal nutrition during the first year of life. Use of formula is indicated for newborns in the following situations (AAP Committee on Nutrition, 2003):

- When their mother chooses not to breastfeed or not to breastfeed exclusively

- In the presence of maternal infections caused by organisms that may be transmitted through human milk
- If the newborn is diagnosed with an inborn error of metabolism causing intolerance to components of human milk, such as galactosemia or tyrosinemia
- When the mother has been exposed to foods, medications, or environmental agents that are excreted in human milk and may be harmful to the newborn (eg, drugs of abuse, antineoplastics, mercury, lead)
- After exposure to radioactive compounds requiring temporary cessation of breastfeeding
- As supplementation to breast milk when the newborn does not demonstrate adequate weight gain

Parents may benefit from an understanding that newborns fed formula have a greater risk of acute and chronic illness, allergies, and obesity. Parents with a family history of allergy or diabetes should be carefully counseled regarding the possible outcomes from the use of formula. Cow's milk; goat's milk; 1%, 2%, or fat-free milk; and evaporated milk are not recommended during the first year of life (AAP Committee on Nutrition, 2003). These milk products do not contain adequate iron concentration, increase the renal solute load because of the amount of protein, sodium, potassium, and chloride, and may result in deficiencies in essential fatty acids, vitamin E, and zinc (AAP Committee on Nutrition, 2003). Direct advertising of infant formulas to the public is a violation of the World Health Organization code and discouraged by the AAP. This important information should be provided to the woman in an objective manner. Some women may choose not to breastfeed. The purpose of the discussion is not to make them feel guilty about their choice.

Composition of Formula

Commercially prepared formula can never totally duplicate the hormones, immunologic agents, enzymes, and live cells found in human milk. In 1980, Congress passed the first Infant Formula Act, which was later revised in 1986. This legislation set minimum and maximum levels of certain nutrients and required that manufactures analyze all batches of formula and state on the labels the concentration of specific nutrients.

The concentrations of nutrients in formula vary slightly between manufacturers and are usually slightly higher in formula than in breast milk to compensate for the possible lower bioavailability (AAP Committee on Nutrition, 2003). Although formula companies may be able to provide a rationale for their individual differences, large, randomized clinical trials supporting their conclusions do not exist. Most formulas use cow's milk as the protein base. Because some newborns develop formula intolerance and some families are aware of existing milk intolerance, formula companies manufacture alternative formulas of special composition for newborns with gastrointestinal or metabolic disturbances.

Milk-Based Formula

Formula development and improvement is an ongoing challenge. Recent changes have been made to make the formulas more closely resemble breast milk. For example, there have been changes in the whey:casein ratio, the quantity of nucleotides, and the addition of long-chain polyunsaturated fatty acids (Schuman, 2003). Animal fat in cow's milk has been replaced with vegetable oils in order to improve digestibility and absorption, eliminate cholesterol, increase the concentration of essential fatty acids, and reduce environmental pollutants (AAP Committee on Nutrition, 2003). The major source of carbohydrate in human milk and formula is lactose. The presence of lactose in the bowel is responsible for proliferation of acidophilic bacterial flora necessary to prevent the growth of pathogenic organisms. Most formulas are fortified with iron, minerals, and electrolytes such as calcium, phosphorus, magnesium, sodium, potassium, and chloride. Cow's milk is the source of most minerals and electrolytes, although some are added as inorganic salts.

Milk-based formulas are available for newborns with special needs. Newborns requiring a lower renal solute load, such as those with cardiovascular or renal disease, can use formulas containing low levels of minerals and electrolytes. Newborns who experience lactose intolerance or a family history of lactose intolerance can be given a lactose-free formula in which glucose rather than lactose is the carbohydrate source. Because this formula contains very small amounts of lactose, it should not be given to newborns with galactosemia. There are also milk-based formulas in which the fat content has been lowered for newborns with fat malabsorption, bile duct obstruction, or severe cholestasis. Newborns who cannot digest protein (eg, cystic fibrosis, short gut syndrome, biliary atresia, cholestasis, and protracted diarrhea) or are severely allergic to cow's milk protein can receive formula in which the protein has been treated with heat and enzymes, decreasing the potential allergic response.

Soy Formulas

Soy formulas are used for newborns allergic to cow's milk proteins and by vegetarians. Although the major source of protein is soy, it is possible for a newborn allergic to cow's milk protein to also demonstrate an allergic reaction to soy protein. Soy formulas are also free of lactose and are recommended for newborns

with lactase deficiency or galactosemia. The carbohydrate source in these formulas is sucrose.

Preterm Human Milk Modifiers

A recent achievement is the development of human milk modifiers to feed preterm and very-low-birth-weight infants (Schuman, 2003). The APA Policy Statement on Breastfeeding and the Use of Human Milk (2005) recommends the use of human milk fortifiers containing protein, minerals, and vitamins to ensure preterm human milk meets the nutritional needs for very-low-birth-weight newborns.

Mechanics of Formula Feeding

The perinatal nurse should ensure that parents who choose to use commercially prepared formula have sufficient information and are doing so safely. Display 13–10

D I S P L A Y   1 3 - 1 0

Guidelines for Parents Using Formula

- Parents should be cautioned to read the formula package labels carefully. On occasion, parents have accidentally diluted ready-to-feed formula or fed concentrated formula without first diluting it.
- The American Academy of Pediatrics recommends boiling water before mixing it in milk (or using sterile bottled water).
- Purchase cans that are not damaged. Check the expiration date and wash the top of the can before opening.
- Wash bottles and artificial nipples in hot, soapy water or a dishwasher. Scrub bottles and nipples with a brush to loosen formula residue that adheres to crevices where bacteria may grow.
- Do not prop bottles or use products that hold a bottle in the newborn's mouth. This practice may contribute to ear infections, dental caries, choking, and aspiration.
- Newborns should be held during feedings.
- Formula does not need to be heated. It can be prepared and used at room temperature.
- Heating formula in a microwave oven can be dangerous. The microwave does not heat evenly, causing "hot spots" in the milk. The bottle should be shaken gently after heating so the temperature of the milk is evenly dispersed, and sprinkling a few drops on the wrist should test the temperature of the milk.
- Once a can of formula has been opened or a bottle of powder formula mixed, it should be stored in the refrigerator and used within 48 hours.
- Formula remaining in a bottle after the newborn has finished drinking should be discarded, because it is an excellent medium for bacterial growth.

contains instructions for parents who choose to feed their newborns with formula. The primary healthcare provider can recommend the most appropriate formula. Formula is available as ready-to-feed, concentrated preparation to be diluted with water or as a powder to be mixed with water. Powdered mixes are more economical than ready-to-feed solutions, although it has been suggested that mixing water into the feeding may not always be done properly. In one trial, less than half of the mothers mixed the feeding correctly, and 26% offered overly concentrated feedings, with the potential for serious consequence such as diarrhea (Lucas, Lockton, & Davies, 1992). Oral water intoxication can be the outcome of mixing too much water with the formula to stretch its availability or of offering water bottles to extend feeding times or to calm a fussy baby. These babies may present to the emergency room with seizures and apnea (Keating, Schears, & Dodge, 1991).

For a long time the AAP felt municipal water supplies did not require boiling prior to mixing with formula. However, due to the contamination of Milwaukee's water in 1993, recommendations were changed and the Academy now recommends boiling water when preparing infant formulas. Use of bottled water is also possible, as long as it is sterile (not all bottled water is sterilized; AAP Committee on Nutrition, 2003).

Standard commercially prepared formula contains 20 kcal/ounce and can be offered to newborns on demand. During the first 3 months of life, intake is approximately 150 to 200 mL/kg each day (AAP Committee on Nutrition, 2003). This provides 100 to 135 kcal/kg per day. Weight gain should be approximately 25 to 30 g/day. Additional water is not necessary in the diet of a newborn.

Parents can begin feeding 0.5 ounce of formula at each feeding during the first 24 hours of life. During the next 24 hours, the feedings can be increased by 0.5-ounce increments, feeding the same volume for two to three feedings before increasing. Parents should not force the baby to finish the bottle and should feed on cue when the baby shows signs of hunger. The newborn should be burped after every 0.5 ounces or halfway through the feeding. The baby should be held at about a 45-degree angle, making sure to keep the nipple full of formula. After a can of formula has been opened, the contents should be stored in the refrigerator and used within 48 hours. Any formula remaining in the feeding bottle should be discarded, because it is an excellent medium for bacterial growth.

There is evidence that feeding position may be responsible for the increased incidence of otitis media in bottle-fed newborns (Tully, 1998). Supine feeding, positioning the newborn in a horizontal position, or propping the bottle for feeding has been associated with reflux of milk into the Eustachian tubes. Researchers have identified a significant difference in the number of abnormal postfeeding tympanogram results when infants were fed in the supine position compared with those fed in the semi-upright position (Tully, Bar-Haim, & Bradley, 1995). Information such as this should be shared with parents choosing to bottle feed along with the following recommendations (Tully, 1998):

- Sit in a comfortable armchair while feeding to reduce arm fatigue.
- Rest the newborn's head in the crook of the elbow, with its head facing the nipple (a position similar to the breastfeeding newborn).
- Avoid putting the newborn to bed with a bottle.
- Do not prop bottles.
- Keep the newborn upright after feeding for about 15 minutes before placing him or her in a supine position to sleep.

The perception of formula intolerance by parents and healthcare providers is usually related to symptoms of constipation, fussiness, abdominal cramps, and excessive spit-up or vomiting (Lloyd et al., 1999). In one study, the concentration of palm oil was reported to be responsible for perception of constipation. Using two different formulas to wean newborns from breast milk, the group receiving the formula containing palm oil had a decreased total number of stools, and they were firmer (Lloyd et al.). Specific formula also influences the color of stools, making them more yellow and green, unlike breast-milk stools, which are usually brown.

LACTATION SUPPRESSION

In postpartum women who are not breastfeeding, milk leakage and breast pain begin 1 to 3 days postpartum, and engorgement begins between 1 to 4 days postpartum. Considerable pain may be experienced during this time. Various interventions have been suggested for many years to decrease milk leakage and pain associated with lactation suppression, but no interventions are supported by randomized, controlled clinical research. However, several interventions may make women more comfortable during this period. Women should be advised to:

- Wear a well-fitting bra or sport bra 24 hours each day until the breasts are soft and nontender. (Historically, breast binding has been recommended for this purpose. However, there is evidence that breast binding may lead to greater tenderness, leakage, and pain [Swift & Janke, 2003]).
- Apply cold packs to the breasts.
- Use mild over-the-counter analgesics taken according to manufacturers' recommendations.

• Avoid nipple or breast stimulation (however, in extreme situations, putting the baby to breast, hand expressing, or pumping a small amount of milk may provide relief).

Restricting fluids is neither necessary nor desirable. The breasts return to normal and tenderness decreases within 48 to 72 hours after engorgement occurs.

SUMMARY

The abundance of research on breastfeeding and human lactation clearly shows the importance of breastfeeding, the side effects of newborn formula use, and the evidence that many traditional newborn feeding practices have no scientific or physiologic validity. Parents and health professionals should be aware of this information. Healthcare professionals have an obligation to support changes in practice that have been shown to remove institutional barriers to breastfeeding. Clinical nurse specialists, educators, nurse managers, lactation consultants, hospital administra-

tors, and physicians can take steps to see that breastfeeding is supported in their institution.

The Association of Women's Health, Obstetric and Neonatal Nurses (2007) supports breastfeeding as the optimal method of feeding and challenges its membership to foster environments that support breastfeeding. Display 13–11 identifies the responsibilities of nurses who care for women and newborns in the prenatal and postpartum periods. Many hospitals have chosen to model their policies and protocols after the Ten Steps to Successful Breastfeeding (Display 13–12; Saadeh & Akre, 1996). This set of recommendations can facilitate successful breastfeeding by all women. In 2006, there were 52 hospitals and birthing centers in the United States, and in 2005 there were four hospitals and birthing centers in Canada that were designated "baby-friendly hospitals."

The AAP Committee on Nutrition (2003) recommends the introduction of solid foods for all infants between 4 and 6 months of age. Breast milk and formula should continue until the infant reaches 1 year of age. Ideally, the decision about the feeding method is a health decision. This choice has a significant effect on

---

DISPLAY 13-11

Role of the Nurse in the Promotion of Breastfeeding

• Attain knowledge about the benefits of breastfeeding. This should include anatomy and physiology of lactation, initiation of lactation, and management of common concerns and problems.
• As part of preconception counseling, review the benefits of breastfeeding.
• Provide breastfeeding education to all women during the prenatal period. This education should explore concerns, fears, and myths that may inhibit successful breastfeeding.
• Work in collaboration with lactation specialists and other healthcare providers to optimize the breastfeeding experience for the mother and infant.
• Integrate culturally appropriate and sensitive information into all breastfeeding education.
• Ensure that breastfeeding is initiated in the immediate postpartum period whenever possible.
• Promote nonseparation of mother and baby during the postpartum period.
• Provide information about breastfeeding resources in the community at the time of hospital or birthing center discharge.
• Use and conduct research related to breastfeeding.

From Association of Women's Health, Obstetric and Neonatal Nursing. (1999). *The role of the nurse in the promotion of breastfeeding.* Washington, DC: Author.

DISPLAY 13-12

Ten Steps to Successful Breastfeeding

1. Have a written breastfeeding policy that is routinely communicated to all healthcare staff.
2. Educate healthcare providers in skills necessary to implement this policy.
3. Inform all pregnant women about the benefits and management of breastfeeding.
4. Help mothers initiate breastfeeding within one-half hour of birth.
5. Show mothers how to breastfeed and how to maintain lactation even when they are separated from their newborns.
6. Give newborns no food or drink other than breast milk, unless medically indicated.
7. Allow mothers and newborns to remain together 24 hours each day.
8. Encourage breastfeeding on demand.
9. Give no artificial teats or pacifiers to breastfeeding newborns.
10. Foster the establishment of breastfeeding support groups, and refer mothers to them on discharge from the hospital or clinic.

WHO/UNICEF Joint Statement. (1989). *Protecting and supporting breastfeeding: The special role of maternity services.* Geneva: World Health Organization.

the health and development of the newborn, health of the mother, and cost of illness to the healthcare system. Breastfeeding saves millions of dollars each year by preventing disease. The perinatal nurse's interactions with families should reflect promotion, protection, and support of breastfeeding as the normal and natural way to feed a newborn.

REFERENCES

Aarts, C., Hornell, A., Kylberg, E., Hofvander, Y., & Gebre-Medhin, M. (1999). Breastfeeding patterns in relation to thumb sucking and pacifier use. *Pediatrics, 104*(4), E50.

Alexander, J. M., Grant, A. M., & Campbell, M. J. (1992). Randomized controlled trial of exercises for inverted and non-protractile nipples. *British Medical Journal, 304*(6833), 1030–1032.

Almroth, S. G. (1978). Water requirements of breastfed infants in a hot climate. *American Journal of Clinical Nutrition, 31*(7), 1154–1157.

American Academy of Pediatrics. (1993). Routine evaluation of blood pressure, hematocrit and glucose in newborns. *Pediatrics, 92*(3), 474–476.

American Academy of Pediatrics Committee on Nutrition. (2003). *Pediatric nutrition handbook* (5th ed.). Elk Grove Village, IL: Author.

American Academy of Pediatrics Task Force on Sudden Infant Death Syndrome. (2005). The changing concept of Sudden Infant Death Syndrome: Diagnostic coding shifts, controversies regarding the sleeping environment, and new variables to consider in reducing risk. *Pediatrics, 116*(5), 1245–1255.

American Academy of Pediatrics Workgroup on Breastfeeding. (2005). Breastfeeding and the use of human milk. *Pediatrics, 115*(2), 496–506.

American Academy of Family Physicians. (2006). Breastfeeding. (Position paper). Retrieved March 22, 2006, from http:/www.aafp.org/x6633.xml?printxml

American College of Obstetricians and Gynecologists [ACOG]. (2000). *Breastfeeding: Maternal and infant aspects.* Washington, DC: Author.

Anderson, G. C., Moore, E., Hepworth, J., & Bergman, N. (2005). Early skin-to-skin contact for mothers and their healthy newborn infants. Cochrane Database of Systematic Reviews. *Cochrane Collaboration, 4.*

Anderson, J. W., Johnstone, B. M., & Remley, D. T. (1999). Breastfeeding and cognitive development: A meta-analysis. *American Journal of Clinical Nutrition, 70*(4), 525–535.

Angelsen, N. K., Vik, T., Jacobsen, G., & Bakketeig, L.S. (2001). Breast feeding and cognitive development at age 1 & 5 years. *Archives of Diseases in Childhood., 85*(3), 183–188.

Aniansson G, Alm B., & Andersson, B. (1994). A prospective cohort study on breastfeeding and otitis media in Swedish infants. *Pediatric Infectious Disease Journal, 13*(6), 183–188.

Arifeen, S., Black, R. E., Antelman, G., Baqui, A., Caulfield, L., & Becker, S. (2001). Exclusive breastfeeding reduces acute respiratory infection and diarrhea deaths among infants in Dhaka slums. *Pediatrics, 108*(4), E67.

Arnold L. D. (2002). The cost-effectiveness of using banked donor milk in the neonatal intensive care unit: Prevention of necrotizing enterocolitis. *Journal of Human Lactation, 18*(2), 172–177.

Armstrong, J., Reilly, J. J., Child Health Information Team. (2002). Child Health Information Team: Breastfeeding and lowering the risk of childhood obesity. *Lancet, 359*(9322), 2003–2004.

Arthur, P. G., Kent, J. C., & Hartmann, P. E. (1994). Metabolites of lactose synthesis in milk from diabetic and non-diabetic women during Lactogenesis II. *Journal of Pediatric Gastroenterology and Nutrition, 19*(1), 100–108.

Association of Women's Health Obstetric and Neonatal Nursing. (1999). *The role of the nurse in the promotion of breastfeeding.* Washington, DC: Author.

Bachrach, V. R., Schwarz, E., & Bachrach, L. R. (2003). Breastfeeding and the risk of hospitalization for respiratory disease in infancy: A meta analysis. *Archives of Pediatrics & Adolescent Medicine, 157*(3), 237–243.

Baker, J. L., Michaelsen, K. F., Rasmussen, K., & Sorensen, T. I. (2005). Maternal prepregnant body mass index, duration of breastfeeding, and timing of complementary food introduction are associated with infant weight gain. *American Journal Clinical Nutrition, 80*(6), 1579–1588.

Ball, T. M., & Wright, A. L. (1999). Health care costs of formula-feeding in the first year of life. *Pediatrics, 103*(4, Pt. 2), 870–876.

Balcazar, H., Trier, C. M., & Cobas, J. A. (1995). What predicts breastfeeding intention in Mexican-American and non-Hispanic white women: Evidence from a national survey. *Birth, 22*(2), 74–80.

Ballard, J. L., Auer, C. E., & Khoury, J. C. (2002) Ankyloglossia: Assessment, incidence, and effect of frenuloplasty on the breastfeeding dyad. *Pediatrics, 110*(5), e63.

Benis, M. M. (2002). Critically appraised topic: Are pacifiers associated with early weaning from breastfeeding. *Advances in Neonatal Care, 2*(5), 259–266.

Bentley, M, E., Caulfield, L. E., Gross, S. M., Bronner, Y., Jensen, J., Kessler, L. A., & Paige, D. M. (1999). Sources of influence on intention to breastfeed among African-American women at entry to WIC. *Journal of Human Lactation, 15*(1), 27–34.

Bhandari, N., Bahl, R., Mazumdar, S., Martines, J., Black, R.E., & Bhan, M.K. (2003). Effect of community-based promotion of exclusive breastfeeding on diarrheal illness and growth: A cluster randomized controlled trial. *Lancet, 361*(9367), 1418–1423.

Biancuzzo, M. (2000). Not enough milk: Reasons, rationale and remedies. Advance for Nurse Practitioners [On-line]. Available at www.advanceforNP.com.

Bier, J. A., Oliver, T., Ferguson, A. E., & Vohr, B. R. (2002). Human milk improves cognitive and motor development of premature infants during infancy. *Journal of Human Lactation, 18*(4), 361–367

Blaymore Bier, B. J., Oliver, T., Ferguson, A., & Vohr, B. R. (2002). Human milk reduces outpatient upper respiratory symptoms in premature infants during their first year of life. *Journal of Perinatology, 22*(5), 354–359.

Bliss, M. C., Wilkie, J., Acredolo, C., Berman, S., & Tebb, K. P. (1997). The effect of discharge pack formula and breast pumps on breastfeeding duration and choice of infant feeding method. *Birth, 24*(2), 90–97.

Brent, N., Rudy, S. J., Redd, B., Rudy, T. E., & Roth, L. A. (1998). Sore nipples in breastfeeding women: A clinical trial of wound dressings vs. conventional care. *Archives in Pediatric Adolescent Medicine, 152*(11), 1077–1082.

Briggs G. G., Freeman R. K., & Yaffee S. J. (Ed.). *Drugs in pregnancy and lactation,* 6th ed. Philadelphia: Lippincott Williams & Wilkins.

British Columbia Reproductive Care Program. (2001). Breastfeeding the health preterm infant ≤37 weeks. Retrieved March 2006 from http://www.rcp.gov.bc.ca/guidelines/Master.NutritionPartII.PremBreastfeeding.October.2001.pdf)

Buchko, B. L., Pugh, L. C., Bishop, B. A., Chochran, J. F., Smith, L. R., & Lerew, D. J. (1994). Comfort measures in breastfeeding, primiparous women. *Journal of Obstetric Gynecologic and Neonatal Nursing, 23*(1), 46–52.

Bulkow, L. R., Singleton, R. J., Karron, R. A., Harrison, L. H. & Alaska RSV study group. (2002). Risk factors for severe respiratory syncytial virus infection among Alaska native children. *Pediatrics, 109*(2), 210–216.

Callen, J., & Pinnelli, J. (2004). Incidence and duration of breast-feeding for term infants in Canada, United States, Europe and Australia: a literature review. *Birth, 31*(4), 285–292.

Center for Disease Control (CDC). (2004). Breastfeeding practices—results from the 2004 National Immunization Survey. Retrieved January 20, 2006, from http://www.cdc.gov/breastfeeding/data/NIS_data/data_2004.htm

Centuori, S., Burmaz, T., Ronfani, L., Franiacomo, M., Quintero, S., Pavan, C., Davanzo, R., & Cattaneo, A. (1999). Nipple care, sore nipples, and breastfeeding: A randomized trial. *Journal of Human Lactation, 15*(2), 125–130.

Chantry, C. J., Howard, C. R., & Auinger, P. (2002). Full breast-feeding duration and associated decrease in respiratory tract infection in US children. *Pediatrics, 117*(2), 425–432.

Chezem, J., Friesen, C., Montgomery, P., Fortman, T., & Clark, H. (1998). Lactation duration: Influences of human milk replacements and formula samples on women planning postpartum employment. *Journal of Obstetric, Gynecologic, and Neonatal Nursing, 27*(6), 646–651.

Cox, D. B., Kent, J. C., Casey, T. M., Owens, R. A., & Hartmann, P. E. (1999). Breast growth and the urinary excretion of lactose during human pregnancy and early lactation: Endocrine relationships. *Experimental Physiology, 84*(2), 421–434.

Cox, D. B., Owens, R. A., & Hartmann, P. E. (1996). Blood and milk prolactin and the rate of milk synthesis in women. *Experimental Physiology, 81*(6), 1007–1020.

Cregan, M. D., & Hartmann, P. E. (1999). Computerized breast measurement from conception to weaning: Clinical implications. *Journal of Human Lactation, 15*(2), 89–96.

Crowell, M. K., Hill, P. D., & Humenick, S. S. (1994). Relationship between obstetric analgesia and time of effective breastfeeding. *Journal of Nurse-Midwifery, 39*(3), 150–155.

Daly, K. A., Brown, J. E., Lindgren, B. R., Meland, M. H., Le, C. T., & Giebink, G. S. (1999). Epidemiology of otitis media onset by six months of age. *Pediatrics, 103*(6, Pt. 1), 1158–66.

Daly, S. E. J., Kent, J. C., Owens, R. A., & Hartmann, P. E. (1996). Frequency and degree of milk removal and the short-term control of human milk synthesis. *Experimental Physiology, 81*(5), 861–875.

Daly, S. E. J., Owens, R. A., & Hartmann, P. E. (1993). The short-term synthesis and infant-regulated removal of milk in lactating women. *Experimental Physiology, 78*(2), 209–220.

Davis, M. K. (2001). Breastfeeding and chronic disease in childhood and adolescence. *Pediatric Clinics of North America, 48*(1), 125–141.

Dennis, C. L., Hodnett, E., Gallop, R., & Chalmers, B. (2002). The effect of peer support on breastfeeding duration among primiparous women: A randomized controlled trial. *Canadian Medical Association Journal, 166*(1), 21–28.

de Silva, A., Jones, P.W., Spencer, S. A. (2004). Does human milk reduce infection rates in preterm infants? A systematic review. *Archives of Diseases of Childhood Neonatal Edition, 89*(6), F509–F513.

Dixit, R., & Gartner, L. M. (1999). The jaundiced newborn: Minimizing the risks. *Contemporary Pediatrics, 16*(4), 166–183.

Donnelly, A., Snowden, H. M., Renfrew, M. J., & Woolridge, M. W. (2000). Commercial hospital discharge packs for breastfeeding women. *Cochrane Database Systematic Review, 2*, CD002075.

Duddridge, E. (2000). The influence of grandparents on infant feeding choice. *British Journal of Midwivery, 8*(5), 302–304.

Dungy, C. I., Losch, M. E., Russell, D., Romitti, P., & Dusdieker, L. B. (1997). Hospital infant formula discharge packages: Do they affect the duration of breastfeeding? *Archives in Pediatric Adolescent Medicine, 151*(7), 724–729.

Dykes, F., & Williams, C. (1999). Falling by the wayside: A phenomenological exploration of perceived breast milk inadequacy in lactating women. *Midwifery, 15*(4), 232–246.

Dyson, L., McCormick, F., & Renfrew M. J. (2005) Intervention for promoting the initiation of breastfeeding. *Cochrane Database of Systematic Reviews, 2*, CD001688.

Earle, S. (2002). Factors affecting the initiation of breastfeeding: implications for breastfeeding promotion. *Health Promotion International, 17*(3), 205–214.

Eidelman, A., Hoffman, N., & Kaitz, M. (1993). Cognitive deficits in women after childbirth. *Obstetrics and Gynecology, 81*(5, Pt. 1), 764–767.

Ekstrom, A., Widstrom, A.M., & Nissen, E. (2003). Duration of breastfeeding in Swedish primiparous and multiparous woman. *Journal of Human Lactation, 19*, 172–178.

Gartner, L. M. (1994). Neonatal jaundice. *Pediatric Review, 15*(11), 422–432.

Gartner, L. M., & Greer, F. R. Section of Breastfeeding and Committee on Nutrition American Academy of Pediatrics. (2003). Prevention of rickets and vitamin D deficiency: New guidelines for vitamin D intake. *Pediatrics, 111*(4, Pt. 1), 908–910.

Gianino, P., Mastretta, E., Longo, P., Laccisaglia, A., Sartore, M., Russo, R., & Mazzaccara, A. (2002). Incidence of nosocomial rotavirus infections, symptomatic and asymptomatic in breastfed and non breastfed infants. *Journal of Hospital Infection, 50*(1), 13–27.

Gillman M. W., Rifas-Shiman S. L., Camargo, C. A., Berkey, C. S., Frazier, A. L., Rockett, H. R., et al. (2001). Risk of overweight among adolescents who were breastfed as infants. *Journal of the American Medical Association. 285*(19), 246–2467.

Goer, M. W., Davis, M.W., & Hemphill, J. (2002).Postpartum stress: Current concepts and the possible protective role of breastfeeding. *Journal of Obstetrics Gynecology and Neonatal Nursing, 31*(4), 411–417.

Greene, L. C., Lucas, A., Livingstone, M. B., Harland, P. S., & Baker, B. A. (1995). Relationship between early diet and subsequent cognitive performance during adolescence. *Biochemical Society Transactions, 23*(2), 376S.

Grummer-Strawn, L. M., & Mei, Z. (2004). Does breastfeeding protect against pediatric overweight? Analysis of longitudinal data from the Centers for Disease Control and Prevention Pediatric Nutrition Surveillance System. *Pediatrics, 113*(2). Available at www.pediatrics.org/cgi/content/full/113/2/e81

Guise, J. M., Palda, V., Westhoff, C., Chan, B. K., Helfand, M., & Lieu, T. A. (2003). The effectiveness of primary care-based interventions to promote breastfeeding: Systematic evidence review and meta-analysis for the U.S. Preventive Services Task Force. *American Family Medicine, 1*(2), 70–78.

Gulick, E. E. (1986). The effects of breastfeeding on toddler health. *Pediatric Nursing, 12*(1), 51–54.

Guthrie, R. A., & Auerbach, K. G. (1999). Jaundice and the breastfeeding baby. In J. Riordan & K. G. Auerbach (Eds.), *Breastfeeding and human lactation* (2nd ed., pp. 375–391). Boston: Jones & Bartlett.

Hale T. (2004). *Medications and mother milk: A manual of lactational pharmacology* (11th ed.). Amarillo, TX: Pharmasoft Medical Publishing.

Hedberg, N. K., & Ewald, U. (1999). Infant and maternal factors in the development of breastfeeding behaviour and breastfeeding outcome in preterm infants. *Acta Paediatrica, 88*(11), 1194–1203.

Henderson, J. J., Dickinson, J. E., Evans, S. F., McDonald, S. J., & Paech, M. J. (2003). Impact of intrapartum epidural analgesia on breastfeeding duration. *Australian and New Zealand Journal of Obstetrics and Gynecology, 43*(5), 372–377.

Hoover, K. (1999). Breast pain during lactation that resolved with fluconazole: Two case studies. *Journal of Human Lactation, 15*(2), 98–99.

Horwood, L. J., & Fergusson, D. M. (1998). Breastfeeding and later cognitive and academic outcomes. *Pediatrics, 101*(1), E9.

Howard, C. R., Howard, F. M., Lanphear, B., deBlieck, E. A., Eberly, S., & Lawrence, R. A. (1999). The effects of early pacifier use on breastfeeding duration. *Pediatrics, 103*(3), E33.

Howard C. R., Howard, F. M., Lanphear, B., deBlieck, E. A., Oakes, D., & Lawrence, R. A. (2003). Randomized clinical trial of pacifier use and bottle-feeding or cup feeding and their effect on breastfeeding. *Pediatrics, 111*(3), 511–518.

Humenick, S. S., Hill, P. D., & Hart, A. M. (1998). Evaluation of a pillow designed to promote breastfeeding. *Journal of Perinatal Education, 7*(3), 25–31.

Humphreys, A. M., Thompson, N. J., & Miner, K. R. (1998). Intention to breastfeed in low-income pregnant women: The role of social support and previous experience. *Birth, 25*(3), 169–174.

Insel, T. R. (1997). A neurobiological basis of social attachment. *American Journal of Psychiatry, 154*(6), 726–735.

Jain. A., Concato, J., & Leventhal, J. M. (2002). How good is the evidence linking breastfeeding and intelligence. *Pediatrics, 109*(6), 1044–1053.

Jensen, D., Wallace, S., & Kelsey, P. (1994). LATCH: A breastfeeding charting system and documentation tool. *Journal of Obstetric, Gynecologic, and Neonatal Nursing, 23*(1), 27–32.

Joann Briggs Institute. (2005). Early childhood pacifier use in relation to breastfeeding, SIDS, infection and dental malocclusion. *Best Practice: Evidence Based Practice Information Sheets for Health Professionals, 9*(3), ISSN 1329–1984.

Johnson, T. S. (2003). Hypoglycemia and the term newborn: How well does birth weight for gestational age predict risk? *Journal of Obstetric, Gynecologic, and Neonatal Nursing, 32*(1), 48–57.

Jordan, S., Emery, S., Bradshaw, C., Watkins, A., & Friswell, W. (2005). The impact of intrapartum analgesia on infant feeding. *British Journal of Obstetrics & Gynecology, 112*(7), 927–934.

Keating, J. P., Schears, G. J., & Dodge, P. R. (1991). Oral water intoxication in infants. *American Journal of Diseases in Children, 145*(9), 985–990.

Kistin, N., Abramson, R., & Dublin, P. (1994). Effect of peer counselors on breastfeeding initiation, exclusivity, and duration among low-income urban women. *Journal of Human Lactation, 10*(1), 11–15.

Klement, E., Cohen, R.V., Boxman, J., Joseph, A., & Reif, S. (2004). Breastfeeding and risk of inflammatory bowel disease: A systematic review with meta analysis. *American Journal of Clinical Nutrition, 80*(5), 1342–1352.

Kramer, M. S., Barr, R. G., Dagenais, S., Yang, H., Jones, P., Ciofani, L., & Jane, F. (2001). Pacifier use, early weaning, and cry/fuss behavior: A randomized controlled trial. *Journal of the American Medical Association, 286*(3), 322–326.

Kramer, M. S., Guo, T., Platt, R. W., Sevkovskaya, Z., Dzikovich, I., Collet, J. P., et al. (2003). Infant growth and health outcomes associated with 3 compared with 6 months exclusive breastfeeding. *American Journal of Clinical Nutrition, 78*(2), 291–295.

Kuhr, M., & Paneth, N. (1982). Feeding practices and early neonatal jaundice. *Journal of Pediatric Gastroenterology and Nutrition, 1*(4), 485–488.

Kull, I., Wickman, M., Lilja, G., Nordvall, S. L., & Pershagen, G. (2002). Breast feeding and allergic diseases in infants—a prospective birth cohort study. *Archives of Disease in Childhood, 87*(6), 478–481.

Lawrence, R. A., & Lawrence, R. M. (2005). *Breastfeeding: A guide for the medical profession* (6th ed., pp. 255–258). St. Louis: Mosby.

Lloyd, B., Halter, R. J., Kuchan, M. J., Baggs, G. E., Ryan, A. S., & Masor, M. L. (1999). Formula tolerance in post breastfed and exclusively formula-fed infants. *Pediatrics, 103*(1), E7.

Lucas, A., & Cole, T. J. (1990). Breast milk and neonatal necrotizing enterocolitis. *Lancet, 336*(8730), 1519–1523.

Lucas, A., Lockton, S., & Davies, P. S. (1992). Randomized trial of a ready-to-feed compared with powdered formula. *Archives of Diseases of Children, 67*(7), 935–939.

Martens, P., Derkesen, S., Gupta, S. (2004). Predictors of hospital readmission of Manitoba newborns within six weeks post birth discharge: A population based study. *Pediatrics, 114*(3), 708–713

Martin, R. M., Ness, A. R., Gunnell, D., Emmett, P., Smith, G. D., & ALSPAC Study Team. (2004). Does breastfeeding in infancy lower blood pressure in childhood? The Avon Longitudinal Study of Parents and Children (ALSPAC). *Circulation, 109*(10), 1259–1266.

Masaitis, N. S., & Kaempf, J. W. (1996). Developing a frenectomy policy at one medical centre: A case study approach. *Journal of Human Lactation, 12*(3), 229–232.

Matthews, M. K. (1989). The relationship between maternal labor analgesia and delay in the initiation of breastfeeding in healthy neonates in the early neonatal period. *Midwifery, 5*(1), 3–10.

Mayer, E. J., Hamman, R. F., Gay, E., C., Lezotte, D. C., & Klingensmith, G. J. (1988). Reduced risk of IDDM among breastfed children. The Colorado IDDM Registry. *Diabetes, 37*(12), 1625–1632.

McCleod, D., Pullon, S., & Cookson, T. (2002). Factors influencing continuation of breastfeeding in a cohort of women. *Journal of Human Lactation, 18*(4), 335–343.

McVea, K. L., Turner, P. D., Peppler, D. K. (2000). The role of breastfeeding in sudden infant death syndrome. *Journal of Human Lactation, 16*(1), 13–20.

Messner, A. H., Lalakea, M. L., Aby, J., Macmahon, J., & Blair, E. (2000). Ankyloglossia: Incidence and associated feeding difficulties. *Archives of Otolaryngology–Head & Neck Surgery, 126*(1), 36–39.

Meyerink, R. O., & Marquis, G. S. (2002). Breastfeeding initiation and duration among low income women in Alabama: The importance of personal and familial experiences in making infant feeding choices. *Journal of Human Lactation, 19*(1), 38–50.

Morland-Schultz, K., & Hill, P. (2005). Prevention of and therapies for nipple pain: A systematic review. *Journal of Obstetric, Gynecologic, and Neonatal Nursing, 34*(4), 4288–4437.

Morrow, A. L., Ruiz-Palacios, G. M., Altaye, M., Jiang, X., Guerrero, M. L., Meinzen-Derr, J. K., et al. (2004). Human milk oligosaccharides are associated with protection against diarrhea in breastfed infants. *Journal of Pediatrics, 145*(3), 297–303.

Mortensen, E. L., Fleishcer, M. K., Sanders, S. A., & Reinisch, J. M. (2002). The association between duration of breastfeeding and adult intelligence. *Journal of the American Medical Association, 287*(22), 2365–2371.

Neifert, M. R. (1999). Clinical aspects of lactation. Promoting breastfeeding. *Clinical Perinatology, 26*(2), 281–306.

Neifert, M. R., McDonough, S. L., & Neville, M. C. (1981). Failure of lactogenesis associated with placental retention. *American Journal of Obstetrics and Gynecology, 140*(4), 477–478.

Nelson, E. E., & Panksepp, J. (1998). Brain substrates of infant–mother attachment: Contributions of opioids, oxytocin, and norepinephrine. *Neuroscience and Biobehavioral Reviews, 22*(3), 437–452.

Nelson, E. A., Yu, L., & Williams, S. (2005). International child care practices study: Breastfeeding and pacifier use. *Journal of Human Lactation, 21*(3), 289–295.

Neubauer, S. H., Ferris, A. M., Chase, C. G., Fanellim, J., Thompson, C. A., Lammi-Keefe, C. J., et al.(1993). Delayed lactogenesis in women with insulin-dependent diabetes mellitus. *American Journal of Clinical Nutrition, 58*(1), 54–60.

Nvqvist, K. H., Rubertsson, C., Ewald, U., & Sjoden, P. O. (1996). Development of the preterm infant breastfeeding behavior scale (PIBBS): A study of nurse-mother agreement. *Journal of Human Lactation, 12*(3), 207–219.

O'Campo, P., Faden, R. R., Gielen, A. C., & Wang, M. C. (1992). Prenatal factors associated with breastfeeding duration: Recommendations for prenatal interventions. *Birth, 19*(4), 195–201.

Oddy, W. H., Garth, E., Kendall, E., Blair, E., Klerk, N. H., Stanley, F. J., et al. (2003). Breast feeding and cognitive development in childhood: A prospective birth cohort study. *Pediatric and Perinatal Epidemiology, 17*(1), 81–90.

Oddy, W. H., Holt, P. G., Sly, P. D., Read, A. W., Landau, L. I., Stanley, F. J., et al. (1999). Association between breastfeeding and asthma in 6 year old children: Findings of a prospective birth cohort study. *British Medical Journal, 319*(7213), 815–819.

Oddy, W. H., Peat, J. K., & de Klerk, N. H. (2002). Maternal asthma, infant feeding, and the risk of asthma in childhood. *Journal of Allergy and Clinical Immunology, 110*(1), 65–67.

Oddy, W. H., Sly, P. D., de Klerk, N. H., Landau, L. I., Kendall, G. E., Holt, P. G., et al. (2003). Breast feeding and respiratory morbidity in infancy: A birth cohort study. *Archives of Disease in Childhood, 88*(3), 224–228.

Owens, C. G., Martin, R. M., Whincup, P. H., Smith, G. D., & Cook, D. G. (2005). Effect of infant feeding on the risk of obesity across the life course: A quantitative review of published evidence. *Pediatrics, 115*(50), 1367–1377.

Owens, C. G., Whincup, P. H., Odoki, K., Gilg, J. A., Cook, D. G. (2002). Infant feeding and blood cholesterol: A study in adolescents and a systematic review. *Pediatrics, 110*(3), 597–608.

Phares, T. M., Morrow, B., Lansky, A., Barfield, W. D., Prince, C. B., Marchi, K. S., et al. (2004). Surveillance for disparities in maternal health-related behaviors—Selected states, Pregnancy Risk Assessment Monitoring Systems (PRAMS), 2000-2001. *Morbidity and Mortality Weekly Report, 53*(4), 1–13.

Piper, S., & Parks, P. L. (1996). Predicting the duration of lactation: Evidence from a national survey. *Birth, 23*(1), 7–12.

Pugh, L. C., Buchko, B. L., Bishop, B. A., Cochran, J. F., Smith, L. R., & Lerew, D. J. (1996). A comparison of topical agents to relieve nipple pain and enhance breastfeeding. *Birth, 23*(2), 88–93.

Ransjo-Arvidson, A. B., Matthiesen, A. S., Lilja, G., Nissen, E., Widstrom, A. M., & Uvnas-Moberg, K. (2001). Maternal analgesia during labor disturbs newborn behavior: Effects on breastfeeding, temperature, and crying. *Birth, 28*(1), 5–12.

Rasmussen, K. M., & Kjolheda, C. L. (2004). Prepregnant overweight and obesity diminish the prolactin response to suckling in the first week postpartum. *Pediatrics, 113*(5), 465–471.

Renfrew, M. J., Lang, S., Martin, L., & Woolridge, M. W. (2000). Feeding schedules in hospitals for newborn infants. *Cochrane Database Systematic Review, 2,* CD000090.

Righard, L. (1998). Are breastfeeding problems related to incorrect breastfeeding technique and the use of pacifiers and bottles? *Birth, 25*(1), 40–44.

Righard, L., & Alade, M. O. (1992). Sucking technique and its effects on success of breastfeeding. *Birth, 19*(4), 185–189.

Righard, L., & Alade, M. O. (1997). Breastfeeding and the use of pacifiers. *Birth, 24*(2), 116–120.

Riordan, J. (2005). *Breastfeeding and human lactation* (3rd ed.). London: Jones & Bartlett Publication.

Riordan, J. M., & Koehn, M. (1997). Reliability and validity testing of three breastfeeding assessment tools. *Journal of Obstetric Gynecologic and Neonatal Nursing, 26*(2), 181–187.

Saadeh, R., & Akre, J. (1996). Ten steps to successful breastfeeding: A summary of the rationale and scientific evidence. *Birth, 23*(3), 154–160.

Scariati, P. D., Grummer-Strawn, L. M., & Fein, S. B. (1997). A longitudinal analysis of infant morbidity and the extent of breastfeeding in the United States. *Pediatrics, 99*(6), E5.

Schafer, E., Vogel, M. K., Viegas, S., & Hausafus, C. (1998). Volunteer peer counselors increase breastfeeding duration among rural low-income women. *Birth, 25*(2), 101–106.

Schanler, R. J. (2001). The use of human milk for premature infants, *Pediatric Clinics of North America, 48*(1), 207–219.

Schuman, A. J. (2003). A concise history of infant formula (twists and turns included). *Contemporary Pediatrics.* Retrieved March 20, 2006, from http://www.contemporarypediatrics.com/contpeds/article/articleDetail.jsp?id=111702

Shrago, L. C., Reifsnider, E., & Insel, E. (2006). The neonatal bowel output study: Indicators of adequate breast milk intake in neonates. *Pediatric Nursing, 32*(3), 195–201.

Sikorski, J., Renfrew, M J., Rindoria, S., & Wade, A. (2002). Support for breastfeeding mothers. *Cochrane Database of Systematic Reviews, 2,* CD001141.

Singhal, A., Cole, T. J, Fewtrell, M., & Lucas, A. (2004). Breastmilk feeding and lipoprotein profile in adolescents born preterm: Follow-up of a prospective randomized study. *Lancet 363*(9421), 1571–1578.

Swift, K., & Janke, J. (2003). Breast binding … is it all that it's wrapped up to be? *Journal of Obstetric, Gynecologic, and Neonatal Nursing, 32*(3), 332–339.

Tarkka, A. T., Paunonen, M., & Laippala, P. (1999). Factors related to successful breast feeding by first time mothers when the child is 3 months old. *Journal of Advanced Nursing, 29*(1), 113–118.

Taylor, J. S., Kacmar, J. E., Nothnagle, M., & Lawrence, R. (2005). A systematic review of literature associating breastfeeding with type 2 diabetes and gestational diabetes. *Journal of American College of Nutrition, 24*(5), 320–326.

Trado, M. G., & Hughes, R. B. (1996). A phenomenological study of breastfeeding WIC recipients in South Carolina. *Advanced Practice Nursing Quarterly, 2*(3), 31–41.

Tully, S. (1998). The right angle: Otitis media and infant feeding position. Advance for Nurse Practitioners [On-line]. Available at www.advanceforNP.com

Tully, S. B., Bar-Haim, Y., & Bradley, R. L. (1995). Abnormal tympanography after supine bottle feeding. *Journal of Pediatrics, 126*(6), S105–111.

United States Department of Health and Human Services [USDHSS]. (2000). *Healthy People 2010.* (Conference edition in two volumes). Washington, DC: Author.

Uvnas-Moberg, K. (1997). Physiological and endocrine effects of social contact. *Annals of the New York Academy of Sciences, 807*(1), 146–163.

Vaarala, O., Knip, M., Paronen, J., Hamalainen, A. M., Muona, P., Vaatainen, M., et al. (1999). Cow's milk formula feeding induces primary immunization to insulin in infants at genetic risk for type I diabetes. *Diabetes, 48*(7), 1389–1394.

Van den Driessche, M., Peeters, K., Marien, P., Ghoos, Y., Devlieger, H., & Veereman-Wauters, G. (1999). Gastric emptying in formula-fed and breastfed infants measured with the C-octanoic acid breath test. *Journal of Pediatric Gastroenterology and Nutrition, 29*(1), 46–51.

Victora, C. G., Behague, D. P., Barros, F. C., Olinto, M. T., & Weiderpass, E. (1997). Pacifier use and short breastfeeding duration: Cause, consequence, or coincidence? *Pediatrics, 99*(3), 445–453.

Vio, F., Salazar, G., & Infante, C. (1991). Smoking during pregnancy and lactation: Its effects on breast milk volume. *American Journal of Clinical Nutrition, 54*(6), 1011–1016.

Vittoz, J. P., Labarere, J., Castell, M., Durand, M., & Pons, J. C. (2004). Effect of a training program for maternity ward professionals on duration of breastfeeding. *Birth, 31*(4), 302–307.

von Kries, R., Koletzko, B., Sauerwald, T., von Mutius, E., Barnert, D., Grunert, V., et al. (1999). Breast feeding and obesity: Cross sectional study. *British Medical Journal, 319*(7203), 147–150.

Walker, M. (1999). Epidurals and breastfeeding. *Birth, 26*(4), 275–276.

Weimer, J. (2001). The economic benefits of breastfeeding: A review and analysis. *ERS Food Assistance and Nutrition Research Report No. 13*. Washington, DC: USDA Economic Research Service.

Widstrom, A. M., Ransjo-Arvidsson, A. B., Christensson, K., Matthiesen, A. S., Winberg, J., & Uvnas-Moberg, K. (1987). Gastric suction in healthy newborn infants: Effects on circulation and developing feeding behavior. *Acta Paediatrica Scandinavica, 76*(4), 566–572.

Wight, N. E. 2001. Donor human milk for preterm infants. *J Perinatal, 21*(4), 249–254,

Wilde, C. J., Addey, C. V., Boddy, L. M., & Peaker, M. (1995). Autocrine regulation of milk secretion by a protein in milk. *Biochemical Journal, 305*(Pt. 1), 51–58.

WHO/UNICEF Joint Statement. (1989). *Protecting and supporting breastfeeding: The special role of maternity services.* Geneva: World Health Organization.

WHO. (2002). Global strategy on infant and young child feeding (Document A55/15). Geneva: Author.

Wright, A., Rice, S., & Wells, S. (1996). Changing hospital practices to increase the duration of breastfeeding. *Pediatrics, 97*(5), 66–675.

Young, T. K, Martens P. J., Taback, S. P., Sellers, E. A., Dean, H. J., Cheang, M., et al. (2002). Type 2 diabetes mellitus in children: prenatal and early infancy risk factors among native Canadians. *Archives of Pediatric and Adolescent Medicine 156*(7), 651–655.

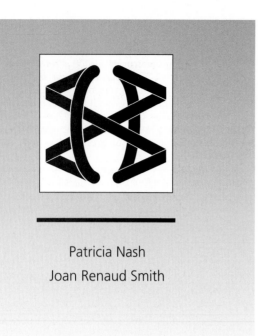

CHAPTER **14**

Common Neonatal Complications

Patricia Nash

Joan Renaud Smith

M OST newborns with complications are identified and cared for in community hospitals or level II perinatal centers. Perinatal nurses must have a thorough understanding of pathophysiology and clinical signs of illness during the immediate newborn period. The length of stay limits the time to identify behavioral cues or subtle changes that could potentially compromise newborn well-being.

Common complications discussed in this chapter include respiratory distress, congenital heart lesions, hyperbilirubinemia, hypoglycemia, and sepsis. Neonatal abstinence syndrome and care of the child with prenatal/antenatal exposure to HIV-1 infection are included because of continuing data about chemical dependency and HIV-1 infection among women during the childbearing years. New to the literature, late-preterm infants, also known as near-term infants, are defined and a section discussing this unique population of infants is included. The chapter concludes with a discussion of neonatal transport because, in some cases, the severity of the disease process necessitates transfer to a tertiary-care center.

RESPIRATORY DISTRESS

Respiratory distress is a major cause of neonatal morbidity and mortality despite significant technologic and pharmacologic advances during the past 30 years. Respiratory distress is one of the most common neonatal complications seen by the perinatal nurse and is a principal indication for neonatal transfer to tertiary-care units. Table 14-1 lists the perinatal events and associated respiratory diseases. The pathophysiology or causative factors of respiratory distress varies, but the result is decreased ability to exchange the oxygen and carbon dioxide necessary to ensure perfusion of well-oxygenated blood to vital organs and to remove metabolic waste products. Respiratory distress may be caused by obstruction or malformation, can develop as a consequence of acute lung injury, reflects prolonged transition to extrauterine life, and may occur in the presence of other medical or systemic problems. Five of the most common respiratory diseases occurring during the neonatal period are respiratory distress syndrome (RDS), meconium aspiration syndrome (MAS), pneumonia, transient tachypnea of the newborn (TTN), and persistent pulmonary hypertension of the newborn (PPHN).

Respiratory Distress Syndrome

RDS primarily occurs in preterm newborns. The incidence varies inversely with advancing gestational age. In the United States, approximately 24,000 newborns each year develop RDS; the incidence of RDS is inversely related to gestational age: 60% of infants born at less than 28 weeks; 30% of those born at 28 to 34 weeks' gestation, and less than 5% of those born after 34 weeks are affected (American Lung Association, 2003). The mortality rate for RDS is 37 deaths per 100,000 live births (Malloy & Freeman, 2002). RDS is caused by insufficient amounts of surfactant or delayed or impaired surfactant synthesis. Surfactant is a mixture of phospholipids and proteins synthesized, packaged, and excreted by alveolar type II cells that lowers surface tension in the alveoli and functions as a stabilizer to prevent atelectasis and alveolar collapse at

TABLE 14–1 ■ CLINICAL CORRELATES OF PERINATAL HISTORY

History	Associated Respiratory Disease
Premature birth Maternal diabetes Maternal hemorrhage Perinatal asphyxia	Respiratory distress syndrome (RDS)
Multiple gestation	RDS more common in second twin
Postmature birth	Meconium aspiration syndrome
Nonreassuring fetal heart rate pattern Meconium-stained amniotic fluid Perinatal asphyxia	Persistent pulmonary hypertension
Oligohydramnios	Pulmonary hypoplasia
Cesarean birth	Transient tachypnea
Prolonged rupture of membranes Maternal fever	Pneumonia
Traumatic delivery Narcotics in labor	Poor respiratory effort

end-expiration (Cole, Nogee, & Hamvas, 2006). Without surfactant, atelectasis (alveolar collapse) occurs, resulting in a series of events that progressively increase disease severity. These events include hypoxemia (decreased concentration of oxygen), hypercapnea (increased concentration of carbon dioxide), acidosis, pulmonary vasoconstriction, alveolar endothelial and epithelial damage, and subsequent protein-rich interstitial and alveolar edema. This cascade of events further decreases surfactant synthesis, storage, and release and worsens respiratory distress.

Meconium Aspiration Syndrome

Passage of meconium in utero is primarily seen in small for gestational age and postmature newborns as well as in those with cord complications or factors that compromise the uteroplacental circulation (Miller, Fanaroff, & Martin, 2002). Under normal intrauterine conditions, amniotic fluid does not enter the fetal lung. However, when the fetus experiences hypoxemia, gasping may result in aspiration of meconium-stained amniotic fluid. Eight to 20% of newborns are exposed to amniotic fluid stained by meconium; of these, rates as high as 10% have been reported for those infants who go on to develop MAS (ACOG, 2006; Miller, Fanaroff, & Martin, 2002). Passage of meconium in utero occurs

as a physiologic maturational event, response to acute hypoxic events, and response to chronic intrauterine hypoxia. The amount and thickness of the meconium appear to directly affect the severity of respiratory distress. Amnioinfusion has been used as a technique to prevent MAS and to improve neonatal outcomes, and recent recommendations for routine prophylactic use of amnioinfusions for the dilution of meconium-stained amniotic fluid is not warranted (ACOG, 2006). However, ACOG also acknowledges that amnioinfusion does appear to be a reasonable treatment of repetitive variable decelerations regardless of the amniotic meconium fluid status (ACOG). When aspirated by the fetus before or during birth, meconium can obstruct the airways, leading to severe hypoxia, inflammation, and infection, and cause significant respiratory difficulties. Some evidence suggest that intrapartum suctioning before the first breath may decrease the risk of MAS; however, subsequent evidence from a large multicentered randomized trial did not show such an effect, and recommendations to discontinue routine intrapartum oropharyngeal and nasopharyngeal suction were made (Velaphi & Vidyasagar, 2006). The American Academy of Pediatrics (AAP) and American Heart Association (AHA) through the Neonatal Resuscitation Program no longer recommend that all meconium-stained babies routinely receive intrapartum suctioning (AAP & AHA, 2006).

Pneumonitis is an inflammatory response likely secondary to bile salts. Pneumonitis results in acute lung injury with protein-rich interstitial and alveolar edema. In situations where meconium only partially obstructs the airway, a ball-valve effect results. Air enters the lower airways on inspiration but cannot escape on expiration. This causes over distention of alveoli, leading to alveolar rupture and pulmonary air leaks. Pneumonitis and airway obstruction result in hypoxemia and acidosis, which cause increased pulmonary vascular resistance and subsequent PPHN (Miller, Fanaroff, & Martin, 2002). Figure 14–1 shows the pathogenesis of MAS.

Pneumonia

Pneumonia is acquired through vertical or horizontal transmission. Vertical transmission occurs in utero from the rupture of membranes for more than 24 hours, chorioamnionitis, intraamniotic infection, transplacental transmission of organisms, or aspiration of infected amniotic fluid or meconium. Horizontal transmission occurs in the nursery as pathogenic organisms are spread from hospital personnel, equipment, and parents. Horizontal transmission also includes secondary infections as a result of some other primary infection. Display 14–1 lists organisms that may cause pneumonia in the newborn. Pneumonia, like MAS, causes an inflammatory process, disrupting the normal barrier

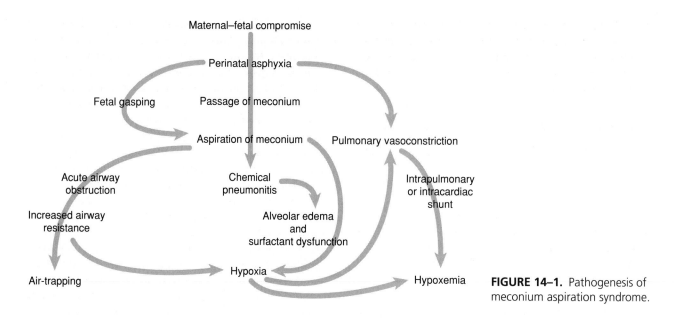

FIGURE 14–1. Pathogenesis of meconium aspiration syndrome.

D I S P L A Y   1 4 - 1

Common Organisms Associated with Neonatal Pneumonia

TRANSPLACENTAL

Rubella

Cytomegalovirus

Herpes simplex virus

Adenovirus

Mumps virus

Toxoplasma gondii

Listeria monocytogenes

Mycobacterium tuberculosis

Treponema pallidum

AMNIOTIC FLUID

Cytomegalovirus

Herpes simplex virus

Enteroviruses

Genital mycoplasma

L. monocytogenes

Chlamydia trachomatis

M. tuberculosis

Group B Streptococcus (GBS)

Escherichia coli

Haemophilus influenzae (nontypeable)

AT DELIVERY

GBS

E. coli

Staphylococcus aureus

Klebsiella sp.

Other streptococci

H. influenzae (nontypeable)

Candida sp.

C. trachomatis

NOSOCOMIAL

S. aureus

Staphylococcus epidermidis

GBS

Klebsiella sp.

Enterobacter

Pseudomonas

Influenza viruses

Respiratory syncytial virus

Enteroviruses

From Hansen, T. N., Cooper, T. R., & Weisman, L. E. (Eds.). (1998). *Contemporary diagnosis and management of neonatal respiratory diseases* (2nd ed., p. 131). Newtown, PA: Handbooks in Health Care.

function of the pulmonary endothelium and epithelium, leading to abnormal protein permeability and edema of lung tissue. Hypoxemia and acidosis result, causing increased pulmonary vascular resistance and PPHN (Miller, Fanaroff, & Martin, 2002).

Transient Tachypnea of the Newborn

TTN occurs in approximately 11 of 1,000 live births (Whitsett, Pryhuber, Rice, Warner, Wert, 1999). Generally, TTN is a mild, self-limiting disorder lasting from 12 to greater than 72 hours. Fetal lungs have a fluid volume of approximately 25 to 30 mL/kg at term, which is maintained by continuous secretion of lung fluid at a rate of about 5 mL/kg/hour. At birth, fluid secretion ceases, and with the onset of breathing, this fluid is absorbed from the air spaces through blood vessels, lymphatics, and upper airways.

Several pathophysiology mechanisms have been suggested for TTN. Historically, this condition was thought to be related to delayed reabsorption of lung fluid by the pulmonary lymphatic system. Retained fluid causes bronchiolar collapse with air trapping or hyperinflation of the alveoli. Hypoxia results when poorly ventilated alveoli are perfused. Hypercarbia is caused by mechanical interference with alveolar ventilation by fluid. Decreased lung compliance results in tachypnea and increased energy needed to do the work of breathing. A second mechanism has to do with the fact that labor causes the active transport of chloride from plasma into the fetal lung fluid to cease. As the concentration of chloride becomes higher in the plasma, fetal lung fluid begins to be reabsorbed. Two-thirds of the fetal lung fluid is absorbed before birth. Newborns without the benefit of labor and those born prematurely do not have the same amount of time to reabsorb lung fluid as those born after a normal course of labor. Infants delivered by elective cesarean section also have a higher incidence of TTN (Hook, Kiwi, Amini, Fanaroff, & Hack, 1995; Jain & Eaton, 2006). Some authorities suggest that TTN could result from mild immaturity of the surfactant system. This idea is supported by lack of phosphatidylglycerol in amniotic fluid samples from newborns with TTN (Whitsett, Pryhuber, Rice, Warner, & Wert, 1999).

Persistent Pulmonary Hypertension of the Newborn

PPHN is defined as a failure of the pulmonary vasculature to relax at birth, resulting in unoxygenated blood to be shunted to the systemic circulation (Perreault, 2006). In fetal circulation, pulmonary blood vessels are constricted, causing most blood flow to bypass the lungs. This is appropriate for the fetus because the placenta rather than the fetal lung acts as the organ of gas exchange. PPHN is the result of a sustained elevation of the pulmonary vascular resistance (PVR) after birth, preventing transition to the normal pattern of circulation. When the PVR remains elevated, blood bypasses the lungs by flowing through the foramen ovale or ductus arteriosus. This pattern of circulation is referred to as right-to-left shunting because blood is diverted from the venous circulation on the right side of the heart to the arterial circulation on the left side of the heart without going through the pulmonary vascular system. Chapter 11 compares fetal and adult circulations. Severe, prolonged hypoxemia (decreased oxygen in the blood) progresses to hypoxia (decreased oxygen in the tissues) and results in metabolic acidosis and worsening pulmonary vasoconstriction. A vicious cycle ensues. PPHN may be idiopathic, caused by abnormal development of pulmonary vessels, or result from pathophysiology events such as asphyxia, MAS, pneumonia, and RDS (Miller, Fanaroff, & Martin, 2002; Zahka & Chandrakant, 2002).

Assessment of Respiratory Distress

Clinical signs of respiratory distress may be present at birth or occur at any time in the early neonatal period. These signs include tachypnea, grunting, retractions, nasal flaring, and cyanosis. Tachypnea is defined as a respiratory rate greater then 60 breaths per minute. Tachypnea develops when the newborn attempts to improve ventilation. Because of the very compliant chest wall, especially in the preterm newborn, it is more energy efficient for the newborn to increase the respiratory rate, breathing at rates greater than 100 breaths per minute for sustained periods, rather than increase the depth of respiration.

On expiration, a grunting sound is heard in newborns with respiratory distress. Grunting is the result of expired air passing through a partially closed glottis. The glottis closes in an effort to increase intrapulmonary pressure and to keep alveoli open. Keeping alveoli open during expiration is a compensatory response to decreased partial pressure of oxygen (pO2). It allows more time for the passage of oxygen into the circulatory system. Grunting develops in an attempt to prevent atelectasis and to improve oxygenation and ventilation abnormalities.

Retractions are depressions observed between the ribs, above the sternum, or below the xiphoid process during inhalation. Retractions are the result of a very compliant chest wall and noncompliant lung. Compliance refers to the stiffness or distensibility of the chest wall and lung parenchyma. As the amount of negative intrathoracic pressure increases on inspiration, the rib cage expands until the soft tissue of the thorax and weak intercostal muscles are pulled inward toward the spine. The result is worsening atelectasis with marked oxygenation and ventilation abnormalities (Cifuentes, Segars, & Carlo, 2003).

Nasal flaring occurs with respiratory distress as the newborn attempts to decrease airway resistance and increase the inflow of air.

Cyanosis results from inadequate oxygenation caused by atelectasis, poor lung compliance, and right-to-left shunting. Although the newborn's color is an indication of oxygenation, it is more appropriately monitored by using pulse oximetry or intermittently monitored by arterial or capillary blood–gas determinations.

Interventions for Respiratory Distress

Care for newborns with respiratory distress focuses on oxygenation and ventilation, warmth, nourishment, and protection from harm. Adequate oxygenation and ventilation requires supportive mechanisms ranging from supplemental oxygen only to supplemental oxygen with mechanical ventilation. Pulse oximetry, arterial catheterization, and blood gas monitoring are methods for ensuring adequate gas exchange. In a preterm newborn, delivery of oxygen should be sufficient to maintain arterial oxygen tension at 50 to 80 mm Hg, which corresponds to a pulse oximetry reading of approximately 88% to 92%. Because oxygen may be toxic to some tissue, care should be taken to avoid excessive tissue oxygenation. Excessive tissue oxygenation increases the risk of developing chronic lung disease and retinopathy of prematurity (Hey & Bell, 2000). In a term newborn at risk for PPHN, oxygen delivery should be sufficient to maintain an arterial oxygen tension of more than 100 mm Hg and an oxygen saturation of 99% to 100%. Hypoxia must be avoided in term newborns because it is one of the most powerful stimuli for pulmonary vasoconstriction and the cycle of PPHN (Cifuentes, Segars, & Carlo, 2003). Infants with suspected PPHN will need to be transferred to a tertiary-care center for further evaluation and management. Recent advances in the delivery of inhaled nitric oxide (i-NO), to provide selective pulmonary vasodilation, and high-frequency ventilation (HFOV) are two of many therapies commonly used in treating PPHN before resorting to extracorporeal membrane oxygenation (ECMO).

A neutral thermal environment is crucial in the care of a newborn with respiratory distress. Hypothermia or hyperthermia increase metabolic demands, leading to decreased oxygenation, metabolic acidosis, and worsening respiratory distress (Kenner, 2003). Newborns with respiratory distress are cared for under a radiant warmer or in an Isolette. Chapter 11 discusses thermoregulation.

Adequate nutrition frequently requires the administration of intravenous fluids during the early neonatal period. Care is taken to prevent hypoglycemia that may occur from respiratory distress and increased metabolic demands.

CONGENITAL HEART DISEASE

Cardiovascular System

The cardiovascular system begins to develop in the third week of gestation and is fully functioning by the end of the eighth week. It is the first major organ system to function in the embryo. This fact may be one of the reasons why congenital heart disease (CHD) is so common, with an incidence of 8 per 1,000 live births (Lott, 2003). Heart defects are among the most common birth defects and are the leading cause of birth defect-related deaths. However, the overall mortality has significantly declined over the past few decades (American Heart Association, 2006). The cause of CHD cannot be ascribed to any single factor. Most cases are probably multifactorial, involving genetic predisposition, familial recurrence, and environmental factors. CHD can also be associated with chromosomal abnormalities (ie, Trisomy 21, 18, 13; Chromosome deletion syndromes; DiGeorge deletion 22q, Turner syndrome, and Cornelia de Lange), and maternal–environmental factors, such as drugs (ie, Thalidomide, anticonvulsants, Lithium, Retonic acid) and alcohol exposure or diseases (insulin-dependent diabetes or maternal lupus erythematosus) or infection (ie, Rubella; Carey, 2002; Lott, 2003). Cardiac lesions are classified as cyanotic, acyanotic, or according to the hemodynamic characteristics related to pulmonary blood flow. Five of the most commonly occurring cardiac lesions presenting in the early neonatal period include ventricular septal defect (VSD), tetralogy of Fallot (TET), patent ductus arteriosus (PDA), atrial septal defect (ASD), and transposition of the great arteries (TGA).

The assessment to exclude CHD includes the following:

- Close observation of cardiorespiratory status
- Palpation of peripheral pulses
- Blood pressures of the four extremities
- Chest radiograph to evaluate heart size and pulmonary vascularity
- Blood gas determinations to evaluate oxygenation and metabolic status
- Evaluation of response to oxygen

The newborn with CHD or persistence of a fetal shunt may present shortly after birth or within the first weeks of life with cyanosis or symptoms of congestive heart failure (CHF). The newborn becomes cyanotic when gas exchange is impaired by pulmonary edema, blood flow to the lungs is restricted as a result of a structural abnormality, or blood flow is shunted away from the lungs. In newborns with normal hemoglobin values, central cyanosis occurs when 5 gm/dL of desaturated hemoglobin is present in the circulating blood volume and usually indicates an arterial hemoglobin saturation of less than 85% (Lott, 2003). Several clinical signs indicate CHF:

- Tachypnea
- Respiratory distress
- Tachycardia
- Hepatomegaly
- Poor feeding

A murmur, if present, varies in quality and intensity, depending on the particular cardiac lesion present. Table 14–2 describes chest radiographic findings for each CHD. If a VSD or ASD is present, allowing mixing of oxygenated and unoxygenated blood, only mild cyanosis occurs. If there is no intracardiac shunt, severe cyanosis is observed. With the exception of cyanosis, the physical examination is often otherwise unremarkable. In the newborn with a large VSD or ASD, signs of CHF develop over time as the PVR falls and the pulmonary blood flow increases. In newborns without an intracardiac shunt, severe hypoxemia and metabolic acidosis develop, followed by a rapid demise if emergency measures are not instituted.

Ventricular Septal Defect

Pathophysiology

Separation of the ventricles begins near the middle of the fourth week of gestation and is completed by the end of the seventh week (Witt, 1997). A VSD is present when there is incomplete division of the right and left ventricles. VSDs are classified by their anatomic location; perimembranous and muscular are the two most

---

TABLE 14–2 ■ CONGENITAL HEART DEFECTS AND CHEST RADIOGRAPHY

Defect	Findings
Ventricular septal defects	Cardiomegaly and congestion (Wood, 1997)
Tetralogy of Fallot	Pulmonary hypoperfusion and a boot-shaped heart (Paul, 1995)
Patent ductus arteriosus	Cardiomegaly and congestion (Wood, 1997)
Atrial septal defect	Cardiomegaly and congestion (Wood, 1997)
Transposition of the great arteries	Heart position described as an egg on a string (Paul, 1965; Witt, 1998)

---

common types. A perimembranous VSD is located just below the aortic valve and accounts for 80% of all VSDs. A muscular VSD is located in the muscular septum. Seventy-five percent to 80% of membranous and muscular VSDs close spontaneously. A VSD is considered an acyanotic lesion with increased pulmonary blood flow. The size and location of the defect, as well as the pulmonary-to-systemic vascular resistance ratio, determine the degree of left-to-right shunt. The timing of the onset of symptoms is directly related to the normal fall in the PVR after birth (Lott, 2003).

Assessment

The onset of symptoms resulting from a VSD is related to the size of the defect and PVR. A newborn with a small defect may appear well and have few or no symptoms other than a harsh holosystolic murmur. The murmur develops as the PVR falls and is best heard over the left lower sternal border. A newborn with a large defect may present with symptoms of CHF at approximately 2 to 4 weeks of life. As with the smaller defects, the murmur is holosystolic and heard over the left lower sternal border. Preterm newborns with large VSDs present with symptoms sooner.

Tetralogy of Fallot

Pathophysiology

TET consists of a large perimembranous VSD, pulmonary stenosis, an overriding aorta, and right ventricle hypertrophy (Lott, 2003). This lesion is a result of disordered embryonic cardiac functioning. TET occurs during the embryonic stage of development, when some unknown factor influences functioning of the heart at the cellular level. This alteration in cellular function is partly responsible for determining development. Any transient change in work can alter cardiac tissue growth or distribution, causing this defect to occur (Witt, 1997). TET is generally considered a cyanotic lesion with decreased pulmonary blood flow, but the hemodynamics vary widely, depending on the severity of pulmonary stenosis, the size of the VSD, and the pulmonary and systemic vascular resistance. Newborns present with varying degrees of cyanosis at birth that worsens over the course of the first year of life (Lott).

Assessment

TET is the most common cyanotic heart disease seen in the first year of life. Newborns with TET present with cyanosis and symptoms of right-sided heart failure. The timing and degree of cyanosis depend on the severity of the pulmonary stenosis and may not be noticed until closure of the ductus arteriosus. In the case of pulmonary atresia and hypoplasia of the pulmonary arteries, marked cyanosis may be observed immediately after birth. The clinical signs of right-sided heart failure include hepatomegaly, tricuspid valve regurgitation, and a murmur best heard over the left lower sternal border.

Patent Ductus Arteriosus

Pathophysiology

The ductus arteriosus is a normal component of fetal circulation. The ductus arteriosus connects the pulmonary artery to the aorta, allowing blood to bypass the lungs. During fetal life, PVR is greater than systemic vascular resistance. After birth, with spontaneous respiration, the arterial oxygen level increases and PVR decreases, causing the ductus to close. If the ductus arteriosus does not close, blood begins to flow left to right through the patent ductus as the PVR decreases. A PDA is an acyanotic lesion with increased pulmonary blood flow. It presents with signs and symptoms of congestive heart failure. It occurs much more commonly in preterm newborns, with the incidence inversely proportional to gestational age (Lott, 2003).

Assessment

The manifestation of PDA depends on the gestational age and the degree of lung disease. Preterm newborns generally develop signs associated with CHF at 3 to 7 days of life, but it can develop sooner in the smaller preterm newborn treated with surfactant. The development of clinical signs is related to the normal fall in the PVR. The classic murmur detected with a PDA is continuous and best heard over the left upper sternal border, radiating to the back.

Atrial Septal Defect

Pathophysiology

The separation of the atrium begins near the middle of the fourth week of gestation and is completed by the end of the sixth week, leaving the foramen ovale open between the two atria. An abnormality occurring during atrial separation can result in an ASD. An ASD is considered an acyanotic lesion with increased pulmonary blood flow. Approximately 10% of newborns with an ASD develop CHF as the PVR decreases (Wood, 1997).

Assessment

Newborns with an uncomplicated ASD are generally asymptomatic. However, about 10% present with signs of CHF, poor feeding, and poor growth. These symptoms develop as the PVR falls over the first few weeks of life. Associated with an ASD is a soft, systolic murmur best heard over the second intercostal space at the left upper sternal border.

Transposition of the Great Arteries

Pathophysiology

The truncus arteriosus begins to divide during the fifth week of gestation. As the cardiac tube folds, the vessel twists on itself and divides into two separate vessels. Transposition occurs because of a failure of the aorticopulmonary septum to grow in a spiral fashion, resulting in inappropriate migration of the vessels (Witt, 1997). The aorta arises from the right ventricle, and the pulmonary artery arises from the left ventricle, resulting in two parallel circulations. When these two arteries are transposed, unoxygenated blood returning from the body enters the right side of the heart and returns to the body, and oxygenated blood returning from the lung enters the left side of the heart and returns to the lungs. TGA is considered a cyanotic lesion with increased pulmonary blood flow. The degree of cyanosis depends on the amount of mixing of oxygenated and unoxygenated blood through the VSD (if present), patent foramen ovale, or PDA (Witt, 1998).

Assessment

The newborn with TGA presents with cyanosis, the degree of which depends on the presence or absence of other defects, such as a VSD or ASD. If a VSD or ASD is present, allowing mixing of oxygenated and unoxygenated blood, only mild cyanosis occurs. If there is no intracardiac shunt, severe cyanosis occurs. With the exception of cyanosis, the physical examination findings are often otherwise unremarkable. With a large VSD or ASD, signs of CHF develop over time as the PVR falls and the pulmonary blood flow increases. In the absence of an intracardiac shunt, severe hypoxemia and metabolic acidosis develop, followed by a rapid demise if emergency measures are not instituted.

Interventions for Congenital Heart Disease

Newborns with known or suspected CHD usually require transfer to a tertiary center for treatment and follow-up. The complete diagnostic workup and subsequent repairs or palliative surgery are performed in centers with pediatric cardiac capabilities. Before transport, close observation and supportive care and treatment are warranted. Nursing care for newborns with known or suspected CHD includes the following:

- Cardiorespiratory monitoring
- Pulse oximetry

- Blood work, including blood gas determinations
- Ongoing assessment of color, perfusion, and degree of distress
- Maintaining a neutral thermal environment
- Intravenous hydration and nutrition
- Oxygen therapy, if appropriate, and mechanical ventilation, if required

Metabolic acidosis is treated with sodium bicarbonate, pulmonary edema with respiratory distress is treated with diuretics, and shock is treated with vasopressors and calcium gluconate. A lesion such as TGA without an intracardiac shunt is treated with prostaglandin E1 to maintain patency of the ductus arteriosus until surgical correction takes place (Lott, 2003; Witt, 1998).

HYPOGLYCEMIA

During the neonatal period, transient low glucose levels are not only common but also considered to be a normal adaptation to extrauterine life (Williams, 2005). Consequently, establishing the incidence of symptomatic and asymptomatic neonatal hypoglycemia is difficult. One of the major difficulties associated with defining hypoglycemia is the lack of correlation between a given blood glucose level and clinical signs. Whether symptomatic or asymptomatic, hypoglycemia can be life threatening and can result in serious neurologic sequelae, such as brain injury, learning disabilities, and cerebral palsy (Kalhan & Parimi, 2002). However, in most circumstances, the clinical effects of hypoglycemia remain poorly defined. Neuropathology is available in only a few infants who have died after severe hypoglycemia. In term infants, symptomatic hypoglycemia may be associated with developmental delay or seizures, but many infants are reported to have normal outcomes (McGowan & Perlman, 2006). Follow-up studies of high-risk infants with recurrent episodes of hypoglycemia resulting from congenital hyperinsulinism have shown that 50% have long-term neurological deficits (Meissner, Wendel, Burgard, Schaetzle, & Mayatepek, 2003; Menni et al., 2001). Additionally, follow-up studies of high-risk infants suggest that adverse neurodevelopmental outcomes are more prevalent in infants with a history of asymptomatic hypoglycemia in the newborn period (McGowan & Perlman, 2006).

The most current data regarding neonatal hypoglycemia discuss operational thresholds rather than clear-cut definitions. Data suggest that treatment should be based on these operational thresholds and guided by clinical assessment, rather than by plasma glucose concentrations alone. More importantly, there is no absolute threshold applicable to all babies, and there is no glucose concentration, which absolutely determines clinical risk or predicts sequelae. Glucose concentrations must be looked at in conjunction with clinical features (Cornblath et al., 2000; Williams, 2005). Most investigators would consider the operational threshold to be 36 mg/dL; therefore, hypoglycemia could be defined as glucose <36 mg/dL.

Pathophysiology

During fetal life, insulin is secreted by the fetal pancreas in response to glucose that readily crosses the placenta. At birth, the newborn's blood glucose level is approximately 70% to 80% that of the mother. After removal of placental circulation, the newborn must maintain glucose homeostasis. This requires initiation of various metabolic processes, including gluconeogenesis (ie, forming glucose from noncarbohydrate sources such as protein and fat) and glycogenolysis (ie, conversion of glycogen stores to glucose), as well as an intact regulatory mechanism and an adequate supply of substrate (Kalhan & Parimi, 2002). The cause of hypoglycemia is overuse of glucose, underproduction of glucose, or a combination of both. Table 14–3 shows clinical situations associated with overuse or underproduction of glucose.

TABLE 14–3 ■ ETIOLOGY OF NEONATAL HYPOGLYCEMIA

Condition	Causes
Increased use of glucose, hyperinsulinemia	Infant of a diabetic mother Islet cell hyperplasia Beckwith–Weidemann syndrome Insulin-producing tumors Maternal tocolytic therapy Hypothermia Malpositioned umbilical artery catheter Exchange transfusion Excessive maternal fluid administration in labor Rapid tapering of high glucose infusion Macrosomic infant
Decreased production or stores of glucose	Prematurity Small for gestational age Maternal starvation
Increased use and/or decreased production of glucose	Asphyxia Sepsis Shock Defects in carbohydrate or amino acid metabolism Endocrine deficiency Polycythemia

Hypoglycemia develops at various hours of life, depending on cause. Transient symptomatic hypoglycemia usually occurs within the first 24 hours after birth but may not manifest until 72 hours or later. Symptomatic hypoglycemia, secondary to maternal or intrapartum causes, generally occurs during the first 2 hours after birth. Hypoglycemia occurring after the first few hours after birth is most commonly caused by hyperinsulinemia, as in the infant of a diabetic mother (Kalhan & Parimi, 2002).

Breastfed term infants have lower concentrations of blood glucose but higher concentrations of ketone bodies than formula-fed infants (Hawdon, Ward Platt, & Aynsley-Green, 1992; Sweene, Ewald, Gustafsson, Sandberg, & Ostenson, 1994). These data suggest that the provision of alternate fuels constitutes a normal adaptive response to transiently low nutrient intake during the establishment of breastfeeding. Therefore, breastfed infants may well tolerate lower plasma glucose levels without significant clinical manifestations or sequelae (Cornblath et al., 2000).

Assessment

Identification of those at risk for developing neonatal hypoglycemia facilitates planning and implementation of appropriate nursing care. This process begins with a review of maternal prenatal and intrapartum history for risk factors associated with neonatal hypoglycemia and a careful physical examination. Signs of hypoglycemia are nonspecific and not easily differentiated from many other common neonatal conditions (Display 14–2). Glucose values in normal term newborns fall after birth; the transition period lasting for 2 to 3 hours after birth (Kalhan & Parimi, 2002).

Universal blood glucose screening before clinical signs develop is not recommended by the American

DISPLAY 14-2

Symptoms of Hypoglycemia

Jitteriness, tremors
Tachypnea, grunting
Diaphoresis
Cyanosis
Lethargy
Hypotonia
Irritability
Temperature instability
Apnea
Seizures, coma

DISPLAY 14-3

Criteria for Routine Screening for Hypoglycemia

Weight <2,500 g or >4,082 g
Small for gestational age
Large for gestational age
<37 weeks' gestation
Infants of diabetic mothers

Academy of Pediatrics (AAP, 1993). Selective screening of at-risk newborns is more appropriate and does not appear to decrease quality of care or result in adverse outcomes. Display 14–3 describes newborns at high risk for hypoglycemia that may benefit from routine screening.

Newborns at risk should be screened within 30 to 60 minutes after birth. Use of proper screening techniques is one of the most important nursing functions. Testing is performed using a bedside glucose oxidase stick method, such as the Chemstrip or a glucometer, approved by the U.S. Food and Drug Administration for use with newborns. Although glucose oxidase sticks are widely used, results depend on the hematocrit, blood source, and operator's skill (Halamek, Benaron, & Stevenson, 1997). They have been shown to have considerable variance from actual blood glucose levels (Kalhan & Parimi, 2002) and to lack reproducibility, especially for blood glucose levels less than 50 mg/dL (Halamek, Benaron, & Stevenson). One reason for variance is the source of the blood used for testing. Venous blood samples have blood glucose levels that are approximately 10% less than capillary or arterial specimens (Deshpande & Ward Platt, 2005). Another possible reason for variance and lack of reproducibility is improper storage or outdated shelf-life of test strips, which may result in inaccurate results. A third potential problem is contamination with isopropyl alcohol, which falsely elevates the results. To increase accuracy of blood glucose determination, isopropyl alcohol should be allowed to dry thoroughly before the skin is punctured, and the first drop of blood should be wiped away before a blood drop is placed on the test strip. It has also been recommended that color blindness testing be done on all staff that routinely perform glucose measurements read by eye and compared with a color chart (Brooks, 1997).

Interventions

Newborns with asymptomatic hypoglycemia should be fed immediately and then retested within 4 hours. Invasive interventions on the basis of low values detected by screening are not warranted as long as infants are assessed and are found to be without clinical features attributing to hypoglycemia. If the blood glucose is 36 mg/dL, the infant should be offered a breastfeeding or given expressed breast milk or formula. The infant should be further assessed within 4 hours and laboratory plasma glucose estimation is repeated. If the glucose remains <36 mg/dL for two consecutive measurements, the infant should be fed again. It may be sufficient to increase the amount of milk offered, and breastfed infants should be offered frequent feedings on demand (Canadian Paediatric Society, 2004; Cornblath et al., 2000; Williams, 2005). If results continue to be low (<36 mg/dL), they should be corroborated by laboratory determination and intravenous therapy started.

The timing of laboratory measurements may also result in inaccurate values, because failure to run the test promptly after blood sampling results in red blood cell oxidation of glucose and produces falsely low values. Blood samples should be transported on ice and analyzed within 30 minutes (Kalhan & Parimi, 2002). Newborns that have had a glucose level less than 36 mg/dL are at risk for subsequent episodes of hypoglycemia and should have a bedside screening performed before feedings and when symptoms occur. When feeding interventions are offered for low blood glucose, levels should be rechecked in 60 minutes to ensure that there has been a response (Canadian Paediatric Society, 2004).

Newborns with symptomatic hypoglycemia, particularly those with neurological signs and low bedside blood glucose, should be treated immediately with an intravenous infusion of glucose, and a blood sample should be drawn and sent to the laboratory for glucose evaluation. Infusion rates should be similar to endogenous hepatic production (approximately 5 mg/kg/min depending on maturity and weight for gestation—equivalent to 10% dextrose at approximately 70–80 mL/kg/day) and titrated based on response. Gradual increases in glucose infusion rate should not exceed 2 mg/kg/min each hour. Newborns who are unable to nipple feed and those whose blood glucose levels do not respond to oral feedings or have glucose level <20 mg/dL are given a 200 mg/kg (2 mL/kg) bolus of 10% dextrose in water intravenously over 1 minute, followed by a continuous infusion starting at the rates given above, until the blood glucose level is stabilized (Cornblath et al., 2000; Williams, 2005). Correction of hypoglycemia should result in resolution of the symptoms. Intravenous administration is tapered off slowly, and the blood glucose level is monitored every 1 to 4 hours initially and then intermittently before feedings until stable.

Newborns that experience persistent hypoglycemia may require an increased concentration of glucose, such as 12.5%, 15%, or 20%; dextrose solutions with concentrations greater than 12.5% require placement of a central line because of the risk of tissue extravasation. Other treatments for persistent or refractory hypoglycemia include glucagon, which promotes glycogenolysis and requires adequate stores; and corticosteroids, which induce gluconeogenic enzyme activity (Kalhan & Parimi, 2002).

Hypoglycemia severe enough to warrant intravenous therapy, or which persists or recurs, requires further investigation to rule out underlying pathology, particularly infection or metabolic and endocrine disease (Deshpande & Ward Platt, 2005). The focus of nursing care is to prevent hypoglycemia when possible. Newborns should be fed within the first 2 hours of life. Care is taken to avoid cold stress and to recognize signs of respiratory distress and sepsis that can increase the newborn's risk for developing hypoglycemia.

HYPERBILIRUBINEMIA

Unconjugated or indirect hyperbilirubinemia resulting in clinical jaundice is detected in up to 60% of term and 80% of preterm newborns (Juretschke, 2005). Typically, healthy newborns are discharged from the hospital before the usual peak of total serum bilirubin (72–120 hours). Most jaundice is benign and resolves within 7–10 days in term newborns. Because of the potential of bilirubin toxicity, newborns are monitored to identify those who may develop severe hyperbilirubinemia and in rare cases bilirubin encephalopathy or kernicterus. Unconjugated hyperbilirubinemia results from physiologic (Display 14–4) or pathologic causes (Display 14–5).

Pathophysiology

Bilirubin is produced from the breakdown of heme-containing proteins (Juretschke, 2005). The major

D I S P L A Y   1 4 - 4

Mechanisms Attributed to Physiologic Unconjugated Hyperbilirubinemia

Increased bilirubin related to relative polycythemia and short (80- to 90-day) life span of fetal red blood cells

Decreased uptake of bilirubin by the liver

Decreased enzyme activity and ability to conjugate bilirubin

Decreased ability to excrete bilirubin

Breastfeeding

Causes of Pathologic Unconjugated Hyperbilirubinemia

Hemolytic disease of the newborn
Bruising, extravascular blood
Polycythemia
Intestinal obstruction
Metabolic conditions
Prematurity
Infection
Respiratory distress

heme-containing protein is hemoglobin, which is the source of approximately 75% of the bilirubin produced. Heme is acted on by the enzyme heme oxygenase, releasing carbon monoxide and biliverdin. Biliverdin is then reduced to bilirubin through the activity of the enzyme biliverdin reductase. The degradation of every 1 gram of hemoglobin produces 34 to 35 mg of bilirubin. Bilirubin binds with albumin for transport to the liver. Bilirubin, but not albumin, diffuses into the liver cytoplasm, where it is transported to the endoplasmic reticulum for conjugation. Bilirubin combines with glucuronate with the help of glucuronyl transferase, the conjugating enzyme. Conjugated bilirubin is water soluble and excreted into bile and subsequently into the small intestine through the common bile duct. In the gut, conjugated bilirubin is excreted from the body or converted to unconjugated bilirubin by a gut enzyme (β-glucuronidase). If conversion to unconjugated bilirubin occurs, it is reabsorbed into the enterohepatic circulation.

Excretion of conjugated bilirubin is facilitated by bacteria in the gut. Meconium contains large amounts of bilirubin, but excretion is inhibited in the newborn because of the sterility of the gut. Normal colonization of bacteria occurs over time and is facilitated by early and frequent feeding. Feeding introduces bacteria into the gut. Lack of bacterial flora allows conversion of conjugated bilirubin back to an unconjugated form. This, along with greater red cell mass per kilogram in the newborn than in the adult and a shortened red cell life span, sets the stage for development of physiologic unconjugated hyperbilirubinemia. Newborns produce twice as much bilirubin as adults (Halamek & Stevenson, 2002; Juretschke, 2005).

In a term newborn, physiologic unconjugated hyperbilirubinemia is characterized by a progressive increase in serum bilirubin to a peak of 5 to 8 mg/dL at 72 hours of age. Bilirubin levels slowly decline over the first 2 weeks of life to less than 1 mg/dL (Wheeler, 2000). In a preterm newborn, bilirubin continues to rise until the fifth postnatal day, reaching a peak of 10 to 12 mg/dL (Halamek & Stevenson, 2002).

Pathologic, unconjugated hyperbilirubinemia occurs in term and preterm newborns. Pathologic hyperbilirubinemia is most commonly associated with isoimmune hemolytic disease; blood group incompatibility results in an increased bilirubin load. Other causes include extravascular blood, polycythemia, intestinal obstruction, various metabolic conditions, prematurity, infection, and RDS (Juretschke, 2005). Table 14–4 lists maternal and newborn risk factors for hyperbilirubinemia.

If bilirubin levels continue to rise, severe hyperbilirubinemia and bilirubin encephalopathy or kernicterus may develop. Recent reports indicate that kernicterus, although rare, is still occurring and is almost always preventable (AAP, 2004a). The term *kernicterus* is used interchangeably with the acute and chronic findings of bilirubin encephalopathy. The AAP subcommittee on hyperbilirubinemia recommends acute bilirubin encephalopathy to be used when describing the acute manifestations of toxicity seen in the first weeks after birth and kernicterus reserved for the chronic and permanent clinical sequelae (AAP, 2004a). Permanent damage to the central nervous system (CNS) results from deposition of unconjugated bilirubin in the brain, specifically in the basal ganglia, hippocampal cortex, subthalamic nuclei, and cerebellum (Juretschke, 2005).

During the early phase of acute bilirubin encephalopathy, severely jaundiced infants become lethargic and hypotonic and have a poor suck. The intermediate phase is characterized by moderate stupor, hypertonia,

TABLE 14–4 ■ RISK FACTORS FOR HYPERBILIRUBINEMIA

Newborn	Maternal
Birth weight <1,500 g	Oxytocin
Preterm delivery	Forceps or vacuum delivery
Male sex	Diabetes
Hypothermia	East Asian heritage
Asphyxia	Native American heritage
Hypoalbuminemia	Pregnancy-induced
Sepsis	hypertension
Meningitis	Family history of jaundice,
Polycythemia (Hct >65%)	liver disease, anemia, or
Drugs that affect	splenectomy
albumin binding	Blood incompatibilities
Congenital hypothyroidism	
Bruising	
Poor feeding	
Inborn error of metabolism	

and irritability. The infant may also develop a fever and high-pitched cry that alternates with drowsiness and hypotonia. The hypertonia is characterized by backward arching of the trunk (opisthotonos) and of the neck (retrocollis). CNS damage may in some cases be reversed during this phase with a combination of intensive phototherapy and an emergent exchange transfusion. The advanced phase is characterized by pronounced retrocollis and opisthotonos, shrill cry, inability to feed, apnea, fever, deep stupor to coma, seizures, and death. In the chronic form, kernicterus, surviving infants may develop severe athetoid cerebral palsy, auditory dysfunction, dental-enamel dysplasia, paralysis of upward gaze, as well as intellectual and other handicaps (AAP, 2004a). There is no absolute level at which bilirubin encephalopathy occurs in all newborns. Gestational age, postnatal age, clinical condition, and the pathophysiologic process involved all play a part in determining what level of unconjugated bilirubin causes encephalopathy in a particular newborn (Juretschke, 2005).

Assessment

Clinical jaundice is apparent at serum bilirubin levels of 5 to 7 mg/dL (Juretschke, 2005; Lund & Kuller, 2003). Jaundice progresses in a caudal direction from head to the lower extremities. Visual recognition of jaundice is inaccurate, unreliable, and unsafe and varies with the experience and level of training of the observer (AAP, 2004a). A careful physical examination of any newborn presenting with jaundice aids in determining the cause of hyperbilirubinemia. The newborn should be examined for signs of prematurity, small-for-gestational age, microcephaly, and extravascular blood such as bruising and cephalohematoma, petechiae, and hepatosplenomegaly. In conjunction with the clinical examination, transcutaneous bilirubin (TcB) assessment and a number of laboratory tests may be done to evaluate and determine the cause of hyperbilirubinemia (Display 14–6).

New guidelines published in July 2004 and further outlined by a sentinel event alert in August 2004 have been established for the management of hyperbilirubinemia in the newborn infant ≥35 weeks' gestation (AAP, 2004a; JCAHO, 2004). These guidelines stress the importance of universal systematic assessment while the newborn is hospitalized, close follow-up, and prompt intervention when indicated. The key elements of the recommendation suggest that the clinician should:

1. Promote and support successful breastfeeding.
2. Establish nursery protocols for the identification and evaluation of hyperbilirubinemia.
3. Measure the total serum bilirubin (TSB) or TcB level on infants jaundiced in the first 24 hours.

DISPLAY 14-6

Laboratory Tests to Evaluate the Cause of Jaundice

Total and direct bilirubin
Blood type
Coombs
Hematocrit
Peripheral smear for red blood cell morphology
Liver enzymes
Viral and/or bacterial cultures
pH
Serum albumin

4. Recognize that visual estimation of the degree of jaundice can lead to errors, particularly in darkly pigmented infants.
5. Interpret all bilirubin levels according to the infant's age in hours.
6. Recognize that infants at less than 38 weeks' gestation, particularly those who are breast-fed, are at higher risk of developing hyperbilirubinemia and require closer surveillance and monitoring.
7. Perform a systematic assessment on all infants before discharge for the risk of severe hyperbilirubinemia.
8. Provide parents with written and verbal information about newborn jaundice.
9. Provide appropriate follow-up based on the time of discharge and the risk assessment.
10. Treat newborns, when indicated, with phototherapy or exchange transfusion.

Interventions

In supporting adequate breastfeeding, clinicians should instruct mothers to nurse their infants 8 to 12 times per day over the first several days. This not only promotes adequate hydration and caloric intake but also decreases the likelihood of subsequent significant hyperbilirubinemia. Nurseries should have established protocols for the assessment of jaundice. Newborns should be assessed with vital signs, but no less than every 8 to 12 hours. Any infant jaundiced in the first 24 hours after birth should have a TcB or TSB measured. Assessment should be done in a well-lit room; however, it is important to remember that safety data have demonstrated that visual assessment of jaundice is unreliable and unsafe (Johnson, Bhutani, & Brown,

2002; Soorani-Lunsing, Woltil, & Hadders-Algra, 2001). A low threshold should be used for measuring bilirubin. Noninvasive TcB devices have proven to be very useful as screening tools. It has also been recommended that protocols allow nurses access to bilirubin testing either TcB or TSB, without a physician's order.

Every newborn should be assessed for the risk of developing severe hyperbilirubinemia before discharge. The risk of kernicterus increases incrementally with rising levels of TSB >19 mg/dL (Smitherman, Stark, & Bhutani, 2006). In the Pilot Kernicterus Registry, the causes for kernicterus were attributed to the following three categories in equal proportions: hemolytic disorders (mostly ABO immunization); G6PD deficiency (associated with hemolysis and impaired bilirubin conjugation); and idiopathic causes (presumably from delayed or impaired function of the glucuronyl transferase enzyme system), coupled with breastfeeding and inadequate nutritional intake (Bhutani, Johnson, & Shapiro, 2004). All nurseries should establish protocols for assessing this risk. This is particularly important if the infant is discharged before 72 hours of age. This risk can be assessed by predischarge measurement of bilirubin and/or assessment of clinical risk factors. Regardless of how risk is assessed, appropriate follow-up is essential. The need for and timing of a repeat TcB or TSB measurement will depend on the zone in which the TSB falls on the nomogram (Fig. 14–2). Predischarged TSBs are plotted on this hour-specific nomogram. The infant is then assigned a low, intermediate, or high risk for developing clinically significant hyperbilirubinemia on subsequent bilirubin levels (Bhutani, Johnson, & Sivievri, 1999).

The risk factors most frequently associated with severe hyperbilirubinemia are predischarge TSB or TcB levels in the high-risk zone of the nomogram, jaundice with the first 24 hours, blood group incompatibility with a positive direct antiglobulin (or other known hemolytic diseases), gestational age between 35 and 36 weeks, previous sibling who received phototherapy, cephalhematoma or significant bruising, East Asian race, and exclusive breastfeeding (particularly if nursing is not going well and weight loss is excessive; AAP, 2004a). Written and verbal information must be provided to parents at discharge. This should include an explanation of jaundice, the need to monitor infants for jaundice, and advice on how monitoring should be done. Newborn jaundice resource materials are available for parents in multiple languages (English, Spanish, Chinese, and Italian) and include a frequently asked question sheet from the AAP (2004b). All infants should be examined by a qualified healthcare professional in the first days after discharge. Infants discharged should be seen by age (AAP, 2004a):

Before 24 hours	72 hours
Between 24 and 47.9 hours	96 hours
Between 48 and 72 hours	120 hours

Phototherapy

In the late 1940s, exchange transfusion was the only available treatment for newborns with hyperbilirubinemia. In the mid 1950s, an observant nurse noticed that newborns exposed to sunlight had less clinical jaundice over exposed areas and decreased serum bilirubin levels. This observation led to the use of phototherapy, which remains the primary treatment for hyperbilirubinemia. In nearly all newborns, phototherapy decreases or blunts the rise in serum-unconjugated bilirubin regardless of gestational age, race, or presence or absence of hemolysis. Phototherapy is used for treatment and prophylaxis of hyperbilirubinemia. No serious long-term side effects have been reported. Recommendations for treatment in infants born at ≥35 weeks gestation are found in Figure 14–3.

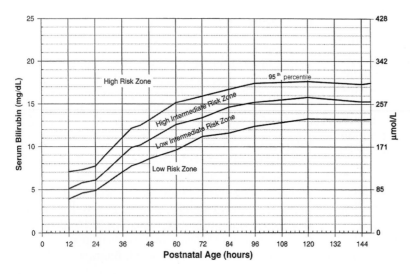

FIGURE 14–2. Nomogram for designation of risk of developing hyperbilirubinemia. (Used with permission from Bhutani, V. K., Johnson, L. H., & Sivievri, E. M. [1999]. Predictive ability of a predischarge hour-specific serum bilirubin for subsequent significant hyperbilirubinemia in healthy term and near-term newborns. *Pediatrics, 103*[1], 6–14.)

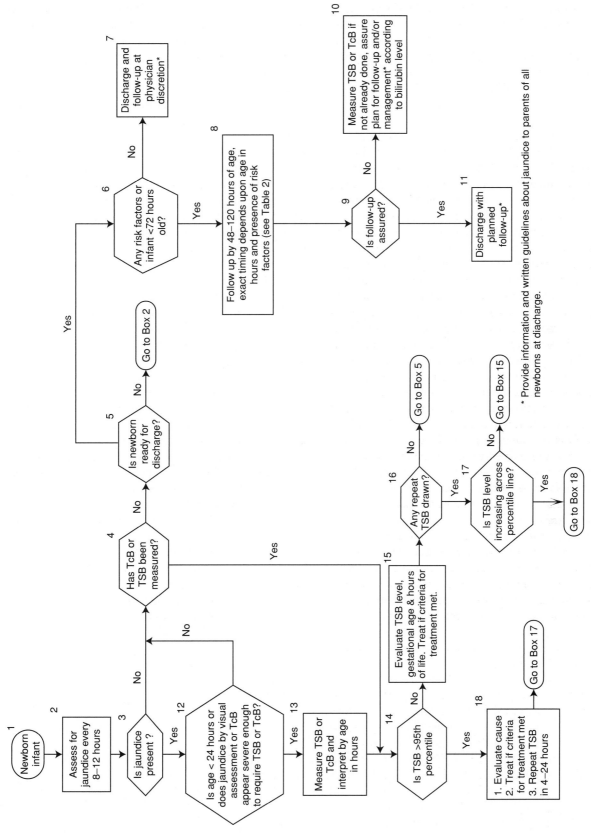

FIGURE 14–3. Algorithm for the management of jaundice in the newborn nursery. (From American Academy of Pediatrics Clinical Practice Guideline Subcommittee on Hyperbilirubinemia. [2004a]. Management of hyperbilirubinemia in the newborn infant 35 or more weeks' gestation. *Pediatrics 114*[1], 297–316.)

There is no consensus or recommendation regarding the discontinuation of phototherapy.

The goal of phototherapy is to decrease the level of unconjugated bilirubin. Phototherapy accomplishes this goal by means of the following:

- Absorption of light by bilirubin
- Photoconversion of bilirubin by photochemical reaction, restructuring the molecule
- Excretion of bilirubin through urine and bile

For phototherapy to be effective, there must be illumination of an adequate area of exposed skin at a sufficiently short distance. Several types of phototherapy lamps are available: daylight, cool white fluorescent, fluorescent green, special blue fluorescent, quartz halogen, and high-intensity gallium nitride light-emitting diodes (AAP, 2004a). Phototherapy can also be delivered using a fiberoptic blanket (McFadden, 1991). Although any light source with irradiance between 400 and 500 nm can be used, the most effective light sources currently available are those that use special blue fluorescent tubes or a specially designed light-emitting diode light (AAP, 2004a). There is a direct relationship between the irradiance used and the rate of bilirubin decline with phototherapy. Irradiance should be monitored and is measured with a radiometer as $\mu W/cm^2/nm$. Standard phototherapy units deliver 8 to 10 $\mu W/cm^2/nm$ (AAP, 2004). A fiberoptic blanket generally delivers irradiance of 15 to 20 $\mu W/cm^2/nm$ (McFadden, 1991). Intensive phototherapy requires >30 $\mu W/cm^2/nm$. Intensive phototherapy can be provided with special blue tubes placed 10 to 15 cm above the infant (AAP, 2004). To expose the maximum surface area of the infant, overhead phototherapy can be used with a fiberoptic blanket. The newborn is placed naked under the phototherapy light and repositioned at least every 2 hours to ensure adequate light exposure to all areas. If a fiberoptic blanket is used, the blanket is wrapped around the newborn's trunk, and clothing is placed over the blanket.

Although phototherapy has not been associated with any serious long-term effects, short-term side effects exist. The focus of nursing care is to prevent or minimize side effects. Newborns receiving phototherapy from phototherapy lamps are placed in a bassinet or under a radiant heat source, and axillary temperature is monitored at least every 2 hours to assess for hyperthermia. Hyperthermia can result in tachycardia and increased insensible water loss and dehydration. Loose stools are an unavoidable effect of phototherapy and can also result in increased insensible water loss and dehydration. Intake, output, and urine-specific gravity are measured accurately and documented. Meticulous skin care is necessary to prevent skin breakdown resulting from loose stools. A generalized macular rash frequently develops and resolves spontaneously when phototherapy is discontinued.

The newborn's eyes are covered at all times while under phototherapy lamps to prevent retinal damage. An advantage of the fiberoptic blanket is that eye protection is unnecessary. Eye patches should be removed during feedings or at least every 4 hours to observe for drainage and to promote social stimulation and visual development. Corneal abrasions can result from eye patches that apply excessive pressure to the eyes (Shaw, 2003). Although human studies have not shown irradiance effects on the developing gonads, animal studies have shown DNA strand breaks and chromatid exchanges and mutations. Diapers or small diaper-like devices are used as a shield for the testicles or ovaries (Blackburn, 1995).

Techniques are being investigated to aid in the identification of rising bilirubin levels, especially in those patients with hemolysis. Knowing that carbon monoxide and biliverdin are produced in equal amounts has led researchers to investigate the possibility of noninvasive carbon monoxide monitoring. Identifying levels of carbon monoxide in blood and breath could be used as an index of heme degradation and thus rising bilirubin levels (Juretschke, 2005). Methods to replace traditional treatment are also being investigated. In 1980, it was discovered that certain metalloporphyrins (ie, family of compounds of which heme belongs) readily bind to heme oxygenase, inhibiting the enzyme's activity and resulting in decreased degradation of heme and bilirubin production. Tin–protoporphyrin and tin–mesoporphyrin are two such compounds that are potent inhibitors of heme oxygenase. There currently is evidence that hyperbilirubinemia can be effectively treated or even prevented with tin–mesoporphyrin. At this time, this drug is not approved by the U.S. Food and Drug Administration. If approved, this drug could find immediate application in infants not responding to phototherapy (AAP, 2004a).

NEONATAL SEPSIS

The incidence of neonatal sepsis is approximately 1 to 5 cases per 1,000 live births (Edwards, 2002). Variations in reported morbidity and mortality rates are related to methodological factors such as healthcare institution practice, risk status of the population or community investigated, and clinical factors such as gestational age and birth weight. Diagnosis of neonatal sepsis is based on clinical signs and evidence of a positive blood culture (Edwards, 2002).

Pathophysiology

Many microorganisms are responsible for infection during the neonatal period (Display 14–7). The most common causative bacterial agents are *group B hemolytic Streptococcus* (GBS) and *Escherichia coli* (Schuchat

DISPLAY 14-7

Organisms Responsible for Neonatal Infection

Toxoplasma gondii
Rubella
Cytomegalovirus
Herpes
Human immunodeficiency virus
Treponema pallidum
Chlamydia trachomatis
Enterovirus
Other bacteria
Hepatitis B
Human papillomavirus

- All pregnant women should be screened at 35 to 37 weeks' gestation for vaginal and rectal colonization.
- Women with GBS bacteriuria during the current pregnancy should automatically receive chemoprophylaxis; no screening culture is needed.
- Women who have had a previous infant with invasive GBS disease should automatically receive chemoprophylaxis; no screening culture is needed.
- At the onset of labor or rupture of membranes, chemoprophylaxis should be given to all women identified as GBS carriers.
- Chemoprophylaxis should be given at the onset of labor or rupture of membranes if the GBS status is unknown and there are risk factors.
- For chemoprophylaxis, IV penicillin is preferred, although IV ampicillin can be used as an alternative. Chapter 6 reviews prevention strategies for early-onset GBS and current intrapartum antimicrobial treatment for mothers.

et al., 2000). Infection occurs as a result of the following conditions:

- Intrauterine exposure by means of ascending infection from one or more of the endogenous flora of the cervix or vagina or, less commonly, by a transplacental route from maternal circulation
- Cutaneous transmission as the fetus passes through the birth canal
- Environmental contamination after the birth

Two patterns of development, early onset and late onset, are observed in neonatal sepsis. Early-onset sepsis occurs within 7 days of life. Frequently, inoculation occurred in utero. If symptoms are not present immediately after birth, most newborns become symptomatic within 12 hours. Development of signs in early-onset sepsis is generally very sudden and may rapidly progress to septic shock. Late-onset infection may occur as early as 1 week of age, or as late as 3 months of life, but more commonly after the first week of life. Late-onset infection usually results from exposure during the birth process or is the result of nosocomial transmission after birth from caregivers or invasive procedures. Because of immaturity of the newborn immune system and inability to localize infection, the most common clinical manifestations of sepsis are septicemia, pneumonia, and meningitis.

GBS acquired from the mother is the most common Gram-positive organism causing sepsis in the newborn. Most of these infections could be prevented by use of prophylactic antimicrobials in at-risk women. The Centers for Disease Control and Prevention (CDC), AAP, and American College of Obstetricians and Gynecologists (ACOG) have recommendations for prevention of early-onset infection (ACOG, 2002; AAP, 2003; Schrag, Gorwitz, Fultz-Butts, & Schuchat, 2002).

Assessment

As with all neonatal complications, early identification of newborns at risk and prompt recognition of developing signs decreases morbidity and increases the chances of survival. Recognizing multiple risk factors is the first step in identifying newborns whose early days may be complicated by infection. Risk factors can be categorized as maternal, neonatal, and environmental. A thorough review of antepartum and intrapartum history should specifically look for conditions that increase the risk of early-onset sepsis (Display 14–8). If different nurses care for the mother and newborn, communication among healthcare team members is

DISPLAY 14-8

Maternal Factors Predisposing Newborns to Sepsis

Preterm labor
Premature rupture of the membranes
Prolonged rupture of membranes
Maternal sepsis
Chorioamnionitis
Intraamniotic infection
Vaginal colonization with group B streptococci (GBS)
Perineal colonization with *Escherichia coli*
Prior birth of an infant with GBS
Chemical dependency or substance abuse
Urinary tract infection
Foul-smelling amniotic fluid

essential to ensure that maternal complications with potential impact on the newborn are not overlooked. The nurse caring for the mother during the postpartum period should notify the neonatal care provider if fever or other symptoms of infection develop.

The primary neonatal factors influencing development of sepsis are gestational age and birth weight. Gestational age and birth weight vary inversely with morbidity and mortality from sepsis. Preterm newborns may be exposed to the same organisms as term newborns, but their ability to fight infection is lessened. Other factors associated with increased risk of sepsis are resuscitation at birth and low Apgar scores. Congenital anomalies in which the skin or mucous membrane is not intact increase the risk of sepsis because a cutaneous port of entry is available for microorganisms. A history of a nonreassuring fetal heart rate pattern during labor, with or without meconium in the amniotic fluid, may identify fetuses at risk for infection. More male than female newborns develop sepsis, suggesting that the susceptibility may be sex linked (Edwards, 2002).

The most obvious environmental risk for developing sepsis is admission to a newborn intensive care unit (NICU). Newborns in the NICU are compromised because of the original reason for admission along with being subjected to manipulation and invasive procedures that frequently puncture the skin, the first line of defense against infection. Environmental risks of nosocomial infection include use of equipment; indwelling catheters and chest tubes; inadequate hand-washing or cleaning procedures; breaks in skin integrity, oxygen therapy, and mechanical ventilation, and surgical procedures.

Overcrowding in the nursery or inadequate attention to isolation precautions increases the risk of cross-contamination. In addition to reviewing antepartum and intrapartum history, identifying the newborn with neonatal sepsis requires a thorough physical examination, evaluation of vital signs and laboratory data, and recognition of signs consistent with the diagnosis of sepsis. Like many conditions complicating the newborn period, the early signs of neonatal sepsis are vague and frequently nonspecific. Clinical indicators such as apnea, tachypnea, temperature instability, tachycardia, lethargy, and poor feeding may be early symptoms of sepsis. Figure 14–4 shows the clinical symptoms associated with neonatal sepsis.

A full diagnostic evaluation includes a complete blood cell (CBC) count with a differential cell count, aerobic and anaerobic blood cultures, and a tracheal aspirate, if intubated. If there are no CNS signs, some

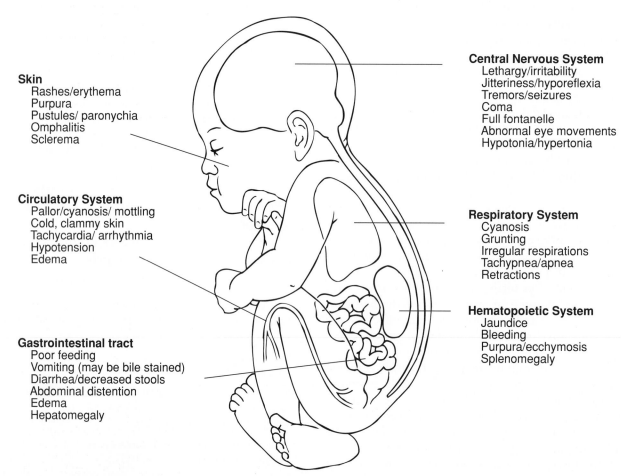

Skin
Rashes/erythema
Purpura
Pustules/ paronychia
Omphalitis
Sclerema

Central Nervous System
Lethargy/irritability
Jitteriness/hyporeflexia
Tremors/seizures
Coma
Full fontanelle
Abnormal eye movements
Hypotonia/hypertonia

Circulatory System
Pallor/cyanosis/ mottling
Cold, clammy skin
Tachycardia/ arrhythmia
Hypotension
Edema

Respiratory System
Cyanosis
Grunting
Irregular respirations
Tachypnea/apnea
Retractions

Hematopoietic System
Jaundice
Bleeding
Purpura/ecchymosis
Splenomegaly

Gastrointestinal tract
Poor feeding
Vomiting (may be bile stained)
Diarrhea/decreased stools
Abdominal distention
Edema
Hepatomegaly

FIGURE 14–4. Clinical signs of neonatal sepsis. (From Wasserman, R. L. [1982] Neonatal sepsis: The potential of granulocyte transfusion. *Hospital Practice, 17*[5], 98.)

believe a lumbar puncture can be postponed while awaiting the blood culture results, although this is controversial (Edwards, 2002). Anaerobic and aerobic blood cultures should be obtained before the initiation of antibiotic therapy from any newborn suspected of being septic. A positive blood culture is the only way to make a definitive diagnosis of bacterial sepsis. Superficial cultures from sites such as the nares, ear, throat, axillary, and umbilicus and cultures of gastric aspirate are rarely performed because they document colonization with a particular organism rather than with bacteremia or sepsis. Other studies may include evaluation of acute-phase reactants such as C-reactive protein (CRP). Acute-phase reactants increase in response to inflammation or tissue necrosis, theoretically indicating of disease such as infection (Edwards, 2002).

Interventions

Many institutions have developed protocols for evaluations to exclude sepsis, including laboratory data and frequency of vital signs and clinical assessment. The CDC, AAP, and ACOG have also published certain recommendations for the management of a neonate born to a mother who received intrapartum antimicrobial prophylaxis for GBS. If there are signs of sepsis, the newborn should receive a full diagnostic evaluation and antimicrobial therapy. If there are no signs of sepsis and the newborn is less than 35 weeks' gestation, a CBC and blood culture should be obtained and the newborn observed for 48 hours or longer. If the newborn is greater than or equal to 35 weeks' gestation and the mother received less than two doses of an antimicrobial agent, a CBC and blood culture should also be obtained and the newborn observed for 48 hours or longer. If the mother received two or more doses of an antimicrobial agent, no evaluation or therapy is required, although the newborn must still be observed for 48 hours or longer. This approach does not allow for early discharge (AAP, 2003). Figure 14–5 is an algorithm for management of infants born to mothers who received intrapartum chemoprophylaxis for GBS infection.

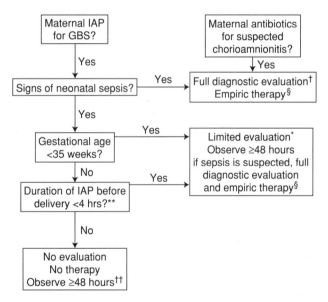

* If no maternal intrapartum prophylaxis for GBS was administered despite an indication being present, data are insufficient on which to recommend a single management strategy.

† Includes complete blood cell count and differential, blood culture, and chest radiograph if respiratory abnormalities are present. When signs of sepsis are present, a lumbar puncture, if feasible, should be performed.

§ Duration of therapy varies depending on results of blood culture, cerebrospinal fluid findings, if obtained, and the clinical course of the infant. If laboratory results and clinical course do not indicate bacterial infection, duration may be as short as 48 hours.

** Applies only to penicillin, ampicillin, or cefazolin and assumes recommended dosing regimens (Box 2).

†† A healthy-appearing infant who was ≥38 weeks' gestation at delivery and whose mother received ≥4 hours of intrapartum prophylaxis before delivery may be discharged home after 24 hours if other discharge criteria have been met and a person able to comply fully with instructions for home observation will be present. If any one of these conditions is not met, the infant should be observed in the hospital for at least 48 hours and until criteria for discharge are achieved.

FIGURE 14–5. Algorithm for infants of mothers who received antepartum antimicrobial agents for prevention of group B streptococcus or suspected chorioamnionitis. (From Schrag, S., Gorwitz, R., Fultz-Butts, K., & Schuchat, A. [2002]. Prevention of perinatal group B streptococcal disease: Revised guidelines from the CDC. *Morbidity and Mortality Weekly Report, 51*[RR11], 1–22.)

After the diagnostic evaluation has been completed, antimicrobial agents are initiated. For early-onset sepsis, ampicillin, a broad-spectrum antimicrobial that is bactericidal for gram-positive and gram-negative bacteria, is used in combination with an aminoglycoside such as gentamicin. The usual dosage of ampicillin is 50 to 100 mg/kg every 8 to 12 hours. When sepsis is complicated by meningitis, the dosage is increased to 100 to 200 mg/kg. The dose of gentamicin effective against *Pseudomonas, Klebsiella,* and *E. coli* has changed and depends on the gestational age and day of life. Treatment for sepsis continues for 7 to 10 days. If a diagnosis of meningitis is made, treatment may continue for 14 days. A spinal tap is usually done by day 10; if results remain positive, antimicrobials are continued for 21 days or until two sterile spinal fluid specimens are obtained. Antimicrobials are changed if results of blood cultures indicate a different medication would be more effective against the involved organism or less toxic to the newborn. After 48 to 72 hours, if the culture result is negative, antimicrobials may be discontinued. Hand hygiene remains a key component for controlling infections in the nursery. Other potentially beneficial infection control practices include adequate staffing, avoiding overcrowding, nursery design, workload capacity, appropriate staff-to-infant ratios, and catheter management teams (Benjamin & Stoll, 2006; Harbarth, Sudre, Dharan, Cadenas, & Pittet, 1999).

NEONATAL ABSTINENCE SYNDROME

Intrauterine exposure to illicit drugs may lead to neonatal intoxication or withdrawal. The incidence has been reported to be 3% to 50%, depending on the population, community setting, and individual hospital sampling practices. Even though studies show that drug use among women of childbearing age is declining, a recent survey found that 5.5% of women use illicit drugs during pregnancy (Rosen & Bateman, 2002). Commonly abused drugs include alcohol, marijuana, cocaine and crack, heroin, amphetamine and methamphetamine, inhalants, and the "club drugs" (Rosen & Bateman, 2002). Drugs associated with neonatal abstinence syndrome (NAS) can be divided into four groups: CNS depressants, opioids, CNS stimulants, and hallucinogens (Display 14–9).

Pathophysiology

Maternal drug use in pregnancy has been associated with higher rates of fetal distress and demise, lower Apgar scores, growth retardation, adverse neurodevelopmental outcomes that may not manifest until later in infancy, and acute withdrawal during the neonatal period (Rosen & Bateman, 2002). It is difficult to know whether substance abuse alone or (more likely)

DISPLAY 14-9

Drugs Associated With Neonatal Abstinence Syndrome

CNS DEPRESSANTS

Alcohol
Barbiturates
Benzodiazepines
Cannabinoids (ie, marijuana, hashish)
Opioids
Morphine

CODEINE

Methadone
Meperidine
Oxycodone
Propoxyphene (Darvon)

Hydromorphone (Dilaudid)
Fentanyl
Heroin
Naloxone (Narcan)
Pentazocine (Talwin)
Nalbuphine (Nubain)
Butorphanol (Stadol)

CNS STIMULANTS

Amphetamines
Cocaine
Methylphenidate (Ritalin)

HALLUCINOGENS

LSD
Ecstasy
Methamphetamines
Inhalants (ie, solvents and aerosols)

American Academy of Pediatrics Committee on Drugs. (1998). Neonatal drug withdrawal. *Pediatrics, 101*(6), 1079–1086.

the multifactorial influence of drug abuse and social problems is responsible. Many pregnant women who use illicit drugs also use tobacco and alcohol, which also pose risks to unborn babies, making it difficult to determine which health problems are caused by a specific illicit drug. Drug abuse in pregnancy is frequently associated with poverty and family disruption, increasing the risk that women will place less value on seeking early and consistent prenatal care. The general health of these women may be poor, predisposing them to suboptimal weight gain and anemia. The CDC reported that 12.3% of pregnant women smoke during pregnancy (Matthews, 2001). Smoking during pregnancy increases the risk of low-birth-weight infants (Guyer et al., 1999). The metabolites of cigarette smoke cause vasoconstriction in intrauterine growth retardation (Ganapathy, Prasad, Ganapathy, & Leibach, 1999), and the nicotine present in cigarettes disrupts the normal development of the fetal brain (Nau, Hansen, & Steldinger, 1985; Slotkin, 1998). Infants exposed to tobacco may demonstrate symptoms such as excitability and hypertonia, and require more handling to keep them in a quiet alert state (Law et al., 2003).

Complete information on transmission of illicit drugs to the fetus is unavailable, but most appear to pass easily through the placenta. Based on animal studies, it is known that rates of transmission and metabolism vary from drug to drug and depend on fetal age. Increased maternal blood flow in later gestation appears to increase transport of substances to the fetus. The vasoconstricting effects of these substances cause abruptio placentae, elevated blood pressure, precipitous labor, inadequate contraction patterns, decreased fetal oxygenation, and decreased length and head circumference. Use of cocaine and heroin, amphetamine, and marijuana is associated with intrauterine growth restriction. Some studies have shown a higher incidence of genitourinary abnormalities in infants of cocaine-using mothers. Cocaine is also thought to increase fetal vasoconstricting hormones, leading to increased blood pressure and an elevated heart rate. These physiologic responses increase risk of cerebral ischemia and hemorrhagic lesions (Rosen & Bateman, 2002).

Assessment

Neonatal abstinence syndrome describes a range of symptoms the newborn experiences during withdrawal (Table 14–5). It is often a multisystem disorder that frequently involves the central nervous and gastrointestinal systems. Although the most severe withdrawal symptoms are seen in the newborn exposed to opioids, symptoms can also occur after exposure to other drugs. Depending on the chemical agent the mother used, after several weeks or months, symptoms no longer

TABLE 14–5 ■ SYMPTOMS OF NEONATAL ABSTINENCE SYNDROME

Site Affected	Symptoms
Central nervous system	Irritability and restlessness Shrill, high-pitched cry Tremors Hyperreflexia Altered sleep patterns Seizures
Gastrointestinal system	Vomiting Diarrhea Excessive sucking Poor feeding
Respiratory system	Tachypnea Stuffy nose Cyanosis Flaring Retractions Apnea
Autonomic nervous system	Yawning Sneezing Mottled skin Sweating Fever
Skin	Excoriations

represent withdrawal but the long-term effects of intrauterine drug exposure.

Clinical signs of opioid withdrawal usually begin 24 to 48 hours after birth, but they may not appear for as long as 10 days. Symptoms generally last for less than 2 weeks, but some infants show mild signs for up to 6 months (Fike, 2003). The severity of the abstinence syndrome depends on the drug or combination of drugs used. Withdrawal symptoms are more severe when the drug exposure is closer to the time of birth. Methadone withdrawal is more severe than any other narcotic (Rosen & Bateman, 2002). Approximately 75% of newborns with prenatal exposure to methadone develop withdrawal symptoms. Time of onset is variable. The newborn may have early withdrawal beginning at 24 to 48 hours or may have one or two types of late withdrawal, in which symptoms may appear shortly after birth, improve, and then reappear in 2 to 4 weeks, or there may be no symptoms until 2 to 3 weeks of age.

Heroin withdrawal begins within the first 2 weeks after birth, with an average onset at 72 hours. The incidence of withdrawal has been associated with maternal dosage of heroin, duration of maternal addiction, and time of the last maternal dose (Rosen & Bateman, 2002).

There is no clearly defined abstinence syndrome associated with in utero cocaine exposure (Fike, 2003). Several neurobehavioral abnormalities frequently occur after intrauterine cocaine exposure:

- Hypertonia
- Hyperactive startle reflex
- Irritability
- Tremulousness
- Tachypnea
- Loose stools
- State disorganization
- Poor feeding

These symptoms usually occur on day 2 or 3 and are more consistent with the cocaine effect itself, rather than with withdrawal.

Preterm newborns are at lower risk for drug withdrawal, presumably because their CNS immaturity prevented damage from exposure to the drug or because of the decreased amount of time in utero they were exposed to maternal substance abuse (AAP, 1998). It is difficult to accurately assess the severity of abstinence in preterm newborns because the tools available were originally developed for use with term newborns. Many of the characteristics seen in neonatal drug withdrawal are common in preterm newborns, such as tremors, high-pitched cry, tachypnea, and poor feeding.

Interventions

Appropriate care of drug-exposed newborns begins with early identification and recognition of maternal drug abuse. Careful prenatal and postnatal maternal screening for substance abuse is essential. All women, regardless of racial or social background and perceived risk status, should be asked directly in a nonjudgmental manner about drug and alcohol use during pregnancy. Illicit drug use should be considered as potentially complicating all pregnancies. The level of suspicion should increase when the pregnant woman

- Has received no prenatal care
- Has a history of sexually transmitted diseases
- Insists on leaving the hospital shortly after birth
- Demonstrates signs of drug use such as needle marks and malnutrition
- Demands medication frequently and in large doses

Laws regulating toxicology screens without maternal consent vary from state to state, and the perinatal nurse should be aware of the laws in her state. When indicated, a maternal urine toxicology screen can be included as part of laboratory tests routinely ordered during the hospital admission process. If results are positive or not obtained, a urine toxicology screen or meconium assay is performed with a sample collected from the newborn's first void or stool (Rosen & Bateman, 2002).

DISPLAY 14-10

Interventions to Support the Newborn Experiencing Withdrawal

Swaddling
Rocking
Decrease tactile stimulation
Dark room
Decrease environmental noise and stimulation
Water bed
Small, frequent feedings
Use of a pacifier

All newborns should be observed for signs of neonatal abstinence syndrome.

Many withdrawal symptoms can be successfully treated with basic supportive care (Display 14–10). These interventions increase the newborn's ability to regulate behavioral state, improve neuromotor control, and promote maternal newborn attachment. Minimal handling, swaddling, and a variety of positioning interventions have been used in an attempt to console and quiet the irritable, narcotic-withdrawing newborn. They can easily become overstimulated during the acute period of withdrawal (Fike, 2003). Using a neonatal abstinence scoring system, narcotic-withdrawing newborns placed in a prone position demonstrated lower scores than narcotic-withdrawing newborns placed in other positions (Fike, 2003).

Newborns who do not respond to symptomatic treatment alone may need medication. Ideally, the decision to begin medication is based on an objective assessment of symptoms such as the Neonatal Abstinence Scoring System (NASS; Fig. 14–6). The newborn is assessed and scored every 2 hours for the first 48 hours and then every 8 hours while symptoms of withdrawal persist. Points are given for all behaviors or symptoms observed during the scoring interval. The newborn must be awake and calm to assess muscle tone, respirations, and Moro reflex. Observations should be made after feeding whenever possible, because hunger can mimic withdrawal. Temperature recorded on the scoring sheet should be obtained rectally, although an axillary temperature 2°F cooler may also indicate withdrawal. If the average of any three successive scores exceeds 8 points and is not reduced by nursing interventions, medications are initiated (Weiner & Finnegan, 1998). A simplified scoring system, the Neonatal Withdrawal Inventory (NWI), has been developed based on the NASS (Zahorodny et al., 1998).

CENTRAL NERVOUS SYSTEM DISTURBANCES													
SIGNS AND SYMPTOMS	SCORE	AM						PM					
Excessive High-Pitched Cry	2												
Continuous High-Pitched Cry	3												
Sleeps <1 Hour After Feeding	3												
Sleeps <2 Hours After Feeding	2												
Sleeps <3 Hours After Feeding	1												
Hyperactive Moro Reflex	2												
Markedly Hyperactive Moro Reflex	3												
Mild Tremors Disturbed	1												
Moderate–Severe Tremors Disturbed	2												
Mild Tremors Undisturbed	1												
Moderate–Severe Tremors Undisturbed	4												
Increased Muscle Tone	2												
Excoriation (Specify Area):	1												
Myoclonic Jerks	3												
Generalized Convulsions	5												
METABOLIC/VASOMOTOR /RESPIRATORY DISTURBANCES													
Sweating													
Fever <101(99–100.8°F/37.2–38.2°C)	1												
Fever >101(38.2°C and Higher)	2												
Frequent Yawning (>3–4 times/interval)	1												
Mottling	1												
Nasal Stuffiness	1												
Sneezing (>3–4 times/interval)	1												
Nasal Flaring	2												
Respiratory Rate >60/Min.	1												
Respiratory Rate >60/Min. with Retractions	2												
GASTROINTESTINAL DISTURBANCES													
Excessive Sucking	1												
Poor Feeding	2												
Regurgitation	2												
Projectile Vomiting	3												
Loose Stools	2												
Watery Stools	3												
TOTAL SCORE													

FIGURE 14–6. Neonatal abstinence scoring system. (From Cloherty, J.P., & Stark, A.R. [1998]. *Manual of neonatal case* [4th ed., pp. 26–27]. Boston: Little, Brown.)

TABLE 14–6 ■ MEDICATIONS USED TO TREAT INFANTS WITH NEONATAL ABSTINENCE SYNDROME

Dilute tincture of opium (10 mg/mL) diluted to 0.4 mg/mL	Starting dose 0.1 mL/kg PO every 4 hours with feedings. Dosing may be increased by 0.1 mL every 4 hours until symptoms are controlled. Once symptoms are controlled, continue that dose for 3–5 days and then slowly decrease the dose every 4 hours without changing the frequency. Preferred over paregoric; 25-fold dilution contains same concentration of morphine found in paregoric without the additives or high alcohol content of paregoric.
Paregoric (0.4 mg/mL of morphine)	Starting dose 0.1 mL/kg PO every 4 hours with feedings. Dosing may be increased by 0.1 mL/kg every 3–4 hours until symptoms are controlled. Once symptoms are controlled, continue that dose for 3–5 days; can be tapered by decreasing the dose slowly without changing the frequency.
Phenobarbital	Starting dose 16 mg/kg IM or PO as loading dose, then change to 2–8 mg/kg/day divided every 12 hours. Once symptoms are controlled, the dose should be weaned slowly. Phenobarbital is a good choice for non-narcotic-related withdrawal, but does not relieve GI symptoms.
Methadone	Starting dose 0.05–0.1 mg/kg/day PO divided every 6 hours. The dose can be increased by 0.05 mg/kg until symptoms are controlled. Maintenance dose should be given every 12–24 hours. Once symptoms are controlled, wean slowly until dose of 0.05 mg/kg/day is reached, when it can be discontinued. Methadone is used to treat NAS from opioid withdrawal.
Diazepam	Dose with 1–2 mg every 8 hours as needed to control symptoms.

A variety of medications are used to treat neonatal abstinence syndrome and the choice of medication varies with individual nurseries (Table 14–6). In a recent Cochrane Review, opiates (used with caution) are the preferred initial therapy for NAS, especially for infants of mothers who used opioids during pregnancy (Osborn, Cole, & Jeffery, 2005). Naloxone use is contraindicated in infants born to narcotic addicted mothers due to the risk or seizures and/or the precipitation of severe signs and symptoms of withdrawal (Rosen & Bateman, 2002). Sedation is the most common potential complication related to treatment. Tapering and discontinuation of medications are best achieved using the NASS. After medication has been initiated, the newborn should be scored every 8 hours and reevaluated on a daily basis. If all scores are 8 or less, or the mean of any three successive scores is 7 or less, the dose should be maintained for 72 hours. If, after 72 hours, the scores are consistently 8 or less, or the mean of three successive scores is 7 or less, the dose should be decreased by 10%. This dose is maintained for 24 hours. If the mean score remains less than 8, the dose is decreased by 10% every 24 hours. After the medication has been discontinued, scoring continues until scores are 8 or less for 72 hours.

Because the symptoms of neonatal abstinence may not be completely resolved at the time of discharge, the parents need education to successfully care for the newborn. Parents should spend extended periods observing and interacting with their newborn in the presence of the nurse. These opportunities can be used by the nurse to observe parental interaction. Because drug-exposed newborns are discharged into an environment where drug use may still be a factor, families are followed after discharge to ensure that growth and development is adequate and that parents are aware of and receive available community resources.

HUMAN IMMUNODEFICIENCY VIRUS

HIV-1 infection in women of childbearing years is a growing problem. The ACOG and the CDC recommend offering all women of childbearing age the opportunity for preconception counseling and care as a component to routine medical care (ACOG, 2005; CDC, 2006a). The ACOG and the AAP recommend HIV testing and counseling, with consent, for all pregnant women in the United States and advocate preconception counseling as part of a comprehensive healthcare program for all women (AAP, 2004c; ACOG, 2005; CDC, 2006b; Public Health Service Task Force Recommendations, 2006). HIV testing must be voluntary and free from coercion. No woman should be tested without her knowledge, and each woman has the option to decline or opt out of the HIV screening (CDC, 2006b).

Many women with HIV-1 infection enter pregnancy with a known diagnosis and are already receiving antiretroviral therapy, although adjustment to their regimen may be necessary (Public Health Service Task Force, 2006). Decisions regarding therapy should be the same for pregnant and nonpregnant women with HIV-1 infection, with the additional consideration of the potential impact of therapy on the fetus and infant. The three-part ZDV chemoprophylaxis regimen alone or in combination with other antiretroviral drugs should be discussed and offered. Discussions regarding the treatment of HIV should not be coercive, and the woman is ultimately responsible for the final decision.

Healthcare providers who treat HIV-1-infected pregnant women and their newborns are strongly advised to report all instances of prenatal exposure to antiretroviral drugs to the Antiretroviral Pregnancy Registry. This is an observational epidemiologic project assessing the potential teratogenicity of these drugs (Public Health Service Task Force, 2006).

Antiretroviral Pregnancy Registry
Research Park
1011 Ashes Dr.
Wilmington, NC 28405
1-800-258-4263
1-800-800-1052 (fax)
www.APRegistry.com

Any recommendations provided here have been developed for the United States only. Although perinatal HIV-1 transmission is a worldwide problem, alternate strategies may be appropriate in other countries (Public Health Service Task Force, 2006).

Chemoprophylaxis for Perinatal HIV-1 Transmission

Studies show nearly a 70% reduction in HIV-1 transmission in infants whose mothers received ZDV prophylaxis. The mechanism by which ZDV reduces transmission is not fully defined; protection is likely multifactorial but may be unique to ZDV due to the fact that is metabolized within the placenta itself. The current recommendations for use of antiretroviral chemoprophylaxis to reduce the risk of perinatal transmission of the HIV-1 infection are guidelines only, and flexibility should be exercised according to individual circumstances. The current standard dosing of ZDV for adults is 200 mg PO TID or 300 mg PO BID (Public Health Service Task Force, 2006).

If a woman does not receive ZDV as a component of her antenatal antiretroviral regimen, intrapartum and newborn ZDV is still recommended. If a woman has not received prior therapy, initiation of an antiretroviral regimen may be delayed until after the first trimester, due to the potential of teratogenic effects related to therapy. If a woman is already on drug therapy, ZDV

should be added in the first trimester whenever possible followed by a 6-week newborn course of ZDV. There are several recommendations for HIV-1–infected women who present in labor and have had no prior therapy (Public Health Service Task Force, 2006).

1. Intrapartum IV ZDV followed by 6 weeks of PO ZDV for the newborn
2. PO ZDV and 3TC during labor followed by 1 week of PO ZDV-3TC for the newborn
3. A single dose of nevirapine at the onset of labor followed by a single dose of nevirapine for the newborn at 48 hours of age
4. A single dose of nevirapine at the onset of labor combined with intrapartum IV ZDV and 6 weeks PO ZDV for the newborn

Although intrapartum antiretroviral therapy will not prevent perinatal transmission that occurs before labor, most transmission occurs near or during labor and delivery. Therefore, preexposure prophylaxis is recommended to give antiretroviral drug levels in the fetus during the intensive exposure to HIV-1 in maternal genital secretions and blood during birth (Public Health Service Task Force, 2006).

Mode of Delivery

Optimal medical management should focus on minimizing the risk of both perinatal transmission of HIV-1 and the potential for maternal and neonatal complications (Public Health Service Task Force, 2006). A meta-analysis looking at 15 studies found that the rate of perinatal HIV-1 transmission in women undergoing elective C-section was significantly lower than in those women undergoing nonelective C-section or vaginal delivery regardless of whether they received ZDV prophylaxis (Public Health Service Task Force, 2006). The ACOG Committee on Obstetric Practice recommends considering an elective C-section for HIV-1-infected women with HIV-1 RNA levels >1,000 copies/mL near the time of delivery (ACOG, 2003). If an elective C-section is performed, it is recommended to be done at 38 weeks' gestation; IV ZDV should begin 3 hours before surgery.

Care of the Newborn

Immediate care of the newborn should limit exposure to maternal fluids. A bath should be given once the infant's temperature is stable. Infants born to HIV-1–infected mothers should have an HIV DNA PCR and CBC with manual differential as part of their admission labs (AAP, 2006; Public Health Task Force, 2006). Chemoprophylaxis should begin within 8 to 12 hours after birth and continue for 6 weeks. The recommended ZDV dosage for infants was derived from pharmacokinetic studies performed on full-term infants. ZDV is primarily cleared through the liver by glucuronidation. This enzyme system is immature in neonates leading to a prolonged half-life. Prolongation of clearance of ZDV is expected in preterm infants due to even greater immaturity of hepatic function. Thus, there are different dosing regimens of ZDV for term and preterm infants. Infants born at ≥35 weeks' gestation should receive 1.5 mg/kg/dose q 12 hours IV or 2 mg/kg/dose (syrup) PO q 12 hours, advancing to q 8 hours at 2 weeks of age if ≥30 weeks' gestation at birth or at 4 weeks of age if <30 weeks' gestation at birth. The dosing for full-term infants is 2 mg/kg/dose (syrup) PO q 6 hours or 1.5 mg/kg/dose IV q 6 hours (AAP, 2006; Public Health Task Force, 2006).

Anemia is the primary complication of the 6-week course of ZDV in the neonate (CDC, 2002b). Therefore, at a minimum, a hemoglobin level should be obtained at the end of the 6-week ZDV course. Infants with negative virologic test results during the first 6 weeks of life should have a repeat HIV DNA PCR after completion of antiretroviral treatment. To prevent *Pneumocystis carinii* pneumonia, all infants born to HIV-1-infected mothers should begin prophylaxis after completion of the ZDV prophylaxis regimen (Public Health Task Force, 2006).

In the United States, HIV-1 infected women are counseled not to breast-feed to avoid postnatal transmission of HIV-1 to their infants, regardless of whether the woman is on antiretroviral therapy (AAP, 2004c; Public Health Task Force, 2006).

LATE-PRETERM INFANTS

Prematurity is the major determinant of neonatal mortality and morbidity. In 2004, 12.5% of the births in the United States were premature (<37 completed weeks of gestation), a 31% increase in the rate of prematurity since 1981 (Martin et al., 2006). This dramatic rise in prematurity has largely been due to the increase in the deliveries between 34 and 36 completed weeks of gestation. More than 71% of all singleton preterm births are between 34 and 36 completed weeks of gestation (Fig. 14–7). There has been a shift from higher to lower gestational ages, leading to the most frequent length of gestation in the United States to shift from 40 to 39 weeks (Davidoff et al., 2006; Martin et al., 2006). These near-term infants (NTI) are often referred to as late-preterm infants, the latter referring to the vulnerability of this unique population. This population of infants is often treated like full-term newborns. However, they have the same risk of complications as infants born prematurely. The

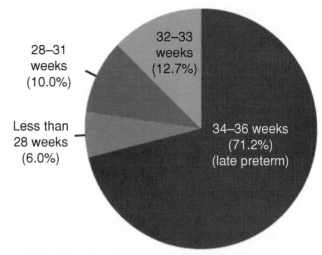

FIGURE 14–7. Percentage distribution of preterm birth: United States, 2004. (From Schrag, S., Gorwitz, R., Fultz-Butts, K., & Schuchat, A. [2002]. Prevention of perinatal group B streptococcal disease: Revised guidelines from the CDC. *Morbidity and Mortality Weekly Report, 51*[RR11], 1–22.

magnitude of their morbidities and their impact on public health has not been well studied. Professional organizations including the Association of Women's Health, Obstetric and Neonatal Nurses (AWHONN), and the National Institute of Child Health and Human Development of the National Institutes of Health (NICHD) have led the way in defining and educating healthcare providers and the public on the distinct needs of the late-preterm infant. In 2005, the NICHD convened a multidisciplinary taskforce which summarized the current state of knowledge on late-preterm births and published a special, two-part supplement summarizing the findings from the meetings in Seminars in Perinatology (National Institutes of Child Health and Human Development Workshop, 2005; Raju, Higgins, Stark, & Leveno, 2006). This multidisciplinary team of experts discussed the definition and terminology, epidemiology, etiology, biology of maturation, clinical care, surveillance, and public health aspects of late-preterm infants. Knowledge gaps were identified and research priorities listed. The NICHD panel recommended that births between 34 completed weeks (thirty-four 0/7 weeks or day 239) and less than 37 completed weeks (thirty-six 6/7 weeks or day 259) of gestation be referred to as late preterm (Raju et al., 2006). Also in 2005, AWHONN launched a multiyear initiative to address the unique physiological and developmental needs of the late-preterm infant. AWHONN developed a conceptual framework for optimizing the health of late-preterm infants and designed goals to emphasize the importance of developing evidence-based guidelines to provide resources to assist nurses and physicians in accurately assessing and managing this high-risk population

(Medoff-Cooper, Bakewell-Sachs, Buus-Frank, & Santa-Donato, 2005).

Obstetrical and Neonatal Issues

Obstetricians face many challenges when managing a woman in preterm labor (Mi Lee, Cleary-Goldman, & D'Alton, 2006; Sibai, 2006; Hankins & Longo, 2006). Continuous assessment of anticipated risks for both the mother and the fetus is crucial. Although a baby born prematurely increases neonatal morbidity and mortality, a fetus left in a suboptimal intrauterine environment can lead to fetal demise. Although there are specific medical indications for delivering a late-preterm infant (placental abruption, placenta previa, bleeding, infection, hypertension, preeclampsia, idiopathic preterm labor, preterm premature rupture of membranes [PPROM], intrauterine growth restriction, and multiple gestation), many babies are being born electively between 35 and 37 weeks resulting from miscalculation or by choice by those who want to avoid the perceived inconvenience of spontaneous labor (Raju et al., 2006; Simpson, 2006). Because estimations of the "due date" can often be miscalculated by up to 2 weeks, to avoid iatrogenic preterm birth, ACOG and AAP recommend that gestational age of 39 completed weeks of gestation be confirmed by at least two methods before elective labor induction, repeat cesarean birth, or nonmedically indicated cesarean birth (AAP & ACOG, 2002; ACOG, 1999; National Institutes of Health, 2006).

Pathophysiology

Late-preterm infants are often referred to as great imposters because their initial size and presentation closely resemble the term newborn (Buus-Frank, 2005). Many times within hours of birth, the late-preterm infant will appear to be functionally term allowing for management decisions to be made accordingly. Despite the fact that these infants are biologically and functionally premature by 3 to 8 weeks, they are often transferred to the regular nursery.

The third trimester is a critical period of rapid growth, development, and biologic maturation. The last few weeks of gestation are vital for fetal development and maturation including surfactant production; control and regulation of breathing; and brain maturation resulting in the infant's ability to coordinate sucking, swallowing, and breathing. Also, during the last trimester, dramatic growth ensues with an increase in body mass and fat stores which enhance thermal and glucose regulation.

Late-preterm infants, compared to term, have a higher frequency of respiratory distress, temperature instability, hypoglycemia, hyperbilirubinemia, kernicterus, apnea, seizures, feeding difficulties, symptoms prompting a sepsis evaluation, need for intravenous infusions; and higher rates of rehospitalization and a potential increase risk for long-term behavior and learning problems (Raju et al., 2006; Wang, Dorer, Fleming, & Catlin, 2004). Table 14–7 identifies the gestational and frequency these complications effect late-preterm infants. Compared to term infants, late-preterm infants have not only significantly more medical problems but also increased hospital costs (Wang et al., 2004).

Hypothermia and Hypoglycemia

Late-preterm infants are at risk for hypothermia and early hypoglycemia. Eighty percent of the fetal energy consumption is provided by glucose. The fetus is solely dependent on maternal glucose that is supplied transplacentally by a process of facilitative diffusion (Garg & Devaskar, 2006). Once the cord is clamped, newborns are required to swiftly adapt to a life of independence and learn to produce endogenous glucose. The risk of hypoglycemia increases for late-preterm infants because metabolic reserves are low, and further energy demands increase because of coexisting conditions of sepsis, birth asphyxia, or cold stress (Halamek et al., 1997; Laptook & Jackson, 2006). Cold stress and hypoglycemia are very common in late-preterm infants, especially soon after birth, during the early transitional period of adaptation (Laptook & Jackson, 2006).

Hyperbilirubinemia

Late-preterm infants are more prone to developing hyperbilirubinemia and its sequelae and to require hospital readmission for treatment (Wang et al., 2004). These vulnerable infants are 2.4 times more likely to develop significant hyperbilirubinemia and have significantly higher total serum bilirubin levels. Elevated bilirubin levels are primarily due to immature liver function and diminished capacity for bilirubin conjugation. These physiologic risks, coupled with more difficult feeding patterns and lower oral intake, exacerbate increased enterohepatic recirculation of bilirubin and may explain the correlation among decreased postmenstrual age, hyperbilirubinemia, and the increased risk for kernicterus (Sarici et al., 2004). Although the incidence of kernicterus in late preterms is unknown, compared to term infants, these infants are at increased risk for bilirubin neurotoxicity and kernicterus (Bhutani et al., 2004; Sarici et al., 2004).

Respiratory Distress

Studies have shown the high incidence of respiratory distress and NICU admissions in the late-preterm infants (Clark, 2005; Escobar et al., 2005; Roth-Kleiner,

TABLE 14–7 ■ ADVERSE OUTCOMES IN LATE-PRETERM INFANTS

Variables	Comments
RDS	12% at 33–34 weeks, 2% at 35–36 weeks, and 0.11% at term
TTN	11.6% at 33–34 weeks, 5% at 35–36 weeks, and 0.7% at term
Pulmonary infection	0.16% at 35–36 weeks and 0.08% at term
Unspecified respiratory failure	3% at 33–34 weeks, 2.48% at 35–36 weeks, and 0.24% at term
Recurrent apnea	4%–5% at 34–36 weeks versus 0% at term
Temperature instability	10% at 35–36 weeks versus 0% at term
Jaundice as cause for discharge delay	16.3% at 35–36 weeks versus 0.03% at term
Bilirubin-induced brain injury	Late-preterm infants represent a large fraction of infants in kernicterus registries
Hypoglycemia	18% at 35–36 weeks versus 4% at term
Clinical problem with ≥1 diagnoses	77.8% at 35–36 weeks versus 45.3% at term
Rehospitalization for all causes	5.3%–9.6% for infants at 33–37 weeks versus 3.6–4.4% at 38–48 weeks
Rehospitalization for dehydration	Odds ratio at gestational age of <39 versus >39 weeks: 2.0 (95% confidence interval: 1.2–3.5)
Brain	It is estimated that the brain size at 34–35 weeks of gestation is ~60% of term, in late-preterm infant autopsies, significant periventricular leukomalacia has been found
Mortality	Death from all causes for births at 34–36 versus ≥37 weeks; early neonatal death relative risks: 5.2; late neonatal death: 2.9; postneonatal death: 2.0; total infant mortality: 2.5; in Canada, the respective rates for relative risk are 7.9, 3.6, 3.0, and 4.5; the 95% confidence intervals ranged from 1.9 to 9.2 for data from both the United States and Canada
Feeding difficulties	Difficulty in initiating and continuing breast-feeding; difficulty in coordinated suck and swallow
Long-term behavioral problems	Higher incidence of learning and behavioral problems at school age

National Institutes of Child Health and Human Development Workshop (2005). Optimizing care and long-term outcome of near-term pregnancy and near-term newborn infant. Workshop held July 18–19, 2005, Bethesda, MD.

Wagner, Bachmann, & Pfenninger, 2003). These infants have a higher incidence of TTN, RDS, PPHN, and hypoxic respiratory failure than term infants (Clark). Nearly 50% of infants born at 34 weeks' gestation require intensive care; this number drops to 15% at 35 weeks and 8% at 36 weeks' gestation (Dudell & Jain, 2006). The last few weeks of gestation are critical for fetal development and maturation specifically related to surfactant and lung maturity. Biochemical and hormonal changes that accompany spontaneous labor and vaginal delivery also play an important role in the newborn's ability to transition smoothly to an extrauterine environment (Dudell & Jain, 2006). For effective gas exchange to occur, alveolar spaces must be cleared of excess fluid and ventilated, and pulmonary blood flow must be increased to match ventilation with perfusion. Failure of either of these events may jeopardize neonatal transition and cause respiratory distress. A significant number of late-preterm infants are delivered by cesarean section, and this number continues to rise steadily, reported at an all-time high in the United States at 29.1% in 2004 (Martin et al., 2006). A higher occurrence of respiratory morbidity in late-preterm and term infants delivered by elective cesarean section has been observed (Annibale, Hulsey, Wagner, & Southgate, 1995; Heritage & Cunningham, 1985; Hook et al., 1997; Keszler, Carbone, Cox, & Schumacher, 1992; Parilla, Dooley, Jansen, & Sucol, 1993; Morrison, Rennie,

Milton, 1995). One study showed that infants born by elective cesarean section at 37 to 38 weeks are 120 times more likely to receive ventilatory support for RDS than those born at 39 to 41 weeks. These infants are known to develop PPHN and become seriously ill and require significant clinical interventions such as i-NO, HFOV, vasopressor support, and ultimately may progress to ECMO. The inability to clear lung fluid, the relative deficiency of pulmonary surfactant, and birth in the absence of labor all contribute to pulmonary dysfunction (Jain & Eaton, 2006).

Apnea of Prematurity

Between 32 and 34 weeks of gestation, the fetus develops synchrony and control of breathing. This period of breathing pattern maturation decreases the risk of apnea of prematurity. The pathogenesis of apnea is multifactorial and includes immature lung volume and upper airway control, ventilatory responses to hypoxia and carbon dioxide, and feeding, as well as physiologic and iatrogenic anemia (Darnall, Ariagno, & Kinney, 2006). It is important to remember that infants born between 33 and 38 weeks' gestation continue to have apnea and are at risk for the resulting periods of bradycardia and hypoxia (Hunt, 2006).

Brain and Long-term Outcomes

Compared to term newborns, late-preterm infants have a more immature brain. It is estimated that an infant at 35 weeks' gestation has fewer sulci and that the weight of the brain is approximately 60% that of the term infant. The degree of significant periventricular leukomalacia has also been found to be higher in this population (Kinney, 2006). The brainstem development of infants born between 33 and 38 weeks' gestation is less mature than that of a term newborn more research on this specific population of infants is needed (Darnall et al., 2006). Few studies have examined the long-term neurodevelopmental status of late-preterm infants and the prevalence rates for subtle neurologic abnormalities, learning and behavioral difficulties, and scholastic achievement (Raju et al., 2006).

Gastrointestinal Tract

The gastrointestinal tract continues to develop throughout gestation, but the late-preterm infant adapts quickly to enteral feedings, including the digestion and absorption of lactose, protein, and fats (Neu, 2006). However, peristaltic functions and sphincter controls in the esophagus, stomach, and intestines are less likely to be mature and fully functional in late-preterm infants which may lead to difficulty in coordinating suck and swallowing, gastroesophageal reflux,

a delay in successful breastfeeding, poor weight gain, and dehydration during early postnatal weeks (Escobar et al., 2002; Neu, 2006; Tomaschek et al., 2006).

The physiologic organization of sucking is almost fully organized by 36 weeks' gestation, whereas swallow rhythm is established by 32 weeks' gestation (Gewolb, Vice, Schweiter-Kenney, Taciak, & Bosma, 2001). Precise timing for the activation of several upper airway muscles is critical for suck–swallow coordination, but unlike sucking, swallowing interrupts breathing, allowing protection of the airway and decreasing the risk for aspiration (Thach, 2005). Overall, minute ventilation decreases during nipple feeding, and this is more pronounced in the preterm infant (Shivpuri, Martin, Carlo, & Fanaroff, 1983). As the infant matures the sequence of breathing and swallowing becomes more consistent. It is likely that the etiology of the frequent feeding issues encountered by late-preterm infants stems from the immaturity of the coordination of sucking, swallowing, and breathing (Darnall et al., 2006). It is important to remember that less energy is required to feed from the breast than from the bottle, as the peristaltic activity of the tongue provokes the peristaltic movement of the GI tract and stimulates deglutition (swallowing; Aguayo, 2001).

Pharmacology and Drug Therapy

Few studies exist describing the drug clearance of a late-preterm infant. Despite the limited evidence, many dosing guidelines used to treat late-preterm infants are based on term data, allowing for inappropriate drug dosing because of the immaturity of the liver and kidney, which can reduce drug clearance in late-preterm infants (Ward, 2006). Additional drug clearance studies are needed.

Immunologic System

Late-preterm infants do have unique susceptibilities to infection including the closed setting of a NICU and the immunologic immaturity of premature infants sets the stage for development of nosocomial infections (Benjamin & Stoll, 2006). There are little data on the host-defense capabilities of late-preterm infants. Recent advances provide a framework for understanding the mechanisms underlying the propensity of infections in this at-risk population. Compared with term and extremely preterm infants, late-preterm infants are intermediate with regard to immunologic maturity (Clapp, 2006).

Assessment

Late-preterm infants masquerade as term infants, making it difficult to determine their potential immediately following delivery. Pathological signs and symptoms of late-preterm infants transitioning to extrauterine life may be subtle or may be considered normal transition (Askin, 2002). Depending on their presentation at delivery, late-preterm infants may be triaged to the newborn nursery and/or room in with their parents. An astute assessment of the infant is critical. It is important to focus on the infant's gestational age and behavior, rather than on weight and APGARS. A conceptual framework for care of the late-preterm infant includes physiologic functional status, nursing care practices, care environment, and family role (Fig. 14–8).

Physiologic Functional Status

Prior to discharge, late-preterm infants must be medically stable and able to spontaneously breathe room air without apnea, bradycardia, or episodes of significant desaturation. Infants must be able to maintain a normal body temperature without the use of adjunctive heating devices. Infants should be assessed for immature feeding behaviors such as failing to feed and difficulty coordinating oral feedings. Establishing breastfeeding prior to discharge is critical in this vulnerable population. Early attention to establishing a good milk supply and frequent feeding opportunities and signs of real milk transfer, along with the ongoing involvement of a lactation consultant who has experience with premature infants, will promote breastfeeding success (Wight, 2003). This unique population should also be assessed for hypoglycemia, jaundice, respiratory dis-

tress, and sepsis. Because it is not unusual for late-preterm infants to require additional thermoregulatory support, feeding support, and/or respiratory support, late-preterm infants require greater vigilance in the frequency and type of nursing assessments performed, and it is important not to misapply guidelines or routines that are designed for normal newborns; one size may not fit all (Medoff-Cooper et al., 2006).

Intervention

Nursing Care Practices

There is a paucity of research focusing on the specific needs of the late-preterm infant. Evidence-based guidelines and assessment parameters for late-preterm infants are lacking, resulting in a variation of how nurses and healthcare providers care for these infants To improve the care delivery to late-preterm infants, by perinatal and neonatal nurses, evidence-based clinical practice guidelines and educational resources need to be developed (Medoff-Cooper et al., 2006).

Care Environment

Determining the most appropriate level of care that late-preterm infants require is critical. NICU or well-baby, nursery-care environments may not be appropriate and may fail this at-risk population. Nurses in the NICU may consider these infants low risk, and well-baby nurses may expect these infants to function like term newborns, both of which may be inappropriate. Currently, no practice guideline is available to establish a clear standard of care for either environment (Medoff-Cooper et al., 2006). Appropriate staffing may not be provided in well-baby nurseries or rooming-in environments. Many times these nurses have multiple mother–baby pairings, and the time required to perform vigilant assessments, establish lactation, and provide detailed discharge instruction is not available.

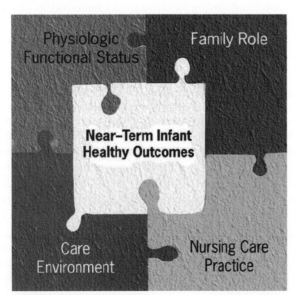

FIGURE 14–8. Conceptual framework for the care of the late-preterm infant. (From Medoff-Cooper, B., Bakewell-Sachs, S., Buus-Frank, M. E., & Santa- Donato, A. [2005]. The AWHONN near-term infant initiative: A conceptual framework for optimizing health for near-term infants. *JOGNN, 34*[6], 666–671.)

Family Role

Parents need to be confident and competent about their ability to care for their baby prior to discharge. However, the lack of evidence-based information specific to this population affects the ability of the nurse to prepare families. Families need to be equipped and empowered with the knowledge to appropriately and effectively care for this population of infants and their potential risks after discharge. The AAP supports early discharge (<48 hours) to infants of singleton births between 38 and 42 weeks' gestation, who are of birth weight appropriate for gestational age, and who meet specific physiologic criteria (AAP, 2004d). However, late-preterm infants are often discharged within 48 hours of age and are 1.8 times more likely to be readmitted than term (Tomashek et al., 2006). Risk factors that have been identified for hospital readmission include maternal complications during labor and delivery, families receiving support from a public payer, parents who are of Asian/Pacific Islander ethnicity, a firstborn infant, and an infant being breast-fed at discharge (Escobar, Clark, Green, 2006; Escobar et al., 2002; National Center for Health Statistics, 2005; Shapiro-Medoza et al., 2006; Tomashek et al., 2006). Jaundice, proven or suspected infections, feeding and respiratory difficulties (including gastroesophageal reflux disease), sepsis, and failure to thrive were the most common diagnoses at readmission (Escobar et al., 2006; Jain & Cheng, 2006). In a recent review, 17.7% of late-preterm infants were seen in the emergency department and were rehospitalized. Over half of these infants were born at 36 weeks' gestation (Jain & Cheng, 2006). Parents need to be informed about the risks associated with late-preterm infants and higher readmission rates.

One of the challenges families confront is the inability of the late-preterm infant to provide behavioral cues. Cues, normally displayed by term newborns, alert the parent to the baby's needs and may be lacking or limited in late-preterm infants. Cues lacking in these infants may include the ability to maintain a robust alert state or demonstrate hunger and satiety. The inability to display appropriate cues can interrupt the parent–infant relationship based on the parent's ability to read and appropriately respond to their infant's behaviors and cues. Parental frustration and a sense of failure or inadequacy may ensue when late-preterm infants are expected to perform like their term counterparts (Medoff-Cooper et al., 2006).

These infants are at risk for breastfeeding hypernatremia related to poor milk transfer and dehydration secondary to poor breastfeeding establishment. breastfeeding-associated hypernatremia is a completely irreversible complication that appears to be common. Primiparas need additional support, education, and follow-up in order to ensure successful lactation and avoid potentially dangerous complications related to insufficient lactation (Moritz, Manole, Bogen, & Avus, 2005). Pediatricians and pediatric/family nurse practitioners need to be equipped with the basic knowledge of breastfeeding this at-risk population. Additionally, it is essential to be able to refer mothers and infants in a timely manner to a trained lactation professional for more complicated breastfeeding problems. A lactation referral should be viewed with the same medical urgency as any other acute medical referral (Adamkin, 2006).

Hyperbilirubinemia discharge teaching and postdischarge management are critical for vigilant follow-up. Late-preterm infants have been reported to be higher TSB levels than term newborns but not until day-of-life 5 to 7, much later after the typical 48 to 72 hours after delivery discharge (Sarici et al., 2004). Experienced visiting nurses coupled with frequent outpatient visits may be necessary depending on the needs of each infant.

Families and primary caregivers need sudden infant death syndrome (SIDS) prevention education. Compared to term infants, late-preterm infants are at a twofold higher risk of developing SIDS (Kramer et al., 2000; Malloy & Freeman, 2000; Thompson & Hunt, 2005). Despite the dramatic reduction in SIDS over the past decade, SIDS continues to be responsible for more infant deaths in the United States during infancy beyond the neonatal period (Arias, MacDorman, Strobino, & Guyer, 2003). Healthcare providers need to educate families about infants' increased risk for SIDS and demonstrate appropriate SIDS prevention strategies within the nurseries prior to discharge so families can mimic appropriate caregiving behaviors. The AAP recommends infants be placed supine (wholly on the back) for every sleep, the use of firm sleep surfaces (soft materials or objects should not be placed under a sleeping infant), keeping soft objects and loose bedding out of crib, avoiding maternal smoking during pregnancy and newborn exposure to secondhand smoke, and a separate but proximate sleep environment (no bed sharing). Also to be considered are the following: offering a pacifier at bed time or nap time once breastfeeding has fully been established, avoiding overheating and commercial devices products marketed to reduce the risk of SIDS, not using home monitors as a strategy to reduce the incidence of SIDS, avoiding developmental positional plagiocephaly (ie, asymmetrical skull), and encouraging "tummy time" when the infant is awake and observed (AAP, 2005).

Research is still needed to understand the etiology of late-preterm births. As the rate of preterm births increase, so does the impact on the burden of disease and the healthcare cost to society. The economic burden caused by preterm births in the United States in 2005 was close to $26.2 billion, or $51,600 per preterm infant (Berhman & Butler, 2006). Any decrease in the rate of prematurity, at any gestation, would reduce the burden of disease and lead to a significant cost savings. Late-preterm infants require diligent evaluation, monitoring, referral, and early return appointments, not only for postneonatal evaluation but also for long-term follow-up (Raju et al., 2006).

TRANSPORT AND RETURN TRANSPORT

Many conditions complicating the neonatal period do not begin with dramatic clinical symptoms. Experience and well-developed assessment skills allow perinatal nurses to recognize subtle changes and intervene before the newborn's condition worsens. Occasionally, the condition of the newborn and services available at a particular perinatal center necessitate transport to a level III NICU. The goal of neonatal transport is to bring a sick newborn to a tertiary-care center in stable condition. The availability of neonatal intensive care has improved outcomes in high-risk newborns, although no standard definitions exist for graded levels of complexity of care that NICUs provide, making it difficult to compare outcomes (AAP, 2004e). Stabilization is ongoing, beginning with the referring hospital through consultation with the tertiary center as needed until the arrival and eventual departure of the transport team. Stabilization takes many forms because of the diversity in the disease process and gestational age. Basic care needs of newborns requiring transport to a tertiary center include adequate oxygenation, prevention of hypothermia, prevention of hypoglycemia, conservation of energy, and maintenance of physiologic integrity.

After the newborn's condition is no longer critical, if an extended hospitalization is anticipated, the decision may be made to move the newborn back to the hospital in which he or she was born. This decision is made with input from neonatology staff at the level III center, the primary care provider who will care for the newborn in the level II hospital, nursing representatives of the level II institution, and the parents. The decision also is influenced by the parents' insurance carrier or managed care providers. Research on the impact of return transport has demonstrated inconsistent results. Several studies have shown that return transport of stable newborns to level II hospitals is safe and cost effective, improving the efficacy and use of level I and II beds and helping to eliminate acute shortages of NICU beds (Bagwell et al., 2003).

Return transport also offers many advantages to family members of the high-risk newborn (Display 14–11). But to be successful, it requires involvement of personnel from the transferring and the receiving hospital, as well as adequate parent preparation. Family involvement is essential to success of back transport; the idea should be presented when the infant is initially transferred to the level III center. Back transports should also be presented as a milestone and a positive step toward discharge (Bagwell et al., 2003).

To provide newborns with the best care possible, healthcare professionals within the referring hospital and between the referring hospital and the tertiary center must communicate and work together as a team. The decision to transport back to the level II hospital first depends on whether the care needs of the newborn can be met at that institution. Communication between the level III and the level II hospitals when a return transport is anticipated should begin several days before the actual transfer. This assists in

DISPLAY 14-11

Advantages of Return Transport to a Level II Nursery

The newborn is usually closer to home, increasing the amount of time family members can spend with the newborn.

Transport allows better use of beds in the level III intensive care unit.

Cost of providing care in a level II hospital is generally less than that in a level III institution.

Ongoing communication is maintained between level II and level III institutions.

preparing the parents, and the receiving hospital has time to anticipate staffing and equipment needs. Using a formal documentation system provides the receiving hospital with information about the current condition of the newborn.

SUMMARY

Most newborns are born in level II hospitals. They are healthy at birth, develop no complications during the neonatal period, and are discharged to their homes with their mothers. Small minorities of newborns are born with complications or develop complications immediately after birth. It is the newborn who develops complications that poses the challenge to the perinatal nurse. The nurse in a level II hospital must strive to identify complications in a timely fashion, care for the infant appropriately, stabilize the infant before transport to a level III facility, and be prepared to accept the patient as a return transfer when he or she is no longer in need of intensive care.

REFERENCES

Adamkin, D. H. (2006). Feeding problems in the late preterm infant. *Clinics in Perinatology, 33*(4), 831–837.

Aguayo, J. (2001). Maternal lactation for preterm newborn infants. *Early Human Development, 65*(Suppl.), S19–S29.

American Academy of Pediatrics. (1993). Routine evaluation of blood pressure, hematocrit and glucose in newborns. *Pediatrics, 92*(3), 474–476.

American Academy of Pediatrics. (2004a). Management of hyperbilirubinemia in the newborn infant 35 or more weeks of gestation. *Pediatrics, 114*(1), 297–316.

American Academy of Pediatrics. (2004b). Questions and answers on jaundice and your newborn. Washington, DC. http://www.aap.org/family/jaundicefaq.htm

American Academy of Pediatrics (2004c). Evaluation and treatment of the human immunodeficiency virus-1-exposed infant. *Pediatrics, 114*(2), 497–505.

American Academy of Pediatrics Committee on Drugs. (1998). Neonatal drug withdrawal. *Pediatrics, 101*(6), 1079–1086.

American Academy of Pediatrics. (2004d). Committee on fetus and newborn. Hospital stay for healthy term newborns. *Pediatrics, 113*(5), 1434–1436.

American Academy of Pediatrics. (2004e). Committee on fetus and newborn. Levels of neonatal care. *Pediatrics, 114,* 1341–1347.

American Academy of Pediatrics & American College of Obstetricians and Gynecologists. (2002). *Guidelines for perinatal care* (5th ed.). Elk Grove Village, IL: Author.

American Academy of Pediatrics Committee on Infectious Diseases. (2006). *Red book* (26th ed.). Elk Grove Village, IL: Author.

American Academy of Pediatrics Task Force on Sudden Infant Death Syndrome. (2005). The changing concept of sudden infant death syndrome: Diagnostic coding shifts, controversies regarding sleep environment, and new variables to consider in reducing risk. *Pediatrics, 116*(5):1245–1255.

American College of Obstetricians and Gynecologists (ACOG). (1999). *Induction of labor.* (Practice Bulletin No. 10). Washington, DC: Author.

American College of Obstetricians and Gynecologists (ACOG). (2002). *Prevention of early-onset group B streptococcal disease in newborns.* (Committee Opinion No. 279). Washington, DC: Author.

American College of Obstetricians and Gynecologists (ACOG). (2003). *Scheduled cesarean delivery and the prevention of vertical transmission of HIV infection.* (Committee Opinion No. 234). Washington, DC: Author.

American College of Obstetricians and Gynecologists (ACOG). (2005). *The importance of preconception care in the continuum in women's health.* (Committee Opinion No. 313). Washington, DC: Author.

American College of Obstetricians and Gynecologists (ACOG). (2006). *Amnioinfusion does not prevent meconium aspiration syndrome.* (Committee Opinion No. 346). Washington, DC: Author.

American Heart Association. (2006). Heart Disease and Stroke Statistics 2006 Update: A report from the American Heart Association Statistics Committee and Stroke Statistics Subcommittee. *Circulation, 113,* e85–e151.

American Heart Association & American Academy of Pediatrics (AHA & AAP). (2006). *Textbook of neonatal resuscitation* (5th ed.). Elk Grove Village, IL: American Heart Association.

American Lung Association. (2003). *American lung association fact sheet: Respiratory distress syndrome of the newborn.* New York: Author.

Annibale, D. J., Hulsey, T. C., Wagner, C. L., & Southgate, W. M. (1995). Comparative neonatal morbidity of abdominal and vaginal deliveries after uncomplicated pregnancies. *Archives of Pediatric and Adolescent Medicine, 149*(8), 862–867.

Arias, E., MacDorman, M. F., Strobino, D. M., & Guyer, B. (2003). Annual summary of vital statistics 2002. *Pediatrics, 112*(6, Pt. 1), 1215–1230.

Askin, D. F. (2002). Complications in the transition from fetal to neonatal life. *Journal of Obstetric, Gynecologic, and Neonatal Nursing, 31*(3), 318–327.

Bagwell, G. A., Acree, C. M., Karlsen, K. A., Sheets, A., Shaw, J., Sandman, K., Routzon, K. L., Waechter, L., Vetter, M. D., Shelley, K., & Kwiecinski, S. (2003). Recognition of today's health care delivery system. In C. Kenner & J. W. Lott (Eds.), *Comprehensive neonatal nursing a physiologic perspective* (3rd ed., pp. 16–38). St. Louis: Saunders.

Benjamin, D. K., & Stoll, B. J. (2006). Infection in late preterm infants. *Clinics in Perinatology, 33*(4), 871–882.

Berhman, R. E., Butler, A. S. (2006). *Preterm birth: Causes, consequences and prevention.* Washington, DC: Institute of Medicine of the National Academies.

Bhutani, V. K., Johnson, L. H., & Shapiro, S. M. (2004). Kernicterus in sick and preterm infants (1999-2002): A need for an effective preventive approach. *Seminars in Perinatology, 28*(5), 319–325.

Bhutani, V. K., Johnson, L. H., & Sivievri, E. M. (1999). Predictive ability of a predischarge hour-specific serum bilirubin for subsequent significant hyperbilirubinemia in healthy term and near-term newborns. *Pediatrics, 103*(1), 6–14.

Blackburn, S. (1995). Hyperbilirubinemia and neonatal jaundice. *Neonatal Network, 14*(7), 15–25.

Brooks, C. (1997). Neonatal hypoglycemia. *Neonatal Network, 16*(2), 15–21.

Buus-Frank, M. (2005). The great imposter (editorial). *Advances in Neonatal Care, 5*(5), 233–236.

Canadian Paediatric Society. (2004). Screening guidelines for newborns at risk for low blood glucose. Fetus and newborn committee. *Paediatrics and Child Health, 9*(10), 723–729.

Carey, B. (2002). Incidence and epidemiology of congenital cardiovascular malformations in the newborn and infant. *Newborn and Infant Nursing Reviews, 2*(2), 54–59.

Centers of Disease Control and Prevention (CDC). (2006a). Preconception care for workgroup. Recommendations to improve preconception health and health care—United States. *Morbidity and Mortality Weekly Report, 55*(RR6), 1–30.

Centers of Disease Control and Prevention (CDC). (2006b). Revised recommendations for HIV testing of adults, adolescents, and pregnant women in health-care settings. *Morbidity and Mortality Weekly Report, 55*(RR14), 1–17.

Centers of Disease Control and Prevention (CDC). (2006c). Achievements in Public Health: Reduction in Perinatal Transmission of HIV Infection United States, 1985–2005. *Morbidity and Mortality Weekly Report, 55*(RR21), 592–597.

Cifuentes, J., Segars, A. H., & Carlo, W. A. (2003). Respiratory system management and complications. In C. Kenner & J. W. Lott (Eds.), *Comprehensive neonatal nursing: A physiologic perspective* (3rd ed., pp. 348–375). St. Louis: Saunders.

Clapp, D. W. (2006). Developmental regulation of the immune system. *Seminars in Perinatology, 30*(2), 48–51.

Clark, R. H. (2005). The epidemiology of respiratory failure in neonates born at an estimated gestational age of 34 weeks or more. *Journal of Perinatology, 25*(4), 251–257.

Cole F. S., Nogee, L. M., & Hamvas, A. (2006). Defects in surfactant synthesis: clinical implications. *Pediatrics Clinics of North America, 53*(5), 911–927.

Cornblath, M., Hawdon, J. M., Williams, A. F., Aynsley-Green, A., Ward Platt, M. P., Swartz, R., et al. (2000). Controversies regarding definition of neonatal hypoglycemia: suggested operational thresholds. *Pediatrics, 105*(5), 1141–1145.

Darnall, R. A., Ariagno, R. L., & Kinney, H. C. (2006). The late preterm infant and the control of breathing, sleep, and brainstem development: A review. *Clinics in Perinatology, 33*(4), 883–914.

Davidoff, M. J., Dias, T., Damus, K., Russell, R., Bettegowda, V. R., Dolan, S., et al. (2006). Changes in the gestational age distribution among U.S. singleton births: Impact on rates of late preterm birth, 1992-2002. *Seminars in Perinatology, 30*(1), 8–15.

Deshpande, S., & Ward Platt, M. W. (2005). The investigation and management of neonatal hypoglycaemia. *Seminars in Fetal and Neonatal Medicine, 10*(4), 351–361.

Dudell, G. G., & Jain, L. (2006). Hypoxic respiratory failure in the late preterm infant.*Clinics in Perinatology, 33*(4), 803–830.

Edwards, M. S. (2002). The immune system. In A. A. Fanaroff & R. J. Martin (Eds.), *Neonatal-perinatal medicine diseases of the fetus and infant* (7th ed., pp. 676-802). St. Louis: Mosby, Inc.

Escobar, G. J., Gonzales, V. M., Armstrong, M. A., Flock, B. F., Xiong, B., & Newman, T. B. (2002). Rehospitalization for neonatal dehydration: A nested case-control study. *Archives of Pediatric and Adolescent Medicine, 156*(2), 155–161.

Escobar, G. J., Clark, R. H., & Green, J. D. (2006). Short-term outcomes of infants born at 35 and 36 weeks gestation: We need to ask more questions. *Seminars in Perinatology, 30*(1), 28–33.

Escobar, G. J., Greene, J. D., Hulac, P., Kincannon, E., Bischoff, K., Gardner, M. N., et al. (2005). Rehospitalisation after birth hospitalization: Patterns among infants of all gestations. *Archives of Disease in Childhood, 90*(2), 124–131.

Fike, D. L. (2003). Assessment and management of the substance exposed newborn and infant. In C. Kenner & J. W. Lott (Eds.), *Comprehensive neonatal nursing: A physiologic perspective* (3rd ed., pp. 773–802). St. Louis: Saunders.

Ganapathy, V., Prasad, P. D., Ganapathy, M. E., & Leibach, F. H. (1999). Drugs of abuse and placental transport. *Advance Drug Delivery Review, 38*(1), 99–110.

Garg, M., & Devaskar, S. U. (2006). Glucose metabolism in the late preterm infant. *Clinics in Perinatology, 33*(4), 853–870.

Gewolb, I. H., Vice, F. L., Schweiter-Kenney, E. L., Taciak, V. L., Bosma, J. F. (2001). Developmental patterns of rhythmic suck and swallow in preterm infants. *Developmental Medicine and Child Neurology, 43*(1), 22–37.

Guyer, B., Hoyert, D. L., Martin, J. A., Ventura, S. J., MacDorman, M. P., & Strobino, D. M. (1999). Annual summary of vital statistics–1998. *Pediatrics, 104*(6), 1229–1246.

Halamek, L. P., Benaron, D. A., & Stevenson, D. K. (1997). Neonatal hypoglycemia, part I: Background and definition. *Clinical Pediatrics, 36*(12), 675–680.

Halamek, L. P., & Stevenson, D. K. (2002). Neonatal jaundice and liver disease. In A. A. Fanaroff & R. J. Martin (Eds.), *Neonatal-perinatal medicine diseases of the fetus and infant* (7th ed., pp. 1309–1350). St. Louis: Mosby.

Hansen, T. N., Cooper, T. R., & Weisman, L. E. (Eds.). (1998). *Contemporary diagnosis and management of neonatal respiratory diseases* (2nd ed.). Newton, PA: Handbooks in Health Care.

Hankins, G. D. V., & Longo, M. (2006). The role of stillbirth prevention and late preterm (near-term) births. *Seminars in Perinatology, 30*(1), 20–23.

Harbarth, S., Sudre, P., Dharan, S., Cadenas, M., & Pittet, D. (1999). Outbreak of enterobacter cloacae related to understaffing, overcrowding, and poor hygiene practices. *Infection Control and Hospital Epidemiology, 20*(9), 598–603.

Hawdon, J. M., Ward Platt, & Aynsley-Green, M. P. (1992). Patterns of metabolic adaptation for preterm and term infants in the first neonatal week. *Archives of Disease in Childhood, 67*(4 Spec No.), 357–365.

Heritage, C. K., & Cunningham, M. D. (1985). Association of elective repeat cesarean delivery and persistent pulmonary hypertension of the newborn. *American Journal of Obstetrics and Gynecology, 152*(6, Pt. 1), 627–629.

Hey, W. W., & Bell, E. F. (2000). Oxygen therapy, oxygen toxicity, and the STOP-ROP trial. *Pediatrics, 105*(2), 424–425.

Hook, B., Kiwi, R., Amini S. B., Fanaroff, A., & Hack, M. (1997). Neonatal morbidity after elective repeat cesarean section and trial of labor. *Pediatrics, 100*(3, Pt. 1), 348–353.

Hunt, C. E. (2006). Ontogeny of automatic regulation in late preterm infants born at 34–37 weeks postmenstrual age. *Seminars in Perinatology, 30*(2), 73–76.

Jain, S., & Cheng, J. (2006). Emergency department visits and rehospitalizations in late preterm infants. *Clinics in Perinatology, 33*(4), 935–945.

Jain, L., & Eaton, D. C. (2006). Physiology of fetal lung fluid clearance and effect of labor. *Seminars in Perinatology, 30*(1), 34–43.

Johnson, L., Bhutani, V. K., & Brown, A. K. (2002). System-based approach to management of neonatal jaundice and prevention of kernicterus. *Journal of Pediatrics, 140*(4), 39–403.

Joint Commission on Accreditation of Healthcare Organizations. (August 31, 2004). Sentinel event alert: Revised guidance to help prevent kernicterus. Retrieved January 12, 2007, from http://www.jointcommission. org

Juretschke, L. J. (2005). Kernicterus: Still a concern. *Neonatal Network, 24*(2), 7–19.

Kalhan, S. C., & Parimi, P. S. (2002). Metabolic and endocrine disorders. In A. A. Fanaroff & R. J. Martin (Eds.), *Neonatal-perinatal medicine diseases of the fetus and infant* (7th ed., pp. 1351–1376). St. Louis: Mosby.

Kenner, C. (2003). Resuscitation and stabilization of the newborn. In C. Kenner & J. W. Lott (Eds.), *Comprehensive neonatal nursing: A physiologic perspective* (3rd ed., pp. 210–227). St. Louis: Saunders.

Keszler, M., Carbone, M. T., Cox, C., & Schumacher, R. E. (1992). Severe respiratory failure after elective repeat cesarean delivery: A potentially preventable condition leading to extracorporeal membrane oxygenation. *Pediatrics, 89*(4, Pt. 1), 670–672.

Kinney, H. C. (2006). The near-term (late preterm) human brain and risk for periventricular leukomalacia: A review. *Seminars in Perinatology, 30*(2), 81–88.

Kramer, M. S., Demissie, K., Yang, H., Platt, R W., Sauve, R., & Liston, R. (2000). The contribution of mild and moderate preterm birth to infant mortality. Fetal and Infant Health Study Group of the Canadian Perinatal Surveillance System. *JAMA, 284*(7), 843–849.

Laptook, A., & Jackson, G. L. (2006). Cold stress and hypoglycemia in the late preterm ("near-term") infant: Impact on nursery of admission. *Seminars in Perinatology, 30*(1), 24–27.

Law, K. L., Stroud, L. R., LaGasse, L., Niaura, R., Liu, J., & Lester, B. M. (2003). Smoking during pregnancy and newborn neurobehavior. *Pediatrics, 111*(6), 1318–1323.

Lott, J. W. (2003). Assessment and management of the cardiovascular system. In C. Kenner & J. W. Lott (Eds.), *Comprehensive neonatal nursing a physiologic perspective* (3rd ed., pp. 376–408). St. Louis: Saunders.

Lund, C. H., & Kuller, J. M. (2003). Assessment and management of integumentary system. In C. Kenner & J. W. Lott (Eds.), *Comprehensive neonatal nursing a physiologic perspective* (3rd ed., pp. 700–724). St. Louis: Saunders.

Malloy, M. H., & Freeman, D. H. (2000). Birth weight and gestational age-specific sudden infant death syndrome mortality: United States, 1991 versus 1995. *Pediatrics, 105*(6), 1227–1231.

Malloy, M. H., & Freeman, D. H. (2002). Respiratory distress syndrome mortality in the United States 1987-1995. *Journal of Perinatology, 20*(7), 414–420.

Martin, J. A., Hamilton, B. E., Sutton, P. D., Ventura, S. J., Menacker, F., & Kirmeyer, S. (2006). Births: Final data for 2004. *National Vital Statistics Reports, 55*(1), 1–102.

Matthews, T. J. (2001). Smoking during pregnancy in the 1990's. *National Vital Statistic Report, 49*(7), 1–14.

McFadden, E. A. (1991). The Wallaby phototherapy system: A new approach to phototherapy. *Journal of Pediatric Nursing, 6*(3), 206–208.

McGowan, J. E., & Perlman, J. M. (2006). Glucose management during and after intensive delivery room resuscitation. *Clinics in Perinatology, 33*(4), 184–196.

Medoff-Cooper, B., Bakewell-Sachs, S., Buus-Frank, M. E., & Santa-Donato, A. (2005). The AWHONN near-term infant initiative: A conceptual framework for optimizing health for near-term infants. *Journal of Obstetric, Gynecologic, and Neonatal Nursing, 34*(6), 666–671.

Menni, F., De Lonely, P., Sevin, C., Touati, G., Peigne, C., Barbier, V., et al. (2001). Neurologic outcomes of 90 neonates and infants with persistent hyperinsulinemic hypoglycemia. *Pediatrics, 107*(3), 476–479.

Meissner, T., Wendel U., Burgard, P., Schaetzle, S., & Mayatepek, E. (2003). Long-term follow-up of 114 patients with congenital hyperinsulinism. *European Journal of Endocrinology, 149*(1), 43–51.

Mi Lee, Y., Cleary-Goldman, J., & D'Alton, M. E. (2006). Multiple gestations and late preterm (near-term) deliveries. *Seminars in Perinatology, 30*(2), 103–112.

Miller, M. J., Fanaroff, A. A., & Martin, R. J. (2002). The respiratory system. In A. A. Fanaroff & R. J. Martin (Eds.), *Neonatal-perinatal medicine diseases of the fetus and infant* (7th ed., pp. 1025–1049). St. Louis: Mosby.

Moritz, M. L., Manole, M. D., Bogen, D. L., & Avus, J. C. (2005). Breastfeeding-associated hypernatremia: Are we missing something? *Pediatrics, 116*(3), 343–347.

Morrison, J. J., Rennie, J. M., & Milton, P. J. (1995). Neonatal respiratory morbidity and mode of delivery at term: Influence of timing of elective caesarean section. *British Journal of Obstetrics Gynaecology, 102*(2), 101–106.

National Center for Health Statistics. (2005). *Public use data tapes. Natality data set: 1992–2002.* Hyattsville, MD: U.S. Department of Health and Human Services, Centers for Disease Control and Prevention.

National Institutes of Child Health and Human Development Workshop (2005). Optimizing care and long-term outcome of near-term pregnancy and near-term newborn infant. Workshop held July 18–19, 2005, Bethesda, MD.

National Institutes of Health. (2006). *State of the science conference statement: Cesarean delivery on maternal request.* Bethesda, MD: Author.

Neu, J. (2006). Gastrointestinal maturation and feeding. *Seminars in Perinatology, 30*(2),77–80.

Neu, H., Hansen, R., & Steldinger, R. (1985). Extent of nicotine and cotinine transfer to the human fetus, placenta and amniotic fluid of smoking mothers. *Developmental Pharmacology and Therapeutics, 8*(6), 384–395.

Osborn, D. A., Cole, M. J., & Jeffery, H. E. (2005). Opiate treatment for opiate withdrawal in newborn infants. *Cochrane Database Systematic Review, 3,* CD002053.

Parilla, B. V., Dooley, S. L., Jansen, R. D., & Sucol, M. L. (1993). Iatrogenic respiratory distress syndrome following elective repeat cesarean delivery. *Obstetrics and Gynecology, 81*(3), 392–395.

Paul, D. E. (1995). Recognition, stabilization, and early management of infants with critical congenital heart disease presenting in the first days of life. *Neonatal Network, 14*(5), 13–20.

Perreault, T. (2006). Persistent pulmonary hypertension of the newborn. *Paediatric Respiratory Reviews, 7*(Suppl.), S175–S176.

Public Health Service Task Force. (2006). Recommendations for use of antiretroviral drugs in pregnant HIV-1-infected women for maternal health and interventions to reduce perinatal HIV-1 transmission in the United States. October 2006. U.S. Public Health Service. Retrieved January 4, 2006, from http://www.aidsinfo.nih.gov, 1–65.

Raju, T. N., Higgins, R. D., Stark, A. R., & Leveno, K. J. (2006). Optimizing care and outcome for late-preterm (near-term) infants: A summary of the workshop sponsored by the national institute of child heath and human development. *Pediatrics, 118*(3), 1207–1214.

Rosen, T. S., & Bateman, D. A. (2002). Infants of addicted mothers. In A. A. Fanaroff & R. J. Martin (Eds.), *Neonatal-perinatal medicine diseases of the fetus and infant* (7th ed., pp. 661–673). St. Louis: Mosby.

Roth-Kleiner, M., Wagner, B. P., Bachmann, D., & Pfenninger, J. (2003). Respiratory distress syndrome in near-term babies after caesarean section. *Swiss Medical Weekly, 133*(19–20), 283–288.

Sarici, S. U., Serdar, M. A., Korkmaz, A., Erdem, G., Oran, O., Tekinalp, G., et al. (2004). Incidence, course, and prediction of hyperbilirubinemia in near-term and term newborns. *Pediatrics, 113*(4), 775–780.

Schivpuri, C. R., Martin, R. J., Carlo, W. A., & Fanaroff, A. A. (1983). Decreased ventilation in preterm infants during oral feeding. *Journal of Pediatrics, 103*(2), 285–289.

Schrag, S., Gorwitz, R., Fultz-Butts, K., & Schuchat, A. (2002). Prevention of perinatal group B streptococcal disease: Revised guidelines from the CDC. *Morbidity and Mortality Weekly Report, 51*(RR11), 1–22.

Schuchat, A., Zywicki, S. S., Dinsmoor, M. J., Mercer, B., Romaguera, J., O'Sullivan, M., et al. (2000). Risk factors and opportunities for prevention of early-onset neonatal sepsis: A multicenter case-control study. *Pediatrics, 105*(1), 21–26.

Shapiro-Mendoza, C. K., Tomashek, K. M., Kotelchuck, M., Barfield, W., Weiss, J., & Evans, S. (2006). Risk factors for neonatal morbidity and mortality among "healthy," late preterm newborns. *Seminars in Perinatology, 30*(2), 54–60.

Shaw, N. M. (2003). Assessment and management of the hematologic system. In C. Kenner & J. W. Lott (Eds.), *Comprehensive neonatal nursing: A physiologic perspective* (3rd ed., pp. 580–623). St. Louis: Saunders.

Sibai, B. M. (2006). Preeclampsia as a cause of preterm and late preterm (near-term) births. *Seminars in Perinatology, 30*(1), 16–19.

Simpson, K. R. (2006). Elective preterm birth. *Perinatal Patient Safety, 31*(1), 68.

Slokin, T. A. (1998). Fetal nicotine or cocaine exposure. Which one is worse. *Journal of Pharmacology & Experimental Therapeutics, 285*(3), 931–945.

Smitherman, H., Stark, A. R., & Bhutani, V. K. (2006). Early recognition of neonatal hyperbilirubinemia and its emergent management. *Seminars in Fetal and Neonatal Medicine, 11*(3), 214–224.

Soorani-Lunsing, I., Woltil, A., & Hadders-Algra, M. (2001). Are moderate degrees of hyperbilirubinemia in health term neonates really safe for the brain? *Pediatric Research, 50*(6), 701–715.

Sweene, I., Ewald U., Gustafsson, J., Sandberg, F., & Ostenson, C. (1994). Inter-relationship between serum concentrations of glucose, glucagon and insulin during the first two days of life in healthy newborns. *Acta Paediatrica, 83*(9), 915–919.

Thach B. T. (2005). Can we breathe and swallow at the same time? *Journal of Applied Physiology, 99*(5), 1633.

Thompson, M. W., & Hunt, C. E. (2005). Control of breathing: Development, apnea of prematurity, apparent life-threatening events, sudden infant death syndrome. In M. G. MacDonald, M. D. Mullett, & M. M. K. Seshia (Eds.), *Avery's neonatology pathophysiology and management of the newborn* (6th ed., pp. 535–552). Philadelphia, PA: Lippincott Williams & Wilkins.

Tomashek, K. M., Shaprio-Mendoza, C. K., Weiss, J., Kotelchuck, M., Barfield, W., Evans, S., et al. (2006). Early discharge among late preterm and term newborns and risk of neonatal morbidity. *Seminars in Perinatology, 30*(2), 61–68.

Velaphi, S. V., & Vidyasagar, D. (2006). Intrapartum and postdelivery management of infants born to mothers with meconium-stained amniotic fluid: Evidence-based recommendations. *Clinics in Perinatology, 33*(4), 29–42.

Wang, M. L., Dorer, D. J., Fleming, M. P., & Catlin, E. A. (2004). Clinical outcomes of near-term infants. *Pediatrics, 114*(2), 373–376.

Ward, R. M. (2006). Drug disposition in the late preterm ("near-term") newborn. *Seminars in Perinatology, 30*(1), 48–51.

Weiner, S. M., & Finnegan, L. P. (1998). Drug withdrawal in the neonate. In B. B. Merenstein & S. L. Gardner (Eds.), *Handbook of neonatal intensive care* (4th ed.). St. Louis: Mosby.

Wheeler, B. J. (2000). Kernicterus: Ancient history or ongoing threat. *Mother-Baby Journal, 5*(2), 21–30.

Whitsett, J. A., Pryhuber, G. S., Rice, W. R., Warner, B. B., & Wert, S. E. (1999). Acute respiratory disorders. In G. B. Avery, M. A. Fletcher, & M. G. MacDonald (Eds.), *Neonatology, pathophysiology and management of the newborn* (4th ed., pp. 429–451). Philadelphia: J.B. Lippincott.

Wight, M E. (2003). Breastfeeding the borderline (near-term) preterm infant. *Pediatric Annals, 32*(5), 329–336.

Williams, A. F. (2005). Neonatal hypoglycaemia: Clinical and legal aspects. *Seminars in Fetal and Neonatal Medicine, 10*(4), 363–368.

Witt, C. (1997). Cardiac embryology. *Neonatal Network, 16*(1), 43–49.

Witt, C. (1998). Cyanotic heart lesions with increased pulmonary blood flow. *Neonatal Network, 17*(7), 7–16.

Wood, M. K. (1997). Acyanotic lesions with increased pulmonary blood flow. *Neonatal Network, 16*(3), 17–25.

Zahka, K. G., & Chandrakant, R. P. (2002). The cardiovascular system. In A. A. Fanaroff & R. J. Martin (Eds.), *Neonatal-perinatal medicine diseases of the fetus and infant* (7th ed., pp. 1140–1163). St. Louis: Mosby.

Zahorodny, W., Rom, C., Whitney, W., Giddens, S., Samuel, M., Maichuk, G., et al. (1998). The neonatal withdrawal inventory: A simplified score of newborn withdrawal. *Journal of Developmental and Behavioral Pediatrics, 19*(2), 89–93.

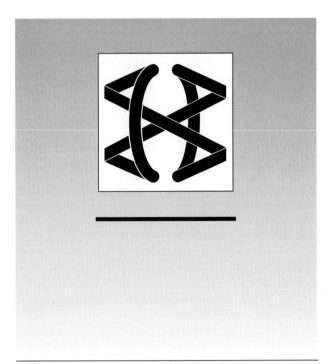

Item Bank Questions and Answer Key

QUESTIONS

Chapter 1

Multiple Choice

1. Inpatient obstetric care results in approximately what percentage of malpractice claims in obstetrics and gynecology?

   a. 25%
   b. 50%
   c. 75%

2. Guidance for ethical nursing care is provided by the

   a. American Nurses Association *Code of Ethics for Nurses*.
   b. American College of Obstetricians and Gynecologists (ACOG) *Patient Ethics Standards*.
   c. Association of Women's Health, Obstetric and Neonatal Nurses (AWHONN) *Ethical Guidelines*.

3. Disruptive clinician behavior

   a. is often directly linked to clinical practice issues.
   b. rarely involves clinical practice issues.
   c. should be handled separately from clinical practice issues.

4. The best approach for addressing disruptive clinician behavior is

   a. immediate intervention.
   b. monitoring trends.
   c. peer review.

5. Successful defense of malpractice claims is enhanced by following

   a. community standards.
   b. national professional standards.
   c. trends in practice.

6. When a sentinel event occurs, according the Joint Commission on Accreditation of Healthcare Organizations (JCAHO),

   a. a root-cause analysis should be conducted.
   b. it must be reported to JCAHO within 45 days.
   c. those involved should be placed on administrative leave pending an investigation.

7. Based on JCAHO criteria, which of the following clinical situations is a sentinel event?

   a. any intrapartum fetal death
   b. any intrapartum maternal death
   c. birth of a baby with previously undiagnosed congenital abnormalities

8. The purpose of the root-cause analysis process is to

   a. determine fault of the healthcare provider or hospital.
   b. examine institutional liability.
   c. review potentially contributing systems.

9. Professional nursing liability is most commonly increased by the absence of

   a. adequate medical record documentation.
   b. annual competency validation.
   c. current unit policies and procedures.

10. An incident-management program will

    a. include "near misses" with potential for adverse outcomes.
    b. identify and discipline those at fault.
    c. increase institutional and nursing liability.

11. Nurse/physician difference of opinion about patient management should be

    a. considered unprofessional behavior.
    b. discussed with the patient's family.
    c. focused on the issue in question.

12. Despite repeated requests to a physician to come to the bedside to evaluate a deteriorating maternal condition, the physician has failed to respond. The nurse appropriately

    a. consults with another physician in the unit.
    b. institutes the chain of command.
    c. provides the intervention indicated.

13. Outcome measures of patient safety include

    a. how care is delivered.
    b. policies and procedures.
    c. rates of maternal morbidity and mortality.

14. Structure measures of patient safety include

    a. the number of elective inductions of labor prior to 39 completed weeks' gestation.
    b. the rates of third- and fourth-degree lacerations.
    c. unit protocols.

15. Process measures of patient safety include

    a. how hyperstimulation is identified and treated.
    b. number of nurses who are certified in fetal monitoring.
    c. rates of cesarean birth for nonreassuring fetal status.

16. Qualitative measures of patient safety include

    a. focus groups.
    b. number of sentinel events per year.
    c. policies and procedures consistent with national standards and guidelines.

Fill in the Blank

17. Essential criteria for safe care include

    _____

    _____

    _____

    _____

18. The areas of clinical practice that are most commonly involved in perinatal patient harm are

    _____

    _____

    _____.

19. In a high-reliability unit, there is an agreement that

    _____.

20. Standards and guidelines from professional organizations and regulatory agencies should guide clinical practice. These include

    _____

    _____

    _____

    _____

    _____.

21. According to ACOG, misoprostol is contraindicated for women _____.

22. According to ACOG, election labor induction should not occur prior to _____.

23. According to ACOG, the preferred method of fetal assessment during labor for women with high-risk conditions is _____.

24. Second-stage pushing should be initiated when _____, or when more than 2 hours have passed since complete dilation for _____ women, or more than 1 hour has passed since complete dilation for _____ women.

25. ACOG and AWHONN recommend use of the _____ definitions for fetal assessment during labor.

26. Triage for pregnant women who present for care should be based on guidelines from the _____.

27. Communication between patients and healthcare providers can be protective against _____.

28. During clinical emergencies, the timing of medical record documentation is often _____.

29. The practice of duplicate documentation on the fetal monitoring strip and the medical record is _____, and it contributes to _____.

30. A serious adverse event is defined by JCAHO as a _____.

31. The recommended nurse-to-patient ratio during oxytocin administration is _____.

32. The recommended nurse-to-patient ratio in the second stage of labor is _____.

33. Notifying the charge nurse when the staff nurse remains concerned about a physician's plan of care, after appropriate attempts to resolve the issues, is an example of implementing the _____.

Chapter 2

Multiple Choice

1. A 25-year-old Vietnamese woman admitted to the birthing unit requests that her husband stay in the waiting area until after she gives birth. The appropriate response is based on the nurse's knowledge that

   a. all husbands should be present during labor and birth.
   b. the husband may fear his response to his wife giving birth.
   c. the woman's request should be honored.

2. Wang Din Wah, a Laotian mother who is 24 hours postpartum, rejects the nurse's instructions to bring the newborn back to the clinic by the 7th day of life for a phenylketonuria test. Wang's reasons for this refusal are most likely based on

   a. her lack of recognition of appropriate health-care for the baby.
   b. the baby's early care being provided largely by the maternal grandmother.
   c. the first month after birth being considered a time for confinement and rest.

3. Berta Wolf Creek is 4 hours postpartum and requests permission to take her placenta home with her. Appropriate instruction by the nurse would include

   a. keeping the placenta in a leakproof container.
   b. requiring disposal of the placenta by internment (burial).
   c. keeping the placenta frozen until burial.

4. Maria Ochoa, a 23-year-old Filipino-American, is 18 weeks pregnant. After receiving a prescription for prenatal vitamins, she tells the nurse that her mother has warned her to take only herbal medication during pregnancy. The nurse appropriately

   a. advises Maria that the pills are only vitamins and not considered medication.

   b. assesses the significance of Maria's mother's advice.
   c. reminds her that the vitamins were ordered by the nurse-midwife.

5. The percentage of the U.S. population who are African-American or black is nearly

   a. 6%.
   b. 13%.
   c. 20%.

6. An African-American/black woman who believes she should not swallow her saliva and carries a spit cup with her during pregnancy is most likely from

   a. Barbados.
   b. Haiti.
   c. West Indies.

7. A major cultural group of childbearing women at increased risk for alcoholism, heart disease, cirrhosis of the liver, and diabetes mellitus is the population of women who are

   a. African American/black.
   b. American Indian/Alaskan native.
   c. Asian American/Pacific Islander.

8. According to the hot/cold theory, pregnancy is thought to be which kind of a condition?

   a. cold
   b. hot
   c. lukewarm

9. Match the sacred day of worship with the religious group.

   a. Sunday   1. Jewish or Seventh-Day
   b. sunset Friday to   Adventists
      sunset Saturday   2. Most Christians
   c. sunset Thursday   3. Muslims
      to sunset Friday

10. Ethnocentrism is the belief that

    a. cultural values are major determiners of one's behavior.
    b. every cultural group has a core or center of common beliefs.
    c. values and practices of one's own culture are superior.

11. A woman whose discharge plan includes her mother-in-law caring for her and her newborn during the postpartum period by tradition is most likely from which of the following cultures?

    a. Korean
    b. Laotian
    c. Tongan

12. What percentage of nurses come from racial or ethnic minority backgrounds?

    a. 9%
    b. 13%
    c. 17%

13. Goals each nurse can set to increase cultural competence while caring for culturally diverse childbearing women and their families are described as

    a. culturally driven.
    b. externally based.
    c. self-generated.

Fill in the Blank

14. Identify three strategies to increase the cultural competence of the nurse.

    1) _____
    2) _____
    3) _____

Chapter 3

Multiple Choice

1. By 28 to 34 weeks' gestation in a normal pregnancy, blood volume has increased by approximately

    a. 10%–20%.
    b. 30%–50%.
    c. 60%–80%.

2. During pregnancy, the position for optimum maternal cardiac output is

    a. lateral.
    b. semi-Fowler's.
    c. supine.

3. During labor, maternal cardiac output

    a. decreases slightly.
    b. increases progressively.
    c. remains the same.

4. An intravenous fluid bolus is given before epidural anesthesia to prevent

    a. hypotension.
    b. renal hypoperfusion.
    c. sympathetic blockade.

5. Normally during pregnancy, maternal sitting and standing diastolic blood pressure readings

    a. decrease, then increase.
    b. increase progressively.
    c. remain unchanged.

6. The volume of the maternal autotransfusion immediately after birth is approximately

    a. 600 mL.
    b. 800 mL.
    c. 1,000 mL.

7. What happens to maternal PaO_2 and $PaCO_2$ levels during pregnancy?

    a. Both decrease.
    b. Both increase.
    c. PaO_2 increases and $PaCO_2$ decreases.

8. The slight increase in pH that occurs during pregnancy is due to

    a. a decrease in hemoglobin and hematocrit.
    b. a decrease in renal excretion of bicarbonate.
    c. an increase in ventilatory rate.

9. During pregnancy, serum urea and creatine levels

    a. decrease.
    b. increase.
    c. remain constant.

10. Heartburn is common during pregnancy due primarily to

    a. decreased gastric motility.
    b. increased secretion of hydrochloric acid.
    c. relaxation of the lower esophageal sphincter.

11. A physical finding that may occur during pregnancy in response to normal cardiovascular changes is

    a. decreased heart rate.
    b. dependent edema.
    c. elevated blood pressure.

12. The average blood loss during vaginal birth is

    a. 300–400 mL.
    b. 500–600 mL.
    c. 700–800 mL.

13. The average blood loss during cesarean birth is

    a. 600 mL.
    b. 800 mL.
    c. 1,000 mL.

14. During pregnancy, cardiac output increases approximately

    a. 10%–25%.
    b. 30%–50%.
    c. 60%–75%.

15. Cardiac output is greatest during which period of the birth process?

    a. first stage, active phase
    b. immediately after birth
    c. second stage

16. A cardiovascular parameter which normally decreases during pregnancy is

    a. heart rate.
    b. stroke volume.
    c. systemic vascular resistance.

17. An expected white cell count during labor and the early postpartum is

    a. 8,000–10,000 mm^3.
    b. 13,000–15,000 mm^3.
    c. 20,000–22,000 mm^3.

18. Which of the following coagulation factors does not increase during pregnancy?

    a. fibrin
    b. platelets
    c. fibrinogen

19. Which of the following increases during pregnancy?

    a. colloid oncotic pressure
    b. glomerular filtration rate
    c. serum osmolality

20. By term, blood flow to the uterus is approximately

    a. 200 mL/min.
    b. 500 mL/min.
    c. 800 mL/min.

21. During pregnancy, the pigmented line in the skin that traverses the abdomen longitudinally from the sternum to the symphysis is called the

    a. linea nigra.
    b. spider nevus.
    c. striae gravidarum.

22. Which of the following is a change occurring in the respiratory system during pregnancy?

    a. Oxygen consumption increases.
    b. Respiratory rate decreases.
    c. Tidal volume decreases.

23. A normal finding during pregnancy is

    a. glycosuria.
    b. hematuria.
    c. proteinuria.

24. The respiratory system parameter that decreases during pregnancy is the

    a. functional residual capacity.
    b. minute ventilation.
    c. vital capacity.

25. A metabolic change characteristic of late pregnancy is decreased

    a. blood free fatty acid levels.
    b. insulin sensitivity.
    c. serum glucose levels after meals.

Fill in the Blank

26. Metabolic changes are characterized by _____ during the first half of pregnancy and _____ during the second half.

27. The greater increase in plasma volume than in red blood cell volume results in _____.

28. Maternal weight gain during the first half of pregnancy is primarily due to changes in the weight of the _____.

29. Both maternal metabolic rate and thyroid hormone levels _____ during pregnancy.

30. The primary determinant of volume hemostasis is _____.

31. The renal clearance of many substances is increased during pregnancy due to the _____.

32. Normal stretching of the skin and hormonal changes during gestation may produce "stretch marks" that are called _____.

33. The hormone released from the anterior pituitary that is responsible for initiating lactation is _____.

34. The increased maternal intestinal absorption of calcium is due to increased _____.

35. Compared to nonpregnant women, a pregnant woman in the third trimester has a _____ initial fasting blood glucose.

36. The hormone responsible for maintaining progesterone and estrogen production by the ovaries until the placenta is established is _____.

37. Placental production of the hormone _____ requires interaction of the mother, fetus, and placenta.

38. Increases in plasma volume and red cell mass result in an increase in _____ during pregnancy.

39. Cardiac output progressively decreases postpartum and returns to nonpregnant levels by _____.

40. The _____ accommodates one-third of the additional maternal blood volume at term.

41. The hormone _____ produces relaxation of smooth muscle and vasodilation.

42. Blood pressure reaches its lowest point at _____ weeks.

43. During pregnancy, the woman becomes resistant to the pressor effects of _____.

44. Pregnancy is considered a _____ state, due to the increases of several essential coagulation factors.

45. The pregnant woman is at increased risk for venous thrombus formation, due to _____ and _____.

46. _____ are potent vasodilators that affect smooth muscle contractility and play an important role in labor onset, myometrial contractility, and cervical ripening.

47. Irregularly shaped brown blotches on the face are known as _____, or the "mask of pregnancy."

48. The bluish discoloration of the cervix occurring during pregnancy is known as _____ sign.

Chapter 4
Multiple Choice

1. The developmental task of the first trimester is
   a. identification of the maternal role.
   b. movement from conflict and ambivalence to acceptance.
   c. resolution of the approach–avoidance conflict related to childbirth and loss of control.

2. A necessary element for the development of a therapeutic relationship with a perinatal client is
   a. establishment of healthy, clear boundaries between the woman and the nurse.
   b. kind and sympathetic judgments to guide the woman toward an appropriate maternal role.
   c. sharing of relevant personal information that demonstrates the empathy of the perinatal nurse.

3. The changes and transitions affecting the mind, body, and soul during pregnancy are best defined using a
   a. holistic model.
   b. physiologic model.
   c. psychosocial model.

4. A major issue during the third trimester is
   a. the physical changes of pregnancy.
   b. fetal well-being.
   c. ambivalence about the maternal role.

5. Symptoms of postpartum depression include
   a. agitation and anger.
   b. anxiety and irritability.
   c. hallucinations and delusions.

6. When the length of postpartum hospitalization is short, discharge planning should include
   a. a brief psychiatric assessment to rule out potential for postpartum psychosis.
   b. directing the new mother to look up the telephone numbers of postpartum resources.
   c. identifying with the new mother and her partner/key support people.

7. Reva Rubin suggests that during the postpartum period it is helpful for the new mother to

   a. accept constructive criticism from the nurse so that she can learn to correctly care for her infant.
   b. be encouraged to focus on the infant's needs exclusively so that she can provide care following discharge.
   c. put meaning into the childbirth experience by verbalizing her reality.

8. The estimated percentage of new mothers who experience "baby blues" is

   a. 30%–40%.
   b. 50%–60%.
   c. 70%–80%.

9. Discharge teaching for the new mother and family includes information that labile moods should stabilize and organization and confidence should increase by

   a. 4 weeks.
   b. 8 weeks.
   c. 12 weeks.

Fill in the Blank

10. Ten elements of a comprehensive psychosocial assessment include

    1) _____
    2) _____
    3) _____
    4) _____
    5) _____
    6) _____
    7) _____
    8) _____
    9) _____
    10) _____

11. Participants included in the psychosocial assessment are _____, _____, and _____.

12. The data obtained during a psychosocial assessment are used to develop _____, _____, and _____.

13. There is a strong correlation between mood and anxiety disorders before pregnancy and _____.

14. A critical aspect of holistic care planning for the perinatal client involves coordination of _____.

15. During the second trimester, women are increasingly vulnerable to _____.

16. When conducting a psychosocial assessment, it is important to determine the _____, _____, and _____ of mood or emotional disturbances.

17. Most women do not seek help with depressive disorders following birth because _____.

18. Becoming a mother is a process of _____ over the maternal–child relation.

19. The mother is better able to meet the needs of her infant when _____.

Chapter 5
Multiple Choice

1. Over the past 40 years, the incidence of preterm birth in the United States has

   a. declined.
   b. increased.
   c. remained the same.

2. An appropriate recommendation for weight gain for an underweight pregnant woman would be

   a. 20 lbs.
   b. 25 lbs.
   c. 30 lbs.

3. The best time to encourage a woman to stop smoking is

   a. before pregnancy.
   b. as soon as she knows she is pregnant.
   c. by the end of the first trimester.

4. The time during pregnancy when blood pressure is lowest in the normotensive woman is the

   a. first trimester.
   b. second trimester.
   c. third trimester.

5. The time when measurement of fundal height in centimeters should correlate with gestational age is

   a. after 20 weeks' gestation.
   b. near term.
   c. before 20 weeks' gestation.

6. Planning culturally specific care includes

   a. making sure that a translator is available when requested.
   b. noting patterns of decision making in the family.
   c. using a translator at each visit.

7. A nonreactive nonstress test at 39 weeks' gestation is an indication for

   a. expedited delivery.
   b. further testing.
   c. reassurance about fetal status.

8. Health promotion and education to improve pregnancy outcome in the next generation should begin when

   a. children are in elementary school.
   b. pregnancy occurs in the peer group.
   c. teens are sexually active.

9. An appropriate gestational age for a glucose screening test is at

   a. 23 weeks' gestation.
   b. 26 weeks' gestation.
   c. 29 weeks' gestation.

10. Risk assessment for all women during the initial prenatal visit should include

    a. a complete health history.
    b. a triple screen.
    c. an ultrasound for fetal anomalies.

11. Which of the following puts a woman at risk for nutritional problems during pregnancy?

    a. advanced maternal age
    b. cigarette smoking
    c. Gravida III, Term I, Preterm 0, Abortion I, Living Child I

12. An effect of cigarette smoking during pregnancy is increased incidence of

    a. low birth weight and prematurity.
    b. neonatal transient tachypnea of the newborn.
    c. pregnancy-induced hypertension.

13. Maternal serum alpha-fetoprotein specifically screens for

    a. heart defects.
    b. neural tube defects.
    c. placental defects.

14. If both parents are affected by sickle cell disease, the risk of their children being affected by sickle cell disease is

    a. 25%.
    b. 50%.
    c. 100%.

15. A primary method of fetal surveillance during pregnancy is

    a. fetal kick counts.
    b. nonstress testing.
    c. ultrasonography.

16. The most significant food shortages for low-income women occur

    a. at the end of the month, when federal/local resources diminish.
    b. before Women, Infants, and Children (WIC) eligibility is determined.
    c. postpartum, when fatigue prevents appointments with WIC.

17. A key component of preterm birth prevention education is

    a. discussing the hospital admission criteria.
    b. empowering the woman to act on her own instincts and self-knowledge.
    c. involving the significant other in the teaching.

18. True/False   With low income, the risk of perinatal morbidity increases after the age of 35, but with adequate income and healthcare, women had only a slight increase in gestational diabetes or pregnancy-induced hypertension.

Fill in the Blank

19. The monitoring of fetal activity by kick counts is initiated at _____ weeks' gestation.

20. It is recommended that every woman have an initial serology and gonorrhea culture, and that the tests be repeated at _____ weeks.

21. The recommended weight gain for an obese woman during pregnancy is _____.

22. Approximately _____ % of human malformations are caused by genetic factors alone.

23. A _____ is an agent that causes congenital malformations.

24. A biophysical profile summative score of _____ or greater is considered a sign of fetal well-being.

25. Male and female genitalia are recognizable by _____ weeks' gestation.

26. Tay-Sachs disease is a recessive disorder common in families of _____ ancestry.

27. The anticoagulant drug _____ is a known teratogen.

28. Folic acid requirements are increased to _____ times normal during pregnancy.

29. List three basic components of prenatal care.

    1) _____
    2) _____
    3) _____

30. Moderate physical activity during an uncomplicated pregnancy maintains _____ and _____ fitness.

31. Diagnosis of gestational diabetes mellitus is made when a glucose tolerance test result has _____.

32. Maternal serum screening is offered between _____ and _____ weeks' gestation.

33. A healthy fetus usually has _____ perceivable movements in 1 hour.

34. List the five parameters assessed in the biophysical profile.

    1) _____
    2) _____
    3) _____
    4) _____
    5) _____

Chapter 6

Hypertensive Disorders

Multiple Choice

1. A diagnosis of severe preeclampsia is consistent with a 24-hour urine showing protein excretion of

   a. 1 g/L.
   b. 3 g/L.
   c. 5 g/L.

2. An indication of impending magnesium sulfate toxicity in the patient being treated for preeclampsia is the absence of

   a. deep tendon reflexes.
   b. fetal movement.
   c. urine output.

3. The therapeutic range of serum magnesium during magnesium sulfate therapy to prevent eclamptic seizures is

   a. 1–4 mg/dL.
   b. 5–8 mg/dL.
   c. 9–12 mg/dL.

4. The first priority in the care of a patient during an eclamptic seizure is to

   a. administer an anticonvulsant agent.
   b. ensure a patent airway.
   c. establish IV access.

5. Diagnosis of preeclampsia requires the presence of hypertension and

   a. edema.
   b. headaches.
   c. proteinuria.

6. Severe preeclampsia can be diagnosed in the presence of

   a. excretion of 4,500 g protein in a 24-hour urine collection.
   b. serial diastolic blood pressures of at least 110 mm Hg.
   c. serum blood urea nitrogen of 10 with a serum creatinine of 1.

Fill in the Blank

7. _____ disorders are the most common medical complication of pregnancy.

8. A diastolic blood pressure of _____ mm Hg on two occasions least 6 hours apart is necessary for diagnosis of severe preeclampsia.

9. The blood pressure should be recorded with the pregnant woman in the _____ position.

10. _____ is the drug of choice to prevent seizure activity in the patient with preeclampsia.

11. Maternal morbidity from hypertension in pregnancy results from

    1) _____
    2) _____
    3) _____
    4) _____

12. The goals of antihypertensive therapy in the woman with preeclampsia are to _____ and to _____.

13. Laboratory markers for HELLP syndrome are _____, _____, and _____.

14. A leading cause of maternal morbidity following an eclamptic seizure is _____.

Bleeding

Multiple Choice

1. Invasion of the trophoblastic cells into the uterine myometrium is termed *placenta*

   a. *accreta.*
   b. *increta.*
   c. *percreta.*

2. Prostaglandin $F_{2\alpha}$ (Hemabate) may fail to control hemorrhage in women with

   a. chorioamnionitis.
   b. multiple gestation.
   c. previous cesarean section.

3. Painless, bright red vaginal bleeding at 28 weeks' gestation is most likely due to

   a. abruptio placentae.
   b. placenta previa.
   c. uterine rupture.

4. A clinical finding associated with a dehiscence of a uterine scar during a trial of labor after cesarean birth (TOLAC) is

   a. cessation of uterine contractions.
   b. fetal heart rate (FHR) with variable decelerations.
   c. sudden decrease of intrauterine pressure.

5. The initial drug of choice for excessive bleeding in the immediate postpartum period is

   a. Methergine IM.
   b. oxytocin IV infusion.
   c. prostaglandin 15-$MF_{2\alpha}$ suppository.

6. The most common cause of postpartum hemorrhage is

   a. an atonic uterus.
   b. a cervical laceration.
   c. a placenta accreta.

Fill in the Blank

7. Vasa previa is the result of a _____ insertion of the cord.

8. For the fetus to maintain adequate oxygenation, the maternal oxygen saturation must be at least _____%.

9. _____ is a late sign of hypovolemia in the woman experiencing bleeding during pregnancy.

Preterm Labor and Birth

Multiple Choice

1. Which of the following is not a common symptom of preterm labor?

   a. headache
   b. menstrual-like cramps
   c. pelvic pressure

2. One of the three most common risk factors predictive of preterm birth is

   a. low prepregnancy weight.
   b. smoking during pregnancy.
   c. history of preterm birth.

3. When considering nursing care of the woman in preterm labor, which of the following is true?

   a. Maternal transport to a high-risk center has improved outcome over neonatal transport to a special care nursery.
   b. The effect of antenatal glucocorticoid treatment is immediate.
   c. Tocolysis has great effectiveness in delaying preterm birth by 7 days.

4. A drug that is used for tocolysis but is not classified as a beta-mimetic is

   a. Procardia.
   b. ritodrine.
   c. terbutaline.

5. To accurately be considered preterm, an infant must be

   a. born at gestational age <37 weeks.
   b. <10th percentile in weight.
   c. small for gestational age.

6. Teaching pregnant women about the symptoms of preterm labor

    a. has been shown to prevent preterm birth.
    b. should be ongoing throughout pregnancy.
    c. should only be done on a one-to-one basis.

7. When beginning IV hydration for a woman with preterm contractions, the nurse must remember that

    a. IV fluids should be administered with the expectation for tocolysis with a beta-mimetic.
    b. preterm labor contractions usually diminish within one hour of initiation of IV hydration.
    c. the first liter of IV fluid should be administered within the first hour of the admission.

8. Antenatal glucocorticoid administration for acceleration of fetal lung maturation is appropriate

    a. for all women who could deliver preterm.
    b. in two doses given 24 hours apart.
    c. once a week from the time of the first preterm symptoms until delivery.

9. Bed rest has been shown by research to

    a. allow the pregnant woman to gain appropriate amounts of weight.
    b. cause bone demineralization.
    c. inhibit preterm labor contractions.

10. Smoking during pregnancy

    a. has been shown to decrease if cessation programs are offered.
    b. is best eradicated using the 2As program.
    c. has nothing to do with preterm birth.

Fill in the Blank

11. Preterm birth in the United States is _____ among African-Americans than among whites.

12. During the past several decades, rates of preterm birth have _____.

13. We now know that the term *Braxton-Hicks contractions* should be _____ from prenatal care teaching.

Diabetes
Multiple Choice

1. An indication to initiate insulin in a pregnant woman with gestational diabetes is

    a. fasting blood sugar (FBS) = <95 mg/dL on two or more occasions.
    b. FBS = normal, but 2-hour, postprandial = >100 mg/dL.
    c. FBS = >95 mg/dL, and 2-hour, postprandial = >120 mg/dL.

2. Hypoglycemia is defined as a plasma blood glucose of

    a. 60 mg/dL.
    b. 80 mg/dL.
    c. 90 mg/dL.

3. To assist in controlling blood glucose, the recommendation for pregnant women with well-controlled diabetes is to exercise

    a. daily for less than 20 minutes.
    b. every other day for 45 minutes.
    c. at least three times a week for 20 minutes.

4. Women with a history of gestational diabetes with a normal postpartum follow-up test should be tested for overt diabetes

    a. every 3 years.
    b. before a subsequent pregnancy.
    c. a and b.

5. Intensive management of diabetes in women with pregestational diabetes should begin

    a. prior to conception.
    b. postpartum.
    c. only if planning to breastfeed.

6. In women with diabetes, medical nutrition therapy

    a. is not necessary.
    b. has no effect on glycemic control.
    c. is a vital component of care.

7. For women with diabetes, breastfeeding

    a. can prevent pregnancy.
    b. is contraindicated; a baby should be bottle-fed.
    c. has been associated with reduced incidence of childhood obesity and diabetes later in life.

8. Diagnostic testing for gestational diabetes includes 3-hour oral glucose tolerance test after administration of

   a. 28 jelly beans.
   b. 50-gram glucose solution.
   c. 100-gram glucose solution.

9. Insulin dosage during periods of nausea and vomiting in pregnant women should be

   a. administered with no adjustment.
   b. based on a sliding scale.
   c. withheld until nausea is resolved.

10. Weekly nonstress testing should be initiated in women with vascular disease beginning at the gestational age of

    a. 28 weeks.
    b. 30 weeks.
    c. 32 weeks.

Fill in the Blank

11. _____ diabetes results due to an autoimmune reaction directed at the pancreas following an environmental trigger.

12. Metabolic changes during the first half of pregnancy characterized by fat storage is called the _____ phase.

13. List five diabetogenic hormones of pregnancy.

    1) _____
    2) _____
    3) _____
    4) _____
    5) _____

14. Preterm labor in women with diabetes should be treated with _____.

15. Three specific symptoms of hyperglycemia are

    1) _____
    2) _____
    3) _____

Cardiac Disease

Multiple Choice

1. The incidence of congenital cardiac disease is

   a. 1:100 live births.
   b. 1:500 live births.
   c. 1:1,000 live births.

2. Maternal outcomes in pregnancies of women with Marfan's syndrome are related to

   a. cardiac dysrhythmias.
   b. degree of aortic root dilation.
   c. hypervolemia of pregnancy.

3. Coronary artery disease during pregnancy is rare due to

   a. hormonal protection against atherosclerosis.
   b. maternal production of relaxin.
   c. progesterone-mediated vasodilation.

4. The incidence of myocardial infarction during pregnancy is

   a. 1:1000.
   b. 1:10,000.
   c. 1:100,000.

5. Peripartum cardiomyopathy is categorized as

   a. dilated cardiomyopathy.
   b. hypertrophic cardiomyopathy.
   c. restrictive cardiomyopathy.

6. A pregnant woman with New York Heart Association (NYHA) class II cardiac disease is symptomatic with

   a. bed rest.
   b. mild exertion.
   c. moderate exertion.

7. The drug of choice to treat epidural analgesia–related hypotension for a pregnant woman with a cardiac disorder would be

   a. dopamine.
   b. ephedrine.
   c. phenylephrine.

8. The time during labor and birth when the greatest cardiac stress occurs is

   a. immediately postpartum.
   b. late first stage (transition).
   c. second stage with descent.

9. The release of catecholamines, which occurs with stimulation of the sympathetic nervous system,

   a. has no effect on uteroplacental perfusion.
   b. increases uteroplacental perfusion.
   c. limits uteroplacental perfusion.

10. An initial sign of inadequate cerebral perfusion is

    a. low pulse oximeter readings.
    b. restlessness.
    c. unequal pupil dilation.

Fill in the Blank

11. _____ regulate the distribution of extracellular fluid.

12. Mitral and aortic stenosis are examples of cardiac diseases caused by _____.

13. Severe consequences from myocardial infarction are _____ during pregnancy.

14. Current risk counseling for pregnant women with cardiac disease is based on the _____ and the _____.

15. The NYHA classification system for cardiac disease categorizes patients by _____.

Pulmonary Complications

Multiple Choice

1. During pregnancy, predicted values of peak expiratory flow rates are

    a. decreased.
    b. increased.
    c. unchanged.

2. The mainstay of asthma therapy is

    a. beta-2 agonists.
    b. corticosteroids.
    c. immunotherapy.

3. Moderate–severe asthma is apparent when respiratory rate is greater than

    a. 20/minute.
    b. 30/minute.
    c. 40/minute.

4. During an exacerbation of asthma, there is

    a. decreased functional residual capacity.
    b. increased expiratory airflow.
    c. increased peripheral vascular resistance.

5. A breath sound rarely auscultated in asthmatics is

    a. rales.
    b. rhonchi.
    c. wheezes.

6. The most commonly seen pneumonia of pregnancy is

    a. aspiration.
    b. bacterial.
    c. viral.

7. A complication seen in up to 26% of women with varicella pneumonia is

    a. intrauterine infection.
    b. pneumothorax.
    c. small for gestational age fetus.

8. When aspiration pneumonia occurs during pregnancy, it is most commonly a result of

    a. bronchitis.
    b. general anesthesia.
    c. smoking.

9. Initial arterial blood gases in the pregnant woman with pneumonia usually reflect significant

    a. acidosis.
    b. hypercapnia.
    c. hypoxia.

10. Hypoxia should be suspected when a pregnant woman is noted to have

    a. hypotension.
    b. increased urine output.
    c. restlessness.

Fill in the Blank

11. Exacerbations of asthma will occur during the intrapartum period _____ % of the time.

12. Oxygen saturation of greater than _____ % by pulse oximetry is vital for a pregnant woman with pneumonia.

13. Following delivery, _____ % of women will return to the prepregnancy status of their asthma.

14. A lifestyle risk factor that may increase a woman's risk of acquiring pneumonia during pregnancy is _____.

15. The most common bacterial pathogen in pneumonia during pregnancy is _____.

16. The maternal position that best supports maximum oxygenation is _____.

17. Common inhalation irritants for many asthmatics are _____.

18. Markers for potentially fatal asthma are _____.

19. Maternal complications of pneumonia during pregnancy are _____.

20. During pregnancy, _____% of women with asthma will experience worsening of symptoms.

Multiple Gestation

Multiple Choice

1. Multiple birth rates have increased most dramatically in which maternal age group?

    a. 25 to 30 years
    b. 30 to 35 years
    c. 45 to 54 years.

2. The likelihood of monozygotic twinning is affected by

    a. older maternal age.
    b. use of assisted reproductive technologies.
    c. black maternal race.

3. The lambda sign, a triangle-shaped ultrasound marker seen at the junction of the chorions and amnions, indicates

    a. monozygotic gestation.
    b. dizygotic gestation.
    c. trizygotic gestation.

4. The dermatologic condition that is more common in multiple gestations than in singletons is

    a. pruritic folliculitis of pregnancy.
    b. herpes gestationis.
    c. pruritic urticarial papules and plaques of pregnancy syndrome.

5. A practice that appears to be effective in preterm birth prevention in multiple gestations is

    a. prophylactic betamimetic tocolytic agents.
    b. routine cervical assessment.
    c. bed rest starting at 28 weeks.

6. The greatest complication of tocolytic therapy for women with multiple gestations is

    a. pulmonary edema.
    b. maternal tachycardia.
    c. hyperreflexia.

7. The risk for fetal death in twin gestations is highest at

    a. 24 weeks.
    b. 35 weeks.
    c. 40 weeks.

8. Effective treatment for severe twin-to-twin transfusion syndrome includes all except

    a. expectant management.
    b. serial amniocentesis.
    c. fetoscopic laser therapy.

9. The prenatal diagnostic screening test most accurate in multiple gestations is

    a. second trimester maternal serum testing.
    b. nuchal translucency.
    c. maternal age risk calculation.

10. Maternal weight gain has the greatest effect on fetal growth and birth weight when gains occur

    a. during the first 20 weeks.
    b. during the third trimester.
    c. evenly throughout pregnancy.

11. The recommended mode of delivery for twins presenting Twin A: vertex/Twin B: vertex without other indications is

    a. vaginal/vaginal.
    b. cesarean/cesarean.
    c. vaginal/cesarean.

12. A contraindication for cobedding of preterm multiples in the neonatal intensive care unit is

    a. gavage feeding.
    b. phototherapy.
    c. infection in one infant.

13. A sign of abnormal parent–infant interaction with multiples is

    a. initial unit attachment.
    b. ongoing preferential attention.
    c. alternating eye contact among infants.

14. After delivery of multiples, breastfeeding or pumping should begin

    a. within 1 to 2 hours.
    b. by 24 hours.
    c. when the mother's milk comes in.

15. When part of a set of multiples dies, parents often

    a. begin grieving immediately.
    b. are able to bond effectively with the survivor.
    c. experience paradoxical feelings.

Fill in the Blank

16. The greatest predictors of infant morbidity and mortality in multiples are _____ and _____.

17. The term for similarity in FHR accelerations, baseline oscillations and periodic changes with contractions in healthy twins is _____ _____.

True or False

18. True/False   Hypertensive disorders in multiple gestations follow a classic pattern of signs and symptoms.

19. True/False   Prenatal education for parents expecting multiples should begin in the second trimester.

20. True/False   The increased prevalence of cerebral palsy in multiple-birth infants is explained by the greater proportion of low birth weight and preterm births.

21. True/False   The increased prevalence of sudden infant death syndrome in multiple birth infants is explained by the greater proportion of low-birth-weight infants.

22. True/False   Mothers of multiples should be shown positions for simultaneous breastfeeding before hospital discharge.

Chapter 7
Multiple Choice

1. According to AWHONN and the American College of Obstetricians and Gynecologists (ACOG), in the absence of risk factors, FHR should be assessed during second stage labor every

    a. 5 minutes.
    b. 15 minutes.
    c. 30 minutes.

2. An appropriate lubricant to use for vaginal examinations during labor is

    a. povidone–iodine gel.
    b. sterile water.
    c. water-soluble jelly.

3. According to the American Society of Anesthesiologists (ASA) *Guidelines For Obstetrical Care*, an elective cesarean could be done when the woman has been NPO for at least

    a. 4 hours.
    b. 5 hours.
    c. 6 hours.

4. An involuntary urge to push is most likely a sign of

    a. low fetal station.
    b. occiput posterior fetal position.
    c. transition.

5. An appropriate solution to use for amnioinfusion is

    a. 5% dextrose in lactated Ringer's solution (D5/LR).
    b. 5% dextrose in water (D5W).
    c. lactated Ringer's solution.

6. An increased risk for shoulder dystocia is associated with

    a. maternal diabetes.
    b. post-date pregnancy.
    c. TOLAC.

7. The primary factor that would allow second-stage labor to continue beyond 2 hours is that

    a. epidural anesthesia is in place with level <T10.
    b. FHR is reassuring as the presenting part descends.
    c. maternal pushing efforts result in progress.

8. Using the Zavanelli maneuver to resolve shoulder dystocia involves

    a. assisting the woman to a knee–chest position.
    b. elevating the fetal head back through the vagina.
    c. sweeping an arm to deliver the posterior shoulder.

9. ACOG defines *uterine hyperstimulation* as

    a. contraction duration of >60 seconds.
    b. contraction frequency of every 2–3 minutes.
    c. contractions >five in 10 minutes.

10. A high probability of successful induction of labor is associated with a Bishop score of

    a. >4.
    b. >6.
    c. >8.

11. Appropriate treatment of hyperstimulation after dinoprostone administration is

    a. IV bolus of D5W.
    b. terbutaline 0.25 mg SQ.
    c. vaginal irrigation with normal saline.

12. In the absence of complications, immediate postpartum maternal vital signs should be assessed every

    a. 5 minutes for 30 minutes.
    b. 15 minutes for 1 hour.
    c. 30 minutes for 2 hours.

13. ACOG recommends a dosing interval for misoprostol of every

    a. 1–2 hours.
    b. 3–6 hours.
    c. 7–12 hours.

14. The most common reason for hospital readmission following operative birth is

    a. endometritis.
    b. hemorrhage.
    c. wound infection.

15. Vacuum extractor cup placement on the fetal head should not exceed

    a. 5 minutes.
    b. 10–15 minutes.
    c. 20–30 minutes.

16. Anesthesia personnel are required to remain with a postanesthesia care unit (PACU) patient until the

    a. monitoring equipment has been applied.
    b. PACU nurse accepts responsibility for the patient.
    c. patient is alert and oriented.

17. The normal length of the pregravid cervix is

    a. 2.5–3 cm.
    b. 3.5–4 cm.
    c. 4.5–5 cm.

18. True labor is characterized by

    a. effacement and/or dilation of the cervix.
    b. painful uterine contractions.
    c. suprapubic discomfort at regular intervals.

19. One liter of D5/LR provides

    a. 100 calories.
    b. 225 calories.
    c. 500 calories.

20. Facilitating a family-centered birth experience involves

    a. allowing immediate family members to participate.
    b. providing a waiting area for siblings.
    c. supporting family as defined by the childbearing woman.

Fill in the Blank

21. Diastolic blood pressure measurements taken from an automatic blood pressure device are typically _____ than diastolic measurements utilizing a stethoscope and a mercury cuff.

22. The enzyme oxytocinase facilitates plasma clearance of oxytocin via the maternal _____ and _____.

23. During the second stage of labor, an alternative to squatting that provides the same benefits is _____.

24. Bearing down efforts accompanied by prolonged breath-holding typifies _____ pushing, which has associated negative maternal and fetal _____ effects.

25. AWHONN's second-stage labor nursing management protocol for a woman with epidural anesthesia encourages rest until the occurrence of _____.

26. The McRoberts maneuver is used to facilitate birth when there is an occurrence of _____, and requires the nurse to assist the woman to _____ her legs at the _____ and at the _____.

27. Adverse outcomes associated with episiotomy include

    1) _____
    2) _____
    3) _____

28. Measures to aid perineal stretching and aid in the goal to avoid episiotomy include

    1) _____
    2) _____
    3) _____

29. Women who have a support person with them in labor have been found to have

    1) _____
    2) _____
    3) _____

30. Before the use of a cervical ripening or labor induction agent, the following should be assessed:

    1) _____
    2) _____
    3) _____

31. Risks associated with stripping of membranes include

    1) _____
    2) _____
    3) _____

32. An interval of _____ hours is recommended between the final dose of dinoprostone and oxytocin administration.

33. Nursing documentation following amniotomy should include

    1) _____
    2) _____
    3) _____

34. A _____ degree laceration extends into the rectal lumen.

35. The maternal landmarks that must be identified to determine fetal stations are the _____.

36. With a physician or certified nurse midwife order, nurses with appropriate training may administer the cervical ripening agents _____ and _____.

37. _____ is a contraindication for the use of misoprostol and Cervidil.

38. A nursing measure to use before forcep application to help prevent maternal trauma is _____.

39. The recommendations for use of the vacuum extractor device state that the pressure should not exceed _____ mm Hg.

40. Requirements for post-anesthesia recovery care include availability of

    1) _____
    2) _____
    3) _____
    4) _____
    5) _____
    6) _____
    7) _____

41. According to ACOG, selection criteria for women who are candidates for vaginal birth after cesarean (VBAC) include

    1) _____
    2) _____
    3) _____
    4) _____
    5) _____

42. _____ is a sign of impending uterine rupture in women experiencing a trial of labor after prior cesarean delivery.

43. Four maternal factors proposed as being responsible for initiation of labor are

    1) _____
    2) _____
    3) _____
    4) _____

44. If any of the following findings are present in a pregnant woman, the perinatal provider should be notified promptly.

    1) _____
    2) _____
    3) _____
    4) _____
    5) _____
    6) _____

45. The Bishop score evaluates these five parameters:

    1) _____
    2) _____
    3) _____
    4) _____
    5) _____

46. Unnecessary interventions during labor increase the risk of _____.

47. Informed consent for VBAC correctly includes discussion about

    1) _____
    2) _____
    3) _____

Chapter 8

Multiple Choice

1. When auscultation is used for fetal assessment during labor for a low-risk woman, the FHR should be auscultated in the first stage of labor every

   a. 5 minutes.
   b. 15 minutes.
   c. 30 minutes.

2. For a low-risk woman in the second stage of labor, the FHR should be auscultated every

   a. 5 minutes.
   b. 10 minutes.
   c. 15 minutes.

3. The normal FHR baseline

   a. decreases during labor.
   b. fluctuates during labor.
   c. increases during labor.

4. Bradycardia in the second stage of labor following a previously normal tracing may be caused by fetal

   a. hypoxemia.
   b. rotation.
   c. vagal stimulation.

5. A likely cause of fetal tachycardia with moderate variability is

   a. fetal hypoxemia.
   b. maternal fever.
   c. vagal stimulation.

6. Loss of FHR variability can result from

   a. fetal scalp stimulation.
   b. medication administration.
   c. vaginal examination.

7. The primary goal in treatment for late decelerations is to

   a. correct cord compression.
   b. improve maternal oxygenation.
   c. maximize uteroplacental blood flow.

8. The most frequently observed type of FHR deceleration is

   a. early.
   b. late.
   c. variable.

9. Amnioinfusion may be useful in alleviating decelerations that are

   a. early.
   b. late.
   c. variable.

10. Findings indicative of progressive fetal hypoxemia are

    a. late decelerations, moderate variability, and stable baseline rate.
    b. prolonged decelerations recovering to baseline and moderate variability.
    c. rising baseline rate and absent variability.

11. Fetal metabolic acidemia is indicated by an arterial cord gas pH of 7.18 and a base deficit of

    a. 3.
    b. 6.
    c. 12.

12. Fetal bradycardia can result during

    a. the sleep state.
    b. umbilical vein compression.
    c. vagal stimulation.

13. While caring for a 235-lb laboring woman who is HIV-seropositive, the external FHR tracing is difficult to obtain. An appropriate nursing action would be to

    a. apply a fetal scalp electrode.
    b. auscultate for presence of FHR variability.
    c. notify the attending midwife or physician.

14. FHR decelerations that are benign and do not require intervention are

    a. early.
    b. late.
    c. variable.

15. FHR decelerations that result from decreased uteroplacental blood flow are

    a. early.
    b. late.
    c. variable.

16. FHR decelerations that result from umbilical cord compression are

    a. early.
    b. late.
    c. variable.

17. A FHR pattern likely to develop with severe fetal anemia is

    a. lambda.
    b. saltatory.
    c. sinusoidal.

18. A workup for maternal systemic lupus erythematosus would likely be ordered in the presence of

    a. complete fetal heart block.
    b. premature fetal ventricular contractions.
    c. fetal supraventricular tachycardia.

Fill in the Blank

19. Late decelerations are characterized by decelerations of the FHR that begin at the _____ of the contraction, do not return to the baseline rate until _____ the contraction ends, and occur with every contraction.

20. Variable decelerations are characterized by decelerations that have _____ timing in relation to the contractions, but always have a(n) _____ change in rate.

21. Early decelerations are characterized by a drop in FHR that begins at the _____ of a contraction and recovers to the _____ by the end of the contraction. Early decelerations are _____ and do not require intervention.

22. Nursing interventions for late decelerations include _____ the oxytocin if it is infusing.

23. Reassuring FHR tracings have an absence of decelerations and may show accelerations and/or _____ variability.

24. Whenever a FHR pattern occurs that cannot be easily characterized, the possibility of a fetus with _____ should be considered.

25. Most fetal dysrhythmias are not life-threatening, except for _____, which may lead to fetal congestive heart failure.

26. Minimal baseline variability may be caused by multiple factors including _____, _____, and _____.

27. In the presence of variable decelerations, progressive hypoxemia may be characterized by an increasing _____ and loss of _____.

28. Late decelerations associated with acute conditions may be caused by uterine _____.

29. If the FHR tracing does not revert to a reassuring tracing following interventions for late decelerations, administration of _____ to stop or decrease uterine activity may be indicated.

30. Uterine resting tone and the intensity of contractions are measured in mm Hg only when a/an _____ is being used.

31. A sinusoidal pattern may develop in the Rh-sensitized fetus or the fetus who is _____.

32. In the absence of maternal and/or fetal risk factors, auscultation of the fetal rate should occur every _____ minutes in the active phase of the first stage of labor and every _____ minutes in the second stage of labor.

33. Moderate baseline variability is defined as _____ bpm.

34. Correcting variable decelerations can best be accomplished by _____.

35. In the presence of late or variable decelerations, two parameters that reassure the nurse of adequate fetal oxygenation are _____ and _____.

36. Evidence shows that when an electronic fetal monitoring tracing is interpreted as nonreassuring or indicative of fetal stress, a well-oxygenated newborn is delivered at least _____% of the time.

37. In the presence of FHR accelerations greater than 15 bpm above baseline and lasting more than 15 seconds, the fetal condition is comparable to the fetal blood gas pH of at least _____ and is considered _____.

38. To correctly interpret a baseline FHR as tachycardic or bradycardic, the rate must persist for a minimum of _____ minutes.

39. In assessing fetal well-being, the most important characteristic of the FHR is _____.

40. Nursing interventions to maximize uteroplacental blood flow include

    1) _____
    2) _____
    3) _____
    4) _____
    5) _____

41. The normal FHR baseline range is _____ bpm to _____ bpm.

Chapter 9

Multiple Choice

1. Pain during the first stage of labor is caused by

   a. cervical and lower uterine segment stretching and traction on ovaries, fallopian tubes, and uterine ligaments.
   b. pressure on the urethra, bladder, and rectum by the descending fetal presenting part.
   c. uterine muscle hypoxia, lactic acid accumulation, and distention of the pelvic floor muscles.

2. The release of maternal catecholamines during labor results in

   a. fetal tachycardia.
   b. decreased metabolic rate and oxygen consumption.
   c. uterine hypoperfusion and decreased blood flow to the placenta.

3. The purpose for administration of medications such as hydroxyzine hydrochloride (Vistaril), and propiomazine (Largon) during early labor is to

   a. decrease pain of contractions.
   b. potentiate effects of narcotics.
   c. provide sedation and relieve anxiety.

4. Intradermal injections of sterile water provide pain relief for up to

   a. 1 hour.
   b. 2 hours.
   c. 3 hours.

5. A medication commonly given to women who are experiencing prolonged latent labor to produce a period of sleep is

   a. butorphanol (Stadol).
   b. morphine.
   c. promethazine hydrochloride (Phenergan).

6. Neonatal respiratory depression could result from the maternal administration of IV opioids if birth occurs within

   a. 1 hour or after 4 hours following administration.
   b. 2–3 hours of administration.
   c. 12 hours of administration.

7. Ephedrine is used to correct which side effect of epidural anesthesia/analgesia?

   a. hypotension
   b. nausea and vomiting
   c. pruritus

8. A medication given to reverse the symptom of a distended bladder during a continuous epidural infusion is

   a. bupivacaine.
   b. epinephrine.
   c. naloxone.

9. Touch/massage is thought to decrease or interrupt the pain of labor by

   a. activating large myelinated nerve fibers.
   b. activating the same type of nerve fibers that would transmit sensations of pain from the uterus.
   c. interrupting the habituation that occurs when labor is prolonged.

10. When pruritus occurs in the presence of an opioid in the epidural infusion, the nurse can correctly tell the patient that this symptom will most likely subside in about

    a. 15 minutes.
    b. 45 minutes.
    c. 1–2 hours.

11. Advantages of combined spinal epidural technique are

    a. decreased hypotension, decreased motor blockade, and increased maternal satisfaction.
    b. decreased hypotension, faster onset of pain relief, and decreased pruritus.
    c. faster onset of pain relief, decreased motor blockade, and increased maternal satisfaction.

12. Meperidine (Demerol) is used less frequently as an analgesia during labor because

    a. it cannot be given intravenously.
    b. it causes neonatal neurobehavioral depression, which may last for several days.
    c. most women receive epidural analgesia.

13. To decrease the transfer of medication to the fetus, IV push narcotics should be given when in relation to the time of uterine contractions?

    a. after
    b. before
    c. during

14. The epidural catheter for labor pain management is generally placed between the

    a. 2nd and 3rd lumbar vertebrae.
    b. 3rd and 4th lumbar vertebrae.
    c. 4th and 5th lumbar vertebrae.

15. Epinephrine may be added to the epidural to

    a. decrease the amount of narcotic needed.
    b. lessen pruritus associated with epidural narcotic.
    c. prevent hypotension.

16. A test dose of a local anesthetic mixed with epinephrine may be injected to determine that the catheter is not in the epidural vein. Injection of epinephrine into an epidural vein causes almost immediate

    a. decreased blood pressure.
    b. increased blood pressure.
    c. increased heart rate.

17. When the epidural catheter is properly placed, a bolus of anesthetic medication is injected. Depending on the specific medications used, women begin to feel relief in

    a. 1 to 2 minutes.
    b. 5 to 10 minutes.
    c. 15 to 20 minutes.

18. Unlike the RN, the doula

    a. has minimal or no contact with the parents after the birth.
    b. meets the woman for the first time in labor.
    c. provides continuous labor support.

19. When a tub is used during labor, water should be maintained at a temperature of

    a. 34–35°C.
    b. 36–37°C.
    c. 38–39°C.

20. One of the contraindications to neuraxial analgesia is that the woman received her last dose of low-molecular-weight heparin within

    a. 1 hour.
    b. 6 hours.
    c. 12 hours.

21. The initial intervention for a woman experiencing pain on one side during a continuous epidural infusion is to

    a. maintain the woman in a lateral position, off the painful side.
    b. request that an anesthesiologist reevaluate the woman.
    c. turn the woman toward the side with pain.

22. The current recommendation from the ASA regarding nourishment during labor is that solid foods

    a. and liquids do not need to be avoided during labor because of superior anesthesia techniques available today, which do not increase the risk for complications should cesarean section become necessary.
    b. and liquids need to be avoided after the patient has reached 3 cm, due to the potential for cesarean section and the potential risk of respiratory complications when any patient receives anesthesia.
    c. should be avoided, but clear liquids increase maternal comfort and satisfaction and do not increase maternal complications.

23. According to AWHONN, nonanesthetist registered nurses can

    a. increase/decrease the rate of a continuous epidural infusion.
    b. re-initiate an epidural infusion once it has been stopped.
    c. remove an epidural catheter after successfully completing an educational program.

24. Maintaining a horizontal position in labor promotes

    a. descent of the presenting part.
    b. increased perception of pain.
    c. maternal oxygenation and comfort.

Fill in the Blank

25. A major limitation for recommending most of the nonpharmacologic methods of pain relief for use in labor is the lack of large _____.

26. Women who labor with the baby's head in the occipitoposterior postion report significantly less back pain when using _____ positioning.

27. Counterpressure requires application of enough force to meet the intensity of pressure from the fetal occipital bone against the _____.

28. _____ pressure equalizes the pressure exerted on all parts of the body below the water surface.

Questions 29–33 relate to the following statement:

Using the Gate Control Theory, explain how each nonpharmacologic pain management strategy interrupts the transmission of painful stimuli (options a–c).

a. auditory or visual stimulation of the cerebral cortex to prevent passage of painful stimuli
b. cutaneous stimulation to block or alter painful stimuli
c. supports the neuromatrix and ultimately how the individual perceives pain

29. _____ hydrotherapy

30. _____ focal point

31. _____ breathing techniques

32. _____ relaxation

33. _____ intradermal injections of sterile water

34. Following administration of an opioid during labor, frequency and duration of contractions and FHR variability may _____.

35. A fluid bolus should be administered before the initiation of regional analgesia/anesthesia to decrease the potential for maternal _____.

36. The advantages of bupivacaine (Marcaine) and ropivacaine (Naropin) over lidocaine (Xylocaine) and chloroprocaine (Nescaine) for use in epidural analgesia/anesthesia is less _____.

37. The failure to obtain complete pain relief despite proper placement of the epidural catheter may be due to the presence of _____ in the epidural space, which limit areas of the epidural space that can be reached by the medication infused.

38. _____ avoids continued pressure on one single area of the body and decreases the risk of unilateral blocks.

39. Supine position is associated with decrease _____ and _____.

Chapter 10

Multiple Choice

1. A normal hemodynamic/hematologic change occurring during the immediate postpartum period is
   a. decreased white blood cell count.
   b. elevated blood pressure.
   c. increased cardiac output.

2. During the postpartum period, normal respiratory and acid-base changes include
   a. decreased base excess.
   b. hypercapnia.
   c. increased PCO_2.

3. Postpartum teaching about sexual activity includes the information that
   a. interest in sexual activity may increase due to hormonal changes.
   b. lubricants will not be needed due to increased vaginal mucus.
   c. sexual intercourse should be avoided until vaginal bleeding has ceased.

4. A normal physiologic finding during the immediate postpartum period is
   a. dizziness when sitting up from a reclining position.
   b. saturation of the peripad every 15 minutes.
   c. urinary output of 25 mL/hour.

5. An appropriate nursing intervention for postpartum hemorrhage is
   a. bimanual pressure.
   b. bladder catheterization.
   c. continuous fundal massage.

6. On the second postpartum/postoperative day following her cesarean delivery, a woman exhibits hypotension, dyspnea, hemoptysis, and abdominal/chest pain. The nurse recognizes these as signs and symptoms of
   a. endometritis.
   b. pulmonary embolism.
   c. sepsis.

7. Normal metabolic changes during the postpartum period include increased levels of
   a. blood glucose.
   b. plasma renin and angiotensin II.
   c. prolactin.

8. The most significant factor influencing a woman's successful transition to motherhood is

   a. emotional support and physical involvement in child care by a significant other.
   b. regular attendance at parent support group meetings.
   c. resumption of a positive and satisfying sexual relationship with her partner.

9. Postpartum endometritis is

   a. associated with internal monitoring, amnioinfusion, prolonged labor, and prolonged rupture of membranes.
   b. effectively treated with a single dose of ampicillin or cephalosporin.
   c. less frequent following cesarean birth, due to sterile technique used during surgery.

10. Disruptions in the integrity of the anal sphincter, third-degree tears, and sphincter weakness are

    a. associated with increased incidence of incontinence of flatus/stool.
    b. prevented through the judicious use of operative delivery.
    c. problems freely discussed by women with their healthcare providers.

11. The nurse can positively affect a new mother's self-concept and mothering abilities by encouraging

    a. establishment of a feeding schedule that the mother finds satisfying.
    b. supportive family and friends to participate in learning opportunities and infant care during the mother's hospitalization.
    c. the mother to provide as much of the infant care as possible.

12. Appropriate fundal massage for postpartum uterine atony involves using

    a. continuous two-handed pressure on the uterus until bleeding stops.
    b. firm one-handed pressure on the fundus until clots are expressed.
    c. two hands and the force needed to effect uterine contraction.

13. Stress incontinence during the postpartum period is more likely to be associated with the techniques used to manage which stage of labor?

    a. first
    b. second
    c. third

14. No more than 800 mL of urine should be removed during postpartum catheterization to minimize the potential for

    a. bladder spasm.
    b. hypertension.
    c. hypotension.

15. The most effective prevention of endometritis is

    a. use of early pericare.
    b. handwashing.
    c. use of intrapartum antibiotics.

16. The most likely cause of a decline in sexual interest/activity during the postpartum period is

    a. bleeding from the vagina.
    b. fatigue.
    c. vaginal dryness.

17. Postpartum hemorrhage is associated with administration of

    a. dicloxacillin.
    b. methadone.
    c. terbutaline.

18. Peak cardiac output after birth occurs at

    a. 1–5 minutes.
    b. 10–15 minutes.
    c. 30 minutes.

19. A normal hematologic change during the postpartum period is a/an

    a. drop in hematocrit between days 2 and 4.
    b. increase in the sedimentation rate.
    c. leukocytosis of 25–30,000/μL.

20. Nutritional counseling for women who breastfeed should include increasing caloric intake by

    a. 300 calories.
    b. 400 calories.
    c. 500 calories.

Fill in the Blank

21. To increase venous return during postpartum hemorrhage, the woman should be positioned with _____.

22. A white blood cell count of 28,000/mm^3 on postpartum day 2 would be considered _____.

23. Vital signs within normal limits do not rule out hypovolemic shock in a woman who has experienced a postpartum hemorrhage, because alterations in vital signs do not occur until _____.

24. _____ is an assessment technique for identification of deep vein thrombosis.

25. When a postpartum woman displays dyspnea and chest pain, the nurse most appropriately suspects _____.

26. The first blood pressure response to hypovolemia would be decreased _____.

27. Counseling regarding contraceptive methods must include information about the _____, _____, and _____.

28. Symptoms of postpartum blues include

    1) _____
    2) _____
    3) _____
    4) _____
    5) _____

29. During the initial postpartum period, the nurse should assess _____, _____, and _____ every 15 minutes for at least 1 hour, or more often if indicated.

30. Typically, postpartum blues occur at _____ days postpartum and continue for no more than a few days.

31. The normal postpartum physiologic diuresis begins within _____ hours of delivery and continues up to _____ days.

32. The acronym BUBBLERS, used to organize postpartum assessment, stands for

    1) _____
    2) _____
    3) _____
    4) _____
    5) _____
    6) _____
    7) _____
    8) _____

33. For each 500 cc of blood loss, the hematocrit will decrease _____% and the hemoglobin will decrease _____ g/dL.

34. Assessment findings suggesting the development of mastitis include

    1) _____
    2) _____
    3) _____
    4) _____

35. Essential topics to be discussed during postpartum teaching are

    1) _____
    2) _____
    3) _____
    4) _____

36. A major factor affecting emotional adjustment during the postpartum period in low-risk women is _____.

37. The first hour after birth is the time of greatest risk for postpartum hemorrhage because _____.

38. Symptoms indicating the development of postpartum preeclampsia are

    1) _____
    2) _____
    3) _____

39. It is important that the nurse has the drug _____ readily available when patients are receiving heparin therapy for thrombophlebitis.

40. Symptoms of impending postpartum eclamptic seizure are

    1) _____
    2) _____
    3) _____
    4) _____
    5) _____

Chapter 11

Multiple Choice

1. The newborn's metabolism of brown fat occurs

    a. immediately after birth.
    b. in response to cold stress.
    c. when oxygen saturation is below 90.

2. A 10-minute Apgar is assigned when the

    a. 1-minute Apgar is less than 8.
    b. 5-minute Apgar is less than 7.
    c. newborn has required resuscitation.

3. During the first week of life, newborns are at risk for bleeding because

   a. milk intake is inadequate to supply vitamin K requirements.
   b. several clotting factors are being under-produced by the spleen.
   c. the liver is immature and not yet producing several clotting factors.

4. According to the American Academy of Pediatrics (AAP), vitamin K should be administered

   a. after the infant is weighed and measured.
   b. after 2 hours of life.
   c. within 1 hour of birth.

5. After administration of eye prophylaxis, excess erythromycin ophthalmic ointment is correctly

   a. left in place until absorbed.
   b. removed using sterile water.
   c. wiped away after 1 minute.

6. According to research, there is an association between shorter separation time and umbilical cord care using

   a. alcohol.
   b. sterile water.
   c. triple antibiotic dye.

7. The key to infant abduction prevention is a

   a. carefully obtained set of newborn footprints.
   b. state of the art electronic infant abduction alert.
   c. systematic infant safety program.

8. Vitamin K is produced by the newborn as

   a. a normal compensatory mechanism whenever bleeding occurs.
   b. a response to the parenteral administration of vitamin K.
   c. the gastrointestinal tract becomes colonized with bacteria following initiation of feeding.

9. As part of the algorithm for performing neonatal resuscitation, medications are administered when the

   a. code team physician orders them.
   b. heart rate is below 60 after PPV with 100% oxygen.
   c. heart rate is 60–80 and not increasing.

10. Initiation of respirations is triggered in the brain by decreased concentration of

    a. carbon dioxide.
    b. oxygen.
    c. surfactant.

11. Fetal pulmonary vascular resistance is

    a. equal to neonatal.
    b. higher than neonatal.
    c. lower than neonatal.

12. In the fetus, blood is shunted into the inferior vena cava through the

    a. ductus arteriosus.
    b. ductus venosus.
    c. foramen ovale.

13. Clamping the umbilical cord at birth causes

    a. decreased blood pressure and decreased systemic vascular resistance.
    b. increased blood pressure and decreased systemic vascular resistance.
    c. increased blood pressure and increased systemic vascular resistance.

14. The major factor contributing to closure of the ductus arteriosus is sensitivity to

    a. decreasing arterial carbon dioxide concentration.
    b. decreasing left ventricular pressure.
    c. increasing arterial oxygen concentration.

15. In the majority of healthy newborns, the ductus arteriosus will have closed or will be closing by

    a. 1–6 hours of life.
    b. 12–24 hours of life.
    c. 48–72 hours of life.

16. The premature infant is more susceptible to evaporative heat loss because of

    a. decreased body surface area.
    b. decreased muscle tone.
    c. increased permeability of skin.

17. Hemorrhagic disease of the newborn is prevented by administration of

    a. vitamin A.
    b. vitamin D.
    c. vitamin K.

18. To protect newborns from infection with hepatitis B virus, all newborns

    a. born to mothers with unknown hepatitis B surface antigen (HBsAg) status should receive one dose of vaccine within 12 hours of birth.
    b. should be screened for HBsAg within 12 hours of birth.
    c. should receive the first dose of hepatitis vaccine within 12 hours of birth.

19. Intrauterine infection should be suspected when the newborn has elevated

    a. immunoglobulin (Ig) A.
    b. IgG.
    c. IgM.

20. An infant born to a group B streptococcus (GBS) positive mother who did not receive antibiotics during labor is at risk for

    a. hyperbilirubinemia.
    b. hypoglycemia.
    c. pneumonia.

Fill in the Blank

For questions 21–24, the following nursing interventions support the newborn's transition to extrauterine life by interrupting what mechanism of heat loss (a–d)?

    a. evaporation
    b. convection
    c. conduction
    d. radiation

21. _____ dry newborn thoroughly, remove wet linen

22. _____ when necessary use humidified, warmed oxygen

23. _____ place cover between newborn and metal scale

24. _____ preheat radiant warmer

25. Maternal intrauterine transmission of _____ antibodies protects the newborn from bacterial and viral infections for which the mother has already produced antibodies.

26. The action that best protects newborns from infection is _____.

27. A 2,000-g infant should receive _____ mg of vitamin K.

28. Erythromycin ophthalmic ointment protects newborns from the organisms _____ and _____.

29. Immediately following birth, in the absence of spontaneous respirations, a nurse begins giving the newborn positive pressure ventilation. The second nurse should _____.

30. Respiratory adaptations during the transition to extrauterine life are dependent on _____, _____, and _____ stimuli to the brain.

31. In utero, oxygenated blood flows from the placenta to the fetus through the _____.

32. During fetal life, the placenta is an organ of _____ vascular resistance.

33. The vessels in the umbilical cord are two _____ and one _____.

34. The four main mechanisms of heat loss in the neonate are _____, _____, _____, and _____.

35. Nonshivering thermogenesis generates heat in the newborn through _____.

36. Hypothermia in the neonate increases _____ consumption.

37. The action of surfactant is to _____ in the alveoli.

38. In neonatal resuscitation, chest compressions should be initiated if the heart rate is below _____ bpm.

39. Women who are positive for GBS infection should be treated with _____ during labor.

40. Postpartum practices that increase breast-feeding duration include _____ and _____.

Chapter 12
Multiple Choice

1. In a newborn with hypospadias, the urinary meatus is located on the

    a. anterior surface of the glans.
    b. posterior surface of the glans.
    c. tip of the glans.

2. A nevus simplex "stork bite"

   a. is usually elevated, rough, and dark red.
   b. most often appears on the neck, forehead, and eyelids.
   c. will not blanch with pressure.

3. Tears are usually absent in a baby until the age of

   a. 2–4 weeks.
   b. 2–3 months.
   c. 4–6 months.

4. Newborn femoral pulses would characteristically be decreased or absent in

   a. congenital heart abnormalities.
   b. hip dysplasia.
   c. sepsis.

5. A persistent newborn heart rate of less than 100 bpm is consistent with

   a. congenital heart block.
   b. congestive heart failure.
   c. vagal stimulation.

6. In dark-skinned newborns, jaundice is more easily observed in the

   a. feet and hands.
   b. nail beds.
   c. sclera and buccal mucosa.

7. In the neonate, blood pressure in the lower extremities is usually

   a. higher than in the upper extremities.
   b. lower than in the upper extremities.
   c. no different than in the upper extremities.

8. The normal umbilical cord contains

   a. one artery and one vein.
   b. two arteries and one vein.
   c. two veins and one artery.

9. Jaundice within the first 24 hours of life may be related to

   a. asphyxia.
   b. cardiac disease.
   c. liver disease.

10. Edema over the presenting part of a newborn's head that feels spongy and resolves within a few days of life is characteristic of

    a. caput succedaneum.
    b. cephalhematoma.
    c. trauma during birth.

11. A gestational age assessment indicating the greatest degree of physical maturity is

    a. labia majora covering clitoris and labia minora.
    b. labia majora large and labia minora small.
    c. prominent clitoris and enlarging labia minora.

12. Newborn jaundice appears initially on the

    a. head and face.
    b. trunk and extremities.
    c. sclera.

13. To measure fontanelles accurately, a ruler or measuring tape is placed

    a. across the widest diameter.
    b. diagonally from bone to bone.
    c. from suture line to suture line.

14. A crossed-eyed appearance in a newborn is called

    a. hypertelorism.
    b. nystagmus.
    c. strabismus.

15. Bowel sounds are expected to be present in the newborn

    a. after passage of first meconium stool.
    b. immediately after birth.
    c. within 1 hour of birth.

16. A prominent xiphoid process identified during a newborn physical assessment is

    a. a normal finding.
    b. associated with intrauterine growth retardation.
    c. indicative of respiratory distress.

17. The most common finding in assessment of the newborn's skin is a

    a. hemangioma.
    b. Mongolian spot.
    c. nevus simplex.

18. Permanent eye color is present by the age of

    a. 2 months.
    b. 4 months.
    c. 6 months.

19. In a newborn, the skin lesion that has discrete borders and does not blanch to pressure or lighten with age is a

    a. hemangioma.
    b. Mongolian spot.
    c. port wine stain.

20. The presence of the red reflex in the newborn indicates

    a. congenital cataracts.
    b. intact cornea and lens.
    c. weak eye musculature.

21. Umbilical hernias are more commonly seen in newborns who are

    a. African-American.
    b. Native American.
    b. South East Asian.

22. Screening programs evaluating newborns at high risk for hearing loss will potentially miss what percentage of newborns with hearing loss?

    a. 25%
    b. 50%
    c. 75%

23. The most common abnormal neck finding in newborns is

    a. cystic hygroma.
    b. torticollis.
    c. webbing.

24. The Moro reflex should disappear by the age of

    a. 2 months.
    b. 4 months.
    c. 6 months.

25. A genitourinary finding in a gestational age assessment of a newborn male at 36 weeks' gestation is

    a. rugae becoming visible.
    b. pendulous scrotum.
    c. testes in the upper scrotum.

26. During the first few days of life, the percentage of newborns with developmental hip dysplasia that is identified during physical assessment is

    a. 40%.
    b. 60%.
    c. 80%.

27. A scrotal mass that does not transilluminate is a/an

    a. hydrocele.
    b. inguinal hernia.
    c. testis.

Fill in the Blank

28. When examining the clavicles, _____ is felt by the examiner if there is a fracture present.

29. At birth, newborns are covered with an odorless, white, cheesy substance called _____.

30. Epstein's pearls are composed of _____ cells.

31. Popping sensations (similar to indenting a ping-pong ball) felt when palpating the parietal or occipital bones of a newborn are called _____.

32. The anterior fontanelle normally closes at about _____ months.

33. The posterior fontanelle normally closes at about _____ months.

34. Apnea refers to pauses in respirations that last _____ seconds or longer.

35. Newborns can see an object clearly when the object is _____ inches away.

36. _____ describes the inability to completely retract the foreskin of the penis.

37. _____ is an asymmetric neck deformity in which the head is noted to be pulled toward the effected side, with the chin pointing toward the opposite shoulder, due to injury to the _____ muscle.

38. Acrocyanosis is the result of _____ and tends to worsen if the newborn becomes chilled.

39. _____ is a compensatory mechanism that decreases upper airway resistance, allowing more air to enter the nasal passages.

40. Newborn _____ are involuntary protective neuromuscular responses.

Chapter 13

Multiple Choice

1. A woman who presents with a history of minimal increase in breast tissue during pregnancy should be informed that

   a. the amount of breast tissue influences milk production.
   b. breast growth during pregnancy does not influence milk production.
   c. breast tissue will increase as she nurses.

2. The onset of milk production in a postpartum woman is triggered by the

   a. periodic stimulation of oxytocin.
   b. rapid rise in prolactin.
   c. sudden decrease in progesterone.

3. A pregnant woman who asks what she should do to prepare her nipples for breastfeeding is correctly informed that nipple exercises

   a. do little to prevent nipple soreness.
   b. improve nipple erectility.
   c. reduce the incidence of engorgement.

4. Frequent breastfeeding during the first 24 hours postpartum increases newborn

   a. immunity.
   b. sleep cycles.
   c. weight gain.

5. Breast engorgement in the breastfeeding mother is minimized by

   a. avoiding unnecessary nipple stimulation.
   b. nursing without time limits.
   c. pumping after nursing.

6. As maternal prolactin levels decline over time, what is responsible for continued milk production?

   a. newborn sucking
   b. maternal ingestion of adequate fluids
   c. return of normal estrogen levels

7. During a home visit to a 4-day-old breastfeeding newborn, the nurse observes jaundice. Which of the following interventions should be suggested to the mother?

   a. increasing the frequency of breastfeeding
   b. supplementing breast-feeds with water
   c. temporarily pumping and discarding her breast milk

8. A newborn is reported to have breastfed very well during the first hour after birth. The baby is now 12 hours old and has not had a second successful feeding. The nurse should

   a. advise the mother to give water every 2–3 hours.
   b. review newborn sleep cycles and hunger cues.
   c. teach the mother to pump her breasts.

9. A woman calls the hospital asking what she should do for her 10-day-old breastfeeding newborn who wants to nurse "all the time." The nurse should recommend that the mother

   a. continue breastfeeding based on the newborn's cues.
   b. offer formula if the newborn is still hungry after breastfeeding.
   c. use other comforting techniques to space feedings at least 2 hours apart.

10. A bottle-feeding mother asks whether she should give her baby water. The nurse should instruct her to

    a. add a little extra water to the formula on hot days.
    b. feed the newborn properly mixed formula.
    c. give the newborn water between feedings if fussy.

11. The hormone responsible for milk ejection is

    a. oxytocin.
    b. progesterone.
    c. prolactin.

12. Mothers can encourage newborns to open their mouths wider while nursing by

    a. applying a small amount of downward pressure on newborns' chin.
    b. guiding the newborns' head toward the breast.
    c. leaning forward, toward the newborn.

13. Compared to mature milk, colostrum is higher in

    a. fat.
    b. IgG.
    c. protein.

14. As human milk matures, the concentration of immunoglobins and proteins

    a. decreases.
    b. increases.
    c. remains the same.

15. A mother holds her breast with her thumb on top and fingers below; she is using the

    a. C hold.
    b. circle hold.
    c. cup hold.

16. Formula feeding is recommended for newborns with

    a. galactosemia.
    b. jaundice.
    c. thalassemia.

17. After opening a can or bottle of formula, the contents should be used within

    a. 24 hours.
    b. 48 hours.
    c. 72 hours.

18. The most economic formula preparation is

    a. concentrate.
    b. powder.
    c. ready-to-feed.

19. Methods to increase comfort while suppressing lactation include

    a. applying heat to the breast.
    b. limiting fluid intake for 48 hours.
    c. wearing a firm-fitting bra.

20. Which of the following breastfeeding positions is MOST useful for the mother recovering from a c-section?

    a. cradle
    b. cross cradle
    c. clutch hold

21. Which of the following statements regarding supplementation of the breastfeeding infant is false?

    a. Mothers on a vegan diet, which excludes dairy products, may need supplemental vitamin B12.
    b. The AAP recommends breastfed infants receive a vitamin D supplement.
    c. Most infants need iron supplementation before 6 months of age.

22. Promotion of breastfeeding for preterm infants should include

    a. frequent pumping of both breasts simultaneously.
    b. skin-to-skin contact.
    c. all of the above.

23. Prenatal physical preparation of the breasts to prevent sore nipples should include

    a. nipple rolling.
    b. expression of colostrums.
    c. none of the above.

24. Breastfed infants may have inadequate intake if they

    a. have uric acid crystals during the first week.
    b. fail to regain birth weight by 2 weeks.
    c. have two to three wet diapers by day 2.

25. Which of the following is a true statement about pacifier use?

    a. They have been used effectively to correct sucking problems.
    b. Early introduction has been, shown to prevent sore nipples.
    c. Introduction of a pacifier, after breastfeeding is well established, during sleep time may prevent SIDS.

26. Ankyloglossia can lead to

    a. yeast infections.
    b. nipple pain.
    c. a reliance on pacifiers.

Fill in the Blank

27. Healthy People 2010's target for percentage of women breastfeeding at discharge is _____.

28. A hard, tender area in the breast of a breastfeeding woman should be treated with _____ and _____.

29. When the breastfeeding baby is correctly latched onto the mother's breast, the tongue covers the _____.

30. Hunger cues can be observed for up to _____ minutes before the newborn begins sustained crying.

31. General guidelines for newborn weight gain during the first few weeks of life are regaining birth weight by _____ weeks and gaining _____ ounces a week or at least _____ pound(s) a month.

32. Current thinking is that newborns will lose _____% of their birth weight in their first few days of life.

33. The easiest, most economic treatments for nipple pain are _____.

34. Alternate breast massage is used to _____.

35. Instructions for alternate breast massage are to _____.

36. Feeding the infant in the _____ position may decrease the risk of otitis media.

Chapter 14
Multiple Choice

1. Transient tachypnea develops more often in the newborn who is born

   a. by cesarean section.
   b. after a prolonged first stage of labor.
   c. small for gestational age.

2. In a newborn, tachypnea is defined as a respiratory rate greater than

   a. 40/minute.
   b. 60/minute.
   c. 80/minute.

3. A cardiac lesion considered to be cyanotic is

   a. atrial septal defect (ASD).
   b. patent ductus arteriosus (PDA).
   c. transposition of great arteries (TGA).

4. A cardiac lesion which results in decreased pulmonary blood flow is

   a. ASD.
   b. TET.
   c. PDA.

5. A medication used to maintain patency of the ductus arteriosus is

   a. caffeine.
   b. indomethacin.
   c. prostaglandin E_1.

6. Hypoglycemia in the infant born to an insulin-dependent diabetic mother occurs after birth between

   a. 1 and 3 hours.
   b. 5 and 7 hours.
   c. 8 and 10 hours.

7. One etiology of hypoglycemia is decreased production of glucose, which should be suspected in the newborn who is

   a. cold-stressed.
   b. the infant of a diabetic mother.
   c. small for gestational age.

8. Clinical jaundice is first apparent at serum bilirubin levels of

   a. 1–3 mg/dL.
   b. 5–7 mg/dL.
   c. 9–11 mg/dL.

9. In a full-term newborn, physiologic hyperbilirubinemia is characterized by a progressive increase in serum bilirubin that peaks at

   a. 24 hours.
   b. 48 hours.
   c. 72 hours.

10. Gastrointestinal symptoms associated with neonatal abstinence syndrome include

    a. constipation.
    b. diarrhea.
    c. flatulence.

11. Which drug, when used alone, is responsible for the most severe withdrawal symptoms in the newborn?

    a. cocaine
    b. heroin
    c. methadone

12. When ruling out sepsis in the newborn, the broad-spectrum antimicrobial agents most commonly initiated after cultures have been obtained are

    a. ampicillin/cephalosporin.
    b. ampicillin/gentamicin.
    c. penicillin/gentamicin.

13. IV antibiotic treatment for neonatal sepsis should continue for

    a. 3–5 days.
    b. 7–10 days.
    c. 12–14 days.

14. Hypothermia can cause

    a. decreased metabolic demand.
    b. hypoglycemia.
    c. metabolic alkalosis.

15. A sign of hypoglycemia in the newborn is

    a. decreased skin turgor.
    b. increased appetite.
    c. temperature instability.

16. An indication to screen for hypoglycemia is an infant who is

    a. a second twin weighing 3,000 g.
    b. born at 38 weeks' gestation.
    c. small for gestational age.

17. In the newborn, physiologic hyperbilirubinemia is characterized by a progressive increase in serum bilirubin to a peak of

    a. 5 mg/dL at 72 hours of age.
    b. 8 mg/dL at 72 hours of age.
    c. 10 mg/dL at 48 hours of age.

18. Infants undergoing phototherapy should have axillary temperatures monitored at least every

    a. 30 minutes.
    b. 1 hour.
    c. 2 hours.

19. Infants born to cocaine-addicted mothers frequently exhibit

    a. constipation.
    b. feeding difficulties.
    c. lethargy.

20. Which of the following interventions is useful to support an infant experiencing abstinence syndrome?

    a. massage
    b. music
    c. rocking

21. The diagnosis of neonatal sepsis is made in the presence of a positive culture of

    a. blood.
    b. both blood and urine.
    c. urine.

22. ACOG and the AAP recommend HIV testing and counseling with consent for

    a. pregnant women in at-risk populations.
    b. all pregnant teenagers.
    c. all pregnant women.

Fill in the Blank

23. Surfactant _____ surface tension in the alveoli function as a stabilizer to prevent collapse during expiration.

24. When meconium only partially obstructs the airway, a _____ effect results in which air enters the lower airways on inspiration but cannot _____ on expiration.

25. The _____ is the first major organ system to function in the embryo.

26. A ventricular septal defect (VSD) is considered to be a(n) _____ lesion with _____ pulmonary blood flow.

27. The three pathophysiologic findings in tetralogy of Fallot are

    1) _____
    2) _____
    3) _____

28. The incidence of the congenital heart defect, _____, is inversely proportional to gestational age.

29. An ASD is considered to be a(n) _____ lesion with _____ pulmonary blood flow.

30. With transposition of the great arteries in two _____ circulations; the degree of cyanosis present depends on the amount of mixing through the _____, if present, _____ or _____.

31. Glucose homeostasis requires the initiation of various metabolic processes including _____ , forming glucose from noncarbohydrate sources, and _____, conversion of glycogen stores to glucose.

32. As bilirubin levels rise, there is concern that bilirubin encephalopathy, also known as _____, will develop.

33. In nearly all newborns, phototherapy decreases or blunts the rise in serum _____ bilirubin regardless of gestational age, race, or presence or absence of hemolysis.

34. _____ is the one common side effect of all of the medications used to treat neonatal abstinence.

35. The two bacterial agents most commonly associated with neonatal sepsis are _____ and _____.

36. The primary neonatal factors influencing the development of sepsis are _____ and _____.

37. Intrapartum administration of prophylactic antibiotics has proven to be beneficial in preventing _____.

38. Heroin withdrawal in a newborn may last _____ weeks.

39. Skin care is important during phototherapy because the infant often has _____.

40. An infant born to a mother who received tocolytic therapy would be prone to _____. .

41. Narcotics used to manage labor pain may result in _____ respiratory effort in the newborn.

42. The mortality rate associated with neonatal sepsis increases as birth weight _____.

43. Studies show a nearly _____ reduction in HIV-1 transmission in infants whose mothers received azidothymidine (ZDV) prophylaxis.

44. ACOG recommends considering an _____ for HIV-1 infected women with HIV-1 RNA levels >1,000 copies/mL near the time of delivery.

45. Newborn chemoprophylaxis should begin _____ hours after birth.

46. _____ is the primary complication of the 6-week course of ZDV in the neonate.

47. In the United States, HIV-1 infected women are counseled not to _____ to avoid postnatal transmission.

ANSWER KEY

Chapter 1

1. b.
2. a.
3. a.
4. a.
5. b.
6. a.
7. a.
8. c.
9. a
10. a
11. b
12. a
13. c.
14. c.
15. a.
16. a.
17. effective leadership; shared philosophy; professional behavior; excellence in key clinical practices
18. fetal assessment; labor induction; second-stage labor management
19. clinical practice will be based on the cumulative body of evidence and national standards and guidelines
20. Association of Women's Health, Obstetric and Neonatal Nurses (AWHONN); American College of Nurse Midwives (ACNM); American College of Obstetricians and Gynecologists (ACOG); American Academy of Pediatrics (AAP); American Society of Anesthesiologists (ASA); Joint Commission on Accreditation of Healthcare Organizations (JCAHO); Centers for Disease Control and Prevention (CDC); Food and Drug Administration (FDA)
21. attempting vaginal birth after cesarean birth
22. 39 completed weeks' gestation
23. electronic fetal monitoring
24. the woman feels the urge to push; nulliparous; multiparous
25. NICHD
26. Emergency Medical Treatment and Active Labor Act
27. lawsuits/litigation/"suits"
28. retrospective
29. outdated, error
30. sentinel event
31. 1:2
32. 1:1
33. chain of command

Chapter 2

1. c
2. a
3. a
4. b
5. b
6. b
7. c
8. b
9. a-2, b-1, c-3
10. c
11. a
12. b
13. c
14. enhance communication skills, develop linguistic skills, determine who the family decision-makers are, understand that agreement may not indicate comprehension, utilize nonverbal communication, use appropriate names and titles, and use culturally appropriate teaching techniques

Chapter 3

1. b
2. a
3. b
4. a
5. a
6. c
7. c
8. c
9. a
10. c
11. b
12. b
13. c
14. b
15. b
16. c
17. c
18. b
19. b
20. b
21. a
22. a
23. a
24. a
25. b
26. anabolism, catabolism
27. hemodilution
28. mother
29. increase
30. renal sodium
31. increased glomerular filtration rate
32. striae gravidarum
33. prolactin
34. vitamin D (or calciferol)
35. lower
36. human chorionic gonadotropin
37. estriol
38. blood volume
39. 6–12 weeks' postpartum
40. uterus
41. progesterone
42. 24 to 32
43. angiotensin II
44. hypercoagulable
45. coagulation changes, venous stasis
46. prostaglandins
47. melasma
48. Chadwick's

Chapter 4

1. b
2. a
3. a
4. b
5. b
6. c
7. c
8. c
9. a
10. 1) family and social history
    2) psychiatric history
    3) mental status
    4) self-concept/self-esteem
    5) support systems
    6) stressors
    7) coping strategies
    8) spirituality
    9) neurovegetative signs
    10) knowledge of the pregnancy experience
11. pregnant woman, family, nurse
12. nursing diagnoses, care plans, and strategies for nursing care delivery
13. exacerbation or recurrence in the postpartum period
14. the multidisciplinary team providing care for the woman and her family
15. emotional nuances in relationships with family and professionals
16. frequency, duration, and intensity

17. they believe it is a normal reaction secondary to the stress of becoming a mother
18. transition
19. her own physical and psychological needs have been met

Chapter 5

1. b
2. c
3. a
4. b
5. a
6. b
7. b
8. a
9. b
10. a
11. b
12. a
13. b
14. c
15. a
16. a
17. b
18. True
19. 28
20. 36
21. 15 lbs
22. 10
23. teratogen
24. 8
25. 12
26. Jewish
27. Coumadin
28. 5–10
29. 1) early and continuing risk assessment
    2) health promotion
    3) medical and psychosocial intervention
30. cardiorespiratory, muscular
31. two or more abnormally elevated values
32. 15, 20
33. 10
34. 1) fetal tone

2) fetal reflex movement
3) fetal breathing
4) amniotic fluid volume
5) nonstress test

Chapter 6

Hypertensive Disorders

1. c
2. a
3. b
4. b
5. c
6. b
7. hypertensive
8. 110
9. semi-Fowler's
10. magnesium sulfate
11. 1) abruptio placentae
    2) disseminated intravascular coagulation
    3) hepatic failure
    4) acute renal failure
12. prevent maternal cerebral vascular accident, maintain uteroplacental perfusion
13. hemolysis, elevated liver enzymes, low platelets
14. aspiration

Bleeding

1. b
2. a
3. b
4. b
5. b
6. a
7. velamentous
8. 95
9. hypotension

Preterm Labor and Birth

1. a
2. c
3. a

4. b
5. a
6. b
7. a
8. b
9. b
10. a
11. 1.6% higher
12. risen
13. eliminated

Diabetes

1. c
2. a
3. c
4. c
5. a
6. c
7. c
8. c
9. a
10. a
11. type 1
12. anabolic
13. 1) prolactin
    2) estrogen
    3) progesterone
    4) human placental lactogen
    5) cortisol
14. magnesium sulfate
15. 1) polyuria
    2) polyphagia
    3) polydipsia

Cardiac Disease

1. a
2. b
3. a
4. b
5. a
6. c
7. c
8. a
9. c
10. b
11. capillaries
12. rheumatic fever
13. rare
14. type of cardiac disorder, the secondary complications
15. functional ability

Pulmonary Complications

1. c
2. b
3. b
4. c
5. a
6. b
7. a
8. b
9. b
10. c
11. 10
12. 95
13. 75
14. illicit drug use, cigarette smoking, alcohol abuse, chronic illness
15. *Streptococcus pneumoniae*
16. high Fowler's
17. pollens, molds, dust mites, animal dander, cockroach antigens, air pollutants, strong odors, food additives, tobacco smoke
18. systemic steroid therapy >4 weeks; three visits for asthma recently; history of multiple hospitalizations for asthma; history of hypoxic seizure, hypoxic syncope, or intubation; history of admission to ICU for asthma
19. preterm labor, empyema, bacteremia, pneumothorax, atrial fibrillation, respiratory failure
20. 33

Multiple Gestation

1. c
2. b
3. b
4. c

5. b
6. a
7. c
8. a
9. b
10. a
11. a
12. c
13. b
14. a
15. c
16. low birth weight and preterm birth
17. fetal synchrony
18. False
19. True
20. False
21. True
22. True

Chapter 7

1. b
2. c
3. c
4. a
5. c
6. a
7. b
8. b
9. c
10. c
11. b
12. b
13. b
14. c
15. c
16. b
17. b
18. a
19. b
20. c
21. lower
22. kidneys, liver
23. sitting on the toilet
24. closed glottis, hemodynamic
25. spontaneous bearing-down efforts (urge to push)
26. shoulder dystocia, flex, knee, hip
27. blood loss, infection, pain, third- and fourth-degree laceration, delayed healing, sexual dysfunction, scarring.
28. 1) open glottis—gentle pushing
    2) spontaneous rather than directed pushing
    3) upright position in second stage
29. 1) fewer perinatal complications
    2) shorter labors
    3) fewer neonatal intensive care unit admissions
30. 1) maternal status
    2) fetal well-being
    3) cervical status
31. bleeding, infection, rupture of membranes, umbilical cord prolapse
32. 6–12 hours
33. color and amount of fluid, FHR before procedure, fetal response to procedure
34. fourth
35. ischial spines
36. misoprostol, Cervidil
37. prior cesarean birth or uterine scar
38. emptying the maternal bladder
39. 500–600
40. 1) oxygen delivery system
    2) continuous and intermittent suction
    3) blood pressure monitoring equipment
    4) ECG monitoring equipment
    5) pulse oximeter
    6) adjustable lighting
    7) means to ensure patient privacy
41. 1) one or two prior low transverse cesarean births
    2) clinically adequate pelvis
    3) no prior uterine surgery or rupture
    4) physician immediately available and capable of performing emergent cesarean birth
    5) surgical team and anesthesia personnel available for emergent cesarean birth
42. pain at the prior incision site
43. 1) stretching of uterine muscles
    2) pressure on the cervix
    3) endogenous oxytocin
    4) change in estrogen:progesterone ratio
44. 1) vaginal bleeding
    2) acute abdominal pain
    3) temperature of 100.4°F or higher
    4) preterm labor
    5) premature preterm rupture of membranes
    6) hypertension
45. 1) dilation
    2) effacement
    3) station
    4) consistency
    5) position
46. iatrogenic injuries to the mother and/or fetus
47. 1) risks
    2) benefits
    3) alternative approaches

Chapter 8

1. b
2. a
3. b
4. c
5. b
6. b
7. c
8. c
9. c
10. c
11. c
12. c
13. c
14. a
15. b
16. c
17. c
18. a
19. peak, after
20. variable, abrupt
21. beginning, baseline rate, benign
22. decreasing or discontinuing
23. moderate
24. congenital anomalies
25. supraventricular tachycardia
26. three of the following: medications, prematurity, fetal sleep, fetal dysrhythmia, anesthetic agents, cardiac anomaly
27. baseline rate, variability
28. hyperstimulation
29. tocolytics
30. intrauterine pressure catheter
31. anemic
32. 15, 5
33. 6–25
34. changing maternal position
35. variability, normal baseline rate
36. 50
37. 7.20, reassuring
38. 10
39. variability
40. 1) increasing IV fluids
    2) maintaining lateral maternal position
    3) administering O_2 by mask

4) decreasing or discontinuing oxytocin

5) delaying the next dose of Prepidil, Cervidil, or Cytotec

41. 110, 160

Chapter 9

1. a
2. c
3. c
4. b
5. b
6. a
7. a
8. c
9. a
10. b
11. c
12. a
13. c
14. c
15. a
16. c
17. b
18. c
19. b
20. c
21. c
22. c
23. c
24. b
25. hands and knees
26. sacrum
27. hydrostatic pressure
28. randomized controlled clinical trials
29. b
30. a
31. a
32. c
33. b
34. decrease
35. hypotension
36. motor block
37. connective tissue bands
38. turning
39. maternal cardiac output and lower fetal oxygen saturation

Chapter 10

1. c
2. c
3. c
4. a
5. b
6. b
7. b
8. a
9. a
10. a
11. b
12. c
13. b
14. c
15. b
16. b
17. c
18. b
19. c
20. c
21. legs elevated 20–30 degrees
22. nonpathologic leukocytosis.
23. a loss of 15%–20% of the total blood volume
24. measurement of the affected leg circumference
25. pulmonary embolism
26. pulse pressure to 30 mm Hg or less
27. advantages, disadvantages, prevention of sexually transmitted diseases
28. 1) insomnia
    2) weepiness
    3) anxiety
    4) irritability
    5) poor concentration
29. vital signs, lochia, uterine tone/position
30. 3–6
31. 12, 5
32. 1) breast
    2) uterus
    3) bladder
    4) bowel
    5) lochia
    6) episiotomy/ incision

7) emotional response
8) Homans' sign
33. 2–4, 1–1.5
34. 1) fever and chills
    2) localized tenderness
    3) palpable, hard, reddened mass
    4) tachycardia
35. 1) pelvic floor exercises
    2) postpartum exercise
    3) sexuality
    4) contraception
36. fatigue
37. large venous areas are exposed after placental expulsion
38. 1) blood pressure of 140/90
    2) headache
    3) decreased urine output
39. protamine sulfate
40. 1) severe persistent headache
    2) scotomata
    3) blurred vision
    4) photophobia
    5) epigastric or right upper quadrant pain

Chapter 11

1. b
2. b
3. c
4. c
5. c
6. b
7. c
8. c
9. b
10. b
11. b
12. a
13. c
14. c
15. c
16. c
17. c
18. a

19. c
20. c
21. a
22. b
23. c
24. c
25. IgG
26. handwashing
27. 1
28. chlamydia, gonococcus
29. evaluate the heart rate
30. chemical, mechanical, sensory
31. umbilical vein
32. low
33. arteries, vein
34. evaporation, convection, conduction, radiation
35. brown fat
36. oxygen
37. lower surface tension
38. 60
39. antibiotics
40. early suckling, uninterrupted contact between mother and newborn

Chapter 12

1. b
2. b
3. c
4. b
5. a
6. c
7. a
8. b
9. c
10. a
11. a
12. a
13. b
14. c
15. a
16. a
17. c
18. c
19. c
20. b
21. a
22. b

23. a
24. c
25. c
26. b
27. b
28. crepitus
29. vernix
30. epithelial
31. craniotabes
32. 18
33. 2–4
34. 20
35. 8–10
36. phimosis
37. torticollis; sternoclei-
    domastoid
38. vasomotor instability
39. flaring
40. reflexes

Chapter 13

1. b
2. c
3. a
4. c
5. b
6. a
7. a
8. b
9. a
10. b
11. a
12. a
13. c

14. a
15. a
16. a
17. a
18. b
19. c
20. c
21. c
22. c
23. c
24. b
25. c
26. b
27. 75%
28. warm compresses,
    frequent feedings
29. lower gum
30. 30 minutes
31. 2, 4–7, 1
32. 7
33. colostrum or breast
    milk on nipples after
    feeding; letting
    nipples air dry;
    warm, moist
    compresses
34. increase milk supply
35. massage the base of
    the breast when the
    infant stops sucking,
    alternate massaging
    of the breast
    between periods of
    sucking
36. semi-upright

Chapter 14

1. a
2. b
3. c
4. b
5. c
6. a
7. c
8. b
9. c
10. b
11. c
12. b
13. b
14. b
15. c
16. c
17. b
18. c
19. b
20. c
21. a
22. c
23. decreases
24. ball–valve, escape
25. cardiovascular
    system
26. acyanotic,
    increased
27. 1) VSD
    2) pulmonary stenosis
    3) overriding aorta
       and right ventric-
       ular hypertrophy

28. PDA
29. acyanotic,
    increased
30. parallel,
    VSD,
    PDA,
    patent foramen
    ovale (PFO)
31. gluconeogenesis,
    glycolysis
32. kernicterus
33. unconjugated or
    indirect
34. sedation
35. GBS & *E. coli*
36. gestational age,
    birth weight
37. early-onset GBS
    sepsis
38. 8–16 weeks
39. loose stools
40. hypoglycemia
41. poor
42. decreases
43. 70%
44. elective c-section
45. 8–12
46. anemia
47. breastfeed

INDEX

Note: Page numbers followed by "*f*" refer to figures; page numbers followed by "*t*" refer to tables.